Mosby's

2001-2002 Medical Drug Reference

Allan J. Ellsworth, Pharm.D.

Professor of Pharmacy and Family Medicine,
University of Washington Schools of Pharmacy and Medicine,
Seattle, Washington

Daniel M. Witt, Pharm.D.

Supervisor,
Clinical Phamacy, Anticoagulation Service,
Kaiser Permanente, Rocky Mountain Division,
Westminster, Colorado

David C. Dugdale, M.D.

Associate Professor of Medicine,
University of Washington School of Medicine,
Seattle, Washington

Lynn M. Oliver, M.D.

Assistant Professor of Family Medicine,
University of Washington School of Medicine,
Seattle, Washington

M Mosby

A Harcourt Health Sciences Company

St. Louis   London   Philadelphia   Sydney   Toronto

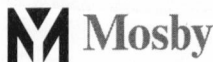
Mosby

A Harcourt Health Sciences Company

Editor: Liz Fathman
Project Manager: Carol Sullivan Weis
Project Specialist: Pat Joiner
Designer: Mark Oberkrom
Cover Art: Adam Cohen

Copyright © 2001 by Mosby, Inc.

NOTICE

Pharmacology is an ever-changing field. Standard safety precautions must be followed, but as new research and clinical experience broaden our knowledge, changes in treatment and drug therapy may become necessary or appropriate. Readers are advised to check the most current product information provided by the manufacturer of each drug to be administered to verify the recommended dose, the method and duration of administration, and contraindications. It is the responsibility of the licensed prescriber, relying on experience and knowledge of the patient, to determine dosages and the best treatment for each individual patient. Neither the publisher nor the editor assumes any liability for any injury and/or damage to persons or property arising from this publication.

Mosby, Inc.
A Harcourt Health Sciences Company
11830 Westline Industrial Drive
St. Louis, Missouri 63146

Printed in the United States of America

ISSN 1089-3202
ISBN 0-8151-3657-9

00   01   02   03   04   GW/FF   9   8   7   6   5   4   3   2   1

Instructions for Use

Mosby's Medical Drug Reference was conceived in response to the demands of physicians and other healthcare providers who require an up-to-date, authoritative, comprehensive, portable drug prescribing reference for use at the point of care. This compact, easily accessible manual has been created in part from the renowned and objective drug database, *Mosby's GenRx,* which is updated quarterly to provide timely drug information for accurate and efficient prescribing. As a standard reference, *Mosby's GenRx* is indispensable in its print and CD-ROM formats; for those situations when the demands of patient care require a more portable drug prescribing guide, we proudly present *Mosby's 2001-2002 Medical Drug Reference.*

Mosby's 2001-2002 Medical Drug Reference is organized into several highly functional parts. The body of the book is a listing, by generic name, of nearly 900 drugs in common clinical use, representing over 2600 products. An appendix of the book contains tables of comparative drug data and other information useful for choosing drug therapy. The comprehensive index provides rapid reference by listing all generic and trade names; index searches are further aided by the colored index paper. The inside front and back covers contain formulas for calculating drug dosages and useful conversion information. The comprehensive Therapeutic Index, which allows prescribers to locate drugs appropriate for a broad range of clinical indications, has been updated for this edition.

Drug monographs in *Mosby's 2001-2002 Medical Drug Reference* are organized in a uniform fashion as follows (when there is no information in a category applicable to a given drug, the category has been deleted entirely):

> Drug name (generic)
> Pronunciation (phonetic)
> Trade Names
> Chemical Class
> Therapeutic Class
> DEA Schedule (if applicable, see p. ix)
> Clinical Pharmacology (including information about the mechanism of action and pharmacokinetics of the drug)
> Indications and Uses (non–FDA-approved uses marked with *
> if applicable)
> Dosage
> Available Forms and Cost of Therapy (average wholesale prices [AWPs] of brands are given)

Contraindications (if the only contraindication is hypersensitivity, this category has been deleted)

Precautions

Pregnancy and Lactation (see p. x)

Side Effects/Adverse Reactions (listed by organ system; *common side effects* [greater than 5% incidence] italicized, ***potentially life-threatening side effects*** bold and italicized)

Drug Interactions, if applicable. The clinical significance of each drug interaction is derived from data presented in Hansten PD, Horn JR: Drug interactions analysis and management. Interactions are classified by potential severity as: ▲—Avoid combination, risk always outweighs benefit; ❷—Usually avoid combination, use combination only under special circumstances; or ❸—Minimize risk, take action as necessary to reduce risk of adverse outcome as a result of drug interaction. Interactions of lesser significance, either because they are minor or poorly documented, are not included. If no drug interactions are known, or if the interactions are of minimal risk, this category has been deleted.

Lab Test Interactions (if applicable). Only laboratory interactions that are well documented and are analytical in nature are included. Changes in lab results that reflect the physiologic action of the drug or an adverse metabolic effect of the drug are not included. If no lab interactions are known, this category has been deleted.

Special Considerations (if applicable) such as patient education or monitoring or information about the place of the drug in therapy.

Every possible effort has been made to ensure the accuracy and currency of the information contained within *Mosby's 2001-2002 Medical Drug Reference*. However, drug information is constantly changing and is subject to interpretation. The authors, editors, or publishers cannot be responsible for information that has either changed or been erroneously published or for the consequences of such errors. Decisions regarding drug therapy for a specific patient must be based on the independent judgment of the clinician.

Allan J. Ellsworth
Daniel M. Witt
David C. Dugdale
Lynn M. Oliver

ACKNOWLEDGMENTS

We are grateful for the support, stimulus, and suggestions of our colleagues in the Departments of Family Medicine, Medicine, and Pharmacy, University of Washington, Seattle, Washington, and the Medical and Pharmacy Staff of Kaiser Permanente of Colorado, Denver, Colorado. We especially appreciate the technical and organizational contributions of Ryan North, a Pharm.D. student at the University of Washington School of Pharmacy, and Erin Ellsworth, a senior dietetics student at Brigham Young University. Finally, to our families and friends, whose support, patience, love, and understanding allowed many things to go undone during the completion of the project, we thank you all.

Abbreviations

ABG arterial blood gas
ac before meals
ACE angiotensin-converting enzyme
ACTH adrenocorticotropic hormone
AD right ear
ADH antidiuretic hormone
aer aerosol
AIDS acquired immunodeficiency syndrome
ALT alanine aminotransferase, serum
ANA antinuclear antibody
aPTT activated partial thromboplastin time
AS left ear
AST aspartate aminotransferase, serum
AU each ear
AUC area under curve
AV atrioventricular
bid twice a day
BP blood pressure
BUN blood urea nitrogen
c-AMP cyclic adenosine monophosphate
cap capsule
°C degrees Celsius (centigrade)
Ca calcium
CAD coronary artery disease
cath catheterize
cc cubic centimeter
CBC complete blood count
chew tab tablet, chewable
CHF congestive heart failure
Cl chloride
cm centimeter
CMV cytomegalovirus
CNS central nervous system
CO₂ carbon dioxide
COPD chronic obstructive pulmonary disease
CPAP continuous positive airway pressure

CPK creatine phosphokinase
CrCl creatinine clearance
cre cream
Creat creatinine
CSF cerebrospinal fluid
CV cardiovascular
CVA cerebrovascular accident
CVP central venous pressure
CXR chest x-ray
D5W 5% dextrose in water
DIC disseminated intravascular coagulation
dL deciliter
D$_L$CO diffusing capacity of carbon monoxide
DNA deoxyribonucleic acid
DUB dysfunctional uterine bleeding
ECG electrocardiogram
EDTA ethylenediaminetetraacetic acid
EEG electroencephalogram
EENT eye, ear, nose, throat
elix elixir
ESR erythrocyte sedimentation rate
ET via endotracheal tube
EXT REL extended release
°F degrees Fahrenheit
FEV₁ forced expiratory volume in 1 second
FSH follicle stimulating hormone
g gram
G6PD glucose-6-phosphate dehydrogenase
GGTP gamma glutamyl transpeptidase
GI gastrointestinal
gtt drop
GU genitourinary
H₂ histamine₂
Hct hematocrit

HCG	human chorionic gonadotropin
HEME	hematologic
Hgb	hemoglobin
5-HIAA	5-hydroxyindoleacetic acid
HIV	human immunodeficiency virus
H$_2$O	water
HMG CoA	3-hydroxy-3-methylglutaryl coenzyme A
HPA	hypothalamic-pituitary-adrenal
hr	hour
hs	at bedtime
HSV	herpes simplex virus
IgG	immunoglobulin G
IM	intramuscular
in	inch
INF	infusion
INH	inhalation
inj	injection
INR	international normalized ratio
IO	intraosseous
IPPB	intermittent positive pressure breathing
IU	international units
IV	intravenous
K	potassium
kg	kilogram
L	liter
L-A	long acting
lb	pound
LDH	lactate dehydrogenase
LDL	low density lipoprotein
LFTs	liver function tests
LH	luteinizing hormone
liq	liquid
LMP	last menstrual period
loz	lozenge
lyphl	lyophilized
m	meter
m^2	square meter
MAOI	monoamine oxidase inhibitor
µg	microgram
MDI	metered dose inhaler
mEq	milliequivalent
mg	milligram
Mg	magnesium
MI	myocardial infarction
min	minute
ml (mL)	milliliter
mm	millimeter
mmol	millimole
mo	month
MS	musculoskeletal
Na	sodium

neb	nebulizer
NPO	nothing by mouth
NS	normal saline
NSAID	nonsteroidal antiinflammatory drug
O$_2$	oxygen
OD	right eye
oint	ointment
OS	left eye
OTC	over the counter
OU	each eye
oz	ounce
PaCO$_2$	arterial partial pressure of carbon dioxide
PaO$_2$	arterial partial pressure of oxygen
pc	after meals
PCWP	pulmonary capillary wedge pressure
P$_i$	inorganic phosphorus
po	by mouth
PO$_4$	phosphate
pr	per rectum
prn	as needed
PT	prothrombin time
PTH	parathyroid hormone
PTT	partial thromboplastin time
PVC	premature ventricular contraction
q	every
qAM	every morning
qd	every day
qh	every hour
qid	four times a day
qod	every other day
qPM	every night
q2h	every 2 hours
q3h	every 3 hours
q4h	every 4 hours
q6h	every 6 hours
q8h	every 8 hours
q12h	every 12 hours
RAIU	radioactive iodine uptake
RBC	red blood cell or count
RESP	respiratory
RNA	ribonucleic acid
sc	subcutaneous
sl	sublingual
sol	solution
SO$_4$	sulfate
ss	one half
supp	suppository

sus rel	sustained release	**U**	unit
susp	suspension	**UA**	urinalysis
sust	sustained	**URI**	upper respiratory infection
syr	syrup	**UTI**	urinary tract infection
T_3	triiodothyronine	**UV**	ultraviolet
T_4	thyroxine	**vag**	vaginal
tab	tablet	**VMA**	vanillylmandelic acid
tid	three times a day	**vol**	volume
tinc	tincture	**VS**	vital signs
top	topical	**WBC**	white blood cell or count
trans	transdermal	**wk**	week
TSH	thyroid stimulating hormone	**yr**	year
TT	thrombin time		

Federal Controlled Substances Act Schedules

SCHEDULE I: No accepted medical use in the United States and a high abuse potential. Examples include heroin, marijuana, LSD, peyote, mescaline, psilocybin, and methaqualone.

SCHEDULE II: High abuse potential with severe dependence liability. Examples include opium, morphine, codeine, fentanyl, hydromorphone, methadone, meperidine, oxycodone, oxymorphone, cocaine, amphetamine, methamphetamine, phenmetrazine, methylphenidate, phencyclidine, amobarbital, pentobarbital, and secobarbital.

SCHEDULE III: Lesser abuse potential with moderate dependence liability. Examples include compounds containing limited quantities of certain narcotic or nonnarcotic drugs, such as barbiturates, glutethimide, methyprylon, nalorphine, benzphetamine, chlorphentermine, clortermine, phendimetrazine, and paregoric; suppository dosage form containing amobarbital, secobarbital, or pentobarbital.

SCHEDULE IV: Low abuse potential. Examples include barbital, phenobarbital, mephobarbital, chloral hydrate, ethchlorvynol, ethinamate, meprobamate, paraldehyde, methohexital, fenfluramine, diethylpropion, phentermine, chlordiazepoxide, diazepam, oxazepam, clorazepate, flurazepam, clonazepam, prazepam, lorazepam, alprazolam, halazepam, temazepam, triazolam, mebutamate, dextropropoxyphene, and pentazocine.

SCHEDULE V: Low abuse potential. These products contain limited quantities of certain narcotic drugs generally for antitussive or antidiarrheal purposes.

FDA Pregnancy Categories

A: Adequate studies in pregnant women have not demonstrated a risk to the fetus in the first trimester of pregnancy, and there is no evidence of risk in later trimesters.

B: Animal studies have not demonstrated a risk to the fetus, but there are no adequate studies in pregnant women; OR animal studies have shown an adverse effect, but adequate studies in pregnant women have not demonstrated a risk to the fetus during the first trimester of pregnancy, and there is no evidence of risk in later trimesters.

C: Animal studies have shown an adverse effect on the fetus, but there are no adequate studies in humans; OR there are no animal reproduction studies and no adequate studies in humans.

D: There is evidence of human fetal risk, but the potential benefits from the use of the drug in pregnant women may be acceptable despite its potential risks.

X: Studies in animals or humans demonstrate fetal abnormalities or adverse reaction; reports indicate evidence of fetal risk. The risk of use in a pregnant woman clearly outweighs any possible benefit.

Contents

abacavir

(ah-bah′cah-veer)
Rx: Ziagen
Chemical Class: Nucleoside analog
Therapeutic Class: Antiretroviral

CLINICAL PHARMACOLOGY
Mechanism of Action: Converted intracellularly to carbovir then phosphorylated to carbovir triphosphate; carbovir triphosphate interferes with HIV reverse transcriptase thus inhibiting viral replication
Pharmacokinetics
PO: Peak 1 hr; oral bioavailability 83%; 50% protein bound; extensively metabolized by liver (primary routes are alcohol dehydrogenase and glucuronyl transferase; metabolism by cytochrome P450 enzymes is insignificant), inactive metabolites excreted in urine (1% excreted unchanged); $t_{1/2}$ 1.5 hr; crosses placenta, excreted in breast milk, CSF level 18-33% of plasma level
INDICATIONS AND USES: HIV infection
DOSAGE
Adult and Child >16 yr
• PO 300 mg bid
• For latest treatment guidelines, see www.hivatis.org
Child 3 months-16 yr
• PO 8 mg/kg (max 300 mg) bid
• For latest treatment guidelines, see www.hivatis.org
⑤   AVAILABLE FORMS/COST OF THERAPY
• Tab—Oral: 300 mg, 60's: **$349.20**
• Liq—Oral: 20 mg/ml, 240 ml: **$91.79**
CONTRAINDICATIONS: Hypersensitivity to carbovir
PRECAUTIONS: Use as monotherapy (rapid resistance develops), prior resistance to antiretroviral agents, pregnancy, hepatic insufficiency
PREGNANCY AND LACTATION: Pregnancy category C; breast feeding not recommended due to drug secretion and potential for HIV transmission
SIDE EFFECTS/ADVERSE REACTIONS
CNS: Dizziness (16%), headache (41%), insomnia (18%)
GI: Hepatic steatosis, *nausea (57%)*
METAB: **Lactic acidosis**
SKIN: Rash
MISC: **Hypersensitivity (fever, rash in 2-5%; rechallenge may be fatal)**
INTERACTIONS
Drugs
③ *Amprenavir:* Mild increase in amprenavir plasm level with co-administration
SPECIAL CONSIDERATIONS
PATIENT/FAMILY EDUCATION
• May administer without regard for food
• If you miss a dose: take the missed dose as soon as you remember, then go back to your normal dosing schedule; skip the missed dose if it is time for your next dose; do not take 2 doses at the same time
MONITORING PARAMETERS
• CBC, metabolic panel, CD4 lymphocyte count, HIV RNA level

abciximab

(ab-six′ih-mab)
Rx: ReoPro
Chemical Class: Glycoprotein (GP) IIb/IIIa inhibitor
Therapeutic Class: Antiplatelet agent

CLINICAL PHARMACOLOGY
Mechanism of Action: Reversibly prevents fibrinogen, von Wille-

brand's factor, and other adhesion ligands from binding to platelet GP IIb/IIIa receptors, thereby inhibiting platelet aggregation

Pharmacokinetics: Duration of action on platelets approximately 48 hr although abciximab remains in the circulation for up to 10 days in a platelet-bound state; initial $t_{1/2}$ <10 min, second phase $t_{1/2}$ 30 min

INDICATIONS AND USES: Adjunct to percutaneous transluminal coronary angioplasty (PCTA) for the prevention of acute cardiac ischemic complications in patients at high risk for abrupt closure of the treated coronary vessel

DOSAGE

Adult

• IV 0.25 mg/kg bolus 10-60 min prior to start of PCTA, followed by a continuous INF of 10 mcg/min for 12 hr

💲 AVAILABLE FORMS/COST OF THERAPY

• Inj, Sol—IV: 2 mg/ml, 5 ml: **$540.02**

CONTRAINDICATIONS: Active internal bleeding; recent (within 6 wk) GI or GU bleeding of clinical significance; history of CVA within 2 yr or CVA with a significant residual neurological deficit; bleeding diathesis; administration of oral anticoagulants within 7 days unless prothrombin time is <1.2 × control; thrombocytopenia (<100,000 cells/μl); recent (within 6 wk) major surgery or trauma; intracranial neoplasm, arteriovenous malformation or aneurysm; severe uncontrolled hypertension; presumed or documented history of vasculitis; use of IV dextran before PCTA or intent to use it during PCTA; hypersensitivity to murine proteins

PRECAUTIONS: Elderly, children, weight <75 kg, prior thrombolytic therapy, history of GI disease; IM injections, urinary catheters, nasotracheal intubation, nasogastric tubes

PREGNANCY AND LACTATION: Pregnancy category C; excretion into breast milk unknown, use caution in nursing mothers

SIDE EFFECTS/ADVERSE REACTIONS

CNS: Hypesthesia, confusion

CV: Hypotension, bradycardia, ***bleeding*** (major bleeding 11.1%-14%)

EENT: Abnormal vision

GI: Nausea, vomiting

HEME: Anemia, leukocytosis, ***thrombocytopenia***

RESP: Pleural effusion, pneumonia

MISC: Pain, peripheral edema, human anti-chimeric antibody development, ***anaphylaxis***

INTERACTIONS

Drugs

🔢 *Antithrombotics* (aspirin, heparin, warfarin, ticlopidine, clopidogrel): Increased risk of bleeding

SPECIAL CONSIDERATIONS

PATIENT/FAMILY EDUCATION

• Fab fragment of the chimeric human-murine monoclonal antibody 7E3

• Intended to be used with aspirin and heparin

• In the event of serious bleeding that cannot be controlled by compression, discontinue abciximab and heparin

• In patients with failed PCTAs, stop INF

• Eptifibitide, tirofiban, and abciximab can all decrease the incidence of cardiac events associated with acute coronary syndromes; direct comparisons are needed to establish which, if any, is superior; for angioplasty, until more data become available, abciximab appears to be the drug of choice

---

* = non-FDA-approved use

MONITORING PARAMETERS
- Baseline platelet count, prothrombin time, aPTT; during INF closely monitor platelet count and aPTT (heparin therapy)

---

acarbose
(a-car'bose)
Rx: Precose
Chemical Class: α-amylase/α-glucosidase inhibitor
Therapeutic Class: Antidiabetic

CLINICAL PHARMACOLOGY
Mechanism of Action: Inhibits intestinal α-glucosidase, the enzyme responsible for digesting complex starches to oligosaccharides; delays postprandial absorption of glucose; attenuates postprandial plasma glucose peaks; does not increase insulin secretion
Pharmacokinetics
PO: Minimally absorbed in unchanged form; 35% of dose is absorbed as metabolites; biotransformation by intestinal microorganisms; metabolites excreted by urinary and fecal routes; $t_{1/2}$ 2.7-9 hr
INDICATIONS AND USES: Diabetes mellitus, type 1 and 2: adjunctive therapy in those insufficiently managed with other antidiabetic agents

DOSAGE
Adult
- PO 25 mg tid, taken at beginning of each meal; increase after 6-8 wk to 50-100 mg tid

💲 AVAILABLE FORMS/COST OF THERAPY
- Tab—Oral: 25 mg, 100's: **$51.71;** 50 mg, 100's: **$51.71;** 100 mg, 100's: **$66.68**

CONTRAINDICATIONS: Inflammatory bowel disease, colonic ulceration, partial intestinal obstruction, chronic intestinal disease associated with marked disorders of absorption or digestion, cirrhosis
PREGNANCY AND LACTATION: Pregnancy category B; excreted into breast milk in rats; no human data available

SIDE EFFECTS/ADVERSE REACTIONS
GI: Abdominal distension, borborygmus, diarrhea, elevated transaminases (15%), flatulence (70%)
METAB: Potential for hypoglycemia only with insulin or sulfonylureas

INTERACTIONS
Drugs
☒ *Charcoal, digestive enzyme preparations:* Reduced effects of acarbose
☒ *Cholestyramine:* Enhanced side effects of acarbose
☒ *Neomycin:* Enhanced reduction of postprandial blood glucose and exacerbation of adverse effects
☒ *Metformin:* Decreased metformin peak serum and AUC concentrations

SPECIAL CONSIDERATIONS
- Does not cause hypoglycemia
- Reduces HbAlc 0.5-1%

MONITORING PARAMETERS
- Self-monitored blood glucose; glucose, HbAlc 3-6 mo
- Consider ALT/AST during first yr

PATIENT/FAMILY EDUCATION
- Take glucose rather than complex carbohydrates to abort hypoglycemic episodes
- Decrease adverse GI effects by reducing dietary starch content

---

acebutolol

(a-se-byoo′-toe-lole)
Rx: Sectral
Chemical Class: β₁-selective (cardioselective) adrenoreceptor blocker
Therapeutic Class: Antihypertensive; antianginal

CLINICAL PHARMACOLOGY

Mechanism of Action: Competitive beta-adrenergic antagonist at β_1-receptor sites (cardioselective at usual doses; β_2-receptor blockade noted at higher doses); produces negative inotropic and chronotropic responses; slows AV nodal conduction; decreases heart rate; decreases myocardial oxygen consumption; antiarrhythmic effects (class II); reduction in platelet aggregation and blood viscosity; suppression of renin release; inhibition of central sympathetic outflow; decreases presynaptic receptor neurotransmitter release; no intrinsic sympathomimetic or membrane stabilizing activity; low lipid solubility

Pharmacokinetics

PO: Incomplete GI absorption (40%-60% bioavailable); peak serum concentrations, 2-4 hr; not metabolized by liver; excreted unchanged in urine and feces; $t_{1/2}$ 6-7 hr; crosses placenta in measurable, but not significant concentrations

INDICATIONS AND USES: Angina pectoris,* anxiety,* performance anxiety,* arrhythmia (class II), congestive heart failure,* hypertension, migraine headache,* post myocardial infarction,* alcohol withdrawal syndrome,* esophageal varices with cirrhosis*

DOSAGE

Adult

• *Hypertension:* PO 400 mg qd or in 2 divided doses; increase to desired response; usual range 400-800 mg/day

• *Ventricular premature beats:* PO 200 mg bid, may increase gradually; usual range 600-1200 mg daily

💲   **AVAILABLE FORMS/COST OF THERAPY**

• Cap, Gel—Oral: 200 mg, 100's: **$84.11-$123.49;** 400 mg, 100's: **$114.38-$164.20**

CONTRAINDICATIONS: Cardiogenic shock, heart block (2nd, 3rd degree), sinus bradycardia, CHF

PRECAUTIONS: Anesthesia/surgery (myocardial depression), avoid abrupt withdrawal, bronchospastic airways, congestive heart failure, diabetes mellitus, hyperthyroidism/thyrotoxicosis (acebutolol, unlike propranolol does not decrease T_3 levels), concurrent clonidine (discontinue acebutolol several days prior to withdrawal of clonidine), peripheral vascular disease, renal disease

PREGNANCY AND LACTATION: Pregnancy category D; frequently used in the third trimester for treatment of hypertension (many studies of efficacy and safety of atenolol in pregnancy induced hypertension); long-term use has been associated with intrauterine growth retardation; excreted into breast milk; observe for signs of beta-blockade

SIDE EFFECTS/ADVERSE REACTIONS

CNS: Catatonia, depression, *dizziness*, drowsiness, *fatigue,* hallucinations, *headache*, insomnia, lethargy, memory loss, strange dreams
CV: Bradycardia, **CHF**, cold extremities, postural hypotension, **2nd or 3rd degree heart block, shock**
EENT: Dry burning eyes, sore throat
GI: Diarrhea, elevated transaminases, **ischemic colitis, mesenteric arterial thrombosis,** nausea, vomiting
GU: Impotence
HEME: **Agranulocytosis,** positive

ANA, ***purpura, thrombocytopenia***
METAB: Hyperglycemia, increased hypoglycemic response to insulin
RESP: **Bronchospasm,** dyspnea, wheezing
SKIN: Alopecia, fever, rash

INTERACTIONS

Drugs

▪ *Alpha-1 adrenergic blockers:* Potential enhanced first dose response (marked initial drop in blood pressure, particularly on standing [especially prazocin])

▪ *Amiodarone:* Bradycardia/ventricular dysrhythmia

▪ *Anesthetics, local:* Enhanced sympathomimetic effects, hypertension due to unopposed α-receptor stimulation

▪ *Antacids:* May reduce β-blocker absorption

▪ *Antidiabetics:* Delayed recovery from hypoglycemia, hyperglycemia, attenuated tachycardia during hypoglycemia, hypertension during hypoglycemia

▪ *Digoxin:* Additive prolongation of atrioventricular (AV) conduction time

▪ *Dihydropyridine calcium channel blockers:* Severe hypotension or impaired cardiac performance; most prevalent with impaired left ventricular function, cardiac arrhythmias, or aortic stenosis

▪ *Diltiazem:* Severe hypotension or impaired cardiac performance; most prevalent with impaired left ventricular function, cardiac arrhythymias, or aortic stenosis

▪ *Dipyridamole:* Bradycardia

▪ *Disopyramide:* Additive decreases in cardiac output

▪ *Epinephrine:* Enhanced pressor response resulting in hypertension

▪ *Neostigmine:* Bradycardia

▪ *Neuroleptics:* Increased serum levels of both resulting in accentu-

ated pharmacologic response to both drugs

▪ *NSAIDs:* Reduced hypotensive effects

▪ *Phenylephrine:* Acute hypertensive episodes

▪ *Prazosin:* First-dose hypotensive response enhanced

▪ *Tacrine:* Additive bradycardia

❷ *Theophylline:* Antagonist pharmacodynamics

▪ *Verapamil:* Severe hypotension or impaired cardiac performance; most prevalent with impaired left ventricular function, cardiac arrhythmias, or aortic stenosis

SPECIAL CONSIDERATIONS

• Properties of low lipid solubility and competitive cardioselectivity yields less CNS and bronchospastic adverse effects

MONITORING PARAMETERS

• Angina: Reduction in nitroglycerin usage; frequency, severity, onset, and duration of angina pain; heart rate

• Arrhythmias: Heart rate

• Congestive heart failure: Functional status, cough, dyspnea on exertion, paroxysmal nocturnal dyspnea, exercise tolerance, and ventricular function

• Hypertension: Blood pressure

• Migraine headache: Reduction in the frequency, severity, and duration of attacks

• Postmyocardial infarction: Left ventricular function, lower resting heart rate

• Toxicity: Blood glucose, bronchospasm, hypotension, bradycardia, depression, confusion, hallucination, sexual dysfunction

PATIENT/FAMILY EDUCATION

• Do not discontinue abruptly; may require taper; rapid withdrawal may produce rebound hypertension or angina

---

italic = common side effects **bold italic** = life-threatening reactions

acetaminophen (APAP)

(ah-seet'ah-min-oh-fen)

OTC: Acephen, Apacet, Arthritis Pain Formula, Aspirin Free Pain Relief, Feverall, Genapap, Liquiprin, Neopap, Panadol, Tapanol Tempra, Tylenol

Combinations

Rx: with butalbital (Phrenilin); with butalbital and caffeine (Fioricet, Esgic, Isocet); with butalbital, caffeine and codeine (Amaphen, Fioricet w/codeine); with codeine (Tylenol, Phenaphen No. 2,3,4); with dichloralphenazone and isometheptene (Midrin, Midchlor); with hydrocodone (Vicodin, Lorcet, Lortab); with oxycodone (Percocet, Roxicet, Tylox); with pentazocine (Talacen); with propoxyphene (Wygesic, Darvocet-N)

OTC: with pamabrom ± pyrilamine (Midol PMS, Pamprin); with antihistamine and decongestant (Actifed Plus, Drixoral Cold & Flu, Benadryl Sinus, Sine-Off, Sinarest); with decongestant, antihistamine, dextromethorphan (Nyquil)

Chemical Class: Nonsalicylate, para-aminophenol derivative

Therapeutic Class: Nonnarcotic analgesic; antipyretic

CLINICAL PHARMACOLOGY

Mechanism of Action: Potent inhibitor of cyclo-oxygenase in the CNS; analgesic and antipyretic properties; no antiinflammatory properties

Pharmacokinetics

PO: Onset 10-30 min, peak ½-2 hr, duration 3-4 hr; 60%-70% bioavailable

PR: Onset slow, peak 1-2 hr, duration 3-4 hr; 30%-40% bioavailable; widely distributed; $t_{\frac{1}{2}}$ 3-4 hr; 85%-90% metabolized by liver, excreted by kidneys

INDICATIONS AND USES: Analgesia, antipyresis; arthritic and rheumatic conditions involving musculoskeletal pain; diseases accompanied by discomfort and fever (i.e., common cold, flu, and other bacterial and viral infections); headache, dysmenorrhea, toothaches, vaccine reaction prophylaxis

DOSAGE

Adult and Child >14 yr

• PO 325-1000 mg q4h prn, not to exceed 4 g/day; PR 325-1000 mg q4h prn, not to exceed 4 g/day

Child

• 10-15 mg/kg q4h, not to exceed 5 doses/24h

$ **AVAILABLE FORMS/COST OF THERAPY**

• Cap—Oral: 500 mg, 100's: **$1.95-$6.99**; 650 mg, 24's: **$3.20**

• Drops—Oral: 80 mg/0.8 ml, 15 ml: **$1.25-$4.34**

• Elixir—Oral: 160 mg/5 ml, 120 ml: **$1.04-$3.78**; 500 mg/15 ml, 240 ml: **$2.60-$3.78**

• Supp—Rect: 80 mg, 6's: **$4.56**; 120 mg, 12's: **$3.95-$6.50**; 325 mg, 12's: **$5.06-$12.73**; 650 mg, 12's: **$3.11-$11.75**

• Tab—Oral: 325 mg, 100's: **$1.40-$10.35**; 500 mg, 100's: **$1.70-$19.42**; 650 mg, 100's: **$9.93**

• Tab, Chewable—Oral: 80 mg, 30's: **$.60-$7.15**; 160 mg, 24's: **$1.63-$4.10**

PRECAUTIONS: Hepatic disease, renal disease, chronic alcoholism (≥3 drinks/day), elderly

PREGNANCY AND LACTATION:
Pregnancy category B; low concentrations in breast milk (1%-2% of maternal dose); compatible with breast feeding

SIDE EFFECTS/ADVERSE REACTIONS

HEME: Hemolytic anemia (long-term use), leukopenia, neutropenia, pancytopenia, thrombocytopenia
MISC: Overdosage: ***acute hepatic and renal failure,*** confusion, ***delirium followed by vascular collapse, convulsions, coma, death,*** drowsiness, jaundice, nausea, vomiting
SKIN: ***Angioedema,*** rash, urticaria

INTERACTIONS

Drugs

⌷ *Anticoagulants:* Enhanced hypoprothrombinemic response

⌷ *Anticonvulsants, Barbiturates, Rifabutin, Rifampin:* Enhanced hepatoxic potential in overdose

⌷ *Cholestyramine/Colestipol:* Reduced acetaminophen levels and response

⌷ *Ethanol:* Increased hepatoxicity in chronic, excessive alcohol ingestion

⌷ *Isoniazid:* Increased acetaminophen levels & hepatotoxicity

Overdosage

• Specific antidote is acetylcysteine; administer as serum level of acetaminophen indicates high risk of hepatotoxicity. Minimal toxic dose 10g (140 mg/kg), can occur with less, ≥20-25g potentially fatal

Labs

• *False decrease:* Amylase
• *False increase:* Urine 5-HIAA
• *Interference:* Cannot assay ticarcillin levels

SPECIAL CONSIDERATIONS
PATIENT/FAMILY EDUCATION

• Many OTC drugs contain acetaminophen; additive dosage may exceed 4 gm/day maximum and increase risk of hepatotoxicity

---

acetazolamide
(a-set-a-zole'a-mide)
Rx: AK-Zol, Diamox, Storzolamide
Chemical Class: Sulfonamide derivative; carbonic anhydrase inhibitor
Therapeutic Class: Diuretic, anticonvulsant; antiglaucoma agent; acute mountain sickness

CLINICAL PHARMACOLOGY

Mechanism of Action: *Kidney:* increased excretion of sodium, potassium, bicarbonate, and water—alkaline diuresis; *CNS:* reduction in rate of aqueous humor formation—decreased intraocular pressure (IOP); *Resp:* resultant metabolic acidosis yields compensatory enhanced ventilatory oxygenation at high altitude

Pharmacokinetics

PO: Onset 1-1½ hr, peak 2-4 hr, duration 6-12 hr
PO-SUS REL: Onset 2 hr, peak 8-12 hr, duration 18-24 hr
IV: Onset 2 min, peak 15 min, duration 4-5 hr
65% absorbed if fasting (oral), 75% absorbed if given with food; $t_{1/2}$ 2½-5½ hr; excreted unchanged by kidneys (80% within 24 hr); crosses placenta

INDICATIONS AND USES: Open-angle glaucoma, narrow-angle glaucoma (preoperatively, if surgery delayed), epilepsy (petit mal, grand mal, mixed), edema in CHF, drug-induced edema, acute mountain sickness (prevention and treatment)

DOSAGE

Adult

• *Narrow-angle glaucoma:* PO/IV 250 mg q4h or 250 mg bid, to be used for short-term therapy
• *Open-angle glaucoma:* PO/IV

---

italic = common side effects   ***bold italic*** = life-threatening reactions

250-1000 mg/day in divided doses for amounts over 250 mg

• *Seizures:* PO/IV 8-30 mg/kg/day, usual range 375-1000 mg/day

• *Mountain sickness:* Treatment: PO 250 mg q8-12h; Prophylaxis: PO 125 mg bid; Periodic breathing at altitude: PO 62.5-125 mg with dinner or hs

Child

• *Seizures:* PO/IV 8-30 mg/kg/day in divided doses tid or qid, or 300-900 mg/m^2/day, not to exceed 1.5 g/day

💲 AVAILABLE FORMS/COST OF THERAPY

• Tab, Uncoated—Oral: 125 mg, 100's: **$9.05-$32.56;** 250 mg, 100's: **$4.00-$48.44**

• Cap, Gel, Sus Action—Oral: 500 mg, 100's: **$120.36**

CONTRAINDICATIONS: Hypersensitivity to sulfonamides, severe renal disease, severe hepatic disease, electrolyte imbalances (hyponatremia, hypokalemia), hyperchloremic acidosis, Addison's disease, long-term use in narrow-angle glaucoma

PRECAUTIONS: Hypercalciuria

PREGNANCY AND LACTATION: Pregnancy category C; premature delivery and congenital anomalies in humans; teratogenic (defects of the limbs) in mice, rats, hamsters, and rabbits; not recommended for nursing mothers

SIDE EFFECTS/ADVERSE REACTIONS

CNS: Anxiety, confusion, depression, dizziness, drowsiness, fatigue, headache, nervousness, paresthesia, sedation, *seizures,* stimulation

EENT: Myopia, tinnitus

GI: Anorexia, constipation, diarrhea, *hepatic insufficiency,* melena, *nausea,* taste alterations, *vomiting,* weight loss

GU: Crystalluria, glucosuria, *hypo-kalemia,* polyuria, renal calculi, ***uremia***

HEME: **Agranulocytosis, aplastic anemia, hemolytic anemia, leukopenia, pancytopenia, purpura, thrombocytopenia**

METAB: Hyperglycemia

SKIN: Fever, photosensitivity, pruritus, *rash,* **Stevens-Johnson syndrome,** urticaria

MISC: Loss of taste of carbonated beverages

INTERACTIONS

Drugs

❸ *Cyclosporine:* Increased trough cyclosporine levels with potential for neurotoxicity and nephropathy

❸ *Flecainide, quinidine:* Alkalinization of urine increases quinidine serum levels

❸ *Methenamine compounds:* Alkalinization of urine decreases antibacterial effects

❸ *Phenytoin:* Increased risk of osteomalacia

❸ *Primidone:* Decreased primidone levels

❷ *Salicylates:* Increased serum levels of acetazolamide—CNS toxicity

Labs

• *False increase:* 17 hydroxysteroid

SPECIAL CONSIDERATIONS
PATIENT/FAMILY EDUCATION

• Carbonated beverages taste flat

• If GI symptoms occur, take with food

MONITORING PARAMETERS

• Intraocular pressure, reduction in AMS symptoms, serum electrolytes, creatinine, CO_2

---

* = non-FDA-approved use

acetic acid

(a-cee'tic)

Rx: Acetasol, Burow's Otic, VoSol

Combinations

Rx: with hydrocortisone (VoSol HC Otic, AA HC Otic, Acetasol HC) with oxyquinolone (Aci-Jel)

Chemical Class: Organic acid
Therapeutic Class: Antibacterial, antifungal

CLINICAL PHARMACOLOGY
Mechanism of Action: Bacteriostatic, fungistatic; penetrates bacterial cells, disrupts cell membrane; restores normal vaginal acidity
INDICATIONS AND USES: Prophylactically in surgical dressings, burns; bladder/urinary catheter irrigant; therapeutically for otitis externa (particularly *Pseudomonas* sp., *Candida* sp., and *Aspergillus* sp.) and to maintain vaginal acidity in vaginitis
DOSAGE
Adult
• *Otitis externa:* Instill 4-5 drops to affected ear tid
• *Urinary bladder catheter irrigant:* 30-50 ml flush
• *Vaginitis:* 1 applicatorful intravaginally bid
Child
• *Otitis externa:* Instill 4-5 drops to affected ear tid
$ AVAILABLE FORMS/COST OF THERAPY
• Gel—Vaginal: 0.92%, 85 g: **$28.20**
• Sol, bladder irrigation: 0.25%, 1000 ml: **$3.08-$4.86**
• Otic drops: 2%, 15 ml: **$1.87-$42.28**
PREGNANCY AND LACTATION:
Pregnancy category C when combined with oxyquinoline

SIDE EFFECTS/ADVERSE REACTIONS
EENT: Burning on instillation, irritation
GU: Irritation, local burning and stinging

acetohexamide

(a-seat-oh-hex'a-mide)

Rx: Dymelor
Chemical Class: Sulfonylurea (1st generation)
Therapeutic Class: Oral hypoglycemic

CLINICAL PHARMACOLOGY
Mechanism of Action: Decreases blood sugar via stimulation of insulin secretion and increased tissue responsiveness to insulin; initial hypoglycemic effects due to stimulation of pancreatic islets (dependent upon functioning beta-cells); extrapancreatic effect predominantly due to inhibition of hepatic glucose production, but may also facilitate improved insulin-insulin receptor binding
Pharmacokinetics
PO: Completely absorbed, onset 1 hr, peak 2-4 hr, duration 12-24 hr, $t_{1/2}$ 6-8 hr; metabolized in liver, excreted in urine (active metabolites, unchanged drug)
INDICATIONS AND USES: Diabetes mellitus, type 2
DOSAGE
Adult
• PO 250 mg-1.5 g/day; before breakfast. At 1.5 g/day divide bid
$ AVAILABLE FORMS/COST OF THERAPY
• Tab, Uncoated—Oral: 250 mg, 100's: **$26.38-$26.42;** 500 mg, 100's: **$26.42-$37.48**
CONTRAINDICATIONS: Diabetes type 1, ketoacidosis

---

italic = common side effects   ***bold italic*** = life-threatening reactions

PRECAUTIONS: Elderly, cardiac disease, renal disease, hepatic disease, thyroid disease, severe hypoglycemic reactions

PREGNANCY AND LACTATION: Pregnancy category; inappropriate for use during pregnancy due to inadequate blood glucose control, potential for prolonged neonatal hypoglycemia, and risk of congenital abnormalities; insulin is the drug of choice for control of blood sugars during pregnancy; breast milk secretion, unknown—the potential for neonatal hypoglycemia dictates caution in nursing mothers

SIDE EFFECTS/ADVERSE REACTIONS

CNS: Dizziness, fatigue, headache, tinnitus, vertigo, weakness

GI: Elevated transaminases, heartburn, jaundice, nausea

GU: Uricosuria

HEME: **Agranulocytosis, aplastic anemia, hemolytic anemia, leukopenia, thrombocytopenia**

METAB: **Hypoglycemia,** hyponatremia (SIADH)

SKIN: Allergic reactions, eczema, erythema, photosensitivity, pruritus, rash, urticaria

INTERACTIONS

Drugs

🔳 *β-adrenergic blockers:* Altered response to hypoglycemia; may increase blood glucose

🔳 *Clofibrate:* Enhanced hypoglycemic effects

🔳 *Clonidine:* Diminished symptoms of hypoglycemia

🔳 *Corticosteroids:* Steroids increase blood glucose in diabetics

🔳 *Cyclosporine:* Increased cyclosporine concentrations (possible nephrotoxicity)

⚠ *Ethanol:* Excessive alcohol increases risks of hypoglycemia; disulfiram-like reactions

🔳 *Halofenate:* May increase acetohexamide serum level

🔳 *H_2 blockers:* Possible altered glycemic response (increased or decreased glucose)

🔳 *MAOIs:* Increased risk of hypoglycemia

❷ *Phenylbutazone:* Increased acetohexamide serum level and hypoglycemic effects

🔳 *Potassium:* Enhanced hypoglycemic effect

🔳 *Rifampin/Rifabutin:* Possible increased glucose levels

🔳 *Sulfonamides:* Possible enhanced hypoglycemic effects

🔳 *Thiazide diuretics:* May increase blood glucose

⚠ *Tricyclic antidepressants:* Increased risk of hypoglycemia

Labs

• *False increase:* BUN, creatinine

SPECIAL CONSIDERATIONS

PATIENT/FAMILY EDUCATION

• Symptoms of hypoglycemia: tingling lips/tongue, nausea, confusion, fatigue, sweating, hunger, visual changes (spots)

• Multiple drug interactions, including alcohol and salicylates

MONITORING PARAMETERS

• Self-monitored blood glucose; HbAlc q3-6 mo

---

acetohydroxamic acid (AHA)

(a-set′oh-hye-drox-am′ic)

Rx: Lithostat

Chemical Class: Hydroxylamine, ethyl acetate compound
Therapeutic Class: Urinary tract product

CLINICAL PHARMACOLOGY

Mechanism of Action: Inhibits bacterial enzyme urease, which decreases conversion of urea to ammonia; the reduced ammonia levels and decreased pH increase the effectiveness of concurrent urinary antimicrobial agents

Pharmacokinetics
PO: Peak 15-60 min, $t_{1/2}$ 3½-10 hr; hepatic metabolism, excreted in urine as unchanged drug (15%-60%)
INDICATIONS AND USES: Adjunctive treatment in chronic urinary tract infections due to urea-splitting organisms
DOSAGE
Adult
• PO 250 mg q6-8h when stomach is empty, not to exceed 1.5 g/day
Child
• PO 10 mg/kg/day in 2-3 divided doses
§ AVAILABLE FORMS/COST OF THERAPY
• Tab—Oral: 250 mg, 100's: **$100.61**
CONTRAINDICATIONS: Severe renal disease, infection by nonurease-producing organisms
PRECAUTIONS: Deep vein thrombosis, hepatic disease, renal disease, lactation
PREGNANCY AND LACTATION: Pregnancy category X; teratogenic (retarded and clubbed rear leg at 750 mg/kg and above and exencephaly and encephalocele at 1500 mg/kg) when given intraperitoneally to rats
SIDE EFFECTS/ADVERSE REACTIONS
CNS: Anxiety, depression, headache, malaise, *nervousness, restlessness*
CV: Deep vein thrombosis, palpitations, phlebitis, pulmonary embolism
GI: Anorexia, nausea, vomiting
*HEME: **Hemolytic anemia (Coombs' negative; 15%)***
SKIN: Alopecia, rash on face, arms

SPECIAL CONSIDERATIONS
PATIENT/FAMILY EDUCATION
• Avoid alcohol: Promotes skin rash
• Concurrent contraception recommended during treatment

---

acetylcholine
(a-se-teel-koe′leen)
Rx: Miochol-E
Chemical Class: Quaternary ammonium derivative
Therapeutic Class: Miotic, ophthalmic cholinergic

CLINICAL PHARMACOLOGY
Mechanism of Action: Intense, immediate miosis by causing contraction of sphincter muscle of iris
Pharmacokinetics
OPHTH: Miosis occurs immediately, duration 10 min
INDICATIONS AND USES: Miosis during anterior segment surgery, cataract surgery, peripheral iridectomy, cyclodialysis
DOSAGE
Adult and Child
• INSTILL 0.5-2 ml of a 1% sol in anterior chamber of eye (instillation by provider)
§ AVAILABLE FORMS/COST OF THERAPY
• Kit—Ophth: 1%, 2 ml: **$28.55**
CONTRAINDICATIONS: When miosis is undesirable
PRECAUTIONS: Acute cardiac failure, bronchial asthma
SIDE EFFECTS/ADVERSE REACTIONS
CV: Bradycardia, hypotension
EENT: Blurred vision, lens opacities

---

acetylcysteine
(a-see-til-sis'tay-een)
Rx: Mucomyst, Mucosil;
Chemical Class: Amino acid,
L-cysteine
Therapeutic Class: Mucolytic;
acetaminophen antidote

CLINICAL PHARMACOLOGY
Mechanism of Action: Decreases
viscosity of secretions by breaking
disulfide links of mucoproteins; increases hepatic glutathione, which
is necessary to inactivate toxic metabolites in acetaminophen overdose
Pharmacokinetics
NEB/INSTILL: Onset 1 min, duration
5-10 min
PO: Peak levels within 1-2 hr (0.35-4
mg/L); 50% protein binding; terminal $t_{1/2}$ 6.25 hr; metabolized by liver,
excreted in urine
INDICATIONS AND USES: Antidote for acetaminophen overdose;
mucolytic: adjuvant therapy for
abnormal, viscid, or inspissated mucus secretions in chronic broncho-
pulmonary disease; diagnostic bronchial scans (bronchograms, bron-
chospirometry, bronchial wedge
catheterization); keratoconjunctivitis sicca* (as ophthalmic solution);
bowel obstruction due to meconium
ileus* (as an enema)
DOSAGE
Adult and Child
• *Mucolytic:* Instill 1-2 ml (10%-
20% sol) q1-4h prn; neb 3-5 ml
(20% sol) or 6-10 ml (10% sol) tid
• *Acetaminophen toxicity*: PO 140
mg/kg, then 70 mg/kg q4h × 17
doses to total of 1330 mg/kg; (dilute 20% solution to concentration
of 5%; dilutions should be freshly
prepared and utilized within 1 hr)

💲 **AVAILABLE FORMS/COST
   OF THERAPY**
• Sol, INH—Oral: 10%, 4 ml, 10
ml, 30 ml: **$2.53-$9.64**/4 ml
• Sol, INH—Oral: 20%, 4 ml, 10
ml, 30 ml: **$3.66-$11.57**/4 ml
PRECAUTIONS: Asthma, hepatic
disease, renal disease, COPD, alco-
holism
PREGNANCY AND LACTATION:
Pregnancy category B
**SIDE EFFECTS/ADVERSE REAC-
   TIONS**
CNS: Chills, dizziness, drowsiness,
fever, headache
EENT: Rhinorrhea
GI: Anorexia, nausea, stomatitis,
vomiting
RESP: Bronchospasm, chest tight-
ness
SKIN: Clamminess, fever, rash, ur-
ticaria
INTERACTIONS
• Avoid use with iron, copper, rub-
ber
SPECIAL CONSIDERATIONS
• Disagreeable odor may be noted
• Solution in opened bottle may
change color, of no significance

acitretin
(a-si-tre'tin)
Rx: Soriatane
Chemical Class: Retinoid
Therapeutic Class: Antipsori-
atic agent

CLINICAL PHARMACOLOGY
Mechanism of Action: Unknown;
accelerated reappearance of stratum
corneum and inhibition of neutrophil migration from dermal capil-
laries are among proposed mechanisms
Pharmacokinetics
PO: Peak serum level 3-4 hr; bioavailability enhanced by food; 99%
protein bound, not stored in adipose

* = non-FDA-approved use

tissue; metabolized by liver to active metabolites, excreted equally in bile and urine; $t_{1/2}$ 50-100 hr

INDICATIONS AND USES: Psoriasis, cutaneous lupus erythematosus*; Darier's disease*; lichen planus*; lichen sclerosis et atrophicus*; X-linked ichthyosis*

DOSAGE

Adult

• *Psoriasis:* PO 25-50 mg qd with food

• *Nonpsoriatic dermatoses:* PO 25-50 mg qd with food

Child

• *Psoriasis:* PO 1 mg/kg qd with food

• *Nonpsoriatic dermatoses:* PO 1 mg/kg qd with food

$ AVAILABLE FORMS/COST OF THERAPY

Caps—Oral: 10 mg, 30's: **$199.10**; 25 mg, 30's: **$261.97**

CONTRAINDICATIONS: Pregnancy, alcohol, concurrent use of vitamin A preparations

PRECAUTIONS: Women of childbearing age should use contraception during therapy and for 3 yr after therapy; renal insufficiency, liver disease, hyperlipidemia, pancreatitis

PREGNANCY AND LACTATION: Pregnancy category X; breast milk excretion unknown

SIDE EFFECTS/ADVERSE REACTIONS

CNS: Dizziness, dysesthesia, fatigue, headache, pseudotumor cerebri

EENT: Cheilitis (80%), conjunctivitis (40%), decreased night vision, *dry eyes (40%), dry nose (50%),* epistaxis, *stomatitis (6%), xerostomia (50%)*

GI: Increased transaminase levels (16%), nausea

HEME: Thrombocytosis

METAB: Hypertriglyceridemia, hyperglycemia

MS: Arthralgia, hyperostosis, *myalgia*

SKIN: Alopecia, dry skin (70%), nail fragility, pruritus, rash

MISC: Chills, diaphoresis (25%)

INTERACTIONS

Drugs

❷ *Methotrexate:* Increased potential for hepatotoxicity

❷ *Ethanol:* Drastically increases the $t_{1/2}$ of acitretin metabolite, etretinate

SPECIAL CONSIDERATIONS
PATIENT/FAMILY EDUCATION

• Avoid low dose (levonorgestrel 0.03 mg) progestin contraceptives

MONITORING PARAMETERS

• Transaminase levels monthly for first 6 mo then every 3 mo

• Lipid levels monthly for first 4 mo then every 2-3 mo

• Yearly radiographs to monitor for drug-induced vertebral abnormalities

• In children, measure PO_4, Ca levels in blood and urine and vitamin D and PTH levels every 6 mo

---

acyclovir

(ay-sye'kloe-ver)

Rx: Zovirax

Chemical Class: Acyclic purine nucleoside analog
Therapeutic Class: Antiviral

CLINICAL PHARMACOLOGY

Mechanism of Action: Interferes with DNA synthesis by conversion to acyclovir triphosphate, causing decreased viral DNA replication

Pharmacokinetics

IV: Onset unknown, peak 1 hr

PO: Onset unknown, peak 1½-2 hr, bioavailability 10%-20%; $t_{1/2}$ 3½ hr; distributed widely, CSF concentrations are 50% of plasma, crosses placenta; metabolized by liver, excreted by kidneys as unchanged drug (95%)

INDICATIONS AND USES

• *PARENTERAL:* Initial and recurrent mucosal and cutaneous HSV-1, HSV-2, herpes zoster in immunocompromised patients; HSV encephalitis in patients >6 months; severe initial clinical episodes of genital herpes in patients who are not immunocompromised

• *Oral:* Initial and recurrent genital herpes, acute treatment of herpes zoster and chicken pox; CMV and HSV following bone marrow or renal transplant*; disseminated primary eczema herpeticum*; herpes simplex—associated with erythema multiforme*; herpes simplex—labialis, ocular infections, proctitis, whitlow*; herpes zoster encephalitis*; infectious mononucleosis*; varicella*; pneumonia*

• *Top:* Initial herpes genitalis and limited non-life-threatening mucocutaneous herpes simplex in immunocompromised patients

DOSAGE

Adult

• *Herpes simplex:* IV 500 mg/m^2 over 1 hr q8h × 5 days

• *Genital herpes:* PO 200 mg q4h 5×/day while awake for 10 days, 5 days, or 6 mo depending on whether initial, recurrent, or chronic

• *Genital herpes, suppressive therapy:* 400 mg bid × 12 mos, then reevaluate need off drug

• *Herpes simplex encephalitis:* IV 10 mg/kg over 1 hr q8h × 10 days

• *Herpes zoster:* PO 800 mg q4h 5×/day × 7-10 days; IV 500 mg/m^2 over 1 hr q8h

• *Chicken pox:* PO 20 mg/kg (not to exceed 800 mg) orally, qid for 5 days at the earliest sign or symptom. With immunosuppression IV 10 mg/kg over 1 h q8h × 10 days

• *Renal failure:* IV CrCl 25-50 ml/

min/1.73m^2: give dose q12h; CrCl 10-25: give dose q24h; CrCl 0-10: reduce dose 50%, give q24h

• *Renal failure:* PO CrCl <10 ml/ min/1.73m^2: give dose q12h

Child

• *Herpes simplex:* IV 250 mg/m^2 over 1 hr q8h × 5 days

• *Herpes simplex encephalitis:* Child >6 mo: IV 500 mg/m^2 q8h × 10 days; child >2 yr with immunosuppression: 20 mg/kg qid × 5 days

• *Chicken pox:* 20 mg/kg orally up to 800 mg qid for 5 days

💲 AVAILABLE FORMS/COST OF THERAPY

• Inj, Powder—IV: 500 mg: **$21.88-$49.00**

• Susp—Oral: 200 mg/5 ml, 480 ml: **$83.26**

• Tab, Uncoated—Oral: 400 mg, 100's: **$189.60;** 800 mg, 100's: **$368.65**

• Cap, Gel—Oral: 200 mg, 100's: **$97.70**

• Oint—Top: 5%, 3 g: **$18.71**

PRECAUTIONS: Hepatic disease, renal disease, electrolyte imbalance, dehydration

PREGNANCY AND LACTATION: Pregnancy category C; excreted into breast milk; compatible with breast feeding

SIDE EFFECTS/ADVERSE REACTIONS

CNS: Confusion, dizziness, hallucinations, headache, lethargy, *seizures,* tremors

EENT: Gingival hyperplasia

GI: Abdominal pain, diarrhea, nausea, transaminase elevation, vomiting

GU: **Acute renal failure,** *elevated BUN/Creat (5-10%),* **glomerulonephritis,** hematuria, oliguria, proteinuria

MS: Joint pain, leg pain, muscle cramps

SKIN: Pain or phlebitis at IV site

---

* = non-FDA-approved use

SPECIAL CONSIDERATIONS
• In recurrent herpes genitalis and herpes labialis in non-immunocompromised patients, no evidence of clinical benefit from topical acyclovir

---

adapalene
(a-dap'pa-leen)
Rx: Differin
Chemical Class: Naphthoic acid derivative (retinoid-like)
Therapeutic Class: Antiacne agent

CLINICAL PHARMACOLOGY
Mechanism of Action: Modulates DNA transcription and thereby cell differentiation; causes comedolysis and reduces inflammation
Pharmacokinetics
TOP: Minimal absorption; primarily biliary excretion
INDICATIONS AND USES: Acne vulgaris
DOSAGE
Adult
• Apply thin film to affected area after washing in the evening at bedtime
💲 AVAILABLE FORMS/COST OF THERAPY
• Gel—Top: 0.1%, 15, 45 g: **$27.31/15 g**
• Sol—Top, 0.1%, 30 ml: **$59.19**
PRECAUTIONS: May aggravate acne early in treatment; do not use if sunburned or if using topical preparations containing sulfur, resorcinol, or salicylic acid
PREGNANCY AND LACTATION: Pregnancy category C; excretion in breast milk unknown
SIDE EFFECTS/ADVERSE REACTIONS
SKIN: Burning, dryness, erythema, pruritus, scaling (most common during first month of therapy; one or more adverse effects in 30-60% with solution, 10-40% with gel)
SPECIAL CONSIDERATIONS
• Avoid excessive exposure to sunlight
• Do not apply to lips or mucous membranes, or to cut, abraded, or sunburned skin
• May aggravate acne early in course of therapy
• Therapeutic results noticed in 8-12 wks

---

adenosine
(ah-den'oh-seen)
Rx: Adenocard
Chemical Class: Endogenous nucleoside
Therapeutic Class: Antidysrhythmic

CLINICAL PHARMACOLOGY
Mechanism of Action: Slows conduction through AV node; interrupts reentry pathways through AV node
Pharmacokinetics
IV: Cleared from plasma in <30 sec, $t_{1/2}$ 10 sec
INDICATIONS AND USES: PSVT, including PSVT associated with Wolff-Parkinson-White syndrome; does *not* convert atrial flutter, atrial fibrillation, or ventricular tachycardia to normal sinus rhythm; symptomatic relief of varicose vein complications with stasis dermatitis
DOSAGE
Adult
• *PSVT:* IV bolus 6 mg; if conversion to normal sinus rhythm does not occur within 1-2 min, give 12 mg by rapid IV bolus; may repeat 12 mg dose again in 1-2 min
• *Varicose veins:* IM 25 mg once or twice daily until relief is obtained and then 25 mg 2 or 3 times weekly for maintenance

---

italic = common side effects   ***bold italic*** = life-threatening reactions

Child
• *PSVT:* IV bolus 0.05 mg/kg; if not effective within 2 min, increase dose in 0.05 mg/kg increments every 2 min to a maximum of 0.25 mg/kg or until termination of PSVT; median dose, 0.15 mg/kg; do not exceed 12 mg/dose

$ AVAILABLE FORMS/COST OF THERAPY
• Inj, Sol—IM: 25 mg/ml, 10 ml: **$7.19-$17.85**
• Inj, Sol—IV: 3 mg/ml, 2 ml: **$31.76-$33.60**

CONTRAINDICATIONS: Second or third degree heart block, AV block, sick sinus syndrome, atrial flutter, atrial fibrillation, ventricular tachycardia

PRECAUTIONS: Asthma

PREGNANCY AND LACTATION: Pregnancy category C; fetal effects unlikely

SIDE EFFECTS/ADVERSE REACTIONS
CNS: Apprehension, arm tingling, blurred vision, dizziness, headache, lightheadedness, numbness
*CV: **Atrial tachydysrhythmia,** chest pain, facial flushing (18%),* hypotension, palpitations, sweating
GI: Groin pressure, metallic taste, nausea, throat tightness
RESP: Chest pressure, dyspnea, hyperventilation

INTERACTIONS
Drug
3 *β-blockers:* Bradycardia
3 *Dipyridamole:* Increased serum adenosine levels, potentiates pharmacologic effects of adenosine
3 *Nicotine:* Greater hemodynamic response to adenosine (hypotension, chest pain)
3 *Theophylline/caffeine:* Inhibits hemodynamic effects of adenosine

albendazole
(al-ben′da-zole)
Rx: Albenza
Chemical Class: Benzimidazole derivative
Therapeutic Class: Anthelminthic

CLINICAL PHARMACOLOGY
Mechanism of Action: Causes selective degeneration of cytoplasmic microtubules in cells of intestinal helminths and their tissue-dwelling larvae

Pharmacokinetics
PO: Onset 30 min, peak 2 hr, elimination $t_{1/2}$ 8 hr; absorption less than 5% of oral dose (serum level increased 4-fold with fatty meal); rapidly metabolized by liver, excreted in urine; active metabolite, albendazole sulfoxide, penetrates hydatid cyst fluid and CSF and is 70% protein bound

INDICATIONS AND USES: Hydatid disease, neurocysticercosis, infestations by susceptible protozoa* and helminths*

DOSAGE
Adult
• *Capillariasis:* PO 200 mg bid × 10 days
• *Clonorchiasis:* PO 400 mg qd × 7 days
• *Cysticercosis, neurocysticercosis (echinococciasis):* PO 7.5 mg/kg bid with food × 8-30 days, maximum dose 400 mg bid
• *Filariasis (loiasis):* PO 400 mg bid × 21 days
• *Giardiasis, Hymenolepsis nana, cutaneous larva migrans (toxocariasis):* PO 400 mg qd × 3 days
• *Hookworm (ancylostomiasis), pinworm (enterobiasis), roundworm (ascariasis), whipworm (trichuria-*

---

* = non-FDA-approved use

sis): PO 400 mg, may repeat dose in 3 wk

• *Hydatid cyst disease (echinococciasis):* PO 7.5 mg/kg bid with food × 28 days, maximum dose 400 mg bid; repeat after 14 drug-free days for total of 3 cycles

• *Microsporidiosis:* PO 400 mg qd × 30 days, maintenance therapy may be required in HIV-infected persons

• *Opisthorchiasis:* PO 400 mg bid × 3 days

• *Strongyloidiasis, tapeworm (taeniasis):* PO 400 mg qd × 3 days, may repeat treatment in 3 wk

• *Trichinosis:* PO 400 mg bid × 15 days

• *Trichostrongyliasis:* PO 400 mg

• *Visceral larva migrans (toxocariasis):* PO 10 mg/kg/day in 2-3 divided doses × 5 days

Child

• *Capillariasis:* Age 1-12 yr: PO 200 mg bid × 10 days

• *Clonorchiasis:* Age 2-12 yr: PO 400 mg qd × 7 days

• *Giardiasis, Hymenolepsis nana, cutaneous larva migrans (toxocariasis):* Age 2-12 yr: PO 400 mg qd × 3 days

• *Hookworm (ancylostomiasis), pinworm (enterobiasis), roundworm (ascariasis), whipworm (trichuriasis):* Age 2-12 yr: PO 400 mg, repeat dose in 3 wk; Age 0-2 yr: PO 200 mg, may repeat dose in 3 wk

• *Hydatid cyst disease (echinococciasis):* Age 2-12 yr: PO 7.5 mg/kg bid with food × 28 days, maximum dose 400 mg bid; repeat after 14 drug-free days for total of 3 cycles

• *Neurocysticercosis (echinococciasis):* Age 1-12 yr: PO 7.5 mg/kg bid with food × 8-30 days, maximum dose 400 mg bid

• *Opisthorchiasis:* Age 2-12 yr: PO 400 mg bid × 3 days

• *Strongyloidiasis, tapeworm (tae-*

niasis): Age 2-12 yr: PO 400 mg qd × 3 days, may repeat treatment in 3 wk; Age 0-2 yr: PO 200 mg qd × 3 days, may repeat treatment in 3 wk

• *Trichinosis:* Age 2-12 yr: PO 400 mg bid × 15 days

• *Trichostrongyliasis:* Age 1-12 yr: PO 400 mg

• *Visceral larva migrans (toxocariasis):* Age 0-12 yr: PO 10 mg/kg/day in 2-3 divided doses × 5 days

💲 AVAILABLE FORMS/COST OF THERAPY

• Tab, Uncoated—Oral: 200 mg, 112's: **$101.80**

PRECAUTIONS: Administer with corticosteroids in patients with neurocysticercosis, avoid during pregnancy

PREGNANCY AND LACTATION: Pregnancy category C, excreted in breast milk

SIDE EFFECTS/ADVERSE REACTIONS

CNS: Dizziness, headache

GI: Abdominal pain, *abnormal LFTs* anorexia, constipation, diarrhea, dry mouth, hepatotoxicity (5%, high dose only), nausea, vomiting

HEME: Eosinophilia, neutropenia (5%, high dose only)

SKIN: Alopecia, pruritus, rash

MISC: Fever

INTERACTIONS

Drugs

3 *Dexamethasone:* 56% increase in serum level of albendazole

3 *Praziquantel:* 50% increase in serum level of albendazole

SPECIAL CONSIDERATIONS

• For appropriate infections, retest stool 3 wk after treatment to detect residual ova

• Patients treated for neurocystircercosis should receive steroid and anticonvulsant therapy

---

italic = common side effects   ***bold italic*** = life-threatening reactions

albuterol

(al-byoo'ter-ole)

Rx: Airet, Albuterol, Proventil, Proventil-HFA, Proventil Repetabs, Respirol, Ventolin, Ventolin Rotacaps, Volmax

Combinations

Rx: with ipratropium (Combivent)

Chemical Class: Sympathomimetic amine; β_2- adrenergic agonist

Therapeutic Class: Antiasthmatic, bronchodilator

CLINICAL PHARMACOLOGY

Mechanism of Action: Causes bronchodilation by β_2-stimulation, resulting in relaxation of bronchial smooth muscle; inhibits mast cell degranulation; stimulates cilia to remove secretions

Pharmacokinetics

PO: Onset ½ hr, peak 2½ hr, duration 4-6 hr

PO EXT REL: Onset ½ hr, peak 2-3 hr, duration 12 hr

INH: Onset 5-15 min, peak 1-1½ hr, duration 4-6 hr

Metabolized in liver to inactive sulfate; 28% appears unchanged in urine; $t_{1/2}$ 2½-4 hr

INDICATIONS AND USES: Relief and prevention of bronchospasm in reversible airway disease; exercise-induced bronchospasm

DOSAGE

Adult

• *Prevention of exercise-induced bronchospasm:* MDI 2 puffs, 15 min before exercising

• *Bronchospasm:* MDI 1-2 puffs q4-6h; neb 2.5 mg (3 ml of 0.083% soln) tid-qid; PO 2-4 mg tid-qid, not to exceed 8 mg qid

Child (6-12 yr)

• *Prevention of exercise-induced bronchospasm:* MDI: 2 puffs 15 min before exercising

• *Bronchospasm:* PO 2 mg qid, not to exceed 24 mg per day (given in divided doses); MDI 1-2 puffs q4-6h; neb 2.5 mg (3 ml of .083% soln) tid-qid

Child (4-6 yr)

• *Bronchospasm:* PO initial, 0.1 mg/kg of body weight tid, not to exceed 2 mg tid; increase to 0.2 mg/kg of body weight tid, but not to exceed a maximum of 4 mg tid; neb 0.1-0.15 mg/kg (0.12-0.18 ml/kg of .083% soln) q1h initially then q4-6h

💲 AVAILABLE FORMS/COST OF THERAPY

• Sol—INH: 0.083%, 3 ml: **$0.60-$1.71**; 0.5%, 20 ml: **$12.50-$20.52**

• Syr—Oral: 2 mg/5 ml, 480 ml: **$5.33-$38.51**

• MDI—INH: 0.09 mg/puff, 17 g (200 puffs): **$7.47-$31.80**

• Cap, Gel—INH: puffs: 200 µg, 100's: **$37.55**

• Tab, Uncoated—Oral: 2 mg, 100's: **$2.67-$46.34;** 4 mg, 100's: **$3.78-$69.11**

• Tab, Coated, Sus Action—Oral: 4 mg, 100's: **$77.62-$79.11;** 8 mg, 100's: **$146.87**

CONTRAINDICATIONS: Tachydysrhythmias, severe cardiac disease

PRECAUTIONS: Ischemic heart disease, cardiac dysrhythmias, hyperthyroidism, diabetes mellitus, hypertension, prostatic hypertrophy

PREGNANCY AND LACTATION: Pregnancy category C

SIDE EFFECTS/ADVERSE REACTIONS

CNS: Anxiety, *dizziness,* flushing, hallucinations, *headache,* insomnia, irritability, restlessness, *stimulation, tremors*

---

* = non-FDA-approved use

CV: Angina, dysrhythmias, hypertension, hypotension, *palpitations, tachycardia*

EENT: Dry nose, irritation of nose and throat

GI: Heartburn, *nausea,* vomiting

METAB: Hypokalemia

MS: Inhibition of uterine contractions, muscle cramps

RESP: Cough

INTERACTIONS

Drugs

3 β*-blockers:* Decreased action of albuterol, cardioselective beta-blockers preferable if concurrent use necessary

3 *Furosemide:* Potential for additive hypokalemia

SPECIAL CONSIDERATIONS
• Inhalation technique critical
• Consider spacer devices

PATIENT/FAMILY EDUCATION
• See clinician if using ≥4 inhalations/day on regular basis or >1 canister (200 inhalations) in 8 wks

---

alclometasone
(al-clo-met′a-sone)

Rx: Aclovate

Chemical Class: Glucocorticoid

Therapeutic Class: Topical corticosteroid, low potency

CLINICAL PHARMACOLOGY

Mechanism of Action: Depresses formation, release, and activity of endogenous mediators of inflammation such as prostaglandins, kinins, histamine, liposomal enzymes, and the complement system resulting in decreased edema, erythema, and pruritus

Pharmacokinetics

TOP: Approximately 3% absorbed during 8 hr of contact with intact, normal skin; metabolized primarily in liver and then excreted by kidneys and into bile

INDICATIONS AND USES: Psoriasis, eczema, contact dermatitis, pruritus of corticosteroid responsive dermatoses

DOSAGE

Adult and Child
• TOP: Apply to affected area bid, rub completely into skin

§ **AVAILABLE FORMS/COST OF THERAPY**
• Cre/Oint—Top: 0.05%, 15, 45, 60 g: **$14.11**/15 g

PRECAUTIONS: Viral infections, bacterial infections, children

PREGNANCY AND LACTATION: Pregnancy category C; unknown whether topical application could result in sufficient systemic absorption to produce detectable amounts in breast milk (systemic corticosteroids are secreted into breast milk in quantities not likely to have detrimental effects on infant)

SIDE EFFECTS/ADVERSE REACTIONS

SKIN: Acne, allergic contact dermatitis, atrophy, burning, dryness, folliculitis, hypertrichosis, hypopigmentation, irritation, itching, miliaria, perioral dermatitis, secondary infection, striae

MISC: Systemic absorption of topical corticosteroids has produced reversible HPA axis suppression (more likely with occlusive dressings, prolonged administration, application to large surface areas, liver failure, and in children)

SPECIAL CONSIDERATIONS
PATIENT/FAMILY EDUCATION
• Apply sparingly only to affected area
• Avoid contact with the eyes
• Do not put bandages or dressings over treated area unless directed by clinician

---

• Discontinue drug, notify clinician if local irritation or fever develops
• Do not use on weeping, denuded, or infected areas

---

alendronate
(a-len'dro-nate)
Rx: Fosamax
Chemical Class: Synthetic analog of pyrophosphate
Therapeutic Class: Bisphosphonate

CLINICAL PHARMACOLOGY
Mechanism of Action: Highly selective binding to hydroxyapatite at sites of bone resorption, inhibits normal and abnormal bone resorption ("crystal poison"); minimal secondary reduction in bone formation (resorption coupled to formation); bone formation exceeds bone resorption at these remodeling sites, leading to progressive gains in bone mass
Pharmacokinetics
PO: Onset 3-4 wk; bioavailability <1%, food decreases bioavailability by 40%; protein binding 78%; t$_{1/2}$ (*in bone*) up to 10 yr
INDICATIONS AND USES: Treatment and prophylaxis of osteoporosis in postmenopausal women; Paget's disease of bone; prevention of glucocorticoid-induced osteoporosis, hyperparathyroidism,* bone pain in prostatic carcinoma and metastatic breast cancer,* hypercalcemia of malignancy*
DOSAGE
Adult
• *Osteoporosis (prophylaxis):* PO 5 mg qd (Treatment): PO 10 mg qd
• *Paget's disease:* PO 40 mg qd for 6 mo
Child
• Safety and efficacy not established

* = non-FDA-approved use

💲 AVAILABLE FORMS/COST OF THERAPY
• Tab—Oral: 5 mg, 100's: **$202.96;** 10 mg, 100's: **$202.96;** 40 mg, 30's: **$159.01**
CONTRAINDICATIONS: Hypocalcemia, esophageal abnormalities, delayed esophageal emptying, patient unable to stand or sit upright for at least 30 min after administration
PRECAUTIONS: CrCl <35 ml/min; uncorrected mineral deficiencies (i.e., calcium, vitamin D)
PREGNANCY AND LACTATION: Pregnancy category C; contraindicated in nursing mothers
SIDE EFFECTS/ADVERSE REACTIONS
CNS: Headache
GI: Abdominal distention, *abdominal pain,* acid regurgitation, dysphagia, esophageal ulcer, flatulence, gastritis
METAB: Hypocalcemia, hypophosphatemia
MS: Musculoskeletal pain
SKIN: Erythema, rash
MISC: Drug fever
INTERACTIONS
Drugs
🔟 *Antacids:* Calcium, magnesium and aluminum bind alendronate and reduce absorption
🔟 *Food (including coffee and orange juice):* Decreases bioavailability of alendronate by 40%-60%
🔟 *Aspirin:* Increased risk of upper GI adverse effects
SPECIAL CONSIDERATIONS
PATIENT/FAMILY EDUCATION
• Patients should receive supplemental calcium and vitamin D if dietary intake is inadequate
• Administer 30 min before the first food/beverage/medication of the day with 6-8 oz plain water; avoid lying down for at least 30 min

alitretinoin
(ah-lee-tret′-i-noyn)
Rx: Panretin
Chemical Class: Vitamin A derivative
Therapeutic Class: Antineoplastic

CLINICAL PHARMACOLOGY
Mechanism of Action: Binds intracellularly to retinoic acid and retinoid X receptors, leading to selective modulation of gene transcription and change in cell proliferation and apoptosis
Pharmacokinetics
• *TOP:* Negligible absorption; onset of action 2 wk; full effect may take up to 14 wk
INDICATIONS AND USES: Cutaneous lesions in patients with AIDS-related Kaposi's sarcoma
DOSAGE
Adult
• *TOP:* Apply generously to lesion bid; allow to dry for 5 min
💲 AVAILABLE FORMS/COST OF THERAPY
• Gel—0.1%: 60 g: **$2439.31**
CONTRAINDICATIONS: Hypersensitivity to retinoids, pregnancy
PRECAUTIONS: Breast feeding, concomitant vitamin A supplements, concurrent systemic therapy for Kaposi's sarcoma, more than 10 new Kaposi's sarcoma lesions in the month prior to starting treatment, symptomatic lymphedema
PREGNANCY AND LACTATION: Pregnancy category D; breast feeding not recommended
SIDE EFFECTS/ADVERSE REACTIONS
SKIN: Photosensitivity, *rash (localized to site of application, 10%)*

SPECIAL CONSIDERATIONS
PATIENT/FAMILY EDUCATION
• Onset of action 2 wk; full effect may take up to 14 wk; response rate 36%
• Let dry for 5 min before covering area with clothing
• Do not use occlusive dressings
• Do not use near eyes, mouth, nose, vagina, or rectum
• Do not use with insect repellents containing DEET
MONITORING PARAMETERS
• CBC, pregnancy test prior to use

allopurinol
(al-oh-pure′i-nole)
Rx: Aloprim, Lopurin, Zurinol, Zyloprim
Chemical Class: Enzyme (xanthine oxidase) inhibitor
Therapeutic Class: Antigout agent

CLINICAL PHARMACOLOGY
Mechanism of Action: Xanthine oxidase inhibitor; reduces uric acid synthesis
Pharmacokinetics
PO: Peak 2-4 hr; excreted in feces and urine; $t_{1/2}$ 2-3 hr, active metabolite $t_{1/2}$ 18-30 hr
INDICATIONS AND USES: Chronic primary or secondary gout (prevention of acute attacks, tophi, joint destruction, uric acid lithiasis or nephropathy), hyperuricemia associated with malignancies, recurrent calcium oxalate calculi, prevention of fluorouracil-induced stomatitis (as mouthwash 1 mg/ml in methylcellulose*)
DOSAGE
Adult
• *Gout/hyperuricemia:* PO 200-600 mg qd depending on severity, not to exceed 800 mg/day
• *Impaired renal function:* PO 200

---

italic = common side effects   ***bold italic*** = life-threatening reactions

mg qd when CrC1 is 10-20 ml/min;
100 mg qd when CrCl 3-10 ml/min;
100 mg qod when CrCl <3 ml/min
• *Recurrent urinary calculi:* PO 200-
300 mg qd
• *Uric acid nephropathy prevention:* PO 600-800 mg qd × 2-3 days
Child (6-10 yr)
• PO 300 mg qd
Child (<6 yr)
• PO 150 mg qd

[$] AVAILABLE FORMS/COST OF THERAPY
• Inj, Sol—IV: 500 mg/vial: **$500**
• Tab, Uncoated—Oral: 100 mg,
100's: **$5.21-$19.70;** 300 mg, 100's:
$21.00-$63.72

PRECAUTIONS: Renal disease, hepatic disease, children

PREGNANCY AND LACTATION:
Pregnancy category C; allopurinol
and oxypurinol have been found in
the milk of a mother who was receiving allopurinol

SIDE EFFECTS/ADVERSE REACTIONS
CNS: Drowsiness, headache, neuritis, paresthesia
EENT: Cataracts, epistaxis, retinopathy
GI: Anorexia, cholestatic jaundice,
cramps, diarrhea, hepatomegaly, hepatotoxicity, malaise, metallic taste,
nausea, peptic ulcer, stomatitis, vomiting
GU: Renal failure
HEME: Bone marrow suppression
MS: Arthralgia, myopathy
SKIN: Alopecia, ecchymosis, erythema, dermatitis, pruritus, purpura,
Stevens-Johnson syndrome
MISC: Chills, fever

INTERACTIONS
Drugs
❷ *Angiotensin-converting enzyme inhibitors:* Predisposed to hypersensitivity reactions including Stevens-Johnson syndrome, skin eruptions,
fever, and arthralgias

❸ *Antacids:* Aluminum hydroxide
inhibits the response to allopurinol
❷ *Azathioprine:* Increased toxicity of azathioprine; requires dose
adjustment
❸ *Cyclophosphamide:* May increase cyclophosphamide toxicity
❸ *Cyclosporine/tachrolimus:* Increased toxicity of immunosuppressive drug
❷ *Mercaptopurine:* Increased effect of mercaptopurine with increased risk of toxicity
❸ *Oral anticoagulants:* Enhanced
hypoprothrombinemic response
❸ *Theophylline:* Large doses may
increase serum theophylline levels

SPECIAL CONSIDERATIONS
• Increased acute attacks of gout
during early stages of allopurinol
administration—cover with colchicine (see next bullet)
• Maintenance doses of colchicine
(0.6 mg qd-bid) should be given
prophylactically along with starting
with low doses of allopurinol
• Parenteral formulation available
as orphan drug and in Canada
• Gel formulation FDA-approved,
not yet marketed

---

alprazolam
(al-pray'zoe-lam)
Rx: Xanax
Chemical Class: Benzodiazepine
Therapeutic Class: Anxiolytic

CLINICAL PHARMACOLOGY
Mechanism of Action: CNS depressants via facilitation of inhibitory GABA at benzodiazepine receptor sites (BZ_1—associated with
sleep; BZ_2—associated with memory, motor, sensory, and cognitive
function); effects include muscle relaxation (spinal cord), anticonvulsant activity (brain stem), ataxia (cer-

ebellum), emotional behavior (limbic and cortical areas), and anxiolytic effects (separate from general CNS depression); other effects include sedative, appetite-stimulating, and weak analgesic actions

Pharmacokinetics

PO: Onset 30 min, peak serum conc 1-2 hr, duration 4-6 hr, therapeutic response 2-3 days, metabolized by liver, excreted by kidneys; crosses placenta; $t_{1/2}$ 12-15 hr

INDICATIONS AND USES: Anxiety, panic disorder, anxiety with depressive symptoms, agoraphobia with social phobia (2-8 mg/day),* depression,* premenstrual syndrome*

DOSAGE

Adult

• *Anxiety:* PO 0.25-0.5 mg tid, up to 4 mg/day in divided doses

• *Panic disorder:* PO 0.5 mg tid; increase dose q3-4 days in 1 mg/day increments to 10 mg/day

• *Geriatric:* PO 0.25 mg bid-tid

💲 AVAILABLE FORMS/COST OF THERAPY

• Tab, Plain Coated—Oral: 0.25 mg, 100's: **$50.55-$79.44;** 0.5 mg, 100's: **$14.04-$98.96;** 1 mg, 100's: **$85.12-$132.04;** 2 mg, 100's: **$145.65-$224.49**

• Sol—Oral: 0.5 mg/5ml, 500 ml: **$51.75;** 1 mg/ml w/dropper, 30 ml: **$37.50**

CONTRAINDICATIONS: Untreated narrow-angle glaucoma, psychosis, concurrent treatment with itraconazole, ketaconazole, nefazadone (FDA recommendation)

PRECAUTIONS: Elderly, debilitated, hepatic disease, renal disease, suicidal patients

PREGNANCY AND LACTATION: Pregnancy category D; children born of a mother receiving benzodiazepines may be at risk for withdrawal symptoms; neonatal flaccidity and respiratory problems have been reported; chronic administration of diazepam to nursing mothers has been reported to cause infants to become lethargic and lose weight

SIDE EFFECTS/ADVERSE REACTIONS

CNS: Anxiety, ataxia, confusion, depression, *dizziness, drowsiness,* fatigue, hallucinations, headache, insomnia, stimulation, tremors

CV: Bradycardia, hypertension, *orthostatic hypotension,* tachycardia

EENT: Blurred vision, mydriasis, tinnitus

GI: Anorexia, constipation, diarrhea, dry mouth, hepatic dysfunction, nausea, vomiting

SKIN: Dermatitis, itching, rash

INTERACTIONS

Drugs

3 *Cimetidine:* Cimetidine inhibits metabolism, increases plasma levels

3 *Digoxin:* Inconsistently raises dig levels

3 *Erythromycin, clarithromycin, troleandomycin:* Possible increased sedation

3 *Ethanol:* Enhanced adverse psychomotor effects; difficulty performing tasks that require alertness

3 *Fluoxetine, fluvoxamine, ketoconazole, itraconazole, nefazadone (see contraindications):* Increases alprazolam plasma concentrations; increases in psychomotor impairment

3 *Grapefruit juice:* Increased alprazolam levels due to inhibition of presystemic (intestinal) enzyme CYP34A

3 *Phenytoin, carbamazepine:* Decreased benzodiazepine effect

SPECIAL CONSIDERATIONS
PATIENT/FAMILY EDUCATION

• Not for "everyday" stress or longer than 3 mo; avoid driving, activities that require alertness

• Caution when medication discon-

---

italic = common side effects   ***bold italic*** = life-threatening reactions

tinued abruptly after long-term (>4 wks) use—may precipitate withdrawal syndrome

---

alprostadil
(al-pros′ta-dil)
Rx: Caverject, Edex, Muse, Prostin VR Pediatric
Chemical Class: Prostaglandin E_1 (PGE$_1$)
Therapeutic Class: Anti-impotence agent; patent ductus arteriosus

---

CLINICAL PHARMACOLOGY
Mechanism of Action: Relaxes vascular smooth muscle, especially of ductus arteriosus and corpus cavernosum
Pharmacokinetics
INTRACAVERNOSAL (Caverject): Peak 5-20 min; INTRAURETHRAL (Muse): onset 5-10 min, duration 30-60 min: 80% metabolized in lungs, excreted in urine (metabolites)
INDICATIONS AND USES: Temporary maintenance of patency of the ductus arteriosus until definitive surgery can be performed, erectile dysfunction, primary pulmonary hypertension,* severe peripheral arterial occlusive disease*
DOSAGE
Adult
• *Erectile dysfunction:* Intracavernosal 2.5 μg prior to intercourse, increase by 2.5-5 μg depending on response. Mean dose 20 μg; Intraurethral-administer pellet via applicator (supplied) with at least 24 hr between uses
Infants
• IV INF 0.1 μg/kg/min, until desired response, then reduce to lowest effective amount; 0.4 μg/kg/min not likely to produce greater beneficial effects

* = non-FDA-approved use

$ AVAILABLE FORMS/COST OF THERAPY
• Inj, Sol—IV: 500 μg/ml, 1 ml: **$187.50**
• Kit-IV: 10 μg: **$20.11**; 20 μg: **$25.90**
• *Pellet, urethral:* 125 μg, 6's: **$118.50**; 250 μg, 6's: **$124.13**; 500 μg, 6's: **$127.50**; 1000 μg, 6's: **$132.75**
CONTRAINDICATIONS: Conditions that might predispose to priapism (e.g., sickle-cell anemia/trait, multiple myeloma, leukemia), patients with anatomical deformation of penis (e.g., Peyronie's disease), penile implants, for sexual intercourse with a pregnant woman (unless a condom is used)
PRECAUTIONS: Bleeding disorders; men for whom sexual activity is inadvisable
SIDE EFFECTS/ADVERSE REACTIONS
CNS: **Cerebral bleeding,** *fever,* hyperextension of the neck, hyperirritability, hypothermia, jitteriness, lethargy, *seizures,* stiffness
CV: *Bradycardia,* **CHF,** edema, *flushing,* **hypotension (4%),** tachycardia, **ventricular fibrillation**
GI: Diarrhea, hyperbilirubinemia, regurgitation
GU (Penile administration): Injection site hematoma, *penile fibrosis,* (3-8%), *penile pain,* (36%), prolonged erection
HEME: **Bleeding, DIC, thrombocytopenia**
METAB: Hyperkalemia, hypoglycemia, hypokalemia
MS: Cortical proliferation of the long bones
RESP: **Apnea** (10% of neonates), **bradypnea,** hypercapnia, tachypnea, wheezing
SPECIAL CONSIDERATIONS
• For intracavernosal use administer 1st dose under medical supervi-

sion. Use ½-inch 27-30 gauge needle along dorso-lateral aspect of proximal third of penis. Alternate sides

• Urinate prior to intraurethral use to disperse pellet

• Use lowest dose allowing satisfactory erection lasting ≥1 h

MONITORING PARAMETERS

• Infant ABG's, arterial pH, arterial pressure, continuous ECG

---

alteplase
(al-teep'lase)
Rx: Activase
Chemical Class: Tissue plasminogen activator (tPA)
Therapeutic Class: Thrombolytic

CLINICAL PHARMACOLOGY
Mechanism of Action: Promotes thrombolysis by promoting conversion of plasminogen to plasmin
Pharmacokinetics
IV: Cleared by liver, 80% cleared within 10 min after infusion is terminated

INDICATIONS AND USES: Acute myocardial infarction; pulmonary embolism; acute ischemic stroke within 3h of onset; unstable angina pectoris*; peripheral arterial thromboembolism*

DOSAGE
Adult

• *Acute MI:* IV 15 mg bolus, then 0.75 mg/kg over 30 min (max 50 mg), then 0.5 mg/kg over 60 min (max 35 mg)

• *Pulmonary embolism:* IV 100 mg over 2 hr

• *Acute ischemic stroke:* IV 0.9 mg/kg (max 90 mg) over 60 min with 10% of total dose administered as an initial IV bolus over 1 min; initiate treatment within 3 hr after onset of stroke symptoms after exclusion of intracranial hemorrhage by CT scan

§ AVAILABLE FORMS/COST OF THERAPY

• Inj, Lyphl-Sol—IV: 1 mg/ml, 50 mg: **$1375.00**; 1 mg/ml, 100 mg: **$2750.00**

CONTRAINDICATIONS: Active bleeding, hemorrhagic stroke, severe uncontrolled hypertension, intracranial/intraspinal surgery/ trauma, aneurysm, arteriovenous malformation, brain tumor

PRECAUTIONS: Recent (within 10 days) major surgery (e.g., coronary artery bypass graft, obstetrical delivery, organ biopsy); previous puncture of noncompressible vessels; cerebrovascular disease; recent gastrointestinal or genitourinary bleeding (within 10 days); recent trauma (within 10 days); hypertension (systolic BP ≥ 180 mm Hg and/or diastolic BP ≥ 110 mm Hg); high likelihood of left heart thrombus (e.g., mitral stenosis with atrial fibrillation); acute pericarditis; bacterial endocarditis; hemostatic defects including those secondary to severe hepatic or renal disease; significant liver dysfunction; pregnancy; diabetic hemorrhagic retinopathy, or other hemorrhagic ophthalmic conditions; septic thrombophlebitis or occluded arteriovenous cannula at seriously infected site; advanced age (>75 yr); patients currently receiving oral anticoagulants (e.g., warfarin); any other condition in which bleeding constitutes a significant hazard or would be particularly difficult to manage because of its location; readministration

PREGNANCY AND LACTATION: Pregnancy category C. Unknown if excreted in breast milk

---

italic = common side effects   **bold italic** = life-threatening reactions

SIDE EFFECTS/ADVERSE REACTIONS

*CV: **Accelerated idioventricular rhythm, sinus bradycardia, ventricular tachycardia***

*HEME: **Intracranial, retroperitoneal, surface, GI, GU bleeding;*** increased PT, aPTT, TT

SKIN: Rash, urticaria

INTERACTIONS

Drugs

3 *Heparin, oral anticoagulants, drugs that alter platelet function (i.e., aspirin, dipyridamole, abciximab, eptifibitide, tirofiban):* May increase the risk of bleeding

Labs

• *Decrease:* Fibrinogen (mitigated by collecting blood in presence of aprotinin)

SPECIAL CONSIDERATIONS

• Heparin (in doses sufficient to prolong the aPTT to 1.5-2 times control value) is usually administered in conjunction with thrombolytic therapy; aspirin may also be administered to inhibit platelet aggregation during and/or following post-thrombolytic therapy

• Compress arterial puncture sites at least 30 min

MONITORING PARAMETERS

• Prior to initiation of therapy: coagulation tests, hematocrit, platelet count

• During therapy: ECG, mental status, neurological status, vital signs

---

aluminum acetate
(aloo'min-um aas'a-tate)

OTC: Bluboro Powder, Boropak Powder, Burow's Solution, Domeboro, Pedi-Boro Soak Paks

Chemical Class: Aluminum salt

Therapeutic Class: Astringent

CLINICAL PHARMACOLOGY

Mechanism of Action: Maintains skin acidity, which is protective to skin surface

INDICATIONS AND USES: Skin irritation, athlete's foot, insect bites, poison ivy, eczema, acne, bruises, pruritus ani

DOSAGE

Adult and Child

• TOP apply for 15-30 min, q4-8h (1:10-1:40 dilution)

• GARGLE prn (1:10 dilution)

$ **AVAILABLE FORMS/COST OF THERAPY**

• Powder Packets—Top: 100's: **$32.05-68.93**

• Tab—Top: 12's: **$6.95-$8.56**

• Sol—Top: 480 ml: **$2.38-$4.35**

CONTRAINDICATIONS: Tight, occlusive dressing

SIDE EFFECTS/ADVERSE REACTIONS

SKIN: Increasing inflammation, irritation

SPECIAL CONSIDERATIONS
PATIENT/FAMILY EDUCATION

• Soap decreases the astringent actions of aluminum acetate; 1 packet or tab in 1 pint water produces a modified 1:40 Burow's solution

---

aluminum chloride hexahydrate

Rx: Drysol (20%), Xerac AC (6.25%)

Chemical Class: Aluminum salt

Therapeutic Class: Antihidrotic

CLINICAL PHARMACOLOGY

Mechanism of Action: Astringent or increased permeability of the sweat duct causing reabsorption of sweat

INDICATIONS AND USAGE: Hyperhidrosis

DOSAGE

Adult

• TOP: Apply to affected area at bedtime; to help prevent irritation, area should be completely dry prior to application; wash treated area the following morning; excessive sweating may be stopped after 2 or more treatments; thereafter, apply once or twice weekly or as needed

$ AVAILABLE FORMS/COST OF THERAPY

• Sol—Top: 6.25%, 35, 60 ml: **$6.00/** 35 ml; 20%, 35, 60 ml: **$6.85**/35 ml

PRECAUTIONS: Broken, irritated, or recently shaved skin

SIDE EFFECTS/ADVERSE REACTIONS

SKIN: Burning or prickling sensation, transient stinging or itching

SPECIAL CONSIDERATIONS
PATIENT/FAMILY EDUCATION

• Do not apply to broken or irritated skin

• For maximum effect, cover treated area with saran wrap held in place by snug-fitting shirt, mitten or sock (never hold saran wrap in place with tape)

• Avoid contact with eyes

aluminum salts

OTC: *Aluminum hydroxide:* AlternaGEL, Alu-Cap, Alu-Tab, Amphojel

Aluminum carbonate: Basaljel

Combinations:

   OTC: with magnesium hydroxide (Maalox, Rulox, Mylanta, Gelusil, Aludrox)

Chemical Class: Aluminum salt

Therapeutic Class: Antacid; phosphate adsorbent

CLINICAL PHARMACOLOGY

Mechanism of Action: Neutralizes gastric acidity; binds phosphates in GI tract; enhances phosphate excretion

Pharmacokinetics

PO: Onset 20-40 min; non-absorbable; excreted in feces

INDICATIONS AND USES: Antacid (symptomatic relief of hyperacidity, GERD, peptic ulcer disease); phosphate renal stones (prevention); phosphate binder, reduction of hyperphosphatemia in chronic renal failure

DOSAGE

ALUMINUM CARBONATE GEL

Adult

• *Urinary phosphate stones:* Susp 5-10 ml 1 hr pc, hs; extra str susp 2.5-5 ml 1 hr pc, hs; PO 2-6 tabs 1 hr pc, hs

• *Antacid:* Susp 15-45 ml 1 hr pc, hs; extra str susp 5-15 ml 1 hr pc, hs; PO chew 1-2 tabs or caps as needed

ALUMINUM HYDROXIDE

Adult

• *Antacid:* PO susp 5-15 ml 1 hr pc, hs; PO tab 600 mg 1 hr pc, hs, chewed with milk or water

• *Hyperphosphatemia in renal failure:* PO susp 5-30 ml bid-qid; PO

---

italic = common side effects   **bold italic** = life-threatening reactions

tab 600-1800 mg bid-qid; titrate to normal serum phosphorus
Child
• *Hyperphosphatemia in renal failure:* PO susp 50-150 mg/kg/24 hr in divided doses q4-6 hr; titrate to normal serum phosphorus

$ AVAILABLE FORMS/COST OF THERAPY
ALUMINUM CARBONATE GEL
• Cap—Oral: 500 mg, 100's: **$16.99**
• Tab—Oral: 500 mg, 100's: **$15.89**
ALUMINUM HYDROXIDE
• Cap—Oral: 475 mg, 100's: **$17.82**
• Tab—Oral: 300 mg, 100's: **$6.94;** 600 mg, 100's: **$10.99**
• Susp—Oral: 320 mg/5 ml, 480 ml: **$5.74-$6.94;** 600 mg/5 ml, 480 ml: **$8.10**

CONTRAINDICATIONS: Appendicitis

PRECAUTIONS: Elderly, fluid restriction, decreased GI motility, GI obstruction, dehydration, sodium-restricted diets

PREGNANCY AND LACTATION: Pregnancy category C

SIDE EFFECTS/ADVERSE REACTIONS
GI: Anorexia, ***bowel obstruction, constipation,*** fecal impaction
METAB: Hypophosphatemia, hypercalciuria
MISC: Aluminum intoxication, osteomalacia

INTERACTIONS
Drugs
▪ *Allopurinol, atenolol, ketoconazole, itraconazole* (not fluconazole): Aluminum hydroxide inhibits GI absorption
▪ *Cefpodoxime, cefuroxime:* Reduced bioavailability and serum concentration of cefpodoxime
▪ *Cyclosporine:* Reduced cyclosporine blood concentrations possible
▪ *Glipizide, glyburide:* Enhanced absorption of hypoglycemic agent

▪ *Iron:* Reduced GI absorption of iron; separate doses by 1-2 hr
▪ *Isoniazid:* Some antacids reduce plasma concentration of isoniazid
▪ *Penicillamine:* Reduced penicillamine bioavailability
▪ *Quinolones:* Antacids reduce the serum concentration of all the quinolone antibiotics and may inhibit their efficacy
▪ *Salicylates:* Decreased serum salicylate concentrations
▪ *Sodium polystyrene sulfonate resin:* Combined use may result in systemic alkalosis
▪ *Tetracycline:* Reduced serum concentration and efficacy of tetracycline
▪ *Vitamin C:* Increases aluminum absorption

SPECIAL CONSIDERATIONS
PATIENT/FAMILY EDUCATION
• Thoroughly chew chewable tablets before swallowing, follow with a glass of water
• May impair absorption of many drugs; do not take other drugs within 1-4 hr of aluminum hydroxide administration
• Stools may appear white or speckled

MONITORING PARAMETERS
• Monitor for hypophosphatemia: anorexia, weakness, fatigue, bone pain, hyporeflexia; urinary pH, Ca^{++}, electrolytes

---

amantadine
(a-man'ta-deen)
Rx: Symmetrel
Chemical Class: Tricyclic amine
Therapeutic Class: Antiviral; antiParkinson's agent

CLINICAL PHARMACOLOGY
Mechanism of Action: Prevents uncoating of nucleic acid in viral cell,

preventing penetration of virus to host; causes release of dopamine from dopaminergic terminals in the substantia nigra

Pharmacokinetics

PO: Onset 48 hr (Parkinson's disease), $t_{1/2}$ 15-17 hr; 67% protein bound, 90% excreted unchanged in urine; excretion increased with acidic urine

INDICATIONS AND USES: Influenza A prophylaxis or treatment, Parkinson's disease, drug-induced extrapyramidal reactions

DOSAGE

Adult

• *Influenza type A:* PO 200 mg/day in single dose or divided bid; start treatment as soon as possible after onset of symptoms and continue for 24-48 hr after symptoms disappear; start prophylaxis in anticipation of contact or as soon as possible after exposure, continue at least 10 days following a known exposure

• *Parkinson's disease:* PO 100 mg qd for 1 wk then increase gradually to 400 mg/day in divided doses if needed

• *Drug-induced extrapyramidal reactions:* PO 100 mg bid, increase to 300 mg/day in divided doses if needed

• *Dosage with renal impairment* (based on CrCl in ml/min/1.73m^2): CrCl 30-50: PO 200 mg 1st day followed by 100 mg qd thereafter; CrCl 15-29: PO 200 mg 1st day followed by 100 mg qod thereafter; CrCl <15: PO 200 mg every 7 days

Elderly

• *Influenza type A:* 100-200 mg/day

Child

• *Influenza type A:* (1-9 yr) PO 4.4-8.8 mg/kg/day divided bid, do not exceed 150 mg/day; (9-12 yr) PO 100 mg bid

$ **AVAILABLE FORMS/COST OF THERAPY**

• Cap—Oral: 100 mg, 100's: **$16.88-$90.94**

• Syr—Oral: 50 mg/5 ml, 480 ml: **$29.90-$90.56**

CONTRAINDICATIONS: Child <1 yr

PRECAUTIONS: Seizure disorder, CHF, orthostatic hypotension, psychiatric disorders, hepatic disease, renal disease, peripheral edema, eczematoid rash, abrupt discontinuation

PREGNANCY AND LACTATION: Pregnancy category C; excreted in human milk, exercise caution when administering to nursing mothers because of potential for urinary retention, vomiting, and skin rash

SIDE EFFECTS/ADVERSE REACTIONS

CNS: Anorexia, anxiety, ataxia, confusion, depression, fatigue, hallucinations, headache, *insomnia, lightheadedness,* psychosis, **seizures**

CV: **CHF,** orthostatic hypotension, peripheral edema

EENT: Blurred vision

GI: Constipation, dry mouth, *nausea,* vomiting

GU: Increased BUN, urinary retention

HEME: **Leukopenia**

SKIN: Eczematoid dermatitis, livedo reticularis, photosensitivity, rash

INTERACTIONS

Drugs

3 *Benztropine:* Potentiation of amantadine's CNS side effects

3 *Triamterene:* Increased amantadine toxicity

3 *Trihexyphenidyl:* Potentiation of amantadine's CNS side effects

SPECIAL CONSIDERATIONS

PATIENT/FAMILY EDUCATION

• Administer at least 4 hr before bedtime to prevent insomnia

• Take with meals for better absorp-

---

italic = common side effects   ***bold italic*** = life-threatening reactions

tion and to decrease GI symptoms
• Arise slowly from a reclining position; avoid hazardous activities if dizziness or blurred vision occurs
• Do not discontinue abruptly in Parkinson's disease

---

ambenonium
(am-be-noe'nee-um)
Rx: Mytelase
Chemical Class: Synthetic quaternary ammonium derivative
Therapeutic Class: Cholinergic

CLINICAL PHARMACOLOGY
Mechanism of Action: An acetylcholinesterase inhibitor, inhibits destruction of acetylcholine, facilitating transmission of impulses across myoneural junction
Pharmacokinetics
PO: Onset 20-30 min, duration 3-8 hr
INDICATIONS AND USES: Myasthenia gravis (particularly useful in patients sensitive to bromides)
DOSAGE
Adult
• PO 5 mg q3-4h while awake, gradually increased q1-2 days to optimal muscle strength and no GI disturbances (range 5-75 mg per dose), doses above 200 mg/day require close supervision to avoid overdosage
💲 **AVAILABLE FORMS/COST OF THERAPY**
• Tab, Scored—Oral: 10 mg, 100's: **$91.80**
CONTRAINDICATIONS: Urinary or intestinal obstruction
PRECAUTIONS: Seizure disorder, asthma, coronary occlusion, hyperthyroidism, dysrhythmias, peptic ulcer, bradycardia, hypotension, children, presence of other cholinergics (atropine sulfate should be available for cholinergic crisis)
PREGNANCY AND LACTATION: Pregnancy category C; would not be expected to cross placenta or be excreted into breast milk because it is ionized at physiologic pH; although apparently safe for the fetus, may cause transient muscle weakness in the newborn
SIDE EFFECTS/ADVERSE REACTIONS
CNS: Dizziness, drowsiness, headache, incoordination, *loss of consciousness, paralysis, seizures*
CV: AV block, bradycardia, *cardiac arrest, dysrhythmias, hypotension,* non-specific ECG changes, tachycardia
EENT: Blurred vision, conjunctival hyperemia, diplopia, lacrimation, miosis, spasm of accommodation, visual changes
GI: Cramps, diarrhea, dysphagia, flatulence, *increased gastric secretions,* increased peristalsis, *increased salivation, nausea, vomiting*
GU: Frequency, incontinence, urgency
MS: Arthralgia, fasciculation, muscle cramps and spasms, weakness
RESP: Bronchospasm, dyspnea, increased secretions, *laryngospasm, respiratory arrest, respiratory depression*
SKIN: Rash, sweating, urticaria
INTERACTIONS
Drugs
3 *Tacrine:* Increased cholinergic effects
SPECIAL CONSIDERATIONS
PATIENT/FAMILY EDUCATION
• Notify clinician of nausea, vomiting, diarrhea, sweating, increased salivation, irregular heartbeat, muscle weakness, severe abdominal pain or difficulty in breathing
• Administer on an empty stomach

---

* = non-FDA-approved use

MONITORING PARAMETERS
• Therapeutic response: Increased muscle strength, improved gait, absence of labored breathing (if severe)
• Appearance of side effects: Narrow margin between 1st appearance of side effects and serious toxicity
• Symptoms of increasing muscle weakness may be due to cholinergic crisis (overdosage) or myasthenic crisis (increased disease severity); if crisis is myasthenia, patient will improve after 1-2 mg edrophonium; if cholinergic, withdraw ambinonium and administer atropine

---

amcinonide
(am-sin'oh-nide)
Rx: Cyclocort
Chemical Class: Synthetic fluorinated glucocorticoid
Therapeutic Class: Topical corticosteroid, high potency

CLINICAL PHARMACOLOGY
Mechanism of Action: Depresses formation, release, and activity of endogenous mediators of inflammation such as prostaglandins, kinins, histamine, liposomal enzymes, and the complement system resulting in decreased edema, erythema, and pruritus
Pharmacokinetics
Absorbed through skin (increased by inflammation and occlusive dressings); metabolized primarily in the liver
INDICATIONS AND USES: Psoriasis, eczema, contact dermatitis, pruritus
DOSAGE
Adult and Child
• Apply to affected area bid; rub completely into skin

$ AVAILABLE FORMS/COST OF THERAPY
• Cre—Top: 0.1%, 15, 30 and 60 g: **$17.26**/15 g
• Oint—Top: 0.1%, 15, 30 and 60 g: **$17.26**/15 g
CONTRAINDICATIONS: Fungal infections, use on face, groin, or axilla
PRECAUTIONS: Viral infections, bacterial infections, children
PREGNANCY AND LACTATION: Pregnancy category C; unknown whether topical application could result in sufficient systemic absorption to produce detectable amounts in breast milk (systemic corticosteroids are secreted into breast milk in quantities unlikely to have detrimental effects on breastfeeding infant)
SIDE EFFECTS/ADVERSE REACTIONS
SKIN: Acne, allergic contact dermatitis, atrophy, burning, dryness, folliculitis, hypertrichosis, hypopigmentation, irritation, itching, miliaria, perioral dermatitis, secondary infection, striae
MISC: Systemic absorption of topical corticosteroids has produced reversible HPA axis suppression (more likely with occlusive dressings, prolonged administration, application to large surface areas, liver failure, and in children)
SPECIAL CONSIDERATIONS
PATIENT/FAMILY EDUCATION
• Apply sparingly only to affected area
• Avoid contact with eyes
• Do not put bandages or dressings over treated area unless directed by clinician
• Do not use on weeping, denuded, or infected areas
• Discontinue drug, notify clinician if local irritation or fever develops

---

italic = common side effects   ***bold italic*** = life-threatening reactions

amikacin
(am-i-kay´sin)
Rx: Amikin
Chemical Class: Aminoglycoside
Therapeutic Class: Antibiotic

CLINICAL PHARMACOLOGY
Mechanism of Action: Interferes with protein synthesis in bacterial cell by binding to ribosomal subunit, which causes misreading of genetic code; inaccurate peptide sequence forms in protein chain, causing bacterial death
Pharmacokinetics
IM: Onset rapid, peak 1-2 hr
IV: Onset immediate
Plasma $t_{1/2}$ 2-3 hr; not metabolized, excreted unchanged in urine
INDICATIONS AND USES: Severe systemic infections of CNS, respiratory, GI, urinary tract, bone, skin, soft tissues caused by susceptible organisms
Antibacterial spectrum usually includes:
• Gram-positive organisms: *Staphylococcus* sp. including methicillin-resistant strains (in general has a low order of activity against other Gram-positive organisms)
• Gram-negative organisms: *Pseudomonas* sp.; *E. coli, Proteus* sp. (indole-positive and indole-negative); *Providencia* sp.; *Klebsiella, Enterobacter,* and *Serratia* sp.; *Acinetobacter* sp.; *Citrobacter freundii*
DOSAGE
Adult
• *Severe systemic infections:* IV INF 15 mg/kg/day (use ideal body weight) in 2-3 divided doses q8-12h in 100-200 ml diluent over 30-60 min, not to exceed 1.5 g/day; decreased doses are needed in poor renal function as determined by blood levels and renal function studies; IM 15 mg/kg/day in divided doses q8-12h
• *Uncomplicated urinary tract infections:* IM 250 mg bid
• *Decreased renal function:* 7.5 mg/kg initially, then adjusted as determined by blood levels and renal function studies
Child
• *Severe systemic infections:* Same as adult
Neonate
• IV INF 10 mg/kg initially, then 7.5 mg/kg q12h in diluent over 1-2 hr
AVAILABLE FORMS/COST OF THERAPY
• Inj, Sol—IM, IV: 50 mg/ml, 2 ml: **$32.50-$317.10;** 250 mg/ml, 2 ml: **$16.54-$105.84**
CONTRAINDICATIONS: Long-term therapy (ototoxic and nephrotoxic)
PRECAUTIONS: Neonates, renal disease, myasthenia gravis, hearing deficits, Parkinson's disease, elderly, sulfite sensitivity (contains sodium bisulfite), dehydration
PREGNANCY AND LACTATION: Pregnancy category C; although fetal ototoxicity has occurred after in utero exposure to other aminoglycosides, 8th cranial nerve toxicity has not been reported with amikacin; excreted into breast milk in low concentrations; poor oral bioavailability reduces potential for ototoxicity for the infant
SIDE EFFECTS/ADVERSE REACTIONS
CNS: Confusion, depression, dizziness, muscle twitching, neurotoxicity, numbness, *seizures,* tremors, vertigo
CV: Hypotension or hypertension, palpitations
EENT: Ototoxicity: hearing loss,

deafness; tinnitus, visual disturbances

GI: Nausea, vomiting

GU: Azotemia, hematuria, ***nephrotoxicity,*** oliguria, ***renal failure***

HEME: ***Agranulocytosis,*** anemia, eosinophilia, ***leukopenia, thrombocytopenia***

SKIN: Alopecia, dermatitis, *rash,* urticaria

INTERACTIONS
Drugs

⬛ *Amphotericin B:* Synergistic nephrotoxicity

❷ *Atracurium:* Amikacin potentiates respiratory depression by atracurium

⬛ *Carbenicillin:* Potential for inactivation of amikacin in patients with renal failure

⬛ *Carboplatin:* Additive nephrotoxicity or ototoxicity

⬛ *Cephalosporins:* Increased potential for nephrotoxicity in patients with preexisting renal disease

⬛ *Cisplatin:* Additive nephrotoxicity or ototoxicity

⬛ *Cyclosporine:* Additive nephrotoxicity

❷ *Ethacrynic acid:* Additive ototoxicity

⬛ *Indomethacin:* Reduced renal clearance of amikacin in premature infants

⬛ *Methoxyflurane:* Additive nephrotoxicity

⬛ *Neuromuscular blocking agents:* Amikacin potentiates respiratory depression by neuromuscular blocking agents

⬛ *NSAIDs:* May reduce renal clearance of amikacin

⬛ *Pencillins (extended spectrum):* Potential for inactivation of amikacin in patients with renal failure

⬛ *Piperacillin:* Potential for inactivation of amikacin in patients with renal failure

❷ *Succinylcholine:* Amikacin potentiates respiratory depression by succinylcholine

⬛ *Ticarcillin:* Potential for inactivation of amikacin in patients with renal failure

⬛ *Vancomycin:* Additive nephrotoxicity or ototoxicity

❷ *Vecuronium:* Amikacin potentiates respiratory depression by vecuronium

Labs

• *False increase:* Urine amino acids

• *False decrease:* Bilirubin, cholesterol, serum creatine kinase, serum glucose, LDH, BUN

• *False positive:* Urine oligosaccharides

• *Interference:* Serum tobramycin, kanamycin

SPECIAL CONSIDERATIONS
PATIENT/FAMILY EDUCATION

• Report headache, dizziness, loss of hearing, ringing, roaring in ears, or feeling of fullness in head

MONITORING PARAMETERS

• Urine output, serum creat

• Serum peak, drawn 30-60 min after IV INF or 60 min after IM inj; trough level drawn just before next dose; adjust dosage per levels (usual therapeutic plasma levels; peak 20-35 mg/L, trough ≤10 mg/L)

---

amiloride

(a-mill'oh-ride)
Rx: Midamor
Combinations:
  Rx: with hydrochlorothiazide (Moduretic)

Chemical Class: Pyrazine
Therapeutic Class: Potassium-sparing diuretic, antihypertensive

---

CLINICAL PHARMACOLOGY
Mechanism of Action: Inhibits renal sodium reabsorption in exchange

---

for potassium and hydrogen ions directly in the distal renal tubule; weak diuretic and antihypertensive effects when used alone

Pharmacokinetics

PO: Onset 2 hr, peak 6-10 hr, duration 24 hr; excreted unchanged in urine (60%), feces (40%); t$_{1/2}$ 6-9 hr

INDICATIONS AND USES: Adjunctive treatment with thiazide or loop diuretics in congestive heart failure or hypertension to help restore potassium balance; lithium-induced polyuria*; aerosolized administration (drug dissolved in 0.3% saline delivered by nebulizer) in cystic fibrosis*

DOSAGE

Adult

• PO 5 mg qd, may be increased to 10-20 mg qd if needed

AVAILABLE FORMS/COST OF THERAPY

• Tab, Uncoated—Oral: 5 mg, 100's: **$43.90-$52.85**

CONTRAINDICATIONS: Hyperkalemia (serum potassium >5.5 mEq/L), impaired renal function, anuria, severe renal disease, antikaliuretic therapy (including angiotensin converting enzyme inhibitors, angiotensin II receptor blockers, and potassium supplements)

PRECAUTIONS: Dehydration, diabetes, acidosis, hepatic function impairment, children

PREGNANCY AND LACTATION: Pregnancy category B; therapy for preexisting hypertension can be continued throughout pregnancy with minimal risk; initiating for simple edema not recommended; few unequivocal indications for diuretic therapy in pregnancy except for pulmonary edema or congestive heart failure; excretion into breast milk unknown; use caution in nursing mothers

SIDE EFFECTS/ADVERSE REACTIONS

CNS: Anxiety, decreased libido, depression, dizziness, encephalopathy, fatigue, *headache,* insomnia, mental confusion, nervousness, paresthesias, tremor, vertigo, weakness

CV: Angina, **dysrhythmias,** orthostatic hypotension

EENT: Blurred vision, increased intraocular pressure, loss of hearing, nasal congestion, tinnitus

GI: Abdominal pain, anorexia, constipation, cramps, *diarrhea,* dry mouth, dyspepsia, flatulence, GI bleeding, jaundice, *nausea, vomiting*

GU: Dysuria, frequency, impotence, polyuria

*HEME: **Agranulocytopenia, leukopenia, thrombocytopenia*** (rare)

METAB: Acidosis, hyperkalemia, hypochloremia, hyponatremia

MS: Cramps, joint pain

SKIN: Alopecia, pruritus, rash, urticaria

INTERACTIONS

Drugs

3 *ACE inhibitors:* Hyperkalemia in predisposed patients

3 *Angiotensin II receptor antagonists:* Concurrent mechanisms to decrease potassium excretion; increased risk of hyperkalemia

2 *Potassium preparations:* Hyperkalemia in predisposed patients

3 *Quinidine:* Increased ventricular arrhythmias

SPECIAL CONSIDERATIONS

PATIENT/FAMILY EDUCATION

• Notify clinician of muscle weakness, fatigue, flaccid paralysis

• Take with food or milk for GI symptoms

• Take early in day to prevent nocturia

• Avoid large quantities of potas-

sium-rich foods: oranges, bananas, salt substitutes
MONITORING PARAMETERS
• Blood pressure, edema, urine output, ECG (if hyperkalemia exists), urine electrolytes, BUN, creatinine, gynecomastia, impotence

---

aminocaproic acid
(a-mee-noe-ka-proe'ik)
Rx: Amicar
Chemical Class: Synthetic monoaminocarboxylic acid
Therapeutic Class: Hemostatic

CLINICAL PHARMACOLOGY
Mechanism of Action: Inhibits fibrinolysis by inhibiting plasminogen activators and, to a lesser degree, by antiplasmin activity
Pharmacokinetics
PO: Rapidly absorbed, peak 2 hr; excreted by kidneys as unmetabolized drug; $t_{1/2}$ 2 hr
INDICATIONS AND USES: Hemorrhage from systemic hyperfibrinolysis and urinary fibrinolysis; adjunctive therapy in hemophilia*; recurrent subarachnoid hemorrhage*; amegakaryocytic thrombocytopenia,* proposed for topical treatment of traumatic hyphema of the eye*
DOSAGE
Adult
• IV 4-5 g in 250 ml NS, D_5W, or LR, infused over 1 hr, followed by continuous infusion at the rate of 1-1.25 g/hr diluted in 50-100 ml of compatible solution, not to exceed 30 g/day; use infusion pump; do not give by direct IV; PO 5 g loading dose during first hour, then 1-1.25 g qh if needed, not to exceed 30 g/day
Child
• IV 100 mg/kg or 3 g/m^2 loading dose followed by continuous infusion at the rate of 33.3 mg/kg/hr or

1 g/m^2/hr; do not exceed 18 g/m^2/day; PO 100-200 mg/kg loading dose followed by 100 mg/kg/dose q6h, not to exceed 30 g/day
⑤ AVAILABLE FORMS/COST OF THERAPY
• Inj, Sol—IV: 250 mg/ml, 20 ml: **$2.68-$16.24**
• Syr—Oral: 1.25 g/5 ml, 480 ml: **$430.40**
• Tab, Uncoated—Oral: 500 mg, 100's: **$172.43**
CONTRAINDICATIONS: DIC, upper urinary tract bleeding, neonates (injectable contains benzyl alcohol)
PRECAUTIONS: Renal disease, hepatic disease, thrombosis, cardiac disease
PREGNANCY AND LACTATION: Pregnancy category C; excretion in milk unknown; use caution in nursing mothers
SIDE EFFECTS/ADVERSE REACTIONS
CNS: **Cerebral ischemia,** delirium, *dizziness,* hallucinations, *headache,* psychosis, **seizures** (in treatment of subarachnoid hemorrhage)
CV: Bradycardia, **dysrhythmias,** hypotension
EENT: Conjunctival suffusion, nasal congestion, tinnitus
GI: Abdominal cramps, diarrhea, nausea, vomiting
GU: Dysuria, ejaculatory failure, frequency, menstrual irregularities, myoglobinuria, oliguria, **renal failure**
HEME: Thrombosis
MS: Fatigue, malaise, myopathy, rhabdomyolysis, weakness
SKIN: Rash
INTERACTIONS
Labs
• *False increase:* Urine amino acids
SPECIAL CONSIDERATIONS
PATIENT/FAMILY EDUCATION
• Report any signs of bleeding or myopathy

---

italic = common side effects   ***bold italic*** = life-threatening reactions

• Change position slowly to decrease orthostatic hypotension

MONITORING PARAMETERS

• Do **not** administer without a definite diagnosis and laboratory findings indicative of hyperfibrinolysis

• Blood studies including coagulation factors, platelets, fibrinolysin; CPK, urinalysis

---

aminoglutethimide

(a-meen-noe-gloo-teth'i-mide)

Rx: Cytadren

Chemical Class: Hormone
Therapeutic Class: Adrenal steroid inhibitor; antineoplastic, adjuvant

CLINICAL PHARMACOLOGY

Mechanism of Action: Inhibits the enzymatic conversion of cholesterol to Δ^5-pregnenolone, resulting in a decrease in the production of adrenal glucocorticoids, mineralocorticoids, androgens, and estrogens

Pharmacokinetics

PO: Peak 1.5 hr, $t_{1/2}$ 13 hr; metabolized in liver, excreted in urine

INDICATIONS AND USES: Suppression of adrenal function in Cushing's syndrome (usually as an interim measure until surgery or in cases where more definitive therapy is not appropriate); postmenopausal patients with advanced breast cancer*; metastatic prostate cancer*

DOSAGE

Adult

• PO 250 mg qid at 6 hr intervals, may increase by 250 mg/day q1-2 wk, not to exceed 2 g/day

$ AVAILABLE FORMS/COST OF THERAPY

• Tab, Uncoated—Oral: 250 mg, 100's: **$134.70**

PREGNANCY AND LACTATION:
Pregnancy category D; not recommended in breastfeeding

SIDE EFFECTS/ADVERSE REACTIONS

CNS: Dizziness, drowsiness (33%), headache, lethargy

CV: Hypotension, tachycardia

GI: Anorexia and nausea (12%, usually resolves within 2 wk), hepatotoxicity

HEME: **Agranulocytosis, leukopenia,** (Rare) **neutropenia, pancytopenia, thrombocytopenia**

METAB: Adrenal insufficiency, hypothyroidism

SKIN: Hirsutism, *pruritus, rash (17%)*

INTERACTIONS

Drugs

▣ *Corticosteroids:* Enhanced elimination leading to reduction in corticosteroid response; accelerates dexamethasone metabolism, if glucocorticoid replacement needed give hydrocortisone

▣ *Digitoxin:* Reduced serum digitoxin concentration

▣ *Medroxyprogesterone:* Reduced plasma medroxyprogesterone concentrations

▣ *Oral anticoagulants:* Reduced hypoprothrombinemic response

▣ *Tacrolimus:* Reduced tacrolimus concentration

❷ *Tamoxifen:* Reduced serum tamoxifen concentration

▣ *Theophylline:* Reduced theophylline levels

SPECIAL CONSIDERATIONS

• May cause adrenal cortical hypofunction, especially under stressful conditions (trauma, surgury, acute illness)

MONITORING PARAMETERS

• BUN, serum uric acid, urine CrCl, electrolytes, liver function tests (bilirubin, AST, alkaline phosphatase) before, during therapy

---

* = non-FDA-approved use

- CBC
- TSH
- Blood pressure (hypotension secondary to aldosterone suppression)

---

aminophylline (theophylline ethylenediamine)

(am-in-off'i-lin)
Rx: Truphylline
Chemical Class: Xanthine derivative; ethylenediamine
Therapeutic Class: Antiasthmatic bronchodilator; COPD agent

CLINICAL PHARMACOLOGY

Mechanism of Action: Activity due to theophylline; directly relaxes bronchial and pulmonary smooth muscle; stimulates CNS; induces diuresis; increases gastric acid secretion, decreases lower esophageal sphincter pressure; is a central respiratory stimulant; exact mechanism unproven but may involve antagonism of pulmonary adenosine receptors

Pharmacokinetics

PO: Well absorbed, onset ¼ hr, peak 1-2 hr, duration 6-8 hr

PO-EXT REL: Onset unknown, peak 4-7 hr, duration 8-12 hr

IV: Onset rapid, duration 6-8 hr

PR: Absorption slow and erratic, onset erratic, peak 3-5 hr, duration 6-8 hr

Metabolized by liver; excreted in urine; $t_{1/2}$ 3-12 hr, $t_{1/2}$ increased in geriatric patients, hepatic disease, cor pulmonale, and CHF, $t_{1/2}$ decreased in children and smoking

INDICATIONS AND USES: Asthma, reversible bronchospasm associated with chronic bronchitis and emphysema; apnea and bradycardia of prematurity*

DOSAGE
Adult and Child

- *PO acute therapy (patients not currently receiving theophylline products):* Following a 6.3 mg/kg loading dose, maintenance dose follows: children age 1-9 yr, 5.1 mg/kg q6h; children age 9-16 yr and smokers, 3.8 mg/kg q6h; otherwise healthy non-smoking adults, 3.8 mg/kg q8h; older patients/patients with CHF, cor pulmonale, 2.5 mg/kg q8h

- *PO acute therapy (patients currently receiving theophylline products):* Defer loading dose if serum theophylline concentration can be rapidly obtained; base loading dose on the principle that each 0.63 mg/kg of aminophylline will increase serum theophylline concentration by 1 µg/ml; if this is not possible and sufficient respiratory distress is present (without signs of theophylline toxicity), use 3.1 mg/kg of a rapidly available form of aminophylline; will likely increase serum theophylline concentration 5 µg/ml; maintenance dosage as described above

- *PO chronic therapy:* Initial dose 20.3 mg/kg/24 hr or 500 mg/24 hr (whichever is less) divided q6-8h; increase q 3 days by 25% as tolerated until clinical response or maximum dose is reached (below); monitor serum theophylline concentrations; do not exceed the following (or 1140 mg, whichever is less without serum level monitoring): Age 1-9 yr, 30.4 mg/kg/day; age 9-12 yr, 25.3 mg/kg/day; age 12-16 yr, 22.8 mg/kg/day; age 16 yr and older, 16.5 mg/kg/day

- *IV (patients not currently receiving theophylline products):* Following a 6.3 mg/kg IV loading dose, maintenance dose follows: Children age 1-9 yr, 1 mg/kg/hr; children age 9-16 yr and smokers, 0.8 mg/kg/hr; otherwise healthy non-

---

italic = common side effects   ***bold italic*** = life-threatening reactions

smoking adults, 0.5 mg/kg/hr; older patients/patients with cor pulmonale, 0.3 mg/kg/hr; patients with CHF, 0.1-0.2 mg/kg/hr

• *IV (patients currently receiving theophylline products):* Defer loading dose if serum theophylline concentration can be rapidly obtained. Base loading dose on the principle that each 0.63 mg/kg of aminophylline will increase serum theophylline concentration by 1 μg/ml; if this is not possible and sufficient respiratory distress is present, use 3.1 mg/kg of aminophylline; will likely increase serum theophylline concentration 5 μg/ml (administer only if theophylline toxicity is not present); maintenance dosage as described above

🔋 **AVAILABLE FORMS/COST OF THERAPY**

• Inj, Sol—IV: 25 mg/ml, 10 ml: **$2.14-$15.54**
• Sol—Oral: 105 mg/5 ml, 240 ml: **$12.13-$14.00**
• Tab, Uncoated—Oral: 100 mg, 100's: **$3.32-$6.05;** 200 mg, 100's: **$3.30-$7.55**
• Supp—Rect: 250 mg, 10's: **$14.50-$17.33;** 500 mg, 10's: **$17.00-$19.25**

CONTRAINDICATIONS: Hypersensitivity to xanthines or ethylenediamine; underlying seizure disorder (not on anticonvulsant therapy); suppositories are contraindicated in the presence of irritation or infection of the rectum or lower colon

PRECAUTIONS: Elderly, CHF, corpulmonale, hepatic disease, pre-existing dysrhythmias, hypertension, infants <1 yr, hypoxemia, sustained high fever, history of peptic ulcer, alcoholism

PREGNANCY AND LACTATION: Pregnancy category C; pharmacokinetics of theophylline may be altered during pregnancy, monitor serum concentrations carefully; excreted into breast milk; may cause irritability in the nursing infant, otherwise compatible with breast feeding

SIDE EFFECTS/ADVERSE REACTIONS

CNS: Anxiety, *dizziness,* headache, insomnia, lightheadedness, muscle twitching, reflex hyperexcitability, restlessness, seizures

CV: **Circulatory failure,** flushing, hypotension, *palpitations, sinus tachycardia,* **ventricular dysrhythmias**

GI: Anal irritation (suppositories), anorexia, bitter taste, black stools, diarrhea, dyspepsia, epigastric pain, esophageal reflux, hematemesis, *nausea, vomiting*

GU: Proteinuria, urinary frequency

METAB: Hyperglycemia, SIADH

RESP: Tachypnea

SKIN: Urticaria, alopecia

INTERACTIONS

Drugs

🔳 *Adenosine:* Decreased hemodynamic effects of adenosine

🔳 *Allopurinol, Amiodarone, Cimetidine, Ciprofloxacin, Disulfiram, Erythromycin, Interferon alfa, Isoniazid, Methimazole, Metoprolol, Norfloxacin, Pefloxacin, Pentoxifylline, Propafenone, Propylthiouracil, Radioactive iodine, Tacrine, Thiabendazole, Ticlopidine, Verapamil:* Increased theophylline concentrations

🔳 *Aminoglutethamide, Barbiturates, Carbamazepine, Moricizine, Phenytoin, Rifampin, Ritonavir, Thyroid hormone:* Reduced theophylline concentrations; decreased serum phenytoin levels

🔳 *Beta-blockers:* Reduced bronchodilating response to theophylline

❷ *Enoxacin; Fluvoxamine, Mexiletine, Propranolol, Troleandomy-*

cin: Markedly increased theophylline concentrations

3 *Imipenem:* Some patients on theophylline have developed seizures following addition of imipenem

3 *Lithium:* Reduced lithium concentrations

3 *Smoking:* Increased aminophylline dosing requirements

SPECIAL CONSIDERATIONS

PATIENT/FAMILY EDUCATION

• Avoid large amounts of caffeine-containing products

• If GI upset occurs, take with 8 oz water

• Notify clinician if nausea, vomiting, insomnia, jitteriness, headache, rash, palpitations occur

MONITORING PARAMETERS

• Serum theophylline concentrations (therapeutic level is 10-20 µg/ml); toxicity may occur with small increase above 20 µg/ml, especially in the elderly

• Serious side effects (ventricular dysrhythmias, seizures, death) may occur without preceding signs of less serious toxicity (nausea, restlessness)

---

aminosalicylate

(a-mee-noe-sal-i'si-late)

Rx: P.A.S. Sodium

Chemical Class: Salicylate derivative

Therapeutic Class: Antituberculosis agent

CLINICAL PHARMACOLOGY

Mechanism of Action: Prevents synthesis of folic acid by competitively blocking the conversion of aminobenzoic acid to dihydrofolic acid; bacteriostatic against *Mycobacterium tuberculosis;* inhibits onset of bacterial resistance to isoniazid and streptomycin

Pharmacokinetics

PO: Peak 0.5-1 hr; concentrates in pleural and caseous tissue; metabolized by liver, excreted in urine; $t_{1/2}$ 1 hr

INDICATIONS AND USES: Alternative treatment of tuberculosis (always in combination with streptomycin, isoniazid, or both), Crohn's disease*

DOSAGE

Adult

PO 14-16 g/day in 2-3 divided doses

Child

PO 275-420 mg/kg/day in 3-4 divided doses

$ AVAILABLE FORMS/COST OF THERAPY

• Tab, Coated—Oral: 500 mg, 100's: **$30.00**

CONTRAINDICATIONS: Severe renal disease; G-6-PD deficiency

PRECAUTIONS: Impaired renal or hepatic function, acidic urine, gastric ulcer, CHF, and other situations in which excess sodium is potentially harmful

PREGNANCY AND LACTATION: Pregnancy category C; excreted into breast milk; use caution in nursing mothers

SIDE EFFECTS/ADVERSE REACTIONS

GI: Abdominal pain, diarrhea, hepatitis, jaundice, *nausea, vomiting*

GU: Crystalluria

*HEME: **Agranulocytosis, hemolytic anemia,** increased PT, **leukopenia, thrombocytopenia***

METAB: Goiter with or without myxedema

SKIN: Skin eruptions

MISC: Encephalopathy, fever, infection, Loeffler's syndrome, mononucleosis-like syndrome, vasculitis

---

italic = common side effects   ***bold italic*** = life-threatening reactions

INTERACTIONS
Drugs
🗓 *Rifampin:* Reduced serum rifampin concentrations
Labs
• *False increase:* BUN, CSF protein serum bilirubin, serum glucose, serum phosphate, urine bile, urine phenylketones, urine porphobilinogen, urine protein, urine vanillylmandelic acid

SPECIAL CONSIDERATIONS
PATIENT/FAMILY EDUCATION
• Administer with food to decrease stomach upset
• Protect from moisture, light, and extremes of temperature
• Notify clinician if fever, sore throat, unusual bleeding, bruising, or skin rashes occur
• 500-mg tablet contains 54.5 mg sodium

---

amiodarone
(a-mee′oh-da-rone)
Rx: Cordarone
Chemical Class: Iodinated benzofuran derivative
Therapeutic Class: Antidysrhythmic (class III)

CLINICAL PHARMACOLOGY
Mechanism of Action: Prolongs action potential duration and effective refractory period; noncompetitive α- and β-adrenergic inhibition
Pharmacokinetics
PO: Slowly and variably absorbed, onset 1-3 wk; extensive distribution; $t_{1/2}$ 26-107 days; eliminated via hepatic excretion into bile
INDICATIONS AND USES: Life-threatening recurrent ventricular fibrillation and hemodynamically unstable ventricular tachycardia unresponsive to adequate doses of other antiarrhythmics; refractory-sustained or paroxysmal atrial fibrillation and paroxysmal supraventricular tachycardia,* symptomatic atrial flutter,* CHF (low dose)*
DOSAGE
Adult
• PO loading dose 800-1600 mg/day for 1-3 wk; then 600-800 mg/day for 1 mo; maintenance 200-600 mg/day (lower doses effective for supraventricular arrhythmias)
Child
• PO loading dose 10-15 mg/kg/day or 600-800 mg/1.73 m²/day for 4-14 days or until adequate control of dysrhythmia or prominent adverse effects occur; maintenance 5 mg/kg/day or 200-400 mg/1.73 m²/day qd for several weeks; reduce to lowest effective dosage possible
• IV 5 mg/kg over 30 min followed by PO 800 mg qd × 7 days, then 600 mg qd × 3 days, then 200-400 mg qd maintenance; IV load allows shorter time to arrhythmic control than PO load; *or* IV 5 mg/kg bolus followed 15 min later by continuous IV infusion of 20 mg/kg/day for 3-5 days

🗓 **AVAILABLE FORMS/COST OF THERAPY**
• Tab, Uncoated—Oral: 200 mg, 100's: **$277.20-$354.90**
• Inj, Sol—intravenous-50 mg/ml, 3 ml: **$84.03**

CONTRAINDICATIONS: Severe sinus-node dysfunction, with resultant marked sinus bradycardia; 2nd and 3rd degree AV block; syncope caused by episodes of bradycardia (except when used in conjunction with a pacemaker); hypersensitivity
PRECAUTIONS: Thyroid disease, 2nd or 3rd degree AV block, electrolyte imbalances, bradycardia, pulmonary disease (poorer prognosis should pulmonary toxicity develop)
PREGNANCY AND LACTATION: Pregnancy category D; due to a very long $t_{1/2}$, amiodarone should be dis-

continued several months prior to conception to avoid early gestational exposure, reserve for refractory dysrhythmias; newborns exposed to amiodarone should have TFTs; excreted into breast milk; contains high proportions of iodine; breast feeding not recommended

SIDE EFFECTS/ADVERSE REACTIONS

Adverse reactions occur in about 75% of patients receiving doses ≥400 mg/day and cause discontinuation of drug in 7%-18% of patients

CNS: Ataxia, *dizziness,* fatigue, *headache,* insomnia, involuntary movements, lack of coordination, malaise, paresthesias, peripheral neuropathy, tremors

CV: Bradycardia, **cardiac conduction abnormalities,** CHF, **dysrhythmias,** hypotension, **sinoatrial node dysfunction, sinus arrest**

EENT: Blurred vision, corneal microdeposits, dry eyes, halos, loss of vision, optic neuritis, optic neuropathy, photophobia

GI: Abdominal pain, anorexia, constipation, diarrhea, hepatotoxicity, nausea, vomiting

METAB: Hyperthyroidism or hypothyroidism

MS: Pain in extremities, weakness

RESP: Cough, dyspnea, **pulmonary fibrosis($^1/_{1000}$),** pulmonary inflammation

SKIN: Alopecia, angioedema, blue-gray skin discoloration, photosensitivity, rash, spontaneous ecchymosis

MISC: Abnormal salivation, abnormal taste or smell, coagulation abnormalities, edema, flushing

INTERACTIONS
Drugs

3 *Aprinidine:* Increased aprinidine concentrations

3 β-*adrenergic blockers:* Bradycardia, cardiac arrest, or ventricular arrhythmia shortly after initiation of β-adrenergic blockers that undergo extensive hepatic metabolism (propranolol, sotalol, metoprolol)

3 *Calcium channel blockers:* Cardiotoxicity with bradycardia and decreased cardiac output with diltiazem and, potentially, verapamil

3 *Cholestyramine, Colestipol:* Decreased amiodarone plasma concentrations

3 *Cimetidine:* Increased amiodarone plasma concentrations (other H_2 blockers likely have no effect)

3 *Cyclosporine, Tacrolimus:* Increased cyclosporine, tacrolimus concentrations

3 *Digitalis glycosides:* Accumulation of digoxin

3 *Flecainide, Ecainide:* Increased flecainide, ecainide serum concentrations

3 *Oral anticoagulants:* Enhanced hypoprothrombinemic response to warfarin

3 *Phenytoin:* Increased serum phenytoin concentrations, decreased amiodarone concentrations

3 *Procainamide:* Increased procainamide concentrations

3 *Quinidine:* Increased quinidine plasma concentrations

3 *Theophylline:* Increased theophylline levels

Labs

• *Increase:* Serum T4 and serum reverse T3

• *Decrease:* Serum T3

SPECIAL CONSIDERATIONS
Should be administered only by clinicians experienced in treatment of life-threatening dysrhythmias who are thoroughly familiar with the risks and benefits of amiodarone therapy

PATIENT/FAMILY EDUCATION
• Take with food and/or divide doses if GI intolerance occurs

---

italic = common side effects   ***bold italic*** = life-threatening reactions

- Use sunscreen or stay out of sun to prevent burns
- Report side effects immediately
- Skin discoloration is usually reversible

MONITORING PARAMETERS

- Chest x-ray and PFTs (baseline and q3 mo)
- Electrolytes
- LFTs
- ECG (measure PR, QRS, QT intervals; check for PVCs, other dysrhythmias); QT interval prolongation of 10%-15% suggests therapeutic effect
- TFTs
- CNS symptoms

---

amitriptyline

(a-mee-trip′ti-leen)

Rx: Elavil

Combinations:

  Rx: with chlordiazepoxide (Limbitrol); with perphenazine (Triavil)

Chemical Class: Tertiary amine Dibenzocycloheptadiene derivative

Therapeutic Class: Antidepressant; anxiolytic; antineurolgic

CLINICAL PHARMACOLOGY

Mechanism of Action: Inhibits reuptake of norepinephrine and serotonin (blocking activity moderate and very high, respectively) at the presynaptic neuron, prolonging neuronal activity; inhibits histamine and acetylcholine activity; mild peripheral vasodilator effects and possible "quinidine-like" actions on cardiac conduction; high anticholinergic and sedative, moderate orthostatic hypotensive side effects

Pharmacokinetics

PO/IM: Onset 45 min, peak 2-4 hr, therapeutic response 2-4 wk once

adequate dosage achieved; metabolized by liver (active metabolite, nortriptyline), excreted in urine/feces; crosses placenta; $t_{1/2}$ 10-50 hr

INDICATIONS AND USES: Depression, chronic pain (chronic tension headache, migraine, diabetic neuropathy, cancer pain, postherpetic neuralgia),* panic disorder,* eating disorders,* myofacial pain syndromes*

DOSAGE

Adult

- PO 50-100 mg hs, may increase to 200 mg/day, not to exceed 300 mg/day (chronic pain doses usually at lower end of range)
- IM (do not administer IV) 20-30 mg qid, or 80-120 mg hs

Adolescent/Geriatric

- PO 30 mg/day in divided doses, may be increased to 150 mg/day

Child

- *Chronic pain management:* PO 0.1 mg/kg/day in 3 divided doses initially, advance as tolerated over 2-3 weeks to 0.5-2 mg/kg qhs
- *Depression:* PO 1 mg/kg/day in 3 divided doses initially with increases to 1.5 mg/kg/day

$ **AVAILABLE FORMS/COST OF THERAPY**

- Inj, Sol—IM: 10 mg/ml, 10 ml: **$0.33-$10.80**
- Tab, Coated—Oral: 10 mg, 100's: **$2.25-$22.56;** 25 mg, 100's: **$2.75-$45.24;** 50 mg, 100's: **$3.25-$116.45;** 75 mg, 100's: **$3.75-$110.21;** 100 mg, 100's: **$6.00-$230.00;** 150 mg, 100's: **$7.75-$198.29**

CONTRAINDICATIONS: Acute recovery phase of MI, concurrent use of MAOIs

PRECAUTIONS: Suicidal patients, convulsive disorders, prostatic hypertrophy, psychiatric disease, severe depression, increased intraocular pressure, narrow-angle glau-

---

* = non-FDA-approved use

coma, urinary retention, cardiac disease (2nd or 3rd degree heart block or sick sinus syndrome), hepatic disease/renal disease, hyperthyroidism, electroshock therapy, elective surgery, elderly, abrupt discontinuation

PREGNANCY AND LACTATION: Pregnancy category D; excreted into breast milk; effect on nursing infant unknown but may be of concern

SIDE EFFECTS/ADVERSE REACTIONS

CNS: Anxiety, confusion (especially in elderly), *dizziness, drowsiness,* extra-pyramidal symptoms (elderly), fatigue, headache, increased psychiatric symptoms, insomnia, memory impairment, nervousness, nightmares, panic, stimulation, tremors, weakness

CV: **Dysrhythmias,** hypertension, *orthostatic hypotension,* palpitations, syncope, tachycardia

EENT: *Blurred vision,* mydriasis, nasal congestion, ophthalmoplegia, tinnitus

GI: *Constipation,* cramps, diarrhea, *dry mouth,*epigastric distress, hepatitis, increased appetite, jaundice, nausea, paralytic ileus, stomatitis, vomiting, weight gain

GU: *Urinary retention*

HEME: **Agranulocytosis, eosinophilia, leukopenia, thrombocytopenia**

SKIN: Photosensitivity, pruritus, rash, sweating, urticaria

INTERACTIONS

Drugs

③ *Altretamine:* Orthostatic hypotension

③ *Amphetamines:* Theoretical increase in effect of amphetamines, clinical evidence lacking

③ *Anticholinergics:* Excessive anticholinergic effects

③ *Barbiturates:* Reduced serum concentrations of cyclic antidepressants

② *Bethanidine:* Reduced antihypertensive effect of bethanidine

③ *Carbamazepine:* Reduced antidepressant serum concentrations

③ *Cimetidine* (other H_2 blockers less likely to have effect): Inhibition of TCA metabolism

② *Clonidine:* Reduced antihypertensive response to clonidine; enhanced hypertensive response with abrupt clonidine withdrawal

② *Epinephrine, norepinephrine:* Enhanced pressor response

③ *Ethanol:* Additive impairment of motor skills; abstinent alcoholics may eliminate cyclic antidepressants more rapidly than non-alcoholics

③ *Fluoxetine, paroxetine:* Marked increases in cyclic antidepressant plasma concentrations

③ *Guanabenz, guanfacine, debrisoquin:* Inhibition of antihypertensive effect

② *Guanethidine, guanadrel:* Inhibited antihypertensive response to guanethidine

③ *Hypoglycemics:* Enhanced hypoglemic effects

③ *Isoproterenol:* Increased cardiac arrhythmias

③ *Lithium:* Increased risk of neurotoxicity

② *MAOIs:* Excessive sympathetic response, mania, or hyperpyrexia possible

② *Moclobemide:* Potential association with fatal or non-fatal serotonin syndrome

③ *Neuroleptics:* Increased therapeutic and toxic effects of both drugs

② *Norepinephrine:* Markedly enhanced pressor response to norepinephrine

3 *Phenylephrine:* Enhanced pressor response

3 *Propoxyphene:* Enhanced effect of cyclic antidepressants

3 *Quinidine:* Increased cyclic antidepressant serum concentrations

3 *Rifampin:* Possible decreased TCA levels

3 *Ritonavir, indinavir:* Increased TCA levels

Labs

• *False increase:* Carbamazepine levels

SPECIAL CONSIDERATIONS
PATIENT/FAMILY EDUCATION

• Therapeutic effects may take 2-3 wk

• Use caution in driving or other activities requiring alertness

• Avoid rising quickly from sitting to standing, especially elderly

• Avoid alcohol ingestion, other CNS depressants

• Do not discontinue abruptly after long-term use

• Wear sunscreen or large hat to prevent photosensitivity

• Increase fluids, bulk in diet if constipation occurs

• Gum, hard sugarless candy, or frequent sips of water for dry mouth

MONITORING PARAMETERS

• Mental status: mood, sensorium, affect, suicidal tendencies

• Determination of amitriptyline plasma concentrations is not routinely recommended but may be useful in identifying toxicity, drug interactions, or noncompliance (adjustments in dosage should be made according to clinical response not plasma concentrations)

• Therapeutic plasma levels 125-250 µg/L (including active metabolites)

amlexanox
(am-lex'a-nox)
Rx: Aphthasol
Chemical Class: Benzopyrano-bipyridine carboxylic acid derivative
Therapeutic Class: Antiallergic, antiinflammatory

CLINICAL PHARMACOLOGY
Mechanism of Action: Accelerates healing probably via inhibition of formation or release of inflammatory mediators

INDICATIONS AND USES: To reduce the duration, pain, size and erythema of aphthous ulcers

DOSAGE
Adult

• *Aphthous ulcers:* TOP apply qid after oral hygiene until ulcer heals

$ AVAILABLE FORMS/COST OF THERAPY

• Top—5% paste: 5 g: **$18.75**

PRECAUTIONS: History of contact dermatitis

SIDE EFFECTS/ADVERSE REACTIONS

SKIN: Contact mucositis; transient pain, stinging, or burning at the site of application

amlodipine
(am-low'di-peen)
Rx: Norvasc
Combinations:
   Rx: with benazepril (Lotrel)
Chemical Class: Dihydropyridine
Therapeutic Class: Calcium channel blocker: antihypertensive; antianginal

CLINICAL PHARMACOLOGY
Mechanism of Action: Inhibits calcium ion influx across cell mem-

brane in vascular smooth muscle and cardiac muscle; produces relaxation of coronary and peripheral vascular smooth muscle; hemodynamics: increases myocardial contractility and cardiac output; significantly decreases peripheral vascular resistance

Pharmacokinetics

PO: Peak serum conc 6-9 hr, bioavailability 60%-65% $t_{1/2}$ 30-50 hr, metabolized by liver, excreted in urine (5%-10% unchanged)

INDICATIONS AND USES: Chronic stable angina pectoris,* hypertension, vasospastic (Prinzmetal's or variant) angina,* CHF*

DOSAGE

Adult

• *Angina:* PO 5-10 mg qd
• *Hypertension:* PO 5 mg qd initially, may increase up to 10 mg/day (small, fragile, or elderly patients or patients with hepatic insufficiency may be started on 2.5 mg qd)

$ **AVAILABLE FORMS/COST OF THERAPY**

• Tab, Uncoated—Oral: 2.5 mg, 90's: **$119.16;** 5 mg, 90's: **$119.16;** 10 mg, 90's: **$195.70**

PRECAUTIONS: CHF, hypotension, hepatic insufficiency, aortic stenosis, elderly

PREGNANCY AND LACTATION: Pregnancy category C; unknown if excreted into milk; use caution in nursing mothers

SIDE EFFECTS/ADVERSE REACTIONS

CNS: Anxiety, asthenia, depression, dizziness, lightheadedness, fatigue, headache (7.5%), insomnia, malaise, nervousness, paresthesia, somnolence, tremor

CV: Bradycardia, **dysrhythmia,** hypotension, palpitations, *peripheral edema,* syncope, tachycardia

GI: Abdominal cramps, constipation, diarrhea, dry mouth, flatulence, gastric upset, nausea (3%), vomiting

GU: Nocturia, polyuria

SKIN: Hair loss, pruritus, rash, urticaria1

MISC: Cough, epistaxis, flushing, muscle cramps, nasal congestion, sexual dysfunction, shortness of breath, sweating, tinnitus, weight gain

INTERACTIONS

Drugs

3 *Barbiturates:* Reduced plasma concentrations of amlodipine

3 *Diltiazem:* Reduced clearance of amlodipine

3 *Erythromycin:* Reduced clearance of amlodipine

3 *Fentanyl:* Severe hypotension or increased fluid volume requirements

3 *Grapefruit juice:* Reduced clearance of amlodipine

3 *H₂ blockers:* Increased plasma concentration of amlodipine possible

3 *Proton pump inhibitors:* Increased plasma concentration of amlodipine possible

3 *Quinidine:* Increased plasma concentration of amlodipine; reduced plasma quinidine level

3 *Rifampin:* Reduced plasma concentration of amlodipine

3 *Vincristine:* Reduced vincristine clearance

SPECIAL CONSIDERATIONS
PATIENT/FAMILY EDUCATION

• Notify clinician of irregular heart beat, shortness of breath, swelling of feet and hands, pronounced dizziness, hypotension

---

italic = common side effects   **bold italic** = life-threatening reactions

ammonium chloride
Rx: injection
OTC: oral
Chemical Class: Ammonium ion
Therapeutic Class: Urinary and systemic acidifier; expectorant

CLINICAL PHARMACOLOGY
Mechanism of Action: Lowers urinary pH; conversion to urea by the liver liberates hydrogen and chloride ions in blood and extracellular fluid with decreased pH and correction of alkalosis

Pharmacokinetics
PO: Absorption occurs in 3-6 hr; metabolized in liver to urea and HCl, excreted in urine and feces

INDICATIONS AND USES: Hypochloremic states and metabolic alkalosis, systemic and urinary acidifier, expectorant (usually in combination with other expectorants and cough mixtures)

DOSAGE
Adult
• *Alkalosis:* IV add contents of 1-2 vials (100-200 mEq) to 500 or 1000 ml of 0.9% sodium chloride inj, do not exceed concentration of 1%-2% ammonium chloride or an infusion rate of 5 ml/min; monitor dosage by repeated serum bicarbonate determinations
• *Acidifier:* PO 4-12 g/day in divided doses
• *Expectorant:* PO 250-500 mg q2-4h as needed
Child
• *Acidifier:* PO 75 mg/kg/day in 4 divided doses

⚡ AVAILABLE FORMS/COST OF THERAPY
• Granules—Oral 500 g: **$8.90-$41.25**

• Tab—Oral: 500 mg, 100's: **$3.04**
• Inj, Conc-Sol—IV: 5.35 g/20 ml (100 mEq), 20 ml: **$1.49**

CONTRAINDICATIONS: Severe hepatic disease, severe renal disease, metabolic alkalosis due to vomiting of hydrochloric acid when accompanied by loss of sodium (excretion of sodium bicarbonate in the urine)

PRECAUTIONS: Severe respiratory disease, cardiac edema, respiratory acidosis, infants, children, elderly

PREGNANCY AND LACTATION: Pregnancy category C; when consumed in large quantities near-term may cause acidosis in mother and fetus; no data available regarding use in nursing mothers

SIDE EFFECTS/ADVERSE REACTIONS
CNS: Coma, confusion, drowsiness, headache, *hyperreflexia,* stimulation, tetany, *tonic convulsions,* tremors, *twitching*
CV: Bounding pulse, bradycardia, *dysrhythmias*
GI: Anorexia, diarrhea, *gastric irritation, nausea,* thirst, *vomiting*
GU: Glycosuria, *hypercalciuria, polyuria*
METAB: Hyperchloremia, hyperglycemia, *hypokalemia, hypomagnesemia, metabolic acidosis*
RESP: Apnea, hyperventilation, irregular respirations
SKIN: Pallor; rash, pain, and irritation at infusion site (minimized by slow infusion); sweating

INTERACTIONS
Drugs
3 *Flecainide:* Increased urinary clearance of flecainide
3 *Spironolactone:* Enhanced acid retention

---

* = non-FDA-approved use

SPECIAL CONSIDERATIONS
PATIENT/FAMILY EDUCATION
• Administer with meals if GI symptoms occur
MONITORING PARAMETERS
• Serum electrolytes
• Urine pH, urinary output, urine glucose, specific gravity during beginning treatment
• ABGs

---

ammonium lactate
Rx: Lac-Hydrin
Chemical Class: Alpha hydroxy acid
Therapeutic Class: Emollient

CLINICAL PHARMACOLOGY
Mechanism of Action: Natural skin humectant; reduces excessive epidermal keratinization (e.g., ichthyosis)
INDICATIONS AND USES: Dry, scaly skin (xerosis); ichthyosis vulgaris; itching associated with these conditions
DOSAGE
Adult and Child
TOP rub in thoroughly to affected areas bid
💲 AVAILABLE FORMS/COST OF THERAPY
• Cre, Top—12%, 140, 280, 385 g: **$34.04**/280 g
• Lotion, Top—12%, 225, 240, 400, 420 g: **$8.75-$31.91**/225 g; **$14.45-$50.23**/400 g
• Lotion, Top—5%, 120, 240 ml: **$5.81**/120 ml
• Sol—500, 2500 ml: **$27.85**/500 ml
PREGNANCY AND LACTATION: Pregnancy category C; unknown if excreted in breast milk; lactic acid is a normal constituent of blood and tissues

SIDE EFFECTS/ADVERSE REACTIONS
SKIN: Burning, erythema, hyperpigmentation, irritation, peeling, stinging
SPECIAL CONSIDERATIONS
• Side effects greater in fair-skinned individuals, if applied to abraded or inflamed areas, and in ichthyosis (where incidence of burning, stinging, and erythema is 10%)

---

amobarbital
(am-oh-bar′bi-tal)
Rx: Amytal
Combinations:
Rx: with secobarbital (Tuinal)
Chemical Class: Barbituric acid derivative
Therapeutic Class: Sedative/hypnotic
DEA Class: Schedule II

CLINICAL PHARMACOLOGY
Mechanism of Action: CNS depressant: depresses the sensory cortex, decreases motor activity, alters cerebellar function, produces drowsiness, sedation, and hypnosis; little analgesic action at subanesthetic doses (may increase reaction to painful stimuli); anticonvulsant activity in anesthetic doses; dose-dependent respiratory depression (hypnotic doses produce respiratory depression similar to physiologic sleep)
Pharmacokinetics
PO: Onset 45-60 min, duration 6-8 hr
IV: Onset 5 min, duration 3-6 hr
Metabolized by liver, excreted by kidneys (inactive metabolites), highly protein bound; $t_{1/2}$ 16-40 hr
INDICATIONS AND USES: Sedation, preanesthetic sedation, short-term (up to 2 wk) treatment of insomnia, anticonvulsant (status epilepticus),* adjunct in psychiatry*

---

italic = common side effects   ***bold italic*** = life-threatening reactions

DOSAGE

Adult

• *Preanesthetic sedation:* PO/IM 200 mg 1-2 hr preoperatively

• *Anticonvulsant/psychiatry:* IV 65-500 mg given over several min, not to exceed 100 mg/min; not to exceed 1 g

• *Insomnia:* PO/IM 65-200 mg hs

Child >6 yr

• *Sedation:* PO 2 mg/kg/day in 4 divided doses

• *Anticonvulsant/psychiatry:* IV 65-500 mg given over several min, not to exceed 100 mg/min; not to exceed 1 g

• *Insomnia:* IM 2-3 mg/kg hs

💲 AVAILABLE FORMS/COST OF THERAPY

• Inj, Lyphl-Sol—IM, IV: 0.5 g/vial: **$8.52-$9.30**

CONTRAINDICATIONS: Hypersensitivity to barbiturates, respiratory depression, severe liver impairment, porphyria

PRECAUTIONS: Anemia, addiction to barbiturates, hepatic disease, COPD/emphysema, renal disease, hypertension, elderly, acute/chronic pain, mental depression, history of drug abuse, abrupt discontinuation

PREGNANCY AND LACTATION: Pregnancy category D; small amount excreted in breast milk, use caution in nursing mothers

SIDE EFFECTS/ADVERSE REACTIONS

CNS: CNS depression, dizziness, *drowsiness, hangover,* headache, *lethargy,* lightheadedness, mental depression, physical dependence, slurred speech, stimulation in the elderly and children, vertigo

CV: Bradycardia, hypotension

GI: Constipation, diarrhea, nausea, vomiting

HEME: **Agranulocytosis, megaloblastic anemia** (long-term treatment), ***thrombocytopenia***

RESP: **Apnea, bronchospasm, depression, laryngospasm**

SKIN: Abscesses at injection site, angioedema, erythema multiforme, pain, *rash,* **Stevens-Johnson syndrome,** thrombophlebitis, urticaria

MISC: Osteomalacia (prolonged use), rickets

INTERACTIONS

Drugs

🔳 *Acetaminophen:* Enhanced hepatotoxic potential of acetaminophen overdoses

🔳 *Antidepressants:* Reduced serum concentration of cyclic antidepressants

🔳 *β-adrenergic blockers:* Reduced serum concentrations of β-blockers which are extensively metabolized

🔳 *Calcium channel blockers:* Reduced serum concentrations of verapamil and dihydropyridines

🔳 *Chloramphenicol:* Increased barbiturate concentrations; reduced serum chloramphenicol concentrations

🔳 *Corticosteroids:* Reduced serum concentrations of corticosteroids; may impair therapeutic effect

🔳 *Cyclosporine:* Reduced serum concentration of cyclosporine

🔳 *Digitoxin:* Reduced serum concentration of digitoxin

🔳 *Disopyramide:* Reduced serum concentrations of disopyramide

🔳 *Doxycycline:* Reduced serum doxycycline concentrations

🔳 *Estrogen:* Reduced serum concentration of estrogen

🔳 *Ethanol:* Excessive CNS depression

🔳 *Griseofulvin:* Reduced griseofulvin absorption

🔳 *Methoxyflurane:* Enhanced nephrotoxic effect

🔳 *MAOIs:* Prolonged effect of barbiturates

🔳 *Narcotic analgesics:* Increased toxicity of meperidine; reduced effect of methadone; additive CNS depression

3 *Neuroleptics:* Reduced effect of either drug

2 *Oral anticoagulants:* Decreased hypoprothrombinemic response to oral anticoagulants

3 *Oral contraceptives:* Reduced efficacy of oral contraceptives

3 *Phenytoin:* Unpredictable effect on serum phenytoin levels

3 *Propafenone:* Reduced serum concentration of propafenone

3 *Quinidine:* Reduced quinidine plasma concentrations

3 *Tacrolimus:* Reduced serum concentration of tacrolimus

3 *Theophylline:* Reduced serum theophylline concentrations

3 *Valproic acid:* Increased serum concentration of amobarbital

2 *Warfarin:* See oral anticoagulants

SPECIAL CONSIDERATIONS
PATIENT/FAMILY EDUCATION
• Indicated only for short-term treatment of insomnia; probably ineffective after 2 wk; physical dependency may result when used for extended time (45-90 days depending on dose)
• Avoid driving or other activities requiring alertness
• Avoid alcohol ingestion or CNS depressants
• Do not discontinue medication abruptly after long-term use

MONITORING PARAMETERS
• Serum folate, vitamin D (if on long-term therapy)
• PT in patients receiving anticoagulants

amoxapine
(a-mox'a-peen)
Rx: Asendin
Chemical Class: Dibenzoxazepine derivative: secondary amine
Therapeutic Class: Tricyclic antidepressant

CLINICAL PHARMACOLOGY
Mechanism of Action: Inhibits reuptake of norepinephrine and serotonin (blocking activity high and moderate, respectively); blocks postsynaptic dopamine receptors; inhibits activity of histamine and acetylcholine; mild peripheral vasodilator effects and possible "quinidine-like" actions; high anticholinergic, moderate sedative, and slight orthostatic hypotension side effects

Pharmacokinetics
PO: Steady state 7 days; metabolized by liver, excreted by kidneys; $t_{1/2}$ 8 hr

INDICATIONS AND USES: Depression in patients with neurotic or reactive depressive disorders; endogenous and psychotic depressions; depression accompanied by anxiety or agitation

DOSAGE
Adult
• PO 50 mg bid-tid, may increase to 100 mg bid-tid by the end of the 1st wk, not to exceed 300 mg/day unless lower doses have been given for at least 2 wk; may be given daily dose hs; not to exceed 600 mg/day in hospitalized patients

Adolescents
• PO 25-50 mg/day, increase gradually to 100 mg/day (divided or as single hs dose)

Child
• Not recommended for patients <16 yr

---

italic = common side effects   ***bold italic*** = life-threatening reactions

$ AVAILABLE FORMS/COST OF THERAPY

• Tab, Uncoated—Oral: 25 mg, 100's: **$46.70-$61.51;** 50 mg, 100's: **$76.48-$99.95;** 100 mg, 100's: **$128.99-$166.95;** 150 mg, 30's: **$60.95-$93.00**

CONTRAINDICATIONS: Acute recovery phase of MI, concurrent use of MAOIs

PRECAUTIONS: Suicidal patients, severe depression, increased intraocular pressure, narrow-angle glaucoma, urinary retention, cardiac disease, hepatic disease, hyperthyroidism, electroshock therapy, elective surgery, elderly, convulsive disorders, prostatic hypertrophy

PREGNANCY AND LACTATION: Pregnancy category C; excreted into breast milk; effect on nursing infant unknown but may be of concern

SIDE EFFECTS/ADVERSE REACTIONS

CNS: Anxiety, ataxia, confusion, *dizziness, drowsiness,* EPS, headache, impairment of sexual functioning, increased psychiatric symptoms, insomnia, **neuroleptic malignant syndrome,** nightmares, paresthesia, **seizures,** stimulation, syncope, tardive dyskinesia, tremor, weakness

CV: Hypertension, *orthostatic hypotension,* palpitations, *tachycardia*

EENT: Blurred vision, mydriasis, ophthalmoplegia, tinnitus

GI: Constipation, cramps, diarrhea, *dry mouth,* epigastric distress, hepatitis, increased appetite, jaundice, nausea, paralytic ileus, peculiar taste, stomatitis, vomiting

GU: Urinary retention

HEME: **Agranulocytosis, eosinophilia, leukopenia, thrombocytopenia**

METAB: Breast enlargement, galactorrhea, menstrual irregularity, SIADH

SKIN: Photosensitivity, pruritus, rash, sweating, urticaria

INTERACTIONS

Drug

3 *Barbiturates:* Reduced serum concentrations of cyclic antidepressants

2 *Bethanidine:* Reduced antihypertensive effect of bethanidine

3 *Carbamazepine:* Reduced serum concentrations of cyclic antidepressants

3 *Cimetidine:* Increased serum concentrations of cyclic antidepressants

3 *Clonidine:* Reduced antihypertensive effect of clonidine; enhanced hypertensive response with abrupt clonidine withdrawal

3 *Debrisoquin:* Reduced antihypertensive effect of debrisoquin

3 *Dilitiazem:* Increased serum concentrations of cyclic antidepressants

2 *Epinephrine:* Markedly enhanced pressor response to IV epinephrine

3 *Ethanol:* Additive impairment of motor skills; abstinent alcoholics may eliminate cyclic antidepressants more rapidly than nonalcoholics

3 *Fluoxetine:* Marked increases in serum concentrations of cyclic antidepressants

3 *Fluvoxamine:* Marked increases in serum concentrations of cyclic antidepressants

3 *Guanabenz, guanadrel, guanethidine, guanfacine:* Reduced antihypertensive effect

3 *Lithium:* Increased risk of neurotoxicity

2 *Moclobemide:* Potential association with fatal or non-fatal serotonin syndrome

A *MAOIs:* Excessive sympathetic response, mania, or hyperpyrexia possible

---

* = non-FDA-approved use

3 *Neuroleptics:* Increased therapeutic and toxic effects of both drugs

2 *Norepinephrine:* Markedly enhanced pressor response to IV norepinephrine

3 *Paroxetine:* Marked increases in serum concentrations of cyclic antidepressants

3 *Propoxyphene:* Increased serum concentrations of cyclic antidepressants

3 *Quinidine:* Increased serum concentrations of cyclic antidepressants

3 *Rifampin:* Reduced serum concentrations of cyclic antidepressants

3 *Ritonavir:* Marked increases in serum concentrations of cyclic antidepressants

3 *Sulfonylureas:* Cyclic antidepressants may increase hypoglycemic effect

SPECIAL CONSIDERATIONS
PATIENT/FAMILY EDUCATION
• Therapeutic effects may take 2-3 wk
• Use caution in driving or other activities requiring alertness
• Avoid rising quickly from sitting to standing, especially elderly
• Avoid alcohol ingestion, other CNS depressants
• Do not discontinue abruptly after long-term use
• Wear sunscreen or large hat to prevent photosensitivity
• Increase fluids, bulk in diet if constipation occurs
• Use gum, hard sugarless candy, or frequent sips of water for dry mouth
• Potential for tardive dyskinesia

MONITORING PARAMETERS
• Mental status: mood, sensorium, affect, suicidal tendencies

---

amoxicillin
(a-mox'i-sill-in)
Rx: Amoxil, Moxilin, Senox, Trimox, Wymox
Chemical Class: Aminopenicillin
Therapeutic Class: Antibiotic

CLINICAL PHARMACOLOGY
Mechanism of Action: Inhibits bacterial wall synthesis, bactericidal
Pharmacokinetics
PO: Peak 1 hr, duration 6-8 hr, $t_{1/2}$ 1-1.3 hr; excreted largely unchanged in urine by glomerular filtration and active tubular secretion (can be delayed by concomitant administration of probenecid)

INDICATIONS AND USES: Infections of the ear, nose, throat, GU tract, skin and soft tissues, lower respiratory tract caused by susceptible organisms; gonococcal infections; prevention of bacterial endocarditis; *Chlamydia trachomatis* in pregnancy*

Antibacterial spectrum usually includes:
• Gram-positive organisms: Streptococci (including *S. faecalis, S. pyogenes, S. pneumoniae*) and nonpenicillinase-producing staphylococci
• Gram-negative organisms: *Haemophilus influenzae, E. coli, Proteus mirabilis,* and *Neisseria gonorrhoeae*

DOSAGE
Adult
• *Systemic infections:* PO 250-500 mg q8h or PO 875 mg q12h
• *Gonorrhea:* PO 3 g given with 1 g probenecid as a single dose (not first line); follow with doxycycline
• *Bacterial endocarditis prophylaxis:* PO 3 g 1 hr before proce-

---

dure, then 1.5 g 6 hr after initial dose

Child

• *Systemic infections:* PO 20-40 mg/ kg/day in divided doses q8h or 25-45 mg/kg/day in divided doses q12h

💲 AVAILABLE FORMS/COST OF THERAPY

• Cap, Gel—Oral: 250 mg, 100's: **$6.52-$82.00;** 500 mg, 100's: **$8.73-$58.75;** 875 mg, 100's: **$96.90**

• Powder, Reconst—Oral: 125 mg/5 ml, 150 ml: **$2.78-$9.55;** 200 mg/5 ml, 100 ml: **$10.15;** 250 mg/5 ml, 150 ml: **$2.87-$10.36;** 400 mg/5 ml; 100 ml: **$10.90**

• Tab, Chewable—Oral: 125 mg, 100's: **$11.00;** 200 mg, 100's: **$50.75;** 250 mg, 100's: **$23.05-$25.35;** 400 mg, 100's: **$62.00**

PRECAUTIONS: Hypersensitivity to cephalosporins, renal insufficiency, prolonged or repeated therapy, mononucleosis

PREGNANCY AND LACTATION: Pregnancy category B; excreted into breast milk in low concentrations; no adverse effects have been observed, but potential exists for modification of bowel flora and allergy/sensitization in nursing infant

SIDE EFFECTS/ADVERSE REACTIONS

CNS: Fever, headache

GI: Abdominal pain, colitis, *diarrhea,* glossitis, increased AST, ALT, *nausea,* pseudomembranous colitis, *vomiting*

HEME: **Bone marrow depression,** eosinophilia, increased bleeding time

RESP: **Anaphylaxis,** respiratory distress

MISC: Hypersensitivity reactions (rashes, urticaria, erythema multiforme, **exfoliative dermatitis, anaphylaxis**)

INTERACTIONS

Drugs

3 *Atenolol:* Reduced serum concentration of atenolol

3 *Chloramphenicol:* Inhibited antibacterial activity of amoxicillin; administer amoxicillin 3 hours before chloramphenicol

3 *Macrolide antibiotics:* Inhibited antibacterial activity of amoxicillin; administer amoxicillin 3 hours before macrolides

3 *Methotrexate:* Increased serum methotrexate concentrations

3 *Oral contraceptives:* Occasional impairment of oral contraceptive efficacy; consider use of supplementary contraception during cycles in which amoxicillin is used

3 *Tetracyclines:* Inhibited antibacterial activity of amoxicillin; administer amoxicillin 3 hours before tetracycline

SPECIAL CONSIDERATIONS
PATIENT/FAMILY EDUCATION

• May administer on a full or empty stomach

• Administer at even intervals

• Shake oral suspensions well before administering; discard after 14 days

• High rates of rash in patients on allopurinol, with mononucleosis, lymphatic leukemia

---

amoxicillin/ clavulanate

(a-mox'i-sill-in clav-u-lan'ate)

Rx: Augmentin

Chemical Class: Aminopenicillin; β-lactamase inhibitor

Therapeutic Class: Antibiotic

CLINICAL PHARMACOLOGY

Mechanism of Action: Inhibits bacterial wall synthesis; bactericidal; clavulanate protects amoxicillin from degradation by β-lactamase enzymes, extending the spectrum of activity

Pharmacokinetics

PO: Peak 2 hr, duration 6-8 hr, t½ 1-1.3 hr; excreted largely unchanged in urine

INDICATIONS AND USES: Infections of the lower respiratory tract, ear, sinuses, skin and soft tissues, urinary tract caused by susceptible organisms

Antibacterial spectrum usually includes:

• Gram-positive organisms: *Staphylococcus aureus, S. epidermidis, S. saprophyticus, Enterococcus, S. pneumoniae, S. pyogenes, S. viridans*

• Gram-negative organisms: *Hemophilus influenzae, Moraxella catarrhalis, Escherichia coli, Klebsiella* sp., *Enterobacter* sp., *Proteus mirabilis, P. vulgaris, Neisseria gonorrhoeae, Legionella* sp.

• Anaerobes: *Clostridium* sp., *Peptococcus* sp., *Peptostreptococcus* sp., *Bacteroides* sp., including *B. fragilis*

DOSAGE

Adult

• PO 250-500 mg (amoxicillin) q8h depending on severity of infection or 875 mg bid

Child

• PO 20-40 mg/kg/day (amoxicillin) in divided doses q8h; use chewable tablets under 40 kg for correct clavulanate dose

💲 AVAILABLE FORMS/COST OF THERAPY

• Powder, Reconst—Oral: 125 mg/ 31.25 mg/5 ml, 150 ml: **$35.20-$44.46;** 250 mg/62.5 mg/5 ml, 150 ml: **$53.37-$80.88;** 200 mg/28.5 mg/5 ml 100 ml: **$30.95;** 400 mg/57 mg/5 ml, 100 ml: **$58.95**

• Tab, Chewable—Oral: 125 mg/ 31.25 mg, 30's: **$36.58;** 200 mg/ 28.5 mg, 20's: **$30.95;** 250 mg/62.5

mg, 30's: **$76.09-$82.51;** 400 mg/57 mg, 20's: **$58.95**

• Tab, Uncoated—Oral: 250 mg/ 125 mg, 30's: **$67.67-$79.78;** 500 mg/125 mg, 20's: **$66.38;** 875 mg/ 125 mg, 20's: **$88.60-$107.56**

• Note: due to clavulanate strength, 2×250 mg tabs do not equal a 500 mg tab

CONTRAINDICATIONS: Hypersensitivity to penicillins

PRECAUTIONS: Hypersensitivity to cephalosporins, renal insufficiency, prolonged or repeated therapy, mononucleosis

PREGNANCY AND LACTATION: Pregnancy category B; excreted into breast milk in low concentrations; no adverse effects have been observed

SIDE EFFECTS/ADVERSE REACTIONS

CNS: Fever, headache

GI: Abdominal pain, black tongue, colitis, *diarrhea,* (9%) glossitis, increased AST, ALT, nausea, pseudomembranous colitis, vomiting

GU: Moniliasis, vaginitis

HEME: **Bone marrow depression,** eosinophilia, increased bleeding time

METAB: Alkalosis, hyperkalemia, hypernatremia, hypokalemia

MISC: Hypersensitivity reactions (rash, urticaria, erythema multiforme, **exfoliative dermatitis, anaphylaxis**)

INTERACTIONS

Drugs

3 *Atenolol:* Reduced serum concentration of atenolol

3 *Chloramphenicol:* Inhibited antibacterial activity of amoxicillin; administer amoxicillin 3 hours before chloramphenicol

3 *Macrolide antibiotics:* Inhibited antibacterial activity of amoxicillin; administer amoxicillin 3 hours before macrolides

---

italic = common side effects   ***bold italic*** = life-threatening reactions

3 *Methotrexate:* Increased serum methotrexate concentrations

3 *Oral contraceptives:* Occasional impairment of oral contraceptive efficacy; consider use of supplementary contraception during cycles in which amoxicillin is used

3 *Tetracyclines:* Inhibited antibacterial activity of amoxicillin; administer amoxicillin 3 hours before tetracycline

SPECIAL CONSIDERATIONS
PATIENT/FAMILY EDUCATION
• Administer with food to decrease GI side effects
• Administer at even intervals
• Shake oral suspensions well before administering; discard after 14 days; must be refrigerated

---

amphetamine
(am-fet′a-meen)
Combinations:
  Rx: with
    dextroamphetamine:
    (Adderall)
Chemical Class:
β-phenylisopropylamine (racemic)
Therapeutic Class: CNS stimulant
DEA Class: Schedule II

CLINICAL PHARMACOLOGY
Mechanism of Action: Sympathomimetic amines with CNS stimulant activity; increases release of norepinephrine from central noradrenergic neurons; at higher doses dopamine may be released in the mesolimbic system; peripheral alpha and beta activity includes elevation of systolic and diastolic blood pressures and weak bronchodilator and respiratory stimulation action; heart rate reflexly slowed at standard doses, arrhythmias with overdose

Pharmacokinetics
PO: Onset 30 min, peak 1-3 hr, duration 4-20 hr; metabolized by liver, excreted by kidneys, crosses placenta; $t_{1/2}$ dependent on urinary pH; at urinary pH <5.6, $t_{1/2}$ is 7-8 hr (increases with alkalinization of urine)
INDICATIONS AND USES: Narcolepsy; short-term adjunct to caloric restriction in exogenous obesity **(high potential for abuse, use only when alternative therapies have failed);** attention deficit disorder
DOSAGE
Adult
• *Narcolepsy:* PO 5-60 mg qd in divided doses
• *Obesity:* PO 5-30 mg in divided doses 30-60 min before meals
Child
• *Narcolepsy:* >12 yr: PO 10 mg qd increasing by 10 mg/day at weekly intervals; 6-12 yr: PO 5 mg qd increasing by 5 mg/wk (max 60 mg/day)
• *Attention deficit disorder:* ≥6 yr: PO 5 mg qd-bid increasing by 5 mg/day at weekly intervals (will rarely exceed 40 mg/day); 3-5 yr: PO 2.5 mg qd increasing by 2.5 mg/day at weekly intervals (usual range 0.1-0.5 mg/kg/dose)
$ **AVAILABLE FORMS/COST OF THERAPY**
• Tab, Combination—Oral: 10 mg 100's: **$55.08;** 20 mg 100's: **$94.38**
CONTRAINDICATIONS: Hyperthyroidism, moderate to severe hypertension, glaucoma, severe arteriosclerosis, history of drug abuse, cardiovascular disease, agitated states, within 14 days of MAOI administration
PRECAUTIONS: Mild hypertension, child <3 yr, Tourette's syndrome, motor and phonic tics
PREGNANCY AND LACTATION: Pregnancy category C; use of amphetamine for medical indications

---

* = non-FDA-approved use

not a significant risk to the fetus for congenital anomalies, mild withdrawal symptoms may be observed in the newborn; illicit maternal use presents significant risks to the fetus and newborn, including intrauterine growth retardation, premature delivery, and the potential for increased maternal, fetal, and neonatal morbidity; concentrated in breast milk; contraindicated during breast feeding

SIDE EFFECTS/ADVERSE REACTIONS

CNS: Addiction, aggressiveness, changes in libido, chills, dependence, dizziness, dyskinesia, dysphoria, euphoria, headache, *hyperactivity, insomnia,* irritability, overstimulation, psychotic episodes, *restlessness, talkativeness,* tremor

CV: **Dysrhythmias** (at larger doses), hypertension, *palpitations,* reflex decrease in heart rate, *tachycardia*

GI: Anorexia, constipation, cramps, diarrhea, dry mouth, metallic taste, nausea, vomiting, weight loss

GU: Impotence

METAB: Reversible elevations in serum thyroxine (T_4) with heavy use

SKIN: Urticaria

INTERACTIONS

Drugs

3 *Antacids:* May inhibit amphetamine excretion

3 *Furazolidone:* Hypertensive reactions

3 *Guanadrel:* Inhibits antihypertensive response to guanadrel

3 *Guanethidine:* Inhibits antihypertensive response to guanethidine

⚠ *MAOIs:* Severe hypertensive reactions possible

2 *Selegiline:* Severe hypertensive reactions possible

3 *Sodium bicarbonate:* May inhibit amphetamine excretion

Labs

• *False positive:* Urine amino acids

• Take early in the day
• Do not discontinue abruptly
• Avoid hazardous activities until stabilized on medication

---

amphotericin B, amphotericin B cholesteryl, amphotericin B lipid complex (ABLC), liposomal amphotericin B

(am-foe-ter'i-sin)

Rx: Abelcet (ABLC); AmBisome, Amphotec, Fungizone (IV and topical)

Chemical Class: Amphoteric polyene; lipid complex (ABLC)

Therapeutic Class: Antifungal

CLINICAL PHARMACOLOGY

Mechanism of Action: Binds to sterols in the cell membrane of susceptible fungi with a resultant change in cell permeability allowing leakage of intracellular components; fungistatic or fungicidal depending on concentration obtained in body fluids and the susceptibility of the fungus

Pharmacokinetics

IV: Peak 1-2 hr, initial plasma $t_{1/2}$ 24 hr, elimination $t_{1/2}$ 15 days; metabolic pathways are not known, very slowly excreted by the kidneys (metabolites), highly bound to plasma proteins; poorly penetrates CSF, bronchial secretions, aqueous humor, muscle, bone, brain, pancreas; not removed by hemodialysis

ABLC: Metabolic pathways unknown, pharmacokinetics not linear; clearance from blood increases with increasing doses; terminal elimination t$_{1/2}$ approx 173 hr; effect of hepatic and renal impairment on disposition unknown

INDICATIONS AND USES: TOP: Cutaneous and mucocutaneous mycotic infections caused by *Candida* sp. IV: Potentially life-threatening fungal infections: aspergillosis *(A. fumigatus),* cryptococcosis (torulosis), North American blastomycosis, systemic candidiasis, coccidioidomycosis and histoplasmosis, mucormycosis due to susceptible species of the genera *Absidia* sp., *Mucor* sp., *Rhizopus* sp., *Entomophthora* sp., and *Basidiobolus* sp., sporotrichosis *(S. schenckii);* American mucocutaneous leishmaniasis (not drug of choice as primary therapy); empirical therapy for presumed fungal infection in febrile neutropenic patients

ABLC: Treatment of aspergillosis in patients refractory to or intolerant of conventional amphotericin B therapy (may have less nephrotoxicity) **Do not use IV form of amphotericin B to treat noninvasive fungal infections, such as oral thrush, vaginal candidiasis and esophageal candidiasis in patients with normal neutrophil counts**

DOSAGE

Adult and Child

• TOP bid-qid for 7-21 days or longer if needed

• IV INF (minimum dilution 0.1 mg/ml) infuse 1 mg test dose slowly over 20-30 min to determine patient tolerance; initial therapeutic dose (if test dose tolerated) 0.25 mg/kg/day over 4-6 hr; individualize subsequent doses by increasing in 0.25 mg/kg/day increments (usual range 0.25-1 mg/kg/day); do not exceed 1.5 mg/kg/day; amphotericin cholesteryl IV INF 3-4 mg/kg/day at a rate of 1 mg/kg/hr; ABLC IV INF 5.0 mg/kg/day at a rate of 2.5 mg/

kg/hr; liposomal amphotericin B IV INF 3-5 mg/kg/day over 2 hr; INTRATHECAL 25-100 µg q48-72 hr; increase to 500 µg as tolerated; BLADDER IRRIGATION 5-15 mg/ 100 ml of sterile water irrigation solution at 100-300 ml/day; instill into bladder, clamp catheter for 60-120 minutes then drain; repeat 3-4 times/day for 2-5 days

$ **AVAILABLE FORMS/COST OF THERAPY**

• Cre—Top: 3%, 20 g: **$30.43**
• Lotion—Top: 3%, 30 ml: **$41.74**
• Oint—Top: 3%, 20 g: **$29.25**
• Inj, Lyphl, Sol—IV: 50 mg vial, 1's: **$16.88-$42.30**
• Susp—Oral: 100 mg/ml, 24 ml, 1's: **$25.30**
• ABLC Susp—IV: 5 mg/ml, 20 ml, 1's: **$173.33**
• ABLC Inj, Lyphl—IV: 50 mg vial, 1's: **$93.33;** 100 mg vial, 1's: **$160.00**

PRECAUTIONS: Renal disease, rapid IV infusion, prior total body irradiation, leukocyte infusions, avoid eye contact

PREGNANCY AND LACTATION: Pregnancy category B; excretion in human milk unknown: due to the potential toxicity, consider discontinuing nursing

SIDE EFFECTS/ADVERSE REACTIONS

Severe reactions may be lessened by giving acetaminophen, antihistamines, and antiemetics before infusion and by maintaining sodium balance; meperidine or hydrocortisone may also help

CNS: Chills, dizziness, *fever, headache,* paresthesias, peripheral nerve pain, peripheral neuropathy, *seizures*

CV: **Cardiac arrest, dysrhythmias,** hypertension, hypotension, ***ventricular fibrillation***

---

* = non-FDA-approved use

EENT: Blurred vision, deafness, diplopia, tinnitus

*GI: **Acute liver failure,** anorexia,* cramps, diarrhea, epigastric pain, hemorrhagic gastroenteritis, *nausea, vomiting*

*GU: **Anuria,** azotemia, hypokalemia,* hyposthenuria, nephrocalcinosis, oliguria, ***permanent renal impairment (especially with doses >5 g),*** renal tubular acidosis

*HEME: **Agranulocytosis,** eosinophilia,* hypomagnesemia, hyponatremia, ***leukopenia,*** normochromic, normocytic anemia, ***thrombocytopenia***

MS: Arthralgia, generalized pain, myalgia, weakness, weight loss

SKIN: Burning, irritation, pain, necrosis at injection site with extravasation; contact dermatitis, dry skin, erythema, flushing, pruritus, staining of nail lesions, stinging, urticaria

INTERACTIONS

Drugs

3 *Aminoglycosides:* Synergistic nephrotoxicity

3 *Cyclosporine:* Increased nephrotoxicity of both drugs

3 *Neuromuscular blocking agents:* Prolonged muscle relaxation due to hypokalemia

Labs

Increase: Serum bilirubin, serum conjugated bilirubin, serum cholesterol

Decrease: Serum unconjugated bilirubin

SPECIAL CONSIDERATIONS
PATIENT/FAMILY EDUCATION

• Long-term therapy may be needed to clear infection (2 wk-3 mo depending on type of infection)

MONITORING PARAMETERS

• BUN, serum creatinine; if BUN exceeds 40 mg/dl or serum creatinine exceeds 3 mg/dl, discontinue the drug or reduce dosage until renal function improves

• Regular monitoring of CBC, K, Na, Mg, LFTs

• Total dosage

---

ampicillin

(am′pi-sill-in)

Rx: Marcillin, Principen, Totacillin

Combinations

  Rx: with probenecid (Polycillin PRB, Probampicin)

Chemical Class: Aminopenicillin

Therapeutic Class: Antibiotic

CLINICAL PHARMACOLOGY

Mechanism of Action: Inhibits bacterial wall synthesis; bactericidal

Pharmacokinetics

PO: Peak 2 hr

IV: Peak 5 min

IM: Peak 1 hr

$t_{1/2}$ 50-110 min, excreted largely unchanged in urine by glomerular filtration and active tubular secretion (can be delayed by concomitant administration of probenecid)

INDICATIONS AND USES: Infections of the respiratory tract and soft tissues caused by susceptible organisms; bacterial meningitis caused by susceptible organisms; septicemia; gonococcal infections; prevention of bacterial endocarditis; prophylaxis in cesarean section*

Antibacterial spectrum usually includes:

• Gram-positive organisms: α- and β-hemolytic streptococci, *Streptococcus pneumoniae,* nonpenicillinase-producing staphylococci, *Bacillus anthracis,* and most strains of enterococci and clostridia

• Gram-negative organisms: *Haemophilus influenzae, Neisseria gonorrhoeae, N. meningitidis, N. ca-*

---

italic = common side effects   ***bold italic*** = life-threatening reactions

tarrhalis, *Escherichia coli, Proteus mirabilis, Bacteroides funduliformis, Salmonella* sp. and *Shigella* sp.

DOSAGE

Adult

• *Systemic infections:* PO 250-500 mg q6h; IV/IM 500 mg-3 g q4-6h
• *Meningitis:* IV 8-14 g/day in divided doses q3-4h
• *Gonorrhea:* PO 3.5 g given with 1 g probenecid as a single dose
• *Renal impairment:* CrCl 10-30 ml/min: administer q6-12h; CrCl <10 ml/min: administer q12h

Child

• *Systemic infections:* PO 50-100 mg/kg/day in divided doses q6h; IV/IM 100-200 mg/kg/day in divided doses q4-6h; max 2-3 g/day
• *Meningitis:* IV 200-400 mg/kg/day in divided doses q4-6h; max 12 g/day

💲 AVAILABLE FORMS/COST OF THERAPY

• Inj, Dry-Sol—IM, IV: 125 mg/vial, 1's: **$0.68;** 250 mg/vial, 1's: **$0.80-$1.00;** 500 mg/vial, 1's: **$1.04-$19.42;** 1 g/vial, 1's: **$1.50-$2.45;** 2 g/vial, 1's: **$2.30-$3.46**
• Cap, Gel—Oral: 250 mg, 100's: **$9.60-$18.56;** 500 mg, 100's: **$10.95-$33.12**
• Powder, Reconst—Oral: 125 mg/5 ml, 200 ml: **$2.95-$7.00;** 250 mg/5 ml, 200 ml: **$4.20-$10.95**

PRECAUTIONS: Hypersensitivity to cephalosporins, renal insufficiency, prolonged or repeated therapy, mononucleosis, neonates

PREGNANCY AND LACTATION: Pregnancy category B; excreted into breast milk in low concentrations; no adverse effects have been observed

SIDE EFFECTS/ADVERSE REACTIONS

CNS: Anxiety, ***coma,*** depression, hallucinations, lethargy, ***seizures*** twitching
GI: Black "hairy" tongue, *diarrhea,* glossitis, *nausea,* pseudomembranous colitis, stomatitis, *vomiting,* increased AST/ALT
GU: Glomerulonephritis, hematuria, *moniliasis,* oliguria, proteinuria, *vaginitis*
HEME: **Bone marrow depression,** increased bleeding time, eosinophilia
MISC: Hypersensitivity reactions (rashes, urticaria, erythema multiforme, ***exfoliative dermatitis anaphylaxis***)

INTERACTIONS

Drugs

🔢 *Atenolol:* Reduced serum concentration of atenolol
🔢 *Chloramphenicol:* Inhibited antibacterial activity of ampicillin; administer ampicillin 3 hr before chloramphenicol
🔢 *Macrolide antibiotics:* Inhibited antibacterial activity of ampicillin; administer amoxicillin 3 hr before macrolides
🔢 *Methotrexate:* Increased serum methotrexate concentrations
🔢 *Oral contraceptives:* Occasional impairment of oral contraceptive efficacy; consider use of supplemental contraception during cycles in which ampicillin is used
🔢 *Tetracyclines:* Inhibited antibacterial activity of ampicillin; administer ampicillin 3 hr before tetracycline

Labs

• *False positive:* Urine amino acids
• *Increase:* Urine glucose (Clinitest method), plasma phenyldanine (dried blood spot method), CSF protein (Ektachem method), serum protein (biuret method), serum the-

---

ophylline (3M Diagnostics Theo-Fast method), serum uric acid
• *Decrease:* Serum cholesterol (CHOD-iodide method only), serum folate (bioassay method only), urine glucose (Clinistix and Diastix methods)

SPECIAL CONSIDERATIONS
PATIENT/FAMILY EDUCATION
• Administer on an empty stomach
• Administer at even intervals
• Shake oral suspensions well before administering, discard after 14 days
• High rates of rash in patients on allopurinol, with mononucleosis, lymphatic leukemia
• Amoxicillin is better oral choice given greater ease of dosing and lower incidence of diarrhea

---

ampicillin/sulbactam
(am′pi-sill-in/sul-bac′tam)
Rx: Unasyn
Chemical Class: Aminopenicillin (ampicillin); penicillinate (sulbactam)
Therapeutic Class: Antibiotic

CLINICAL PHARMACOLOGY
Mechanism of Action: Inhibits bacterial cell wall synthesis; sulbactam inhibits β-lactamase; bactericidal
Pharmacokinetics
IV: Immediate peak, serum $t_{1/2}$ 1 hr; 75%-85% excreted unchanged in urine
IM: Peak levels lower than for IV administration
INDICATIONS AND USES: Infections of skin and skin structures; gynecological infections; intra-abdominal infections caused by susceptible organisms
Antibacterial spectrum usually includes:
• Gram-positive organisms: *Staphylococcus aureus, S. epidermidis,*

S. saprophyticus, Enterococcus, Streptococcus pneumoniae, S. pyogenes, S. viridans
• Gram-negative organisms: *Hemophilus influenzae, Moraxella catarrhalis, Escherichia coli, Klebsiella* sp., *Proteus mirabilis, P. vulgaris, Providencia* sp., *Morganella morganii, Neisseria gonorrhoeae*
Anaerobes: *Clostridium* sp., *Peptococcus* sp., *Peptostreptoccoccus* sp., *Bacteroides* sp. including *B. fragilis*
DOSAGE
Adult and Child ≥40 kg
• IV/IM 1.5-3.0 g (ampicillin + sulbactam) q6h
• Child <40 kg, ≥1 yr old, IV 300 mg/kg/day (200 mg ampicillin/100 mg sulbactam) in divided doses q6h
• *Impaired renal function:*

CREATININE CLEARANCE (ML/MIN/1.73M²)	T₁/₂ (hr)	DOSAGE
≥30	1	1.5-3.0 g q6-8h
15-29	5	1.5-3.0 g q12h
5-14	9	1.5-3.0 g q24h

$ **AVAILABLE FORMS/COST OF THERAPY**
Inj, Dry-Sol—IM, IV: 1.5 g, (1 g ampicillin + 0.5 g sulbactam) 1's: **$7.42-$8.60**
Inj, Dry-Sol—IM, IV: 3.0 g, (2 g ampicillin + 1 g sulbactam) 1's: **$14.01-$15.26**
CONTRAINDICATIONS: Hypersensitivity to penicillins
PRECAUTIONS: Mononucleosis (incidence of rash 43%-100%); safety not established in children
PREGNANCY AND LACTATION: Pregnancy category B; animal studies at doses 10× the human dose reveal no evidence of harm; low concentrations excreted in breast milk
SIDE EFFECTS/ADVERSE REACTIONS
CNS: Fatigue, headache, malaise, *seizures* (overdosage)

---

italic = common side effects   **bold italic** = life-threatening reactions

EENT: Epitaxis, glossitis, stomatitis
GI: Abdominal distension, diarrhea
(3%), elevated LFTs, flatulence, gastritis, nausea, ***pseudomembranous colitis,*** vomiting
GU: Dysuria, increased BUN/creatinine, urinary retention
HEME: ***Bone marrow depression***
SKIN: Erythema multiforme, ***exfoliative dermatitis,*** pain at injection site (16% for IM, 3% for IV), rash (2%), thrombophlebitis (3%), urticaria
MISC: ***Anaphylaxis***

INTERACTIONS
Drugs
🔢 *Chloramphenicol:* Inhibited antibacterial activity of ampicillin/sulbactam; administer ampicillin/sulbactam 3 hr before chloramphenicol
🔢 *Macrolide antibiotics:* Inhibited antibacterial activity of ampicillin/sulbactam; administer ampicillin/sulbactam 3 hr before macrolides
🔢 *Methotrexate:* Increased serum methotrexate concentrations
🔢 *Oral contraceptives:* Occasional impairment of oral contraceptive efficacy; consider use of supplemental contraception during cycles in which ampicillin/sulbactam is used
🔢 *Tetracyclines:* Inhibited antibacterial activity of ampicillin/sulbactam; administer ampicillin/sulbactam 3 hr before tetracyclines
Labs
• *False positive:* Urine amino acids
• *Increase:* Urine glucose (Clinitest method), plasma phenyldanine (dried blood spot method), CSF protein (Ektachem method), serum protein (biuret method) serum theophylline (3M Diagnostics TheoFast method), serum uric acid, serum creatinine
• *Decrease:* Serum cholesterol (CHOD-iodide method only), serum folate (bioassay method only)

SPECIAL CONSIDERATIONS
• Do not reconstitute or administer with aminoglycosides (ampicillin inactivates aminoglycosides, may be administered separately)
• Safety and efficacy established for pediatric skin and soft tissue infections only

---

amprenavir
(am-prehn'-eh-veer)
Rx: Agenerase
Chemical Class: HIV protease inhibitor
Therapeutic Class: HIV infection

CLINICAL PHARMACOLOGY
Mechanism of Action: Inhibits HIV protease preventing cleavage of viral polypeptides resulting in the formation of immature noninfectious viral particles
Pharmacokinetics
PO: Peak 1-2 hr; bioavailability 70% with capsule, 60% with liquid; 90% protein bound; metabolized by CYP 3A4 isoenzyme with metabolites found in stool and urine; 3% excreted unchanged in urine; inhibits CYP 3A4 to a degree similar to nelfinavir; t₁/₂ 7-10 hr
INDICATIONS AND USES: HIV infection treatment
DOSAGE
Adult and Child >16 yr
• PO 1200 mg bid
• For hepatic insufficiency, reduce dose: Child-Pugh score 5-8: 450 mg bid; Child-Pugh score 9-12: 300 mg bid
• For latest treatment guidelines, see www.hivatis.org
Child 4-16 yr
• PO CAP 20 mg/kg bid (max 2400 mg per day); LIQ 22.5 mg/kg bid (max 2800 mg per day)

* = non-FDA-approved use

• For latest treatment guidelines, see www.hivatis.org

💲 AVAILABLE FORMS/COST OF THERAPY

• Cap—Oral: 50 mg, 480's: **$201.60**
• Cap—Oral: 150 mg, 240's: **$302.40**
• Liq—Oral: 15 mg/ml, 240 ml: **$30.24**
• Note: Capsules of amprenavir contain 109 IU of vitamin E; liquid contains 46 IU per ml

PRECAUTIONS: Blood coagulation defects related to vitamin K deficiency, child under 4 yrs old, diabetes mellitus, hemophilia A or B, hepatic insufficiency (adjust dose), hypersensitivity to other protease inhibitors, oral contraceptive use, sulfonamide allergy

PREGNANCY AND LACTATION: Pregnancy category C; excreted in breast milk of animals

SIDE EFFECTS/ADVERSE REACTIONS

CNS: Depression or mood disorder (15%), headache (10%), paresthesia (8%), perioral paresthesia (26%)
*GI: Abdominal pain, **diarrhea (10%)**, nausea, vomiting*
METAB: Hyperglycemia, hypertriglyceridemia
SKIN: Rash (10%)

INTERACTIONS

Drugs

3 *Abacavir:* Mild increase in amprenavir plasma level when given with abacavir
⚠ *Astemizole:* Increased plasma levels of astemizole
3 *Barbiturates:* Increased clearance of amprenavir; reduced clearance of barbiturates
2 *Carbamazepine:* Increased clearance of amprenavir; reduced clearance of carbamazepine
⚠ *Cisapride:* Increased plasma levels of cisapride

⚠ *Ergot alkaloids:* Increased plasma levels of ergot alkaloids
3 *Erythromycin:* Reduced clearance of amprenavir; amprenavir reduces clearance of erythromycin
⚠ *Lovastatin:* Amprenavir reduces clearance of lovastatin
⚠ *Midazolam:* Increased plasma levels of midazolam and prolonged effect
3 *Nevirapine:* Reduces plasma amprenavir levels
3 *Oral contraceptives:* Amprenavir may reduce efficacy
3 *Phenytoin:* Increased clearance of amprenavir; reduced clearance of phenytoin
2 *Rifabutin:* Increased clearance of amprenavir; reduced clearance of rifabutin
⚠ *Rifampin:* Increased clearance of amprenavir
3 *Ritonavir:* Decreased clearance of amprenavir
3 *Saquinavir:* Decreased clearance of saquinavir; reduce dose of Fortovase (saquinavir soft gel capsule) to 800 mg tid
3 *Sildenafil:* Decreased clearance of sildenafil
⚠ *Simvastatin:* Amprenavir reduces clearance of simvastatin
⚠ *Terfenadine:* Increased plasma levels of terfenadine
⚠ *Triazolam:* Increased plasma levels of triazolam and prolonged effect

SPECIAL CONSIDERATIONS
PATIENT/FAMILY EDUCATION

• May take with or without food, but do not take with a high-fat meal
• Do not take supplemental vitamin E; capsule and liquid forms have vitamin E in them

MONITORING PARAMETERS

• CBC, metabolic panel, hepatic function panel, CD4 lymphocyte count, HIV RNA level

amrinone

(am′ri-none)
Rx: Inocor
Chemical Class: Bipyrimidine derivative
Therapeutic Class: Cardiac inotropic agent

CLINICAL PHARMACOLOGY

Mechanism of Action: Cardiac inotrope distinct from digitalis glycosides or catecholamines; direct vasodilator, which reduces preload and afterload; not a β-adrenergic agonist; dose-related increases in cardiac output occur (28% at 0.75 mg/kg to about 61% at 3 mg/kg IV bolus); pulmonary capillary wedge pressure, total peripheral resistance, and diastolic and mean arterial pressures show dose-related decreases; heart rate generally unchanged

Pharmacokinetics

Onset of action 2-5 min, peak 10 min, duration variable, $t_{1/2}$ 4-6 hr; metabolized in liver, 60%-90% excreted in urine as drug and metabolites; in patients with compromised renal and hepatic perfusion, plasma levels of amrinone may rise during the infusion period

INDICATIONS AND USES: Short-term management of congestive heart failure unresponsive to other medication

DOSAGE

Adult

• IV bolus 0.75 mg/kg over 2-3 min; start infusion of 5-10 μg/kg/min; may give another 0.75 mg/kg bolus 30 min after start of therapy; daily dose should not exceed 10 mg/kg; the above dosing regimen will yield a plasma concentration of amrinone of 3 μg/ml; increases in cardiac index show a linear relationship to

plasma concentration in a range of 0.5 μg/ml to 7 μg/ml

$ **AVAILABLE FORMS/COST OF THERAPY**

• Inj, Sol—IV: 5 mg/ml, 20 ml vial: **$80.58-$84.42**

CONTRAINDICATIONS: Hypersensitivity to bisulfites, severe aortic or pulmonic obstructive valvular disease, acute MI

PRECAUTIONS: Diuretic therapy (decreased cardiac filling pressure may cause decreased response to amrinone), arrhythmias, aortic or pulmonic valvular disease

PREGNANCY AND LACTATION: Pregnancy category C

SIDE EFFECTS/ADVERSE REACTIONS

CV: Chest pain, *dysrhythmias (3%),* headache, hypotension (1.3%)

GI: Abdominal pain, anorexia, hepatotoxicity, hiccups, nausea, vomiting

HEME: Thrombocytopenia (2.4%); dose dependent

RESP: Pleuritis

SKIN: Allergic reactions, burning at injection site

MISC: Fever, hypersensitivity reaction manifested by pleuritis, pericarditis, myositis, or interstitial pulmonary infiltrates

INTERACTIONS

Drugs

• *Furosemide:* Precipitates when furosemide is injected into an IV line infusing amrinone

Labs

• *Increase:* Serum digoxin (Abbott TdX method)

SPECIAL CONSIDERATIONS

MONITORING PARAMETERS

• BP and pulse q5 min during infusion; if BP drops 30 mm Hg, stop infusion

• Cardiac output and pulmonary capillary wedge pressure

• Monitor platelet count and serum

K, Na, Cl, Ca, BUN, creatinine, ALT, AST, and bilirubin daily

amyl nitrite
(am'il)
Rx: Amyl nitrite
Chemical Class: Organic nitrate
Therapeutic Class: Vasodilator: Anti-anginal; cyanide antidote

CLINICAL PHARMACOLOGY
Mechanism of Action: Stimulation of c-GMP production yields vascular smooth muscle relaxation; venous dilation predominates but dose-dependent dilation of arterial beds occurs; dilation of postcapillary vessels promotes venous pooling, decreases venous return to the heart, reducing left ventricular end-diastolic pressure (preload); arteriolar relaxation reduces systemic vascular resistance and arterial pressure (afterload); myocardial oxygen consumption/demand is decreased; blood pressure decreases with reflex tachycardia; converts hemoglobin to methemoglobin, which binds to cyanide
Pharmacokinetics
INH: Onset 30 sec, duration 3-5 min; metabolized by liver, ⅓ excreted in urine

INDICATIONS AND USES: Acute angina pectoris, cyanide poisoning, diagnostic aid in cardiac auscultation*

DOSAGE
With the patient seated or recumbent, a capsule of amyl nitrite is crushed with the fingers and held to the nostrils for inhalation of the vapors
Adult
• *Angina pectoris, cardiac diagnostic aid:* INH 0.18-0.3 ml cap as needed, 1-6 INH from 1 cap, may repeat in 3-5 min
• *Cyanide poisoning:* INH 0.3 ml cap inhaled for 15 sec until sodium nitrite infusion is ready

💲 AVAILABLE FORMS/COST OF THERAPY
• Sol—INH: 0.3 ml: **$2.90-$6.60**
CONTRAINDICATIONS: Severe anemia, increased intracranial pressure, hypertension, cerebral hemorrhage

PRECAUTIONS: Volatile nitrites abused for sexual stimulation; transient dizziness, weakness, or other signs of cerebral hypoperfusion may develop following inhalation; glaucoma

PREGNANCY AND LACTATION: Pregnancy category: markedly reduces systemic blood pressure and blood flow on maternal side of the placenta

SIDE EFFECTS/ADVERSE REACTIONS
CNS: Dizziness, headache, syncope, weakness
CV: **Cardiovascular collapse,** palpitations, *postural hypotension,* tachycardia
GI: Abdominal pain, nausea, vomiting
GU: Urinary incontinence
HEME: Hemolytic anemia, methemoglobinemia
MS: Muscle twitching
SKIN: Flushing, pallor, sweating
INTERACTIONS
Drugs
3 *Alcohol:* Exaggerated hypotension and cardiac collapse
3 *Calcium channel blockers:* Exaggerated symptomatic orthostatic hypotension
3 *Dihydroertotamine:* Increases the bioavailability of dihydroertotamine with resultant increase in mean standing systolic blood pressure;

---

italic = common side effects   ***bold italic*** = life-threatening reactions

functional antagonism, decreasing effects

3 *Sildenafil:* Excessive hypotensive effects

Labs

• False decrease in cholesterol via Zlatkis-Zak color reaction

SPECIAL CONSIDERATIONS
PATIENT/FAMILY EDUCATION

• Drug should be inhaled while the patient is seated or lying down

• Taking after drinking alcohol may worsen side effects; alert to probable headache, dizziness, or flushing side effects

• Amyl nitrite is very flammable

• Tolerance may develop with repeated use

---

anagrelide

(ah-na' greh-lide)
Rx: Agrylin
Chemical Class: Not available
Therapeutic Class: Antiplatelet agent

CLINICAL PHARMACOLOGY
Mechanism of Action: Reduces blood platelet count, perhaps via a dose-related reduction in platelet production resulting from a decrease in megakaryocyte hypermaturation

Pharmacokinetics
PO: Peak 1 hr, bioavailability reduced by food; extensively metabolized; metabolites eliminated in urine (>70%) and feces (10%); $t_{1/2}$ 1.3 hr, terminal elimination $t_{1/2}$ approximately 3 days

INDICATIONS AND USES: Essential thrombocythemia—secondary to myeloproliferative disorders

DOSAGE
Adult

• PO 0.5 mg qid or 1 mg bid; dose may be adjusted after at least 1 wk to the lowest amount required to maintain platelet count <600,000; do not increase dose by >0.5 mg/day in any 1 wk period; do not exceed 10 mg/day or 2.5 in a single dose

$ **AVAILABLE FORMS/COST**
OF THERAPY

• Cap, opaque—Oral: 0.5 mg, 100's: **$441.00**

PRECAUTIONS: Known or suspected heart disease; renal or hepatic function impairment

PREGNANCY AND LACTATION: Pregnancy category C; not recommended in women who are or may become pregnant; excretion into breast milk unknown

SIDE EFFECTS/ADVERSE REACTIONS

CNS: Dizziness, headache (44.5%)
*CV: **Arrhythmia, cerebrovascular accident,** chest pain, **CHF,** edema,* hemorrhage, *palpitations,* postural hypotension, syncope, *tachycardia,* vasodilation
EENT: Abnormal vision, amblyopia, diplopia, epistaxis, rhinitis, sinusitis, tinnitus
GI: Abdominal pain, anorexia, aphthous stomatitis, constipation, *diarrhea (24.3%), dyspepsia,* elevated liver enzymes, *flatulence,* gastritis, **GI hemorrhage,** melena, *nausea, vomiting*
GU: Dysuria, hematuria
HEME: Anemia, ecchymosis, lymphadenoma, **thrombocytopenia**
MS: Arthralgia, *back pain,* leg cramps, myalgia
RESP: Asthma, *dyspnea*
SKIN: Alopecia, photosensitivity, pruritus, rash
MISC: Asthenia, chills, fever, flu symptoms, *malaise,* neck pain, *pain, paresthesia*

MONITORING PARAMETERS

• Platelet count q2 days during first wk, then weekly thereafter until maintenance dose reached

---

anisindione
(ay-nis-in'die-own)
Rx: Miradon
Chemical Class: Inandione
Therapeutic Class: Oral anti-
coagulant

CLINICAL PHARMACOLOGY
Mechanism of Action: Interferes
with the hepatic synthesis of vitamin K-dependent clotting factors,
causing depression in the activity of
factors II, VII, IX, X and proteins C
and S in a dose-dependent manner;
has no effect on an established
thrombus, but prevents further extension of formed clot
Pharmacokinetics
PO: Peak activity 3-5 days, 97%-
99% protein bound, metabolized by
liver and excreted in the urine and
feces as inactive metabolites; $t_{1/2}$ 3-5
days
INDICATIONS AND USES: Prophylaxis and treatment of deep venous
thrombosis; pulmonary embolism;
prophylaxis of embolism associated
with atrial fibrillation, MI, cardioversion of chronic atrial fibrillation;
prosthetic heart valves*; adjunctive
treatment of coronary occlusion; prevention of recurrent transient ischemic attacks and recurrent MI*
DOSAGE
Adult
• PO 300 mg the 1st day, 200 mg
the 2nd day, 100 mg the 3rd day, and
25-250 mg qd for maintenance based
on the results of INR monitoring
💲 **AVAILABLE FORMS/COST
OF THERAPY**
• Tab, Uncoated—Oral: 50 mg,
100's: **$45.46**
CONTRAINDICATIONS: Active
bleeding; hemorrhagic blood dyscrasias; hemorrhagic tendencies; history of bleeding diathesis; recent cerebral hemorrhage; active ulceration of the GI tract; ulcerative colitis; open traumatic or surgical
wounds; recent or contemplated
brain, eye, spinal cord surgery, or
prostatectomy; regional or lumbar
block anesthesia; continuous tube
drainage of the small intestine; severe renal or hepatic disease; subacute bacterial endocarditis; pericarditis; polyarthritis; diverticulitis;
visceral carcinoma; severe or malignant hypertension; eclampsia or
preeclampsia; threatened abortion;
emaciation; malnutrition; vitamin C
or K deficiencies
PRECAUTIONS: Trauma, infection,
renal insufficiency, hypertension,
vasculitis, indwelling catheters, severe diabetes, active tuberculosis,
postpartum, protein C deficiency, hepatic insufficiency, elderly, children,
hyperthyroidism, hypothyroidism,
CHF, polyarteritis, diverticulitis, antibiotic therapy, malnutrition
PREGNANCY AND LACTATION:
Pregnancy category X; may be excreted in breast milk in amounts sufficient to cause bleeding in the nursing infant; contraindicated in breast-
feeding
**SIDE EFFECTS/ADVERSE REAC-
TIONS**
CNS: Headache
EENT: Blurred vision, paralysis of
accommodation, sore throat
GI: Diarrhea, hepatitis, liver damage, mouth ulcers, nausea, sore
mouth, steatorrhea
GU: Albuminuria, ***anuria, renal tubular necrosis***
HEME: ***Agranulocytosis,*** anemia,
atypical mononuclear cells, eosinophilia, ***hemorrhage,*** leukocyte ag-
glutinins, leukocytosis, ***leukopenia,***
myeloid immaturity, red cell aplasia, ***thrombocytopenia***
SKIN: Alopecia, dermatitis, urticaria

INTERACTIONS

Drugs

• Little is known about interactions with other drugs

SPECIAL CONSIDERATIONS

• Warfarin is generally the oral anticoagulant of choice due to higher incidence of serious adverse reactions with anisindione

PATIENT/FAMILY EDUCATION

• Dosing is highly individual and may have to be adjusted several times based on lab test results

• Strict adherence to prescribed dosage schedule is necessary

• Avoid alcohol, salicylates, and drastic changes in dietary habits

• Consult provider before undergoing dental work or elective surgery

MONITORING PARAMETERS

• INR, CBC, stool guaiac, urinalysis

---

anistreplase (anisoylated plasminogen streptokinase activator complex, APSAC)

(an-ih-strep′layz)

Rx: Eminase

Chemical Class: Anisoylated plasminogen streptokinase activator complex

Therapeutic Class: Thrombolytic

CLINICAL PHARMACOLOGY

Mechanism of Action: Promotes thrombolysis by promoting conversion of plasminogen to plasmin; made *in vitro* from lys-plasminogen and streptokinase

Pharmacokinetics

IV: Onset immediate, $t_{1/2}$ of fibrinolytic activity of circulating anistreplase 70-120 min

INDICATIONS AND USES: Acute myocardial infarction

DOSAGE

Adult

• IV 30 U over 4-5 min as soon as possible after onset of symptoms

💲 **AVAILABLE FORMS/COST OF THERAPY**

• Powder—Inj: 30 U/vial, 1 vial: **$2,511.93**

CONTRAINDICATIONS: History of severe allergic reactions to anistreplase or streptokinase, active internal bleeding, intraspinal or intracranial surgery within 2 mo, neoplasms of CNS, severe hypertension, cerebral embolism/thrombosis/hemorrhage, known bleeding diathesis

PRECAUTIONS:

Recent major surgery, previous puncture of noncompressible vessels, cerebrovascular disease, recent gastrointestinal or genitourinary bleeding, recent trauma; hypertension: systolic BP ≥180 mmHg and/or diastolic BP ≥110 mmHg; high likelihood of left heart thrombosis; acute pericarditis, subacute bacterial endocarditis, hemostatic defects, including those secondary to severe hepatic or renal disease; severe hepatic or renal dysfunction; pregnancy; diabetic hemorrhagic retinopathy or other hemorrhagic ophthalmic conditions; septic thrombophlebitis; advanced age; patients currently receiving oral anticoagulants; any other condition in which bleeding constitutes a significant hazard

Readministration

Because of the increased likelihood of resistance due to antistreptokinase antibody, anistreplase may not be effective if administered between 5 days and 12 mo after prior anistreplase or streptokinase therapy; risk of allergic reactions also increased following readministration

---

* = non-FDA-approved use

PREGNANCY AND LACTATION:
Pregnancy category C
**SIDE EFFECTS/ADVERSE REAC-
TIONS**
CNS: Agitation, dizziness, fever,
headache, paresthesia, sweating,
tremor, vertigo
*CV: **Dysrhythmias and conduction
disorders (38%),** hypotension (10%),*
EENT: Epistaxis
GI: Elevated transaminase levels,
nausea, vomiting
GU: Hematuria
*HEME: GI (2%), GU (2%), **intra-
cranial (1%), retroperitoneal,** or
surface bleeding (total incidence
15%), **thrombocytopenia***
MS: Arthralgia, low back pain
*RESP: **Bronchospasm,** dyspnea, he-
moptysis*
SKIN: Flushing, itching, phlebitis at
infusion site, rash, urticaria
*MISC: **Anaphylaxis (0.2%)***
INTERACTIONS
Drugs
■ *Heparin, oral anticoagulants,
drugs that alter platelet function (i.e.,
aspirin, dipyridamole, abciximab,
eptifibitide, tirofiban):* May increase
the risk of bleeding

---

anthralin

(anth-rah′lin)
Rx: Dritho-Scalp, .
Dritho creme, Micanol
Chemical Class: Anthratriol
derivative
Therapeutic Class: Anti-
psoriatic; keratolytic

CLINICAL PHARMACOLOGY
Mechanism of Action: Reduces the
mitotic rate and proliferation of epidermal cells in psoriasis by inhibiting the synthesis of nucleic protein
Pharmacokinetics
Absorption in humans has not been
determined; appears to be low

INDICATIONS AND USES: Psoriasis
DOSAGE
Adult
Begin with the lowest concentration
(0.1%) and gradually increase until
desired effect is obtained
• *Skin:* TOP apply at bedtime to
plaque sites; wash off remaining
drug in the morning
• *Scalp:* TOP massage into affected
areas; shampoo in the morning
■ **AVAILABLE FORMS/COST
OF THERAPY**
• Cre—Top: 0.1%, 50 g: **$31.13;**
0.25%, 50 g: **$36.29;** 0.5%, 50 g:
$44.24; 1%, 50 g: **$42.93-$43.94**
CONTRAINDICATIONS: Acute
psoriasis (where inflammation is
present)
PRECAUTIONS: Excessive irritation, renal and hepatic impairment,
inflammation, application to face,
genitalia, or intertriginous skin
PREGNANCY AND LACTATION:
Pregnancy category C; excretion
into human milk unknown; because
of the potential for tumorigenicity
shown in animal studies, use with
caution in nursing mothers
**SIDE EFFECTS/ADVERSE REAC-
TIONS**
SKIN: Discoloration of fingernails,
irritation of normal skin, sensitivity
reaction, staining of hair
SPECIAL CONSIDERATIONS
PATIENT/FAMILY EDUCATION
• Use plastic gloves for application
and wear a plastic cap over treated
scalp at bedtime to avoid staining
• Apply a protective film of petrolatum to areas surrounding plaque
• May stain fabrics

---

italic = common side effects   ***bold italic*** = life-threatening reactions

apraclonidine
(ap-raa-kloe′ni-deen)
Rx: Iopidine
Chemical Class: α₂-Adrenergic agonist
Therapeutic Class: Antiglaucoma agent (postsurgical)

CLINICAL PHARMACOLOGY
Mechanism of Action: Reduces intraocular pressure by reducing aqueous formation; exact mechanism of action unknown
Pharmacokinetics
Onset 1 hr, peak 3-5 hr
INDICATIONS AND USES: Controls or prevents elevations of intraocular pressure after laser iridotomy or trabeculoplasty; short-term adjunctive therapy in patients requiring additional reduction of intraocular pressure
DOSAGE
Adult
• INSTILL 1 gtt 1 hr before laser surgery, second gtt at completion of surgery (1%); for short-term adjunctive therapy instill 1-2 gtt 0.5% sol tid
Child
• Safety and efficacy not established
⚕ **AVAILABLE FORMS/COST OF THERAPY**
• Sol—Ophth: 0.5%, 5, 10 ml: **$42.50**/5 ml; 1%, 0.1 ml: **$7.03**
CONTRAINDICATIONS: Hypersensitivity to clonidine
PRECAUTIONS: Severe cardiovascular disease, history of vasovagal attack
PREGNANCY AND LACTATION: Pregnancy category C; excretion into breast milk unknown; consider discontinuing nursing on day apraclonidine is used

SIDE EFFECTS/ADVERSE REACTIONS
CNS: Dream disturbances, headache, insomnia, irritability, restlessness
CV: Bradycardia, orthostatic episode, palpitations, vasovagal attack
EENT: Blurred vision, burning, conjunctival blanching, conjunctival microhemorrhage, dryness, foreign body sensation, itching, mydriasis, nasal dryness/burning, taste abnormalities, *upper lid elevation*
GI: Abdominal pain, cramps, diarrhea, dry mouth, emesis
MISC: Fatigue, head cold sensation, paresthesia, pruritus, shortness of breath, sweaty palms
SPECIAL CONSIDERATIONS
PATIENT/FAMILY EDUCATION
• May cause burning, itching, blurring, dryness of eye area
• Store at room temperature, away from light

aprobarbital
(ape-roh-bar′bi-tal)
Rx: Alurate
Chemical Class: Barbituric acid derivative
Therapeutic Class: Sedative/hypnotic
DEA Class: Schedule III

CLINICAL PHARMACOLOGY
Mechanism of Action: Depresses activity in brain cells primarily in reticular activating system in brain stem; also selectively depresses neurons in posterior hypothalamus, limbic structures; able to decrease seizure activity in hypnotic doses by inhibition of impulses in CNS; depresses REM sleep
Pharmacokinetics
PO: Peak 3 hr; 35% bound to plasma proteins; $t_{1/2}$ 14-40 hr, partially metabolized by liver, excreted in urine

as unchanged drug and inactive metabolites

INDICATIONS AND USES: Routine sedation; hypnotic in the short-term treatment of insomnia for periods up to 2 wk

DOSAGE

Adult

• *Sedative:* PO 40 mg tid

• *Mild insomnia:* PO 40-80 mg before retiring

• *Pronounced insomnia:* PO 80-160 mg before retiring

$ AVAILABLE FORMS/COST OF THERAPY

• Elixir—Oral: 40 mg/5 ml, 480 ml: **$28.11**

CONTRAINDICATIONS: Hypersensitivity to barbiturates, respiratory depression, addiction to barbiturates, severe liver impairment, porphyria

PRECAUTIONS: Anemia, hepatic disease, renal disease, hypertension, elderly, acute/chronic pain, mental depression, history of drug abuse, abrupt discontinuation

PREGNANCY AND LACTATION: Pregnancy category D; small amount excreted in breast milk; use caution in nursing mothers

SIDE EFFECTS/ADVERSE REACTIONS

CNS: CNS depression, dizziness, *drowsiness, hangover,* headache, *lethargy,* lightheadedness, mental depression, physical dependence, slurred speech, stimulation in the elderly and children, vertigo

CV: Bradycardia, hypotension

GI: Constipation, diarrhea, hepatic dysfunction (long-term use), nausea, vomiting

*HEME: **Agranulocytosis, megaloblastic anemia (long-term use), thrombocytopenia***

*RESP: **Apnea,** bronchospasm, depression, **laryngospasm***

*SKIN: **Angioedema,*** erythema

multiforme, pain, *rash,* ***Stevens-Johnson syndrome,*** thrombophlebitis, urticaria

MISC: Osteomalacia (prolonged use), rickets

INTERACTIONS

Drugs

3 *Acetaminophen:* Enhanced hepatotoxic potential of acetaminophen overdoses

3 *Antidepressants, corticosteroids, cyclosporine, digitoxin, disopyramide, doxycycline, estrogens, propafenone, quinidine, tacrolimus, theophylline:* Reduced serum concentration of these drugs

3 *β-adrenergic blockers:* Reduced serum concentrations of β-blockers which are extensively metabolized

3 *Calcium channel blockers:* Reduced concentrations of verapamil and dihydropyridines

3 *Chloramphenicol:* Increased barbiturate concentrations; reduced serum chloramphenicol concentrations

3 *Ethanol:* Excessive CNS depression

3 *Griseofulvin:* Reduced griseofulvin absorption

3 *Methoxyflurane:* Enhanced nephrotoxic effect

3 *MAOIs:* Prolonged effect of barbiturates

3 *Narcotic analgesics:* Increased toxicity of meperidine; reduced effect of methadone; additive CNS depression

3 *Neuroleptics:* Reduced effect of either drug

3 *Oral contraceptives:* Reduced efficacy of oral contraceptives

3 *Phenytoin:* Unpredictable effect on serum phenytoin levels

3 *Valproic acid:* Increase serum concentrations of amobarbital

2 *Warfarin:* Decreased hypoprothrombinemic response to warfarin

---

italic = common side effects   ***bold italic*** = life-threatening reactions

SPECIAL CONSIDERATIONS

• Indicated only for short-term treatment of insomnia and is probably ineffective after 2 wk; physical dependency may result when used for extended time (45-90 days depending on dose)

PATIENT/FAMILY EDUCATION

• Avoid driving or other activities requiring alertness
• Avoid alcohol ingestion or CNS depressants
• Do not discontinue medication abruptly after long-term use

MONITORING PARAMETERS

• Serum folate (long-term therapy)
• LFTs and CBC (long-term therapy)
• Mental status, vital signs

---

ardeparin

(ar-da-pare'in)
Rx: Normiflo

Chemical Class: Depolymerized heparin derivative (low-molecular-weight heparin)
Therapeutic Class: Anticoagulant

CLINICAL PHARMACOLOGY

Mechanism of Action: Enhances the inhibition of Factor Xa and thrombin by binding to and accelerating antithrombin activity; preferentially inhibits Factor Xa; activated partial thromboplastin time (aPTT) not affected

Pharmacokinetics
SC: Peak activity 2.1-3.3 hr; duration 8-12 hr; likely undergoes saturable elimination; $t_{1/2}$ 2.5-3.3 hr

INDICATIONS AND USES: Prevention of deep vein thrombosis (DVT) which may lead to pulmonary embolism (PE) following knee replacement surgery; secondary prophylaxis for recurrent thromboembolic events*

DOSAGE

Adult
• SC 50 anti-Xa units/kg q12h for up to 14 days or until fully ambulatory; begin therapy the evening after surgery or the following morning; for patients ≤100 kg use the 5,000 anti-Xa unit/0.5 ml solution (dose in ml = patient weight [kg] × 0.005 ml/kg); for patients > 100 kg use the 10,000 anti-Xa unit/0.5 ml solution (dose in ml = patient weight [kg] × 0.0025 ml/kg)

💲 AVAILABLE FORMS/COST OF THERAPY

• Sol, inj—SC: 5,000 units/0.5 ml: **$15.45;** 10,000 units/0.5 ml: **$24.50**

CONTRAINDICATIONS: Active major bleeding; hypersensitivity to pork products; thrombocytopenia associated with a positive *in vitro* test for anti-platelet antibody in the presence of ardeparin

PRECAUTIONS: History of heparin-induced thrombocytopenia; increased risk for hemorrhage; hypersensitivity to methylparaben or propylparaben, or sulfite sensitivity; neuraxial anesthesia

PREGNANCY AND LACTATION: Pregnancy category C; teratogenic effects observed following administration of high doses IV in rats and rabbits; excretion in breast milk unknown but likely minimal

SIDE EFFECTS/ADVERSE REACTIONS

CNS: Confusion
GI: Constipation, increased AST and/or ALT, nausea, vomiting
HEME: **Anemia, hemorrhage, thrombocytopenia**
SKIN: Ecchymosis, pruritus, rash
MISC: Fever

INTERACTIONS

Drugs
3 *Aspirin:* Increased risk of hemorrhage

---

* = non-FDA-approved use

3 *Oral anticoagulants:* Additive anticoagulant effects

SPECIAL CONSIDERATIONS
• Cannot be used interchangeably (unit for unit) with unfractionated heparin or other low molecular weight heparins

PATIENT/FAMILY EDUCATION
• Administer by deep SC inj into abdominal wall; alternate inj sites
• Report any unusual bruising or bleeding to clinician

MONITORING PARAMETERS
• CBC with platelets, stool occult blood, urinalysis
• Monitoring aPTT is not required

---

ascorbic acid (vitamin C)

(a-skor'bic)

Rx: injection: Cenolate, CEE-500, Mega-C/A Plus, Ortho/CS

OTC: Ascorbicap, Cecon, Cevi-Bid, Ce-Vi-Sol, C-Crystals, Cebid Timecelles, Dull-C, Flavorcee, N'ice Vitamin C Drops

Chemical Class: Water soluble vitamin
Therapeutic Class: Urinary acidifier; vitamin

CLINICAL PHARMACOLOGY
Mechanism of Action: Needed for wound healing, collagen synthesis, carbohydrate metabolism; antioxidant

Pharmacokinetics
PO: Readily absorbed; metabolized in liver by oxidation and sulfation, unused amounts excreted in urine (unchanged) and as metabolites

INDICATIONS AND USES: Prevention and treatment of scurvy; urinary acidifying agent; dietary supplementation

DOSAGE
Adult
• *Scurvy:* PO/SC/IM/IV 100 mg-500 mg qd for at least 2 wk, then 50 mg or more qd
• *Urinary acidification:* PO/SC/IM/IV 4-12 g qd in divided doses
• *Dietary supplementation:* PO/SC/IM/IV 50-200 mg qd

Child
• *Scurvy:* PO/SC/IM/IV 100-300 mg qd for at least 2 wk, then 35 mg or more qd
• *Urinary acidification:* PO/SC/IM/IV 500 mg q6-8h
• *Dietary supplementation:* PO/SC/IM/IV 35-100 mg qd

$ **AVAILABLE FORMS/COST OF THERAPY**
• Inj, Sol—IM, IV, SC: 250 mg/ml, 2 ml: **$2.40-2.62;** 500 mg/ml, 2 ml: **$3.79-$7.50**
• Syr—Oral: 500 mg/5 ml, 480 ml: **$13.50**
• Sol—Oral: 100 mg/ml, 50 ml: **$11.84**
• Tab—Oral: 100 mg, 100's: **$1.30-$1.75;** 250 mg, 100's: **$1.50-$2.25;** 500 mg, 100's: **$1.80-$10.50;** 1000 mg, 100's: **$3.50-$6.27**
• Tab, Chewable—Oral: 250 mg, 100's: **$1.90-$2.76;** 500 mg, 100's: **$2.70**

PRECAUTIONS: Gout, excessive doses for prolonged periods of time (diabetics, patients with recurrent renal calculi, patients undergoing anticoagulant therapy), tartrazine sensitivity, sulfite sensitivity, G-6-PD deficiency

PREGNANCY AND LACTATION: Pregnancy category A if doses do not exceed the RDA, otherwise pregnancy category C; excreted into breast milk via a saturable process; the RDA during lactation is 90-100 mg; maternal supplementation up to

---

italic = common side effects   ***bold italic*** = life-threatening reactions

the RDA is needed only in those women with poor nutritional status

SIDE EFFECTS/ADVERSE REACTIONS

CNS: Dizziness, fatigue, flushing, headache, insomnia

GI: Anorexia, cramps, diarrhea, heartburn, nausea, vomiting

GU: Crystalluria, oxalate or urate renal stones, polyuria, urine acidification

*HEME: **Hemolysis** (after large doses in patients with G-6-PD deficiency), **sickle-cell crisis***

INTERACTIONS

Drugs

3 *Antacids:* Vitamin C increases the amount of aluminum absorbed from aluminum-containing antacids

Labs

• *False negative:* Amine-dependent stool occult blood, urine bilirubin, blood, leukocyte determinations

• *False positive:* Urine glucose

• *Decrease:* Urine amphetamine, serum AST (Ames Seralyzer method), urine barbiturate (Abbott TDx method) serum bicarbonate (Kodak Ektachem 700 method), serum bilirubin (Jendrassik method), serum cholesterol (Olympus, Abbott TDx, CHOD-PAP methods), serum CK (Kodak Ektachem Systems), serum creatinine (Merck, Wako, Boehringer Mannheim methods), urine glucose (glucose oxidase methods), serum HDL-cholesterol (Kodak Ektachem Systems), urine oxalate (oxalate decarboxylase methods), urine porphobilinogen, serum triglycerides (GPO-PAP, Boehringer Mannheim methods), serum urea nitrogen (Ames Seralyzer), serum uric acid (Ames Seralyzer), urine uric acid (Kodak Ektachem Systems)

• *Increase:* Serum amylase (only at toxic ascorbic acid levels), serum AST (SMA 12/60 method), serum bilirubin (SMA 12/60 method), serum glucose (SMA 12/60 and O-toluidine methods), serum HbAlc (electrophoretic method), urine β-hydroxybutyrate, urine 17-hydroxy corticosteroids, urine iodide, urine 17-ketosteroids, urine oxalate (chromatographic methods), serum phosphate (Boehringer-Mannheim method), CSF and urine protein (Kodak Ektachem Systems), serum uric acid (Klein and phosphotungstate methods)

---

aspirin

(as′pir-in)

Rx: Aspirin CR, Aspirin Delayed Release, Easprin, ZORprin

OTC: Ascriptin, Aspergum, Bayer, Bayer Children's Aspirin, Ecotrin, Ecotrin Maximum Strength, 8-Hour Bayer Extended Release, Empirin, Maximum Bayer, Norwich

Combinations:

　Rx: with butalbital (Fiorinal); with codeine (Empirin); with dihydrocodeine and caffeine (Synalgos DC); with dipyridamole (Aggrenox); with oxycodone (Percodan); with propoxyphene (Darvon)

　OTC: with antacids (Ascriptin, Bufferin, Magnaprin)

Chemical Class: Salicylate derivative

Therapeutic Class: Nonnarcotic analgesic; anti-inflammatory; antiplatelet agent; antipyretic

---

CLINICAL PHARMACOLOGY

Mechanism of Action: Inhibits prostaglandin synthesis and release;

acts on the hypothalamus heat-regulating center to reduce fever; blocks prostaglandin synthetase action, which prevents formation of the platelet-aggregating substance thromboxane A_2

Pharmacokinetics

PO: Well-absorbed, enteric coated product may exhibit erratic absorption, onset 15-30 min (delayed with enteric coated), peak 1-2 hr, duration 4-6 hr

PR: Absorption erratic, onset slow, duration 4-6 hr

Metabolized by liver, metabolites excreted by kidneys; $t_{1/2}$ 3 hr at lower doses (300-600 mg), 5-6 hr (1000 mg) up to 30 hrs in larger doses (due to saturable metabolic pathways)

INDICATIONS AND USES: Mild to moderate pain and fever; inflammatory conditions such as rheumatic fever, rheumatoid arthritis; osteoarthritis; thromboembolic disorders; reducing risk of recurrent transient ischemic attacks; reducing the risk of death or nonfatal MI in patients with previous MI or unstable angina; prevention of systemic embolism in patients with atrial fibrillation or prosthetic heart valves*; low doses may be useful in preventing toxemia of pregnancy*; to reduce the risk of stroke in patients who have had transient ischemia of the brain or completed ischemic stroke due to thrombosis (Aggrenox)

DOSAGE

Adult

• *Arthritis:* PO 2.6-5.2 g/day in divided doses q4-6h

• *Pain/fever:* PO/PR 325-650 mg q4h prn, not to exceed 4 g/day

• *Acute ischemic stroke:* PO (within 48 hours) 160-325 mg qd

• *Transient ischemic attacks:* PO 50-325 mg qd

• Heart disease (stable angina, unstable angina, acute MI, clinical or laboratory evidence of CAD): PO 160-325 mg qd

• *Atrial fibrillation* (<65 yr and no risk factors or unable to take warfarin): PO 75-325 mg qd

• Following CABG with no risk factors: PO 325 mg qd for 1 yr

• *Mechanical caged ball heart valve:* PO 80-100 mg (given with warfarin)

• *Any mechanical heart valve and additional clot risk factors:* PO 80 mg qd (given with warfarin)

• *Mechanical heart valve patients who develop systemic embolism:* PO 80 mg qd (given with warfarin)

• *Bioprosthetic heart valve and sinus rhythm after warfarin for 3 mo:* PO 160 mg qd

Child

• *Arthritis:* PO 60-90 mg/kg/day in divided doses; usual maintenance dose 80-100 mg/kg/day divided q6-8h; maintain serum salicylate level of 150-300 µg/ml

• *Pain/fever:* PO/PR 10-15 mg/kg/dose q4-6h prn

🔋 **AVAILABLE FORMS/COST OF THERAPY**

• Tab, Chewable—Oral: 81 mg, 36's: **$1.00-$2.25**

• Tab, Enteric Coated—Oral: 81 mg, 100's: **$6.89;** 325 mg, 100's: **$1.15-$13.60;** 500 mg, 60's: **$1.55-$6.26;** 650 mg, 100's: **$3.70-$4.51;** 975 mg, 100's: **$8.19-$37.34**

• Gum Tab, Chewable—Oral: 227 mg, 16's: **$1.75**

• Tab, Film Coated—Oral: 325 mg, 100's: **$0.80-$3.70;** 500 mg, 100's: **$1.29-$3.50;** 600 mg, 100's: **$3.50**

• Tab, Sus Action—Oral: 800 mg, 100's: **$8.03-$58.68**

• Supp—Rect: 120 mg, 12's: **$1.80-$3.60;** 300 mg, 12's: **$2.39-$3.59;** 600 mg, 12's: **$2.60-$3.89**

CONTRAINDICATIONS: Hypersensitivity to salicylates, NSAIDs, or tartrazine (FDC yellow dye #5);

GI bleeding; hemophilia; hemorrhagic states

PRECAUTIONS: Anemia, asthma, nasal polyps, nasal allergies, hepatic disease, renal disease, Hodgkin's disease, pre/postoperatively, children or teenagers with flu-like symptoms (may be associated with the development of Reye's syndrome), gout, history of coagulation defects, bleeding disorders

PREGNANCY AND LACTATION: Pregnancy category C (category D if full doses used in 3rd trimester); use in pregnancy should generally be avoided; in pregnancies at risk for the development of pregnancy-induced hypertension and preeclampsia, and in fetuses with intrauterine growth retardation, low-dose aspirin (40-150 mg/day) may be beneficial; excreted into breast milk in low concentrations

SIDE EFFECTS/ADVERSE REACTIONS

CNS: Confusion, dizziness, drowsiness, headache

EENT: Dimness of vision, reversible hearing loss, tinnitus

GI: Acute reversible hepatotoxicity, anorexia, cholestasis, diarrhea, *dyspepsia,* epigastric discomfort, **GI bleeding,** heartburn, increased transaminase levels, *nausea*

HEME: Decreased plasma iron concentration, hyperuricemia (low dose), hyperuricosuria (high dose), **leukopenia,** prolonged bleeding time, shortened erythrocyte survival time, **thrombocytopenia**

METAB: Hypoglycemia, hypokalemia, hyponatremia

RESP: Hyperpnea, wheezing

SKIN: Angioedema, bruising, hives, rash, urticaria

MISC: Fever, thirst

INTERACTIONS
Drugs
3 *ACE inhibitors:* Reduced antihypertensive effect
2 *Acetazolamide:* Increased concentrations of acetazolamide, possibly leading to CNS toxicity
3 *Antacids:* Decreased serum salicylate concentrations; high dose salicylates only
3 *Corticosteroids:* Increased incidence and/or severity of GI ulceration; enhanced salicylate excretion
3 *Diltiazem:* Enhanced antiplatelet effect of aspirin
3 *Ethanol:* Enhanced aspirin-induced GI mucosal damage and aspirin-induced prolongation of bleeding time
3 *Griseofulvin:* Reduced serum salicylate level
3 *Intrauterine contraceptive device:* May reduce contraceptive effectiveness
2 *Methotrexate:* Increased serum methotrexate concentrations and enhanced methotrexate toxicity
2 *Oral anticoagulants:* Increased risk of bleeding by inhibiting platelet function and possibly by producing gastric erosions
3 *Probenecid:* Salicylates inhibit the uricosuric activity of probenecid
3 *Sulfinpyrazone:* Salicylates inhibit the uricosuric activity of sulfinpyrazone
3 *Sulfonylureas:* Enhanced hypoglycemic response to sulfonylureas
2 *Warfarin:* Enhanced hypoprothrombinemic effect of warfarin
3 *Zarfirlukast:* Increased plasma concentrations of zarfirlukast
Labs
• *Increase:* Serum acetaminophen (Glynn-Kendal method), urine acetoacetate (Gerhardt ferric chloride procedure), urine glucose (Ames Clinitest method), serum HbAlc

(chromatographic and electrophoretic, but not colorimetric methods), urine hippuric acid, urine homogentisic acid, urine homovanillic acid, urine ketones (Gerhardt's test), urine phenyl ketones, CSF and urine protein (Folm-Ciocalteu method), serum and urine uric acid (non-specific methods only)

• *Decrease:* Serum albumin, urine glucose (glucose oxidase methods), total serum phenytoin (but not free serum phenytoin)

SPECIAL CONSIDERATIONS
PATIENT/FAMILY EDUCATION

• Administer with food
• Do not exceed recommended doses
• Read label on other OTC drugs, many contain aspirin
• Therapeutic response may take 2 wk (arthritis)
• Avoid alcohol ingestion, GI bleeding may occur
• **Not to be given to children with flu-like symptoms, Reye's syndrome may develop**
MONITORING PARAMETERS
• AST, ALT, bilirubin, creatinine, CBC, hematocrit if patient is on long-term therapy

---

astemizole
(a-stem′mi-zole)
Rx: Hismanal
Chemical Class: Benzimidazole derivative
Therapeutic Class: Antihistamine

CLINICAL PHARMACOLOGY
Mechanism of Action: Competitively antagonizes most of the pharmacologic effects of histamine by preferentially binding to peripheral rather than central H_1-receptors; has little sedative or anticholinergic effects

Pharmacokinetics
PO: Absorption reduced by 60% when taken with food, peak 1-2 hr (does not correlate with onset of effect); 97% bound to plasma proteins; metabolized in the liver; terminal $t_{1/2}$ 7-11 days

INDICATIONS AND USES: Seasonal allergic rhinitis; chronic idiopathic urticaria (should not be used as a prn product for immediate relief of symptoms)

DOSAGE
Adult and Child >12 yr
• PO 10 mg qd on an empty stomach
Child 6-12 yr
• PO 5 mg qd on an empty stomach
Child <6 yr
• PO 0.2 mg/kg qd on an empty stomach

AVAILABLE FORMS/COST OF THERAPY
• Tab, Uncoated—Oral: 10 mg, 100's: **$199.70**

CONTRAINDICATIONS: Hypersensitivity; severe hepatic disease; concomitant erythromycin, ketoconazole, or itraconazole therapy

PRECAUTIONS: Conditions leading to QT prolongation, hepatic dysfunction

PREGNANCY AND LACTATION: Pregnancy category C; to avoid early exposure during pregnancy, remember that metabolites may remain in the body for as long as 4 mo after end of dosing; excretion into breast milk unknown; use caution in nursing mothers

SIDE EFFECTS/ADVERSE REACTIONS
CNS: Drowsiness, fatigue, *headache,* increased appetite, nervousness
CV: **Dysrhythmias** (rare)
EENT: Conjunctivitis, dry mouth, pharyngitis
GI: Abdominal pain, diarrhea, nausea
MISC: Increased weight

---

italic = common side effects   ***bold italic*** = life-threatening reactions

INTERACTIONS
Drugs
⚠ *Erythromycin:* QT interval prolongation and arrhythmia
⚠ *Fluvoxamine:* Increased astemizole concentrations; QT interval prolongation and arrhythmia
⚠ *Ketoconazole:* QT interval prolongation and arrhythmia

SPECIAL CONSIDERATIONS
PATIENT/FAMILY EDUCATION
• Administer on empty stomach, 1 hr before or 2 hr after meals
• Do not increase the dose in an attempt to accelerate the onset of action
• Do not exceed recommended dose, dysrrhythmias may occur
• Do not use as needed for immediate relief of symptoms

---

atenolol
(a-ten'oh-lol)
Rx: Tenormin
Combinations
  Rx: with chlorthalidone (Tenoretic)
Chemical Class: β$_1$-selective (cardioselective) adrenoreceptor blocker
Therapeutic Class: Antihypertensive; antianginal

CLINICAL PHARMACOLOGY
Mechanism of Action: Competitive beta-adrenergic agonist inhibition at β$_1$ receptor sites (cardioselective at usual doses; β$_2$-blockade noted at higher doses); produces negative inotropic and chronotropic responses; slows AV nodal conduction; decreases heart rate; decreases myocardial oxygen consumption; antiarrhythmic effects (class II); reduction in platelet aggregation and blood viscosity; suppression of renin release; inhibition of central sympathetic outflow; decreases presynaptic receptor neurotransmitter release; no intrinsic sympathomimetic, membrane stabilizing activity; low lipid solubility

Pharmacokinetics
PO: Incomplete GI absorption (40%-60% bioavailable); peak serum concentrations, 2-4 hr; not metabolized by liver; excreted unchanged in urine and feces; t$_{1/2}$ 6-7 hr; crosses placenta in measurable, but not significant concentrations

INDICATIONS AND USES: Angina pectoris, anxiety,* performance anxiety,* arrhythmia (class II),* congestive heart failure,* migraine headache,* post myocardial infarction,* alcohol withdrawal syndrome,* esophageal varices with cirrhosis*

DOSAGE
Adult and Child >16 yr
• *Post myocardial infarction:* IV 5 mg over 5 min; repeat in 10 min if initial dose tolerated; start PO 50 mg q12h×2 doses immediately after last IV dose; then 100 mg qd×10 days
• *Hypertension:* PO 50-100 mg qd
• *Angina pectoris:* PO 50-200 mg qd
Child
• PO initial 1-1.2 mg/kg/dose qd; maximum 2 mg/kg/day qd
Renal impairment:

CREATININE CLEARANCE	MAXIMUM DOSE	DOSING INTERVAL
15-35 ml/min	50 mg or 1 mg/kg/dose	Daily
<15 ml/min	50 mg or 1 mg/kg/dose	Every other day

💲 **AVAILABLE FORMS/COST OF THERAPY**
• Tab, Uncoated—Oral: 25 mg, 100's: **$65.30-$107.35;** 50 mg, 100's: **$13.43-$109.54;** 100 mg, 100's: **$89.85-$164.32**

* = non-FDA-approved use

• Inj, Sol—IV, Buffered: 5 mg/10 ml, 10 ml: **$7.16**

CONTRAINDICATIONS: Cardiogenic shock, 2nd or 3rd degree heart block, sinus bradycardia, overt cardiac failure

PRECAUTIONS: Anesthesia/surgery (myocardial depression), avoid abrupt withdrawal, bronchospastic airways, congestive heart failure, diabetes mellitus, hyperthyroidism/thyrotoxicosis (atenolol, unlike propranolol does not decrease T_3 levels), concurrent clonidine (discontinue atenolol several days prior to withdrawal of clonidine), peripheral vascular disease, renal disease

PREGNANCY AND LACTATION Pregnancy category D; frequently used in the third trimester for treatment of hypertension (many studies of efficacy and safety of atenolol in pregnancy-induced hypertension); long-term use has been associated with intrauterine growth retardation; excreted into breast milk; observe for signs of beta-blockade

SIDE EFFECTS/ADVERSE REACTIONS

CNS: Ataxia, depression, *dizziness,* drowsiness, *fatigue,* hallucinations, insomnia, *lethargy,* memory loss, mental changes, strange dreams

CV: Bradycardia, CHF, cold extremities, postural hypotension, profound hypotension, **2nd or 3rd degree heart block, withdrawal angina, rebound hypertension**

EENT: Dry burning eyes, sore throat, visual disturbances

GI: Diarrhea, dry mouth, **ischemic colitis, mesenteric arterial thrombosis,** nausea, vomiting

GU: Impotence, sexual dysfunction

METAB: Hyperglycemia, hyperlipidemia (increase TG, total cholesterol, LDL; decrease HDL), **masked hypoglycemic response** (sweating excepted)

RESP: **Bronchospasm,** dyspnea, wheezing

SKIN: Alopecia, pruritis, rash

INTERACTIONS

Drugs

3 *Adenosine:* Bradycardia aggravated

3 *Alpha-1 adrenergic blockers:* Potential enhanced first dose response (marked initial drop in blood pressure, particularly on standing [especially prazocin])

3 *Amoxicillin, Ampicillin:* Reduced atenolol bioavailability

3 *Antacids:* Reduced atenolol absorption

3 *Calcium channel blockers:* See dihydropyridine and verapamil

3 *Clonidine:* Exacerbation of rebound hypertension upon discontinuation of clonidine

3 *Digoxin:* Additive prolongation of atrioventricular (AV) conduction time

3 *Dihydropyridines:* Additive hemodynamic effects; increased serum concentration of atenolol

3 *Dipyridamole:* Bradycardia aggravated

3 *Disopyramide:* Additive decreases in cardiac output

3 *Lidocaine:* Increased serum lidocaine concentrations possible

3 *Neostigmine:* Bradycardia aggravated

3 *NSAIDs:* Reduced antihypertensive effects of atenolol

3 *Physostigmine:* Bradycardia aggravated

3 *Prazosin:* First-dose response to prazosin may be enhanced by β-blockade

3 *Tacrine:* Bradycardia aggravated

2 *Theophylline:* Antagonistic pharmacodynamic effects

3 *Verapamil:* Enhanced effects of both drugs, particularly AV node conduction slowing; reduced atenolol clearance

SPECIAL CONSIDERATIONS
• Properties of low lipid solubility and competitive cardioselectivity yield less CNS and bronchospastic adverse effects

PATIENT/FAMILY EDUCATION
• Do not discontinue drug abruptly, may precipitate angina
• Report bradycardia, dizziness, confusion, depression, fever, shortness of breath, swelling of the extremities
• Take pulse at home, notify clinician if <50 beats/min
• Avoid hazardous activities if dizziness, drowsiness, lightheadedness are present
• May mask the symptoms of hypoglycemia, except for sweating, in diabetic patients

MONITORING PARAMETERS
• Angina: Reduction in nitroglycerin usage; frequency, severity, onset, and duration of angina pain; heart rate
• Arrhythmias: Heart rate
• Congestive heart failure: Functional status, cough, dyspnea on exertion, paroxysmal nocturnal dyspnea, exercise tolerance, and ventricular function
• Hypertension: Blood pressure
• Migraine headache: Reduction in the frequency, severity, and duration of attacks
• Postmyocardial infarction: Left ventricular function, lower resting heart rate
• Toxicity: Blood glucose, bronchospasm, hypotension, bradycardia, depression, confusion, hallucination, sexual dysfunction

---

atorvastatin
(a-tor′va-sta-tin)
Rx: Lipitor
Chemical Class: Substituted hexahydronaphthalene
Therapeutic Class: Antilipemic (HMG-CoA reductase inhibitor); "statin"

CLINICAL PHARMACOLOGY
Mechanism of Action: Competitively inhibits 3-hydroxy-3-methylglutaryl-coenzyme A (HMG-CoA) reductase, an early rate-limiting step in cholesterol biosynthesis; increases HDL-cholesterol mildly [5%-14%], dramatically decreases total and LDL cholesterol [28%-45%, 27%-60% respectively], and dramatic lowering effect on triglycerides [20%-50%]

Pharmacokinetics
PO: Peak 1-2 hours; 12% bioavailability; food decreases absorption 30% (not clinically significant); >98% protein bound; metabolized via CYP-3A4; $t_{1/2}$ 14 hours

INDICATIONS AND USES: Primary hypercholesterolemia (heterozygous familial and nonfamilial hypercholesterolemia), mixed dyslipidemia (Fredrickson types IIa and IIb), hypertriglyceridemia (includes Fredrickson type IV), primary dysbetalipoproteinemia (Fredrickson type III), and homozygous familial hyperlipidemia

DOSAGE
Adult
• PO: 10-80 mg qd; dose can be administered without regard to meals

§ AVAILABLE FORMS/COST OF THERAPY
Tablet, film-coated—Oral: 10 mg, 90's: **$169.08;** 20 mg, 90's: **$261.41;** 40 mg, 90's: **$314.81**

---

* = non-FDA-approved use

CONTRAINDICATIONS: Active liver disease; unexplained persistent elevations of serum transaminases; pregnancy and lactation

PRECAUTIONS: Liver dysfunction

PREGNANCY AND LACTATION: Pregnancy category X; not recommended for nursing mothers

SIDE EFFECTS/ADVERSE REACTIONS

CNS: Headache

CV: Migraine, palpitation, postural hypotension, syncope, vasodilation

EENT: Amblyopia, dry eyes, taste disturbances, tinnitus

GI: Abdominal pain, constipation, diarrhea, dyspepsia, flatulence, gastroenteritis, LFT abnormalities

HEME: Anemia, ecchymosis, petechia, thrombocytopenia

METAB: Hyperglycemia, increased creatinine phosphokinase

MS: Arthralgia, leg cramps, *myalgia*

SKIN: Pruritus, rash

MISC: Face edema, fever, flu-like syndrome, malaise, photosensitivity

INTERACTIONS

Drugs

🔳 *Azole antifungals* (fluconazole, itraconazole, ketoconazole, miconazole): Increased atorvastatin levels; increased risk of rhabdomyolysis

🔳 *Bile acid sequestrants (cholestyramine, colestipol):* 25% reduction in atorvastatin plasma levels if coadministered

🔳 *Cyclosporine:* Concomitant administration increases risk of severe myopathy or rhabdomyolysis

🔳 *Digoxin:* Elevation of digoxin level (approximately 20%)

🔳 *Erythromycin:* Increased atorvastatin concentrations (approximately 40%); increased risk of rhabdomyolysis

🔳 *Fibric acid:* Increased risk of severe myopathy, especially with high statin doses

🔳 *Nefazodone:* Increased atorvastatin levels; increased risk of rhabdomyolyisis

🔳 *Niacin:* Concomitant administration increases risk of severe myopathy or rhabdomyolysis

🔳 *Oral contraceptives:* Coadministration increases AUC for norethindrone and ethinyl estradiol by approximately 30% and 20%, respectively

SPECIAL CONSIDERATIONS

• Statin selection based on lipid-lowering prowess, cost, and availability

• Potency and ability to lower serum triglycerides is unique among the HMG-CoA reductase inhibitors. However, no outcome data available

PATIENT/FAMILY EDUCATION

• Report symptoms of myalgia, muscle tenderness, or weakness

• Take daily doses in the evening for increased effect

MONITORING PARAMETERS

• Cholesterol (max therapeutic response 4-6 wk)

• LFT's (AST, ALT) at baseline and at 12 wk of therapy: if no change, no further monitoring necessary (discontinue if elevations persist at >3 × upper limit of normal)

• CPK in patients complaining of diffuse myalgia, muscle tenderness, or weakness

---

atovaquone
(a-toe′va-kwone)
Rx: Mepron
Chemical Class: Hydroxy-napthoquinone derivative
Therapeutic Class: Antiprotozoal

CLINICAL PHARMACOLOGY
Mechanism of Action: Inhibits synthesis of nucleic acid and ATP
Pharmacokinetics
PO: Peak 1-8 hr; bioavailability 23% fasting, 47% with food; highly lipophilic, with low aqueous solubility (CSF : plasma ratio <1%); 99.9% protein bound; $t_{1/2}$, 2.2-2.9 days, fecal elimination with enterohepatic circulation
INDICATIONS AND USES: Acute oral treatment of mild to moderate *Pneumocystis carinii* pneumonia (PCP) in patients who are intolerant to co-trimoxazole
DOSAGE
Adult
• PO 750 mg bid with food for 21 days
📳 **AVAILABLE FORMS/COST OF THERAPY**
• Susp—Oral: 750 mg/5 ml, 210 ml: **$612.59-$655.07**
CONTRAINDICATIONS: GI disorders that inhibit absorption
PREGNANCY AND LACTATION: Pregnancy category C; human breast milk studies not available; in rats, concentrations in milk 30% of maternal serum
SIDE EFFECTS/ADVERSE REACTIONS
CNS: Headache, insomnia
GI: Diarrhea, nausea, vomiting
METAB: Fever
RESP: Cough
SKIN: Skin rash

SPECIAL CONSIDERATIONS
• Plasma concentrations have been shown to correlate with the likelihood of successful treatment and survival

atropine
(a′troe-peen)
Rx: Atropine Care, Atropisol, Atrosulf-1, Isopto Atropine, Ocu-Tropine, Sal-Tropine
Chemical Class: Belladonna alkaloid
Therapeutic Class: Anticholinergic; ophthalmic anticholinergic; gastrointestinal antispasmodic; antiasthmatic, bronchodilator; mydriatic

CLINICAL PHARMACOLOGY
Mechanism of Action: Blocks acetylcholine at parasympathetic neuroeffector sites; increases cardiac output and heart rate by blocking vagal stimulation in heart; dries secretions by blocking vagus; blocks response of iris sphincter muscle, muscle of accommodation of ciliary body to cholinergic stimulation, resulting in dilation, paralysis of accommodation
Pharmacokinetics
PO/IM/SC: Well absorbed
PO: Onset ½ hr, peak ½-1 hr, duration 4-6 hr
IM/SC: Onset 15-50 min, peak 30 min, duration 4-6 hr
IV: Peak 2-4 min, duration 4-6 hr
OPHTH: Peak 30-40 min (mydriasis), 60-180 min (cycloplegia), duration 6-12 days, $t_{1/2}$ 13-40 hr; excreted by kidneys unchanged (70%-90% in 24 hr); metabolized in liver, 40%-50% crosses placenta, excreted in breast milk
INDICATIONS AND USES: Bradycardia, bradydysrhythmia; anticholinesterase insecticide poisoning;

* = non-FDA-approved use

blockade of cardiac vagal reflexes; antisialagogue (preanesthetic to prevent or reduce secretions of the respiratory tract and end of life comfort measure); rigidity and tremor of parkinsonism; antispasmodic with GU, biliary surgery; bronchodilator; mydriasis/cycloplegia for iritis, cycloplegic refraction; INH via neb for bronchospasm with COPD* (replaced with ipratropium bromide)

DOSAGE

Adult

• *Bradycardia/bradydysrhythmias:* IV BOL 0.5-1 mg given q3-5 min, not to exceed 2 mg

• *Insecticide poisoning:* IM/IV 2 mg qh until muscarinic symptoms disappear; may need 6 mg qh

• *Pre-surgery:* SC/IM/IV 0.4-0.6 mg before anesthesia

• *Iritis/cycloplegic refraction:* Instill sol 1-2 gtt of a 1% sol qd-tid for iritis or 1 hr before refracting

• Parkinsonism: PO 0.4 mg

Child

• *Bradycardia/bradydysrhythmias:* IV BOL 0.01-0.03 mg/kg up to 0.4 mg or 0.3 mg/m^2; may repeat q4-6h

• *Insecticide poisoning:* IM/IV 2 mg qh until muscarinic symptoms disappear; may need 6 mg qh

• *Pre-surgery:* SC 0.1-0.4 mg 30 min before surgery

• *Iritis/cycloplegic refraction:* Instill sol 1-2 gtt of a 0.5% sol qd-tid for iritis or bid × 1-3 days before exam (cycloplegic refraction); instill oint qd-bid 2-3 days before exam

\$ **AVAILABLE FORMS/COST OF THERAPY**

• Inj, Sol—IM, IV, SC 0.05 mg/ml, 5 ml: **\$11.19;** 0.1 mg/ml, 5 ml: **\$5.91-\$14.22;** 0.4 mg/ml, 1 ml: **\$0.43-\$1.12;** 0.5 mg/ml, 1 ml: **\$1.33;** 1 mg/ml, 1 ml: **\$0.49-\$1.12**

• Oint—Ophth: 1%, 3.5 g: **\$2.42-\$3.02**

• Sol—Ophth: 0.5%, 5 ml: **\$10.00;** 1%, 5 ml: **\$1.40-\$12.75;** 3%, 5 ml: **\$10.00**

• Tab—Oral: 0.4 mg, 100's: **\$26.95**

CONTRAINDICATIONS: Hypersensitivity to belladonna alkaloids, angle-closure glaucoma, GI obstructions, myasthenia gravis, thyrotoxicosis, ulcerative colitis, prostatic hypertrophy, tachycardia/tachydysrhythmias, asthma, acute hemorrhage, myocardial ischemia

PRECAUTIONS: Renal disease, lactation, CHF, hyperthyroidism, COPD, hepatic disease, child <6 yr, hypertension, elderly, intraabdominal infections, Down syndrome, spastic paralysis, gastric ulcer

PREGNANCY AND LACTATION: Pregnancy category C; passage into breast milk still controversial; neonates particularly sensitive to anticholinergic agents; compatible with breast feeding

SIDE EFFECTS/ADVERSE REACTIONS

CNS: Anxiety, **coma,** confusion, dizziness, drowsiness, flushing, headache, insomnia, involuntary movement, psychosis, weakness

CV: Angina, ectopic ventricular beats, hypertension, hypotension, **paradoxical bradycardia,** PVCs, tachycardia

EENT: Blurred vision, eye pain, glaucoma, nasal congestion, photophobia, pupil dilation

GI: Abdominal distension, abdominal pain, altered taste, anorexia, constipation, dry mouth, nausea, **paralytic ileus,** vomiting

GU: Dysuria, hesitancy, impotence, retention

SKIN: Contact dermatitis, dry skin, flushing, rash, urticaria

MISC: Decreased sweating, suppression of lactation

---

italic = common side effects   ***bold italic*** = life-threatening reactions

INTERACTIONS
Drugs
3 *Amantadine:* Enhanced anticholinergic effect of atropine; enhanced CNS effect of amantadine

3 *Neuroleptics:* Reduced neuroleptic effect

3 *Rimantadine:* Enhanced anticholinergic effect of atropine; enhanced CNS effect of rimantadine

3 *Tacrine:* May reduce anticholinergic effect of atropine; atropine may reduce CNS effect of tacrine

---

auranofin
(ah-RAN-oh-fin)
Rx: Ridaura
Chemical Class: Gold compound
Therapeutic Class: Disease-modifying arthritis drug (DMARD)

CLINICAL PHARMACOLOGY
Mechanism of Action: Unknown; best hypothesis relates to uptake of gold by macrophages with resultant inhibition of phagocytosis and activities of lysosomal enzymes; decreases both polymorphonuclear and monocyte function; decreased concentration of rheumatoid factor and immunoglobulins; impairs mitogen-induced proliferation of lymphocytes
Pharmacokinetics
PO: 25% of the gold absorbed by GI tract, peak 2 hr, steady state 8-16 wk; excreted in urine (60% of the absorbed gold) and feces; terminal plasma $t_{1/2}$ (steady state) 26 days; terminal body $t_{1/2}$ 80 days
INDICATIONS AND USES:
Asthma,* rheumatoid arthritis; psoriatic arthritis*

DOSAGE
Adult
• PO 6 mg qd or 3 mg bid, may increase to 9 mg/day after 3 mo
Child
• PO (initial) 0.1 mg/kg/day, (maintenance) 0.15 mg/kg/day, (max) 0.2 mg/kg/day
$ AVAILABLE FORMS/COST OF THERAPY
• Cap, Gel—Oral: 3 mg, 60's: **$94.43**
CONTRAINDICATIONS: Necrotizing enterocolitis, bone marrow aplasia, child <6 yr, lactation, pulmonary fibrosis, exfoliative dermatitis, blood dyscrasias, recent radiation therapy, renal/hepatic disease, marked hypertension, uncontrolled CHF
PRECAUTIONS: Skin rash, renal disease, liver disease
PREGNANCY AND LACTATION: Pregnancy category C; nursing not recommended; gold appears in breast milk
SIDE EFFECTS/ADVERSE REACTIONS
CNS: Confusion, dizziness, EEG abnormalities, hallucinations, *seizures*
EENT: Corneal ulcers, gold deposits in ocular tissues, iritis
GI: Abdominal cramping, anorexia, constipation, *diarrhea,* dyspepsia, *enterocolitis,* flatulence, gingivitis, glossitis, increased AST/ALT, jaundice, melena, metallic taste, *nausea, stomatitis, vomiting*
GU: Hematuria, increased BUN/creatinine, proteinuria, vaginitis
HEME: Agranulocytosis, aplastic anemia, eosinophilia, *leukopenia, neutropenia, thrombocytopenia*
RESP: Cough, dyspnea, *fibrosis, interstitial pneumonitis*
SKIN: Alopecia, *dermatitis, exfoliative dermatitis,* photosensitivity, *pruritus, rash,* urticaria

---

* = non-FDA-approved use

A

MISC: Gold toxicity: decreased Hgb, WBC <4000/mm^3, granulocytes <1500/mm^3, platelets <150,000/mm^3, hematuria, itching, proteinuria, rash, severe diarrhea, stomatitis

SPECIAL CONSIDERATIONS
MONITORING PARAMETERS
• Rheumatoid arthritis: tender, swollen joints, visual analogue scale for pain; acute phase reactants (ESR, C-reactive protein), duration of early morning stiffness, preservation of function; persistence of loose stools and/or severe diarrhea may be a drug effect; pruritus is a warning sign for development of cutaneous reactions, metallic taste may be a warning sign of stomatitis development; CBC with differential, platelet count, urinalysis, renal function, and hepatic function tests should be done prior to treatment; CBC with differential, platelet count, and urinalysis should be done every month during therapy

---

aurothioglucose/gold sodium thiomalate
(aur-oh-thye-oh-gloo'kose/gold sodium thye-oh-maa'late)
Rx: Solganol (aurothioglucose); Aurolate, Myochrysine (gold sodium thiomalate)
Chemical Class: Heavy metal, active gold compound (50%)
Therapeutic Class: Gold salt, slowly-acting antiarthritic drug, disease-modifying arthritis drug (DMARD)

CLINICAL PHARMACOLOGY
Mechanism of Action: Unknown; best hypothesis relates to uptake of gold by macrophages with resultant inhibition of phagocytosis and ac-

tivities of lysosomal enzymes; decreases both polymorphonuclear and monocyte function; decreased concentration of rheumatoid factor and immunoglobulins; impairs mitogen-induced proliferation of lymphocytes

Pharmacokinetics
IM: Peak 4-6 hr; excreted in urine, feces; t$_{1/2}$ 3-27 days, increases up to 168 days with 11th dose
INDICATIONS AND USES: Asthma,* Felty's syndrome, rheumatoid arthritis; Sjögren's syndrome; pemphigus*; psoriatic arthritis
DOSAGE
Adult
• *Aurothioglucose:* IM administer weekly; 1st dose 10 mg; 2nd, 3rd doses 25 mg; then 50 mg q wk up to 0.8-1.0 g; continue 25-50 mg q3-4 wk if improvement without toxicity
• *Gold sodium thiomalate:* IM 10 mg, then 25 mg after 1 wk, then 50 mg q wk for total of 14-20 doses, then 50 mg q2 wk × 4, then 50 mg q3 wk × 4, then 50 mg qmo for maintenance
Child 6-12 yr
• *Aurothioglucose:* IM 1 mg/kg/wk × 20 wk, or ¼ of adult dose
• *Gold sodium thiomalate:* IM 1 mg/kg/wk × 20 wk, then q3-4wk if improvement without toxicity; not to exceed 50 mg/dose
💲 AVAILABLE FORMS/COST OF THERAPY
Aurothioglucose
• Inj, Susp in Oil—IM: 50 mg/ml, 10 ml: **$148.24**
Gold Sodium Thiomalate
• Inj, Sol—IM: 50 mg/ml, 1 ml: **$14.23**
CONTRAINDICATIONS: Systemic lupus erythematosus, uncontrolled diabetes mellitus, marked hypertension, recent radiation therapy, CHF, renal disease, liver disease, agran-

ulocytosis, blood dyscrasias, hemorrhagic diathesis, history of hepatitis, colitis, urticaria, eczema
PREGNANCY AND LACTATION:
Pregnancy category C; gold has been demonstrated in breast milk and in the serum and red blood cells of a nursing infant; the slow excretion and persistence of gold in the mother, even after discontinuing therapy, must also be considered
SIDE EFFECTS/ADVERSE REACTIONS

CNS: Confusion, *dizziness,* EEG abnormalities, ***encephalitis,*** hallucinations
CV: Bradycardia, rapid pulse
EENT: Corneal ulcers, iritis
GI: Cramping, diarrhea, flatulence, hepatitis, jaundice, metallic taste, nausea, stomatitis, vomiting
GU: Hematuria, ***nephrosis,*** proteinuria, ***tubular necrosis***
HEME: ***Agranulocytosis, aplastic anemia,*** eosinophilia, ***leukopenia, neutropenia,*** thrombocytopenia
RESP: Interstitial pneumonitis, pharyngitis, ***pulmonary fibrosis***
SKIN: Alopecia, ***angioedema,*** *dermatitis,* ***exfoliative dermatitis,*** photosensitivity, *pruritus, rash,* urticaria
MISC: ***Anaphylaxis:*** "nitritoid" reaction (vasomotor reaction manifests as nausea, weakness, flushing, tachycardia, and/or syncope in 5% of patients receiving gold sodium thiomalate; not reported with aurothioglucose, hence probably related to vehicle or preservative in alternative product); gold toxicity (decreased Hgb, WBC <4000/mm^3, granulocytes <1500/mm^3, platelets <150,000/mm^3, severe diarrhea, stomatitis, hematuria, rash, itching, proteinuria)

SPECIAL CONSIDERATIONS
• Administer in gluteal muscle with patient recumbent for 10 min after injection
MONITORING PARAMETERS
• Rheumatoid arthritis: tender, swollen joints, visual analogue scale for pain; acute phase reactants (ESR, C-reactive protein), duration of early morning stiffness, preservation of function; persistence of loose stools and/or severe diarrhea may be a drug effect; pruritus is a warning sign for development of cutaneous reactions, metallic taste may be a warning sign of stomatitis development; CBC with differential, platelet count, urinalysis, renal function, and hepatic function tests should be done prior to treatment; CBC with differential, platelet count, and urinalysis should be done every month during therapy

---

azatadine
(a-za′ta-deen)
Rx: Optimine
Chemical Class: Piperidine derivative
Therapeutic Class: Antihistamine

CLINICAL PHARMACOLOGY
Mechanism of Action: Decreases allergic response by blocking histamine at H_1-receptors
Pharmacokinetics
PO: Peak 4 hr; metabolized in liver, excreted by kidneys; crosses placenta, crosses blood-brain barrier; minimally bound to plasma proteins; $t_{1/2}$ 9-12 hr
INDICATIONS AND USES: Perennial and seasonal allergic rhinitis; chronic urticaria

---

DOSAGE
Adult
• PO 1-2 mg bid, not to exceed 4 mg/day
Child >12 yr
• PO 1-2 mg bid
💲 AVAILABLE FORMS/COST OF THERAPY
• Tab, Uncoated—Oral: 1 mg, 100's: **$111.37**

CONTRAINDICATIONS: Concurrent acute asthma attack, lower respiratory tract disease, child <12 yr

PRECAUTIONS: Increased intra-ocular pressure, renal disease, cardiac disease, asthma, seizure disorder, stenosed peptic ulcers, hyperthyroidism, prostatic hypertrophy, bladder neck obstruction, elderly

PREGNANCY AND LACTATION: Pregnancy category B; excretion into breast milk unknown

SIDE EFFECTS/ADVERSE REACTIONS
CNS: Anxiety, chills, confusion, *dizziness, drowsiness,* euphoria, fatigue, neuritis, paresthesia, poor coordination, sweating
CV: Hypotension, palpitations, tachycardia
EENT: Blurred vision; dilated pupils; dry nose, throat; tinnitus
GI: Anorexia, constipation, dry mouth, nausea, vomiting
GU: Dysuria, frequency, impotence, retention
HEME: **Agranulocytosis, hemolytic anemia, thrombocytopenia**
RESP: Chest tightness, increased thick secretions, wheezing
SKIN: Photosensitivity, rash, urticaria

azathioprine
(ay-za-thye'oh-preen)
Rx: Imuran
Chemical Class: Purine analog; derivative of 6-mercaptopurine
Therapeutic Class: Immunosuppressant

CLINICAL PHARMACOLOGY
Mechanism of Action: Immunosuppressive by inhibiting purine synthesis in cells
Pharmacokinetics
PO: Peak 1-2 hr; metabolized in liver (cleaved to mercaptopurine then inactivated by xanthine oxidase); 30% bound to serum proteins; excreted in urine (both parent and metabolite) rapidly; crosses placenta

INDICATIONS AND USES: Renal homotransplantation to prevent graft rejection; refractory rheumatoid arthritis, refractory ITP*; glomerulonephritis*; nephrotic syndrome*; bone marrow transplant*; ulcerative colitis*; myasthenia gravis* (2-3 mg/kg/day); Behçet's syndrome*; Crohn's disease*

DOSAGE
Adult
• *Prevention of rejection:* PO/IV 3-5 mg/kg/day, then maintenance (PO) of at least 1-2 mg/kg/day
• *Refractory rheumatoid arthritis:* PO 1 mg/kg/day; may increase dose after 2 mo by 0.5 mg/kg/day; not to exceed 2.5 mg/kg/day
Child
• *Prevention of rejection:* PO/IV 3-5mg/kg/day, then maintenance (PO) of at least 1-2 mg/kg/day

💲 AVAILABLE FORMS/COST OF THERAPY

• Inj, Lyphl-Sol—IV: 100 mg; **$34.46**
• Tab, Uncoated—Oral: 50 mg, 100's: **$80.64-$163.03**

PRECAUTIONS: Severe leukopenia and/or thrombocytopenia may occur as well as macrocytic anemia and bone marrow depression; fungal, viral, bacterial, and protozoal infections may be fatal; may increase the patient's risk of neoplasia via mutagenic and carcinogenic properties (skin cancer and reticulum cell or lymphomatous tumors); temporary depression in spermatogenesis

PREGNANCY AND LACTATION: Pregnancy category D

SIDE EFFECTS/ADVERSE REACTIONS

GI: Esophagitis, hepatotoxicity, jaundice, nausea, *pancreatitis,* stomatitis, vomiting

HEME: Anemia (macrocytic), *leukopenia, pancytopenia, thrombocytopenia*

MS: Arthralgia, muscle wasting

SKIN: Rash

MISC: Fungal, viral, bacterial, and protozoal infections

INTERACTIONS

Drugs

❷ *Allopurinol:* Allopurinol may increase toxicity of azathioprine; dosage adjustment is necessary

❸ *Warfarin:* Reduced warfarin effect

SPECIAL CONSIDERATIONS

MONITORING PARAMETERS

• Hgb, WBC, platelets monthly
• D/C if leukocytes are <3000/mm^3
• Therapeutic response may take 3-4 mo in rheumatoid arthritis

---

azelaic acid

(a-zuh-lay'ick)
Rx: Azelex
Chemical Class: Dicarboxylic acid
Therapeutic Class: Antiacne agent

CLINICAL PHARMACOLOGY

Mechanism of Action: Normalizes keratinization, resulting in decreased microcomedo formation; antimicrobial activity against *S. epidermidis* and *P. acnes*

Pharmacokinetics

TOP: 4% absorbed systemically; elimination t$_{1/2}$ 12 hr, onset of action within 4 wk; renal excretion, primarily as unchanged azelaic acid

INDICATIONS AND USES: Acne

DOSAGE

Adult and Child >12 yr

• Apply thin film to affected area bid

💲 AVAILABLE FORMS/COST OF THERAPY

Cre—Top: 20%, 30, 50 g: **$35.44/ 30 g**

PREGNANCY AND LACTATION: Pregnancy category B; distributed in breast milk but little absorbed systemically and unlikely that concentrations of this normal dietary consituent would exceed baseline endogenous concentrations

SIDE EFFECTS/ADVERSE REACTIONS

SKIN: Burning and itching (1%-5%), contact dermatitis, dryness and redness (<1%), hypopigmentation (especially in darker-skinned individuals), keratosis pilaris

SPECIAL CONSIDERATIONS

• Wash hands after application; avoid contact with mucous membranes; if drug gets into eyes, wash with large quantities of water

---

• If skin irritation occurs, decrease frequency of application or temporarily discontinue treatment

• Azelaic acid is a naturally occurring substance found in the human diet

---

azelastine
(a'zel-ah-steen)
Rx: Astelin
Chemical Class: Phthalazinone derivative
Therapeutic Class: Antihistamine

CLINICAL PHARMACOLOGY
Mechanism of Action: Decreases allergic response by blocking histamine at H_1-receptors
Pharmacokinetics
Nasal: Onset within 3 hr, duration 12 hr; systemic absorption occurs despite inhaled route; metabolized by hepatic cytochrome P-450 system, metabolites excreted renally
INDICATIONS AND USES: Seasonal allergic rhinitis; perennial rhinitis*
DOSAGE
Adult
• INH 2 sprays in each nostril bid
Child ≥12 yr
• INH 2 sprays in each nostril bid
$ AVAILABLE FORMS/COST OF THERAPY
• Spray, Nasal—INH: 17 ml (twin pack), 1 mg/spray (200 sprays/twin pack): **$44.76**
PREGNANCY AND LACTATION: Pregnancy category C, excretion into breast milk unknown
SIDE EFFECTS/ADVERSE REACTIONS
CNS: Headache, *somnolence*
EENT: Bitter taste
METAB: Weight gain

SPECIAL CONSIDERATIONS
• Low sedating antihistamine nasal spray with first-dose activity; note: onset of action not as fast as decongestant nasal sprays, but appropriate for prn use
PATIENT/FAMILY EDUCATION
• Advise caution with use concomitant with activities that require concentration or while operating machinery; may cause drowsiness

---

azithromycin
(ay-zi-thro-mye'sin)
Rx: Zithromax
Chemical Class: Macrolide (azalide) derivative
Therapeutic Class: Antibiotic

CLINICAL PHARMACOLOGY
Mechanism of Action: Binds to 50S ribosomal subunits of susceptible bacteria and suppresses protein synthesis
Pharmacokinetics
PO: Peak 2.2 hr, duration 24 hr, rapidly absorbed and widely distributed into tissues (higher concentrations in tissues than in plasma), protein binding 51%, bioavailability 40%, $t_{1/2}$ 68 hr; excreted in bile, feces, urine primarily as unchanged drug
INDICATIONS AND USES: Mild to moderate infections of the upper and lower respiratory tract; uncomplicated skin and skin structure infections; nongonococcal urethritis or cervicitis caused by susceptible organisms; gonococcal urethritis*; chancroid; otitis media; prevention of *Mycobacterium avium* complex infection in AIDS patients*
Antibacterial spectrum usually includes:
• Gram-positive organisms: *Staphylococcus aureus, Streptococcus pneumoniae, S. pyogenes, S. aga-*

---

italic = common side effects　　　**bold italic** = life-threatening reactions

lactiae, streptococci (Groups C,F,G), *S. viridans* group streptococci
• Gram-negative organisms: *Moraxella catarrhalis, Haemophilus influenzae, Bordetella pertussi, Campylobacter jejuni, H. ducreyi, Legionella pneumophilia*
• Anaerobes: *Bacteroides bivivu, Clostridium perfringens,* other *Clostridium* sp., *Peptostreptococcus* sp.
• Misc: *Chlamydia trachomatis, Borrelia burgdorferi, Mycoplasma pneumoniae, Treponema pallidum, Ureaplasma urealyticum*

DOSAGE
Adult
• *Pneumonia:* PO 500 mg on day 1, then 250 mg qd on days 2-5 for a total dose of 1.5 g; IV 500 mg qd for 2 days followed by 5-8 days by PO 500 mg qd
• *Nongonococcal urethritis or cervicitis:* 1 g single PO dose for chlamydial infections
• *Chancroid:* 1 g as a single dose
• *Gonococcal urethritis or cervicitis:* 2 g PO as single dose
• *Pelvic inflammatory disease:* 500 mg IV then 250 mg PO qd for 6 days
• *Prevention of Mycobacterium avium complex infection in AIDS patients:* PO 1200 mg once per week
Child
• *Acute otitis media:* PO 10 mg/kg × 1, then 5 mg/kg qd for next 4 days
• *Pharyngitis/tonsillitis:* PO 12 mg/kg qd × 5 days
• *Community-acquired pneumonia:* PO 10 mg/kg × 1, then 5 mg/kg qd for next 4 days

[$] AVAILABLE FORMS/COST OF THERAPY
• Cap—Oral: 250 mg, 6's: **$40.39-$60.74**
• Sachet—Oral: 1 g: **$20.35**
• Susp—Oral: 100 mg/5 ml, 15 ml: **$27.74-$38.69;** 200 mg/5 ml, 15 ml: **$27.74-$38.69**

• Tab—Oral: 600 mg, 30's: **$471.71**
• Inj, Dry-Sol—IV: 500 mg: **$23.71**

CONTRAINDICATIONS: Hypersensitivity to erythromycin

PRECAUTIONS: Hepatic, renal, cardiac disease

PREGNANCY AND LACTATION: Pregnancy category B; excretion into breast milk unknown

SIDE EFFECTS/ADVERSE REACTIONS
CV: Chest pain, palpitations
CNS: Dizziness, headache, somnolence, vertigo
GI: Abdominal pain, cholestatic jaundice, diarrhea, dyspepsia, flatulence, heartburn, hepatotoxicity, melena, nausea, stomatitis, vomiting
GU: Moniliasis, nephritis, vaginitis
SKIN: Photosensitivity, pruritus, rash, urticaria

INTERACTIONS
Drugs
[3] *Penicillins:* Azithromycin may inhibit antibacterial activity of penicillins
Labs
• *Increase:* Serum 17 Hydroxycorticosteroids, 17 ketosteroids
• *Decrease:* Serum folate (bioassay only)

SPECIAL CONSIDERATIONS
PATIENT/FAMILY EDUCATION
• New formulation can be taken without regard to food
• Tablet and capsule may be taken without regard to food. Suspension should be taken on an empty stomach

---

aztreonam
(az-tree'oo-nam)
Rx: Azactam
Chemical Class: Monobactam
Therapeutic Class: Antibiotic

CLINICAL PHARMACOLOGY
Mechanism of Action: Inhibits bacterial wall synthesis; bactericidal

A

Pharmacokinetics

IV: Peak, following single 1 g dose 204 μg/ml; trough, at 8 hr 3 μg/ml; $t_{1/2}$ 1.7 hr, $t_{1/2}$ prolonged in renal disease; protein binding 56%; metabolized by liver, excreted in urine; small amounts appear in breast milk, placenta

INDICATIONS AND USES: Infections of the respiratory, urinary, and gynecologic tracts, skin, muscle, and bone; intra-abdominal septicemia caused by susceptible organisms. Antibacterial spectrum usually includes:

• Gram-negative organisms: *E. coli, Klebsiella pneumoniae, Proteus mirabilis, P. aeruginosa, Enterobacter* sp., *K. oxytoca, Citrobacter* and *S. marcescens, Haemophilus influenzae*

DOSAGE

Adult

• *Urinary tract infections:* IV/IM 500 mg-1 g q8-12h

• *Systemic infections:* IV/IM 1-2 g q8-12h

• *Severe systemic infections:* IV/IM 2 g q6-8h; do not exceed 8 g/day; continue treatment for 48 hr after negative culture or until patient is asymptomatic

Child

• Postnatal age <7 days, <2000 g: IM/IV 30 mg/kg q12h; >2000 g 30 mg/kg q8h

• Postnatal age >7 days, <2000 g: 30 mg/kg q8h; >2000 g: 30 mg/kg q6h

• Children >1 mo: 90-120 mg/kg/day divided q6-8h

• *Cystic Fibrosis:* 50 mg/kg/dose q6-8h (max 6-8 g/day)

💲 AVAILABLE FORMS/COST OF THERAPY

• Inj, Lyphl-Sol—IM, IV: 500 mg/vial: **$8.45;** 1 g/vial: **$16.98;** 2 g/vial: **$34.00**

PRECAUTIONS: Children; impaired renal, hepatic function; elderly; hypersensitivity to penicillins, cephalosporins

PREGNANCY AND LACTATION: Pregnancy category B; excreted in breast milk in concentrations <1% of maternal serum concentrations

SIDE EFFECTS/ADVERSE REACTIONS

CNS: Anxiety, **coma,** depression, hallucinations, lethargy, malaise, **seizures,** twitching

EENT: Diplopia, nasal congestion, tinnitus

GI: Abdominal pain, colitis, *diarrhea,* glossitis, increased AST/ALT, *nausea, vomiting*

GU: Breast tenderness, vaginal candidiasis, vaginitis

HEME: **Bone marrow depression,** increased bleeding time

INTERACTIONS

Drugs

🔳 *Aminoglycosides:* Potential increased nephrotoxicity, ototoxicity

🔳 *Cephalosporins, imipenem:* Antagonism secondary to antibiotic-induced high levels of β-lactamase

SPECIAL CONSIDERATIONS

• Minimal cross-reactivity between aztreonam and penicillins and cephalosporins; aztreonam and aminoglycosides have been shown to be synergistic *in vitro* against most strains of *P. aeruginosa,* many strains of *Enterobacteriaceae,* and other gram-negative aerobic bacilli

---

bacampicillin
(ba-kam'pi-sill'in)
Rx: Spectrobid
Chemical Class: Aminopenicillin
Therapeutic Class: Antibiotic

CLINICAL PHARMACOLOGY
Mechanism of Action: Inhibits bacterial cell wall synthesis, bactericidal, ampicillin class of semisynthetic penicillins
Pharmacokinetics
PO: Peak 30-60 min (400 mg provides peak serum concentrations ampicillin, 7.9 μg/ml), duration 5-6 hr, hydrolyzed to ampicillin during absorption, $t_{1/2}$ ½-1 hr; metabolized in liver, excreted in urine
INDICATIONS AND USES: Infections of the upper and lower respiratory tract, including acute exacerbations of chronic bronchitis, skin and skin structure, urinary tract infections, and gonorrhea (acute uncomplicated urogenital infections) due to susceptible organisms
Antibacterial spectrum usually includes:
• Gram-positive organisms: *Streptococcus faecalis, S. pneumoniae,* β-hemolytic streptococci, *S. pyogenes,* non-penicillinase-producing staphylococci
• Gram-negative organisms: *Neisseria gonorrhoeae, E. coli, Haemophilus influenzae, Proteus mirabilis*
DOSAGE
Adult
• Usual dosage PO 400-800 mg q12h
• *Gonorrhea:* (acute uncomplicated urogenital infections due to *N. gonorrhoeae,* males and females) 1.6 g (4 × 400 mg tablet plus 1 g probenecid) as a single oral dose

Child
• Usual dosage PO 25-50 mg/kg/day in divided doses q12h
$ AVAILABLE FORMS/COST OF THERAPY
• Tab, Uncoated—Oral: 400 mg, 100's: **$232.54**
CONTRAINDICATIONS: Hypersensitivity to penicillins
PRECAUTIONS: Superinfections with mycotic or bacterial pathogens, concomitant mononucleosis (high percentage develop a skin rash)
PREGNANCY AND LACTATION: Pregnancy category B; excreted in milk; milk:plasma ratios up to 0.2
SIDE EFFECTS/ADVERSE REACTIONS
CNS: Anxiety, *coma,* depression, hallucinations, lethargy, *seizures,* twitching
GI: Black "hairy" tongue, *diarrhea,* enterocolitis, gastritis, glossitis, increased AST/ALT, *nausea, pseudomembranous colitis,* stomatitis, *vomiting*
GU: **Glomerulonephritis,** hematuria, *moniliasis,* oliguria, proteinuria, *vaginitis*
HEME: Anemia, **bone marrow depression, granulocytopenia,** increased bleeding time, **thrombocytopenia, thrombocytopenic purpura, eosinophilia, leukopenia, and agranulocytosis** (hypersensitivity phenomena)
MISC: Hypersensitivity reactions (skin rashes, urticaria, erythema multiforme, and an occasional case of exfoliative dermatitis; skin rash when given with allopurinol), serious and occasional fatal hypersensitivity (anaphylactic)
INTERACTIONS
Drugs
3 *Atenolol:* Reduced serum concentration of atenolol

---

* = non-FDA-approved use

3 *Chloramphenicol:* Inhibited antibacterial activity of bacampicillin; administer bacampicillin 3 hours before chloramphenicol

3 *Macrolide antibiotics:* Inhibited antibacterial activity of bacampicillin; administer bacampicillin 3 hours before macrolides

3 *Methotrexate:* Increased serum methotrexate concentrations

3 *Oral contraceptives:* Occasional impairment of oral contraceptive efficacy; consider use of supplemental contraception during cycles in which bacampicillin is used

3 *Tetracyclines:* Inhibited antibacterial activity of bacampicillin; administer bacampicillin 3 hours before tetracycline

Labs

• *False positive:* Urine amino acids
• *Increase:* Urine glucose (Clinitest method), plasma phenylalanine (dried blood spot method), CSF protein (Ektachem method), serum protein (biuret method), serum theophylline (3M Diagnostics THEO-FAST method), serum uric acid
• *Decrease:* Serum cholesterol (CHOD-iodide method only), serum folate (bioassay method only), urine glucose (Clinistix and Diastix methods)

SPECIAL CONSIDERATIONS
• A 400 mg tab of bacampicillin and 125 mg/5 ml of the oral susp is chemically equivalent to 280 mg and 87.5 mg of ampicillin, respectively

PATIENT/FAMILY EDUCATION
• Administer 1 hr before or 2 hr after meals

bacitracin

(bass-i-tray´sin)
Rx: Ak-Tracin, Baci-Rx, Bacticin, Ocu-Tracin, Spectro-Bacitracin
Combinations:
  Rx: with neomycin, polymixin, and hydrocortisone (Cortisporin)
  OTC: with neomycin and polymixin (Neosporin); with polymixin (Polysporin)
Chemical Class: Bacillus subtilis derivative
Therapeutic Class: Antibacterial; ophthalmic antibacterial

CLINICAL PHARMACOLOGY
Mechanism of Action: Inhibits bacterial cell wall synthesis (bactericidal)

Pharmacokinetics
IM: Peak 1-2 hr, duration >12 hr; widely distributed (demonstrable in ascitic and pleural fluids after IM injection); metabolized in liver, excreted in urine

INDICATIONS AND USES: Ophth for superficial ocular infections involving the conjunctiva and/or cornea caused by susceptible organisms; IM for infants with pneumonia and empyema caused by susceptible staphylococci; PO for antibiotic-associated colitis (Orphan Drug status); top treatment of impetigo due to *Staphylococcus aureus*

DOSAGE
Adult
• OPHTH: Apply to conjunctival sac bid-qid
• IM: 20,000-25,000 U q6h × 7-10 days
• PO: 25,000 U qid × 10 days

---

italic = common side effects   ***bold italic*** = life-threatening reactions

Child

- OPHTH: Apply to conjunctival sac bid-qid; IM: infants <2.5 kg 900 U/kg/day in divided doses q8-12h; infants >2.5 kg 1000 U/kg/day in divided doses q8-12h

💲 AVAILABLE FORMS/COST OF THERAPY

- Inj, Lyphl-Sol—IM: 50,000 U/ vial: **$5.25-$9.26**
- Oint—Ophth: 500 unit/g, 3.5 g: **$2.82-$8.00**
- Powder: 7.3 g: **$34.38**

CONTRAINDICATIONS: Severe renal disease

PRECAUTIONS: Overgrowth of non-susceptible organisms; skin sensitivity due to neomycin in combination products

PREGNANCY AND LACTATION: Pregnancy category C

SIDE EFFECTS/ADVERSE REACTIONS

EENT: Poor corneal wound healing, visual haze (temporary)

GI: Diarrhea, nausea, vomiting

GU: Albuminuria, casts, cylindruria, proteinuria, **renal failure due to tubular and glomerular necrosis**

SKIN: Rash

MISC: Pain at injection site

SPECIAL CONSIDERATIONS

- Administer IM in deep muscle mass; rotate injection site; do *not* give IV/SC

---

baclofen

(bak'loe-fen)

Rx: Lioresal, Lioresal Intrathecal

Chemical Class: GABA chlorophenyl derivative

Therapeutic Class: Skeletal muscle relaxant

CLINICAL PHARMACOLOGY

Mechanism of Action: Inhibits synaptic responses at the spinal level by decreasing excitatory neurotransmitter release; decreases frequency, severity of muscle spasms; structural analog of the inhibitory neurotransmitter gamma-aminobutyric acid (GABA); general CNS depressant properties

Pharmacokinetics

PO: Peak 2-3 hr, duration >8 hr

INTRATHECAL: (CSF levels with plasma levels 100 times oral route); bolus: onset ½-1 hr, peak 4 hr, duration 4-8 hr; continuous INF: peak 24-48 hr, $t_{1/2}$ 2½-4 hr; partially metabolized in liver, excreted in urine (unchanged)

INDICATIONS AND USES: Spasticity with spinal cord injury; spasticity in multiple sclerosis; intractable spasticity in children with cerebral palsy* (intrathecal); trigeminal neuralgia*; tardive dyskinesia in combination with neuroleptics*

DOSAGE

Adult

- PO 5 mg tid × 3 days, then 10 mg tid × 3 days, then 15 mg tid × 3 days, then 20 mg tid × 3 days, then titrated to response, not to exceed 80 mg/day
- INTRATHECAL use implantable intrathecal INF pump; use screening trial of 3 separate bolus doses if needed (50 µg/ml, 75 µg/1.5 ml, 100 µg/2 ml); initial: double screening dose that produced result and give over 24 hr, increase by 10%-30% q24h only; maintenance: 12-1500 µg/day (limited experience with doses >1000 µg/day)

Child

- 2-7 yr: initial: PO 10-15 mg/24 hr divided q8h; titrate dose every 3 days in increments of 5-15 mg/day to a max of 40 mg/day
- ≥8 yr: PO max 60 mg/day in 3 divided doses

---

* = non-FDA-approved use

B

AVAILABLE FORMS/COST OF THERAPY

• Tab, Uncoated—Oral: 10 mg, 100's: **$8.00-$61.96**; 20 mg, 100's: **$15.05-$113.42**

• Kit—Intrathecal: 500 µg/ml, 20 ml: **$227.00**; 2000 µg/ml, 5 ml: **$237.00**

PRECAUTIONS: Peptic ulcer disease, renal disease, hepatic disease, stroke, seizure disorder, diabetes mellitus, elderly

PREGNANCY AND LACTATION: Pregnancy category C; present in breast milk, 0.1% of mother's dose; compatible with breast feeding

SIDE EFFECTS/ADVERSE REACTIONS

CNS: Disorientation, *dizziness, drowsiness, fatigue,* headache, insomnia, paresthesias, **seizures** (decreased seizure threshold); tremors; *weakness*

CV: Chest pain, edema, hypotension, palpitations

EENT: Blurred vision, mydriasis, nasal congestion, tinnitus

GI: Abdominal pain, anorexia, constipation, dry mouth, increased AST, alk phosphatase, *nausea,* vomiting

GU: Urinary frequency

METAB: Hyperglycemia

SKIN: Pruritus, rash

SPECIAL CONSIDERATIONS

• Abrupt discontinuation may lead to hallucinations, spasticity, tachycardia; drug should be tapered off over 1-2 wk

---

beclomethasone

(be-kloe-meth'a-sone)

Rx: INH: Beclovent, Vanceril; NASAL: Beconase AQ, Beconase, Vancenase, Vancenase AQ, Vancenase AQ Double Strength

Chemical Class: Halogenated synthetic glucocorticoid
Therapeutic Class: Anti-inflammatory corticosteroid, synthetic

---

CLINICAL PHARMACOLOGY

Mechanism of Action: Anti-inflammatory via inhibition of migration of polymorphonuclear leukocytes, fibroblasts, reversal of increased capillary permeability and lysosomal stabilization

Pharmacokinetics

INH: Despite inhaled routes, systemic absorption occurs; absorption occurs rapidly from all respiratory and gastrointestinal tissues; metabolized in lungs, liver, GI system; excreted in feces (with metabolites), less than 10% excreted in urine; $t_{1/2}$ 3-15 hr, crosses placenta

INDICATIONS AND USES: INH for chronic asthma; nasal for seasonal or perennial rhinitis; prevention of recurrence of nasal polyps; non-allergic (vasomotor) rhinitis

DOSAGE

Adult

• INH 2-4 puffs tid-qid, not to exceed 20 INH/day; NASAL 1-2 sprays in each nostril bid-qid; double strength NASAL 1-2 sprays each nostril qd

Child (6-12 yr)

• INH 1-2 puffs tid-qid, not to exceed 10 INH/day

---

italic = common side effects   ***bold italic*** = life-threatening reactions

Child (>12 yr)
• NASAL 1-2 sprays in each nostril bid-qid

$ AVAILABLE FORMS/COST OF THERAPY
• MDI Aer—INH: 42 µg/INH, 6.7 g: **$17.23-$23.99**; 16.8 g: **$26.72-$38.13**
• MDI Aer—Nasal INH: 6.7-7 g: **$18.01-$39.31**; 16.8 g: **$34.47-$40.61**
• MDI Double Strength Aer—INH: 84 µg/INH, 12.2 g: **$45.46**
• MDI Double Strength Aer—Nasal INH: 84 µg/INH, 19 g: **$44.17**
• Spray—Nasal: 42 µg/spray, 25 g: **$32.40-$42.33**

CONTRAINDICATIONS: Primary treatment for status asthmaticus; nonasthmatic bronchial disease; bacterial, fungal, or viral infections of mouth, throat, or lungs; children <3 yr

PRECAUTIONS: Nasal disease/surgery, children <12 yr (potential reduction in bone growth velocity), nasal ulcers, recurrent epistaxis; suppression of HPA-axis observed when administered at doses of 2000 µg/day by oral aerosol; not a bronchodilator; not indicated for rapid relief of bronchospasm; systemic effects such as mental disturbances, increased bruising, weight gain, cushingoid features, and cataracts

PREGNANCY AND LACTATION: Pregnancy category C; breast milk excretion unknown; other corticosteroids excreted in low concentrations with systemic administration; compatible with breast feeding

SIDE EFFECTS/ADVERSE REACTIONS
CNS: Headache, paresthesia
EENT: Burning, candidal infection, *dryness,* earache, *nasal irritation,* nasal ulcerations, perforation of nasal septum, secretions with blood, *sneezing,* sore throat
GI: Dry mouth, dysphonia
METAB: Adrenal suppression
RESP: **Bronchospasm**
SKIN: Pruritus, urticaria

SPECIAL CONSIDERATIONS PATIENT/FAMILY EDUCATION
• Rinse mouth with water following INH to decrease possibility of fungal infections, dysphonia
• Review proper MDI administration technique regularly
• Systemic corticosteroid effects from inhaled and nasal steroids inadequate to prevent adrenal insufficiency in patients withdrawn from corticosteroids abruptly
• Response to nasal steroids seen in 3 days-2 wk; D/C if no improvement in 3 wk
• For prophylactic use, no role in acute treatment of asthma/allergy

belladonna alkaloids
(bell-a-don'a)
Rx: Belladonna Tincture Combinations
  Rx: with butalbital (Butibel); with ergotamine and phenobarbital (Bellergal-S, Phenerbel-S); with phenobarbital (Donnatal, Donnatal Extentabs)
Chemical Class: Belladonna alkaloid
Therapeutic Class: Anticholinergic; gastrointestinal antispasmodic

CLINICAL PHARMACOLOGY
Mechanism of Action: Belladonna inhibits muscarinic actions of acetylcholine at postganglionic parasympathetic neuroeffector sites including smooth muscle, secretory glands, and CNS sites
Pharmacokinetics
PO: Duration 4-6 hr: metabolized by liver, excreted in urine

* = non-FDA-approved use

INDICATIONS AND USES: Adjunctive therapy in treatment of peptic ulcer, functional digestive disorders, diarrhea, diverticulitis, pancreatitis; dysmenorrhea; nocturnal enuresis; Parkinsonism; motion sickness; nausea and vomiting

DOSAGE

Adult

• PO 0.6-1 ml of tincture tid-qid

Child

• PO 0.03 ml/kg of tincture tid

§ AVAILABLE FORMS/COST OF THERAPY

• Tincture—Oral: 27-33 mg/100 ml, 120 ml: **$8.52**

CONTRAINDICATIONS: Hypersensitivity to anticholinergics, narrow-angle glaucoma, GI obstruction, myasthenia gravis, paralytic ileus, GI atony, toxic megacolon, obstructive uropathy

PRECAUTIONS: Hyperthyroidism, coronary artery disease, dysrhythmias, CHF, ulcerative colitis, hypertension, hiatal hernia, hepatic disease, renal disease, elderly, children, prostatic hypertrophy, chronic lung disease, high environmental temperatures

PREGNANCY AND LACTATION: Pregnancy category C; excretion into breast milk is controversial; neonates may be particularly sensitive to anticholinergic agents; use caution in nursing mothers

SIDE EFFECTS/ADVERSE REACTIONS

CNS: Anxiety, confusion, dizziness, drowsiness, hallucinations, headache, insomnia, nervousness, stimulation in elderly, weakness

CV: Palpitations, tachycardia

EENT: Blurred vision, cycloplegia, increased ocular pressure, mydriasis, photophobia

GI: Altered taste, *constipation, dry mouth,* dysphagia, heartburn, nausea, ***paralytic ileus,*** vomiting

GU: Hesitancy, impotence, *retention*

SKIN: Allergic reactions, anhidrosis, flushing, pruritus, rash, urticaria

INTERACTIONS

Drugs

§ *Amantadine:* Enhanced anticholinergic effect; enhanced CNS effect of amantadine

§ *Neuroleptics:* Reduced neuroleptic effect

§ *Rimantadine:* Enhanced anticholinergic effect; enhanced CNS effect of rimantadine

§ *Tacrine:* May reduce anticholinergic effect of atropine; belladonna may reduce CNS effect of tacrine

SPECIAL CONSIDERATIONS

• Product contains hyoscyamine, atropine, and scopolamine

PATIENT/FAMILY EDUCATION

• Avoid hot environments, heat stroke may occur

• Use sunglasses when outside to prevent photophobia

---

belladonna and opium

(bell-a-don'a)

Rx: B & O Supprettes

Chemical Class: Belladonna alkaloid/opiate

Therapeutic Class: Antispasmodic; narcotic analgesic

DEA Class: Schedule II

CLINICAL PHARMACOLOGY

Mechanism of Action: Belladonna inhibits muscarinic actions of acetylcholine at postganglionic parasympathetic neuroeffector sites including smooth muscle, secretory glands, and CNS sites; opium contains many narcotic alkaloids including morphine, which inhibit gastric motility and provide sedation and analgesic properties

---

italic = common side effects   ***bold italic*** = life-threatening reactions

Pharmacokinetics
PR: Onset 30 min (opium), 1-2 hr (belladonna); opium metabolized in the liver

INDICATIONS AND USES: Ureteral spasm not responsive to non-narcotic analgesics; rectal or bladder tenesmus occurring in postoperative states and neoplastic situations

DOSAGE

Adult

• PR 1 supp 1-2 times daily, up to 4 doses/day

Child

• Not recommended for children <12

💲 AVAILABLE FORMS/COST OF THERAPY

• Supp—Rect: 16.2 mg/30 mg, 12's: **$33.75;** 16.2 mg/60 mg, 12's: **$36.25**

CONTRAINDICATIONS: Hypersensitivity to anticholinergics or opium, narrow-angle glaucoma, severe hepatic or renal disease, bronchial asthma, respiratory depression, seizure disorders, acute alcoholism, delirium tremens, premature labor

PRECAUTIONS: Elderly, debilitated patients, increased intracranial pressure, toxic psychosis, myxedema

PREGNANCY AND LACTATION: Pregnancy category C; excretion of belladonna into breast milk is controversial; neonates may be particularly sensitive to anticholinergic agents, therefore use caution in nursing mothers

SIDE EFFECTS/ADVERSE REACTIONS

CNS: CNS depression, confusion, *drowsiness,* headache, memory loss, sedation, tiredness, weakness

CV: **Dysrhythmias,** bradycardia, flushing, hypotension, increased intracranial pressure, orthostatic hypotension, palpitations, peripheral vasodilation, tachycardia

EENT: Blurred vision, dry mouth, intraocular pain, mydriasis, photophobia

GI: Bloated feeling, *constipation,* nausea, vomiting

GU: Hesitancy, retention

RESP: **Respiratory depression**

SKIN: Decreased sweating, rash

MISC: Physical and psychological dependence

INTERACTIONS

Drugs

🔳 *Amantadine:* Enhanced anticholinergic effect; enhanced CNS effect of amantadine

🔳 *Neuroleptics:* Reduced neuroleptic effect

🔳 *Rimantadine:* Enhanced anticholinergic effect; enhanced CNS effect of rimantadine

🔳 *Tacrine:* May reduce anticholinergic effect; belladonna may reduce CNS effect of tacrine

SPECIAL CONSIDERATIONS

PATIENT/FAMILY EDUCATION

• Moisten finger and suppository with water before inserting

• May cause drowsiness, dry mouth, and blurred vision

• Store at room temperature; DO NOT refrigerate

---

benazepril
(be-naze'a-pril)
Rx: Lotensin
Combinations
  Rx: with hydrochlorothi-
    azide (Lotensin HCT)
  Rx: with amlodipine (Lotrel)
Chemical Class: Nonsulfhy-
dryl, angiotensin-converting
enzyme (ACE) inhibitor
Therapeutic Class: Antihyper-
tensive

CLINICAL PHARMACOLOGY
Mechanism of Action: Antihypertensive, hypoproliferative, and
cardioprotective effects attributable to competitive inhibition
of angiotensin-converting enzyme
(ACE) yielding decreased plasma
concentrations of angiotensin II,
plasma aldosterone concentrations,
systemic vascular resistance, blood
pressure, preload and afterload, not
accompanied by changes in heart
rate, pressor sensitivity to exogenous norepinephrine, or baroreceptor sensitivity

Pharmacokinetics
PO: Peak ½-1 hr, serum protein binding 97%, $t_{1/2}$ 10-11 hr; metabolized
by liver to active metabolite
(benazeprilat), which is excreted by
the kidneys

INDICATIONS AND USES: Hypertension, CHF, MI, erythrocytosis,*
nephropathy,* retinopathy*

DOSAGE
Adult
• PO 10 mg qd initially, increase as
needed to 20-40 mg/day divided bid
or qd
• *Renal impairment:* PO 5 mg qd
with CrCl <30 ml/min/1.73 m²; increase as needed to maximum of
40 mg/day

$ AVAILABLE FORMS/COST
  OF THERAPY
• Tab, Uncoated—Oral: 5 mg, 100's:
$79.04; 10 mg, 100's: **$79.04**; 20
mg, 100's: **$79.04**; 40 mg, 100's:
$79.04

PRECAUTIONS: History of anaphylaxis, renal insufficiency (<30
ml/min), hypotension (CHF, elderly,
volume depletion—diuretics, dialysis, cirrhosis), aortic stenosis, hyperkalemia (potassium supplements,
potassium-sparing diuretics, renal
disease, diabetes), neutropenia (autoimmune diseases, collagen-vas-
cular, febrile illness, immunosupres-
sant drug therapy), proteinuria, renal
artery stenosis, surgery/anesthesia
(excessive hypotension, correctable
with fluids)

PREGNANCY AND LACTATION:
Pregnancy category C (1st trimester), category D (2nd and 3rd trimesters); ACE inhibitors can cause
fetal and neonatal morbidity and
death when administered to pregnant women; detectable in breast
milk in trace amounts, a newborn
would receive <0.1% of the mg/kg
maternal dose; effect on nursing infant has not been determined

**SIDE EFFECTS/ADVERSE REAC-
  TIONS**
CNS: Anxiety, *dizziness, fatigue,
headache,* insomnia, paresthesia
CV: Angina, hypotension, palpitations, postural hypotension, syncope (especially with first dose)
GI: Abdominal pain, constipation,
melena, nausea, vomiting
GU: Decreased libido, impotence,
increased BUN/creatinine, urinary
tract infection
HEME: **Agranulocytosis, neutropenia**
METAB: Hyperkalemia, hyponatremia

---

italic = common side effects   ***bold italic*** = life-threatening reactions

MS: Arthralgia, arthritis, myalgia
RESP: Asthma, bronchitis, *cough,* dyspnea, sinusitis
SKIN: Angioedema, flushing, rash, sweating

INTERACTIONS
Drugs
❷ *Allopurinol:* Combination may predispose to hypersensitivity reactions
❸ *Alpha adrenergic blockers:* Exaggerated first dose hypotensive response when added to benazepril
❸ *Aspirin:* May reduce hemodynamic effects of benazepril; less likely at doses under 236 mg; less likely with nonacetylated salicylates
❸ *Azathioprine:* Increased myelosuppression
❸ *Cyclosporine:* Combination may cause renal insufficiency
❸ *Insulin:* Benazepril may enhance insulin sensitivity
❸ *Iron:* Benazepril may increase chance of systemic reaction to IV iron
❸ *Lithium:* Reduced lithium clearance
❸ *Loop diuretics:* Initiation of benazepril may cause hypotension and renal insufficiency in patients taking loop diuretics
❸ *NSAIDs:* May reduce hemodynamic effects of benazepril
❸ *Potassium-sparing diuretics:* Increased risk of hyperkalemia
❸ *Trimethoprim:* Additive risk of hyperkalemia, especially in patient predisposed to renal insufficiency
Labs
• ACE inhibition can account for approximately 0.5 mEq/L rise in serum potassium

SPECIAL CONSIDERATIONS
PATIENT/FAMILY EDUCATION
• Caution with salt substitutes containing potassium chloride
• Rise slowly to sitting/standing position to minimize orthostatic hypotension
• Dizziness, fainting, lightheadedness may occur during 1st few days of therapy
• May cause altered taste perception or cough; persistent dry cough usually does not subside unless medication is stopped; notify clinician if these symptoms persist

MONITORING PARAMETERS
• BUN, creatinine, potassium within 2 wk after initiation of therapy (increased levels may indicate acute renal failure)

---

bentoquatum
(ben′toe-kwa-tum)
OTC: Ivy Block
Chemical Class: Organoclay compound
Therapeutic Class Rhus dermatitis protectant

CLINICAL PHARMACOLOGY
Mechanism of Action: May interfere with allergen absorption by physical blocking
INDICATIONS AND USES: Prevention of poison ivy, oak, and sumac
DOSAGE
Adult and Child
• TOP apply 15 min prior to potential exposure; wash with soap and water after exposure
💲 **AVAILABLE FORMS/COST OF THERAPY**
• Lotion—Top: 5%, 120 ml: **$7.17**
CONTRAINDICATIONS: Preexisting rash
PRECAUTIONS: Children <6 yr

B

SPECIAL CONSIDERATIONS
PATIENT/FAMILY EDUCATION
• To be used prior to exposure only

benzocaine
(ben'zoe-kane)
Rx: Americaine;
OTC: Anbesol, Bicozene,
Boil-ease, Chigger-tox,
Dermoplast, Foille,
Hurricaine, Orajel, Orabase,
Solarcaine
Combinations
  Rx: with antipyrine (Aller-
    gen, Auralgan, Auroto,
    with benzethonium chlo-
    ride (Americaine, Otocain);
    with phenylephrine (Tym-
    pagesic)
Chemical Class: Aminobenzo-
ate derivative; ester
Therapeutic Class: Topical
local anesthetic

CLINICAL PHARMACOLOGY
Mechanism of Action: Benzocaine
reversibly stabilizes the neuronal
membrane, which decreases its permeability to sodium ions; depolarization of the neuronal membrane is
inhibited thereby blocking the initiation and conduction of nerve impulses, topical anesthetic
Pharmacokinetics
TOP: Peak 1 min, duration 0.5-1 hr
INDICATIONS AND USES: Lubricant and topical anesthetic on intratracheal catheters, nasogastric and
endoscopic tubes, urinary catheters,
laryngoscopes, proctoscopes, sig-
moidoscopes, vaginal specula; topical anesthetic for pharyngeal and
nasal airways to obtund the pharyngeal and tracheal reflexes; relief of
pain and pruritis in acute congestive
and serous otitis media, acute swim-
mer's ear, and other forms of otitis
externa

DOSAGE
Adult and Child >1 yr
• *Anesthetic lubricant:* TOP apply
evenly to exterior of tube or instru-
ment prior to use
• *Cerumen removal:* Instill tid for
2-3 days to help cerumen detach
and facilitate removal
• *Otic drops:* Instill 4-5 gtts in the
external auditory canal, then insert
a cotton pledget into the external
ear; repeat every 1-2 hr if necessary
to relieve pain
**$ AVAILABLE FORMS/COST
OF THERAPY**
• Liq 20%—Top: 30 ml: **$6.24**
• Gel 20%—Top: 30 g: **$6.24**
• Gel 6.3%—Top: 7.5 g: **$4.52**
• Gel 7.5%—Top: 15 g: **$2.92-$3.32**
• Gel 10%—Top 15 g: **$3.23-$3.50**
• Oint 20%—Top: 30 g: **$5.23**
• Spray/Aerosol 20%—Top: 60, 120
ml: **$2.52-$3.70/60 ml**
• Cr 5%—Top: 30 g: **$1.40-$1.60**
• Lotion 2.5%—Top: 15 ml: **$2.09**
• Oint 2%—Rect: 30 g: **$3.70/30 g**
• Oint—Top: 5%, 28 g: **$2.03;** 10%,
30 g: **$11.90;** 20%, 30 g: **$3.81-
$5.44**
• Paste—Top: 20%, 15 g: **$6.38**
• Swab 20%—Oral: 100's: **$36.06**
• Wax 20%—Oral: 1 g: **$2.19**
• Sol—Otic: (with antipyrine) 10
ml-15 ml: **$3.00-$17.04**
CONTRAINDICATIONS: Perfo-
rated tympanic membrane or ear dis-
charge (otic drops)
PREGNANCY AND LACTATION:
Pregnancy category C; excretion in
breast milk unknown; use caution in
nursing mothers
SIDE EFFECTS/ADVERSE REAC-
TIONS
EENT: Irritation in ear, itching
HEME: **Methemoglobinemia in in-
fants**
SKIN: Burning, edema, erythema,
pruritis, rash, stinging, tenderness,
urticaria

---

italic = common side effects   ***bold italic*** = life-threatening reactions

SPECIAL CONSIDERATIONS
PATIENT/FAMILY EDUCATION
• Protect the solution from light and heat, do not use if it is brown or contains a precipitate
• Discard this product 6 mo after dropper is first placed in the drug solution

---

benzonatate
(ben-zoe'na-tate)
Rx: Tessalon Perles
Chemical Class: Tetracaine derivative
Therapeutic Class: Antitussive

CLINICAL PHARMACOLOGY
Mechanism of Action: Acts peripherally by anesthetizing the stretch receptors located in the respiratory passages, lungs, and pleura; reduces cough reflex at its source; has no inhibitory effect on the respiratory center in recommended dosage
Pharmacokinetics
PO: Onset 15-20 min, duration 3-8 hr
INDICATIONS AND USES: Symptomatic relief of cough
DOSAGE
Adult and Child >10 yr
• PO 100 mg tid, not to exceed 600 mg/day
$ AVAILABLE FORMS/COST OF THERAPY
• Cap, Elastic—Oral: 100 mg, 100's: **$36.38-$106.81**
CONTRAINDICATIONS: Hypersensitivity to ester-type local anesthetics
PREGNANCY AND LACTATION: Pregnancy category C; excretion into breast milk unknown; use with caution in nursing mothers
SIDE EFFECTS/ADVERSE REACTIONS
CNS: Dizziness, drowsiness, headache
CV: Chest numbness

EENT: Burning eyes, nasal congestion
GI: Constipation, *nausea,* upset stomach
SKIN: Pruritus, rash, urticaria
SPECIAL CONSIDERATIONS
PATIENT/FAMILY EDUCATION
• Avoid driving, other hazardous activities until stabilized on this medication
• Do not chew or break capsules, will anesthetize mouth

---

benzoyl peroxide
(ben'zoe-ill per-ox'ide)
Rx: Benzac, Benzagel, Benzashave, Benzox, Brevoxyl, Delaqua, Desquam-E, Desquam-X, Pan-Oxyl, Persa-Gel;
OTC: Acetoxyl, Acne-10, Acnomel, Advanced Formula Oxy Sensitive, Ambi-10, Benoxyl, Clearasil, Clear by Design, Dermoxyl, Dryox, Exact, Fostex, Loroxide, Neutrogena, Oxyderm, Oxy-10, Perfectoderm, Solugel
Chemical Class: Benzoic acid derivative
Therapeutic Class: Antiacne agent

CLINICAL PHARMACOLOGY
Mechanism of Action: Antibacterial activity against *Propionibacterium acnes,* the predominant organism in sebaceous follicles and comedones; aided by mild drying action, removal of excess sebum; mild desquamation and sebostatic effects
Pharmacokinetics
TOP: 50% absorbed through skin; metabolized to benzoic acid, excreted in urine as benzoate
INDICATIONS AND USES: Mild to moderate acne

DOSAGE
Adult and Child
• TOP apply to affected area qd or bid

💲 AVAILABLE FORMS/COST OF THERAPY
• Bar—Top: 5%, 10%, 4 oz: **$3.58-$4.94**
• Cre—Top: 5%, 20, 120 g: **$15.37/120g**; 10%, 30, 120 g: **$11.50-$16.77**
• Gel—Top: 2.5%, 30, 45, 60, 90, 120 g: **$4.93-$7.60**/45 g; 4%, 42.5, 90 g: **$11.80**/42.5 g; 5%, 30, 45, 60, 90 g: **$1.73-$7.96**/45 g; 10%, 45, 60, 90 g: **$2.40-$8.37**/45 g
• Liq—Top: 2.5%, 240 ml: **$18.75**; 5%, 120, 150, 240 ml: **$21.25**/240 ml; 10%, 150, 240 ml: **$9.82-$23.44**/240 ml
• Lotion—Top: 5%, 25 30, 50 ml: **$17.32**/25 ml; 10%, 30, 60 ml: **$2.25-$5.48**
• Mask—Top: 5%, 30, 60 ml: **$2.45-$5.23**

PRECAUTIONS: Concurrent use with tretinoin may cause excess skin irritation

PREGNANCY AND LACTATION: Pregnancy category C; excretion into milk unknown

SIDE EFFECTS/ADVERSE REACTIONS
SKIN: Allergic and contact dermatitis, dryness, edema, erythema, local skin irritation, scaling, stinging

SPECIAL CONSIDERATIONS
PATIENT/FAMILY EDUCATION
• Keep away from eyes, mouth, inside of nose and other mucous membranes
• May cause transitory feeling of warmth or slight stinging
• Expect dryness and peeling, discontinue use if rash or irritation develops
• Water-based cosmetics may be used over drug; don't counter-treat dryness with emollients

---

benztropine
(benz'troe-peen)
Rx: Cogentin
Chemical Class: Tertiary amine
Therapeutic Class: Anticholinergic, anti-Parkinson's agent

CLINICAL PHARMACOLOGY
Mechanism of Action: Blocks striatal cholinergic receptors, which helps balance cholinergic and dopaminergic activity

Pharmacokinetics
IM/IV: Onset 15 min, duration 6-10 hr
PO: Onset 1 hr, duration 6-10 hr

INDICATIONS AND USES: Adjunctive treatment of all forms of Parkinson's disease; drug-induced extrapyramidal symptoms

DOSAGE
Adult
• *Parkinsonism:* PO 0.5-6 mg/day in 1-2 divided doses, begin with 0.5 mg/day and increase in 0.5 mg increments at 5-6 day intervals to achieve desired effect
• *Drug-induced extrapyramidal symptoms:* PO/IM/IV 1-4 mg/dose 1-2 times/day; switch to PO as soon as possible

Child >3 yr
• *Drug-induced extrapyramidal symptoms:* PO/IM/IV 0.02-0.05 mg/kg/dose 1-2 times/day

💲 AVAILABLE FORMS/COST OF THERAPY
• Tab, Uncoated—Oral: 0.5 mg, 100's: **$2.22-$19.60**; 1 mg, 100's: **$3.60-$22.40**; 2 mg, 100's: **$3.97-$28.25**
• Inj, Sol—IM, IV: 1 mg/ml, 2 ml: **$7.30**

CONTRAINDICATIONS: Narrow-angle glaucoma, myasthenia gravis, GI/GU obstruction, child <3 yr, pep-

---

tic ulcer, megacolon, prostatic hypertrophy

PRECAUTIONS: Elderly, tachycardia, liver/kidney disease, drug abuse history, dysrhythmias, hypotension, hypertension, psychiatric patients, children, tardive dyskinesia

PREGNANCY AND LACTATION: Pregnancy category C; an inhibitory effect on lactation may occur; infants may be particularly sensitive to anticholinergic effects

SIDE EFFECTS/ADVERSE REACTIONS

CNS: Anxiety, confusion, delusions, depression, dizziness, hallucinations, headache, incoherence, irritability, memory loss, restlessness, sedation
CV: Hypotension, mild bradycardia, palpitations, postural hypotension, tachycardia
EENT: Angle-closure glaucoma, blurred vision, difficulty swallowing, dilated pupils, dry eyes, increased intraocular tension, mydriasis, photophobia
GI: Abdominal distress, *constipation, dry mouth,* epigastric distress, nausea, ***paralytic ileus,*** vomiting
GU: Dysuria, hesitancy, retention
MS: Cramping, muscular weakness
SKIN: Dermatoses, rash, urticaria
MISC: Decreased sweating, erectile dysfunction, flushing, heat stroke, hyperthermia, increased temperature, numbness of fingers

INTERACTIONS

Drugs

3 Anticholinergics: Excess anticholinergic side effects
3 *Amantadine:* Potentiates CNS side effects of amantadine
3 *Neuroleptics:* Inhibition of therapeutic response to neuroleptics; excessive anticholinergic effects
3 *Tacrine:* Reduced therapeutic effects of both drugs

SPECIAL CONSIDERATIONS
PATIENT/FAMILY EDUCATION
• Do not discontinue abruptly
• Administer with or after meals to prevent GI upset
• Drug may increase susceptibility to heat stroke

---

benzylpenicilloyl-polylysine

(ben′zill-pen-i-cill′oyl-poly-ly′seen)
Rx: Pre-Pen
Chemical Class: Penicillin derivative
Therapeutic Class: Penicillin allergy skin test

CLINICAL PHARMACOLOGY
Mechanism of Action: Elicits IgE antibodies that produce type I accelerated urticarial reactions to penicillins

INDICATIONS AND USES: Adjunct in assessing the risk of administering penicillin (benzylpenicillin or penicillin G) when it is the preferred drug of choice in patients who have a history of clinical penicillin hypersensitivity

DOSAGE

Adult and Child

• *Scratch Test* (always perform first): A sterile 20 gauge needle should be used to make a 3-5 mm scratch of the epidermis; apply a small drop of Pre-Pen solution to the scratch and rub gently with an applicator, toothpick, or the side of the needle; a positive reaction consists of the development within 10 min of a pale wheal, usually with pseudopods, surrounding the scratch site and varying in diameter from 5 to 15 mm (or more)

• *Intradermal Test* (use only if scratch test completely negative):

Use a tuberculin syringe with a 26 to 30 gauge, short, bevel needle to inject a volume of 0.01-0.02 ml; use a separate syringe and needle to inject a like amount of saline as a control at least 1.5 in removed from the test site; most skin reactions will develop within 5-15 min; a positive reaction consists of itching and marked increase in size of original bleb; wheal may exceed 20 mm in diameter and exhibit pseudopods; the control site should be completely reactionless

$ AVAILABLE FORMS/COST OF THERAPY

• Inj, Sol—Intradermal: 0.25 ml: **$93.18**

CONTRAINDICATIONS: Extreme hypersensitivity

PRECAUTIONS: Repeated skin testing

PREGNANCY AND LACTATION: Pregnancy category C

SIDE EFFECTS/ADVERSE REACTIONS

SKIN: Edema, erythema, pruritus, urticaria, wheal

MISC: Systemic allergic reactions occur rarely

SPECIAL CONSIDERATIONS

• Does not identify those patients who react to a minor antigenic determinant (i.e., anaphylaxis); does not reliably predict the occurrence of late reactions; patients with a negative skin test may still have allergic reactions to therapeutic penicillin

bepridil
(beh′prih-dill)
Rx: Vascor
Chemical Class: Diarylaminopropylamine ether
Therapeutic Class: Calcium-channel blocker; Antianginal

CLINICAL PHARMACOLOGY

Mechanism of Action: Inhibits both calcium and sodium ion flux across cell membrane during cardiac depolarization; produces relaxation of coronary vascular smooth muscle; dilates coronary arteries; slows SA/AV node conduction times; dilates peripheral arteries; hemodynamics: decreases myocardial contractility, no effect on cardiac output, decreases peripheral vascular resistance

Pharmacokinetics

PO: Peak serum concentration 2-3 hr, 99% bound to plasma proteins, $t_{1/2}$ 24 hr; completely metabolized in the liver, excreted in urine and feces

INDICATIONS AND USES: Chronic stable angina; because of potential side effects (ventricular arrhythmias, agranulocytosis), should be reserved for patients who are unresponsive to, or intolerant of, other antianginal medication; may be used alone or in combination with β-blockers and/or nitrates

DOSAGE

Adult

• PO 200 mg qd initially, increase after 10 days depending on response, max 400 mg/day; most patients maintained on 300 mg/day

$ AVAILABLE FORMS/COST OF THERAPY

• Tab, Plain Coated—Oral: 200 mg, 100's: **$331.57;** 300 mg, 90's: **$330.91**

---

italic = common side effects   ***bold italic*** = life-threatening reactions

CONTRAINDICATIONS: Sick sinus syndrome, 2nd or 3rd degree heart block, Wolff-Parkinson-White syndrome, hypotension <90 mm Hg systolic, uncompensated cardiac insufficiency, history of serious ventricular dysrhythmias, congenital QT interval prolongation or taking other drugs that prolong QT interval

PRECAUTIONS: CHF, renal disease, hepatic disease, children, hypokalemia, left bundle branch block, sinus bradycardia, recent MI

PREGNANCY AND LACTATION: Pregnancy category C; excreted in breast milk; use caution in nursing mothers

SIDE EFFECTS/ADVERSE REACTIONS

CNS: Anxiety, *asthenia,* confusion, depression, *dizziness,* drowsiness, fatigue, *headache,* insomnia, lightheadedness, nervousness, tremor, weakness

CV: **AV block,** bradycardia, CHF, **dysrhythmia (torsades de pointes, ventricular tachycardia),** edema, hypotension, palpitations

EENT: Blurred vision, tinnitus

GI: Constipation, *diarrhea,* dry mouth, *gastric upset,* increased liver function studies, *nausea,* vomiting

GU: Nocturia, polyuria

HEME: **Agranulocytosis** (rare)

RESP: Shortness of breath

SKIN: Rash

INTERACTIONS

Drugs

❸ *Beta-blockers:* Additive depressant effects on myocardial contractility or AV conduction

❸ *Digitalis glycosides:* Reduced clearance; increased digitalis levels; potential toxicity

SPECIAL CONSIDERATIONS

PATIENT/FAMILY EDUCATION

• ECGs will be necessary during initiation of therapy and after dosage changes

• Notify provider immediately for irregular heartbeat, shortness of breath, pronounced dizziness, constipation, or hypotension

• May be taken with food or meals

MONITORING PARAMETERS

• Blood pressure, pulse, respiration, ECG intervals (PR, QRS, QT) at initiation of therapy and again after dosage increases prologation of QT interval by >0.52 sec predisposes to proarrhythmia

• Serum potassium (normalize before initiation)

---

beractant

(ber-akt'ant)

Rx: Survanta

Chemical Class: Phospholipid
Therapeutic Class: Natural bovine lung surfactant

CLINICAL PHARMACOLOGY

Mechanism of Action: Prevents alveoli from collapsing during expiration by lowering surface tension between air and alveolar surfaces

Pharmacokinetics

Most of the dose probably becomes lung-associated within hours of administration; the lipids enter endogenous surfactant pathways of reutilization and recycling

INDICATIONS AND USES: Prevention and treatment (rescue) of respiratory distress syndrome (RDS) in premature infants

DOSAGE

Infant

• Administer through a number 5 French end-hole catheter inserted into the endotracheal tube with the tip protruding just beyond the end of the endotracheal tube, divide each dose into quarters and administer with infant in different positions

• *Prophylactic treatment:* Intratracheal 4 ml/kg as soon as possible (preferably within 15 min of birth); as many as 4 doses may be administered during the first 48 hr of life no more frequently than q6h

• *Rescue treatment:* Intratracheal 4 ml/kg as soon as diagnosis of RDS is made (preferably by 8 hr of age)

$ AVAILABLE FORMS/COST OF THERAPY

• Inj—Intratracheal: 25 mg phospholipid/ml, 8 ml: **$807.00**

PRECAUTIONS: Use in infants <600 g birth weight or >1750 g birth weight has not been evaluated in controlled trials; use only in highly supervised clinical settings with immediate availability of clinicians experienced with intubation, ventilator management, and general care of premature infants

SIDE EFFECTS/ADVERSE REACTIONS

CV: Hypertension, *transient bradycardia,* vasoconstriction

RESP: **Apnea,** endotracheal tube reflux and blockage, hypercarbia, hypocarbia, *oxygen desaturation*

SKIN: Pallor

SPECIAL CONSIDERATIONS

• Refrigerate unopened vials (2-8° C); protect from light

MONITORING PARAMETERS

• Continuous ECG and transcutaneous oxygen saturation monitoring during instillation

• Frequent ABG sampling is necessary to prevent postdosing hyperoxia and hypocarbia

betamethasone

(bay-ta-meth′a-sone)

Rx: *Systemic:* Celestone, Celstone Soluspan

Rx: *Topical:* Alphatrex, Betatrex, Diprolene, Diprosone, Luxiq Qualisone, Maxivate, Valisone

Combinations

Rx: with clotrimazole (Lotrisone)

Chemical Class: Synthetic glucocorticoid

Therapeutic Class: Topical corticosteroid, intermediate potency (benzoate [cream, gel, lotion, ointment], valerate [cream, lotion, ointment, powder]), high potency (dipropionate [cream, lotion, ointment, spray]); systemic corticosteroid

CLINICAL PHARMACOLOGY

Mechanism of Action: Decreases inflammation by depressing migration of polymorphonuclear leukocytes and activity of endogenous mediators of inflammation; has many profound metabolic effects; does not possess mineralocorticoid activity

Pharmacokinetics

Extensive metabolism in liver; $t_{1/2}$ 300+ min, duration 36-54 hr

INDICATIONS AND USES:

Systemic: Antiinflammatory or immunosuppressant agent in the treatment of a variety of diseases of hematologic, allergic, inflammatory, neoplastic, and autoimmune origin; Addison's disease, congenital adrenal hyperplasia, thyroiditis, hypercalcemia, serum sickness; prevention of neonatal respiratory distress syndrome (by administration to mother)*

---

italic = common side effects   ***bold italic*** = life-threatening reactions

Topical: Psoriasis, eczema, contact dermatitis, pruritus, and other corticosteroid responsive dermatoses

DOSAGE

Adult

• PO 0.6-7.2 mg/day; IM 0.5-9 mg/day divided q12h (usually ⅓-½ the oral dose); IM (to mother for prophylaxis of infant lung prematurity) 12.5 mg q24h × 2 doses; IV (sodium phosphate salt only) up to 9 mg; Intra-articular and soft tissue (sodium phosphate/acetate salt): large joints 6-12 mg (1-2 ml), smaller joints 1.5-3 mg (0.25-1 ml), bursitis 6 mg, ganglia 3 mg, tendonitis 1.5-3 mg; TOP apply to affected area bid-tid

Child

• PO 0.0175-0.25 mg/kg/day divided q6-8h or 0.5-7.5 mg/m²/day divided q6-8h; IM 0.0175-0.125 mg base/kg/day divided q6-12h or 0.5-7.5 mg/m²/day divided q6-12h; TOP apply to affected area bid-tid

💲 AVAILABLE FORMS/COST OF THERAPY

• Syr—Oral: 0.6 mg/5 ml, 120 ml: **$44.14**
• Tab—Oral: 0.6 mg, 100's: **$158.67-$176.70**
• Inj, Susp (sodium phosphate)—Intra-articular, Intradermal, IM: 3 mg/ml, 5 ml: **$4.25-$17.95**
• Cre (dipropionate)—Top: 0.05%, 15, 45 g: **$8.95-$43.18**/45 g
• Lotion (dipropionate)—Top: 0.05%, 20, 60 ml: **$11.27-$62.89**/60 ml
• Oint (dipropionate)—Top: 0.05%, 15, 45 g: **$7.50-$47.63**/45 g
• Aer, Spray (dipropionate)—Top: 0.1%, 85 g: **$25.97**
• Cre, Augmented (dipropionate)—Top: 0.05%, 15, 45 g, 50 g: **$30.05**/15 g
• Gel, Augmented (dipropionate)—Top: 0.05%, 15, 50 g: **$69.88**/50 g

• Lotion, Augmented (dipropionate)—Top: 0.05%, 30, 60 ml: **$35.84**/30 ml
• Oint, Augmented (dipropionate)—Top: 0.05%, 15, 45 g, 50 g: **$41.42**/45 g
• Cre (valerate)—Top: 0.1%, 15, 45 g: **$5.59-$35.28**/45 g
• Lotion (valerate)—Top: 0.1%, 20, 60 ml: **$7.80-$47.38**/60 ml
• Oint (valerate)—Top: 0.1%, 15, 45 g: **$2.51-$35.28**/45 g
• Powder (valerate): 5 g: **$106.88**

CONTRAINDICATIONS: Systemic fungal infection; use on face, groin, or axilla (topical)

PRECAUTIONS: Psychosis, diabetes mellitus, glaucoma, osteoporosis, seizure disorders, ulcerative colitis (intestinal perforation), CHF, hypertension, myesthenia gravis (if used with anticholinesterase agents), renal disease, esophagitis, peptic ulcer, latent tuberculosis or amebiasis (reactivation of disease)

PREGNANCY AND LACTATION: Pregnancy category C; used in patients with premature labor at about 24-36 wk gestation to stimulate fetal lung maturation (see dosage); excreted in breast milk, could suppress infant's growth and interfere with endogenous corticosteroid production

SIDE EFFECTS/ADVERSE REACTIONS

CNS: Depression, headache, *mood changes,* **seizures,** vertigo
CV: **CHF,** hypertension, tachycardia, thromboembolism, thrombophlebitis
EENT: Blurred vision, cataracts, increased intraocular pressure
GI: Abdominal distention, diarrhea, **hemorrhage,** increased appetite, *nausea,* **pancreatitis**
METAB: Cushingoid state, decreased glucose tolerance, growth suppression in children, ***HPA suppression***

MS: Aseptic necrosis of femoral and humeral heads, fractures, muscle mass loss, osteoporosis, weakness
SKIN: Acne, allergic contact dermatitis, atrophy, bruising, burning, dryness, ecchymosis, folliculitis, hypertrichosis, hypopigmentation, irritation, itching, miliaria, perioral dermatitis, petechiae, poor wound healing, secondary infection, striae, suppression of skin test reactions

INTERACTIONS

Drugs

3 *Aminoglutethamide:* Enhanced elimination of corticosteroids; marked reduction in corticosteroid response; increased clearance of prednisone; doubling of dose may be necessary

3 *Antidiabetics:* Increased blood glucose

3 *Barbiturates, carbamazepine:* Reduced serum concentrations of corticosteroids; increased clearance of prednisone

3 *Cholestyramine, colestipol:* Possible reduced absorption of corticosteroids

3 *Cyclosporine:* Possible increased concentration of both drugs, seizures

3 *Erythromycin, troleandomycin, clarithromycin, ketoconazole:* Possible enhanced steroid effect

3 *Estrogens, oral contraceptives:* Enhanced effects of corticosteroids

3 *Isoniazid:* Reduced plasma concentrations of isoniazid

3 *IUDs:* Inhibition of inflammation may decrease contraceptive effect

3 *NSAIDs:* Increased risk GI ulceration

3 *Rifampin:* Reduced therapeutic effect of corticosteroids; may reduce hepatic clearance of prednisone

3 *Salicylates:* Subtherapeutic salicylate concentrations possible

Labs

• *False negative:* Skin allergy tests

SPECIAL CONSIDERATIONS

• Recommend single daily doses in AM

• Signs of adrenal insufficiency include fatigue, anorexia, nausea, vomiting, diarrhea, weight loss, weakness, dizziness and low blood sugar; drug-induced secondary adrenocorticoid insufficiency may be minimized by gradual systemic dosage reduction; relative insufficiency may exist for up to 1 yr after discontinuation of therapy; be prepared to supplement in situations of stress

• May mask infections

• Do not give live virus vaccines to patients on prolonged therapy

• Patients on chronic steroid therapy should wear medic alert bracelet

• Do not use topical products on weeping, denuded, or infected areas

MONITORING PARAMETERS

• Serum K and glucose

• Growth of children on prolonged therapy

betaxolol
(bay-tax'oh-lol)
Rx: Betoptic, Betoptic S, Kerlone
Chemical Class: β_1-selective (cardioselective) adrenoreceptor blocker
Therapeutic Class: Antihypertensive; antiglaucoma agent

CLINICAL PHARMACOLOGY
Mechanism of Action: Preferentially competes with β-adrenergic agonists for available β_1-receptor sites inhibiting the chronotropic and inotropic responses to β_1-adrenergic stimulation (cardioselective); blocks

β_2 receptors in bronchial system at higher doses; weak membrane stabilizing activity; lacks intrinsic sympathomimetic (partial agonist) activity; reduces aqueous humor production; slight increase in outflow may be an additional mechanism; little or no effect on pupil size or accommodation

Pharmacokinetics

PO: Peak 1.5-6 hr

OPHTH: Onset 30 min, duration 12 hr 50% protein bound; metabolized by liver, excreted in urine as metabolites and unchanged drug; $t_{1/2}$ 14-22 hr

INDICATIONS AND USES: Hypertension; chronic open-angle glaucoma

DOSAGE

Adult

• PO 10 mg qd, increased to 20 mg qd after 7-14 days if desired response is not achieved; doses >20 mg/day have not produced additional antihypertensive effect

• OPHTH 1 gtt bid

Elderly

• PO reduce initial dose to 5 mg qd

$ AVAILABLE FORMS/COST OF THERAPY

• Susp—Ophth: 0.25%, 2.5, 5, 10, 15 ml: **$24.75/5 ml**

• Sol—Ophth: 0.5%, 2.5, 5, 10, 15 ml: **$24.75/5 ml**

• Tab, Plain Coated—Oral: 10 mg, 100's: **$87.49;** 20 mg, 100's: **$131.20**

CONTRAINDICATIONS: Cardiogenic shock, 2nd or 3rd degree heart block, sinus bradycardia, CHF unless secondary to a tachydysrhythmia treatable with β-blockers

PRECAUTIONS: Major surgery, diabetes mellitus, renal disease, thyroid disease, COPD, asthma, well-compensated heart failure, abrupt withdrawal, peripheral vascular disease; ophthalmic preparations can be absorbed systemically

PREGNANCY AND LACTATION: Pregnancy category C; excretion into breast milk unknown; use caution in nursing mothers

SIDE EFFECTS/ADVERSE REACTIONS

CNS: Depression, *dizziness,* drowsiness, *fatigue,* hallucinations, insomnia, *lethargy,* memory loss, mental changes, strange dreams

CV: Bradycardia, **CHF,** cold extremities, profound hypotension, **2nd or 3rd degree heart block**

EENT: Blepharoptosis, diplopia, dry burning eyes, keratitis, ptosis, sore throat, visual disturbances

GI: Diarrhea, dry mouth, **ischemic colitis, mesenteric arterial thrombosis,** nausea, vomiting

GU: Impotence, sexual dysfunction

HEME: **Agranulocytosis, thrombocytopenia**

METAB: Hyperlipidemia (increase TG, total cholesterol, LDL; decrease HDL), masked hypoglycemic response to insulin (sweating excepted)

RESP: **Bronchospasm,** dyspnea

SKIN: Alopecia, pruritis, rash

INTERACTIONS

Drugs

3 *Adenosine:* Increased risk of bradycardic response

3 *Antacids:* Decreased absorption of oral betaxolol

3 *Antidiabetics:* Altered response to hypoglycemia, prolonged recovery of normoglycemia, hypertension, blockade of tachycardia; may increase blood glucose and impair peripheral circulation

3 *Dipyridamole:* Bradycardia

3 *Neostigmine:* Additive risk of bradycardia

B

3 *NSAIDs:* Reduced hypotensive effects of β-blockers

3 *Tacrine:* Additive bradycardia

3 *Theophylline:* Antagonistic pharmacodynamic effects

3 *Verapamil:* Enhanced effects of both drugs, particularly atrioventricular conduction slowings

SPECIAL CONSIDERATIONS

• Do not discontinue oral drug abruptly, may precipitate angina or MI

• Anaphylactic reactions may be more severe and not be as responsive to usual doses of epinephrine

• Transient stinging/discomfort is relatively common with ophthalmic preparations, notify clinician if severe

MONITORING PARAMETERS

• Blood pressure, pulse, intraocular pressure (ophth)

---

bethanechol

(be-than'e-kole)
Rx: Duvoid, Urecholine
Chemical Class: Synthetic choline ester
Therapeutic Class: Cholinergic stimulant

CLINICAL PHARMACOLOGY

Mechanism of Action: Stimulates muscarinic acetylcholine receptors directly mimicking the effects of parasympathetic nervous system stimulation; stimulates gastric motility and micturition

Pharmacokinetics

PO: Onset 30-90 min, duration 1-6 hr
SC: Onset 5-15 min, duration 1 hr

INDICATIONS AND USES: Acute postoperative and postpartum non-obstructive (functional) urinary retention; neurogenic atony of

the urinary bladder with retention; gastric atony or stasis*; congenital megacolon*; gastroesophageal reflux*

DOSAGE

Adult

• PO 10-50 mg bid-qid; SC 2.5-5 mg tid-qid, up to 7.5-10 mg q4h for neurogenic bladder

Child

• *Abdominal distention or urinary retention:* PO 0.6 mg/kg/day divided tid-qid

• *Gastroesophageal reflux:* PO 0.1-0.2 mg/kg/dose given 30 min to 1 hr before each meal, max qid; SC 0.12-0.2 mg/kg/day divided tid-qid

$ **AVAILABLE FORMS/COST OF THERAPY**

• Tab, Uncoated—Oral: 5 mg, 100's: **$2.75-$39.44**; 10 mg, 100's: **$2.95-$80.88**; 25 mg, 100's: **$3.95-$125.53**; 50 mg, 100's: **$7.25-$194.18**

• Inj, Sol—SC: 5 mg/ml, 1 ml: **$5.44**

CONTRAINDICATIONS: Severe bradycardia, asthma, severe hypotension, hypertension, hyperthyroidism, peptic ulcer, parkinsonism, seizure disorders, coronary artery disease, coronary occlusion, mechanical bladder neck obstruction, possible GI obstruction, peritonitis, recent urinary or GI surgery, atrioventricular conduction defects, vasomotor instability, IM/IV inj

PRECAUTIONS: Child <8 yr, urinary retention due to obstruction; not for IM or IV administrations (severe cholinergic overstimulation)

PREGNANCY AND LACTATION: Pregnancy category C; abdominal pain and diarrhea have been reported in a nursing infant exposed to bethanechol in milk; use caution in nursing mothers

---

italic = common side effects   ***bold italic*** = life-threatening reactions

SIDE EFFECTS/ADVERSE REACTIONS

More common after SC injection

CNS: Dizziness, headache, light-headedness or fainting

CV: Fall in blood pressure with reflex tachycardia, vasomotor response

EENT: Lacrimation, miosis

GI: Abdominal cramps, *belching,* borborygmi, colicky pain, *diarrhea, nausea,* salivation

GU: Urinary urgency

RESP: **Bronchospasm, may precipitate asthmatic attack**

SKIN: Flushing, sweating

MISC: Malaise

INTERACTIONS

Drugs

3 β*-blockers:* Additive bradycardia

3 *Tacrine:* Increased cholinergic effects

SPECIAL CONSIDERATIONS

• Recommend taking on an empty stomach to avoid nausea and vomiting

---

biperiden

(bye-per'i-den)

Rx: Akineton

Chemical Class: Tertiary amine

Therapeutic Class: Anticholinergic; anti-Parkinson's agent

CLINICAL PHARMACOLOGY

Mechanism of Action: Blocks striated cholinergic receptors, which helps balance cholinergic and dopaminergic activity

Pharmacokinetics

PO: Onset 1 hr, duration 6-10 hr

INDICATIONS AND USES: Adjunctive treatment of all forms of Parkinson's syndrome; drug-induced extrapyramidal symptoms

DOSAGE

Adult

• *Parkinson symptoms:* PO 2 mg tid-qid; max 16 mg/24 hr

• *Extrapyramidal symptoms:* PO 2 mg qd-tid

💲 AVAILABLE FORMS/COST OF THERAPY

• Tab, Uncoated—Oral: 2 mg, 100's: **$29.76**

CONTRAINDICATIONS: Narrow-angle glaucoma, myasthenia gravis, GI/GU obstruction, megacolon, stenosing peptic ulcers, prostatic hypertrophy

PRECAUTIONS: Elderly, tachycardia, dysrhythmias, liver or kidney disease, drug abuse, hypotension, hypertension, psychiatric patients; give parenteral dose with patient recumbent to prevent postural hypotension; isolated instances of mental confusion, euphoria, agitation, and disturbed behavior have been reported in susceptible patients

PREGNANCY AND LACTATION: Pregnancy category C; breast milk excretion not known, nursing infants particularly sensitive to anticholinergic effects

SIDE EFFECTS/ADVERSE REACTIONS

CNS: Anxiety, confusion, delusions, depression, dizziness, euphoria, hallucinations, headache, incoherence, irritability, memory loss, restlessness, sedation, tremor

CV: Bradycardia, palpitations, postural hypotension, tachycardia

EENT: Angle-closure glaucoma, blurred vision, difficulty swallowing, dilated pupils, increased intraocular tension, mydriasis, photophobia

GI: Abdominal distress, *constipation, dry mouth,* nausea, **paralytic ileus,** vomiting

GU: Dysuria, hesitancy, retention

MS: Cramping, weakness

---

* = non-FDA-approved use

SKIN: Dermatoses, rash, urticaria
MISC: Decreased sweating, flushing, heat stroke, hyperthermia, increased temperature, numbness of fingers

INTERACTIONS
Drugs
❸ *Amantadine:* Potentiates CNS side effect of amantadine
❸ *Anticholinergics:* Increased anticholinergic effects
❸ *Neuroleptics:* Inhibition of therapeutic response to neuroleptics; excessive anticholinergic effects
❸ *Tacrine:* Reduced therapeutic effects of both drugs

SPECIAL CONSIDERATIONS
PATIENT/FAMILY EDUCATION
• May increase susceptibility to heat-stroke
• Do not discontinue drug abruptly; taper off over 1 wk

---

bisacodyl
(bis-a-koe′dill)
OTC: Bisac-Evac, Bisco-Lax, Dulagen, Dulcolax, Fleet Bisacodyl
Chemical Class: Diphenylmethane derivative
Therapeutic Class: Stimulant laxative

CLINICAL PHARMACOLOGY
Mechanism of Action: Acts directly on intestine by increasing motor activity; irritates colonic intramural plexus
Pharmacokinetics
PO: Onset 6-8 hr
PR: Onset 15-60 min
Absorption is minimal; absorbed drug metabolized by liver; excreted in urine, bile, feces, breast milk

INDICATIONS AND USES: Short-term treatment of constipation; bowel or rectal preparation for surgery, examination

DOSAGE
Adult
• PO 5-15 mg; up to 30 mg for bowel or rect preparation; PR 10 mg, 37.5 ml enema
Child
• PO 5-10 mg (or 0.3 mg/kg) for age >3 yr; PR 5-10 mg for age 2-11 yr; 5 mg for age <2 yr

⚡ AVAILABLE FORMS/COST OF THERAPY
• Tab, Enteric Coated—Oral: 5 mg, 100's: **$2.80-$16.88**
• Supp—Rect: 10 mg, 12's: **$2.63-$8.40**
• Liq—Rect: 10 mg/37.5 ml: **$1.10**

CONTRAINDICATIONS: Rectal fissures, abdominal pain, nausea, vomiting, appendicitis, acute surgical abdomen, ulcerated hemorrhoids, acute hepatitis, fecal impaction, intestinal/biliary tract obstruction

PREGNANCY AND LACTATION: Pregnancy category B; excreted in breast milk

SIDE EFFECTS/ADVERSE REACTIONS
GI: Anorexia, cramps, diarrhea, *nausea,* rectal burning (suppositories), *vomiting*
METAB: Alkalosis, hypokalemia, protein-losing enteropathy, ***tetany***
MS: Muscle weakness

DRUG INTERACTIONS
Labs
• Glucose: Low with Clinistix, Diastix; no effect with Tes-tape

SPECIAL CONSIDERATIONS
PATIENT/FAMILY EDUCATION
• Do not take within 1 hr of antacids or milk

---

bismuth subsalicylate
(bis'meth)

OTC: Pepto-Bismol, Pink Bismuth

Combinations:

Rx: with metronidazole, tetracycline (Helidac)

Chemical Class: Salicylate derivative

Therapeutic Class: Antidiarrheal; gastrointestinal antiulcer agent

CLINICAL PHARMACOLOGY

Mechanism of Action: Inhibits prostaglandin synthesis responsible for GI hypermotility (salicylate moiety); bismuth moiety may have direct antimicrobial effect

Pharmacokinetics

PO: Onset 1 hr, peak 2 hr, duration 4 hr; salicylate moiety absorbed (262 mg bismuth subsalicylate yields 102 mg salicylate)

INDICATIONS AND USES: Diarrhea; indigestion; nausea, abdominal cramps, prevention of travelers' diarrhea; as part of combination therapy for *Helicobacter pylori;* infantile diarrhea*

DOSAGE

Adult

• *Diarrhea:* PO 30 ml or 2 tabs q30-60 min; not to exceed 8 doses for >2 days

• *Prevention of travelers' diarrhea:* PO 30 ml or 2 tabs qid

• *Helicobacter pylori:* PO 2 tabs qid (in combination with other agents)

Child

• *Diarrhea:* Age 9-12 yr PO 15 ml or 1 tab q30-60 min, not to exceed 8 doses for >2 days; Age 6-9 yr PO 10 ml or ⅔ tab q30-60 min, not to exceed 8 doses for >2 days; Age 3-6 yr PO 5 ml or ⅓ tab q30-60 min, not to exceed 8 doses for >2 days

⚡ AVAILABLE FORMS/COST OF THERAPY

• Tab, Chewable—Oral: 262 mg, 30's: **$1.45-$3.15**

• Susp—Oral: 262 mg/15 ml, 240 ml: **$1.50-$2.86**; 524 mg/15 ml, 240 ml: **$1.65-$4.03**

CONTRAINDICATIONS: Child <3 yr

PRECAUTIONS: Anticoagulant therapy; stop use if symptoms do not improve within 2 days or become worse, or if diarrhea is accompanied by high fever or severe abdominal pain

PREGNANCY AND LACTATION: Pregnancy category C; salicylate excreted in breast milk

SIDE EFFECTS/ADVERSE REACTIONS

CNS: Confusion, twitching

EENT: Blue gums, hearing loss, metallic taste, tinnitus

GI: Black tongue, *dark stools,* fecal impaction (high doses)

HEME: Increased bleeding time

INTERACTIONS

Drugs

❷ *Tetracyclines:* Decreased absorption of tetracyclines

Labs

• *Color:* Blackens or discolors stool

• *Glucose (urine):* Interferes with Benedict's reaction

SPECIAL CONSIDERATIONS
PATIENT/FAMILY EDUCATION

• Chew or dissolve in mouth; do not swallow whole

• Shake suspension before using

---

* = non-FDA-approved use

bisoprolol
(bis-ope'pro-lal)
Rx: Zebeta
Combinations
  Rx: with
  hydrochlorothiazide: (Ziac)
Chemical Class: β_1-selective
(cardioselective) adrenoreceptor blocker
Therapeutic Class: Antihypertensive

CLINICAL PHARMACOLOGY
Mechanism of Action: Competitive β-adrenergic antagonist at β_1-
receptor sites (cardioselective at
usual doses; β_2-blockade noted at
doses >20 mg); produces negative
inotropic and chronotropic responses; slow AV nodal conduction; decreses heart rate; decreases
myocardial oxygen consumption;
antiarrhythmic effects (class II); reduction in platelet aggregation and
blood viscosity; suppression of renin release; inhibition of central sympathetic outflow; decreases presynaptic receptor neurotransmitter release; no intrinsic sympathomimetic,
or membrane stabilizing activity;
low to moderate lipid solubility
Pharmacokinetics
PO: Peak plasma level 2-4 hr, plasma
$t_{1/2}$ 9-12 hr; 50% excreted unchanged
in urine; protein binding 30%; metabolized in liver to inactive metabolites; full antihypertensive effect after 1 wk of therapy; if creatinine clearance <40 ml/min, plasma
$t_{1/2}$ tripled; in cirrhotics, plasma $t_{1/2}$ is
8.3 to 21.7 hours
INDICATIONS AND USES: Angina
pectoris,* postmyocardial infarction,* hypertension, migraine
headache,* psychiatric disorders*
(anxiety,* performance anxiety,*

panic attacks,* neuroleptic induced
akathisia*)
DOSAGE
Adult and Child >16 yr
• *Hypertension:* PO 5-20 mg qd;
reduce dose in renal or hepatic impairment
💲 AVAILABLE FORMS/COST OF THERAPY
• Tab, Plain Coated—Oral: 5 mg,
30's: **$33.60;** 10 mg, 30's: **$33.60**
• Tab, Plain Coated—Oral: with hydrochlorothiazide: 2.5 mg/6.25 mg,
100's: **$112.03;** 5 mg/6.25 mg,
100's: **$112.03;** 10 mg/6.25 mg,
30's: **$33.61**
CONTRAINDICATIONS: Cardiogenic shock, heart block (2nd, 3rd
degree), sinus bradycardia, overt cardiac failure
PRECAUTIONS: Anesthesia/
surgery (myocardial depression),
avoid abrupt withdrawal; bronchospastic airways, congestive heart
failure, diabetes mellitus, hyper-
thyroidism/thyrotoxicosis (bisoprolol, unlike propranolol, does not
decrease T_3 levels), concurrent clonidine (discontinue bisoprolol several days prior to withdrawal of clonidine), peripheral vascular disease,
renal disease
PREGNANCY AND LACTATION:
Pregnancy category C; similar
drug, atenolol frequently used in the
third trimester for treatment of hypertension (many studies of efficacy and safety of atenolol in
pregnancy-induced hypertension);
long-term use has been associated
with intrauterine growth retardation; excreted into breast milk; observe for signs of beta-blockade
**SIDE EFFECTS/ADVERSE REAC-
TIONS**
CNS: Catatonia, depression, dizziness, drowsiness, *fatigue,* hallucinations, headache, insomnia, lethargy, memory loss, mental changes,

peripheral neuropathy, strange dreams, vertigo

CV: Bradycardia, *CHF,* cold extremities, postural hypotension, *profound hypotension, 2nd or 3rd degree heart block, ventricular dysrhythmias*

EENT: Dry burning eyes, rhinitis, sinusitis, sore throat

GI: Diarrhea, flatulence, gastric pain, gastritis, increased AST/ALT (1-2 times normal in 4%), ischemic colitis, mesenteric arterial thrombosis, nausea, vomiting

GU: Decreased libido, impotence

HEME: Purpura

METAB: Azotemia, hyperglycemia, hyperkalemia, hypertriglyceridemia, hyperuricemia, increased hypoglycemic response to insulin

MS: Arthralgia, joint pain

RESP: **Bronchospasm,** cough, dyspnea, wheezing

SKIN: Alopecia, fever, pruritus, rash, sweating

MISC: Decreased exercise tolerance, edema, facial swelling, weight gain

INTERACTIONS

Drugs

3 *Adenosine:* Additive bradycardia

3 *Alpha-1 adrenergic blockers:* Potential enhanced first dose response [marked initial drop in blood pressure, particularly on standing (especially prazocin)]

3 *Amiodarone:* Increased bradycardic effect of bisoprolol

3 *Antidiabetics:* Reduced response to hypoglycemia (sweating persists)

3 *Barbiturates:* Enhanced bisoprolol metabolism

3 *Cimetidine:* Plasma levels of β-blocker may be elevated

3 *Cocaine:* Bisprolol potentiates cocaine-induced coronary vasoconstriction

3 *Contrast media:* Increased risk for anaphylaxis

3 *Digoxin, digitoxin:* Potentiation of bradycardia; additive prolongation of atrioventricular (AV) conduction time

3 *Dipyridamole:* Additive bradycardia

3 *Disopyramide:* Additive decreases in cardiac output

3 *Fluoxetine:* Fluoxetine inhibits CYPD26, partially responsible for bisoprolol metabolism; increased β-blocker effects

3 *Lidocaine:* β-blocker-induced reductions in cardiac output and hepatic blood flow may yield increased lidocaine concentrations

3 *Neostigmine:* Additive bradycardia

3 *Neuroleptics:* Decreased bisoprolol metabolism; decreased neuroleptic metabolism

3 *NSAIDs:* Reduced antihypertensive effect

3 *Physostigmine:* Additive bradycardia

3 *Prazosin:* Enhanced 1st-dose response to prazosin

3 *Rifampin:* Increases clearance by 51%, reduced β-blocker effects

3 *Tacrine:* Additive bradycardia

2 *Theophylline:* Bisoprolol reduces clearance of theophylline; antagonistic pharmacodynamics

SPECIAL CONSIDERATIONS

• Property of competitive cardioselectivity yields less bronchospastic adverse effects

MONITORING PARAMETERS

• Arrhythmias: Heart rate
• Hypertension: Blood pressure
• Migraine headache: Reduction in the frequency, severity, and duration of attacks
• Postmyocardial infarction: Left ventricular function, lower resting heart rate
• Toxicity: Blood glucose, bronchospasm, hypotension, bradycardia, de-

---

pression, confusion, hallucination, sexual dysfunction

---

bitolterol
(bye-tole'ter-ol)
Rx: Tornalate
Chemical Class: Sympathomimetic amine; β_2-adrenergic agonist
Therapeutic Class: Antiasthmatic, bronchodilator

CLINICAL PHARMACOLOGY
Mechanism of Action: Causes bronchodilation by β_2-stimulation, resulting in relaxation of bronchial smooth muscle; inhibits mast cell degranulation; stimulates cilia to remove secretions
Pharmacokinetics
INH: Onset 3 min, peak 30-60 min, duration 5-8 hr; bitolterol is a prodrug that is hydrolyzed by esterases in tissue and blood to the active moiety colterol
INDICATIONS AND USES: Prophylaxis and treatment of bronchial asthma and reversible bronchospasm
DOSAGE
Adult and Child >12 yr
• *Bronchospasm:* MDI 1-3 puffs at intervals of 1-3 min, not to exceed 3 puffs q6h or 2 puffs q4h; via neb 1.5-3.5 mg (continuous flow) or 0.5-1.5 mg (intermittent flow) tid-qid, interval between treatments should not be <4 hr
• *Prophylaxis of bronchospasm:* MDI 2 puffs at intervals of 1-3 min q8h
$ **AVAILABLE FORMS/COST OF THERAPY**
• MDI—INH: 0.37 mg/puff, 15 ml in metered dose inhaler: **$43.68**
• Sol—INH: 0.37 mg/0.05 ml, 30 ml: **$15.75;** 0.37 mg/0.05 ml, 60 ml: **$29.85**
PRECAUTIONS: Ischemic heart disease, cardiac dysrhythmias, hyperthyroidism, diabetes mellitus, hypertension
PREGNANCY AND LACTATION: Pregnancy category C; excretion into breast milk unknown
SIDE EFFECTS/ADVERSE REACTIONS
CNS: Dizziness, hallucinations, headache, hyperkinesia, insomnia, lightheadedness, nervousness, *tremors*
CV: Chest discomfort, palpitations, tachycardia
EENT: Throat irritation
GI: Heartburn, nausea
MS: Muscle cramps
RESP: ***Bronchospasm,*** coughing, dyspnea
INTERACTIONS
Drugs
❷ β-*blockers:* Decreased action of bitolterol, cardioselective beta-blockers preferable if concurrent use necessary
❸ *Furosemide:* Potential for additive hypokalemia
SPECIAL CONSIDERATIONS
• No real clinical advantage over less expensive agents (e.g., albuterol, metaproterenol)
PATIENT/FAMILY EDUCATION
• Wash inhaler in warm water and dry qd
• If previously effective dosage regimen fails to provide usual relief, seek medical advice immediately

---

bretylium
(bre-til'ee-um)
Chemical Class: Bromobenzyl quaternary ammonium compound
Therapeutic Class: Antidysrhythmic (class III)

CLINICAL PHARMACOLOGY
Mechanism of Action: Causes an early release of norepinephrine from

---

italic = common side effects   ***bold italic*** = life-threatening reactions

postganglionic nerve terminals, then selectively accumulates in sympathetic ganglia and their postganglionic adrenergic neurons where it inhibits norepinephrine release; suppresses ventricular fibrillation and ventricular dysrhythmias; increases action potential duration and effective refractory period without changes in heart rate

Pharmacokinetics

IV: Onset 5 min for suppression of ventricular fibrillation, onset 20-120 min for suppression of ventricular tachycardia

IM: Onset 20-120 min for suppression of ventricular tachycardia, duration 6-24 hr; 80% excreted unchanged by kidneys in 24 hr

INDICATIONS AND USES: Ventricular tachycardia and other life threatening ventricular dysrhythmias that have failed to respond to 1st-line agents; ventricular fibrillation

DOSAGES

Adult

• *Ventricular fibrillation:* IV bolus 5 mg/kg, then 10 mg/kg repeated q15 min, up to total 30-35 mg/kg; maintenance therapy is IV INF 1-2 mg/min or 5-10 mg/kg over 10 min q6h

• *Ventricular dysrhythmias:* IV INF 500 mg diluted in 50 ml D₅W or NS, infuse over 10-30 min, may repeat in 1 hr, maintain with 1-2 mg/min or 5-10 mg/kg over 10-30 min q6h; IM 5-10 mg/kg undiluted, repeat in 1-2 hr if needed, maintain with same dose q6-8h

Child

• *Ventricular fibrillation:* IV bolus 5 mg/kg, then 10 mg/kg if ventricular fibrillation persists

💲 AVAILABLE FORMS/COST OF THERAPY

• Inj, Sol—IM, IV: 50 mg/ml, 10 ml: **$2.00-$38.71**

CONTRAINDICATIONS: Digitalis toxicity (initial release of norepinephrine caused by bretylium may aggravate digitalis toxicity)

PRECAUTIONS: Renal disease; postural hypotension, hypertension or increased frequency of PVCs and other dysrhythmias may occur transiently in some patients; aortic stenosis, pulmonary hypertension

PREGNANCY AND LACTATION: Pregnancy category C

SIDE EFFECTS/ADVERSE REACTIONS

CNS: Anxiety, confusion, dizziness, psychosis, syncope

CV: Angina, bradycardia, *hypotension, postural hypotension (50%),* PVCs, transient hypertension

GI: Nausea, vomiting

RESP: **Respiratory depression**

INTERACTIONS

Drugs

3 *Catecholamines:* Enhanced pressor effects

3 *Digoxin:* Digitalis toxicity may be aggravated by the initial norepinephrine release

MONITORING PARAMETERS

• ECG, electrolytes, BP

---

brimonidine

(bry-mo'nih-deen)

Rx: Alphagan

Chemical Class: Relatively selective α_2-adrenergic agonist

Therapeutic Class: Antiglaucoma agent

CLINICAL PHARMACOLOGY

Mechanism of Action: Reduces aqueous humor production and increases uveoscleral outflow

Pharmacokinetics

OPHTH: Peak ocular hypotensive effect 2 hr, peak plasma concentration 1-4 hr; metabolized by liver, excreted mainly in urine (74%); $t_{1/2}$ 3 hr

---

INDICATIONS AND USES: Open-angle glaucoma; ocular hypertension; prevention of postoperative increases in intraocular pressure after laser trabeculoplasty

DOSAGE

Adult

OPHTH: 1 gtt in affected eye(s) tid, approximately 8 hr apart

§ AVAILABLE FORMS/COST OF THERAPY

• Sol—Ophth: 0.2%, 5, 10 ml: **$25.94**/5 ml

CONTRAINDICATIONS: Patients receiving MAO inhibitors

PRECAUTIONS: Severe cardiovascular disease, hepatic/renal impairment, depression, cerebral/coronary insufficiency, Raynaud's phenomenon, orthostatic hypotension, thromboangiitis obliterans

PREGNANCY AND LACTATION: Pregnancy category B

SIDE EFFECTS/ADVERSE REACTIONS

CNS: Anxiety, asthenia, depression, dizziness, *drowsiness, fatigue, headache,* insomnia

CV: Hypertension, palpitations, syncope

EENT: Abnormal vision, blepharitis, *blurred vision, burning,* conjunctival blanching, conjunctival discharge, conjunctival edema, conjunctival hemorrhage, corneal staining/erosion, eyelid edema, eyelid erythema, *foreign body sensation,* lid crusting, nasal dryness, ocular ache/pain, ocular dryness, *ocular hyperemia,* ocular irritation, *ocular itching,* photophobia, *stinging,* tearing

GI: Abnormal taste, *dry mouth,* GI symptoms

MS: Muscular pain

SPECIAL CONSIDERATIONS

• Intraocular pressure lowering efficacy tends to wane over time in some patients

PATIENT/FAMILY EDUCATION

• Wait at least 15 min after instilling to insert soft contact lenses (preservative may be adsorbed by soft contact lenses)

---

brinzolamide

(brin-zol'a-mide)

Rx: Azopt

Chemical Class: Sulfonamide derivative

Therapeutic Class: Antiglaucoma agent

CLINICAL PHARMACOLOGY

Mechanism of Action: Inhibition of carbonic anhydrase in ciliary processes of the eye decreases aqueous humor secretion, reducing intraocular pressure

Pharmacokinetics:

OPHTH: Systemically absorbed, amounts below the degree of inhibition anticipated to be necessary for pharmacologic effect on renal function and respiration; 60% bound to plasma proteins; excreted as N-desethyl metabolite and unchanged in urine; $t_{1/2}$ in RBCs, 4 mo

INDICATIONS AND USES: Treatment of elevated intraocular pressure in patients with ocular hypertension or open-angle glaucoma

DOSAGE

Adult

• *OPHTH:* 1 gtt in affected eye(s) tid

§ AVAILABLE FORMS/COST OF THERAPY

• Susp—Ophth: 1%, 5, 10, 15 ml: **$40.75**/10 ml

PRECAUTIONS: Renal/hepatic impairment (severe)

PREGNANCY AND LACTATION: Pregnancy category C; use caution in nursing mothers

---

italic = common side effects   ***bold italic*** = life-threatening reactions

SIDE EFFECTS/ADVERSE REACTIONS

CNS: Headache

EENT: Blurred vision, blepharitis, dry eye, foreign body sensation, ocular discharge, ocular discomfort, ocular keratitis, ocular pain, ocular pruritus, rhinitis

GI: Bitter, sour, or unusual taste

SPECIAL CONSIDERATIONS

• As effective as dorzolamide in lowering intraocular pressure; may be worth trying in patients who complain of burning and stinging with dorzolamide

PATIENT/FAMILY EDUCATION

• Can be administered concomitantly with other top ophth products; separate administration by 10 min

• The preservative in brinzolamide susp, benzalkonium chloride, may be absorbed by soft contact lenses; reinsert lenses>15 min after drug administration

---

bromfenac

(brome-fen-ack′)

Rx: Duract

Chemical Class: Phenylacetic acid derivative

Therapeutic Class: Non-narcotic analgesic, NSAID

CLINICAL PHARMACOLOGY

Mechanism of Action: Inhibits prostaglandin synthetase, inhibiting the inflammatory process

Pharmacokinetics

PO: Onset of analgesia 60 min, duration 6 hrs; 99% protein bound; cleared by kidney; elimination $t_{1/2}$ 30-60 min

INDICATIONS AND USES: Mild to moderate pain, studied in postoperative pain and patients undergoing oral surgery; osteoarthritis and rheumatoid arthritis

DOSAGE

Adult

PO: 25 mg q6-8h

⚡ AVAILABLE FORMS/COST OF THERAPY

• Cap—Oral: 25 mg, 100's: **$103.00**

CONTRAINDICATIONS: Chronic hepatitis

PRECAUTIONS: Renal disease, elderly, diabetes, peptic ulcer disease, GI bleeding

SIDE EFFECTS/ADVERSE REACTIONS

CNS: Dizziness, fatigue, headache, lightheadedness

GI: Abdominal pain, burning in stomach and throat, dry mouth, hepatotoxicity, nausea, vomiting

MISC: Shakiness, sweating, warm feeling in face

DRUG INTERACTIONS

Drugs

❸ *Cholestyramine/Colestipol:* Decreased NSAID absorption

❸ *Cyclosporine, Triamterene:* Enhanced nephrotoxicity

❸ *Lithium:* Increased lithium levels

❷ *Methotrexate:* Increased methotrexate toxicity

❸ *Verapamil:* Reduced verapamil levels

❷ *Oral anticoagulants:* Increased risk GI bleeding

❸ *Aminoglycosides:* Possible increased aminoglycoside levels

❸ β-*blockers, α₁-blockers, Hydralazine:* Possible decreased antihypertensive effect

❸ *Loop Diuretics:* Possible decreased diuretic and antihypertensive efficacy

❸ *ACE Inhibitors:* Possible decreased efficacy ACE inhibitor

❸ *Phenylpropanolamine:* Possible hypertensive reaction

❸ *Corticosteroids:* Increased GI ulceration

SPECIAL CONSIDERATIONS
• Causes less GI blood loss than aspirin, more than placebo; equal analgesia to tramadol, hydrocodone/acetaminophen, naproxen; long-term use (> 10 days) may be limited due to risk of hepatotoxicity

---

bromocriptine
(broe-moe-krip'teen)
Rx: Parlodel
Chemical Class: Ergot alkaloid derivative
Therapeutic Class: Anti-Parkinson's agent; ovulation stimulant; dopaminergic

CLINICAL PHARMACOLOGY
Mechanism of Action: Inhibits prolactin release by activating postsynaptic dopamine receptors; activation of striatal dopamine receptors may be reason for improvement in Parkinson's disease
Pharmacokinetics
PO: Peak 1-3 hr, duration 4-8 hr; 90%-96% protein bound; $t_{1/2}$ 3 hr; metabolized by liver (inactive metabolites), 85%-98% of dose excreted in feces
INDICATIONS AND USES: Hyperprolactinemia-associated dysfunctions (including amenorrhea with or without galactorrhea, infertility, or hypogonadism); prolactin-secreting adenomas (may be used to reduce the tumor mass prior to surgery); female infertility associated with hyperprolactinemia; acromegaly; Parkinson's disease; prevention of physiological lactation* (after parturition when the mother elects not to breast-feed the infant, when breast feeding is contraindicated, after stillbirth or abortion); neuroleptic malignant syndrome,* cocaine addiction*; cyclic mastalgia*

DOSAGE
Adult
• *Hyperprolactinemic indications:* PO 1.25-2.5 mg with meals; may increase by 2.5 mg q3-7 days; usual 5-7.5 mg/day with range from 2.5-15 mg/day
• *Acromegaly:* PO 1.25-2.5 mg qPM with food × 3 days; may increase by 1.25-2.5 mg q3-7 days until optimal therapeutic benefit; usual range 20-30 mg/day; max 100 mg/day (monitor growth hormone levels)
• *Parkinson's disease:* PO 1.25 mg bid with meals; may increase q2-4 wk by 2.5 mg/day; not to exceed 100 mg qd
• *Postpartum lactation:* (After vital signs have stabilized and no sooner than 4 hr after delivery) PO 2.5 mg bid with meals × 14 days; an additional 7 days may be necessary (NOTE: this indication has been withdrawn by the manufacturer)
$ AVAILABLE FORMS/COST OF THERAPY
• Cap, Gel—Oral: 5 mg, 100's: **$268.21-$298.01**
• Tab, Uncoated—Oral: 2.5 mg, 100's: **$156.05-$195.29**
CONTRAINDICATIONS: Severe ischemic disease, uncontrolled hypertension, toxemia of pregnancy, sensitivity to any ergot alkaloids, severe peripheral vascular disease
PRECAUTIONS: Hepatic disease, renal disease, children, pituitary tumors, hypotension, concurrent BP-lowering medications
PREGNANCY AND LACTATION: Pregnancy category D; since it prevents lactation, should not be administered to mothers who elect to breast-feed infants
SIDE EFFECTS/ADVERSE REACTIONS
CNS: Abnormal involuntary movements, anxiety, ataxia, cerebrospinal fluid rhinorrhea (treatment of

prolactinomas), confusion, depression, *dizziness,* drowsiness, fatigue, hallucinations, *headache,* insomnia, nervousness, "on-off" phenomenon, psychosis, restlessness, *seizures,* visual disturbance

CV: Bradycardia, decreased BP, *dysrhythmias,* extrasystole, orthostatic hypotension, palpitation, *shock, stroke*

EENT: Blurred vision, burning eyes, diplopia, nasal congestion

GI: Anorexia, constipation, cramps, diarrhea, dry mouth, *GI hemorrhage, nausea (49%),* vomiting

GU: Diuresis, frequency, incontinence, retention

SKIN: Alopecia, rash on face, arms

INTERACTIONS
Drugs

3 *Erythromycin:* Marked elevations in bromocriptine levels

⚠ *Isometheptene:* Case report of hypertension and ventricular tachycardia with combination

3 *Neuroleptics:* Neuroleptic drugs probably inhibit the ability of bromocriptine to lower serum prolactin concentrations in patients with pituitary adenomas; theoretically, bromocriptine should inhibit the antipsychotic effects of neuroleptic agents, but clinical evidence suggests that this may be uncommon

⚠ *Phenylpropanolamine:* Increased risk of hypertension and seizures

SPECIAL CONSIDERATIONS
• Routine use for suppression of lactation not recommended

PATIENT/FAMILY EDUCATION
• Use measures to prevent orthostatic hypotension

brompheniramine
(brome-fen-ir'a-meen)
Rx: Colhist, ND Stat, Nasahist-B
OTC: Dimetane Extentabs
Combinations
 Rx: with phenylpropanolamine, codeine (Bromanate DC, Bromphen DC with Codeine, Dimetane-DC Cough, Myphetane DC Cough, Polyhistine CS); with pseudoephedrine, dextromethorphan (Bromadine-DM, Bromarest DX, Bromatane DX, Bromfed DM, Bromphen DX, Dimetane DX, Myphetane DX)
 OTC: with phenylpropanolamine (Bromaline, Bromanate, Dimaphen, Dimetane Decongestant, Dimetapp, Vicks DayQuil Allergy); with pseudoephedrine (Bromfed, Drixoral)
Chemical Class: Alkylamine derivative
Therapeutic Class: Antihistamine

CLINICAL PHARMACOLOGY
Mechanism of Action: Decreases allergic response by blocking histamine at H_1-receptors
Pharmacokinetics
PO: Peak 2-5 hr; metabolized in liver, excreted in urine as inactive metabolites; $t_{1/2}$ 12-34 hr

INDICATIONS AND USES: Perennial and seasonal allergic rhinitis (PO); allergic reactions to blood and plasma, adjunctive anaphylactic therapy (parenteral)

DOSAGE
Adult
• PO 4-8 mg tid-qid, not to exceed 24 mg/day; PO TIME REL 8-12 mg bid-tid or 12 mg q12h, not to exceed 24 mg/day; IM/IV/SC 5-20 mg q6-12h, not to exceed 40 mg/day
Child 6-12 yr
• PO 2-4 mg q4-6h, not to exceed 16 mg/day; IM/IV/SC 0.5 mg/kg/day divided q6-8h
Child <6 yr
• PO 0.125 mg/kg/dose q6h, not to exceed 8 mg/day

$ AVAILABLE FORMS/COST OF THERAPY
• Tab, Uncoated—Oral: 4 mg, 100's: **$1.14-$2.95**
• Tab, Ext Rel—Oral: 12 mg, 100's: **$24.38**
• Elixir—Oral: 2 mg/5 ml, 120, 480 ml: **$3.95-$10.28**/480 ml
• Inj, Sol—IM, IV, SC: 10 mg/ml, 10 ml: **$5.50-$14.75**

CONTRAINDICATIONS: Narrow-angle glaucoma, bladder neck obstruction
PRECAUTIONS: Liver disease, elderly, increased intraocular pressure, hyperthyroidism, cardiovascular disease, hypertension, urinary retention, newborn or premature infants, renal disease, stenosed peptic ulcers
PREGNANCY AND LACTATION: Pregnancy category C; an association between 1st trimester exposure and congenital defects has been found in humans; excreted into breast milk, compatible with breast feeding
SIDE EFFECTS/ADVERSE REACTIONS
CNS: Anxiety, confusion, *dizziness, drowsiness,* euphoria, fatigue, neuritis, paresthesia, poor coordination
CV: Hypotension, palpitations, tachycardia

EENT: Blurred vision, dry nose, throat; mydriasis, nasal stuffiness, tinnitus
GI: Anorexia, *constipation,* diarrhea, *dry mouth,* nausea, vomiting
GU: Dysuria, frequency, impotence, retention
HEME: **Agranulocytosis, hemolytic anemia, thrombocytopenia**
RESP: Chest tightness, increased thick secretions, wheezing
SKIN: Photosensitivity
DRUG INTERACTIONS
Labs
• *Aminoacids:* Urine, increase; on thin-layer chromatography
• *Amphetamine:* Urine, increase; false positives
• *False negative:* Skin allergy tests
SPECIAL CONSIDERATIONS
PATIENT/FAMILY EDUCATION
• Do not crush or chew sustained release forms
• Use hard candy, gum, frequent rinsing of mouth for dryness

---

budesonide
(bu-dess'ah-nide)
Rx: Powder INH: Pulmicort Turbuhaler Nasal: Rhinocort Aqua
Chemical Class: Glucocorticoid
Therapeutic Class: Antiasthmatic, antiinflammatory corticosteroid

CLINICAL PHARMACOLOGY
Mechanism of Action: Decreases inflammation by suppression of migration of polymorphonuclear leukocytes, fibroblasts, reversal of increased capillary permeability, and lysosomal stabilization
Pharmacokinetics
INH: 20% of dose reaches systemic circulation; extensive first-pass me-

tabolism, no unchanged drug excreted in urine; peak effect 3-7 days
INDICATIONS AND USES: Management of symptoms of seasonal or perennial rhinitis in adults and children and nonallergic perennial rhinitis in adults (nasal); chronic asthma (oral inhaler)
DOSAGE
Adult
• *Allergic rhinitis:* NASAL INH 2 inh each nostril bid or 4 inh each nostril q AM; when response achieved taper dose q2-4 wks to minimum effective dose
• *Asthma:* ORAL INH 1-4 inh bid
Child ≥6 yr
• Allergic rhinitis: NASAL INH same as adult
• Asthma: ORAL INH 1-2 inh bid
🔳 AVAILABLE FORMS/COST OF THERAPY
• MDI Aer—INH; 200 μg/inh, 200 doses: **$113.42**
• Spray—Nasal INH: 32 μg/inh, 200 doses: **$36.17**
CONTRAINDICATIONS: Treatment of acute asthma
SIDE EFFECTS/ADVERSE REACTIONS
EENT: Dry mouth (nasal use), epistaxsis, nasal irritation, pharyngitis
GI: Difficulty swallowing (oral use), dyspepsia, hoarseness, oral thrush
RESP: Cough
SPECIAL CONSIDERATIONS
• May allow discontinuation of chronic systemic corticosteroids in many patients with asthma
• 3-7 days required for maximum benefit (nasal)
PATIENT/FAMILY EDUCATION
• To be used on regular basis, not for acute symptoms
• Use bronchodilators before oral inhaler (for patients using both)
• Nasal vehicle may cause rhinitis

MONITORING PARAMETERS
• Monitor children for growth as well as for effects on the HPA axis during chronic therapy
• Monitor patients switched from chronic systemic corticosteroids to avoid acute adrenal insufficiency in response to stress

---

bumetanide
(byoo-met′a-nide)
Rx: Bumex
Chemical Class: Sulfonamide derivative
Therapeutic Class: Loop diuretic

CLINICAL PHARMACOLOGY
Mechanism of Action: Inhibits sodium and chloride reabsorption in the ascending limb of the loop of Henle; potassium excretion is increased in a dose-related fashion; more chloruretic than natriuretic; may have an additional action in the proximal tubule
Pharmacokinetics
PO: Onset 0.5-1 hr, duration 4 hr
IM: Onset 40 min, duration 4 hr
IV: Onset 5 min, duration 0.5-1 hr
94-96% bound to plasma proteins; excreted by kidneys; $t_{1/2}$ 1-1.5 hr
INDICATIONS AND USES: Edema (congestive heart failure, hepatic cirrhosis, nephrotic syndrome); hypertension; adult nocturia*
DOSAGE
Adult
• PO 0.5-2.0 mg qd, may give 2nd or 3rd dose at 4-5 hr intervals up to max of 20 mg/day, may be given on alternate days or intermittently; IV/IM 0.5-1.0 mg/day, may give 2nd or 3rd dose at 2-3 hr intervals up to max of 10 mg/day
Child >6 months
• PO/IM/IV 0.015 mg/kg/dose qd

or qod, maximum 0.1 mg/kg/day or 10 mg

💲 AVAILABLE FORMS/COST OF THERAPY

• Inj, Sol—IM, IV: 0.25 mg/ml, 2 ml: **$1.26-$1.88**
• Tab, Uncoated—Oral: 0.5 mg, 100's: **$27.18-$31.91;** 1 mg, 100's: **$38.15-$44.81;** 2 mg, 100's: **$64.53-$75.74**

CONTRAINDICATIONS: Anuria, hepatic coma, severe electrolyte depletion

PRECAUTIONS: Fluid and electrolyte imbalance (including sodium, chloride, potassium, magnesium, calcium), renal disease, hepatic disease (may precipitate hepatic encephalopathy), gout, COPD, lupus erythematosus, diabetes mellitus, hyperparathyroidism, vomiting, diarrhea, elevated cholesterol/triglycerides

PREGNANCY AND LACTATION: Pregnancy category C; cardiovascular disorders such as pulmonary edema, severe hypertension, or CHF are probably the only valid indications for loop diuretics during pregnancy; excretion into breast milk unknown

SIDE EFFECTS/ADVERSE REACTIONS

CNS: Dizziness, fatigue, headache, *vertigo,* weakness
CV: ECG changes, *hypotension*
EENT: Blurred vision, ear pain, ototoxicity, tinnitus
GI: Abdominal pain, anorexia, cramps, diarrhea, dry mouth, *nausea,* upset stomach, vomiting
GU: Glycosuria, *polyuria,* **renal failure,** sexual dysfunction
HEME: **Thrombocytopenia**
METAB: Hyperglycemia, hyperuricemia, hypocalcemia, hypochloremic alkalosis, *hypokalemia,* hypomagnesemia, hyponatremia

MS: Arthritis, hyperuricemia, *muscular cramps,* stiffness, tenderness
SKIN: Photosensitivity, pruritus, purpura, rash, **Stevens-Johnson syndrome,** sweating

INTERACTIONS

Drugs

❷ *Aminoglycosides (gentamicin, kanamycin, neomycin, streptomycin):* Additive ototoxicity (ethacrynic acid > furosemide, torsemide, bumetanide)

❸ *Angiotensin converting enzyme inhibitors:* Initiation of ACEI with intensive diuretic therapy may result in precipitous fall in blood pressure; ACEIs may induce renal insufficiency in the presence of diuretic-induced sodium depletion

❸ *Barbiturates (phenobarbital):* Reduced diuretic response

❸ *Bile acid-binding resins (cholestyramine, colestipol):* Resins markedly reduce the bioavailability and diuretic response of furosemide

❸ *Carbenoxolone:* Severe hypokalemia from coadministration

❸ *Cephalosporins (cephaloridine, cephalothin):* Enhanced nephrotoxicity with coadministration

❷ *Cisplatin:* Additive ototoxicity (ethacrynic acid > furosemide, torsemide, bumetanide)

❸ *Clofibrate:* Enhanced effects of both drugs, especially in hypoalbuminemic patients

❸ *Corticosteroids:* Concomitant loop diuretic and corticosteroid therapy can result in excessive potassium loss

❸ *Digitalis glycosides (digoxin, digitoxin):* Diuretic-induced hypokalemia may increase risk of digitalis toxicity

❸ *Nonsteroidal antiinflammatory drugs (flurbiprofen, ibuprofen, indomethacin, naproxen, piroxicam, sulindac):* Reduced diuretic and antihypertensive effects

---

italic = common side effects   **bold italic** = life-threatening reactions

3 *Phenytoin:* Reduced diuretic response

3 *Serotonin-reuptake inhibitors (fluoxetine, paroxetine, sertraline):* Case reports of sudden death; enhanced hyponatremia proposed; causal relationships not established

3 *Terbutaline:* Additive hypokalemia

3 *Tubocurarine:* Prolonged neuromuscular blockade

Labs
• *Cortisol:* False increases
• *Glucose:* Falsely low urine tests with clinistix and diastix
• *Thyroxine:* Increased serum concentration
• *T_3 uptake:* Interference causes increased serum values

SPECIAL CONSIDERATIONS
• Cross-sensitivity with furosemide rare; may substitute bumetanide at a 1:40 ratio with furosemide in patients allergic to furosemide; may show cross-hypersensitivity to sulfonamides

PATIENT/FAMILY EDUCATION
• Take early in the day

MONITORING PARAMETERS
• Urine volume, creatinine clearance, BUN, electrolytes, reduction in edema, increased diuresis, decrease in body weight, reduction in blood pressure, glucose, uric acid, serum calcium (tetany), tinnitus, vertigo, hearing loss (especially in those at risk for ototoxicity—IV doses >120 mg; concomitant ototoxic drugs; renal disease)

bupivacaine

(byoo-piv′a-caine)

Rx: Marcaine, Marcaine Spinal, Sensorcaine, Sensorcaine-MPF

Combinations
   Rx: with epinephrine (Marcaine with Epinephrine, Sensorcaine with Epinephrine, Sensorcaine-MPF with Epinephrine)

Chemical Class: Amide; aminoacyl derivative
Therapeutic Class: Local anesthetic

CLINICAL PHARMACOLOGY
Mechanism of Action: Blocks the generation and conduction of nerve impulses; the order of loss of nerve function is: (1) pain, (2) temperature, (3) touch, (4) proprioception, and (5) skeletal muscle tone

Pharmacokinetics
INJ: Peak 30-45 min, duration 3-6 hr; 96% bound to plasma proteins; metabolized in liver, excreted in urine; $t_{1/2}$ 3.5 hr

INDICATIONS AND USES: Local or regional anesthesia; analgesia for surgery, oral surgical procedures, diagnostic and therapeutic procedures, obstetrical procedures

DOSAGE
Dose varies with procedure, depth of anesthesia, vascularity of tissues, duration of anesthesia, and condition of patient

Adult
• *Caudal block:* Inj 15-30 ml of 0.25% or 0.5%
• *Epidural block:* Inj 10-20 ml of 0.25% or 0.5%
• *Peripheral nerve block:* Inj 5 ml of 0.25% or 0.5% (12.5-25 mg), max 2.5 mg/kg or 400 mg/day

• *Sympathetic nerve block:* Inj 20-50 ml of 0.25%
Child
• *Caudal block:* Inj 1-3.7 mg/kg
• *Epidural block:* Inj 1.25 mg/kg/dose

💲 AVAILABLE FORMS/COST OF THERAPY
• Inj, Sol—Caudal Block, Epidural: 0.25%, 10 ml: **$3.47-$4.90**; 0.5%, 10 ml: **$3.79-$5.22**; 0.75%, 10 ml: **$3.95-$5.99**

CONTRAINDICATIONS: Obstetrical paracervical block anesthesia
PRECAUTIONS: Obstetrical anesthesia (0.75% concentration), intravenous regional anesthesia, hypotension, heart block, hepatic disease, impaired cardiovascular function, use in head and neck area, retrobulbar blocks, elderly, anaphylaxis
PREGNANCY AND LACTATION: Pregnancy category C; excretion into breast milk unknown; regional use may prolong labor and delivery
SIDE EFFECTS/ADVERSE REACTIONS
CNS: Anxiety, disorientation, drowsiness, *loss of consciousness,* restlessness, *seizures,* shivering, tremors
CV: Bradycardia, *cardiac arrest, dysrhythmias,* fetal bradycardia, hypertension, hypotension, *myocardial depression*
EENT: Blurred vision, miosis, tinnitus
GI: Nausea, vomiting
RESP: Respiratory arrest
SKIN: Allergic reactions, burning, edema, rash, skin discoloration at injection site, tissue necrosis, urticaria
INTERACTIONS
Drugs
3 *β-blockers:* Hypertensive reactions possible, especially with local anesthetics containing epinephrine; acute discontinuation of β-blockers before local anesthesia may increase the risk of side effects due to anesthetic
SPECIAL CONSIDERATIONS
• Amide-type local anesthetic
MONITORING PARAMETERS
• Blood pressure, pulse, respiration during treatment, ECG
• Fetal heart tones if drug is used during labor

---

buprenorphine
(byoo-pre-nor'feen)
Rx: Buprenex
Chemical Class: Semisynthetic opiate (thebaine) derivative
Therapeutic Class: Narcotic agonist-antagonist analgesic
DEA Class: Schedule V

CLINICAL PHARMACOLOGY
Mechanism of Action: Analgesia via binding to µ subclass opiate receptors in the CNS; µ receptors mediate morphinelike supraspinal analgesia, euphoria, and respiratory and physical depression; narcotic antagonist activity is approximately equipotent to naloxone
Pharmacokinetics
IM: Onset 15 min, peak 1 hr, duration 6 hr
IV: Onset 1 min, peak 5 min, duration 2-5 hr
Metabolized by liver, excreted predominantly in feces; 96% bound to plasma proteins; $t_{1/2}$ 2-3 hr
INDICATIONS AND USES: Moderate to severe pain
DOSAGE
Note: Parenteral dose of 0.3 mg equivalent to 10 mg morphine
Adult
• IM/IV 0.3 mg q6h prn (reduce dosage by half in the elderly, debilitated patients, or in the presence of respiratory disease); repeat once (up

---

to 0.3 mg) prn 30-60 min after initial dose
Child >2 yr
• IM/IV 2 µg/kg/dose q6-8h prn
§ AVAILABLE FORMS/COST OF THERAPY
• Inj, Sol—IM, IV: 0.3 mg/ml:1 ml: **$2.67-$3.03**
PRECAUTIONS: Addictive personality, narcotic-dependent patients (may cause withdrawal), increased intracranial pressure, respiratory depression, hepatic disease, renal disease, hypothyroidism, biliary tract dysfunction, prostatic hypertrophy
PREGNANCY AND LACTATION: Pregnancy category C; safe use in labor and delivery has not been established; excretion into breast milk unknown
SIDE EFFECTS/ADVERSE REACTIONS
CNS: **Coma,** confusion, depression, *dizziness,* euphoria, hallucinations, headache, nervousness, paresthesia, psychosis, *sedation,* slurred speech, tremor, weakness
CV: Bradycardia, hypertension, hypotension, tachycardia
EENT: Blurred vision, conjunctivitis, diplopia, miosis, tinnitus
GI: Constipation, dry mouth, dyspepsia, flatulence, loss of appetite, nausea
GU: Urinary retention
RESP: Apnea, cyanosis, dyspnea, *respiratory depression*
SKIN: Injection site reactions, pallor, pruritus, rash, sweating, urticaria
SPECIAL CONSIDERATIONS
• Effective long-acting opioid agonist-antagonist; unconfirmed reported lower physical dependence; no significant advantages
MONITORING PARAMETERS
• Respiration rate

---

bupropion
(byoo-proe'pee-on)
Rx: Wellbutrin, Wellbutrin SR, Zyban
Chemical Class: Aminoketone derivative
Therapeutic Class: Antidepressant

CLINICAL PHARMACOLOGY
Mechanism of Action: Inhibits neuronal reuptake of dopamine and norepinephrine (slight) at the presynaptic neuron; moderate anticholinergic, sedation; slight orthostatic hypotensive activity
Pharmacokinetics
PO: Peak 2 hr, onset 2-4 wk, t$_{1/2}$ 12-14 hr; metabolized by liver
INDICATIONS AND USES: Depression; smoking cessation, bipolar disorder
DOSAGE
Adult
• *Depression:* PO 100 mg bid initially, increase based on clinical response to 100 mg tid no sooner than 3 days after initiating therapy, may increase after 1 month to 150 mg tid; **no single dose should exceed 150 mg; at least 6 hr should elapse between doses;** or PO EXT REL 150 mg bid
• Smoking cessation:150 mg EXT REL qd ×3 days; then 150 mg EXT REL bid × 7-12 weeks (target quit date to follow 1 week of therapy)
§ AVAILABLE FORMS/COST OF THERAPY
• Tab, Coated—Oral: 75 mg, 100's: **$79.30;** 100 mg, 100's: **$105.79**
• Tab, EXT REL—Oral:100 mg, 60's: **$78.13;** 150 mg, 60's: **$83.74**
• Advantage pack—tab, EXT REL—Oral: 150 mg, 60's: **$83.74** plus behavioral modification program

CONTRAINDICATIONS: Seizure disorder, prior or current diagnosis of bulimia or anorexia nervosa (increased risk of seizure), concurrent use of MAOI

PRECAUTIONS: Renal and hepatic disease, recent MI, unstable heart disease, history of drug abuse or dependence, bipolar affective disorder

PREGNANCY AND LACTATION: Pregnancy category B; excretion into breast milk unknown

SIDE EFFECTS/ADVERSE REACTIONS

CNS: Agitation, anxiety, confusion, decreased libido, dizziness, dry mouth, *headache/migraine, insomnia, **seizures,*** sweating, tremor

*CV: **Arrhythmias,*** edema, hypertension, hypotension, palpitations, syncope, tachycardia

EENT: Auditory disturbance, blurred vision

GI: Appetite increase, constipation, dyspepsia, *nausea, vomiting*

GU: Impotence, menstrual complaints, urinary frequency

METAB: Glycosuria, gynecomastia

MS: Arthritis

SKIN: Pruritus, rash

SPECIAL CONSIDERATIONS
• Equal efficacy as tricyclic antidepressants; advantages include minimal anticholinergic effects, lack of orthostatic hypotension, no cardiac conduction problems, absence of weight gain, no sedation
• Prescribe in equally divided doses of 3 or 4 times daily to minimize risk of seizures

PATIENT/FAMILY EDUCATION
• Ability to perform tasks requiring judgment or motor and cognitive skills may be impaired
• Therapeutic effects may take 2-4 wk
• Do not discontinue medication quickly after long-term use

---

buspirone
(byoo-spir'own)
Rx: BuSpar
Chemical Class: Azaspirodecanedione
Therapeutic Class: Anxiolytic

B

CLINICAL PHARMACOLOGY
Mechanism of Action: Anxiolytic activity presumed secondary to high affinity for serotonin ($5-HT_{1A}$) receptors; there is also moderate affinity for brain D_2-dopamine receptors and increases norepinepherine metabolism in the locus ceruleus; the drug has no affinity for benzodiazepine receptors; there are no anticonvulsant, muscle relaxant, or sedative effects

Pharmacokinetics
PO: Peak 40-90 min; 95% bound to plasma proteins; metabolized by liver, excreted in urine and feces; $t_{1/2}$ 2-3 hr

INDICATIONS AND USES: Anxiety disorders, premenstrual syndrome*

DOSAGE
Adult
• PO 5 mg tid, may increase by 5 mg/day q2-3 d, not to exceed 60 mg/day

⑧ AVAILABLE FORMS/COST OF THERAPY
• Tab, Uncoated—Oral: 5 mg, 100's: **$74.54;** 10 mg, 100's: **$130.00;** 15 mg, 60's: **$116.55**

PRECAUTIONS: Liver disease, renal disease, elderly, children <18 yr

PREGNANCY AND LACTATION: Pregnancy category B; excretion into breast milk unknown; use caution in nursing mothers

SIDE EFFECTS/ADVERSE REACTIONS
CNS: Akathisia, confusion, depression, *dizziness, drowsiness,* excite-

---

ment, headache, incoordination, insomnia, involuntary movements, lightheadedness, nervousness, paresthesia, stimulation, tremor

CV: Bradycardia, hypertension, hypotension, non-specific chest pain, palpitations

EENT: Altered taste, smell; blurred vision; nasal congestion; red, itchy eyes; sore throat; tinnitus

GI: Constipation, diarrhea, dry mouth, dyspepsia, flatulence, increased appetite, *nausea,* rectal bleeding

GU: Change in libido, frequency, hesitancy, menstrual irregularity

MS: Muscle cramps, pain, spasms, weakness

RESP: Chest congestion, hyperventilation, shortness of breath

SKIN: Alopecia, dry skin, edema, pruritus, rash

MISC: Fatigue, fever, sweating, weight gain

INTERACTIONS

Drugs

3 *Fluoxetine:* Reduced therapeutic response to both drugs

SPECIAL CONSIDERATIONS

• Advantages include less sedation (preferable in elderly), less effect on psychomotor and psychologic function, minimal propensity to interact with ethanol and other CNS depressants

• Will not prevent benzodiazepine withdrawal

PATIENT/FAMILY EDUCATION

• Optimal results may take 3-4 wk of treatment, some improvement may be seen after 7-10 days

---

butabarbital

(byoo-tah-bar'bi-tal)

Rx: Butisol

Chemical Class: Barbituric acid derivative

Therapeutic Class: Sedative/hypnotic

DEA Class: Schedule III

CLINICAL PHARMACOLOGY

Mechanism of Action: Non-selective CNS depressant: depresses the sensory cortex, decreases motor activity, alters cerebellar function, produce drowsiness, sedation, and hypnosis; little analgesic action at subanesthetic doses (may increase reaction to painful stimuli); anticonvulsant activity in anesthetic doses; dose-dependent respiratory depression (hypnotic doses produce respiratory depression similar to physiologic sleep)

Pharmacokinetics

PO: Onset 0.5-1 hr, $t_{1/2}$ 66-140 hr; metabolized by liver, excreted in urine as metabolites

INDICATIONS AND USES: Hypnotic in the short-term treatment of insomnia for periods up to 2 wk in duration (may lose efficacy for sleep induction and maintenance after this period of time)

DOSAGE

Adult

• *Daytime sedation:* PO 15-30 mg tid-qid

• *Bedtime hypnotic:* PO 50-100 mg

• *Preoperative sedation:* PO 50-100 mg 60-90 min before surgery

Child

• *Preoperative sedation:* PO 2-6 mg/kg; max 100 mg

• *Daytime sedation:* PO 7.5-30 mg; depending on age, weight, and sedation desired

💲 AVAILABLE FORMS/COST OF THERAPY

• Elixir—Oral: 30 mg/5 ml, 480 ml: **$116.77**
• Tab, Uncoated—Oral: 30 mg, 100's: **$82.82**; 50 mg, 100's: **$107.70**

CONTRAINDICATIONS: Respiratory depression, addiction to barbiturates, severe liver impairment, porphyria

PRECAUTIONS: Anemia, hepatic disease, renal disease, hypertension, elderly, acute/chronic pain, mental depression, history of drug abuse, abrupt discontinuation

PREGNANCY AND LACTATION: Pregnancy category D; small amounts excreted in breast milk; use caution in nursing mothers

SIDE EFFECTS/ADVERSE REACTIONS

CNS: CNS depression, dizziness, *drowsiness, hangover,* headache, *lethargy,* light-headedness, mental depression, physical dependence, slurred speech, stimulation in the elderly and children, vertigo

CV: Bradycardia, hypotension

EENT: **Laryngospasm**

GI: Constipation, diarrhea, nausea, vomiting

HEME: **Agranulocytosis,** megaloblastic anemia, (long-term treatment), **thrombocytopenia**

MS: Osteomalacia (prolonged use), rickets

RESP: **Apnea, bronchospasm, respiratory depression**

SKIN: Abscesses at injection site, angioedema, erythema multiforme, pain, *rash,* **Stevens-Johnson syndrome,** thrombophlebitis, urticaria

INTERACTIONS

Drugs

❸ *Acetaminophen:* Enhanced hepatotoxic potential of acetaminophen; reduced therapeutic response to acetaminophen

❸ *Antidepressants:* Reduced serum concentrations and therapeutic response of cyclic antidepressants

❸ *β-adrenergic blockers:* Reduced serum concentrations of β-blockers that are extensively metabolized

❸ *Calcium channel blockers:* Reduced plasma concentrations of verapamil and nifedipine

❸ *Chloramphenicol:* Increased serum barbiturate concentrations; reduced serum chloramphenicol concentrations

❸ *Corticosteroids:* Induced metabolism leads to decreases in steroid levels and therapeutic effect

❸ *Cyclosporine A:* Barbiturates, as inducers of metabolism, reduce cyclosporine levels

❸ *Digitoxin:* Induced hepatic metabolism leads to reduced serum levels of digitoxin

❸ *Disopyramide:* Reduced serum concentrations of disopyramide

❸ *Doxycycline:* Reduced serum doxycycline concentrations

❸ *Ethanol:* Excessive CNS depression

❸ *Furosemide:* Reduced diuretic effect

❸ *Lamotrigine:* Induced metabolism leads to decreased lamotrigine levels and therapeutic effect

❸ *MAOIs:* Prolonged effect of barbiturates

❸ *Methoxyflurane:* Enhanced nephrotoxicity of methoxyflurane

❸ *Narcotic analgesics:* Increased toxicity of meperidine; reduced effect of methadone; excessive CNS depression

❸ *Neuroleptics:* Possible reduction in neuroleptic effect

❷ *Oral anticoagulants:* Inhibited hypoprothrombinemic response to oral anticoagulants; fatal bleeding episodes have occurred when barbiturates were discontinued in patients stabilized on an anticoagulant

---

italic = common side effects **bold italic** = life-threatening reactions

3 *Oral contraceptives:* Reduced efficacy of oral contraceptives; menstrual irregularities and unintended pregnancies may occur

3 *Phenytoin:* Barbiturates usually decrease phenytoin levels; monitor closely when concurrent therapy is stopped, started, or changed

3 *Quinidine:* Reduced serum quinidine plasma concentrations

3 *Theophylline:* Reduced serum theophylline concentrations; potential of reduced therapeutic response to theophylline

3 *Valproic acid:* Increases barbiturate concentrations

Labs

• *Barbiturates:* Positive urine

• *Phenobarbital:* Increased serum levels; significant interference

SPECIAL CONSIDERATIONS
PATIENT/FAMILY EDUCATION

• Not chronic medication; indicated only for short-term treatment of insomnia and is probably ineffective after 2 wk

• Physical dependency may result when used for extended time (45-90 days depending on dose)

• Avoid driving or other activities requiring alertness

• Avoid alcohol ingestion or CNS depressants

• Do not discontinue medication abruptly after long-term use

MONITORING PARAMETERS

• CBC, serum folate, vitamin D (if on long-term therapy)

• PT in patients receiving anticoagulants, LFTs

• Mental status, vital signs

---

butalbital compound
(byoo-tal'bih-tall)

**Rx: Butalbital/
acetaminophen/caffeine:**
Amaphen, Americet, Endolor, Esgic, Ezol, Fioricet, Fiorpap, Geone, Medigesic, Repan, Tencet

**Butalbital/aceta-
minophen/caffeine with
codeine:** Ezol III, Fioricet w/codeine; **Butalbital/
acetaminophen:** Bancap, Phrenilin, Phrenilin Forte, Sedapap-10, Triaprin

**Butalbital/aspirin/
caffeine:** Farbital, Fiorgen PF, Fiorinal, Fiormor Fiortal Fortabs; **Butalbital/aspirin/
caffeine with codeine:**
Fiorinal w/codeine

Chemical Class: Barbituric acid derivative
Therapeutic Class: Nonnarcotic analgesic
DEA Class: Schedule III (aspirin-containing products)

CLINICAL PHARMACOLOGY
Mechanism of Action: Combines the analgesic properties of acetaminophen, aspirin, and caffeine with the anxiolytic and muscle relaxant properties of butalbital

INDICATIONS AND USES: Tension (muscle contraction) headache

DOSAGE

Adult

• PO 1-2 tabs q4h as needed, max 6 tabs/day

$ **AVAILABLE FORMS/COST
OF THERAPY**

*Butalbital/Acetaminophen/
Caffeine*

• Cap, Gel—Oral: 50 mg/325 mg/40 mg, 100's: **$12.23-$129.94**

---

* = non-FDA-approved use

• Tab, Uncoated—Oral: 50 mg/325 mg/40 mg, 30's: **$6.13**
• With Codeine Cap, Gel—Oral: 50 mg/325 mg/40 mg/30 mg, 100's: **$136.18**

Butalbital/Aspirin/Caffeine
• Cap, Gel—Oral: 50 mg/325 mg/40 mg, 100's: **$4.28-$61.35**
• Tab, Uncoated—Oral: 325 mg/50 mg/40 mg, 100's: **$6.95-$61.35**
• With Codeine Cap, Gel—Oral: 50 mg/325 mg/ 40 mg/ 30 mg, 100's: **$136.18**

CONTRAINDICATIONS: Porphyria
PRECAUTIONS: History of drug abuse, elderly, children
PREGNANCY AND LACTATION: Pregnancy category C (category D if used for prolonged periods or in high doses at term); excretion into breast milk unknown (see also aspirin, acetaminophen, and caffeine)
SIDE EFFECTS/ADVERSE REACTIONS (see also aspirin, acetaminophen, and caffeine)
CNS: Chronic daily headache, depression, *dizziness, drowsiness,* lightheadedness, mental confusion
GI: Flatulence, nausea, vomiting
INTERACTIONS
Drugs
❷ *Oral anticoagulants:* Barbiturates inhibit the hypoprothrombinemic response to oral anticoagulants; fatal bleeding episodes have occurred when barbiturates were discontinued in patients stabilized on an anticoagulant (see also aspirin, acetaminophen, and caffeine)
SPECIAL CONSIDERATIONS
PATIENT/FAMILY EDUCATION
• May cause psychological and/or physical dependence
• May cause drowsiness, use caution driving or operating machinery
• Avoid alcohol and other CNS depressants

butenafine
(byoo-ten'a-feen)
Rx: Mentax
Chemical Class: Benzylamine derivative
Therapeutic Class: Antifungal

CLINICAL PHARMACOLOGY
Mechanism of Action: Blocks the biosynthesis of ergosterol, an essential component of fungal cell membranes; fungicidal
Pharmacokinetics
TOP: Slight transdermal absorption; peak 6-15 hr; excreted in urine (metabolites)
INDICATIONS AND USES: Interdigital tinea pedis (athlete's foot); tinea cruris
Antifungal spectrum usually includes:
Epidermophyton floccosum, Trichophyton mentagrophytes, Trichophyton rubrum
DOSAGE
Adult and Child >12 yr
• TOP cover affected and immediately surrounding skin qd for 2-4 wk
🚺 **AVAILABLE FORMS/COST OF THERAPY**
• Cre—Top: 1%, 15, 30 g: **$27.12/ 15 g**
PRECAUTIONS: Sensitivity to allylamine antifungals (cross-reactivity possible)
PREGNANCY AND LACTATION: Pregnancy category B
SIDE EFFECTS/ADVERSE REACTIONS
SKIN: Burning, contact dermatitis, erythema, irritation, itching, stinging
SPECIAL CONSIDERATIONS
Good cutaneous absorption, prolonged skin retention, and fungicidal activity are potential advan-

---

italic = common side effects   ***bold italic*** = life-threatening reactions

tages. Comparative trials with other agents necessary

butoconazole
(byoo-toe-ko′na-zole)
OTC: Femstat-3
Chemical Class: Imidazole derivative
Therapeutic Class: Antifungal

CLINICAL PHARMACOLOGY
Mechanism of Action: Alteration of the fungal cell membrane, which allows leakage of essential intracellular components
Pharmacokinetics
VAG: 5.5% of dose absorbed, peak plasma levels at 24 hr, $t_{1/2}$ 21-24 hr
INDICATIONS AND USES: Local treatment of vulvovaginal candidiasis
DOSAGE
Adult
• VAG 1 applicator hs × 3 days (non-pregnant), 6 days (2nd and 3rd trimester pregnancy)
$ **AVAILABLE FORMS/COST OF THERAPY**
• Cre—Vag: 2%, 3X5 g applicators: **$14.08**
PREGNANCY AND LACTATION: Pregnancy category C; excretion into breast milk unknown
SIDE EFFECTS/ADVERSE REACTIONS
GU: Burning, discharge, finger itching, rash, soreness, stinging, swelling, vulvovaginal itching

butorphanol
(byoo-tor′fa-nole)
Rx: Stadol
Chemical Class: Synthetic opiate derivative—morphinian congener
Therapeutic Class: Narcotic agonist-antagonist analgesic

CLINICAL PHARMACOLOGY
Mechanism of Action: Analgesia via μ subclass opiate receptor binding in CNS; μ receptors mediate morphinelike supraspinal analgesia, euphoria, and respiratory and physical depression; narcotic antagonist activity is approximately 30 × pentazocine or 1/40 naloxone
Pharmacokinetics
IM: Onset 10-30 min, peak ½ hr, duration 3-4 hr
IV: Onset 1 min, peak 5 min, duration 2-4 hr
PR: Onset slow, duration 4-6 hr
NASAL: Onset 15 min, peak 30-60 min 80% protein bound; extensively metabolized by liver, excreted by kidneys (reduce dose to 75% for CrCl 10-50 ml/min, to 50% for CrCl <10 ml/min); $t_{1/2}$ 2½-3½ hr
INDICATIONS AND USES: Moderate to severe pain, including postoperative analgesia; preoperative or preanesthetic medication, as a supplement to balanced anesthesia; relief of pain during labor
DOSAGE
Adult
Note: 2 mg IM is equivalent to 10 mg morphine
• IV 0.5-2 mg q3-4h prn; NASAL 1 mg (1 spray in one nostril); may repeat in 60-90 minutes if adequate pain relief is not achieved; initial 2-dose sequence outlined above may be repeated in 3-4 hr as needed; depending on the severity of the pain,

an initial dose of 2 mg (1 spray in each nostril) may be given

• *Geriatric:* Half the usual dose at twice the usual interval

💲 AVAILABLE FORMS/COST OF THERAPY

• Aer, Spray—Nasal: 10 mg/ml, 2.5 ml: **$69.66**

• Inj, Sol—IM, IV: 1 mg/ml, 1 ml: **$8.04**; 2 mg/ml, 1 ml: **$9.40**

CONTRAINDICATIONS: Narcotic addiction (may precipitate withdrawal), CHF, MI

PRECAUTIONS: Hypotension, addictive personality, head injuries, increased intracranial pressure, respiratory depression, hepatic disease, renal disease, child <18 yr

PREGNANCY AND LACTATION: Pregnancy category B; crosses placenta; excreted in breast milk, though probably clinically insignificant

SIDE EFFECTS/ADVERSE REACTIONS

CNS: Asthenia/lethargy, confusion, dizziness (19%), drowsiness (43%), drug abuse and dependence, *euphoria,* hallucinations, *headache, sedation*

CV: Bradycardia, hypertension, hypotension, palpitations

EENT: Blurred vision, diplopia, *epistaxis,* miosis, *nasal congestion, nasal irritation, sinus congestion* (nasal spray), tinnitus

GI: Anorexia, constipation, cramps, *dry mouth,* increased amylase, *nausea, vomiting*

GU: Dysuria, increased urinary output, urinary retention

RESP: Pulmonary hypertension, ***respiratory depression***

SKIN: Bruising, *diaphoresis,* flushing, pruritus, rash, urticaria

INTERACTIONS

Drugs

• *Nasal vasoconstrictors:* Slower onset of action of butorphanol (nasal spray)

SPECIAL CONSIDERATIONS

• Chronic use can precipitate withdrawal symptoms of anxiety, agitation, mood changes, hallucinations, dysphoria, weakness, and diarrhea

• Although not classified as a controlled substance by the FDA, prolonged use can result in habituation and drug-seeking behavior

• 2 mg=1 spray in each nostril

---

cabergoline

(kab-er´go-leen)
Rx: Dostinex
Chemical Class: Synthetic ergoline derivative
Therapeutic Class: Antiparkinson's agent, dopaminergic

CLINICAL PHARMACOLOGY

Mechanism of Action: D_2 receptor agonist; inhibits prolactin

Pharmacokinetics

PO: Well absorbed, peak 0.5-4 hr, $t_{1/2}$ 63-68 hr; extensively metabolized to inactive metabolites, excreted mostly in feces, <14% in urine; 41% protein bound

INDICATIONS AND USES: Hyperprolactinemia, Parkinson's disease,* inhibition of lactation,* prolactinomas acromegaly,* polycystic ovary syndrome*

DOSAGE

Adult

• PO 0.25 mg 2 × per wk; increase by 0.25 mg 2 × per wk to desired prolactin level or 1 mg 2 × per wk

💲 AVAILABLE FORMS/COST OF THERAPY

• Tab—Oral: 0.5 mg, 8's: **$229.33**

CONTRAINDICATIONS: Sensitivity to ergot derivatives, uncontrolled hypertension, pregnancy-induced hypertension

PREGNANCY AND LACTATION: Pregnancy category B; unknown if excreted in breast milk

---

SIDE EFFECTS/ADVERSE REACTIONS

CNS: Confusion, *dizziness (25%),* dyskinesias, *fatigue, headache (43%),* somnolence, vertigo, visual hallucinations

CV: Edema, orthostatic hypotension

EENT: Nasal stuffiness

GI: Abdominal pain, *constipation (16%),* nausea *(45%),* vomiting

SPECIAL CONSIDERATIONS

• More potent with longer half-life than bromocriptine or pergolide, allowing for less frequent dosing

• Initial treatment produces dramatic response; as disease progresses response duration decreases

---

caffeine

(kaf´een)

OTC: Caffedrine, No-Doz, QuickPep, Stay Awake, Vivarin

Chemical Class: Xanthine derivative

Therapeutic Class: Analeptic; CNS stimulant

CLINICAL PHARMACOLOGY

Mechanism of Action: Increases calcium permeability in sarcoplasmic reticulum; promotes accumulation of cAMP; competitively blocks adenosine receptors; stimulates the CNS; produces diuresis; relaxes bronchial smooth muscle

Pharmacokinetics

PO: Onset 15 min, peak ½-1 hr; metabolized by liver, less than 5% excreted unchanged by kidneys; crosses placenta; $t_{1/2}$ 3-4 hr

INDICATIONS AND USES: Respiratory depression associated with overdose (IM); aid in staying awake and restoring mental alertness; adjuvant with analgesics; neonatal apnea*; headaches associated with spinal puncture,* orthostatic hypotension*

DOSAGE

Adult

• PO 100-200 mg q4h prn; TIME REL 200 mg q3-4h; IM 250-500 mg

Child

• *Neonatal apnea:* IV/IM/PO 5-10 mg/kg loading dose followed by 2.5-5 mg/kg qd; adjust maintenance dose based on response and serum levels

💲 **AVAILABLE FORMS/COST OF THERAPY**

• Tab chewable—Oral: 200 mg, 16's: **$1.00-$2.50**

• Tab, EXT REL—Oral: 200 mg, 16's: **$1.66-$2.40**

• Caps—Oral: 250 mg, 100's: **$3.90**

• Inj, Sol—IM, IV: 125 mg/ml, 2 ml: **$9.70-$21.39** (Rx only)

PRECAUTIONS: Dysrhythmias, Gilles de la Tourette's disorder, psychologic disorders, depression (large parenteral doses can cause further depression in an already depressed patient), ulcers, diabetes mellitus

PREGNANCY AND LACTATION: Pregnancy category B; amounts in breast milk after maternal ingestion of caffeinated beverages not clinically significant; accumulation can occur in heavy-using mothers

SIDE EFFECTS/ADVERSE REACTIONS

CNS: Aggressiveness, dizziness, headache, *hyperactivity, insomnia,* irritability, mild delirium, *restlessness,* scintillating scotoma, *stimulation, talkativeness,* tinnitus, tremors, twitching

CV: **Dysrhythmias,** extrasystole, palpitations, tachycardia

GI: Anorexia, diarrhea, gastric irritation, nausea, vomiting

GU: Diuresis

---

* = non-FDA-approved use

METAB: Hyperglycemia
SKIN: Hyperesthesia

INTERACTIONS

Drugs

3 *β-adrenergic agents:* Enhanced beta-adrenergic stimulating effects

3 *Cimetidine:* Impairs caffeine metabolism resulting in excessive CNS or cardiovascular effects

3 *Clozapine:* Caffeine inhibits CYP1A2, with elevations of clozapine levels

3 *Contraceptives, oral:* Impair caffeine metabolism resulting in excessive CNS or cardiovascular effects

3 *Disulfiram:* Impairs caffeine metabolism resulting in excessive CNS or cardiovascular effects

3 *Fluroquinolone antibiotics:* Increases caffeine concentrations and may enhance its side effects

3 *Fluconazole:* Increased caffeine concentrations

3 *Mexiletine:* 30%-50% reduction in caffeine clearance; potentially increased risk of CNS or cardiovascular effects

3 *Phenylpropanolamine:* Additive effects

3 *Phenytoin:* Induced hepatic metabolism of caffeine; decreased caffeine effects

3 *Pipemidic acid:* Produces a large increase in caffeine concentrations and may increase side effects

3 *Terbinafine:* Impairs caffeine metabolism resulting in excessive CNS or cardiovascular effects

3 *Theophylline:* Caffeine reduces theophylline clearance by 30%; may affect serum theophylline levels

Labs

• *False positive elevations:* Serum uric acid levels, urine levels of VMA, catecholamines, 5-hydroxyindoleacetic acid

SPECIAL CONSIDERATIONS
PATIENT/FAMILY EDUCATION

• Gradual taper if used long-term to prevent withdrawal syndrome, especially headache

• Most authorities believe caffeine and other analeptics should not be used in overdose with CNS depressants and recommend other supportive therapy

---

calcifediol
(kal-si-fe-dye'ole)
Rx: Calderol
Chemical Class: Sterol derivative
Therapeutic Class: Vitamin D analog

CLINICAL PHARMACOLOGY
Mechanism of Action: Same as 25-hydroxy-vitamin D; product of first metabolic step to biologic activity; relatively inactive before renal hydroxylation to calcitriol; increases intestinal absorption of calcium; increases renal tubular absorption of phosphate; increases rate of accretion and resorption of minerals in bone; regulates calcium homeostasis

Pharmacokinetics
PO: Peak 4 hr, duration 15-20 days; rapid absorption from small intestine; activated in kidneys, stored in liver and fat; excreted via bile in feces; $t_{1/2}$ 12-22 days

INDICATIONS AND USES: Management of metabolic bone disease or hypocalcemia in patients on chronic renal dialysis

DOSAGE
Adult

• PO 300-350 µg q wk divided into qd or qod doses, may increase q4 wk

---

🖺 **AVAILABLE FORMS/COST OF THERAPY**
• Cap, Elastic—Oral: 20 µg, 60's: **$59.20;** 50 µg, 60's: **$134.98**
CONTRAINDICATIONS: Hyperphosphatemia, hypercalcemia, vitamin D toxicity
PRECAUTIONS: Renal calculi, CV disease
PREGNANCY AND LACTATION: Pregnancy category C; excreted in breast milk and may cause infant hypercalcemia

SIDE EFFECTS/ADVERSE REACTIONS
CNS: Drowsiness, fever, headache, lethargy, vertigo
CV: **Dysrhythmias**
EENT: Conjunctivitis, photophobia, rhinorrhea, tinnitus
GI: Anorexia, constipation, cramps, diarrhea, dry mouth, jaundice, metallic taste, nausea, vomiting
GU: Hematuria, hypercalciuria, hyperphosphatemia, polyuria
MS: Arthralgia, decreased bone development, myalgia

SPECIAL CONSIDERATIONS
PATIENT/FAMILY EDUCATION
• Adequate dietary calcium is necessary for clinical response to vitamin D therapy
MONITORING PARAMETERS
• Blood Ca, P determinations must be made every 2 wk or more frequently if necessary
• Vitamin D levels also helpful, although less frequently
• Height and weight in children

calcipotriene
(kal-sip′oh-tri-een)
Rx: Dovonex
Chemical Class: Synthetic vitamin D_3 analog
Therapeutic Class: Antipsoriatic

CLINICAL PHARMACOLOGY
Mechanism of Action: Vitamin D_3 receptors occur in many parts of the body, including keratinocytes; the scaly red patches of psoriasis are caused by abnormal growth and production of keratinocytes; calcipotriene regulates skin cell production and development
Pharmacokinetics
TOP: 6% of applied dose absorbed systemically (mostly converted to inactive metabolites within 24 hr); transported in blood bound to specific plasma proteins; recycled via the liver and excreted in the bile; systemic disposition expected to be similar to the naturally occurring vitamin
INDICATIONS AND USES: Treatment of moderate plaque psoriasis
DOSAGE
Adult
• TOP apply thin layer to affected skin qd or bid

🖺 **AVAILABLE FORMS/COST OF THERAPY**
• Cre—Top: 0.005%, 30, 60, 100 g: **$43.72/** 30 g
• Oint—Top: 0.005%, 30, 60, 100 g: **$43.72**/30 g
• Sol—Top: 0.005%, 60 ml: **$84.04**
CONTRAINDICATIONS: Demonstrated hypercalcemia, evidence of vitamin D toxicity, use on the face
PRECAUTIONS: Elderly, children
PREGNANCY AND LACTATION: Pregnancy category C

SIDE EFFECTS/ADVERSE REACTIONS

METAB: Hypercalcemia

SKIN: Burning, dermatitis, dry skin, erythema, folliculitis, hyperpigmentation, *itching,* peeling, rash, skin atrophy, *skin irritation (10% to 15%);* worsening of psoriasis (including development of facial/scalp psoriasis)

SPECIAL CONSIDERATIONS
MONITORING PARAMETERS

• Serum calcium (if elevated discontinue therapy until normal calcium levels are restored); topical administration can yield systemic effects with excessive use

---

calcitonin (salmon)

(kal-si-toe'nin)

Rx: *Salmon:* Calcimar, Miacalcin (nasal)

Chemical Class: Polypeptide hormone

Therapeutic Class: Hypercalcemia antidote; antiosteoporotic

CLINICAL PHARMACOLOGY

Mechanism of Action: Decreases bone resorption and blood calcium levels; increases deposits of calcium in bones; analgesic effect thought to be related to prostaglandin inhibition

Pharmacokinetics

IM/SC: Onset 15 min, peak 4 hr, duration 8-24 hr; metabolized by kidneys, excreted as inactive metabolites

INTRANASAL: 7.5% bioavailability

INDICATIONS AND USES: Hypercalcemia; postmenopausal osteoporosis; Paget's disease; analgesia secondary to vertebral fracture*

DOSAGE

• *Skin test* (salmon calcitonin): 1 unit/0.1 mg (0.1 ml of 10 IU/ml dilution) intradermally; observe for 15 min for significant erythema

Adult

• *Osteoporosis:* Salmon SC/IM 100 IU qd; intranasal 200 IU qd alternating nostrils

• *Hypercalcemia:* Salmon IM 4-8 IU/kg q6-12h

• *Paget's disease:* Human SC 50-100 IU mg/day initially; maintenance range 50 IU bid to 25-50 IU 2-3 ×/ week; Salmon SC/IM 100 IU qd initially; usual maintenance 50 IU qd or qod

• *Analgesic doses:* Same as above, salmon 100 IU SC/IM qd × 2-4 wk, then 50 IU qod three times weekly as maintenance (effect should be noticeable within 2 wk)

🔢 **AVAILABLE FORMS/COST OF THERAPY**

• Inj, Sol—IM, SC: 200 U/ml, 2 ml: **$31.35-$53.40** (salmon)

• Spray, Sol—Nasal: 200 IU/metered dose, 14 doses/2 ml: **$29.50** (salmon)

CONTRAINDICATIONS: Hypersensitivity (skin test recommended for salmon calcitonin), children

PRECAUTIONS: Hypocalcemia

PREGNANCY AND LACTATION: Pregnancy category C; inhibits lactation in animals

SIDE EFFECTS/ADVERSE REACTIONS

CNS: Chills, dizziness, flushing, headache, tetany, weakness

CV: Chest pressure

EENT: Bleeding (nasal), dryness, itching, nasal irritation, redness, *rhinitis*

GI: Abdominal pain, anorexia, diarrhea, epigastric pain, nausea, salty taste, vomiting

GU: Diuresis

MS: Swelling, tingling of hands

RESP: Dyspnea

---

italic = common side effects   **bold italic** = life-threatening reactions

SKIN: Edema of feet, flushing, pruritus of ear lobes, rash

SPECIAL CONSIDERATIONS
PATIENT/FAMILY EDUCATION
• Before first dose of new bottle of nasal spray pump must be activated by holding upright and pumping nozzle 6 times until a faint spray is emitted
• Human calcitonin for injection (Cibacalcin) Novartis, pharmaceutical orphan drug

---

calcitriol (1,25-dihydroxycholecalciferol)
(kal-si-trye'ole)
Rx: Calcijex, Rocaltrol
Chemical Class: Sterol derivative
Therapeutic Class: Vitamin D analog; antiosteoporotic

CLINICAL PHARMACOLOGY
Mechanism of Action: 1,25-(OH)$2D_3$ (calcitriol), the active form of vitamin D_3; active in regulation of the absorption of calcium from the gastrointestinal tract and its utilization in the body; increases renal tubular resorption of phosphate

Pharmacokinetics
PO: Peak 3-6 hr, duration 3-5 days, $t_{1/2}$ 3-6 hr, rapid oral absorption; metabolized and excreted via bile in feces, 4%-6% excreted in urine

INDICATIONS AND USES: Hypocalcemia and resultant metabolic bone disease in patients on chronic renal dialysis; hypoparathyroidism and pseudohypoparathyroidism; osteoporosis*(congenital, steroid induced, postmenopausal); osteitis fibrosa; osteodystrophy; osteomalacia

DOSAGE
Adult
• *Hypocalcemia:* PO 0.25 µg qd; may increase by 0.25 µg/day q4-8wk; maintenance 0.25-1 µg qd; IV 0.5 µg three times weekly (can be administered through the catheter at the end of dialysis)
• *Hypoparathyroidism/pseudohypoparathyroidism:* PO 0.25 µg qd; may be increased by 0.25 µg/day q2-4wk; maintenance 0.25-2 µg qd
• *Osteoporosis:* 0.25 µg qd

Child >1 yr
• *Hypoparathyroidism/pseudohypoparathyroidism:* PO 0.25 µg qd; may be increased q2-4 wk; maintenance 0.25-0.75 µg qd

💲 AVAILABLE FORMS/COST OF THERAPY
• Cap,Elastic—Oral:0.25µg,100's: **$119.69;** 0.5 µg, 100's: **$191.38**
• Inj, Sol—IV: 1 µg/ml, 1 ml: **$13.50;** 2 µg/ml, 1 ml: **$24.68**

CONTRAINDICATIONS: Hyperphosphatemia, hypercalcemia, vitamin D toxicity

PRECAUTIONS: Renal calculi, CV disease

PREGNANCY AND LACTATION: Pregnancy category C; may be excreted in breast milk

SIDE EFFECTS/ADVERSE REACTIONS
CNS: Drowsiness, fever, headache, lethargy, vertigo
GI: Anorexia, constipation, cramps, diarrhea, dry mouth, jaundice, metallic taste, nausea, vomiting
GU: Hematuria, hypercalciuria, hyperphosphatemia, polyuria
MS: Arthralgia, decreased bone development, myalgia

INTERACTIONS
Drugs
3 *Thiazide diuretics:* Hypercalcemia
3 *Verapamil:* Hypercalcemia may inhibit the activity of verapamil

---

* = non-FDA-approved use

SPECIAL CONSIDERATIONS
PATIENT/FAMILY EDUCATION

• Adequate dietary calcium is necessary for clinical response to vitamin D therapy

MONITORING PARAMETERS

• Blood Ca and P determinations must be made every week until stable, or more frequently if necessary
• Vitamin D levels also helpful, although less frequently
• Height and weight in children

---

calcium salts

Rx: *Calcium acetate:* PhosLo
OTC: *Calcium carbonate:*
Amitone, Cal-Carb Forte,
Calci-Chew, Calci-Mix,
Caltrate 600, Chooz, Florical,
Maalox, Mallamint, Mylanta,
Nephro-Calci, Os-Cal 500,
Oysco 500, Oyst-Cal 500,
Oyster Calcium, Rolaids,
Titralac, Tums, Tums Ex
Calcium citrate: Citracal
Calcium glubionate: Neo-
Calglucon
Tricalcium phosphate:
Posture
Combinations
  Rx: with cholecalciferol
   (Os-Cal-D)
  OTC: with sodium fluoride
   (Caltrate, Florical)

Therapeutic Class: Antacid;
antiosteoporotic; phosphate
adsorbent (acetate)

CLINICAL PHARMACOLOGY

Mechanism of Action: Neutralizes gastric acidity; acetate salt binds phosphate in GI tract, increases elimination; caution needed for maintenance of nervous, muscular, skeletal, enzyme reactions, normal cardiac contractility, coagulation of blood; effects secretory activity of endocrine, exocrine glands

Pharmacokinetics

PO: 30% absorbed (variably) depending on demand; absorption vitamin D dependent; bioavailability not significantly different between different salts
IV: Rapid increase in serum levels, with return to pre-drug level within 30 min-2 hr; 80% excreted in the feces as insoluble salts, urinary excretion accounts for the remaining 20%

INDICATIONS AND USES: Prevention and treatment of hypocalcemia, hypermagnesemia, hypoparathyroidism, osteoporosis; neonatal tetany; cardiac toxicity caused by hyperkalemia; cardiac arrest (adjunct); lead colic; hyperphosphatemia; vitamin D deficiency; hyperacidity (antacid); calcium antagonist toxicity; hypertension during pregnancy

DOSAGE
U.S. RDA is:
Adults: 1000-1500 mg
Children: <4 yrs: 800 mg
Infants: 600 mg
Adult
• Calcium acetate
Hyperphosphatemia: PO initial, 1334 mg (2 tabs) with meals; increase gradually to bring phosphate below 6 mg/dl (usually 3-4 tabs per meal)
• Calcium carbonate
Hyperphosphatemia: 1-17 g qd in divided doses
Hypocalcemia (replenish electrolytes): PO 1.25 g (500 mg Ca^{++}) 4-6 per day, chewed with water
Antacid: PO tabs 500 mg-1 g (250-500 mg Ca^{++}) 1 and 3 hr pc, hs prn; Susp 1.25 g (500 mg Cat^{++}), 1 and 3 hr pc, hs prn
Hypertension in pregnancy: 500 mg tid during third trimester
• Calcium chloride
Hypocalcemia (replenish electrolytes): IV 500 mg-1 g (6.8-13.6 mEq

---

italic = common side effects   ***bold italic*** = life-threatening reactions

Ca^{++}) q1-3 days as indicated by serum calcium levels; give at <1 ml/min

Cardiotonic: IV 500 mg-1 g (6.8-13.6 mEq Ca^{++}); give at <1 ml/min; Intraventricular 200-800 mg (2.72-9.6 mEq Ca^{++}) inj as single dose

• Calcium citrate

Hypocalcemia (replenish electrolytes): PO: 950 mg-1.9 g (200-400 mg Ca^{++}) tid-qid, pc

• Calcium glubionate

Hypocalcemia (replenish electrolytes): 5.4 g (345 mg Ca^{++}) tid-qid

• Calcium gluceptate

Hypocalcemia (replenish electrolytes): IM 440 mg-1.1 g (1.8-4.5 mEq Ca^{++}); IV 1.1-4.4 g (1.8-4.5 mEq Ca^{++}), slowly (rate not to exceed 2 mL/min)

• Calcium gluconate

Hypocalcemia, hyperkalemia, hypermagnesemia (replenish electrolytes): PO 11 g (1 g Ca^{++})/day in divided doses; IV 1 g (4.72 mEq Ca^{++}) at 0.5 ml/min (10% sol)

• Calcium lactate

Hypocalcemia: PO 325 mg-1.3 g (1 g Ca^{++}/day) tid with meals

• Tribasic calcium phosphate

Hypocalcemia: PO 1.6 mg (600 mg Ca^{++}) bid after meals

Child

• Calcium chloride: IV 25 mg/kg over several min

• Calcium glubionate

Infants up to 1 yr PO 1.8 g (115 mg Ca^{++}) 5× daily before meals

Children 1-4 yr PO 3.6 g (230 mg Ca^{++}) tid, ac

Children > 4 yr PO; see adult dose

• Calcium gluceptate

Newborn

Hypocalcemia: IM 440 mg-1.1 g (1.8-4.5 mEq Ca^{++}); IV 440 mg-1.1 g (1.8-4.5 mEq Ca^{++}) as single dose, rate not to exceed 2 mL/min

Exchange transfusions in newborns: IV 110 mg (approx. 0.45 mEq Ca^{++}) after every 100 ml of blood transfused

• Calcium gluconate: PO 500 mg/kg/day in divided doses, pc

• Calcium lactate: PO 500 mg/kg/day in divided doses

$ AVAILABLE FORMS/COST OF THERAPY

Calcium acetate

• Inj, Sol—IV: 0.5 mEq/ml, 10 ml: **$1.01**

• Tab, Uncoated—Oral: 667 mg, 200's: **$18.50-$19.60**

Calcium carbonate (mg of calcium)

• Tab, Uncoated, Chewable—Oral: 500 mg, 100's: **$6.17-$8.94;** 600 mg, 60's: **$3.00-$3.47**

• Tab, Uncoated—Oral: 500 mg, 60's: **$1.25-$6.86;** 600 mg, 60's: **$1.20-$6.34**

• Cap—Oral: 500 mg, 100's: **$10.52**

• Susp—Oral: 500 mg/5 ml, 500 ml: **$9.50**

Calcium chloride

• Inj, Sol—IV: 10%, 10 ml: **$4.93-$13.31**

Calcium citrate (mg of calcium)

• Tab—Oral: 200 mg, 100's: **$3.10-$6.87**

Calcium glubionate (mg of calcium)

• Tab, Effervescent—Oral: 500 mg, 30's: **$4.13**

• Syr—Oral: 115 mg/5 ml, 480 ml: **$22.11-$23.76**

Calcium gluceptate

• Inj, Sol—IM: 90 mg/5 ml, 5 ml: **$1.89**

Calcium gluconate (mg of calcium)

• Inj, Sol—IV: 10%, 10 ml: **$1.75-$1.89**

• Tab: 45 mg, 100's: **$5.00-$6.91;** 58.5 mg, 100's: **$2.16-$3.49;** 87.75 mg, 100's: **$7.95**

Calcium lactate (mg of calcium)

• Tab: 42.25 mg, 100's: **$1.50;** 84.5 mg, 100's: **$1.55-$5.25**

Tribasic calcium phosphate (mg of calcium)

• Tab: 600 mg, 60's: **$7.97**

* = non-FDA-approved use

CONTRAINDICATIONS: Hypercalcemia, hypercalciuria, hyperparathyroidism, bone tumors, digitalis toxicity, ventricular fibrillation, renal calculi, sarcoidosis, renal insufficiency (tribasic calcium phosphate)

PRECAUTIONS: Elderly, fluid restriction, decreased GI motility, GI obstruction, dehydration

PREGNANCY AND LACTATION: Pregnancy category C; some oral supplemental calcium may be excreted in breast milk (chloride, gluconate, unknown); concentrations not sufficient to produce an adverse effect in neonates

SIDE EFFECTS/ADVERSE REACTIONS

CV: Bradycardia, ***cardiac arrest, dysrhythmias,*** heart block, hemorrhage, hypotension, rebound hypertension, shortened Q-T

GI: Anorexia, constipation, diarrhea, eructation, flatulence, nausea, obstruction, rebound hyperacidity, vomiting

GU: Renal dysfunction, ***renal failure,*** renal stones

METAB: Hypercalcemia (drowsiness, lethargy, muscle weakness, headache, constipation, ***coma,*** anorexia, nausea, vomiting, polyuria, thirst); metabolic alkalosis; milk-alkali syndrome (nausea, vomiting, disorientation, headache)

MISC: Burning at IV site, extravasation, necrosis, pain, severe venous thrombosis

INTERACTIONS

Drugs

3 *Calcium channel blockers:* Calcium administration (especially parenteral) may inhibit calcium channel blocker activity

3 *Digoxin, digitoxin:* Elevated calcium concentrations associated with acute digitalis toxicity

3 *Doxycycline, Tetracycline:* Cotherapy with a tetracycline and a divalent or trivalent cation can reduce the serum concentration and efficacy of tetracyclines

3 *Iron:* Some calcium antacids reduce the GI absorption of iron; inhibition of the hematological response to iron has been reported

3 *Itraconazole, Ketoconazole:* Antacids containing calcium may reduce antifungal concentrations

3 *Quinidine:* Calcium antacids capable of increasing urine pH may increase serum quinidine concentrations

3 *Quinolones:* Reduced bioavailability of quinolone antibiotics

3 *Sodium polystyrene sulfonate resin:* Combined use with calcium-containing antacid may result in systemic alkalosis

3 *Thiazides:* Large doses of calcium with thiazides may lead to milk-alkali syndrome

Labs

• *False increase:* Chloride, green color, benzodiazepine (false positive)

• *False decrease:* Magnesium, oxylate, lipase

SPECIAL CONSIDERATIONS

• Percentage elemental calcium content of various calcium salts: calcium acetate (25), calcium carbonate (40), calcium chloride (27.2), calcium citrate (21), calcium glubionate (6.5), calcium gluceptate (8.2), calcium gluconate (9.3), calcium lactate (13), tricalcium phosphate, (39)

MONITORING PARAMETERS

• Serum calcium or serum ionized calcium concentrations (ionized calcium concentrations are preferable to determine free and bound calcium, especially with concurrent low serum albumin)

• Alternatively, ionized calcium can be estimated using the following

---

italic = common side effects   **bold italic** = life-threatening reactions

rule: Total serum calcium will fall by 0.8 mg/dL for each 1.0 g/dL decrease in serum albumin concentration

---

calfactant
(cal-fac'tant)
Rx: Infasurf
Chemical Class: Phospholipid
Therapeutic Class: Lung surfactant

CLINICAL PHARMACOLOGY
Mechanism of Action: Prevents alveoli from collapsing during expiration by lowering surface tension between air and alveolar surfaces in neonates with deficient or ineffective lung surfactant
Pharmacokinetics
Most of dose probably becomes lung-associated within hours of administration; the lipids enter endogenous surfactant pathways of reutilization and recycling
INDICATIONS AND USES: Prevention of respiratory distress syndrome (RDS) in premature infants at high risk for RDS and for the treatment ("rescue") of premature infants who develop RDS
DOSAGE
Infant
• Treatment of RDS: Intratracheally through an endotracheal tube; 3 ml/kg birth weight administered in two aliquots of 1.5 ml/kg each; dose is drawn into a syringe from the single-use vial using a 20-gauge or larger needle with care taken to avoid excessive foaming; administration is made by instillation of the suspension into the endotracheal tube; after each aliquot is instilled, the infant should be positioned with either the right or the left side dependent; administration is made while ventilation is continued over 20-30 breaths for each aliquot, with small bursts timed only during the inspiratory cycles; a pause followed by evaluation of the respiratory status and repositioning should separate the two aliquots; repeat doses of 3 ml/kg of birth weight, up to a total of 3 doses 12 hours apart, have been given in controlled clinical trials if the patient was still intubated
• Prophylaxis of RDS: Administer as above as soon as possible after birth
█ AVAILABLE FORMS/COST OF THERAPY
• Susp—Intratracheal: 6 ml: **$32.12**
PRECAUTIONS: Should be administered under the supervision of clinicians experienced in the acute care of newborn infants with respiratory failure who require intubation
SIDE EFFECTS/ADVERSE REACTIONS
CV: Bradycardia
RESP: Cyanosis; airway obstruction; **apnea;** *reflux of surfactant into endotracheal tube; requirement for manual ventilation;* reintubation
SPECIAL CONSIDERATIONS
• Store refrigerated temperature 2° to 8° C (36° to 46° F) and protect from light; vials are for single use only; after opening, discard unused drug
MONITORING PARAMETERS
• Rapid and substantial increases in blood oxygenation and improved lung compliance often follow Infasurf instillation; close clinical monitoring and surveillance following administration may be needed to adjust oxygen therapy and ventilator pressures appropriately

---

candesartan
(kan-de-sar'-tan)
Rx: Atacand
Chemical Class: Angiotensin II receptor antagonist
Therapeutic Class: Antihypertensive

CLINICAL PHARMACOLOGY
Mechanism of Action: Antihypertensive (inhibition of vasoconstriction and aldosterone secretion), smooth muscle hypoproliferative, and cardioprotective effects are attributable to selective blockade of angiotensin II (AT1) receptors found throughout the cardiovascular and renal systems; effects independent of angiotensin II synthesis
Pharmacokinetics
PO: Onset 2-4 hrs; peak 6-8 hrs; majority of antihypertensive response to a fixed-dose is manifested in 2 wk; full impact present after 4 wk; oral bioavailability 15%, unaffected by meals; >99% protein bound; apparent clearance 0.20-0.25 L/h/kg; candesartan cilexetil, the esterified pro-drug of candesartan completely metabolized during absorption from the intestinal wall (peak metabolite levels 3-4 hrs), 33% renal excreted; 67% recovered in feces; $t_{1/2}$ 5-7 hrs
INDICATIONS AND USES: Hypertension, CHF (left ventricular dysfunction*), myocardial infarction*, diabetic nephropathy
DOSAGE
Adult and child >16 yr
• Hypertension: PO 8-32 mg qd
$ AVAILABLE FORMS/COST OF THERAPY
• Tab, Coated—Oral: 4 mg, 30's: **$37.26;** 8 mg, 30's: **$37.26;** 16 mg, 30's: **$37.26;** 32 mg, 30's: **$50.40**
CONTRAINDICATIONS: Primary hyperaldosteronism; bilateral renal artery stenosis

PRECAUTIONS: Hypovolemic patients (salt and/or volume depleted; diuretic therapy) at greater risk of symptomatic hypotension; concurrent potassium-sparing diuretics, potassium-laden salt substitutes, or other potassium-sparing medications, bilateral renal artery stenosis; aortic or mitral valve stenosis; hypertrophic cardiomyopathy; severe hepatic dysfunction/cholestasis
PREGNANCY AND LACTATION: Pregnancy category C (1st trimester) and D (2nd and 3rd trimester)
SIDE EFFECTS/ADVERSE REACTIONS
CNS: Anxiety, depression, dizziness (2.4%), drowsiness, fatigue (1.4%), headache (3.8%), lightheadedness, parethesia, vertigo
CV: Flushing, palpitations, tachycardia
EENT: Epistaxis
MS: Back pain, myalgia (1.9%)
RESP: Cough (1.8-6.5%), upper respiratory infection
SKIN: Facial edema, angioedema, diaphoresis
MISC: Angioedema
INTERACTIONS
Drugs
3 *Cimetidine:* Increased levels of candesartan
3 *Fluconazole:* Decreased conversion to active metabolite (CYP2C9 inhibition), loss of antihypertensive effects
2 *Lithium:* Increased renal lithium reabsorption at the proximal tubular site due to the natriuresis associated with the inhibition of aldosterone secretion; increased risk of lithium toxicity
3 *Phenobarbital:* Decreased levels of candesartan
3 *Rifampin:* Induced metabolism of losartan and metabolite, resulting in a decrease in the area under the

---

italic = common side effects　　　　**bold italic** = life-threatening reactions

concentration-time curve (AUC) and half-life of both compounds and reduced losartan efficacy

SPECIAL CONSIDERATIONS
• Potentially as or more effective than angiotensin-converting enzyme inhibitors, without cough; no evidence for reduction in morbidity and mortality as first-line agents in hypertension yet; whether they provide the same cardiac and renal protection also still tentative; like ACE inhibitors, less effective in black patients

PATIENT/FAMILY EDUCATION
• Call your clinician immediately if the following side effects are noted: wheezing; lip, throat or face swelling; hives or rash

MONITORING PARAMETERS
• Baseline electrolytes, urinalysis, blood urea nitrogen and creatinine with recheck at 2-4 wk after initiation (sooner in volume-depleted patients); monitor sitting BP; watch for symptomatic hypotension, particularly in volume-depleted patients

---

capreomycin
(kap-ree-oh-mye′sin)
Rx: Capastat
Chemical Class: S. capreolus derivative
Therapeutic Class: Antituberculosis agent

CLINICAL PHARMACOLOGY
Mechanism of Action: Inhibits RNA synthesis, decreases mycobacterial replication
Pharmacokinetics
IM: Peak 1-2 hr, $t_{1/2}$ 4-6 hr (prolonged with decreased renal function); excreted in urine unchanged (small amount in bile)
INDICATIONS AND USES: Pulmonary tuberculosis caused by *Mycobacterium tuberculosis* after failure or intolerability with primary medications; use concurrently with other antituberculars

DOSAGE
Adult
• IM 1 g or 13.9 mg/kg (not to exceed 20 mg/kg/day) qd × 2-4 mo, then 1 g 2-3 ×/wk × 18-24 mo, not to exceed 20 mg/kg/day; *must* be given with another antitubercular medication; dosage reduction necessary with declining renal function, as follows (dose in mg/kg/day designed to achieve steady state levels of 10 mg/L: if CrCl = 50 ml/min, give 7 mg/kg q24h; if CrCl = 20 ml/min, give 3.6 mg/kg q24h; if CrCl = 10 ml/min, give 2.4 mg/kg q24h; if CrCl = 0 ml/min, give 1.3 mg/kg q24h)
Child
• 15-30 mg/kg qd, though safety and efficacy not established

⑧ AVAILABLE FORMS/COST OF THERAPY
• Inj, Sol—IM: 1 g/vial: **$24.33**
PRECAUTIONS: Renal disease, hearing impairment, hepatic disease, myasthenia gravis, Parkinsonism
PREGNANCY AND LACTATION: Pregnancy category C; breast milk excretion is unknown; however, problems in humans have not been documented (poorly absorbed from GI tract)
SIDE EFFECTS/ADVERSE REACTIONS
CNS: Fever, headache, hearing loss, neuromuscular blockade, tinnitus, vertigo
EENT: Deafness, ototoxicity (11%), tinnitus
GU: Albuminuria, alkalosis, decreased CrCl, hematuria, hypokalemia, increased BUN, *nephrotoxicity* (36%), proteinuria, *tubular necrosis*
HEME: Eosinophilia, leukocytosis, *leukopenia*

SKIN: Irritation, pain, rash, sterile abscess at injection site; urticaria

INTERACTIONS

Drugs

3 *Amphotericin B, Cephalosporins, Cyclosporine, Methoxyflurane:* Additive nephrotoxicity risk

3 *Carboplatin:* Additive ototoxicity

2 *Ethacrynic acid:* Additive ototoxicity

2 *Neuromuscular blocking agents:* Potentiate the respiratory suppression produced by neuromuscular blocking agents

3 *Oral anticoagulants:* Enhanced hypoprothrombinemic response

SPECIAL CONSIDERATIONS
• When used in renal insufficiency or pre-existing auditory impairment, risks of additional 8th-nerve impairment or renal injury should be weighed against the benefits of therapy

MONITORING PARAMETERS
• Electrolytes, BUN, creatinine weekly
• Blood levels of drug
• Audiometric testing before, during, after treatment

---

capsaicin
(cap-say'sin)
OTC: Zostrix, Zostrix HP
Chemical Class: Alkaloid derivative of Solanaceae plant family
Therapeutic Class: Topical analgesic

CLINICAL PHARMACOLOGY
Mechanism of Action: Early counterirritant properties, then depletes substance P in sensory neurons
Pharmacokinetics
TOP: Therapeutic effect in 14-28 days
INDICATIONS AND USES: Relief of pain in postherpetic neuralgia, diabetic neuropathy, rheumatoid arthritis, osteoarthritis, mastectomy,* psoriasis*

DOSAGE

Adult and Child ≥2 yrs

TOP: Apply 3-5 times/day, less frequent application not effective; continue for 3-5 months, some pts may require lifelong therapy

AVAILABLE FORMS/COST OF THERAPY
• Cre—Top: 0.025%, 60 g: **$4.69-$21.20;** 0.075%, 60 g: **$7.00-$27.00**
• Balm—Top: 0.025%, 20 g: **$9.56;** 0.075%, 20 g: **$16.09**
• Gel—Top: 0.025%, 60 g: **$4.37-$6.13;** 0.05%, 60 g: **$5.37;** 0.075%, 30 g: **$5.80**
• Lot—Top: 0.025%, 60 ml: **$9.62;** 0.075% 60 ml: **$6.00**

CONTRAINDICATIONS: Application to damaged skin

SIDE EFFECTS/ADVERSE REACTIONS

CNS: Neurotoxicity
SKIN: Burning, itching, local discomfort

SPECIAL CONSIDERATIONS
• Pretreatment with topical lidocaine 5% ointment may relieve burning

PATIENT/FAMILY EDUCATION
• Wash hands following use

---

captopril
(cap-toe-pril)
Rx: Capoten
Combinations
Rx: with hydrochlorothiazide (Capozide)
Chemical Class: Sulfhydryl-containing angiotensin-converting enzyme (ACE) inhibitor
Therapeutic Class: Antihypertensive

CLINICAL PHARMACOLOGY

Mechanism of Action: Antihypertensive, hypoproliferative, and cardioprotective effects atributable to competitive inhibition of angiotensin-converting enzyme (ACE) yielding decreased plasma concentrations of angiotensin II, plasma aldosterone concentrations, systemic vascular resistance, blood pressure, preload, and afterload, not accompanied by changes in heart rate, pressor sensitivity to exogenous norepinephrine, or baroreceptor sensitivity

Pharmacokinetics

PO: Peak 1 hr (presence of food reduces absorption by 3%-40%), duration 2-6 hr, metabolized by liver, excreted in urine (40%-50% unchanged); $t_{1/2}$ <2-3 hr crosses placenta; excreted in breast milk

INDICATIONS AND USES: Hypertension (essential, malignant,* renovascular, associated with pheochromocytoma,* scleroderma*), CHF (left ventricular dysfunction), MI (left ventricular salvage), erythrocytosis,* diabetic and nondiabetic nephropathy, retinopathy with diabetes, hepatorenal syndrome,* polycythemia vera,* Bartter's syndrome,* aldosteronism,* cystinuria,* rheumatoid arthritis,* Kaposi's sarcoma*

DOSAGE

Adult

• *Hypertension:* PO initial: 6.25 mg-12.5 mg tid (patients with low blood pressure, hyponatremia (<130 mEq/L), hypovolemia, or those on diuretics); others 25 mg tid; increase every 1-2 weeks to 50 mg tid; usual maintenance range 25-150 tid; max 450 mg/day

• *Congestive heart failure* (left ventricular dysfunction): PO 3.125-6.25 mg tid (for patients pretreated with diuretics, hypotensive, hypovolemic, or hyponatremic); others 12.5 mg bid-tid; may increase to 50 mg bid-tid (as systolic blood pressure will allow, i.e., >100 mm Hg), generally given with digitalis and diuretics; maximum daily doses, 450 mg/day

• *Myocardial infarction* (left ventricular salvage): PO initial dose of 6.25 mg (to minimize excessive or symptomatic hypotensive responses) given within 3 days of MI; if tolerated, 12.5 mg tid, with titration over the next few days to a goal of 50 mg tid as maintenance

• *Diabetic nephropathy:* PO 50 mg bid or 25 mg tid

Child

• *Hypertension:* PO initial dose, 0.01 mg-0.25 mg/kg q12h (infants); 0.-0.5 mg tid (older children); maintenance dose, 2 mg/kg/dose bid-tid

• *Congestive heart failure* (left ventricular dysfunction): PO initial 2.5 mg/kg/dose, increasing to 3.5 mg/kg/dose, usually tid, with diuretics and digoxin

[$] AVAILABLE FORMS/COST OF THERAPY

• Tab, Uncoated—Oral: 12.5 mg, 100's: **$3.75-$88.03;** 25 mg, 100's: **$5.45-$95.15;** 50 mg, 100's: **$9.90-$163.18;** 100 mg, 100's: **$18.83-$217.30**

PRECAUTIONS: History of anaphylaxis, renal insufficiency (<30 ml/min), hypotension (CHF, elderly, volume depletion—diuretics, dialysis, cirrhosis), aortic stenosis, hyperkalemia (potassium supplements, potassium-sparing diuretics, renal disease, diabetes), neutropenia (autoimmune diseases, collagen vascular, febrile illness, immunosuppressant drug therapy), proteinuria, renal artery stenosis, surgery/anesthesia (excessive hypotension, correctable with fluids)

* = non-FDA-approved use

PREGNANCY AND LACTATION:
Pregnancy category C (1st trimester) and D (2nd and 3rd trimesters—fetal and neonatal hypotension, neonatal skull hypoplasia, anuria, reversible or irreversible renal failure, death, oligohydramnios); excreted into breast milk in small amounts; compatible with breast feeding

SIDE EFFECTS/ADVERSE REACTIONS

CNS: Chills, fever

CV: Chest pain, hypotension, palpitations, postural hypotension, tachycardia

GI: Loss of taste

GU: Acute reversible renal failure, dysuria, frequency, impotence, nephrotic syndrome, nocturia, oliguria, polyuria, proteinuria

HEME: Agranulocytosis, neutropenia

METAB: Hyperkalemia, hyponatremia

RESP: Angioedema, ***bronchospasm,*** *cough,* dyspnea

SKIN: Rash

INTERACTIONS

Drugs

❷ *Allopurinol:* Increased risk of hypersensitivity reactions including Stevens-Johnson syndrome, skin eruptions, fever, and arthralgias

❸ α-*blockers:* Possible exaggerated "first dose" response

❸ *Aspirin:* Reduced hemodynamic effects of captopril; less likely at doses <236 mg qd

❸ *Azathioprine:* Increased myelosuppression

❸ *Cyclosporine:* Increased nephrotoxicity

❸ *Indomethacin:* Inhibits the antihypertensive response to ACE inhibition; other NSAIDs probably have similar effect

❸ *Insulin:* ACE inhibitors enhance insulin sensitivity; hypoglycemia possible

❸ *Iron:* Increased risk of systemic reaction (GI symptoms, hypotension) with parenteral iron

❸ *Lithium:* Increased risk of lithium toxicity

❸ *Loop diuretics:* Initiation of ACE inhibition therapy with concurrent intensive diuretic therapy may cause significant hypotension, renal insufficiency

❸ *Mercaptopurine:* Increased risk of neutropenia

❸ *Potassium, Potassium-sparing diuretics:* ACE inhibition tends to increase potassium; increased risk of hyperkalemia in predisposed patients

❸ *Trimethoprim:* Additive risk of hyperkalemia, especially in patient predisposed to renal insufficiency

Labs

• ACE inhibition can account for approximately 0.5mEq/L rise in serum potassium

• Blood in urine: Decreased reactivity with occult blood test

• Fructosamine: Captopril interferes with assay increasing serum fructosamine

• Ketones in urine: False positive dip-sticks

• *False positive:* Urine acetone

SPECIAL CONSIDERATIONS

PATIENT/FAMILY EDUCATION

• Caution with salt substitutes containing potassium chloride

• Rise slowly to sitting/standing position to minimize orthostatic hypotension

• Dizziness, fainting, lightheadedness may occur during 1st few days of therapy

• May cause altered taste perception or cough; persistent dry cough usually does not subside unless medication is stopped; notify clinician if these symptoms persist

MONITORING PARAMETERS

• BUN, creatinine, potassium within 2 wk after initiation of therapy (increased levels may indicate acute renal failure)

---

carbachol

(kar'ba-kole)

Rx: Carbastat, Carboptic, Miostat, Isopto Carbachol

Chemical Class: Choline ester
Therapeutic Class: Antiglaucoma agent; miotic; ophthalmic cholinergic

CLINICAL PHARMACOLOGY

Mechanism of Action: Cholinergic (parasympathomimetic) agent, stimulates the motor endplate of the muscle cell, and also partially inhibits cholinesterase; contracts sphincter muscle of iris; causes spasms of ciliary muscle, deepening of anterior chamber

Pharmacokinetics

OPHTH: Onset of miosis 10-20 min, peak reduction in intraocular pressure 4 hr; duration of miosis 4-8 hr, decreased intraocular pressure 8 hr

INTRAOCULAR: Peak miosis within 2-5 min, duration miosis 24 hr

INDICATIONS AND USES: Miosis during ocular surgery, glaucoma

DOSAGE

• *Ocular surgery:* Intraocular 0.5 ml 0.01% sol in anterior chamber of eye (done by physician) for miosis during surgery

• *Glaucoma:* Instill 1-2 gtt (top) of 0.75%-3% sol into eye bid-tid

$ AVAILABLE FORMS/COST OF THERAPY

• Sol—Ophth: 0.01%, 1.5 ml: **$27.50;** 0.75%, 15 ml: **$21.25;** 1.5%, 15 ml: **$23.50;** 2.25%, 15 ml: **$23.38;** 3%, 15 ml: **$12.11-$26.25**

CONTRAINDICATIONS: When miosis is undesirable; corneal abrasions

PRECAUTIONS: Bradycardia, CAD, hyperthyroidism, asthma, pregnancy, obstruction of GI or urinary tract, peptic ulcer, parkinsonism, epilepsy, peritonitis; retinal detachment reported in susceptible individuals

PREGNANCY AND LACTATION: Pregnancy category C; transplacental passage in significant amounts not expected

SIDE EFFECTS/ADVERSE REACTIONS

CNS: Headache

CV: Bradycardia, marked hypotension

EENT: Blurred vision, conjunctival hyperemia, decreased visual acuity in dim light, eye ache, myopia

GI: Abdominal discomfort, diarrhea, nausea, salivation, vomiting

RESP: Bronchospasm

SPECIAL CONSIDERATIONS

PATIENT/FAMILY EDUCATION

• Blurred vision will decrease with repeated use of drug

• Caution if driving during first few days of treatment

---

carbamazepine

(kar-ba-maz'e-peen)

Rx: Atretol, Carbatrol, Epitol, Tegretol, Tegretol-XR

Chemical Class: Iminostilbene derivative
Therapeutic Class: Anticonvulsant; antineuralgic; antimanic; antipsychotic

CLINICAL PHARMACOLOGY

Mechanism of Action: Anticonvulsant action by inhibition of influx of sodium ions across nerve cell membrane in motor cortex, reducing polysynaptic response and blocking post-

---

tetanic potentiation; antineuralgic may involve GABA$_B$ receptors, which may be linked to calcium channels; antimanic/antipsychotic effects on neurotransmitter modulator systems

Pharmacokinetics

PO: Anticonvulsant onset varies hours to days; antineuralgic onset 8-72 hr; antimanic onset 7-10 days; peak concentrations: susp 1.5 hr; tabs 4-5 hr; therapeutic serum concentrations 4-12 µg/mL; absorption slow (suspension faster than tablets); metabolized by liver (autoinduction); excreted in urine and feces; crosses placenta; excreted in breast milk; t$_{1/2}$ variable 14-16 hr after repeated dosing

INDICATIONS AND USES: Tonic-clonic, complex-partial, mixed seizures; trigeminal neuralgia, glossopharyngeal neuralgia; manic depressive disorder,* chronic neurogenic pain syndromes,* diabetes insipidus (central),* alcohol withdrawal,* psychotic disorders,* restless legs syndrome*

DOSAGE

Adult

• *Seizures:* PO 200 mg bid; may be increased by 200 mg/day in divided doses q6-8h; maintenance 800-1200 mg/day; max 1200 mg/day

• *Trigeminal neuralgia:* PO 100 mg bid; may increase 100 mg q12h until pain subsides; not to exceed 1.2 g/day; maintenance is 200-400 mg bid

• *Antidiuretic:* 300-600 mg/day, as sole therapy; 200-400 mg/day, if concurrent with other antidiuretic agents

• *Antipsychotic:* PO 200-400 mg/day divided tid-qid; max 1600 mg/day

Child <12 yr

• *Seizures:* PO 10-20 mg/kg/day in 2-3 divided doses

💲 AVAILABLE FORMS/COST OF THERAPY

• Tab, Chewable—Oral: 100 mg, 100's: **$17.45-$23.76**

• Tab, Uncoated—Oral: 200 mg, 100's: **$23.25-$45.26**

• Susp—Oral: 100 mg/5 ml, 450 ml: **$29.15**

• Tab, EXT REL—Oral: 100 mg, 100's: **$22.67;** 200 mg, 100's: **$45.26;** 400 mg, 100's: **$90.46**

• Cap, EXT REL—Oral: 200 mg, 120's: **$53.96;** 300 mg, 120's: **$80.94**

CONTRAINDICATIONS: Hypersensitivity to tricyclic antidepressants, bone marrow depression, concomitant use of MAO inhibitor

PRECAUTIONS: Glaucoma, hepatic disease, renal disease, cardiac disease, psychosis, child <6 yr

PREGNANCY AND LACTATION: Pregnancy category C; concentration in milk approximately 60% of maternal plasma concentration; compatible with breast feeding

SIDE EFFECTS/ADVERSE REACTIONS

CNS: Ataxia, confusion, dizziness, *drowsiness,* fatigue, hallucinations, headache, paralysis

CV: Aggravation of coronary artery disease, ***CHF,*** hypertension, hypotension

EENT: Blurred vision, conjunctivitis, diplopia, dry mouth, nystagmus, tinnitus

GI: Abdominal pain, anorexia, *constipation, diarrhea,* enzymes, glossitis, hepatitis, increased liver enzymes, *nausea,* stomatitis, vomiting

GU: Albuminuria, frequency, glycosuria, impotence, urinary retention

HEME: ***Agranulocytosis, aplastic anemia,*** eosinophilia, ***leukocytosis, neutropenia, thrombocytopenia***

RESP: Pulmonary hypersensitivity (fever, dyspnea, pneumonitis)

*SKIN: Rash, **Stevens-Johnson syndrome,*** urticaria

---

italic = common side effects   ***bold italic*** = life-threatening reactions

INTERACTIONS
Drugs

3 *Acetaminopen:* Enhanced hepatotoxic potential; reduced acetaminophen response

3 *Antidepressants, tricyclic:* Carbamazepine reduces serum concentrations of imipramine and probably other cyclic antidepressants

3 *Benzodiazepines* (alprazolam, diazepam, midazolam, triazolam): Metabolized by CYP3A4; enzyme induced by carbamazepine; reduced benzo effect

2 *Calcium channel blockers:* Verapamil and diltiazem reduce the metabolism of carbamazepine leading to increased carbamazepine toxicity when these CCBs are added to chronic carbamazepine therapy; enzyme induction by carbamazepine can reduce the bioavailability of CCBs that undergo extensive 1st-pass hepatic clearance, like felodipine (94% reduction)

3 *Cimetidine:* Transient (1 week) increases in carbamazepine levels

3 *Corticosteroids:* Carbamazepine reduces levels and therapeutic effect

3 *Cyclosporine:* Carbamazepine reduces cyclosporine blood levels

2 *Danazol:* Increases carbamazepine levels with toxicity expected

3 *Doxycycline:* Carbamazepine reduces doxycycline levels and antibiotic effects

3 *Erythromycin, clarithromycin:* Increased carbamazepine levels

3 *Ethinyl Estradiol, Oral contraceptives:* Carbamazepine-induced metabolic induction may lead to menstrual irregularities and unplanned pregnancies

3 *Felbamate:* Reductions in carbamazepine levels and increases in 10,11-epoxide metabolite, along with decreased felbamate concentrations

3 *Fluoxetine, fluvoxamine:* Inhibits carbamazepine metabolism, increased levels and risk of toxicity

3 *Isoniazid:* Increases carbamazepine levels with increased risk of toxicity

3 *Isotretinoin:* Reduced carbamazepine bioavailability

3 *Lamotrigine:* Increased carbamazepine metab and risk of toxicity; carbamazepine reduces lamotrigine levels

3 *Lithium:* Increased potential for neurotoxicity with normal lithium concentrations; reverses carbamazepine-induced leukopenia; additive antithyroidal effects

3 *Mebendazole:* Carbamazepine decreases mebendazole levels, significant only when large doses given

3 *Methadone:* Carbamazepine reduces levels and therapeutic effect

3 *Metronidazole:* Increases carbamazepine concentrations with toxicity

3 *Neuroleptics:* Reduced concentration of and therapeutic response to these agents when used with carbamazepine

3 *Omeprazole:* May increase carbamazepine concentrations

3 *Oral anticoagulants:* Decreased prothrombin time

3 *Phenytoin:* Concurrent use reduces serum concentrations of both

2 *Propoxyphene:* Increases carbamazepine levels

3 *Theophylline:* Carbamazepine reduces levels and therapeutic effect

3 *Thyroid:* Carbamazepine reduces levels and therapeutic effect

3 *Valproic acid:* Valproic acid can increase, decrease, or have no effect on carbamazepine, monitor serum levels; carbamazepine decreases levels of valproic acid

Labs

• *Chloride, serum:* falsely elevated at elevated carbamazepine concentrations

---

* = non-FDA-approved use

- *Thyroxine (T₄), free serum:* Falsely elevated by certain test methods
- *Tri-iodothyronine (T₃), free serum:* Falsely decreased by certain test methods
- *T₃ uptake:* Carbamazepine interference falsely increases assay
- *Uric acid, serum:* High carbamazepine levels falsely decrease uric acid

SPECIAL CONSIDERATIONS
PATIENT/FAMILY EDUCATION
- Caution about driving and other activities that require alertness, at least initially
- Drug may turn urine pink to brown

MONITORING PARAMETERS
- CBC—aplastic anemia and agranulocytosis have been reported 5-8× greater than in the general public
- Liver function test
- Serum drug levels (therapeutic 4-12 µg/ml) during initial treatment

---

carbamide peroxide
(kar′ba-mide per-ox′ide)
OTC: *Otic:* Debrox, Murine Ear Drops
Oral: Gly-Oxide Liquid, Orajel Perioseptic, Proxigel
Chemical Class: Urea compound and hydrogen peroxide
Therapeutic Class: Cerumenolytic; topical oral anti-inflammatory

CLINICAL PHARMACOLOGY
Mechanism of Action: Foaming action facilitates removal of impacted cerumen; releases oxygen on contact with mouth tissues to provide cleansing effects, reduced inflammation, pain relief, and inhibition of odor-causing bacteria

INDICATIONS AND USES: Impacted cerumen, prevention of cerumenosis; oral inflammation (canker sores, denture irritation, irritated gums)

DOSAGE
Adult and Child
- INSTILL 5-10 gtt affected ear bid × 3-4 days
- PO Place several gtts of undiluted solution on affected area qid (expectorate after 2-3 min); gently massage gel on affected area qid

$ AVAILABLE FORMS/COST OF THERAPY
- Sol—Otic: 6.5%, 15 ml: **$2.00-$5.98**
- Sol—Oral: 10%, 15 ml: **$4.76;** 60 ml: **$8.63**
- Gel—Oral: 10%, 36 g: **$12.42**
- Liq—Oral: 15%, 13.3 ml: **$3.71**

CONTRAINDICATIONS: Otic surgery, perforated eardrum; children <3 yr (PO)

PREGNANCY AND LACTATION: Pregnancy category C

SIDE EFFECTS/ADVERSE REACTIONS
EENT: Irritation in ear, itching, redness

---

carbenicillin
(car-ben′a-sill-in)
Rx: Geocillin
Chemical Class: Semisynthetic penicillin derivative
Therapeutic Class: Antibiotic

CLINICAL PHARMACOLOGY
Mechanism of Action: Inhibits bacterial wall synthesis, bactericidal
Pharmacokinetics
PO: Peak urine concentration within 3 hr (therapeutic concentrations *only* in urine)
Rapidly absorbed PO from the small intestine (40% bioavailable), distributed to bile, 50% protein bound; t₁/₂ 1-1.5 hr; excreted in the urine (85%-90% unchanged); crosses placenta
INDICATIONS AND USES: Acute and chronic infections of the upper

and lower urinary tract and in asymptomatic bacteriuria, prostatitis

Antibacterial spectrum usually includes:

- Gram-negative organisms: *Neisseria gonorrhoeae, Enterobacter* sp., *Enterococcus faecalis, E. coli, Haemophilus influenzae, Klebsiella* sp., *Pseudomonas aeruginosa, Serratia* sp.
- Anaerobes: *Bacteroides* sp.

DOSAGE

Adult

- *UTI:* PO 382-764 mg q6h (use high doses for infections due to *Pseudomonas* and enterococci)
- *Prostatitis:* 764 mg q6h

§ AVAILABLE FORMS/COST OF THERAPY

- Tab, Uncoated—Oral: 382 mg, 100's: **$202.35**

PRECAUTIONS: Severe renal impairment (CrCl <10 ml/min will not achieve therapeutic levels)

PREGNANCY AND LACTATION: Pregnancy category B

SIDE EFFECTS/ADVERSE REACTIONS

CNS: Headache

EENT: Itchy eyes

GI: Bad taste, diarrhea, flatulence, glossitis, mild SGOT elevations, nausea, vomiting

GU: Vaginitis

HEME: Eosinophilia, ***bone marrow suppression***

SKIN: Hypersensitivity reactions (skin rash, urticaria, pruritus)

INTERACTIONS

Drug

3 *Aminoglycosides:* Chemically inactivated by carbenicillin

3 *Methotrexate:* Increased methotrexate serum concentration

3 *Probenecid:* Increased penicillin concentrations

Labs

- *Albumin:* Decreased serum concentrations
- *Amino acids:* Increased urine

- *Bilirubin:* Increased serum bilirubin levels
- *Gentamicin:* 25% increase in serum level
- *Glucose:* False positive using Clinitest
- *Protein:* Increased serum levels
- *Triglycerides:* Increased serum levels

SPECIAL CONSIDERATIONS

- **NOTE:** When high and rapid blood and urine levels of antibiotic are indicated, alternative parenteral therapy should be used

---

carbidopa and levodopa

(kar-bee-doe′pa; lee-voe-doe′pa)

Rx: Sinemet, Sinemet CR

Chemical Class: Catecholamine precursor

Therapeutic Class: Antiparkinson's agent; antidyskinetic

CLINICAL PHARMACOLOGY

Mechanism of Action: Symptoms of Parkinson's disease are related to depleted dopamine in the corpus striatum; carbidopa inhibits peripheral decarboxylation of levodopa; thus, more levodopa is made available for transport to brain and conversion to dopamine, which replenishes dopamine in the corpus striatum

Pharmacokinetics

PO: Peak concentration, 0.7 hr (tabs), 2.4 hr (TIME REL), absorption rapid and complete within 2-3 hr (tabs); gradual and continuous over 4-6 hr (TIME REL); widely distributed, 36% protein bound, $t_{1/2}$ 1-2 hr; excreted in urine (metabolites)

INDICATIONS AND USES: Parkinson's disease, restless legs syndrome,* phenylketonuria,* psoriasis,* shingles,* sleep behavior dis-

---

* = non-FDA-approved use

order,* swallowing disorders,* tardive dyskinesia,* vitiligo*

DOSAGE

Adult

• Sinemet

PO 1 tab of 25 mg carbidopa/100 mg levodopa tid or 10 mg/100 mg tid-qid; increase by 1 tab qd-qod prn until dosage of 8 tabs/day is reached; provide at least 70-100 mg of carbidopa/day

• Sinemet CR

PO 1 tab bid at intervals of not <6 hr; usual dose is 2-8 tabs/day in divided doses at intervals of 4-8 hr while awake; allow at least 3 days between dosage adjustments

• *Restless legs:* PO 1 tab 25 mg/100 mg qhs

⑤ AVAILABLE FORMS/COST OF THERAPY

• Tab, Uncoated—Oral: 10 mg/100 mg, 100's: **$25.53-$68.81;** 25 mg/100 mg, 100's: **$27.54-$77.69;** 25 mg/250 mg, 100's: **$32.55-$99.00**

• Tab, Time-Rel—Oral: 25 mg/100 mg, 100's: **$82.87;** 50 mg/200 mg, 100's: **$166.31**

CONTRAINDICATIONS: Narrow-angle glaucoma, undiagnosed skin lesions

PRECAUTIONS: Renal disease, cardiac disease, hepatic disease, respiratory disease, MI with dysrhythmias, convulsions, peptic ulcer

PREGNANCY AND LACTATION: Pregnancy category C; should not be given to nursing mothers

SIDE EFFECTS/ADVERSE REACTIONS

CNS: Agitation, anxiety, confusion, dizziness, *fatigue,* hallucination, *hand tremors, headache,* hypomania, *insomnia, involuntary choreiform movements, nightmares, numbness,* psychosis, severe depression, *twitching, weakness*

CV: Hypertension, *orthostatic hypotension,* palpitation, tachycardia

EENT: Blurred vision, dilated pupils, diplopia

GI: Abdominal distress, anorexia, bitter taste, constipation, diarrhea, *dry mouth, dysphagia, flatulence, nausea, vomiting*

GU: Dark urine, incontinence, urinary retention

HEME: **Agranulocytosis, hemolytic anemia, leukopenia**

METAB: Weight change

SKIN: Alopecia, rash, sweating

DRUG INTERACTIONS

Drugs

③ *Benzodiazepines:* May exacerbate Parkinsonism in patients receiving levodopa; inhibits antiparkinsonian effects of levodopa

③ *Food:* High protein diets inhibit the efficacy of levodopa

③ *Iron (oral):* Reduces levodopa bioavailability by 50%

③ *MAOIs:* May result in hypertensive response

③ *Methionine:* Inhibits the clinical response to levodopa

② *Neuroleptics:* Phenothiazines block dopamine receptors, can produce extrapyramidal symptoms, and inhibit the antiparkinsonian effect of levodopa

③ *Phenytoin:* May inhibit the antiparkinsonian effect of levodopa

③ *Pyridoxine:* Inhibits the antiparkinsonian effect of levodopa; concurrent carbidopa negates the interaction

③ *Spiramycin:* Reduces the plasma concentration of levodopa, with reduction of antiparkinson efficacy

③ *Tacrine:* May inhibit the effect of levodopa in Parkinsons patients; dosage adjustments may be required

Labs

• *Acid phosphatase:* Increased serum acid phosphatase

• *Amino acids:* Increased urine amino acids

---

italic = common side effects   ***bold italic*** = life-threatening reactions

• *Aspartate aminotransferase:* Increased serum aspartate aminotransferase

• *Bilirubin:* Decreased serum bilirubin at concentrations of 15 mg/dL (Kodak Ektachem systems 2083); increased bilirubin at concentrations above 80 mg/dL (methods of Jendrassik and Grof) and below 5 mg/dL (Kodak Ektachem systems 2083)

• *Bilirubin, conjugated:* Decreased serum levels by 0.3 mg/dL at therapeutic levels of levodopa; minimally increased serum levels at markedly elevated levodopa concentrations (i.e., >60 mg/dL)

• *Catecholamines:* Increased plasma catecholamines, reported as epinephrine and norepinephrine

• *Cholinesterase:* Increased serum cholinesterase activity

• *Sputum:* Brown discoloration reported

• *Creatinine:* Increased serum creatinine

• *Creatinine clearance:* Increased urinary creatinine clearance (Jaffe method)

• *Ferric chloride test:* False positive

• *Glucose:* Decreases serum glucose as measured by GODPERID method, Ames Seralyzer, and glucose oxidase method; increased serum glucose by alkaline ferricyanide procedure, Technicon SMA method, and glucokinase method of Scott; false negative urine glucose (inhibits glucose oxidase method)

• *Guaiacols Spot test:* False negative

• *Hydroxy-methoxymandelic acid:* Increased urinary levels

• *Lithium:* Positive bias on serum lithium levels measured with Kodak Ektachem systems 2083

• *Triglycerides:* Lowered triglyceride levels measured by GPOPAP method

• *Urea nitrogen:* Decreases BUN

• *Uric acid:* Lowers serum urate levels as measured by uricase PAP method

SPECIAL CONSIDERATIONS
• Caution with use until after MAO inhibitors have been discontinued for 2 wk
• If previously on levodopa, discontinue for at least 8 hr before change to carbidopa and levodopa

PATIENT/FAMILY EDUCATION
• Limit protein taken with drug
• Arise slowly from a reclining position

---

carboprost

(kar′boe-prost)
Rx: Hemabate
Chemical Class: Prostaglandin F2α
Therapeutic Class: Abortifacient; uterine stimulant; antihemorrhagic (postpartum and postabortal uterine bleeding)

CLINICAL PHARMACOLOGY
Mechanism of Action: Stimulates uterine contractions, GI and vascular smooth muscle
Pharmacokinetics
IM: Peak 30 min; mean abortion time 16 hr; metabolized in lungs, liver; excreted in urine (metabolites)

INDICATIONS AND USES: Postpartum hemorrhage due to uterine atony that has not responded to conventional methods of management; abortion between 13-20 wk gestation as calculated from the 1st day of the last normal menstrual period and in the following conditions related to 2nd trimester abortion:
• Failure of expulsion of the fetus during the course of treatment by another method

• Premature rupture of membranes using intrauterine methods with loss of drug and insufficient or absent uterine activity

• Requirement of a repeat intrauterine instillation of drug for expulsion of the fetus

• Inadvertent or spontaneous rupture of membranes in the presence of a previable fetus and absence of adequate activity for expulsion

DOSAGE

Adult

• *Abortion:* IM 250 µg, then 250 µg q1½-3½ hr; may increase to 500 µg if no response; not to exceed 12 mg total dose or continuous administration for >2 days

• *Refractory postpartum uterine bleeding:* IM 250 µg single inj (75% response); selected cases, multiple dosing at intervals of 15 to 90 min; max dose 2 mg (total)

$ AVAILABLE FORMS/COST OF THERAPY

• Inj, Sol—IM: 250 µg/ml, 1 ml: **$42.30**

CONTRAINDICATIONS: Severe pulmonary, cardiac, or hepatic disease, acute PID

PRECAUTIONS: Asthma, anemia, jaundice, diabetes mellitus, seizure disorders, past uterine surgery

PREGNANCY AND LACTATION: Pregnancy category C; any dose which produces increased uterine tone could put the embryo or fetus at risk.

SIDE EFFECTS/ADVERSE REACTIONS

CNS: Chills, fever, headache

CV: Chest pain, ***dysrhythmias***

GI: Diarrhea, nausea, vomiting

GU: Endometritis, uterine/vaginal pain

RESP: Coughing, dyspnea, wheezing

SPECIAL CONSIDERATIONS

• Antiemetic, analgesic, and antidiarrheal medications should be considered concurrently to counter adverse GI effects

• In the treatment of uterine atony, IV oxytocin, uterine massage and IM methylergonovine (unless contraindicated) should be used before carboprost

carisoprodol

(kar'i-so-pro'dol)

Rx: Soma, Vanadom

Combinations

Rx: with aspirin (Soma Compound); with aspirin and codeine (Soma Compound with Codeine)

Chemical Class: Meprobamate congener

Therapeutic Class: Skeletal muscle relaxant

CLINICAL PHARMACOLOGY

Mechanism of Action: Muscle relaxation by blocking interneuronal activity in the descending reticular formation and spinal cord; produces sedation

Pharmacokinetics

PO: Onset ½ hr, duration 4-6 hr; metabolized by liver, excreted in urine; $t_{1/2}$ 8 hr

INDICATIONS AND USES: Adjunct to rest, physical therapy, and other measures for the relief of discomfort associated with acute, painful, musculoskeletal conditions; does not directly relax tense skeletal muscles

DOSAGE

Adult and Child >12 yr

• PO 350 mg tid-qid (take last dose hs)

$ AVAILABLE FORMS/COST OF THERAPY

• Tab, Uncoated—Oral: 350 mg, 100's: **$12.22-$240.65**

CONTRAINDICATIONS: Hypersensitivity (including related compounds such as meprobamate, me-

---

italic = common side effects   ***bold italic*** = life-threatening reactions

butamate, or tybamate), child <12 yr, intermittent porphyria

PRECAUTIONS: Renal disease, hepatic disease, addictive personality, elderly

PREGNANCY AND LACTATION: Pregnancy category C; crosses placenta; excreted in breast milk (2-4× maternal plasma)

SIDE EFFECTS/ADVERSE REACTIONS

CNS: Agitation, ataxia, depression, *dizziness, drowsiness,* headache, insomnia, irritability, syncope, tremor, vertigo, *weakness*

CV: Facial flushing, postural hypotension, tachycardia

EENT: Diplopia, temporary loss of vision

GI: Epigastric discomfort, hiccups, *nausea,* vomiting

SKIN: Eosinophilia, erythema multiforme, facial flushing, fever, fixed drug eruptions, pruritus, rash

SPECIAL CONSIDERATIONS
• Caution when used in addiction-prone individuals
• Abused on the street in conjunction with narcotics

PATIENT/FAMILY EDUCATION
• Abrupt cessation may precipitate mild withdrawal symptoms such as abdominal cramps, insomnia, chills, headache, and nausea

---

carteolol
(kar-tee'oe-lole)

Rx: Cartrol, Ocupress

Chemical Class: Nonselective β-adrenergic blocker with intrinsic sympathomimetic activity

Therapeutic Class: Antihypertensive; antiglaucoma agent

CLINICAL PHARMACOLOGY

Mechanism of Action: Nonselective β-adrenergic blocker with intrinsic sympathomimetic activity

Pharmacokinetics

PO: Onset 1-2 hr, peak 2-4 hr, duration 8-12 hr, food slows absorption but does not lower total absorption; metabolized by liver (metabolites inactive); excreted in urine, bile; crosses placenta; $t_{1/2}$ 6-8 hr

INDICATIONS AND USES: Chronic open-angle glaucoma, hypertension

DOSAGE

Adult

• *Hypertension:* PO 2.5-10 mg qd; in renal impairment: CrCl 20-60 ml/min, dosage interval is 48 hr; CrCl <20 ml/min, dosage interval is 72 hr

• *Chronic open-angle glaucoma:* Ophth sol, 1%, 1 gtt in affected eye bid

$ AVAILABLE FORMS/COST OF THERAPY

• Sol—Ophth: 1%, 5, 10, 15 ml: **$36.68/10 ml**

• Tab, Plain Coated—Oral: 2.5 mg, 100's: **$106.18;** 5 mg, 100's: **$106.18**

CONTRAINDICATIONS: Hypersensitivity to β-blockers, heart block (2nd or 3rd degree), sinus bradycardia, overt CHF, bronchial asthma

PRECAUTIONS: Major surgery, diabetes mellitus, renal disease, thyroid disease, COPD, well-compensated heart failure, nonallergic bronchospasm; exacerbation of angina or MI may occur following abrupt discontinuation of β-blockers; ophth carteolol may be absorbed systemically; adverse reactions found with systemic administration may occur with ophth administration

PREGNANCY AND LACTATION: Pregnancy category C; excreted in breast milk

SIDE EFFECTS/ADVERSE REACTIONS

CNS: Anxiety, catatonia, decreased concentration, depression, dizzi-

---

* = non-FDA-approved use

ness, drowsiness, *fatigue (7%)*, headache, insomnia, lethargy, mental changes, nightmares, paresthesia

CV: AV block, bradycardia, chest pain, ***CHF,*** orthostatic hypotension, palpitations, peripheral vascular insufficiency, ***ventricular dysrhythmias***

EENT: Double vision; dry, burning eyes; sore throat, tinnitus, visual changes

GI: Anorexia, constipation, diarrhea, dry mouth, flatulence, nausea, vomiting

GU: Dysuria, ejaculatory failure, impotence, urinary retention

HEME: ***Agranulocytosis, thrombocytopenic purpura (rare)***

MS: Arthralgia, joint pain, muscle cramps

RESP: ***Bronchospasm,*** dyspnea, nasal stuffiness, pharyngitis, wheezing

SKIN: Alopecia, fever, pruritus, rash, urticaria

MISC: Decreased exercise tolerance, facial swelling, Raynaud's syndrome, weight change

INTERACTIONS

Drugs

🖪 *Adenosine:* Increased risk of bradycardic response

🖪 *Amiodarone:* Increased bradycardic effect of carteolol

🖪 *Antacids:* Decreased absorption of oral carteolol

🖪 *Antidiabetics:* Carteolol reduces response to hypoglycemia (sweating excepted)

🖪 *Antipyrine:* Many β-blockers increase serum concentrations of antipyrine; though antipyrine is not used therapeutically, this interaction has implications by other drugs whose metabolism is similarly inhibited

🖪 *Barbiturates, rifampin:* Enhanced carteolol metabolism

🖪 *Bupivacaine:* Potentiates cardiodepression and heart block

🖪 *Cimetidine, Propafenone, Propoxyphene, Quinidine:* Decreased carteolol metabolism

🖪 *Cocaine:* β-Blockade increases angina-inducing potential of cocaine

🖪 *Contrast media:* Increased risk of anaphylaxis

🖪 *Digoxin, digitoxin:* Bradycardia potentiated

🖪 *Dipyridamole:* Bradycardia

🖪 *Epinepherine:* Enhanced pressor response resulting in hypertension and bradycardia

🖪 *Fluoxetine:* Fluoxetine may reduce hepatic metabolism; increased β-blocking activity

🖪 *Isoproterenol:* Reduced effectiveness of isoproterenol in the treatment of asthma

🖪 *Neuroleptics:* Decreased carteolol metabolism; decreased neuroleptic metabolism

🖪 *Nonsteroidal anti-inflammatory drugs:* Reduced antihypertensive effect

🖪 *Physostigmine:* Additive bradycardia

🖪 *Prazosin, terazosin:* Enhanced 1st-dose response to prazosin

🖪 *Tacrine:* Additive bradycardia

🖪 *Theophylline:* Decreased metabolism of theophylline

SPECIAL CONSIDERATIONS

• Does not alter serum cholesterol or triglycerides

PATIENT/FAMILY EDUCATION

• Do not stop drug abruptly; taper over 2 wk

• Do not use OTC products containing α-adrenergic stimulants (nasal decongestants, cold remedies) unless directed by physician

---

italic = common side effects   ***bold italic*** = life-threatening reactions

carvedilol

(kar-vea'die-lole)

Rx: Coreg

Chemical Class: Nonselective β-adrenergic blocker; peripheral α-adrenergic blocker

Therapeutic Class: Antihypertensive; congestive heart failure agent

CLINICAL PHARMACOLOGY

Mechanism of Action: PO: Competitive β-adrenergic and α-adrenergic antagonist; produces negative inotropic and chronotropic responses; slows AV nodal conduction; decreases heart rate; decreases myocardial oxygen consumption; antiarrhythmic effects (class II); reduction in platelet aggregation and blood viscosity; suppression of renin release; inhibition of central sympathetic outflow; decreases presynaptic receptor neurotransmitter release; no intrinsic sympathomimetic; moderate membrane stabilizing activity; high lipid solubility

Pharmacokinetics

PO: Extensive first pass metabolism, 25% to 35% bioavailable; beta blocker effects seen in 30-60 min; terminal elimination $t_{1/2}$ 7-10 hrs; 98% protein bound; extensive hepatic metabolism, metabolite 13 times more potent beta blocker than parent drug, <2% excreted unchanged in urine; metabolites excreted in bile and feces

INDICATIONS AND USES: Hypertension, congestive heart failure, angina pectoris,* arrhythmias,* doxorubicin-induced cardiomyopathy,* nitrate tolerance,* postmyocardial infarction,* anxiety*

DOSAGE

Adult and Child >16 yr

• *Angina pectoris:* PO 25-50 mg

• *Congestive heart failure:* PO: 3.125 mg bid ×2 wk; if tolerated, double dose q2wk to the highest tolerated dose (max 25 mg bid for patients <85 kg; 50 mg bid for patients >85 kg). Administration with food slows absorption and reduces risk of postural hypotension

• *Hypertension:* PO 6.25 mg bid; adjust dose upward to 12.5 mg, then 25 mg bid every 1-2 wk as tolerated (max 50 mg bid)

$ AVAILABLE FORMS/COST OF THERAPY

• Tab—Oral: 3.125 mg, 6.25 mg, 12.5 mg, 25 mg, 100's: **$154.50**

CONTRAINDICATIONS: Bronchial asthma, cardiogenic shock, overt cardiac failure, second and third degree AV block, severe sinus bradycardia

PRECAUTIONS: Anesthesia/surgery (myocardial depression), avoid abrupt withdrawal, bronchospastic airways, congestive heart failure, diabetes mellitus, hyperthyroidism/thyrotoxicosis, concurrent clonidine (discontinue several days prior to withdrawal of clonidine), peripheral vascular disease, renal disease

PREGNANCY AND LACTATION: Pregnancy category C; increased spontaneous abortion in animal studies; highly lipophilic with a large volume of distribution, may accumulate in human breast milk; monitor infant closely

SIDE EFFECTS/ADVERSE REACTIONS

CNS: Dizziness

CV: **AV block,** bradycardia (2%), **CHF,** postural hypotension (1.8%), syncope (0.1%)

GI: Elevated LFTs (1.1%)

RESP: **Bronchospasm**

* = non-FDA-approved use

INTERACTIONS
Drugs

▪ *α-1 adrenergic blockers:* Potential enhanced first dose response (marked initial drop in blood pressure, particularly on standing)

▪ *Amiodarone:* Symptomatic bradycardia and sinus arrest; AV node refractory period prolonged and sinus node automaticity decreased, especially patients with bradycardia, sick sinus syndrome, or partial AV

▪ *Benzodiazepines:* Increased benzodiazepine activity

▪ *Cimetidine:* Via inhibition of hepatic metabolism, cimetidine increases many β-blocker serum concentrations

▪ *Clonidine:* Withdrawal of clonidine abruptly may exaggerate the hypertension due to unopposed alpha stimulation; safer than other beta-blockers, however

▪ *Digoxin:* Additive prolongation of atrioventricular (AV) conduction time

▪ *Dihydropyridine calcium channel blockers:* Severe hypotension or impaired cardiac performance; most prevalent with impaired left ventricular function, cardiac arrhythmias, or aortic stenosis

▪ *Diltiazem:* Potentiates beta-adrenergic effects; hypotension, left ventricular failure, and AV conduction disturbances problematic in elderly, patients with left ventricular dysfunction, aortic stenosis, or with large doses of either drug

▪ *Hypoglycemic agents:* Masked hypoglycemia, hyperglycemia

▪ *Nonsteroidal antiinflammatory drugs:* Reduced antihypertensive effect

▪ *Rifampin:* 70% decrease in carvedilol concentrations

▪ *Verapamil:* Potentiates beta-adrenergic effects; hypotension, left ventricular failure, and AV conduction disturbances problematic in elderly, patients with left ventricular dysfunction, aortic stenosis, or with large doses of either drug

SPECIAL CONSIDERATIONS
PATIENT FAMILY EDUCATION

• Do not discontinue abruptly; may require taper; rapid withdrawal may produce rebound hypertension or angina

• Careful monitoring essential when initiating therapy to detect and correct worsening symptoms of heart failure

• If heart rate drops below 55 beats per minute, reduce dosage

• Initiate therapy with 3.125 mg dosage to decrease risk of synocope

• Take with food

• Avoid driving, hazardous tasks during initiation of therapy

• Response less in African-Americans

MONITORING PARAMETERS

• Angina: Reduction in nitroglycerin usage; frequency, severity, onset, and duration of angina pain; heart rate.

• Arrhythmias: Heart rate

• Congestive heart failure: Functional status, cough, dyspnea on exertion, paroxysmal nocturnal dyspnea, exercise tolerance, and ventricular function

• Hypertension: Blood pressure

• Postmyocardial infarction: Left ventricular function, lower resting heart rate

• Toxicity: Blood pressure, blood glucose, bronchospasm, hypotension, bradycardia, depression, confusion, hallucination, sexual dysfunction

cascara sagrada

(kas-kar'a)
OTC: Cascara Sagrada, Cascara Aromatic
Chemical Class: Anthraquinone derivative
Therapeutic Class: Stimulant laxative

CLINICAL PHARMACOLOGY
Mechanism of Action: Direct chemical irritation in colon; increases propulsion of stool
Pharmacokinetics
PO: Peak 6-12 hr, only slightly absorbed; metabolized by liver, excreted by kidneys and in feces

INDICATIONS AND USES: Constipation; bowel or rectal preparation for surgery or examination
DOSAGE
Adult
• PO 325 mg (1 tab) or 5 ml of fluid extract qd prn
Child
• Age 2-12 yr: PO ½ adult dose; Age <2 yr: PO ¼ adult dose

$ AVAILABLE FORMS/COST OF THERAPY
• Tab—Oral: 325 mg, 100's: **$3.69-$4.72**
• Cap—Oral: 450 mg, 100's: **$5.39**
• Sol (fluid extract)—Oral: 120 ml **$2.10-$5.00**
• Sol (aromatic fluid)—Oral: 480 ml: **$16.29-$17.65**

CONTRAINDICATIONS: GI bleeding, obstruction, appendicitis, acute surgical abdomen
PRECAUTIONS: CHF, abdominal pain, nausea/vomiting, alcoholism (aromatic form)

PREGNANCY AND LACTATION: Pregnancy category C; excreted in breast milk
SIDE EFFECTS/ADVERSE REACTIONS
GI: Anorexia, cramps, diarrhea, melanosis coli, *nausea, vomiting*
GU: Discoloration of urine (pink, red, brown)
METAB: Alkalosis, hypocalcemia, hypokalemia
MS: Tetany
INTERACTIONS
Labs
• *Increase:* Color of urine (brown-acid; yellow-pink- alkaline); porphobilinogen; urobiligen
SPECIAL CONSIDERATIONS
• Stimulant laxatives are habit forming
• Long term use may lead to colonic atony

castor oil

OTC: Emulsoil, Purge
Chemical Class: Fatty acid ester
Therapeutic Class: Stimulant laxative

CLINICAL PHARMACOLOGY
Mechanism of Action: Increases motor activity of small intestine and colon; causes fluid secretion in colon
Pharmacokinetics
PO: Peak effect 2-3 hr; ester hydrolyzed in small intestine and partially absorbed
INDICATIONS AND USES: Constipation; bowel preparation for surgery or examination
DOSAGE
Adult
• PO LIQ 15-60 ml
Child
• Age >2 yr: PO LIQ 5-15 ml; Age <2 yr: PO LIQ 1.25-7.5 ml

---

* = non-FDA-approved use

💲 AVAILABLE FORMS/COST OF THERAPY

• Oil—Oral: 60 ml: **$0.68-$4.58**
• Liq—Oral: 95% oil, 60 ml: **$2.35-$3.00**

CONTRAINDICATIONS: Fecal impaction, GI bleeding, appendicitis, intestinal obstruction

PRECAUTIONS: Abdominal pain, nausea/vomiting, laxative dependence; colonic atony from prolonged use

PREGNANCY AND LACTATION: Pregnancy category X; excreted in breast milk

SIDE EFFECTS/ADVERSE REACTIONS

GI: Anorexia, colon irritation, *cramps,* diarrhea, flatus, *nausea,* rebound constipation, *vomiting*
METAB: Alkalosis; fluid or electrolyte imbalance; hypokalemia

SPECIAL CONSIDERATIONS

• Stimulant laxatives are habit forming
• Long-term use may lead to colonic atony

---

cefaclor

(sef'a-klor)
Rx: Ceclor, Ceclor CD
Chemical Class: Cephalosporin (2nd generation)
Therapeutic Class: Antibiotic

CLINICAL PHARMACOLOGY

Mechanism of Action: Inhibits bacterial cell wall synthesis, bactericidal

Pharmacokinetics
PO: Peak ½-1 hr (15 µg/ml after 500 mg), $t_{1/2}$ 36-54 min; 25% bound by plasma proteins; 60%-85% eliminated unchanged in urine in 8 hr; crosses placenta; when taken with food, peak concentration is 50%-75% of that when taken fasting; serum $t_{1/2}$ slightly prolonged in renal insufficiency; $t_{1/2}$ 2.3-2.8 hr if anephric; hemodialysis shortens $t_{1/2}$ by 25%-30%

INDICATIONS AND USES: Pharyngitis, tonsillitis, otitis media, bronchitis, pneumonia, skin and urinary tract infections caused by susceptible organisms

Antibacterial spectrum usually includes:

• Gram-positive organisms: *S. pneumoniae, S. pyogenes, S. aureus*
• Gram-negative organisms: *H influenzae, Moraxella catarrhalis, E. coli, P. mirabilis, Klebsiella* sp.
• Anaerobes: *Peptococci, Peptostreptococci*
• β-lactamase-producing strains of the above pathogens are usually susceptible

DOSAGE

Adult
• PO 250-500 mg q8h, double dose in serious infections and pneumonia
Child >1 mo
• PO 20-40 mg/kg qd in divided doses q8h, not to exceed 1 g/day (use higher dose in serious infections and otitis media)

💲 AVAILABLE FORMS/COST OF THERAPY

• Cap, Gel—Oral: 250 mg, 100's: **$89.40-$327.57;** 500 mg, 100's: **$127.10-$364.52**
• Powder, Reconst—Oral: 125 mg/5 ml, 150 ml: **$14.20-$37.20;** 187 mg/5 ml, 100 ml: **$28.13-$34.26;** 250 mg/5 ml, 150 ml: **$25.23-$56.38;** 375 mg/5 ml, 100 ml: **$51.80-$56.38**
• Tab, EXT REL—Oral: 375 mg, 60's: **$199.82;** 500 mg, 100's: **$349.70**

CONTRAINDICATIONS: Infants <1 mo

PRECAUTIONS: Hypersensitivity to penicillins, renal disease

---

italic = common side effects   **bold italic** = life-threatening reactions

PREGNANCY AND LACTATION:
Pregnancy category B; excreted in breast milk

SIDE EFFECTS/ADVERSE REACTIONS

CNS: Chills, dizziness, fever, headache, paresthesia, weakness

GI: Abdominal pain, anorexia, bleeding, diarrhea, glossitis, increased LFTs, nausea, ***pseudomembranous colitis,*** vomiting

GU: Candidiasis, ***nephrotoxicity,*** vaginitis

HEME: ***Bone marrow suppression*** eosinophilia, ***hemolytic anemia,*** lymphocytosis, thrombocytosis

RESP: Dyspnea

SKIN: Dermatitis, rash, urticaria

MISC: Serum sickness-like syndrome

INTERACTIONS

Drugs

🔳 *Aminoglycosides:* Additive nephrotoxicity

🔳 *Loop diuretics:* Increased nephrotoxicity

❷ *Warfarin:* Hypoprothrombinemic response enhanced

Labs

• *Creatinine:* Analytical increases and decreases depending on assay

SPECIAL CONSIDERATIONS

• Last choice 2nd generation cephalosporin given relative decreased activity against *S. pneumonia* and increased side effects

---

cefadroxil

(sef-a-drox'ill)
Rx: Duricef
Chemical Class: Cephalosporin (1st generation)
Therapeutic Class: Antibiotic

CLINICAL PHARMACOLOGY
Mechanism of Action: Inhibits bacterial cell wall synthesis; bactericidal

Pharmacokinetics

PO: Peak 1-1½ hr; measurable levels persist for 12 hr; 90% excreted unchanged in urine within 24 hr; $t_{1/2}$ 1-2 hr; 20% bound by plasma proteins

INDICATIONS AND USES: Infections of the urinary tract and skin caused by susceptible organisms; pharyngitis and tonsilitis caused by Group A β-hemolytic streptococci Antibacterial spectrum usually includes:

• Gram-negative bacilli: *E. coli, P. mirabilis, Klebsiella*

• Gram-positive organisms: *S. pneumoniae, S. pyogenes, S. aureus*

DOSAGE

Adult

• PO 1-2 g qd or q12h, give a loading dose of 1 g initially; dosage reduction appropriate in renal impairment (CrCl <50 ml/min)

Child

• PO 30 mg/kg/day

💲 **AVAILABLE FORMS/COST OF THERAPY**

• Cap, Gel—Oral: 500 mg, 100's: **$276.72-$345.92**

• Powder, Reconst—Oral: 125 mg/5 ml, 100 ml: **$16.00;** 250 mg/5 ml, 100 ml: **$30.06-$45.23;** 500 mg/5 ml, 100 ml: **$41.61-$54.62**

• Tab, Uncoated—Oral: 1 g, 100's: **$357.08-$759.91**

• Cap—Oral: 500 mg, 100's: **$284.65-$406.86**

CONTRAINDICATIONS: Infants <1 mo

PRECAUTIONS: Hypersensitivity to penicillins

PREGNANCY AND LACTATION: Pregnancy category B; low concentrations in milk

SIDE EFFECTS/ADVERSE REACTIONS

CNS: Chills, dizziness, fever, headache, paresthesia, weakness

GI: Abdominal pain, *anorexia,* bleed-

---

* = non-FDA-approved use

ing; *diarrhea,* glossitis, increased LFTs, nausea, *pseudomembranous colitis,* vomiting

GU: Candidiasis, *nephrotoxicity,* proteinuria, pruritus, vaginitis

HEME: Bone marrow suppression, eosinophilia, hemolytic anemia, lymphocytosis

RESP: Dyspnea

SKIN: Dermatitis, rash, urticaria

INTERACTIONS

Drugs

3 *Aminoglycosides:* Additive nephrotoxicity

3 *Loop diuretics:* Increased nephrotoxicity

SPECIAL CONSIDERATIONS

• No clinical advantage over less expensive cephalexin

---

cefamandole
(sef-a-man′dole)

Rx: Mandol

Chemical Class: Cephalosporin (2nd generation)

Therapeutic Class: Antibiotic

CLINICAL PHARMACOLOGY

Mechanism of Action: Inhibits bacterial wall synthesis; bactericidal

Pharmacokinetics

IM/IV: Peak 1-1½ hr, $t_{1/2}$, ½-1 hr; 60%-75% bound by plasma proteins; distributed to pleura, joint fluids, bile, and bone; 85% excreted by kidneys over 8 hr

INDICATIONS AND USES: Infections of the lower respiratory tract, urinary tract, skin and skin structure, bone, and joints; peritonitis, septicemia, and presurgical prophylactic therapy caused by susceptible organisms

Antibacterial spectrum usually includes:

• Gram-positive organisms: *S. pneumoniae, S. aureus* (penicillinase and non-penicillinase-producing),

β-hemolytic streptococci, *S. epidermidis, S. pyogenes*

• Gram-negative organisms: *H. influenzae, Klebsiella* sp., *P. mirabilis, E. coli, Proteus* sp., *Enterobacter* sp.

• Anaerobes: *Peptostreptococcus, Peptococcus* sp., *Clostridium* sp.

DOSAGE

Adult

• IM/IV 500 mg-1 g q4-8h, may give up to 2 g q4h for severe infections; 1 or 2 g IM/IV ½-1 hr prior to surgery, followed by 1 or 2 g q6h after surgery for 24-48 hr for prophylaxis

• Dosage reduction indicated in severe renal impairment (CrCl <5 ml/min): 1 g q12h

Child >1 mo

• IM/IV 50-150 mg/kg/day in divided doses q4-8h, not to exceed adult dose; 50 to 100 mg/kg/day in equally divided doses ½-1 hr before surgery and q6h for 24-48 hr after surgery for prophylaxis

$ **AVAILABLE FORMS/COST OF THERAPY**

• Inj, Dry-Sol—IM, IV: 1 g/vial: **$9.06;** 2 g/vial: **$18.13**

CONTRAINDICATIONS: Infants <1 mo

PRECAUTIONS: Hypersensitivity to penicillins, renal disease; hypoprothrombinemia

PREGNANCY AND LACTATION: Pregnancy category B; low milk concentrations

SIDE EFFECTS/ADVERSE REACTIONS

CNS: Chills, dizziness, fever, headache, paresthesia, weakness

GI: Abdominal pain, anorexia, *bleeding; diarrhea,* glossitis, increased LFTs, nausea, *pseudomembranous colitis,* transient hepatitis and cholestatic jaundice, *vomiting*

GU: Candidiasis, *nephrotoxicity,* vaginitis

---

italic = common side effects   ***bold italic*** = life-threatening reactions

HEME: **Bone marrow suppression,** eosinophilia, **hemolytic anemia, hypoprothrombinemia,** lymphocytosis

RESP: Dyspnea

SKIN: Dermatitis, maculopapular rash, urticaria

MISC: Thrombophlebitis (rare)

INTERACTIONS

Drugs

3 *Aminoglycosides:* Potential additive nephrotoxicity

3 *Ethanol:* Disulfiram-like reactions secondary to acetaldehyde accumulation

3 *Loop diuretics:* Increased nephrotoxicity

2 *Oral anticoagulants:* Additive hypoprothrombinemia

Labs

• *Creatinine:* Increases and decreases depending assay

• *Erythromycin:* False positive

• *Metronidazole:* Interferes with assay

SPECIAL CONSIDERATIONS

• Caution with alcohol; disulfiram reaction possible

MONITORING PARAMETERS

• If severe diarrhea occurs, pseudomembranous colitis should be considered

• Bleeding: ecchymosis, bleeding gums, hematuria, stool guaiac daily

---

cefazolin

(sef-a'zoe-lin)

Rx: Ancef, Kefzol

Chemical Class: Cephalosporin (1st generation)

Therapeutic Class: Antibiotic

CLINICAL PHARMACOLOGY

Mechanism of Action: Inhibits bacterial cell wall synthesis; bactericidal

Pharmacokinetics

IM: Peak ½-2 hr

IV: Peak 10 min, $t_{1/2}$ 1½-2¼ hr; distribution (70%-86% protein bound) to bile; without obstructive biliary disease, bile levels can exceed serum levels by up to 5×; with obstructive biliary disease, bile levels considerably lower than serum levels; to synovial fluid, comparable to levels reached in serum at about 4 hr after administration; eliminated unchanged in urine

INDICATIONS AND USES: Infections of the lower respiratory tract, urinary tract, biliary tract, and genitourinary tract; infections of the skin and skin structure, bones and joints; endocarditis, prostatitis, surgical prophylaxis, septicemia

Antibacterial spectrum usually includes:

• Gram-positive organisms: *S. pneumoniae, S. pyogenes, S. aureus*

• Gram-negative bacilli: *E. coli, P. mirabilis, Klebsiella sp, H. influenzae*

DOSAGE

Adult

• *Life-threatening infections:* IM/IV 1-2 g q6h

• *Mild/moderate infections:* IM/IV 250-500 mg q8h

• *Surgical prophylaxis:* IM/IV 1 g ½-1 hr prior to surgery then 500 mg-1 g q6-8 hr × 24 hr postoperatively

Dosage reduction appropriate in renal impairment (CrCl <50 ml/min)

Child >1 mo

• *Life-threatening infections:* IM/IV 100 mg/kg in 3-4 equal doses

• *Mild/moderate infections:* IM/IV 25-50 mg/kg in 3-4 equal doses

$ AVAILABLE FORMS/COST OF THERAPY

• Inj, Dry-Sol—IM, IV: 1 g/vial: **$1.90-$8.87;** 500 mg/vial: **$1.14-$4.06**

---

* = non-FDA-approved use

CONTRAINDICATIONS: Infants <1 mo

PRECAUTIONS: Hypersensitivity to penicillins, renal disease

PREGNANCY AND LACTATION: Pregnancy category B; low milk concentrations

SIDE EFFECTS/ADVERSE REACTIONS

CNS: Chills, dizziness, fever, headache, paresthesia, weakness

GI: Abdominal pain, anorexia, ***bleeding; diarrhea,*** glossitis, increased LFTs, nausea, vomiting, ***pseudomembranous colitis***

GU: Candidiasis, ***nephrotoxicity,*** pruritus, vaginitis

HEME: ***Bone marrow suppression,*** eosinophilia, ***hemolytic anemia,*** lymphocytosis

SKIN: Dermatitis, rash, urticaria

INTERACTIONS

Drugs

❸ *Aminoglycosides:* Additive nephrotoxicity

❸ *Ethanol:* Disulflozm-like reaction

❸ *Chloramphenicol:* Inhibits antibacterial activity of cefazolin

❸ *Loop diuretics:* Increased nephrotoxicity

❷ *Oral Anticoagulants:* Additive hypoprothrombinemia

---

cefepime
(sef'e-peem)
Rx: Maxipime
Chemical Class: Cephalosporin (4th generation)
Therapeutic Class: Antibiotic

CLINICAL PHARMACOLOGY
Mechanism of Action: Inhibits bacterial cell wall synthesis; bactericidal

Pharmacokinetics
IV/IM: Peak 30 min (IV), peak 2 hr (IM); $t_{1/2}$ 2 h; 20% protein bound;

excreted in breast milk; metabolites excreted renally

INDICATIONS AND USES: Infections of the urinary (including pyelonephritis) and lower respiratory (pneumonia) tracts and skin and skin structure infections, including cases associated with bacteremia caused by susceptible organisms, empiric monotherapy for febrile neutropenia in pediatric patients

Antibacterial spectrum usually includes:

• Gram-positive organisms: *S. pnemoniae, S. aureus* (methicillin-susceptible strains only), *S. pyogenes* (Group A streptococci), *S. epidermidis* (methicillin-susceptible strains only), *S. saprophyticus, S. agalactiae* (Group B streptococci)

• Gram-negative organisms: *E. coli, K. pneumoniae, P. mirabilis, Pseudomonas aeruginosa, Enterobacter* sp., *Acinetobacter calcoaceticus, Citrobacter diversus, C. freundii, Haemophilus influenzae* (including β-lactamase-producing strains), *Klebsiella oxytoca, Moraxella catarrhalis* (including β-lactamase-producing strains), *Morganella morganii, Proteus vulgaris, Providencia retteri, P. stuartii, Serratia marcescens*

DOSAGE
Adult

• *Uncomplicated or complicated urinary tract infection:* 0.5-2 g IV/IM q12h × 7-10 days

• *Pneumonia:* 1-2 g IV q12h × 10 days

• *Moderate to severe skin and skin structure infections:* 2 g IV q12h × 10 days

Note: IM route appropriate only for mild to moderate urinary tract infection; doses above appropriate for concurrent bacteremia

• *Maintenance dosing with renal impairment:* If CrCl > 60 ml/min, usual

---

italic = common side effects   ***bold italic*** = life-threatening reactions

dosing; CrCl 30-60 ml/min, usual dose given q24h; CrCl 11-29 ml/min, ½ usual dose given q24h; CrCl ≤10 ml/min, ¼ usual dose given q24h

Child 2 mo-16 yrs

• ≤40 kg: 50 mg/kg IV q12h (q8h for febrile neutropenia) × 7-10 days

💲 AVAILABLE FORMS/COST OF THERAPY

• Inj—IV/IM 500 mg/vial: **$7.71**; 1 g/ml vial; **$15.94-$17.06**; 2 g/ml vial: **$31.63-$32.75**

PRECAUTIONS: Hypersensitivity to penicillins, decreased prothrombin activity

PREGNANCY AND LACTATION: Pregnancy category B; excreted into breast milk in very low concentrations (0.5 µg/ml)

SIDE EFFECTS/ADVERSE REACTIONS

CNS: Encephalopathy (in renally impaired without dosage reduction), *seizures*

CV: Thrombophlebitis

EENT: Oral candidiasis

GI: Abdominal cramps, diarrhea, hepatic dysfunction including cholestasis, nausea, *pseudomembranous colitis,* vomiting

GU: Renal dysfunction, *nephrotoxicity,* vaginitis

HEME: **Bone marrow suppression,** hemolytic anemia, *hemorrhage,* hypoprothrombinemia

SKIN: **Erythema multiforme, Stevens-Johnson syndrome, toxic epidermal necrolysis**

MISC: Serum sickness-like reactions

INTERACTIONS

Drugs

3 *Aminoglycosides:* Additive nephrotoxicity

3 *Loop diuretics:* Increased nephrotoxicity

2 *Oral anticoagulants:* Potential increase in hypoprothrombinemic response to oral anticoagulants

Labs

• *False positive:* Positive direct Coombs test, positive urine glucose test (copper reduction method, i.e., Clinitest)

SPECIAL CONSIDERATIONS

• Broad spectrum, 4th generation cephalosporin demonstrating a low potential for resistance due to lack of β-lactamase induction and low potential for selection of resistant mutant strains; as effective as ceftazidime and cefotaxime in comparative trials; twice daily dosing may add economic advantage

---

cefixime

(sef-ix'ime)

Rx: Suprax

Chemical Class: Cephalosporin (3rd generation)

Therapeutic Class: Antibiotic

CLINICAL PHARMACOLOGY

Mechanism of Action: Inhibits bacterial cell wall synthesis; bactericidal

Pharmacokinetics

PO: Peak 1 hr, $t_{1/2}$ 3-4 hr; 65% bound by plasma proteins; 50% eliminated unchanged in urine; crosses placenta

INDICATIONS AND USES: Infections of the upper and lower respiratory tract (including pharyngitis, tonsillitis), otitis media, genitourinary tract (including uncomplicated UTI and gonorrhea, cervical, and urethral due to *N. gonorrhoeae*)

Antibacterial spectrum usually includes:

• Gram-positive organisms: *S. pneumoniae, S. pyogenes*

• Gram-negative organisms: *E. coli, P. mirabilis, Klebsiella; H. influenzae, M. catarrhalis, Neisseria gonorrhoeae*

---

* = non-FDA-approved use

• Anaerobes: *Peptostreptococcus, Peptococcus* sp.

DOSAGE

Adult

• PO 400 mg qd as a single dose or 200 mg q12h; for uncomplicated cervical/urethral GC infections, single 400 mg oral dose

Child <50 kg or <12 yr

• PO 8 mg/kg/day as a single dose or 4 mg/kg q12h

$ AVAILABLE FORMS/COST OF THERAPY

• Susp—Oral: 100 mg/5 ml, 50 ml: **$30.96-$43.62**

• Tab, Plain Coated—Oral: 200 mg, 100's: **$367.58**; 400 mg, 100's: **$720.39**

CONTRAINDICATIONS: Infants <6 mo

PRECAUTIONS: Hypersensitivity to penicillins

PREGNANCY AND LACTATION: Pregnancy category B; excreted in breast milk

SIDE EFFECTS/ADVERSE REACTIONS

CNS: Chills, confusion, dizziness, fatigue, fever, headache, lethargy, paresthesia

GI: Anorexia, *bleeding;* diarrhea, dysgeusia, flatulence, glossitis, heartburn, increased LFTs; nausea, *pseudomembranous colitis,* vomiting

GU: Candidiasis, *nephrotoxicity,* proteinuria, pruritus, vaginitis

HEME: **Bone marrow suppression** eosinophilia, **hemolytic anemia,** lymphocytosis

RESP: **Bronchospasm,** dyspnea

SKIN: **Exfoliative dermatitis,** rash, urticaria

INTERACTIONS

Drugs

3 *Aminoglycosides:* Additive nephrotoxicity

3 *Loop diuretics:* Increased nephrotoxicity

2 *Oral anticoagulants:* Enhanced hypoprothrombinemia

Labs

• *Cefotaxime:* Interferes with assay

• *Creatinine:* Increases or decreases depending on assay

SPECIAL CONSIDERATIONS

• No *S. aureus* coverage

---

cefmetazole

(sef-met′a-zole)

Rx: Zefazone

Chemical Class: Cephalosporin (2nd generation)

Therapeutic Class: Antibiotic

Note: Removed from the market voluntarily by manufacturer

CLINICAL PHARMACOLOGY

Mechanism of Action: Inhibition of bacterial cell wall synthesis; bactericidal

Pharmacokinetics

IV: Peak, 86 µg/ml after 1 g INF; 68% bound by plasma proteins; excreted by kidneys; $t_{1/2}$ 1-3 hr

INDICATIONS AND USES: Infections of the lower respiratory tract, urinary tract, skin and skin structure, bones and joints; septicemia, intra-abdominal infections, uncomplicated gonorrhea, perioperative prophylaxis

Antibacterial spectrum usually includes:

• Gram-positive organisms: *S. pneumoniae, S. pyogenes, S. agalactiae, S. aureus*

• Gram-negative organisms: *H. influenzae, E. coli, Proteus, Klebsiella, Morganella Morganii, Providencia stuartii, Neisseria gonorrhoeae*

• Anaerobes: *B. fragilis, Clostridium* sp.

---

italic = common side effects   ***bold italic*** = life-threatening reactions

DOSAGE
Adult
• *Uncomplicated gonorrhea:* Single dose IM 1 g (with 1 g of probenecid given by mouth at the same time or up to ½ hour before)
• *UTI:* IV 2 g q12h
• *Mild to moderate infections:* IV 2 g q8h
• *Severe to life-threatening infections:* IV 2 g q6h
• *Perioperative prophylaxis:* For vaginal hysterectomy, abdominal hysterectomy, cesarean section, colorectal surgery, or cholecystectomy (high risk) in adults, 2 g given as a single dose 30-90 min before surgery or 1 g doses given 30-90 min before surgery and repeated 8 and 16 hr later (if surgery lasts more than 4 hours, the preoperative dose should be repeated)

Dosage reduction appropriate with impaired renal function

$ **AVAILABLE FORMS/COST OF THERAPY**
• Inj, Lyphl-Sol—IV: 1 g/vial: **$7.19;** 2 g/vial: **$14.34**

CONTRAINDICATIONS: Infants <1 mo

PRECAUTIONS: Hypersensitivity to penicillins

PREGNANCY AND LACTATION: Pregnancy category B; trace milk concentrations

SIDE EFFECTS/ADVERSE REACTIONS
CNS: Chills, confusion, dizziness, fatigue, fever, headache, lethargy, paresthesia
EENT: Periorbital edema
GI: Anorexia, **bleeding;** diarrhea (4%), flatulence, glossitis, heartburn, increased AST, ALT, bilirubin, LDH, alk phosphatase; nausea, pain, ***pseudomembranous colitis,*** vomiting
GU: Candidiasis, increased BUN, ***nephrotoxicity,*** proteinuria, pruritus, ***renal failure,*** vaginitis
HEME: ***Agranulocytosis,*** anemia, ***eosinophilia, hemolytic anemia, leukopenia, lymphocytosis, neutropenia, pancytopenia, thrombocytopenia***
SKIN: Angioedema, erythema, ***exfoliative dermatitis,*** pruritus, rash, thrombophlebitis, urticaria
MISC: Pain and/or swelling at inj site, phlebitis, superinfection, thrombophlebitis

DRUG INTERACTIONS
Drugs
3 *Aminoglycosides:* Additive nephrotoxicity
3 *Chloramphenicol:* Inhibits antibacterial activity of cefmetazole
2 *Oral anticoagulants:* Additive hypoprothrombinemia; enhanced anticoagulation effect

---

cefonicid
(se-fon'i-sid)
Rx: Monocid
Chemical Class: Cephalosporin (2nd generation)
Therapeutic Class: Antibiotic

CLINICAL PHARMACOLOGY
Mechanism of Action: Inhibits bacterial cell wall synthesis; bactericidal
Pharmacokinetics
IV: Peak 5 min
IM: Peak 1 hr, $t_{1/2}$ 4½ hr; 98% protein bound; although reaches therapeutic levels in bile, levels lower than those seen with other cephalosporins, and amounts released into the GI tract are minute; *not* metabolized, 99% excreted unchanged in the urine in 24 hr

INDICATIONS AND USES: Infections of the lower respiratory and urinary tracts; skin and skin structure infections, septicemia, bone and joint infections, preoperative prophylaxis

Antibacterial spectrum usually includes:

• Gram-positive organisms: *S. aureus, S. epidermidis S. pneumoniae, S. pyogenes*

• Gram-negative organisms: *E. coli, K. pneumoniae, Providencia rettgeri, Proteus vulgaris, Morganella morganii, Proteus mirabilis, H. influenzae, Moraxella catarrhalis, K. oxytoca, Enterobacter aerogenes, N. gonorrhoeae*

• Anaerobes: *C. perfringens, Peptostreptococcus anaerobius, Peptococcus magnus, C. freundii, C. diversus, Fusobacterium* sp.

DOSAGE

Adult

• IM/IV 1-2 g/24 hr (divide in two doses if giving 2 g)

• *Perioperative prophylaxis:* IV 1 g 1 hr prior to procedure

Dosage reduction appropriate in renal impairment (CrCl <50 ml/min)

$ **AVAILABLE FORMS/COST OF THERAPY**

• Inj, Lyphl-Sol—IM, IV: 1 g: **$26.10**

CONTRAINDICATIONS: Infants <1 mo

PRECAUTIONS: Hypersensitivity to penicillins, renal disease

PREGNANCY AND LACTATION: Pregnancy category B; excreted in breast milk in low concentrations

SIDE EFFECTS/ADVERSE REACTIONS

CNS: Chills, dizziness, fever, headache, paresthesia, weakness

GI: Abdominal pain, anorexia, ***bleeding,*** diarrhea; glossitis, increased LFTs, *nausea, vomiting*

GU: Candidiasis, ***nephrotoxicity,*** vaginitis

*HEME: **Bone marrow suppression,*** anemia, eosinophilia, ***hemolytic anemia,*** lymphocytosis

SKIN: Dermatitis, rash, urticaria

INTERACTIONS

Drugs

3 *Aminoglycosides:* Additive nephrotoxicity

3 *Chloramphenicol:* Inhibits the antibacterial activity of cefonicid

3 *Loop diuretics:* Increased nephrotoxicity

---

cefoperazone

(sef-oh-per′a-zone)

Rx: Cefobid

Chemical Class: Cephalosporin (3rd generation)

Therapeutic Class: Antibiotic

CLINICAL PHARMACOLOGY

Mechanism of Action: Inhibits bacterial cell wall synthesis; bactericidal

Pharmacokinetics

IV: Peak 5 min, duration 6-8 hr

IM: Peak 1-2 hr, duration 6-8 hr

$t_{1/2}$ 2 hr; 70%-75% eliminated unchanged in bile, 20%-30% unchanged in urine

INDICATIONS AND USES: Infections of the lower respiratory tract, urinary tract, skin; bone infections, septicemia, peritonitis, PID caused by susceptible organisms

Antibacterial spectrum usually includes:

• Gram-positive organisms: *S. aureus,* (penicillinase and non-penicillinase-producing strains), *S. epidermidis, Streptococcus pneumoniae, S. pyogenes,* Group A β-hemolytic streptococci, *S. agalactiae,* Group B β-hemolytic streptococci, *Enterococcus, Streptococcus faecalis, S. faecium, S. durans*

• Gram-negative organisms: *H. influenzae, E. coli, Proteus mirabilis, P. vulgaris, Klebsiella, Enterobac-*

---

italic = common side effects   ***bold italic*** = life-threatening reactions

ter, Serratia, Citrobacter, Morganella morganii, N. gonorrhoeae, Providencia, Pseudomonas aeruginosa
• Anaerobes: Peptococcus and Peptostreptococcus, Clostridium sp., Bacteroides sp.

DOSAGE
Adult
• *Mild/moderate infections:* IM/IV 1-2 g q12h
• *Severe infections:* IM/IV 6-12 g/day divided in 2-4 equal doses
• *Hepatic disease or biliary obstruction:* Doses >4 g/day generally not necessary

Child
• Neonates 50 mg/kg/dose q12h; children 100-150 mg/kg/day divided q8-12h, up to 12 g/day

⚕ AVAILABLE FORMS/COST OF THERAPY
• Inj, Sol—IM, IV: 1 g: **$16.42;** 2 g: **$32.84; 10g: $157.29**

CONTRAINDICATIONS: Infants <1 mo

PRECAUTIONS: Hypersensitivity to penicillins

PREGNANCY AND LACTATION: Pregnancy category B; low concentrations excreted in human milk

SIDE EFFECTS/ADVERSE REACTIONS
CNS: Chills, dizziness, fever, headache, paresthesia, weakness
GI: Abdominal pain, *anorexia, bleeding;* diarrhea, glossitis, increased LFTs; *nausea, pseudomembranous colitis, vomiting*
GU: Candidiasis, **nephrotoxicity,** proteinuria, vaginitis
HEME: **Bone marrow suppression,** anemia, **bleeding,** eosinophilia, **hemolytic anemia, hypoprothrombinemia,** leukopenia, lymphocytosis,
RESP: Dyspnea
SKIN: Dermatitis, rash, urticaria

INTERACTIONS
Drugs
❸ *Aminoglycosides:* Increased risk of nephrotoxicity
❸ *Ethanol:* Disulfiram-like reactions
❸ *Loop diuretics:* Increased nephrotoxicity
❷ *Oral anticoagulants:* Via hypoprothrombinemia, may enhance anticoagulant effects
Labs
• *Creatinine:* Increased serum values

SPECIAL CONSIDERATIONS
• No dose adjustment necessary in renal failure when usual doses are administered

PATIENT/FAMILY EDUCATION
• Avoid alcohol during and for 3 days after use

---

ceforanide
(sef-or'aa-nide)
Rx: Precef
Chemical Class: Cephalosporin (2nd generation)
Therapeutic Class: Antibiotic

CLINICAL PHARMACOLOGY
Mechanism of Action: Inhibition of bacterial cell wall synthesis; bactericidal
Pharmacokinetics
IV: Peak 5 min
IM: Peak 1 hr, $t_{1/2}$ 2½-3 hr; 80% bound to plasma proteins; reaches therapeutic levels in the gall bladder, myocardium, bone, skeletal muscle, and vaginal tissue, pericardial fluid, and synovial fluid; 90% eliminated unchanged in urine
INDICATIONS AND USES: Infections of the lower respiratory tract, urinary tract, skin; bone infections; septicemia, endocarditis, and perioperative prophylaxis

Antibacterial spectrum usually includes:

- Gram-negative organisms: *H. influenzae, E. coli, P. mirabilis, Klebsiella, Providencia* sp., *Citrobacter* sp., *Salmonella typhi, Neisseria gonorrhoeae*

- Gram-positive organisms: *S. pneumoniae, S. aureus* (including penicillinase-producing strains), Group A and B streptococci, *Streptococcus viridans*

DOSAGE
Adult
- IM/IV 0.5-1 g q12h
- *Perioperative prophylaxis:* IM/IV 0.5-1 g 1 hr prior to surgery

Increased dosage interval is appropriate in renal dysfunction
Child
- IM/IV 20-40 mg/kg/day in 2 equal doses q12h

Dosage reduction appropriate in renal impairment (CrCl <50 ml/min)

AVAILABLE FORMS/COST OF THERAPY
- Inj, Dry-Sol—IM, IV: 500 mg/vial: **$7.25;** 1 g/vial: **$11.94**

CONTRAINDICATIONS: Infants <1 mo

PRECAUTIONS: Hypersensitivity to penicillins, renal disease

PREGNANCY AND LACTATION: Pregnancy category B

SIDE EFFECTS/ADVERSE REACTIONS

CNS: Chills, dizziness, fever, headache, paresthesia, weakness

GI: Abdominal pain, *anorexia, bleeding; diarrhea,* glossitis, increased AST, ALT, bilirubin, LDH, alk phosphatase; *nausea,* pain, *vomiting*

GU: Increased BUN, **nephrotoxicity,** proteinuria, pruritus, **renal failure,** vaginitis

HEME: **Agranulocytosis,** anemia, **eosinophilia, hemolytic anemia, leukopenia, lymphocytosis, neutropenia, pancytopenia, thrombocytopenia**

RESP: Dyspnea

SKIN: Dermatitis, rash, urticaria

INTERACTIONS
Drugs

☒ *Aminoglycosides:* Additive nephrotoxicity

☒ *Chloramphenicol:* Inhibits antibacterial activity of cidal-ceforanide

☒ *Oral anticoagulants:* Hypoprothrombinemia

---

cefotaxime
(sef-oh-taks′eem)
Rx: Claforan
Chemical Class: Cephalosporin (3rd generation)
Therapeutic Class: Antibiotic

CLINICAL PHARMACOLOGY
Mechanism of Action: Inhibits bacterial cell wall synthesis; bactericidal.
Pharmacokinetics
IV: Onset 5 min
IM: Onset 30 min, $t_{1/2}$ 1 hr; 35%-65% protein bound; 40%-65% is eliminated unchanged in urine in 24 hr, 25% metabolized to active and inactive metabolites

INDICATIONS AND USES: Infections of the lower respiratory tract, genitourinary tract (including UTI, uncomplicated gonorrhea, PID, endometritis, pelvic cellulitis), skin and skin structure, bone and joints, CNS, intra-abdominal infections; perioperative prophylaxis (e.g., abdominal or vaginal hysterectomy, gastrointestinal and genitourinary tract surgery)

Antibacterial spectrum usually includes:
- Gram-positive organisms: Group A streptococci, *S. pneumoniae, S. pyogenes, Staphylococcus aureus*

---

italic = common side effects   **bold italic = life-threatening reactions**

(penicillinase and non-penicillinase producing), *Enterococcus* sp., *S. epidermidis*

• Gram-negative organisms: *E. coli, Klebsiella* sp., *H. influenzae* (including ampicillin-resistant strains), *H. parainfluenzae, P. mirabilis, S. marcescens, Enterobacter* sp., indole-positive *Proteus, Citrobacter* sp., *Morganella morganii, Providencia rettgeri, N. gonorrhoeae* (including penicillinase-producing strains), *N. meningitidis*

• Anaerobes: *Bacteroides* sp. (including *Bacteroides fragilis*), *Clostridium* sp., *Peptostreptococcus* sp., *Peptococcus* sp., *Fusobacterium* sp.

DOSAGE
Adult
• IM/IV 1-2 g q8-12h
• *Severe infections:* IM/IV 2 g q4h; not to exceed 12 g/day
• *Uncomplicated gonorrhea:* 1 g IM
• *Perioperative prophylaxis:* IM/IV 1 g 30-90 min prior to start of surgery, followed by doses at 6 and 12 hr postsurgery
Dosage reduction appropriate for severe renal impairment (CrCl <10 ml/min)
Child
• Neonates: 0-1 wk of age 50 mg/kg IV q12h; 1-4 wk of age 50 mg/kg IV q8h (it is not necessary to differentiate between premature and normal gestational-age infants)
• Infants and children (1 mo to 12 yr): <50 kg 50-180 mg/kg IM or IV divided into 4-6 equal doses; >50 kg the usual adult dosage should be used; max daily dosage should not exceed 12 g

$ AVAILABLE FORMS/COST OF THERAPY
• Inj, Dry-Sol—IM, IV: 0.5 g/vial: **$8.62;** 1 g/vial: **$14.40;** 2 g/vial: **$26.39**

PRECAUTIONS: Hypersensitivity to penicillins
PREGNANCY AND LACTATION: Pregnancy category B; low milk concentrations
SIDE EFFECTS/ADVERSE REACTIONS
CNS: Chills, dizziness, fever, headache, paresthesia, weakness
GI: Abdominal pain, anorexia, ***bleeding;*** diarrhea, glossitis, increased AST, ALT, bilirubin, LDH, alk phosphatase; nausea, pain, ***pseudomembranous colitis,*** vomiting
GU: Candidiasis, proteinuria, pruritus, vaginitis, ***nephrotoxicity***
HEME: ***Bone marrow suppression,*** eosinophilia, ***hemolytic anemia,*** lymphocytosis
SKIN: Dermatitis, induration (IM), inflammation (IV), pain, rash, urticaria

INTERACTIONS
Drugs
❸ *Aminoglycosides:* Additive nephrotoxicity
❸ *Chloramphenicol:* Inhibits antibacterial activity of cidal-cefotaxime
❷ *Oral anticoagulants:* Hypoprothrombinemia
Labs
• *False serum increased:* Albumin, alkaline phosphatase, calcium ceftriaxone cholesterol, creatine kinase, creatinine, glucose, iron, iron saturation, metronidazole, potassium, sodium, tetracycline, trimethoprim
• *False serum decreased:* Ammonia, amylase, chloride, γ-glutamyltransferase (GGT), lactate dehydrogenase, magnesium, phosphate, potassium, urea nitrogen, uric acid
• *False positive:* Clindamycin, colistin, erythromycin, polymyxin

cefotetan

(sef'oh-tee-tan)

Rx: Cefotan

Chemical Class: Cephamycin (structurally related to cephalosporins, 2nd generation)

Therapeutic Class: Antibiotic

CLINICAL PHARMACOLOGY

Mechanism of Action: Inhibits bacterial cell wall synthesis; bactericidal

Pharmacokinetics

IM: Peak 1 hr, $t_{1/2}$ 3-5 hr; 88% bound by plasma proteins; wide distribution; no active metabolites, 50%-80% eliminated unchanged in urine over 24 hr

INDICATIONS AND USES: Infections of the lower respiratory tract, urinary tract, skin and skin structure; intra-abdominal, gynecologic, bone and joint infections, as well as perioperative prophylaxis of susceptible organisms

Antibacterial spectrum usually includes:

• Gram-positive organisms: *Streptococcus pneumoniae, S. pyogenes, Staphylococcus aureus* (penicillinase- and non-penicillinase-producing strains), *S. epidermidis*

• Gram-negative organisms: *E. coli, Klebsiella* sp., *Proteus* sp., *H. influenzae* (including ampicillin-resistant strains), *Serratia marcescens, Shigella, N. gonorrhoeae*

• Anaerobes: *Peptococcus* sp; *Peptostreptococcus* sp., *Bacteroides* sp. (excluding *B. distasonis, B. ovatus, B. thetaiotaomicron*), *Fusobacterium* sp.

DOSAGE

Adult

• IV/IM 1-2g q12h, may increase to 3 g q12 hr for life-threatening infections

• *Perioperative prophylaxis:* IV 1-2 g ½-1 hr before surgery

• *Renal failure:* Give usual dose q24 hr for CrCl of 10-30 ml/min; q48 hr for CrCl <10 ml/min

Child

• IV/IM 20-40 mg/kg q12h

\[§\] AVAILABLE FORMS/COST OF THERAPY

• Inj, Lyphl-Sol—IM, IV: 1 g/vial: **$11.58-$12.17;** 2 g/vial: **$22.73-$25.92**

• Inj, Dry-Sol—IM, IV: 10 g: **$122.86**

CONTRAINDICATIONS: Infants <1 mo

PRECAUTIONS: Hypersensitivity to penicillins, renal disease

PREGNANCY AND LACTATION: Pregnancy category B; small amounts excreted into breast milk

SIDE EFFECTS/ADVERSE REACTIONS

CNS: Chills, dizziness, fever, headache, paresthesia, weakness

CV: Hypotension

GI: Abdominal pain, *anorexia,* **bleeding;** *diarrhea,* glossitis, increased LFTs, *nausea,* **pseudomembranous colitis,** *vomiting*

GU: Candidiasis, **nephrotoxicity,** proteinuria, vaginitis

HEME: **Bone marrow suppression,** eosinophilia, **hypoprothrombinemia,** lymphocytosis

SKIN: Dermatitis, **exfoliative dermatitis,** pruritus, rash, thrombophlebitis, urticaria

INTERACTIONS

Drugs

\[3\] *Aminoglycosides:* Additive nephrotoxicity

\[3\] *Ethanol:* Disulfiram-like reaction

\[3\] *Chloramphenicol:* Inhibits antibacterial activity of cidal-cefotetan

\[2\] *Oral anticoagulants:* Additive hypoprothrombinemia; enhanced anticoagulant effects

---

italic = common side effects   ***bold italic*** = life-threatening reactions

SPECIAL CONSIDERATIONS
PATIENT/FAMILY EDUCATION
• Avoid alcohol during and for 3 days after use

---

cefoxitin sodium
(se-fox'i-tin)
Rx: Mefoxin
Chemical Class: Cephamycin (structurally related to cephalosporins, 2nd generation)
Therapeutic Class: Antibiotic

CLINICAL PHARMACOLOGY
Mechanism of Action: Inhibits bacterial cell wall synthesis; bactericidal

Pharmacokinetics
IV: Peak 5 min
IM: Peak 20-30 min
$t_{1/2}$ 1 hr; 55%-75% bound by plasma proteins; passes into pleural and joint fluids and is detectable in antibacterial concentrations in bile; 85% eliminated unchanged in urine; crosses blood-brain barrier

INDICATIONS AND USES: Infections of the lower respiratory tract, urinary tract, skin and skin structure; gynecologic, intra-abdominal, bone, and joint infections as well as perioperative prophylaxis of susceptible organisms; septicemia; uncomplicated gonorrhea

Antibacterial spectrum usually includes:
• Gram-positive organisms: *Streptococcus pneumoniae, S. pyogenes, Staphylococcus aureus* (penicillinase- and nonpenicillinase-producing strains), *S. epidermidis*
• Gram-negative organisms: *E. coli, Klebsiella* sp., *Proteus* sp., *H. influenzae* (including ampicillin-resistant strains), *N. gonorrhoeae, Morganella morganii, Providencia* sp.
• Anaerobes: *Peptococcus* sp., *Peptostreptococcus* sp., *Bacteroides* sp. (excluding *B. distasonis, B. ovatus, B. thetaiotaomicron*).

DOSAGE
Adult
• IM/IV 1-2 g q6-8h
• *Uncomplicated gonorrhea:* 2 g IM as single dose with 1 g PO probenecid
• *Severe infections:* IM/IV 2 g q4h or 3 g q6h
• *Perioperative prophylaxis:* IM/IV 2 g 30-60 min prior to surgery, then 2 g q6h × 24 hr
Dose reduction appropriate in renal impairment (CrCl <50 ml/min)
Child ≥ 3 mo
• IM/IV 80 to 160 mg/kg of body weight per day divided in 4-6 equal doses, not to exceed 12 g/day

💲 **AVAILABLE FORMS/COST OF THERAPY**
• Inj, Dry-Sol—IM, IV: 1 g: **$11.40-$13.48;** 2 g: **$21.79-$23.81;** 10 g: **$104.48**

PRECAUTIONS: Hypersensitivity to penicillins, renal disease

PREGNANCY AND LACTATION: Pregnancy category B; low milk concentrations

SIDE EFFECTS/ADVERSE REACTIONS
CNS: Chills, dizziness, fever, headache, paresthesia, weakness
CV: Hypotension
GI: Abdominal pain, anorexia, ***bleeding;*** *diarrhea,* glossitis, increased LFTs; *nausea,* ***pseudomembranous colitis,*** *vomiting*
GU: Candidiasis, ***nephrotoxicity***, proteinuria, vaginitis
HEME: **Bone marrow suppression,** eosinophilia, **hemolytic anemia, hypoprothrombinemia,** lymphocytosis
SKIN: Dermatitis, ***exfoliative dermatitis,*** pruritus, rash, thrombophlebitis, urticaria

---

* = non-FDA-approved use

INTERACTIONS
Drugs

3 *Aminoglycosides:* Additive nephrotoxicity

3 *Chloramphenicol:* Inhibits antibacterial activity of cidal-cefoxitin

2 *Oral anticoagulants:* Additive hypoprothrombinemia, enhanced anticoagulant effects

Labs
• *False serum increases:* Creatinine (serum and urine), cefuroxime, gentamicin, metronidazole, potassium, tetracycline
• *False urine increases:* 17-hydroxycorticosteroids
• *False serum decreases:* Creatine clearance
• *False positive:* Polymyxin

---

cefpodoxime

(sef-pod'ox-ime)
Rx: Vantin
Chemical Class: Cephalosporin (2nd generation)
Therapeutic Class: Antibiotic

CLINICAL PHARMACOLOGY
Mechanism of Action: Inhibits bacterial cell wall synthesis; bactericidal

Pharmacokinetics
PO: Peak 2-3 hr; absorbed as prodrug; de-esterified to its active metabolite, cefpodoxime (approximately 50% of the administered dose is systemically absorbed); minimal metabolism; $t_{1/2}$ 2-3 hr; 25% bound by plasma proteins; 30% eliminated unchanged in urine in 12 hr

INDICATIONS AND USES: Infections of the upper and lower respiratory tract, skin and skin structure, urinary tract; sexually transmitted diseases (uncomplicated urethral and cervical gonorrhea)

Antibacterial spectrum usually includes:
• Gram-positive organisms: *Streptococcus pneumoniae, S. pyogenes, Staphylococcus aureus* (including penicillinase-producing strains), *S. saprophyticus*
• Gram-negative organisms: *H. influenzae* (some β-lactamase-producing strains), *N. gonorrhoeae* (including penicillinase-producing strains), *Moraxella catarrhalis, E. coli, Klebsiella pneumoniae, Proteus mirabilis*

DOSAGE
Adult
• *Pneumonia:* 200 mg q12h for 14 days
• *Uncomplicated gonorrhea:* 200 mg single dose
• *Skin and skin structure:* 400 mg q12h for 7-14 days
• *Pharyngitis and tonsillitis:* 100 mg q12h for 10 days
• *Uncomplicated UTI:* 100 mg q12h for 7 days
• *Renal failure:* Increase dosing interval to q24h for CrCl <30 ml/min
Child 5-12 yr
• *Acute otitis media:* 10 mg/kg q24h for 10 days (max 400 mg/dose)
• *Pharyngitis/tonsillitis:* 5 mg/kg q12h (max 100 mg/dose) for 10 days

$ **AVAILABLE FORMS/COST OF THERAPY**
• Susp—Oral: 50 mg/5 ml, 100 ml: **$34.45-$39.78;** 100 mg/5 ml, 100 ml: **$65.54-$67.49**
• Tab, Uncoated—Oral: 100 mg, 100's: **$297.73;** 200 mg, 100's: **$391.48-$401.26**

CONTRAINDICATIONS: Infants
PRECAUTIONS: Hypersensitivity to penicillins, renal disease
PREGNANCY AND LACTATION: Pregnancy category B; excreted into breast milk; average 2% of serum levels at 4 hr following 200 mg dose

---

italic = common side effects   ***bold italic*** = life-threatening reactions

SIDE EFFECTS/ADVERSE REACTIONS

CNS: Chills, dizziness, fatigue, fever, headache, lethargy, paresthesia

GI: Anorexia, **bleeding;** *diarrhea,* glossitis, increased LFTs; nausea, **pseudomembranous colitis,** vomiting

GU: Candidiasis, **nephrotoxicity,** vaginitis

HEME: **Bone marrow suppression,** eosinophilia, **hemolytic anemia,** lymphocytosis

RESP: Dyspnea

SKIN: Dermatitis, rash, urticaria

INTERACTIONS
Drugs

3 *Aminoglycosides:* Additive nephrotoxicity

3 *Antacids:* Reduced bioavailability and serum cefpodoxime levels

3 *H$_2$-blockers (cimetidine, famotidine, nizatidine, ranitidine), proton pump blockers (lansoprazole, omeprazole):* Reduced bioavailability and serum cefpodoxime levels

3 *Loop diuretics:* Increased nephrotoxicity

SPECIAL CONSIDERATIONS
• Reserve use for otitis media to infections that fail to respond to less expensive agents (e.g., amoxicillin, co-trimoxazole)

• Suspension tastes very bitter

---

cefprozil
(sef-pro'zil)
Rx: Cefzil

Chemical Class: Cephalosporin (2nd generation)
Therapeutic Class: Antibiotic

CLINICAL PHARMACOLOGY
Mechanism of Action: Inhibits bacterial cell wall synthesis; bactericidal

Pharmacokinetics
PO: Peak serum and urine concentration 1.5 and 4 hr; 95% absorbed (no food effect observed); plasma protein binding 36%; t$_{1/2}$ 1.3 hr

INDICATIONS AND USES: Infections of the upper and lower respiratory tract (pharyngitis, tonsillitis, otitis media, secondary bacterial infection of acute bronchitis, acute bacterial exacerbation of chronic bronchitis); skin and skin structure due to susceptible organisms

Antibacterial spectrum usually includes:

• Gram-positive organisms: *Staphylococcus aureus* (including penicillinase-producing strains), *Streptococcus pneumoniae,* *S. pyogenes*

• Gram-negative organisms: *Moraxella catarrhalis,* *H. influenzae* (including penicillinase-producing strains)

DOSAGE
Adult

• *Upper respiratory infections:* PO 500 mg qd ×10 days

• *Lower respiratory infections:* PO 500 mg bid ×10 days

• *Skin/skin structure infections:* PO 250-500 mg q12h or 500 mg qd × 10 days

Child 6 mo-12 yr

• *Upper respiratory tract infections:* PO 7.5 mg/kg q12h × 10 days

• *Otitis media:* PO 15 mg/kg q12h×10 days

• *Skin/skin structure infections:* PO 20 mg/kg qd × 10 days

$ **AVAILABLE FORMS/COST OF THERAPY**

• Susp—Oral: 125 mg/5 ml, 100 ml: **$31.39-$39.03;** 250 mg/5 ml, 100 ml: **$56.88-$64.93**

• Tab, Uncoated—Oral: 250 mg, 100's: **$275.34-$329.69;** 500 mg, 100's: **$653.82**

PRECAUTIONS: Elderly, hypersensitivity to penicillins

---

* = non-FDA-approved use

PREGNANCY AND LACTATION:
Pregnancy category B
SIDE EFFECTS/ADVERSE REACTIONS
CNS: Chills, dizziness, fever, headache, paresthesia, weakness
GI: Abdominal pain, anorexia, ***bleeding;*** diarrhea, flatulence, glossitis, increased LFTs; ***pseudomembranous colitis,*** vomiting
GU: Candidiasis, genitoanal pruritus, hematuria, ***nephrotoxicity,*** vaginitis
HEME: ***Bone marrow suppression,*** eosinophilia, ***hemolytic anemia,*** lymphocytosis
SKIN: Dermatitis, rash, urticaria
RESP: Dyspnea
INTERACTIONS
Drugs
3 *Aminoglycosides:* Additive nephrotoxicity
3 *Loop diuretics:* Increased nephrotoxicity
SPECIAL CONSIDERATIONS
• Reserve use for otitis media to infections that fail to respond to less expensive agents (e.g., amoxicillin, co-trimoxazole)

---

ceftazidime
(sef-taz'i-deem)
Rx: Ceptaz, Fortaz, Tazicef, Tazidime
Chemical Class: Cephalosporin (3rd generation)
Therapeutic Class: Antibiotic

CLINICAL PHARMACOLOGY
Mechanism of Action: Inhibits bacterial cell wall synthesis; bactericidal
Pharmacokinetics
IM: Peak 1 hr, <10% bound to plasma proteins; 80% eliminated unchanged in urine; t$_{1/2}$ 1.9 hr
INDICATIONS AND USES: Infections of the lower respiratory tract, urinary tract, skin and skin structure; bone and joint, gynecological, intra-abdominal infections; septicemia; meningitis caused by susceptible organisms

Antibacterial spectrum usually includes:
• Gram-positive organisms: *Streptococcus pneumoniae, S. pyogenes,* Group B streptococci, *Staphylococcus aureus*
• Gram-negative organisms: *H. influenzae, E. coli, E. aerogenes, P. aeruginosa, P. mirabilis, P. vulgaris, Klebsiella, Citrobacter, Enterobacter, Salmonella, Shigella, Acinetobacter, Neisseria, Serratia*
DOSAGE
Adult
• *IV/IM* 1 g q8-12h
• *Uncomplicated UTI:* IM/IV 250 mg q12h
• *Complicated UTI:* IM/IV 500 mg q8-12h
• *Bone and joint infections:* IV 2 g q12h
• *Severe infections/meningitis:* IV 2 g q8h
• *Renal disease:* Decrease dose or increase dosing interval in patients with CrCl <30 ml/min
Child 1 mo-12 yr
• IV 30-50 mg/kg q8h, not to exceed 6 g/day
Neonates 0-4 wk
• IV 30 mg/kg q12h
$ AVAILABLE FORMS/COST OF THERAPY
• Inj, Dry-Sol—IV, IM: 500 mg/vial: **$7.11;** 1 g/vial: **$14.59-$21.94;** 2 g/vial: **$28.81-$43.34;** 6 g/vial: **$43.34-$82.80**
PRECAUTIONS: Hypersensitivity to penicillins, renal disease, children
PREGNANCY AND LACTATION: Pregnancy category B; excreted in human milk in low concentrations

---

italic = common side effects   ***bold italic*** = life-threatening reactions

SIDE EFFECTS/ADVERSE REACTIONS

CNS: Chills, dizziness, fever, headache, paresthesia, weakness

GI: Anorexia, *bleeding;* diarrhea, glossitis, increased LFTs, nausea *pseudomembranous colitis,* vomiting

GU: Candidiasis, *nephrotoxicity,* proteinuria, vaginitis

HEME: Bone marrow suppression, eosinophilia, *hemolytic anemia,* lymphocytosis

RESP: Dyspnea

SKIN: Dermatitis, rash, urticaria

INTERACTIONS

Drugs

3 *Aminoglycosides:* Additive nephrotoxicity

3 *Chloramphenicol:* Inhibition of the antibacterial activity of ceftazidime

3 *Loop diuretics:* Increased nephrotoxicity

SPECIAL CONSIDERATIONS

• Especially useful for infections due to *Pseudomonas aeruginosa* (with or without an aminoglycoside)

---

ceftibuten

(cef'te-bute-in)

Rx: Cedax

Chemical Class: Cephalosporin (3rd generation, oral)

Therapeutic Class: Antibiotic

CLINICAL PHARMACOLOGY

Mechanism of Action: Inhibits bacterial cell wall synthesis; bactericidal

Pharmacokinetics

PO: C_{max} 15 mcg/ml 2.6 hr after 400 mg adult dose, 13.4 µg/ml 2 hr after 9 mg/kg pediatric dose; well absorbed (80% bioavailability), capsule and suspension equal; widely distributed, 65%-77% protein bound; renal excretion; $t_{1/2}$ 1.53-2.5 hr

INDICATIONS AND USES: Pharyngitis, tonsillitis, otitis media, acute bacterial exacerbation of chronic bronchitis, gonococcal urethritis* Antibacterial spectrum usually includes:

• Gram-positive organisms: *Streptococcus pyogenes, S. pneumoniae* (penicillin susceptible strains only)

• Gram-negative organisms: Enterobacter sp., *E. coli, Klebsiella* sp., *Morganella morganii, Proteus* sp., *Providencia* sp., *Salmonella* sp., *Serratia* sp., *Haemophilus influenzae, Neisseria* sp., *Moraxella catarrhalis*

DOSAGE

Adult

• PO 400 mg qd × 10 days

• *Renal failure:* CrCl 30-49 ml/min, 4.5 mg/kg or 200 mg qd; CrCl 5-29 ml/min, 2.25 mg/kg or 100 mg qd

Child <12 yr

• PO 9 mg/kg, up to 400 mg qd × 10 days

AVAILABLE FORMS/COST OF THERAPY

• Cap, Gel—Oral: 400 mg, 100's: **$741.40**

• Powder, Reconst—Oral: 90 mg/5 ml, 30, 60, 120 ml: **$36.71**/60 ml; 180 mg/5 ml, 30, 60 ml: **$110.14**/60 ml

PRECAUTIONS: Hypersensitivity to penicillins, renal disease

PREGNANCY AND LACTATION: Pregnancy category B; excreted into breast milk in negligible concentrations

SIDE EFFECTS/ADVERSE REACTIONS

CNS: Chills, dizziness, fever, headache, paresthesia, weakness

GI: Abdominal pain, anorexia, *bleeding,* diarrhea, glossitis, nausea, *pseudomembranous colitis,* vomiting

GU: Candidiasis, *nephrotoxicity,* proteinuria, vaginitis

HEME: **Bone marrow suppression,** anemia, eosinophilia, **hemolytic anemia,** lymphocytosis, thrombocytosis

RESP: Dyspnea

SKIN: Dermatitis, rash, urticaria

INTERACTIONS

Drugs

3 *Aminoglycosides:* Additive nephrotoxicity

3 *Loop diuretics:* Increased nephrotoxicity

SPECIAL CONSIDERATIONS

• Comparable to many other oral cephalosporins; may produce higher serum levels and better penetration, but unsubstantiated

• Clinical application as alternative in respiratory tract infections

• Recommend empty stomach administration for the suspension

---

ceftizoxime

(sef-ti-zox'eem)

Rx: Cefizox

Chemical Class: Cephalosporin (3rd generation)

Therapeutic Class: Antibiotic

CLINICAL PHARMACOLOGY

Mechanism of Action: Inhibits bacterial cell wall synthesis; bactericidal

Pharmacokinetics

IM: Peak 1 hr, 30% bound by plasma proteins; not metabolized, eliminated unchanged in urine in 24 hr; crosses placenta; $t_{1/2}$ 1.7 hr

INDICATIONS AND USES: Infections of the skin and skin structures, bone and joints, lower respiratory tract, urinary tract; gonorrhea, pelvic inflammatory disease, septicemia, meningitis, intra-abdominal infections caused by susceptible organisms

Antibacterial spectrum usually includes:

• Gram-positive organisms: *Streptococcus pneumoniae, S. pyogenes, S. agalactiae, Staphylococcus aureus, S. epidermis*

• Gram-negative organisms: *Acinetobacter, H. influenzae, E. coli, E. aerogenes, P. mirabilis, P. vulgaris, Providencia rettgeri, P. aeruginosa, Serratia, Klebsiella, Enterobacter, Morganella morganii, N. gonorrhoeae*

• Anaerobes: *Bacteroides* sp., *Peptococcus, Peptostreptococcus*

DOSAGE

Adult

• IM/IV 1-2 g q8-12h, may give up to 2g q4h in life-threatening infections

• *PID:* IV 2 g q8h

• *Uncomplicated gonorrhea:* Single, 1 g IM dose

Dosage reduction appropriate in renal impairment (CrCl < 50 ml/min)

Child ≥6 mo

• 150-200 mg/kg/day divided q6-8h

$ **AVAILABLE FORMS/COST OF THERAPY**

• Inj, Sol—IV: 1 g: **$13.98;** 2 g: **$23.74**

CONTRAINDICATIONS: Infants <1 mo

PRECAUTIONS: Hypersensitivity to penicillins, renal disease

PREGNANCY AND LACTATION: Pregnancy category B; excreted in human milk in low concentrations

SIDE EFFECTS/ADVERSE REACTIONS

CNS: Dizziness, fever, headache, paresthesia

GI: Abdominal pain, anorexia, **bleeding;** diarrhea, glossitis, increased LFTs; nausea, **pseudomembranous colitis,** vomiting

GU: Candidiasis, proteinuria, pruritus, vaginitis, **nephrotoxicity**

---

italic = common side effects   **bold italic** = life-threatening reactions

HEME: **Bone marrow suppression,** eosinophilia, **hemolytic anemia**
RESP: Dyspnea
SKIN: Dermatitis, rash, urticaria
INTERACTIONS
Drugs
3 *Aminoglycosides:* Additive nephrotoxicity
3 *Loop diuretics:* Increased nephrotoxicity

---

ceftriaxone
(sef-try-ax′one)
Rx: Rocephin
Chemical Class: Cephalosporin (3rd generation)
Therapeutic Class: Antibiotic

CLINICAL PHARMACOLOGY
Mechanism of Action: Inhibits bacterial cell wall synthesis; bactericidal
Pharmacokinetics
IV: Peak 30 min (123 µg/ml for 1 g)
IM: Peak 1.5-4 hr (83 µg/ml for 1 g)
90% bound by plasma proteins; 35%-60% eliminated unchanged in urine, remainder secreted in bile; crosses placenta; elimination $t_{1/2}$ 7.2 hr, prolonged in elderly, liver disease (9 hr), and renal disease (CrCl <16 ml/min 15 hr, CrCl 16-60 ml/min 11-12 hr.)
INDICATIONS AND USES: Infections of the lower respiratory tract, urinary tract, skin, bone, joint; intra-abdominal infections; septicemia; meningitis caused by susceptible organisms; localized and disseminated gonococcal infections including pelvic inflammatory disease; surgical prophylaxis
Antibacterial spectrum usually includes:
• Gram-positive organisms: *Streptococcus pneumoniae, S. pyogenes, Staphylococcus aureus*
• Gram-negative organisms: *H. in-* *fluenzae, E. coli, E. aerogenes, E. cloacae, P. mirabilis, P. vulgaris, Serratia marcescens, Providencia rettgeri, Klebsiella* sp., *Citrobacter* sp., *Salmonella* sp. (including *S. typhi*), *Shigella* sp., *Acinetobacter* sp., *Neisseria* sp.; some strains of *Pseudomonas aeruginosa*
• Anaerobes: *B. fragilis, B. bivivus, B. melaninogenicus, Peptostreptococcus* sp.
DOSAGE
Adult
• *Infections of the lower respiratory tract, urinary tract, skin, bone, joint; intra-abdominal infections; septicemia:* IM/IV 1-2 g qd
• *Uncomplicated gonorrhea:* IM 125 mg as single dose plus 1 g azithromycin PO or doxycycline 100 mg PO bid × 7 days
• *Meningitis:* IM/IV 100 mg/kg/day in equal doses q12h; not to exceed 4 g qd
• *Surgical prophylaxis:* IV 1 g ½-2 hr preop
Child
• *Acute otitis media:* IM 50 mg/kg (max 1 g) as a single dose
• *Infections of the lower respiratory tract, urinary tract, skin, bone, joint; intra-abdominal infections; septicemia:* IM/IV 50-75 mg/kg/day in equal doses q12h; not to exceed 2 g qd
• *Meningitis:* IM/IV 100 mg/kg/day in equal doses q12h; not to exceed 4 g qd
$ **AVAILABLE FORMS/COST OF THERAPY**
• Inj, Dry-Sol—IM, IV: 250 mg/vial: **$14.51;** 500 mg/vial: **$25.50;** 1 g/vial: **$40.18-$50.08;** 2 g/vial: **$70.57-$87.62**
PRECAUTIONS: Hypersensitivity to penicillins, renal disease
PREGNANCY AND LACTATION: Pregnancy category B; excreted in breast milk

---

SIDE EFFECTS/ADVERSE REACTIONS

CNS: Chills, dizziness, fever, headache, paresthesia, weakness

GI: Abdominal pain, anorexia, bleeding; diarrhea, glossitis, increased LFTs; nausea, *pseudomembranous colitis,* vomiting

GU: Candidiasis, *nephrotoxicity,* vaginitis

HEME: Bone marrow suppression, eosinophilia, *hemolytic anemia,* lymphocytosis, thrombocytosis

RESP: Dyspnea

SKIN: Dermatitis; induration or tenderness at injection site; rash, urticaria

INTERACTIONS
Drugs
3 *Aminoglycosides:* Additive nephrotoxicity

3 *Loop diuretics:* Increased nephrotoxicity

2 *Warfarin:* Hypoprothrombinemic response enhanced

SPECIAL CONSIDERATIONS
• Meningitis the only indication requiring bid dosing; qd sufficient for all other indications in adults

• Often administered in acute care settings for dubious indications due to long $t_{1/2}$, avoid overuse

---

cefuroxime
(sef-yoor-ox′eem)

Rx: Zinacef, Kefurox (as sodium), Ceftin (as axetil)

Chemical Class: Cephalosporin (2nd generation)

Therapeutic Class: Antibiotic

CLINICAL PHARMACOLOGY
Mechanism of Action: Inhibits bacterial cell wall synthesis; bactericidal

Pharmacokinetics

PO: Peak level 2 hr (7 µg/ml after 500 mg); absorption greater after food (absolute bioavailability increases from 37% to 52%); bioavailability of susp 91% of tab; peak plasma concentration for susp 71% of peak plasma concentration for tab

IV: Peak 30 min

IM: Peak 15-60 min; 33%-50% bound by plasma proteins; 70%-100% eliminated unchanged in urine; crosses placenta, blood-brain barrier; not metabolized; $t_{1/2}$ 1-2 hr

INDICATIONS AND USES: Pharyngitis, tonsillitis, otitis media, bronchitis, pneumonia, infections of the skin and urinary tract, localized and disseminated gonococcal infections, bone or joint infections, septicemia, or meningitis caused by susceptible organisms; treatment of early Lyme's disease

Antibacterial spectrum usually includes:

• Gram-positive organisms: *Streptococcus pneumoniae, S. pyogenes, Staphylococcus aureus*

• Gram-negative organisms: *H. influenzae, H. parainfluenzae, Moraxella catarrhalis* (including ampicillin- and cephalothin-resistant strains), *E. coli, P. mirabilis, Neisseria* sp., *Klebsiella* sp.

• Anaerobes: *Peptococcus* and *Peptostreptococcus* sp.; β-lactamase-producing strains of these pathogens are usually susceptible

DOSAGE
Adult
• *Pharyngitis, tonsillitis, bronchitis, skin infections:* PO (tab) 250-500 mg q12h

• *UTI:* PO (tab) 125-250 mg q12h

• *Uncomplicated gonorrhea:* PO 1000 mg single dose; IM 1.5 g single dose, 2 sites, with 1g PO probenecid

• *Early Lyme disease:* PO 500 mg bid × 20 days.

---

italic = common side effects   **bold italic** = life-threatening reactions

• *Uncomplicated urinary tract infections, skin infections, disseminated gonococcal infections, uncomplicated pneumonia:* IM/IV 750 mg-1.5 g q8h

• *Bone and joint infections:* IM/IV 1.5 g q8h

• *Surgical prophylaxis:* IV 1.5 g ½-1 hr preop

• *Severe infections including meningitis:* IM/IV 1.5 g q6h; may give up to 3 g q8h for bacterial meningitis

• *Dosage in renal impairment:* CrCl >20 ml/min, use 750 mg-1.5 g q8h; CrCl 10-20 ml/min, use 750 mg q12h; CrCl <10 ml/min, use 750 mg q24h; since cefuroxime sodium is dialyzable, patients on hemodialysis should be given a further dose at the end of the dialysis

Child

• *Pharyngitis, tonsillitis, bronchitis:* Age >12 yr PO (tab) 250-500 mg q12h; age 3 mo-12 yr PO (susp) 20 mg/kg/day, divided bid, max dose 500 mg daily

• *Skin infections:* Age >12 yr PO (tab) 250-500 mg q12h; age 3 mo-12 yr PO (susp) 30 mg/kg/day, divided bid, max dose 1000 mg daily

• *Otitis media:* Age >12 yr PO (tab) 250 mg bid, age 3 mo-12 yr PO (susp) 30 mg/kg/day, divided bid, max dose 1000 mg daily

• *Uncomplicated urinary tract infections, skin infections, disseminated gonococcal infections, uncomplicated pneumonia:* Age >3 mo IM/IV 50-100 mg/kg qd (not to exceed the max adult dosage) in equally divided doses q8h

• *Bone and joint infections:* Age >3 mo IM/IV 150 mg/kg qd (not to exceed the max adult dosage) in equally divided doses q8h

• *Severe infections including meningitis:* Age >3 mo IM/IV 50-100 mg/kg qd in equally divided doses q6-8h; may give up to 200-240 mg/kg/day IV in divided doses for bacterial meningitis

§ AVAILABLE FORMS/COST OF THERAPY

• Powder, Reconst—Oral: 125 mg/5 ml, 50, 100, 200 ml: **$46.71**/100 ml; 250 mg/5 ml, 50, 100 ml: **$76.15**/100 ml

• Tab, Coated—Oral: 125 mg, 100's: **$205.03;** 250 mg, 100's: **$394.31;** 500 mg, 100's: **$860.25**

• Inj, Dry-Sol—IM; IV: 750 mg/vial: **$6.76-$7.24;** 1.5 g/vial: **$13.46-$13.94**

CONTRAINDICATIONS: Infants <1 mo

PRECAUTIONS: Hypersensitivity to penicillins, renal disease

PREGNANCY AND LACTATION: Pregnancy category B; excreted in breast milk

SIDE EFFECTS/ADVERSE REACTIONS

CNS: Chills, dizziness, fever, headache, paresthesia, weakness

GI: Abdominal pain, anorexia, ***bleeding;*** diarrhea, glossitis, increased LFTs; nausea, ***pseudomembranous colitis,*** vomiting

GU: Candidiasis, ***nephrotoxicity,*** vaginitis

HEME: ***Bone marrow suppression,*** eosinophilia, ***hemolytic anemia,*** lymphocytosis, thrombocytosis

RESP: Dyspnea

SKIN: Rash, urticaria

INTERACTIONS

Drugs

▨ *Aminoglycosides:* Additive nephrotoxicity

▨ *Antacids, H₂-blockers, omeprazole, lansoprazole:* Decreased absorption of cefuroxime axetil

▨ *Loop diuretics:* Increased nephrotoxicity

SPECIAL CONSIDERATIONS

• Oral tabs and oral susp not bioequivalent

- Take with food
- Alternative to amoxicillin or co-trimoxazole for resistant upper respiratory pathogens; expensive, but bid dosing

---

celecoxib
Rx: Celebrex
Chemical Class:
Cyclooxygenase-2 (COX-2) inhibitor
Therapeutic Class: Nonsteroidal antiinflammatory drug (NSAID)

CLINICAL PHARMACOLOGY
Mechanism of Action: Suppression of production of prostaglandin E_2 at inflammation sites via inhibition of the cyclooxygenase-2 (COX-2) isoform. COX-2 is the inducible isoform, responsible for production of the inflammatory prostaglandins. Nonsteroidal antiinflammatory drug (NSAID) (analgesic, antipyretic, antiinflammatory)
Pharmacokinetics
PO: Peak about 3 hr; food enhanced bioavailability; 97% bound to plasma protein; extensively metabolized by liver (via CYP450 2C9-3 inactive metabolites), excreted in urine (27%) and feces (57%); $t_{1/2}$ 9-10 hr; crosses placenta

INDICATIONS AND USES: Signs and symptoms of osteoarthritis and rheumatoid arthritis, dental pain*

DOSAGE
Adult and Child >16 yr
- *Osteoarthritis:* PO 200 mg qd or 100 mg bid
- *Rheumatoid arthritis:* PO 100-200 mg bid

$ AVAILABLE FORMS/COST OF THERAPY
- Cap—Oral: 100 mg, 100's: **$143.00;** 200 mg, 100's: **$242.00**

CONTRAINDICATIONS: Documented allergic-type reaction to sulfonamides, rhinitis, urticaria, asthma, or allergic reactions to aspirin or other antiinflammatory agents

PRECAUTIONS: Late pregnancy (premature closure of ductus arteriosus), liver dysfunction, hypertension, congestive heart failure, previous history of gastrointestinal ulceration, bleeding, or perforation, renal dysfunction, concurrent use of warfarin

PREGNANCY AND LACTATION: Pregnancy category C; breast milk secretion, unknown

SIDE EFFECTS/ADVERSE REACTIONS
CNS: Dizziness, headache
CV: Fluid retention, peripheral edema
EENT: Hypersensitivity reactions in aspirin-sensitive asthma patients
GI: Dyspepsia, diarrhea, abdominal pain, flatulence, ulcer, **gastrointestinal bleed,** LFT elevations
GU: **Acute renal failure**
RESP: Upper respiratory tract infection, sinusitis, pharyngitis, rhinitis

INTERACTIONS
Drugs
3 *Diuretics:* Potential reduction of both diuretic and antihypertensive effects of loop and thiazide diuretics

SPECIAL CONSIDERATIONS
- COX-2 specific inhibition great choice for patients with inflammatory conditions who are at high risk of gastrointestinal adverse effects (e.g., older than 60 years, history of peptic ulcer disease, prolonged, high-dose NSAID therapy, concurrent use of corticosteroids or anticoagulants)

MONITORING PARAMETERS
- Rheumatoid arthritis—Decreased acute phase reactants (ESR, C-reactive protein), pain relief, reduction in number of swollen joints,

---

italic = common side effects   ***bold italic*** = life-threatening reactions

improved range of motion, less fatigue, functional capacity, structural damage, maintenance of normal lifestyle
• Osteoarthritis—Decreased pain and stiffness of affected joints
• Toxicity—Initial hemogram, fecal occult blood, then q 6-12 mo; electrolytes and renal function tests q 6-12 mo; LFT's q 6-12 mo in high-risk patients; query patient for dyspepsia, nausea, vomiting, right upper abdominal pain, anorexia, fatigue, jaundice, edema, weight gain, decreased urine output

---

cellulose sodium phosphate (CSP)

Rx: Calcibind
Chemical Class: Phosphorylated cellulose
Therapeutic Class: Hypercalciuria

CLINICAL PHARMACOLOGY
Mechanism of Action: Decreases hypercalciuria by binding with calcium in bowel; reduces urinary calcium by approximately 50 mg/5 g qd of CSP
Pharmacokinetics
Not absorbed
INDICATIONS AND USES: Absorptive hypercalciuria type I with recurrent calcium oxalate or calcium phosphate renal stones
DOSAGE
Adult
• PO 15 g qd in divided doses with each meal, then 10 g qd (5 g with supper, 2.5 g with each remaining meal) when 24 hr urine Ca excretion <150 mg; for each 15 g qd of CSP, give 1.5 g magnesium gluconate bid (at least 1 hr before or after a dose of CSP)

$ **AVAILABLE FORMS/COST OF THERAPY**
• Powder, Reconst—Oral: 2.5 g/scoop, 300 g: **$103.13**
CONTRAINDICATIONS: Hyperparathyroidism, hypomagnesemia, enteric hyperoxaluria, metabolic bone disease, hypocalcemia
PRECAUTIONS: CHF, ascites, liver disease, children <16, elderly
PREGNANCY AND LACTATION:
Pregnancy category C
SIDE EFFECTS/ADVERSE REACTIONS
GI: Anorexia, diarrhea, dyspepsia, nausea
GU: Hyperoxaluria, hyperphosphaturia, hypomagnesuria
METAB: Depletion of trace metals (copper, zinc, iron), hypomagnesemia
SPECIAL CONSIDERATIONS
PATIENT/FAMILY EDUCATION
• Suspend each dose of CSP powder in glass of water, soft drink or fruit juice
• Injest within 30 min of a meal
MONITORING PARAMETERS
• Serum Ca, Mg, copper, zinc, iron, parathyroid hormone, CBC every 3 to 6 mo
• Serum parathyroid hormone should be obtained at least once between the 1st 2 wk to 3 mo of treatment

---

cephalexin

(sef-a-lex'in)
Rx: Biocef, Keflex, Keftab
Chemical Class: Cephalosporin (1st generation)
Therapeutic Class: Antibiotic

CLINICAL PHARMACOLOGY
Mechanism of Action: Inhibits bacterial cell wall synthesis; bactericidal

Pharmacokinetics
PO: Peak 1 hr (15 µg/ml after 500 mg), duration 6-8 hr, 5%-15% bound by plasma proteins; 90%-100% eliminated unchanged in urine within 8 hr; crosses placenta; $t_{1/2}$ 30-72 min; may be given without regard to meals

INDICATIONS AND USES: Pharyngitis, tonsillitis, otitis media, bronchitis, pneumonia, skin, bone and urinary tract infections caused by susceptible organisms

Antibacterial spectrum usually includes:

• Gram-positive organisms: *Streptococcus pneumoniae, S. pyogenes, Staphylococcus aureus*

• Gram-negative organisms: *H. influenzae, E. coli, P. mirabilis, Moraxella catarrhalis, Klebsiella* sp.

DOSAGE
Adult

• *Bronchitis, pneumonia, urinary tract infections:* PO 250-500 mg q6h

• *Pharyngitis, tonsillitis, cystitis, mild to moderate skin infections:* PO 500 mg q12h

• *Severe infections:* PO 500 mg-1 g q6h

• *Dosage in renal impairment:* CrCl 11-40 ml/min, max adult dose 500 mg q8-12h; CrCl 5-10 ml/min, max adult dose 250 mg q12h; CrCl <5 ml/min, max adult dose 250 mg q12-24h

Child

• *Bronchitis, pneumonia, urinary tract infections:* PO 25-50 mg/kg/day in 4 equal doses

• *Pharyngitis, tonsillitis, cystitis, mild to moderate skin infections:* Age >15 yr PO 500 mg q12h; age >1 yr PO 25-50 mg/kg/day in 2 equal doses

• *Severe infections:* PO 50-100 mg/kg/day in 4 equal doses

• *Otitis media:* PO 75-100 mg/kg/day in 4 equal doses

§ AVAILABLE FORMS/COST OF THERAPY

• Cap, Gel—Oral: 250 mg, 100's: **$10.29-$141.67;** 500 mg, 100's: **$25.00-$266.03**

• Powder, Reconst— 125 mg/5 ml, 200 ml: **$4.65-$27.89;** 250 mg/5 ml, 200 ml: **$7.58-$20.56**

• Tab, Plain Coated—Oral: 250 mg, 100's: **$29.99;** 500 mg, 100's: **$63.51-$206.58**

CONTRAINDICATIONS: Infants <1 mo

PRECAUTIONS: Hypersensitivity to penicillins, renal disease

PREGNANCY AND LACTATION: Pregnancy category B; excreted in breast milk

SIDE EFFECTS/ADVERSE REACTIONS

CNS: Chills, dizziness, fever, headache, paresthesia, weakness
GI: Abdominal pain, anorexia, ***bleeding; diarrhea,*** glossitis, increased LFTs, nausea, ***pseudomembranous colitis,*** vomiting
GU: Candidiasis, ***nephrotoxicity,*** proteinuria, pruritus, vaginitis
HEME: **Bone marrow suppression,** eosinophilia, **hemolytic anemia,** lymphocytosis, thrombocytosis
RESP: Dyspnea
SKIN: Dermatitis, rash, urticaria
MISC: Serum sickness-like syndrome

INTERACTIONS
Drugs

§ *Aminoglycosides:* Additive nephrotoxicity

§ *Loop diuretics:* Increased nephrotoxicity

Labs

• *Increase:* Urinary amino acids
• *False positive:* Urine glucose with Benedict's, Fehlings, Clinitest
• *Decrease:* Urine leukocytes

SPECIAL CONSIDERATIONS

• 1st generation oral cephalosporin of choice

---

italic = common side effects   **bold italic** = life-threatening reactions

cephalothin

(sef-a-loe'thin)
Rx: Keflin
Chemical Class: Cephalosporin (1st generation)
Therapeutic Class: Antibiotic

CLINICAL PHARMACOLOGY
Mechanism of Action: Inhibits bacterial wall synthesis; bactericidal
Pharmacokinetics
IM: Peak 0.5 hr; 65%-80% bound by plasma proteins; excreted by the kidneys (inhibited by probenecid); $t_{1/2}$ ½-1 hr

INDICATIONS AND USES: Infections of the respiratory tract, skin and skin structures, genitourinary tract, gastrointestinal tract, bones and joints; endocarditis, septicemia; perioperative prophylaxis for contaminated or potentially contaminated procedures

Antibacterial spectrum usually includes:

• Gram-positive organisms: Group A β-hemolytic streptococci, staphylococci (including coagulase-positive, coagulase-negative, and penicillinase-producing strains [not MRSA]); *Streptococcus pneumoniae*

• Gram-negative organisms: *Haemophilus influenzae, Escherichia coli, Klebsiella* sp., *Proteus mirabilis, Salmonella* sp., *Shigella* sp.

DOSAGE
Adult
• IM/IV 500 mg-1 g q4-6h
• *Uncomplicated gonorrhea:* IM 2 g as single dose
• *Severe infections:* IM/IV 1-2 g q4h

. Dosage reduction indicated in renal impairment (CrCl <50 ml/min)

• *Preoperative:* IV 1-2 g ½-1 hrs prior to procedure
Child
• IM/IV 14-27 mg/kg q4h or 20-40 mg/kg q6h

$ **AVAILABLE FORMS/COST OF THERAPY**
• Inj, Premix—IV: 1 g/50 ml: **$10.08;** 2 g/50 ml: **$14.30**

PRECAUTIONS: Hypersensitivity to penicillins, renal disease

PREGNANCY AND LACTATION: Pregnancy category B; excreted into breast milk in low concentrations; no adverse effects have been observed

SIDE EFFECTS/ADVERSE REACTIONS
CNS: Chills, dizziness, fever, headache, paresthesia, weakness
GI: Abdominal pain, anorexia, *bleeding; diarrhea,* glossitis, increased LFTs; nausea, *pseudomembranous colitis,* vomiting
GU: Candidiasis, *nephrotoxicity,* proteinuria, pruritus, vaginitis
HEME: Bone marrow suppression, eosinophilia, *hemolytic anemia,* lymphocytosis
RESP: Dyspnea
SKIN: Dermatitis, rash, urticaria

INTERACTIONS
Drugs
3 *Aminoglycosides:* Additive nephrotoxicity
3 *Furosemide:* Increased nephrotoxicity
Labs
• *False positive:* Urinary protein; urinary glucose by Benedict's or Fehling's solution, Clinitest tabs
• *False increase:* Creatinine (serum, urine), urinary 17-KS
• *False decrease:* Urine leukocytes

cephapirin
(sef-a-peer'in)
Rx: Cefadyl
Chemical Class: Cephalosporin (1st generation)
Therapeutic Class: Antibiotic

CLINICAL PHARMACOLOGY
Mechanism of Action: Inhibits bacterial cell wall synthesis; bactericidal

Pharmacokinetics
IM: Peak 30 min, 44-50% bound by plasma proteins; metabolized in liver, 40%-70% eliminated unchanged in urine; $t_{1/2}$ 21-47 min

INDICATIONS AND USES: Infections of the respiratory tract, skin and skin structures, urinary tract; septicemia; endocarditis; osteomyelitis; perioperative prophylaxis for contaminated or potentially contaminated procedures

Antibacterial spectrum usually includes:

• Gram-positive organisms: Group A β-hemolytic streptococci, staphylococci (including coagulase-positive, coagulase-negative, and penicillinase-producing strains [not MRSA]); *Streptococcus pneumoniae*

• Gram-negative organisms: *Haemophilus influenzae, Escherichia coli, Klebsiella* sp., *Proteus mirabilis*

DOSAGE
Adult
• IM/IV 500 mg-1 g q4-6h, maximum 12 g/day
• *Preoperative:* IV/IM 1-2 g ½-1 hr prior to surgery
• *Renal function impairment* (serum creatinine >5 mg/dl): IM/IV 7.5-15 mg/kg q12h

Child
• IM/IV 40-80 mg/kg/day divided q6h

$ **AVAILABLE FORMS/COST OF THERAPY**
• Inj, Dry-Sol—IM; IV: 1 g/vial: **$1.64**

PRECAUTIONS: Hypersensitivity to penicillins, renal disease, prolonged use, colitis

PREGNANCY AND LACTATION: Pregnancy category B; excreted into breast milk in low concentrations; no adverse effects have been observed

SIDE EFFECTS/ADVERSE REACTIONS
CNS: Chills, dizziness, fever, headache, paresthesia, weakness
GI: Abdominal pain, anorexia, ***bleeding;*** *diarrhea,* glossitis, increased LFTs; nausea, ***pseudomembranous colitis,*** vomiting
GU: Candidiasis, ***nephrotoxicity,*** proteinuria, pruritus, vaginitis
HEME: ***Bone marrow suppression,*** eosinophilia, ***hemolytic anemia,*** lymphocytosis
RESP: Dyspnea
SKIN: Dermatitis, rash, urticaria

INTERACTIONS
Drugs
3 *Aminoglycosides:* Additive nephrotoxicity
3 *Loop diuretics:* Increased nephrotoxicity

SPECIAL CONSIDERATIONS
• No advantage over cefazolin; price should guide usage of 1st generation cephalosporins

---

italic = common side effects   ***bold italic*** = life-threatening reactions

cephradine

(sef'ra-deen)
Rx: Velosef
Chemical Class: Cephalosporin (1st generation)
Therapeutic Class: Antibiotic

CLINICAL PHARMACOLOGY
Mechanism of Action: Inhibits bacterial cell wall synthesis; bactericidal
Pharmacokinetics
PO: Peak 1 hr
IM: Peak 1 hr
8%-17% bound to plasma proteins; 80%-90% eliminated unchanged in urine; $t_{1/2}$ 0.75-1.5 hr
INDICATIONS AND USES: Infections of the respiratory tract, skin and skin structure, urinary tract; otitis media; osteomyelitis
Antibacterial spectrum usually includes:
• Gram-positive organisms: Group A β-hemolytic streptococci, staphylococci (including penicillinase-producing strains [not MRSA]); *Streptococcus pneumoniae*
• Gram-negative organisms: *Escherichia coli, Proteus mirabilis, Klebsiella* spp., *Hemophilus influenzae*
DOSAGE
Adult
• *Skin, respiratory infections:* PO 250 mg q6h or 500 mg q12h
• *Lobar pneumonia:* PO 500 mg q6h or 1g q12h
• *UTI:* PO 500 mg q12 (up to 1 g q6h may be administered for severe infections)
• *Renal function impairment:* PO CrCl 5-20 ml/min 250 mg q6h; CrCl <5 ml/min 250 mg q12h
Child >9 mo
• PO 25-50 mg/kg/day divided q6h or q12h
• *Otitis media:* PO 75-100 mg/kg/day divided q6h or q12h; max 4g/day

$ AVAILABLE FORMS/COST OF THERAPY
• Cap, Gel—Oral: 250 mg, 100's: **$30.00-$80.54;** 500 mg, 100's: **$52.00-$201.01**
• Powder, Reconst—Oral: 125 mg/5 ml, 100 ml: **$4.25-$9.73;** 250 mg/5 ml, 100 ml: **$7.98-$18.25**
PRECAUTIONS: Hypersensitivity to penicillins, renal disease
PREGNANCY AND LACTATION: Pregnancy category B; excreted into breast milk in low concentrations; no adverse effects have been observed
SIDE EFFECTS/ADVERSE REACTIONS
CNS: Chills, dizziness, fever, headache, paresthesia, weakness
GI: Abdominal pain, anorexia, *bleeding; diarrhea,* glossitis, increased LFTs; nausea, *pseudomembranous colitis,* vomiting
GU: Candidiasis, *nephrotoxicity,* proteinuria, pruritus, vaginitis
HEME: Bone marrow suppression, eosinophilia, *hemolytic anemia,* lymphocytosis
RESP: Dyspnea
SKIN: Dermatitis, rash, urticaria
INTERACTIONS
Drugs
3 *Aminoglycosides:* Additive nephrotoxicity
3 *Loop diuretics:* Increased nephrotoxicity
SPECIAL CONSIDERATIONS
• No advantage over cephalexin; cost should be major consideration for selection of first generation cephalosporins

* = non-FDA-approved use

cerivastatin
(se-reev′a-stat-in)
Rx: Baycol
Chemical Class: Substituted hexahydronaphthalene
Therapeutic Class: Antilipemic (HMG-CoA reductase inhibitor); statin

CLINICAL PHARMACOLOGY
Mechanism of Action: Competitively inhibits 3-hydroxy-3-methylglutaryl-coenzyme A (HMG-CoA) reductase, an early rate-limiting step in cholesterol biosynthesis; increases HDL cholesterol mildly [10%], moderate decreases in total and LDL cholesterol [17-19%, 25-28% respectively], minimal lowering effect on triglycerides [11-24%]
Pharmacokinetics
PO: Peak 2.5 hrs; well absorbed (PO bioavailability 60%); 99% protein bound; moderately distributed into tissues; metabolized by liver, CYP3A4 and others (two major metabolites, 50, 100% as active as parent); low clearance drug; metabolites excreted in feces; $t_{1/2}$ 2-3 hr
INDICATIONS AND USES: Primary hypercholesterolemia (heterozygous familial and nonfamilial hypercholesterolemia) and mixed dyslipidemia (Fredrickson types IIa and IIb)
DOSAGE
Adult
• PO 0.3 mg qd in the evening; may be taken with or without food; no dosage adjustments necessary for renal function as low as CrCl 60 ml/min; for CrCl <60 ml/min, start with 0.2 mg qd
💲 AVAILABLE FORMS/COST OF THERAPY
• Tab—Oral: 0.2 mg, 100's: **$141.90**; 0.3 mg, 100's: **$141.90**; 0.4 mg, 100's: **$141.90**

CONTRAINDICATIONS: Active liver disease; unexplained persistent elevations of serum transaminases
PRECAUTIONS: Liver dysfunction or heavy alcohol ingestion; renal insufficiency; conditions predisposing to renal failure secondary to rhabdomyolysis (e.g., sepsis, hypotension, trauma, metabolic, endocrine, or electolyte disorders), or uncontrolled epilepsy
PREGNANCY AND LACTATION: Pregnancy category X; present in breast milk 1.3:1, M:P ratio; not recommended for nursing mothers
SIDE EFFECTS/ADVERSE REACTIONS
CNS: Insomnia
CV: Peripheral edema
GI: Diarrhea, dyspepsia, *transaminasemia*
GU: Urinary tract infection
MS: Arthralgia, myalgia
RESP: Cough, pharyngitis, rhinitis, sinusitis
SKIN: Rash
INTERACTIONS
Drugs
3 *Azole antifungals (fluconazole, itraconazole, ketoconazole, miconazole):* Increased cerivastatin levels; increased risk of rhabdomyolysis
3 *Erythromycin:* Increased cerivastatin concentrations; increased risk of rhabdomyolysis
3 *Fibric acid derivatives:* Increased risk of myopathy, especially with high statin doses
3 *Cyclosporine:* Increased cyclosporine concentrations; increased risk of rhabdomyolysis
3 *Nefazodone:* Increased cerivastatin levels; increased risk of rhabdomyolysis
3 *Niacin:* Isolated cases of myopathy and rhabdomyolysis have oc-

curred in patients receiving other "statins" and nicacin

SPECIAL CONSIDERATIONS
• Statin selection based on lipid-lowering prowess, cost, and availability

PATIENT/FAMILY EDUCATION
• Report symptoms of myalgia, muscle tenderness, or weakness
• Take daily doses in the evening for increased effect

MONITORING PARAMETERS
• Cholesterol (max therapeutic response 4-6 wk)
• LFTs (AST, ALT) at baseline and at 12 wk of therapy; if no change, no further monitoring necessary (discontinue if elevations persists at >3× upper limit of normal)
• CPK in patients complaining of diffuse myalgia, muscle tenderness, or weakness

---

cetirizine

(si-tear'a-zeen)
Rx: Zyrtec
Chemical Class: Piperazine derivative
Therapeutic Class: Antihistamine

CLINICAL PHARMACOLOGY
Mechanism of Action: Decreases allergic response by blocking histamine at H_1-receptors; negligible anticholinergic and antiserotonergic activity; negligible brain penetration and interaction with cerebral H_1-receptors

Pharmacokinetics
PO: Peak 1 hr; rapid absorption reduced by food; 93% protein bound; 70% excreted by kidneys (primarily as unchanged drug, 10% in feces); $t_{1/2}$ 8.3 hr

INDICATIONS AND USES: Seasonal and perennial allergic rhinitis; chronic idiopathic urticaria

DOSAGE
Adult
• PO 5-10 mg qd prn; reduce dose to 5 mg qd for patients with decreased renal function (CrCl <30) and in hepatically impaired patients
Child ≥6 yr
• PO 5-10 mg qd prn

🛈 AVAILABLE FORMS/COST OF THERAPY
• Syrup—Oral: 5 mg/5 ml, 480 ml: **$108.69**
• Tab, Coated—Oral: 5, 10 mg 100's: **$185.99**

PRECAUTIONS: Activities requiring mental alertness; coadministration with alcohol and other CNS depressants

PREGNANCY AND LACTATION: Pregnancy category B; excreted into breast milk

SIDE EFFECTS/ADVERSE REACTIONS
CNS: Anorexia, confusion, depression, fatigue, headache, insomnia, nervousness, paresthesia, *somnolence*
CV: **Cardiac failure,** flushing, hypertension, palpitation, tachycardia
EENT: Deafness, earache, epistaxis, ototoxicity, rhinitis, tinnitus
GI: Diarrhea, dry mouth, dyspepsia, flatulence, increased appetite, increased salivation, nausea, vomiting
GU: Breast pain, cystitis, dysmenorrhea, dysuria, hematuria, polyuria, urinary retention
METAB: Dehydration, diabetes mellitus, thirst
MS: Arthralgia, arthritis, arthrosis, muscle weakness, myalgia
RESP: Bronchospasm, coughing, dyspnea
MISC: Lymphadenopathy

SPECIAL CONSIDERATIONS
• H_1 antagonist with minimal effect on CNS; no affinity for other receptors

---

* = non-FDA-approved use

• Very potent antihistamine
• Kinetics allow qd dosing and do not have cytochrome P-450 drug interactions
• Effective versus itching

---

charcoal/activated charcoal

(char'coal)
OTC: *Oral caps:* CharcoCaps *Oral tablets:* Charco Plus DS *Oral Suspensions (activated):* Actidose-Aqua, Liqui-Char, CharcoAide
Combinations
   OTC: with simethicone (Charcoal Plus, Flatulex); with sorbitol (Actidose with sorbitol)
Chemical Class: Carbon
Therapeutic Class:Antiflatulent; antidote (activated); antidiarrheal

---

CLINICAL PHARMACOLOGY
Mechanism of Action: Adsorbent, detoxicant, soothing agent; reduces volume of intestinal gas; binds poisons, toxins, irritants in GI tract; bound toxins inactive until excreted
Pharmacokinetics
PO: Insoluble in water; excreted in feces
INDICATIONS AND USES: Flatulence; emergency treatment in most poisonings; dyspepsia, abdominal distention; deodorant in wounds; diarrhea
DOSAGE
Adult
• *Flatulence/dyspepsia:* PO 520-975 mg pc up to 4.16 g/day
• *Poisoning:* PO 25-100 g (or 1 g/kg or approximately 10× the amount of poison ingested; may give 20-40 g q6h for 1-2 days in severe poisoning

Child <1 yr
• *Poisoning:* 1 g/kg as single dose
Child 1-12 yr
• *Poisoning:* 25-50 g as single dose
💲 AVAILABLE FORMS/COST OF THERAPY
• Susp (activated)—Oral: 15 gm/75 ml, 150 ml: **$3.50** 25 g/120 ml: **$5.38-$6.64**
• Caps—Oral: 260 mg, 120's: **$5.29**
• Tab—Oral: 250 mg, 125's: **$6.60**
• Tab, enteric coated—Oral: 250 mg, 125's: **$13.56**
CONTRAINDICATIONS: Unconsciousness, semiconsciousness; poisoning with cyanide, mineral acids, alkalies
PRECAUTIONS: Absence of bowel sounds
SIDE EFFECTS/ADVERSE REACTIONS
GI: Black stools, constipation, diarrhea, nausea, vomiting
INTERACTIONS
Drugs
❷ *Digitalis glycosides:* Reduced digoxin levels; less effect on digitoxin
SPECIAL CONSIDERATIONS
• Administer activated charcoal for adsorption in emergency management of poisonings as a slurry with water, a saline cathartic, or sorbitol

---

chenodiol

(kee-noe-dye'ole)
Rx: Chenix
Chemical Class: Chenodeoxycholic acid
Therapeutic Class: Cholelitholytic

CLINICAL PHARMACOLOGY
Mechanism of Action: Suppresses hepatic synthesis of cholesterol and cholic acid, replacing cholic acid with drug metabolite; contributes to biliary cholesterol desaturation and

---

gradual dissolution of radiolucent cholesterol gallstones; has no effects on radiopaque (calcified) gallstones or on radiolucent bile pigment stones

Pharmacokinetics

PO: Extensive enterohepatic recirculation; 80% excreted in feces as metabolite

INDICATIONS AND USES: Dissolution of gallstones in patients with radiolucent stones in well-opacifying gallbladders, in whom effective surgery would be undertaken except for the presence of increased surgical risk due to systemic disease or age (the likelihood of successful dissolution is far greater if the stones are floatable or small)

DOSAGE

Adult

• PO 250 mg bid for 2 wk, then increased by 250 mg/day, not to exceed 16 mg/kg/day

$ AVAILABLE FORMS/COST OF THERAPY

• Tab, Plain Coated—Oral: 250 mg, 100's: **$107.98**

CONTRAINDICATIONS: Hepatic disease, bile duct abnormalities, biliary GI fistula

PRECAUTIONS: Children, atherosclerosis, elderly, colon cancer

PREGNANCY AND LACTATION: Pregnancy category X; excretion into breast milk unknown; use extreme caution in nursing mothers

SIDE EFFECTS/ADVERSE REACTIONS

GI: Absence of taste, *biliary pain,* cramps; *diarrhea,* dyspepsia, dysphagia, fecal urgency, flatulence, heartburn, hepatotoxicity, increased ALT, AST, LDH (50% of patients); *nausea,* vomiting

*HEME: **Leukopenia***

METAB: Increased total and LDL-cholesterol

SPECIAL CONSIDERATIONS

• Comparative trials of ursodiol and chenodiol show equivalent efficacy; ursodiol associated with less adverse effects, hence preferred

MONITORING PARAMETERS

• Monthly aminotransferase levels for 3 mo then q3 mo

• Serum cholesterol, cholecystogram or ultrasonogram, CBC

---

chloral hydrate

(klor-al hye′drate)

Rx: Aquachloral, Noctec

Chemical Class: Halogenated alcohol

Therapeutic Class: Sedative/hypnotic

DEA Class: Schedule IV

CLINICAL PHARMACOLOGY

Mechanism of Action: CNS depressant effects are due to active metabolite trichloroethanol: hypnotic doses produce mild cerebral depression and quiet deep sleep with little or no "hangover"; slight blood pressure and respiration depression; uncertain effects on REM sleep

Pharmacokinetics

PO: Onset 30 min-1 hr, duration 4-8 hr

PR: Onset slow, duration 4-6 hr

Metabolized by liver to trichloroethanol, excreted by kidneys and feces; $t_{1/2}$ (trichloroethanol) 8-11 hr

INDICATIONS AND USES: Nocturnal sedation, preoperative sedation, sedation prior to EEG evaluations; adjunct to opiates and analgesics in postoperative care and pain control; alcohol withdrawal

DOSAGE

Adult

• *Sedation:* PO/PR 250 mg tid pc

• *Hypnotic:* PO/PR 500 mg-1 g ½ hr before bedtime or ½ hr before surgery; max 2 g/day

---

* = non-FDA-approved use

Child

• *Sedative:* PO 8 mg/kg tid; not to exceed 500 mg tid

• *Hypnotic:* PO/PR 50 mg/kg in one dose; not to exceed 1 g

💲 AVAILABLE FORMS/COST OF THERAPY

• Cap, Gel—Oral: 500 mg, 100's: **$19.95**

• Supp—Rect: 325 mg, 12's: **$29.13;** 500 mg, 100's: **$125.00-$213.50;** 650 mg, 12's: **$39.75**

• Syr—Oral: 500 mg/5 ml, 480 ml: **$9.41-$13.79**

CONTRAINDICATIONS: Severe renal disease, hepatic disease, or cardiac disease; gastritis

PRECAUTIONS: Cardiac disease, GI conditions, acute intermittant porphyria, history of drug abuse, tartrazine sensitivity, elderly

PREGNANCY AND LACTATION: Pregnancy category C; excreted into breast milk; may cause mild drowsiness in infant, otherwise compatible with breast feeding

SIDE EFFECTS/ADVERSE REACTIONS

CNS: Ataxdisorientation, dizziness, *drowsiness,* hallucinations (rare), hangover (rare), headache, lightheadedness, mental confusion, nightmares, paranoia, somnambulism, stimulation

GI: Diarrhea, flatulence, gastric irritation, nausea, unpleasant taste, vomiting

HEME: Eosinophilia, ***leukopenia***

SKIN: Eczematoid dermatitis, erythema, hives, rash, scarlatiniform exanthems, urticaria

INTERACTIONS

Drugs

3 *Ethanol:* Additive CNS-depressant effects

3 *Warfarin:* Transient increase in the hypoprothrombinemic response to warfarin

Labs

• *Interference:* Urine catecholamines, urinary 17-hydroxycorticosteroids

• *False positive:* Urine glucose (Benedict's reagent)

• *False increase:* Serum urea nitrogen, vitamin B_{12}

SPECIAL CONSIDERATIONS

• Not as effective as benzodiazepines, loses much of effectiveness for inducing and maintaining sleep after 2 weeks of use

• Frequently used preoperatively or preprocedurally in children because less paradoxical excitement (not confirmed by well-controlled studies)

PATIENT/FAMILY EDUCATION

• May cause GI upset, recommend administration with full glass of water or fruit juice, dilute syrup in a half glass of water or fruit juice

---

chloramphenicol

(klor-am-fen'i-kole)

Rx: *Systemic:* Chloromycetin
Ophthalmic: Chloromycetin
Ophthalmic, Chloroptic; *Otic:* Chloromycetin Otic
Combinations

Rx: Topical: with desoxyribonuclease and fibrinolysin (Elase-Chloromycetin); Ophthalmic: Hydrocortisone acetate and polymixin B sulfate (Opthocort); hydrocortisone acetate (Chloromycetin Hydrocortisone)

Chemical Class: Dichloroacetic acid derivative
Therapeutic Class: Antibiotic

CLINICAL PHARMACOLOGY

Mechanism of Action: Reversibly binds to 50S ribosomal subunits of susceptible organisms, thus inhibiting protein synthesis

---

Pharmacokinetics

PO/IV: Peak 1-2 hr, duration 8 hr; 60% bound to plasma proteins; $t_{1/2}$ 1.5-4 hr; conjugated in liver, excreted in urine (up to 15% as free drug) and feces (in neonates, 6%-80% of drug excreted unchanged in the urine; $t_{1/2}$ 10-24 hr)

INDICATIONS AND USES: *Systemic:* Meningitis, paratyphoid fever, Q fever, rickettsial pox, Rocky Mountain spotted fever, septicemia, typhoid fever, typhus infections; serious infections due to organisms resistant to other less toxic antibiotics or when its penetration into the site of infection is clinically superior to other antibiotics to which the organisms are sensitive; *ophthalmic:* superficial ocular infections involving the conjunctiva or cornea (use only in serious infections for which less toxic drugs are ineffective or contraindicated); *otic:* superficial infections involving the external auditory canal; *topical:* infected skin lesions

Antibacterial spectrum usually includes:

• Gram-positive organisms: *Streptococcus pneumoniae* and other streptococci

• Gram-negative organisms: *Haemophilus influenzae, Neisseria meningitidis, Salmonella, Proteus mirabilis, Pseudomonas mallei, P. cepacia, Vibrio cholerae, Francisella tularensis, Yersinia pestis, Brucella, Shigella*

• Anaerobes: *Prevotella melaningogenica, B. fragilis, Clostridium, Fusobacterium, Veillonella*

• Other: *Rickettsia, Chlamydia,* and *Mycoplasma*

DOSAGE

Adult

• PO/IV 50-100 mg/kg/day divided q6h, max 4 g/day; OPHTH apply 1 gtt or small amount of ointment q3-6h, increase interval between applications after 48 hr; OTIC instill 2-3 gtt into the ear tid; TOP apply daily

Child

• *Meningitis:* IV 75-100 mg/kg/day divided q6h; max dose 4 g/day

• *Other infections:* IV 50-75 mg/kg/day divided q6h; max 4 g/day

Neonates

• IV 20 mg/kg loading dose, maintenance dose based on postnatal age (given 12 hr after loading dose); ≤7 days or ≤2000 g 25 mg/kg/day q24h; >7 days and >2000 g 50 mg/kg/day q12h

$ AVAILABLE FORMS/COST OF THERAPY

• Cap—Oral: 250 mg, 100's: **$26.80**
Oint—Ophth: 1%, 3.5 g: **$8.99-$14.94**

• Sol—Ophth: 0.5%, 2.5 ml, 7.5 ml, 15 ml: **$4.86-$7.60/15 ml**

• Sol—Otic: 5 mg/ml, 15 ml: **$22.49**

• Inj, Lyphl-Sol—IV: 1 g: **$5.47**

• Oint—Top: 1% with deoxyribonuclease and fibrinolysin, 30g: **$40.80**

CONTRAINDICATIONS: Trivial infections, prophylaxis

PRECAUTIONS: Neonates (use in reduced dosages to avoid "gray baby syndrome" toxicity), repeated courses, prolonged therapy, impaired hepatic or renal function, acute intermittent porphyria, G-6-PD deficiency, bone marrow depression (drug induced)

PREGNANCY AND LACTATION: Pregnancy category C; use caution at term due to potential for "gray baby syndrome" toxicity; excreted into breast milk; milk levels are too low to precipitate the "gray baby syndrome," but a theoretical risk does exist for bone marrow depression

SIDE EFFECTS/ADVERSE REACTIONS

CNS: Confusion, delirium, headache, mild depression, peripheral neuropathy

CV: ***"Gray baby syndrome" in newborns (failure to feed, pallor, cyanosis, abdominal distention, irregular respiration, vasomotor collapse)***

EENT: Irritation in ear (otic preparations), itching, optic neuritis (prolonged therapy); overgrowth of nonsusceptible organisms (ophthalmic preparations); poor corneal wound healing, temporary visual haze

GI: Diarrhea, enterocolitis, glossitis, *nausea, vomiting*

HEME: **Aplastic anemia, granulocytopenia, hypoplastic anemia, thrombocytopenia**

SKIN: Angioedema, burning, contact dermatitis, itching, rash, stinging, urticaria

INTERACTIONS

Drugs

🔳 *Barbiturates:* Increased serum barbiturate concentrations; reduced serum chloramphenicol concentrations

🔳 *Ceftazidime:* Inhibited antibacterial activity

🔳 *Cimetidine:* Increased risk of myelosuppression

🔳 *Penicillins:* Inhibited antibacterial activity of penicillins

🔳 *Phenytoin:* Predictable increases in serum phenytoin concentrations, toxicity has occurred

🔳 *Rifampin:* Reduced chloramphenicol concentrations

🔳 *Sulfonylureas:* Increased hypoglycemic effects of tolbutamide and chlorpropamide

❷ *Warfarin:* Enhanced hypoprothrombinemic response to warfarin and possibly other oral anticoagulants

Labs

• *False positive:* Urine glucose (copper reduction)

• *False decrease:* Serum folate, serum urea nitrogen, serum uric acid

• *False increase:* 17-ketosteroids, CSF protein, serum protein, serum urea nitrogen

SPECIAL CONSIDERATIONS

• Because of severe adverse effects (e.g. aplastic anemia) not indicated for less serious infections; aplastic anemia reported with topical use

MONITORING PARAMETERS

• CBC with platelets and reticulocytes before and frequently during therapy (discontinue drug if bone marrow depression occurs); serum iron and iron-binding globulin saturation may also be useful

• Serum drug level (peak 10-20 µg/ml, trough 5-10 µg/ml) weekly (more often in impaired hepatic, renal systems)

• Early signs of "gray baby syndrome" (cyanosis, abdominal distention, irregular respiration, failure to feed), ***drug should be discontinued immediately***

---

chlordiazepoxide

(klor-dye-az-e-pox′ide)
Rx: Libritabs, Librium, Mitran, Resposans-10
Combinations
  Rx: with amitriptyline (Limbitrol DS 10-25); with clidinium (Clindex, Librax)
Chemical Class: Benzodiazepine
Therapeutic Class: Anxiolytic
DEA Class: Schedule IV

CLINICAL PHARMACOLOGY

Mechanism of Action: CNS depressants via facilitation of inhibitory GABA at benzodiazepine receptor sites (BZ$_1$ associated with

---

italic = common side effects
bold italic = life-threatening reactions

sleep; BZ_2—associated with memory, motor, sensory, and cognitive function); effects include muscle relaxation (spinal cord), anticonvulsant activity (brain stem), ataxia (cerebellum), emotional behavior (limbic and cortical areas), and anxiolytic effects (separate from general CNS depression); other effects include sedative, appetite-stimulating, and weak analgesic actions

Pharmacokinetics

PO: Onset 30 min, peak ½-4 hr

IM: Slow erratic absorption and lower peak plasma levels than oral or IV administration

Metabolized by liver to active metabolites, excreted by kidneys; $t_{1/2}$ 5-30 hr

INDICATIONS AND USES: Anxiety disorders, acute alcohol withdrawal, preoperative apprehension and anxiety; familial, senile, or essential action tremors*; tension headache,* panic disorders*

DOSAGE

Adult

• *Mild anxiety:* PO 5-10 mg tid-qid

• *Severe anxiety:* PO 20-25 mg tid-qid; IM/IV 50-100 mg initially, then 25-50 mg tid-qid prn

• *Preoperative apprehension and anxiety:* PO 5-10 mg tid-qid on days before surgery; IM 50-100 mg 1 hr before surgery

• *Acute alcohol withdrawal:* PO/IM/IV 50-100 mg initially; repeat in 2-4 hr prn; not to exceed 300 mg/day

Geriatric or debilitated patients

• PO 5 mg bid-qid

Child >6 yr

• PO 5 mg bid-qid, not to exceed 10 mg bid-tid

[$] AVAILABLE FORMS/COST OF THERAPY

• Inj, Conc, w/buf—IM, IV: 100 mg/ampul, 5 ml: **$22.88**

• Cap, Gel—Oral: 5 mg, 100's:

$5.60-$45.63; 10 mg, 100's: **$6.49-$66.38;** 25 mg, 100's: **$6.95-$113.81**

CONTRAINDICATIONS: Narrow-angle glaucoma, psychosis

PRECAUTIONS: Elderly, debilitated, hepatic disease, renal disease, long-term use, history of drug abuse

PREGNANCY AND LACTATION: Pregnancy category D; excreted into breast milk; drug and metabolites may accumulate to toxic levels in nursing infant

SIDE EFFECTS/ADVERSE REACTIONS

CNS: Anterograde amnesia, anxiety, ataxia, *confusion,* depression, dizziness, *drowsiness,* fatigue, hallucinations, headache, hysteria, insomnia, psychosis, slurred speech, stimulation, tremor

CV: Bradycardia, hypertension, hypotension, orthostatic hypotension, *shock,* tachycardia

EENT: Auditory disturbances, blurred vision, mydriasis, nystagmus

GI: Anorexia, constipation, diarrhea, dry mouth, nausea, vomiting

GU: Changes in libido, incontinence, menstrual irregularities, urinary retention

SKIN: Dermatitis, hair loss, hirsutism, itching, rash, urticaria

INTERACTIONS

Drugs

3 *Cimetidine:* Increased plasma levels of chlordiazepoxide and/or active metabolites

3 *Disulfiram:* Increased serum chlordiazepoxide concentrations

3 *Ethanol:* Enhanced adverse psychomotor side effects of benzodiazepines

3 *Fluconazole, itraconazole, ketoconazole:* Increased chlordiazepoxide concentrations

* = non-FDA-approved use

3 *Levodopa:* Potential for exacerbation of Parkinsonism in patients taking levodopa

Labs

• *False increase:* Urine 5-HIAA, urine 17-ketogenic steroids

• *False decrease:* Urine 17-ketogenic steroids

• *False positive:* Urine pregnancy tests

SPECIAL CONSIDERATIONS

• No advantage over diazepam; poor choice for elderly patients

• Do not use for everyday stress or use longer than 4 mo

• Do not discontinue medication abruptly after long-term use

---

chlorhexidine

(klor-hex′ih-deen)

Rx: Peridex, Periogard

Chemical Class: Bis-biguanide

Therapeutic Class: Antimicrobial mouth rinse; antiseptic

CLINICAL PHARMACOLOGY

Mechanism of Action: Adsorbed during oral rinsing on the surfaces of teeth, plaque, and oral mucosa; gradually released from these sites by diffusion for up to 24 hr; adsorbed onto the cell walls of microorganisms, which causes leakage of intracellular components

Pharmacokinetics

PO: Poorly absorbed, 30% retained in oral cavity following rinsing and is slowly released into the oral fluids; excreted primarily through the feces

INDICATIONS AND USES: Gingivitis

DOSAGE

Adult

• Use 15 ml as oral rinse for 30 sec bid after toothbrushing (not intended for ingestion; expectorate after rinsing)

$ AVAILABLE FORMS/COST OF THERAPY

• Mouthwash—Oral: 0.12%, 480 ml: **$5.23-$11.82**

PREGNANCY AND LACTATION: Pregnancy category B; excretion into breast milk unknown; use caution in nursing mothers

SIDE EFFECTS/ADVERSE REACTIONS

GI: Altered taste perception, increase in calculus formation, irritation of oral mucosa, *staining of teeth and other oral surfaces,* transient parotitis

SPECIAL CONSIDERATIONS

• Adjunctive to mechanical toothbrushing and dental prophylaxis, not as a substitute; also used as a topical antiseptic

---

chloroprocaine

(klor-oh-pro′kane)

Rx: Nesacaine, Nesacaine-MPF

Chemical Class: Procaine derivative

Therapeutic Class: Local anesthetic

CLINICAL PHARMACOLOGY

Mechanism of Action: Blocks the generation and the conduction of nerve impulses; the order of loss of nerve function is: (1) pain, (2) temperature, (3) touch, (4) proprioception, and (5) skeletal muscle tone

Pharmacokinetics

INJ: Rapid onset, 6-12 min, duration of anesthesia up to 60 min; widely distributed; metabolized by pseudocholinesterase, excreted renally; $t_{1/2}$ 21-25 sec (adults) (NOTE: Pharmacokinetic parameters may be altered by the presence of hepatic or renal disease, addition of epinephrine, factors affecting urinary pH,

---

renal blood flow, the route of administration, and age)

INDICATIONS AND USES: Infiltration and peripheral nerve block; central nerve block, including lumbar and caudal epidural blocks (without preservatives)

DOSAGE

Dose varies with procedure, depth of anesthesia, vascularity of tissues, duration of anesthesia, and condition of patient

Adult

• Max single recommended doses without epinephrine, 11 mg/kg, not to exceed a max total dose of 800 mg; with epinephrine (1:200,000) 14 mg/kg, not to exceed a max total dose of 1000 mg

• *Lumbar and caudal epidural block:* 15-25 ml of a 2% or 3% preservative-free solution; repeated doses may be given at 40-60 min intervals

• *Infiltration and peripheral nerve block (1-2%):* Mandibular 2-3 ml; infraorbital 0.5-1 ml; brachial plexus 30-40 ml; digital (without epinephrine) 3-4 ml; pudendal 10 ml each side; paracervical 3 per each of up to 4 sites

• *Lumbar epidural anesthesia:* 15-25 ml, repeated doses 10-20 ml at 40-50 min intervals

Child >3 yr

• Max single recommended dose 11 mg/kg

💲 AVAILABLE FORMS/COST OF THERAPY

• Inj, Sol-Caudal Block, Epidural—INF: 1%, 30 ml: **$18.83**; 2%, 30 ml: **$9.50-$19.30**; 3%, 20 ml: **$22.05-$23.88**

CONTRAINDICATIONS: Hypersensitivity to drugs of the PABA ester group

PRECAUTIONS: Lumber and caudal epidural anesthesia should be used with extreme caution in persons with the following conditions: existing neurological disease, spinal deformities, septicemia, and severe hypertension

PREGNANCY AND LACTATION: Pregnancy category C; use caution in nursing mothers

SIDE EFFECTS/ADVERSE REACTIONS

CNS: Anxiety, disorientation, drowsiness, loss of consciousness, restlessness, *seizures,* shivering, tremors

CV: Bradycardia, *cardiac arrest, dysrhythmias,* fetal bradycardia, hypertension, hypotension, *myocardial depression*

EENT: Blurred vision, pupil constriction, tinnitus

GI: Nausea, vomiting

RESP: Respiratory arrest, status asthmaticus

SKIN: Allergic reactions, burning, edema, rash, skin discoloration at inj site, tissue necrosis, urticaria

INTERACTIONS

Drugs

🔢 *Beta-blockers:* Acute discontinuation of β-blockers before local anesthesia may increase the risk of side effects due to anesthetic

SPECIAL CONSIDERATIONS

• Ester-type local anesthetic

---

chloroquine

(klor'oh-kwin)

Rx: Aralen

Chemical Class: Synthetic 4-aminoquinoline derivative
Therapeutic Class: Antimalarial; amebicide

CLINICAL PHARMACOLOGY

Mechanism of Action: Inhibits parasite replication via an interaction with DNA transcription

Pharmacokinetics

PO: Peak 1-6 hr, rapidly and completely absorbed; 55% protein bound; deposited in brain, spinal cord, liver, spleen, kidney, lungs, and leukocytes (from 30×-70× the plasma concentration); metabolized in the liver, excretion slow (enhanced via acidification of urine) in urine, feces; crosses placenta; $t_{1/2}$ 3-5 days

INDICATIONS AND USES: Prophylaxis and treatment of acute attacks of malaria caused by susceptible strains, including *P. vivax, P. malariae, P. ovale, P. falciparum* (some strains); extraintestinal amebiasis

DOSAGE

NOTE: The dosage of chloroquine is often expressed or calculated as the base: 500 mg tab of chloroquine phosphate is equivalent to 300 mg base; 50 mg of chloroquine hydrochloride is equivalent to 40 mg base

Adult

• *Malaria suppression:* PO 300 mg (base)/wk on same day of wk; treatment should begin 1-2 wk before exposure and for 4 wk after; if treatment begins after exposure, 600 mg (base) in 2 divided doses 6 hr apart

• *Acute attack:* PO 600 mg (base) initial dose followed by 300 mg 6-8 hr later, then 300 mg on each of 2 consecutive days (total dose 1.5 g in 3 days); IM 160-200 mg initially, repeat in 6 hr if necessary; begin oral therapy as soon as possible and continue for 3 days until 1.5 g of base has been administered

• *Extraintestinal amebiasis:* IM 200-250 mg qd (HCl) up to 12 days, then substitute or resume PO administration as soon as possible; PO 600 mg (base) qd for 2 days, then 300 mg qd for 2-3 wk

Child

• *Malaria suppression:* PO 5 mg/kg/wk on same day of wk, not to exceed 300 mg (base); treatment should begin 1-2 wk before exposure and for 4 wk after; if treatment begins after exposure, 10 mg/kg (base) in 2 divided doses 6 hr apart

• *Acute attack:* PO 10 mg/kg (base) initial dose (do not exceed 600 mg) followed by 5 mg/kg 6-8 hr later (do not exceed 300 mg) then 5 mg/kg (do not exceed 300 mg) on each of 2 consecutive days (total dose 25 mg/kg in 3 days)

💲 **AVAILABLE FORMS/COST OF THERAPY**

• Tab, Uncoated—Oral (Phosphate salt): 250 mg, (150 mg base) 100's: **$5.61-$17.50;** 500 mg (300 mg base), 100's: **$389.00**

• Inj, Sol—IV, IM (Hydrochloride): 50 mg/ml, 5 ml: **$15.77**

CONTRAINDICATIONS: Retinal field changes, porphyria

PRECAUTIONS: Children, blood dyscrasias, severe GI disease, neurologic disease, alcoholism, hepatic disease, G-6-PD deficiency, psoriasis, eczema, lactation

PREGNANCY AND LACTATION: Pregnancy category C; excreted into breast milk; average infant consumption, considered safe; NOTE: doesn't protect infant against malaria

SIDE EFFECTS/ADVERSE REACTIONS

CNS: Fatigue, headache, psychosis, *seizures,* stimulation

*CV: **Asystole with syncope,*** ECG changes, ***heart block,*** hypotension

EENT: Blurred vision, corneal changes, corneal edema, deafness, *difficulty focusing,* photophobia, *retinal changes,* tinnitus, vertigo

GI: Anorexia, cramps, diarrhea, *nausea, vomiting*

*HEME: **Agranulocytosis, hemolytic anemia, leukopenia, thrombocytopenia***

---

italic = common side effects   ***bold italic*** = life-threatening reactions

SKIN: Eczema, **exfoliative dermatitis,** lichen planus-like eruptions, pigmentary changes, pruritus, skin eruptions

INTERACTIONS
Drugs
3 *Chlorpromazine:* Increased chlorpromazine concentrations
3 *Cyclosporine:* Elevates cyclosporine levels, toxicity possible
3 *Methotrexate:* Decreased methotrexate levels
3 *Praziquantel:* Decreased praziquantel absorption

SPECIAL CONSIDERATIONS
• Certain strains of *P. falciparum* have become resistant to chloroquine

MONITORING PARAMETERS
• Ophthalmic examinations (visual acuity, slit lamp, funduscopic, visual fields) and CBC if long-term treatment or drug dosage >150 mg/day

---

chlorothiazide
(klor-oh-thye′a-zide)
Rx: Diachlor, Diurigen, Diuril
Combinations
  Rx: with methyldopa
  (Aldoclor); with reserpine
  (Chloroserp, Diaserp,
  Diupres)
Chemical Class: Sulfonamide
derivative
Therapeutic Class: Thiazide
diuretic; antihypertensive

CLINICAL PHARMACOLOGY
Mechanism of Action: Inhibits reabsorption of sodium and chloride in cortical thick ascending limb of the loop of Henle and the early distal tubules, increasing the urinary excretion of sodium and chloride; sulfonamide moiety provides some carbonic anhydrase inhibition activity; other actions: increased potassium and bicarbonate excretion; decreased calcium excretion; uric acid retention; antihypertensive action dependent on sodium depletion, drop in peripheral vascular resistance, and reduction in extracellular volume

Pharmacokinetics
PO: Poor oral absorption (33%); onset 2 hr, peak 4 hr, duration 6-12 hr
IV: Onset 15 min, maximal action 30 min
Eliminated unchanged by the kidneys; crosses placenta, but not blood-brain barrier; excreted in breast milk; $t_{1/2}$ 45-120 min

INDICATIONS AND USES: Edema (CHF, hepatic cirrhosis, nephrotic syndrome, acute glomerulonephritis, corticosteroid and estrogen therapy; hypertension; calcium nephrolithiasis*; prevention of osteoporosis*; diabetes insipidus

DOSAGE
NOTE: Equivalent hydrochlorothiazide dose: 50 mg-500 mg.
Adult
• *Edema:* PO/IV 500 mg-1 g/day in 1-2 divided doses
• *Hypertension:* PO 500 mg-1 g/day in 1-2 divided doses; max 2 g/day in divided doses
Child
• *Diuresis/hypertension:* PO 10-20 mg/kg/day in 2 divided doses, not to exceed 375 mg per day in infants up to 2 yr of age or 1 g per day in children 2 to 12 yr of age; infants less than 6 mo of age, up to 30 mg/kg/day in 2 divided doses; IV use generally not recommended

💲 **AVAILABLE FORMS/COST OF THERAPY**
• Tab, Uncoated—Oral: 250 mg, 100's: **$4.00-$15.43;** 500 mg, 100's: **$7.95-$25.30**
• Susp—Oral: 250 mg/5 ml, 237 ml: **$11.25**
• Inj—IV: 500 mg: **$10.13**

---

* = non-FDA-approved use

CONTRAINDICATIONS: Anuria, renal decompensation

PRECAUTIONS: Fluid and electrolyte imbalance (including sodium, potassium, magnesium, calcium), renal disease, hepatic disease, gout, COPD, lupus erythematosus, diabetes mellitus, hyperparathyroidism, vomiting, diarrhea, elevated cholesterol/triglycerides

PREGNANCY AND LACTATION: Pregnancy category C; therapy for preexisting hypertension can be continued throughout pregnancy with minimal risk; initiating for simple edema not recommended; few unequivocal indications for diuretic therapy in pregnancy except for pulmonary edema or congestive heart failure; excreted in low concentrations in breast milk; compatible with breast feeding

SIDE EFFECTS/ADVERSE REACTIONS

CNS: Anxiety, depression, *dizziness,* drowsiness, fatigue, headache, paresthesia, weakness

CV: Arrhythmias, irregular pulse, orthostatic hypotension, palpitations, volume depletion

EENT: Blurred vision

GI: Anorexia, constipation, cramps, diarrhea, GI irritation, hepatitis, *nausea,* pancreatitis, *vomiting*

GU: Frequency, glucosuria, polyuria, uremia, impotence, decreased libido

HEME: **Agranulocytosis, aplastic anemia, hemolytic anemia, leukopenia, neutropenia, thrombocytopenia**

METAB: Hypercalcemia, *hyperglycemia, hyperuricemia;* hypochloremia, *hypokalemia,* hypomagnesemia, lipid abnormalities (increased total and LDL cholesterol, triglycerides) hyponatremia, hypophosphatemia, increased creatinine, BUN

SKIN: Fever, photosensitivity, purpura, rash, urticaria

INTERACTIONS

Drugs

2 *Angiotensin-converting enzyme inhibitors:* Risk of postural hypotension when added to ongoing diuretic therapy; more common with loop diuretics; first-dose hypotension possible in patients with sodium depletion or hypovolemia caused by diuretics or sodium restriction; hypotensive response is usually transient; hold diuretic day of first dose

3 *Calcium* (high doses): Risk of milk-alkali syndrome; monitor for hypercalcemia

3 *Carbenoxolone:* Additive potassium wasting; severe hypokalemia

3 *Cholestyramine/colestipol:* Reduced serum concentrations of thiazide diuretics

3 *Corticosteroids:* Concomitant therapy may result in excessive potassium loss

3 *Diazoxide:* Hyperglycemia

3 *Digitalis glycosides:* Diuretic-induced hypokalemia may increase the risk of digitalis toxicity

3 *Hypoglycemic agents:* Thiazide diuretics tend to increase blood glucose, may increase dosage requirements of antidiabetic drugs

3 *Lithium:* Increases serum lithium concentrations; toxicity may occur

3 *Methotrexate:* Increased bone marrow suppression

3 *Nonsteroidal antiinflammatory drugs:* Concurrent use may reduce diuretic and antihypertensive effects

Labs

• *Interference:* Urine 17-hydroxycorticosteroids

• False decrease: urine estriol

SPECIAL CONSIDERATIONS

• Doses above 250 mg provide no further blood pressure reduction, but

---

italic = common side effects   **bold italic** = life-threatening reactions

are more likely to induce metabolic disturbance (i.e., hypokalemia, hyperuricemia, etc.)

• May protect against osteoporotic hip fractures

• Loop diuretics or metolazone more effective if CrCl <40-50 ml/min

PATIENT/FAMILY EDUCATION

• Will increase urination temporarily (approximately 3 wk); take early in the day to prevent sleep disturbance

• May cause sensitivity to sunlight; avoid prolonged exposure to the sun and other ultraviolet light

• May cause gout attacks; notify clinician if sudden joint pain occurs

MONITORING PARAMETERS

• Weight, urine output, serum electrolytes, BUN, creatinine, CBC, uric acid, glucose, lipids

---

chlorotrianisene

(klor-oh-trye-an'i-seen)
Rx: TACE
Chemical Class: Nonsteroidal synthetic estrogen derivative
Therapeutic Class: Estrogen

CLINICAL PHARMACOLOGY
Mechanism of Action: Needed for adequate functioning of female reproductive system; affects release of pituitary gonadotropins; inhibits bone resorption

Pharmacokinetics
PO: Stored in fat tissues, with delayed and prolonged duration of action; effect persists after the 14th day of discontinuance; metabolized to more active metabolite in liver, excreted in urine; crosses placenta

INDICATIONS AND USES: Moderate to severe vasomotor symptoms associated with menopause, atrophic vaginitis, and kraurosis vulvae,

female hypogonadism, prostatic carcinoma (palliation only)

DOSAGE

Adult

• *Prostatic cancer:* PO 12-24 mg qd

• *Menopause:* PO 12-24 mg qd × 30 days or 3 wk on 1 wk off

• *Female hypogonadism:* PO cycle 12-24 mg × 21 days, then progesterone 100 mg IM or coadminister 5 days of progesterone PO during last 5 days of cycle

• *Vaginitis:* PO 12-24 mg qd × 30-60 days

💲 **AVAILABLE FORMS/COST OF THERAPY**

• Cap, Gel—Oral: 12 mg, 100's: **$107.52**

CONTRAINDICATIONS: Breast cancer, thromboembolic disorders, reproductive cancer, genital bleeding (abnormal, undiagnosed)

PRECAUTIONS: Hypertension, blood dyscrasias, gallbladder disease, CHF, diabetes mellitus, bone disease, depression, migraine headache, convulsive disorders, hepatic disease, renal disease, family history of cancer of the breast or reproductive tract

PREGNANCY AND LACTATION: Pregnancy category X; excreted into milk; associated with shortened duration of lactation, decreased infant weight gain, decreased milk production, decreased nitrogen and protein content of milk

SIDE EFFECTS/ADVERSE REACTIONS

CNS: Depression, dizziness, headache, migraines

CV: Edema, hypotension, *MI, pulmonary embolism, stroke,* thromboembolism, thrombophlebitis

EENT: Astigmatism, contact lens intolerance, increased myopia

GI: Anorexia, cholestatic jaundice, constipation, cramps, diarrhea, in-

creased appetite, increased weight, nausea, pancreatitis, vomiting
GU: Amenorrhea, breakthrough bleeding, breast changes, cervical erosion, dysmenorrhea, *gynecomastia, impotence, testicular atrophy,* vaginal candidiasis
METAB: Folic acid deficiency, hypercalcemia, hyperglycemia
SKIN: Acne, alopecia, hirsutism, melasma, oily skin, purpura, rash, seborrhea, urticaria

SPECIAL CONSIDERATIONS
• Not first line option for treatment of menopausal symptoms due to prolonged duration of effect and cost

PATIENT/FAMILY EDUCATION
• Report unusual vaginal bleeding, edema, headache, blurred vision, abdominal pain, numbness, stiffness or pain in legs, chest pain

MONITORING PARAMETERS
• Women with an intact uterus should be closely monitored for signs of endometrial cancer

---

chloroxine
(klor-ox'ine)
Rx: Capitrol
Chemical Class: Hydroxyquinoline derivative
Therapeutic Class: Antiseborrheic

CLINICAL PHARMACOLOGY
Mechanism of Action: Presumed reduction in scaling via effects on mitotic activity; antibacterial and antifungal role in seborrheic dermatitis speculated as *S. aureus* and *Pityrosporon* spp. are often present in increased numbers
INDICATIONS AND USES: Dandruff and mild to moderately severe seborrheic dermatitis
DOSAGE
Adult
• TOP rub into wet scalp, allow to

remain for 3 min before rinse, repeat; 2 treatments/wk usually sufficient

⑤ AVAILABLE FORMS/COST OF THERAPY
• Shampoo—Top: 120 ml: **$19.57**
CONTRAINDICATIONS: Acute inflammation
PRECAUTIONS: External use only, avoid contact with eyes
PREGNANCY AND LACTATION: Pregnancy category C; excretion into breast milk unknown
SIDE EFFECTS/ADVERSE REACTIONS
SKIN: Discoloration of light-colored (blond, gray, bleached) hair, irritation and burning
SPECIAL CONSIDERATIONS
PATIENT/FAMILY EDUCATION
• Improvement may not occur for 14 days

---

chlorphenesin
(klor-fen'e-sin)
Rx: Maolate
Chemical Class: Carbamate derivative
Therapeutic Class: Skeletal muscle relaxant

CLINICAL PHARMACOLOGY
Mechanism of Action: Unknown; related to central sedative properties; does not directly relax muscle or depress nerve conduction
Pharmacokinetics
PO: Onset ½ hr, peak 1-2 hr, duration 4-6 hr; metabolized by liver, excreted in urine; crosses placenta; $t_{1/2}$ 4 hr
INDICATIONS AND USES: Adjunct for relieving pain in acute, painful musculoskeletal conditions
DOSAGE
Adult
• PO 800 mg tid; maintenance 400

mg qid, not to exceed 8 wk of therapy

💲 **AVAILABLE FORMS/COST OF THERAPY**
• Tab, Uncoated—Oral: 400 mg, 50's: **$39.58**

PRECAUTIONS: Renal disease, hepatic disease, addictive personality, elderly, hypersensitivity to FD&C Yellow No. 5 (tartrazine), aspirin hypersensitivity

PREGNANCY AND LACTATION: Pregnancy category C; excreted in breast milk (large amounts), safety not established

SIDE EFFECTS/ADVERSE REACTIONS
CNS: Confusion, depression, *dizziness, drowsiness,* headache, insomnia, tremor, *weakness*
CV: Postural hypotension, tachycardia
EENT: Diplopia, temporary loss of vision
GI: Hiccups, *nausea,* vomiting
HEME: **Blood dyscrasias**
SKIN: Facial flushing, fever, pruritus, rash

SPECIAL CONSIDERATIONS PATIENT/FAMILY EDUCATION
• Avoid concurrent alcohol, other CNS depressants, hazardous activities if drowsiness/dizziness occurs

chlorpheniramine
(klor-fen-eer´a-meen)
Rx: Chlor-Phen, Prohist-8
OTC: Aller-Chlor, Chlo-Amine, Chlorate, Chlor-Trimeton, Pfeiffer's Allergy, Teldrin
Combinations
  Rx: with hydrocodone (Tussionex); with phenylephrine and pyrilamine (Rynaton); with phenylpropanolamine (Ornade, Resaid S.R.); with pseudoephedrine (Deconamine, Fedahist)
  OTC: with phenylpropanolamine (Allerhist Maximum Strength, Contac 12-Hour Capsules, Triaminic Syrup) with pseudoephedrine (Chlor-Trimeton, Dorcol Children's Cold Formula Liquid, Fedahist)
Chemical Class: Alkylamine derivative
Therapeutic Class: Antihistamine

CLINICAL PHARMACOLOGY
Mechanism of Action: Decreases allergic response by blocking histamine at H_1-receptors
Pharmacokinetics
PO: Onset 20-60 min, duration 8-12 hr; detoxified in liver; excreted by kidneys (metabolites/unchanged drug); $t_{1/2}$ 20-24 hr
INDICATIONS AND USES: Perenial and seasonal allergic rhinitis (PO); allergic reactions to blood and plasma, adjunctive anaphylactic therapy (parenteral)
DOSAGE
Adult
• PO 2-4 mg tid-qid, not to exceed

---

36 mg/day; TIME REL 8-12 mg bid-tid, not to exceed 36 mg/day; IM/IV/SC 5-40 mg/day

Child

• 2-5 yr: PO 1 mg q6h, not to exceed 6 mg/day

• 6-12 yr: PO 2 mg q4-6h, not to exceed 12 mg/day; SUS REL 8 mg hs or qd (not recommended for child <6 yr)

$ AVAILABLE FORMS/COST OF THERAPY

• Tab, Chewable—Oral: 2 mg, 96's: **$14.16**

• Tab, Uncoated—Oral: 4 mg, 100's: **$0.85-$12.23**

• Tab, Sus Action—Oral: 8 mg, 100's: **$20.35;** 12 mg, 100's: **$32.60**

• Cap, Gel, Sus Action—Oral: 4 mg, 100's: **$4.49-$10.77;** 8 mg, 100's: **$6.25-$10.90;** 12 mg, 100's: **$7.15-$11.75**

• Inj, Sol—IV: 100 mg/ml, 10 ml: **$4.00;** 10 mg/ml, 1 ml: **$2.34-$8.00**

• Syr—Oral: 2 mg/5 ml, 120 ml: **$3.27-$4.26**

CONTRAINDICATIONS: Acute asthma attack, lower respiratory tract disease

PRECAUTIONS: Increased intraocular pressure (angle-closure glaucoma), renal disease, cardiac disease, hypertension, bronchial asthma, seizure disorder, stenosed peptic ulcers, hyperthyroidism, prostatic hypertrophy, bladder neck obstruction, elderly

PREGNANCY AND LACTATION: Pregnancy category B

SIDE EFFECTS/ADVERSE REACTIONS

CNS: Anxiety, confusion, *dizziness, drowsiness,* euphoria, fatigue, neuritis, paresthesia, poor coordination

EENT: Blurred vision, dilated pupils, dry nose, throat; tinnitus

GI: Anorexia, diarrhea, *dry mouth,* nausea

GU: Dysuria, frequency, *retention*

HEME: **Agranulocytosis, hemolytic anemia, thrombocytopenia**

RESP: Chest tightness, increased thick secretions, wheezing

SKIN: Photosensitivity

SPECIAL CONSIDERATIONS

• More potent antihistamine than nonsedating agents (e.g., fexofenidine), good first-line choice for allergic rhinitis

PATIENT/FAMILY EDUCATION

• Tolerance develops to sedation with chronic use

---

chlorpromazine

(klor-proe'ma-zeen)
Rx: Thorazine
Chemical Class: Aliphatic phenothiazine derivative
Therapeutic Class: Antipsychotic; antiemetic

CLINICAL PHARMACOLOGY

Mechanism of Action: Dopamine receptor antagonist, with higher affinity for D_2 over D_1 receptors, and variable selectivity among the cortical dopamine tracts; also activity on nondopaminergic sites, i.e., cholinergic, alpha$_1$-adrenergic and histamine receptors (explaining side effects); standard phenothiazine, with high incidence of sedation and orthostatic hypotension, moderate risk of extrapyramidal and anticholinergic effects

Pharmacokinetics

PO: Absorption variable, onset erratic 30-60 min, duration 4-6 hr

PO-ER: Onset 30-60 min, peak unknown, duration 10-12 hr

IM: Well absorbed, peak 15-20 min, duration 4 to 8 hr

IV: Onset 5 min, peak 10 min, duration unknown

REC: Onset erratic, duration 3 hr Widely distributed; metabolized by

---

italic = common side effects   ***bold italic*** = life-threatening reactions

liver, excreted in urine (metabolites); crosses placenta; 95% bound to plasma proteins; elimination $t_{1/2}$ 10-30 hr

INDICATIONS AND USES: Psychotic disorders, mania, schizophrenia, anxiety; intractable hiccups; nausea, vomiting; preoperatively for relaxation; acute intermittent porphyria; behavioral problems in children; adjunct in treatment of tetanus; treatment of 'angel dust' psychosis,* migraine headaches (IM/IV)*

DOSAGE

Adult

• *Psychosis:* PO 10 mg tid-qid or 25 mg bid-tid, increase by 20-50 mg semiweekly, maintenance 200-800 mg/day; IM 25 mg, may repeat dose of 25-50 mg in 1 hr prn, increase gradually over several days up to 400 mg q4-6h in severe cases, substitute PO when possible

• *Nausea and vomiting:* PO 10-25 mg q4-6h prn; IM 25-50 mg q3h prn; Rect 50-100 mg q6-8h prn, not to exceed 400 mg/day; IV 25-50 mg qd-qid

• *Intractable hiccups:* PO 25-50 mg tid-qid; IM 25-50 mg (use only if PO dose does not work); IV 25-50 mg in 500-1000 ml saline (only for severe hiccups)

• *Intermittent porphyria:* PO 25-50 mg tid-qid; IM 25 mg tid-qid

• *Tetanus:* IM 25-50 mg tid-qid; IV 25-50 mg

Child

• Not to exceed 40 mg/day (<5 yr) or 75 mg/day (5-12 yr)

• *Psychosis:* PO 0.5 mg/kg q4-6h prn; IM 0.5 mg/kg q6-8h; Rect 1 mg/kg q6-8h

• *Nausea and vomiting:* PO 0.55 mg/kg q4-6h prn, IM 0.55 mg/kg q6-8h prn; Rect 1.1 mg/kg: q6-8h prn; IV 0.55 mg/kg q6-8h

§ AVAILABLE FORMS/COST OF THERAPY

• Conc—Oral: 30 mg/ml, 120 ml: **$5.95;** 100 mg/ml, 240 ml: **$20.12-$30.17**

• Inj, Sol—IM, IV: 25 mg/ml, 1 ml: **$1.00-$1.80**

• Supp—Rect: 25 mg, 12's: **$40.75**

• Tab, Plain Coated—Oral: 10 mg, 100's, **$6.95-$27.24;** 25 mg, 100's: **$3.00-$46.95;** 50 mg, 100's: **$4.00-$61.76;** 100 mg, 100's: **$7.00-$73.55;** 200 mg, 100's: **$10.00-$94.75**

CONTRAINDICATIONS: Circulatory collapse, liver damage, cerebral arteriosclerosis, coronary disease, severe hypertension/hypotension, blood dyscrasias, coma, child <2 yr, brain damage, bone marrow depression, alcohol and barbiturate withdrawal

PRECAUTIONS: Seizure disorders, hypertension, hepatic disease, cardiac disease, elderly (orthostasis upon arising), COPD

PREGNANCY AND LACTATION: Pregnancy category C; enters breast milk in small concentrations; report of drowsy and lethargic infant who consumed milk with 92 ng/ml concentration

SIDE EFFECTS/ADVERSE REACTIONS

CNS: Extrapyramidal symptoms (pseudoparkinsonism, akathisia, dystonia), headache, *seizures,* tardive dyskinesia

CV: Cardiac arrest, ECG changes, hypertension, *orthostatic hypotension,* tachycardia

EENT: Blurred vision, dry eyes, glaucoma

GI: Anorexia, constipation, diarrhea, dry mouth, jaundice, nausea, vomiting, weight gain

GU: Amenorrhea, breast engorgement, enuresis, gynecomastia, im-

---

* = non-FDA-approved use

potence, urinary frequency, urinary retention

HEME: **Agranulocytosis,** anemia, **leukocytosis, leukopenia**

RESP: Dyspnea, **laryngospasm,** respiratory depression

SKIN: Dermatitis, photosensitivity, rash

MISC: **Neuroleptic malignant syndrome (NMS)**

INTERACTIONS

Drugs

3 *Amodiaquine, chloroquine, sulfadoxine-pyrimethamine:* Increased chlorpromazine concentrations

3 *Anticholinergics:* May inhibit neuroleptic response; excess anticholinergic effects

3 *Antidepressants:* Potential for increased therapeutic and toxic effects from increased levels of both drugs

3 *Barbiturates:* Decreased neuroleptic levels

3 *Clonidine, guanadrel, granethidine:* Severe hypotensive episodes possible

3 *Epinephrine:* Blunted pressor response to epinephrine

3 *Ethanol:* Additive CNS depression

2 *Levodopa:* Inhibited antiparkinsonian effect of levodopa

3 *Lithium:* Lowered levels of both drugs, rarely neurotoxicity in acute mania

3 *Narcotic analgesics:* Hypotension and increased CNS depression

3 *Orphenadrine:* Lower neuroleptic concentrations, excessive anticholinergic effects

3 *Propranolol:* Increased plasma levels of both drugs with accentuated responses

Labs

• *False decrease:* 5-HIAA, vitamin B$_{12}$

• *Interference:* 17-ketogenic steroids

• *False increase:* Urine bilirubin, cholesterol, urine porphobilinogen, CSF protein, urine protein

• *False positive:* Ferric chloride test, guiacols spot test, phenylketones

SPECIAL CONSIDERATIONS

PATIENT/FAMILY EDUCATION

• Orthostasis on rising, especially in elderly

• Avoid hot tubs; hot showers, tub baths

• Meticulous oral hygiene; frequent rinsing of mouth, sugarless gum for dry mouth

• Use a sunscreen and sunglasses

• Urine may turn pink or red

chlorpropamide
(klor-pro'pa-mide)

Rx: Diabinese

Chemical Class: Sulfonylurea (first generation)

Therapeutic Class: Oral hypoglycemic

CLINICAL PHARMACOLOGY

Mechanism of Action: Decreases blood sugar via stimulation of insulin secretion and increased tissue responsiveness to insulin; initial hypoglycemic effects due to stimulation of pancreatic islets (dependent upon functioning β-cells); extrapancreatic effect predominantly due to inhibition of hepatic glucose production, but may also facilitate improved insulin-insulin receptor binding

Pharmacokinetics

PO: Onset 1 hr. peak 3-6 hr. duraton 60 hr; completely absorbed by GI route; 90%-95% plasma protein bound; metabolized in liver, excreted in urine (metabolites and unchanged drug); t$_{1/2}$ 36 hr

INDICATIONS AND USES: Diabetes mellitus, type 2, neurogenic diabetes insipidus*

---

italic = common side effects   **bold italic** = life-threatening reactions

DOSAGE
Adult
• PO 100-250 mg qd initially, then 100-500 mg maintenance according to response, max 750 mg/day

💲 AVAILABLE FORMS/COST OF THERAPY
• Tab, Uncoated—Oral: 100 mg, 100's: **$4.50-$35.00;** 250 mg, 100's: **$4.95-$67.37**

CONTRAINDICATIONS: Diabetes mellitus, type 1; ketoacidosis

PRECAUTIONS: Elderly, cardiac disease, thyroid disease, renal disease, hepatic disease, severe hypoglycemic reactions

PREGNANCY AND LACTATION: Pregnancy category D; inappropriate for use during pregnancy due to inadequate for blood glucose control, potential for prolonged neonatal hypoglycemia, and risk of congenital abnormalities; insulin is the drug of choice for control of blood sugars during pregnancy; breast milk reported at 17% of plasma; the potential for neonatal hypoglycemia dictates caution in nursing mothers

SIDE EFFECTS/ADVERSE REACTIONS
CNS: Dizziness, drowsiness, fatigue, *headache,* tinnitus, vertigo, *weakness*

GI: Anorexia, cholestatic jaundice, diarrhea, hepatotoxicity, hunger, nausea, vomiting

*HEME: **Agranulocytosis, aplastic anemia, hemolytic anemia, leukopenia, pancytopenia, thrombocytopenia***

METAB: Hepatic porphyria, hypoglycemia, hyponatremia, syndrome of inappropriate antidiuretic hormone release

SKIN: Allergic reactions, eczema, erythema multiforme, ***exfoliative dermatitis,*** photo-sensitivity, pruritus, rash, urticaria

INTERACTIONS
Drugs
3 *Anabolic steroids: Chloramphenicol, Fibric acid derivatives, MAOIs, Salicylates, Sulfonamides:* Enhanced hypoglycemic effect

⚠ *Ethanol:* Altered glycemic control, most commonly hypoglycemia; disulfiram-like reaction may occur

3 *Halofenate:* Increased sulfonylurea concentrations

2 *NSAIDs:* Enhanced hypoglycemic effect

3 *Thiazide diuretics:* Increased glucose concentrations, may increase dose requirements

Labs
• *False increase:* Serum calcium

SPECIAL CONSIDERATIONS
PATIENT/FAMILY EDUCATION
• Multiple drug interactions, including alcohol and salicylates
• Symptoms of hypoglycemia: tingling lips/tongue, nausea, confusion, fatigue, sweating, hunger, visual changes (spots)
• Due to potential for prolonged hypoglycemia, other sulfonylureas should be considered before trying chlorpropamide (especially in the elderly)

MONITORING PARAMETERS
• Self-monitored blood glucose; glycosolated hemoglobin q 3-6 mo

---

* = non-FDA-approved use

chlorthalidone
(klor-thal'i-doan)
Rx: Hygroton, Thalitone
Combinations
Rx: with atenolol
(Tenoretic); with clonidine
(Combipres, Chlorpres);
with reserpine (Demi-
Regroton, Regroton)
Chemical Class: Phthalimidine
derivative
Therapeutic Class: Thiazide
diuretic; antihypertensive

CLINICAL PHARMACOLOGY
Mechanism of Action: Inhibits reabsorption of sodium and chloride in cortical thick ascending limb of the loop of Henle and the early distal tubules, increasing the urinary excretion of sodium and chloride; sulfonamide moiety provides some carbonic anhydrase inhibition activity; other actions: increased potassium and bicarbonate excretion; decreased calcium excretion; uric acid retention; antihypertensive action dependent on sodium depletion, drop in peripheral vascular resistance, and reduction in extracellular volume
Pharmacokinetics
PO: Absorption, 65%; onset 2 hr, peak 6 hr, duration 48-72 hr, excreted unchanged by kidneys; crosses placenta; $t_{1/2}$ 51-89 hr
INDICATIONS AND USES: Edema (CHF, hepatic cirrhosis, nephrotic syndrome, acute glomerulonephritis and corticosteroid and estrogen therapy); hypertension; calcium nephrolithiasis*; osteoporosis*; diabetes insipidus prevention
DOSAGE
NOTE: Equivalent hydrochlorothizide dose: 50 mg-50 mg

Adult
• PO 15-100 mg/day or 100 mg every other day
Child
• PO 2 mg/kg 3×/wk
$ AVAILABLE FORMS/COST OF THERAPY
• Tab, Uncoated—Oral: 15 mg, 100's: **$77.78;** 25 mg, 100's: **$5.50-$83.35;** 50 mg, 100's: **$7.50-$92.61;** 100 mg, 100's: **$8.45-$25.98**
CONTRAINDICATIONS: Anuria, renal decompensation
PRECAUTIONS: Fluid and electrolyte imbalance (including sodium, potassium, magnesium, calcium), renal disease, hepatic disease, gout, COPD, lupus erythematosus, diabetes mellitus, hyperparathyroidism, vomiting, diarrhea, elevated cholesterol/triglycerides
PREGNANCY AND LACTATION: Pregnancy category B; therapy for preexisting hypertension can be continued throughout pregnancy with minimal risk; initiating for simple edema not recommended; few unequivocal indications for diuretic therapy in pregnancy except for pulmonary edema or congestive heart failure; compatible with breast feeding
SIDE EFFECTS/ADVERSE REACTIONS
CNS: Anxiety, depression, *dizziness,* drowsiness, *fatigue,* headache, paresthesia, *weakness*
CV: Irregular pulse, orthostatic hypotension, palpitations, volume depletion
EENT: Blurred vision
GI: *Anorexia,* constipation, cramps, diarrhea, GI irritation, hepatitis, *nausea,* pancreatitis, *vomiting*
GU: *Frequency,* glucosuria, impotence, polyuria, *uremia*
HEME: **Agranulocytosis, aplastic anemia, hemolytic anemia, leuko-**

---

italic = common side effects   ***bold italic*** = life-threatening reactions

penia, neutropenia, thrombocyto-penia
METAB: Lipid abnormalities (increased total and LDL-cholesterol, triglycerides), Gout, hypercalcemia, hyperglycemia, hyperuremia; hypochloremia, *hypokalemia,* hypomagnesemia, hyponatremia, increased creatinine, BUN
SKIN: Fever, photosensitivity, purpura, rash, urticaria

INTERACTIONS
Drugs
❷ *Angiotensin-converting enzyme inhibitors:* Risk of postural hypotension when added to ongoing diuretic therapy; more common with loop diuretics; first dose hypotension possible in patients with sodium depletion or hypovolemia due to diuretics or sodium restriction; hypotensive response is usually transient; hold diuretic day of first dose
❸ *Calcium:* Increased risk of milk-alkali syndrome
❸ *Carbenoxolone:* Additive potassium wasting, severe hypokalemia
❸ *Cholestyramine, Colestipol:* Reduced absorption
❸ *Corticosteroids:* Concomitant therapy may result in excessive potassium loss
❸ *Diazoxide:* Hyperglycemia
❸ *Digitalis glycosides:* Diuretic-induced hypokalemia increases risk of digitalis toxicity
❸ *Hypoglycemic agents:* Increased dosage requirements due to increased glucose levels
❸ *Lithium:* Increased lithium levels, potential toxicity
❸ *Methotrexate:* Increased risk of bone marrow depression
❸ *Nonsteroidal antiinflammatory drugs:* Concurrent use may reduce diuretic and antihypertensive effects
Labs
• False decrease: urine esriol

SPECIAL CONSIDERATIONS
• Doses above 25 mg provide no further blood pressure reduction, but are more likely to induce metabolic disturbance (i.e., hypokalemia, hyperuricemia, etc.)
• May protect against osteoporotic hip fractures
• Loop diuretics or metolazone more effective if CrCl <40-50 ml/min
PATIENT/FAMILY EDUCATION
• Will increase urination temporarily (approximately 3 wk); take early in the day to prevent sleep disturbance
• May cause sensitivity to sunlight; avoid prolonged exposure to the sun and other ultraviolet light
• May cause gout attacks; notify clinician if sudden joint pain occurs
MONITORING PARAMETERS
• Weight, urine output, serum electrolytes, BUN, creatinine, CBC, uric acid, glucose, lipids

---

chlorzoxazone
(klor-zox′a-zone)
Rx: Parafon Forte DSC, Remular-S
Chemical Class: Benzoxazole derivative
Therapeutic Class: Skeletal muscle relaxant

CLINICAL PHARMACOLOGY
Mechanism of Action: Inhibition of multisynaptic reflex arcs involved in producing and maintaining skeletal muscle spasm of varied etiology at the level of the spinal cord and subcortical areas of the brain; mode of action may be related to sedative properties
Pharmacokinetics
PO: Onset 30 min, peak 1-2 hr, duration 6 hr; metabolized in liver, excreted in urine (glucuronide metabolites); $t_{1/2}$ 1 hr

---

* = non-FDA-approved use

INDICATIONS AND USES: Adjunct to rest and physical therapy for the relief of discomfort associated with acute, painful musculoskeletal conditions; does not directly relax tense skeletal muscles

DOSAGE

Adult

• PO 250-750 mg tid-qid

Child

• PO 20 mg/kg/day in divided doses bid-tid

💲 AVAILABLE FORMS/COST OF THERAPY

• Tab, Uncoated—Oral: 250 mg, 100's: **$14.86-$34.89**; 500 mg, 100's: **$8.43-$122.20**

CONTRAINDICATIONS: Impaired hepatic function

PRECAUTIONS: Lactation, hepatic disease, elderly

PREGNANCY AND LACTATION: Pregnancy category C

SIDE EFFECTS/ADVERSE REACTIONS

CNS: Dizziness, drowsiness, headache, insomnia, malaise, stimulation

*GI: Anorexia, constipation, diarrhea, **gastrointestinal bleeding, hepatotoxicity,** jaundice, nausea,* vomiting

GU: Urine discoloration

HEME: Anemia, **granulocytopenia**

SKIN: Angioedema, ecchymoses, petechiae, pruritus, rash

SPECIAL CONSIDERATIONS

PATIENT/FAMILY EDUCATION

• Potential for psychologic dependency

---

cholestyramine
(koe-less-tir'a-meen)

Rx: Questran, Questran Light

Chemical Class: Bile acid sequestrant

Therapeutic Class: Anti-lipemic

CLINICAL PHARMACOLOGY

Mechanism of Action: Absorbs, combines with bile acids to form insoluble complex that is excreted via feces; loss of bile acids lowers cholesterol levels

Pharmacokinetics

PO: Excreted in feces, max effect in 2 wk

INDICATIONS AND USES: Primary hypercholesterolemia, pruritus associated with partial biliary obstruction, diarrhea caused by excess bile acid or *Clostridium difficile* toxin,* digitalis toxicity*

DOSAGE

Adult

• PO 4 g 1-6× daily (recommended schedule is bid), not to exceed 32 g/day

Child

• PO 240 mg/kg/day in 3 divided doses

💲 AVAILABLE FORMS/COST OF THERAPY

• Powder—Oral: 4 g/9 g, 60 pkts: **$80.05-$110.71**; 378 g: **$32.65-$73.30** (Questran)

• Powder, Reconst—Oral: 4 g/5 g, 60 pkts: **$82.88-$110.71**; 210 g: 210 g/214 g: **$36.29-$48.49**/210 g (Questran Light)

CONTRAINDICATIONS: Complete biliary obstruction

PRECAUTIONS: Children, constipation

PREGNANCY AND LACTATION: Pregnancy category C

---

italic = common side effects   ***bold italic*** = life-threatening reactions

SIDE EFFECTS/ADVERSE REACTIONS

CNS: Dizziness, drowsiness, headache, tinnitus, vertigo

GI: Abdominal pain, constipation, fecal impaction, flatulence, hemorrhoids, *nausea,* peptic ulcer, steatorrhea, vomiting

MS: Joint pain, muscle

SKIN: Irritation of perianal area, tongue, skin; rash

HEME: Bleeding, decreased protime, decreased vitamin A, D, K, red cell folate content, hyperchloremic acidosis

INTERACTIONS

Drugs

3 *Acetaminophen, Amiodarone, Corticosteroids, Diclofenac, Digitalis glycosides, Furosemide, Methotrexate, Metronidazole, Thiazide diuretics, Thyroid hormones, Valproic acid:* Cholestyramine reduces interacting drug concentrations and probably subsequent therapeutic response

3 *Oral anticoagulants:* Inhibition of hypoprothrombinemic response; colestipol might be less likely to interact

SPECIAL CONSIDERATIONS

• Avoid use in patients with elevated triglycerides

PATIENT/FAMILY EDUCATION

• Give all other medications 1 hr before or 4 hr after cholestyramine to avoid poor absorption

• Mix drug with applesauce or noncarbonated beverage (2-6 oz), let stand for 2 min; do not take dry

choline magnesium trisalicylate

(koe'leen mag-nees'ee-um tri-sal'eh-cye'late)

Rx: CMT, Trilisate, Tricosal, Trisalcid

Chemical Class: Salicylate derivative

Therapeutic Class: Nonnarcotic analgesic; NSAID

CLINICAL PHARMACOLOGY

Mechanism of Action: Inhibits prostaglandin synthesis; analgesic, anti-inflammatory, antipyretic actions

Pharmacokinetics

PO: Onset 15-30 min, peak 1.5-2 hrs, rapid absorption; metabolized by liver; excreted by kidneys

INDICATIONS AND USES: Mild to moderate pain, rheumatoid arthritis, osteoarthritis, related rheumatic disorders

DOSAGE

NOTE: Each 500 mg of choline magnesium trisalicylate contains 500 mg of salicylate (equivalent to 650 mg aspirin); dosage based on total salicylate content

Adult

• PO 1-4.5 g of salicylate daily in single dose or in 2-3 divided doses (based on response, tolerance, and serum salicylate concentration)

Child

• PO 50 mg/kg/day divided into 2 doses

$ AVAILABLE FORMS/COST OF THERAPY

• Liq—Oral: 500 mg/5 ml, 240 ml: **$24.99-$37.58**

• Tab, Uncoated—Oral: 500 mg, 100's: **$27.70-$79.06;** 750 mg, 100's: **$34.40-$98.15;** 1000 mg, 100's: **$45.40-$126.54**

CONTRAINDICATIONS: GI bleed-

---

* = non-FDA-approved use

ing, bleeding disorders, children <3 yr, vitamin K deficiency, children with flu-like symptoms

PRECAUTIONS: Anemia, hepatic disease, renal disease, Hodgkin's disease, lactation

PREGNANCY AND LACTATION: Pregnancy category C; excreted into breast milk

SIDE EFFECTS/ADVERSE REACTIONS

CNS: Coma, confusion, dizziness, drowsiness, flushing, hallucinations, headache, *seizures,* stimulation

CV: Pulmonary edema, rapid pulse

EENT: Hearing loss, tinnitus

GI: Anorexia, *diarrhea,* GI bleeding, *heartburn,* hepatitis, *nausea, vomiting*

HEME: **Agranulocytosis, hemolytic anemia,** increased pro-time (transient), **leukopenia, neutropenia, thrombocytopenia**

METAB: Hypoglycemia, hypokalemia, hyponatremia

RESP: Hyperpnea, wheezing

SKIN: Bruising, *rash,* urticaria

INTERACTIONS

Labs

• *False increase:* Serum bicarbonate, CSF protein, serum theophylline

• *False decrease:* Urine cocaine, urine estrogen, serum glucose, urine 17-hydroxycorticosteroids, urine opiates

• *False positive:* Ferric chloride test

SPECIAL CONSIDERATIONS

• Consider for patients with GI intolerance to aspirin or patients in whom interference with normal platelet function by aspirin or other NSAIDs is undesirable

PATIENT/FAMILY EDUCATION

• Solution may be mixed with fruit juice just before administration; do not mix with antacid

MONITORING PARAMETERS

• Liver and renal function studies,

stool for occult blood and hct if long-term therapy

---

choline salicylate
(koe'leen sa-lis'i-late)
OTC: Arthropan
Chemical Class: Salicylate derivative
Therapeutic Class: Nonnarcotic analgesic; NSAID

C

CLINICAL PHARMACOLOGY
Mechanism of Action: Inhibits prostaglandin synthesis; analgesic, anti-inflammatory, antipyretic actions

Pharmacokinetics

PO: Onset 15-30 min, rapid absorption; metabolized by liver, excreted by kidneys

INDICATIONS AND USES: Mild to moderate pain, rheumatoid arthritis, osteo-arthritis, related rheumatic disorders

DOSAGE

NOTE: Dosage based on total salicylate content

Adult

• *Arthritis:* PO 870-1740 mg (5-10 ml) up to qid

• *Pain/fever:* PO 870 mg (5 ml) q3-4h prn (max 6×/day)

Child

• PO 50 mg/kg/day in 2 divided doses for children weighing up to 37 kg and 2250 mg/day for larger children

$ AVAILABLE FORMS/COST OF THERAPY

• Liq—Oral: 870 mg/5 ml, 480 ml: **$42.74**

CONTRAINDICATIONS: GI bleeding, bleeding disorders, children <3 yr, vitamin K deficiency, children with flu-like symptoms

PRECAUTIONS: Anemia, hepatic

---

italic = common side effects   **bold italic** = life-threatening reactions

disease, renal disease, Hodgkin's disease

PREGNANCY AND LACTATION: Pregnancy category C; excreted into breast milk

SIDE EFFECTS/ADVERSE REACTIONS

CNS: Coma, confusion, dizziness, drowsiness, flushing, hallucinations, headache, *seizures,* stimulation

CV: Pulmonary edema, rapid pulse

EENT: Hearing loss, tinnitus

GI: Anorexia, *diarrhea,* **GI bleeding,** *heartburn,* hepatitis, *nausea, vomiting*

HEME: **Agranulocytosis, hemolytic anemia,** increased pro-time (transient), **leukopenia, neutropenia, thrombocytopenia**

METAB: Hypoglycemia, hypokalemia, hyponatremia

RESP: Hyperpnea, wheezing

SKIN: Bruising, *rash,* urticaria

INTERACTIONS

Labs

• *False increase:* Serum bicarbonate, CSF protein, serum theophylline

• *False decrease:* Urine cocaine, urine estrogen, serum glucose, urine 17-hydroxycorticosteroids, urine opiates

• *False positive:* Ferric chloride test

SPECIAL CONSIDERATIONS

• Consider for patients with GI intolerance to aspirin or patients in whom interference with normal platelet function by aspirin or other NSAIDs is undesirable

MONITORING PARAMETERS

• Liver and renal function studies, stool for occult blood and hct if long-term therapy

---

ciclopirox

(sye-kloe-peer′ox)

Rx: Loprox

Chemical Class: N-hydroxy-pyridinone derivative

Therapeutic Class: Topical antifungal

CLINICAL PHARMACOLOGY

Mechanism of Action: Interferes with fungal cell membrane, which increases permeability, which allows leaking of intracellular material

Pharmacokinetics

TOP: 1.3% absorbed systematically; $t_{1/2}$ 1.7 hr; excreted via kidneys

INDICATIONS AND USES: Topical dermal infections (tinea cruris, tinea corporis, tinea pedis, tinea versicolor, cutaneous candidiasis) caused by susceptible organisms

Antifungal spectrum usually includes: *Trichophyton mentagrophytes, Epidermophyton floccosum, Trichophyton rubrum, Microsporum canis, Candida albicans, Malassezia furfur*

DOSAGE

Adult and Child >10 yr

• TOP apply bid

$ **AVAILABLE FORMS/COST OF THERAPY**

• Cre—Top: 0.77%, 15, 30, 90 g: **$22.20**/30 g

• Lotion—Top: 0.77%, 30, 60 ml: **$46.50**/60 ml

PREGNANCY AND LACTATION: Pregnancy category B; excretion into breast milk unknown

SIDE EFFECTS/ADVERSE REACTIONS

SKIN: Burning, pain, pruritus, rash, stinging, urticaria

SPECIAL CONSIDERATIONS
PATIENT/FAMILY EDUCATION

• Continue medication for several days after condition clears

---

• Consult prescriber if no improvement after 4 wk of treatment

---

cidofovir
(ci-dah'fo-veer)
Rx: Vistide
Chemical Class: Acyclic purine nucleoside analog
Therapeutic Class: Antiviral

CLINICAL PHARMACOLOGY
Mechanism of Action: Metabolite (cidofovir diphosphate) inhibits viral DNA viral polymerase at intracellular concentrations 50- to 1000-fold lower than those required to inhibit cellular DNA synthesis
Pharmacokinetics
IV: Peak serum levels 12 µg/ml following 5 mg/kg INF; concurrent PO high dose probenecid/saline hydration doubles peak levels; minimal protein binding or hepatic systemic metabolism; intracellularly, phosphorylated to active diphosphate form (independent of virus infection); V_d, 300 mL/kg (steady state); $t_{1/2}$ 2.5 hr; 70% urinary excretion; no accumulation with weekly dosing
INDICATIONS AND USES: Cytomegalovirus retinitis in AIDS patients who are unresponsive to, intolerant to, or have relapsed on IV foscarnet or ganciclovir
DOSAGE
Adult
• *Cytomegalovirus retinitis in AIDS patients:* 5 mg/kg IV weekly for 2 wk (induction); 5 mg/kg IV every other week until retinitis progression or therapy-limiting toxicity; (see Special Considerations section); probenecid coadministration considered mandatory; for patients with renal insufficiency, schedule is same but dose reduced: CrCl 41-55 ml/min: 2 mg/kg; CrCl 30-40 ml/min: 1.5 mg/kg; CrCl 20-29 ml/min: 1.0 mg/kg; CrCl ≤19 ml/min: 0.5 mg/kg

💲 AVAILABLE FORMS/COST OF THERAPY
• Inj, Sol—IV: 75 mg/ml; 5 ml; **$727.09**
CONTRAINDICATIONS: Severe hypersensitivity to probenecid or sulfa drugs
PRECAUTIONS: Renal impairment (should administer probenecid/saline hydration concurrently to prevent nephrotoxicity), myelosuppression; do not give within 7 days of drugs listed in Drug Interactions section
PREGNANCY AND LACTATION: Pregnancy category C
SIDE EFFECTS/ADVERSE REACTIONS
GI: Dyspepsia (with probenecid)
GU: **Nephrotoxicity** (proximal tubular dysfunction), **renal insufficiency (29%)**
HEME: **Neutropenia**
SKIN: Rash (with probenecid)
INTERACTIONS
Drugs
🔳 *Aminoglycosides:* Additive nephrotoxicity
🔳 *Amphotericin B:* Additive nephrotoxicity
🔳 *Foscarnet:* Additive nephrotoxicity
🔳 *Pentamidine:* Additive nephrotoxicity (IV route only)
SPECIAL CONSIDERATIONS
• Concurrent high-dose probenecid plus saline hydration reduces nephrotoxicity; procedure: probenecid 2 g 3 hr prior to INF, then 1 g at 2 and 8 hr after INF; normal saline 1000 ml over 1 hr immediately prior to INF
MONITORING PARAMETERS
• Renal function, urinalysis (especially serum creatinine and urine protein prior to each dose), and blood chemistry (to include serum uric acid, phosphate, and bicarbonate),

---

italic = common side effects　　　　*bold italic* = life-threatening reactions

white counts with differential during intravenous therapy

---

cilostazol

(sil-os'tah-zol)
Rx: Pletal
Chemical Class: Quinolinone derivative
Therapeutic Class: Hemorheologic agent

CLINICAL PHARMACOLOGY
Mechanism of Action: Inhibits cAMP phosphodiesterase III; increases levels of cAMP in platelets and blood vessels resulting in vasodilation and inhibition of platelet aggregation
Pharmacokinetics
PO: Peak plasma concentration 3 to 4 hr, duration 48 hr; extensively metabolized by liver, primarily through CYP3A4 and to a lesser extent CYP2C19; 74% renal excreted in urine, 20% in feces; $t_{1/2}$ 11-13 hr (parent compound and active metabolites)
INDICATIONS AND USES: Intermittent claudication, percutaneous transluminal coronary angioplasty,* coronary stent implantation,* graft vs. host disease*
DOSAGE
Adult and Child >16 yr
• *Intermittent claudication:* PO 100 mg bid, consider a decrease in dose to 50 mg bid if coadministration with a CYP3A4 or CYP2C19 inhibitor
$ **AVAILABLE FORMS/COST OF THERAPY**
• Tab, Coated—Oral: 50 mg, 100's: **$89;** 100 mg, 100's: **$89**
CONTRAINDICATIONS: Congestive heart failure
PRECAUTIONS: Congestive heart failure (several drugs with this pharmacologic effect have caused decreased survival compared with placebo in patients with class III-IV CHF), cardiovascular lesions, children
PREGNANCY AND LACTATION: Pregnancy category C; excreted in breast milk
SIDE EFFECTS/ADVERSE REACTIONS
CNS: Dizziness, vertigo, *headache*
CV: Palpitations, tachycardia, peripheral edema
GI: Abnormal stool, diarrhea, dyspepsia, flatulence, nausea
MS: Back pain, myalgia
RESP: Cough, pharyngitis, rhinitis
MISC: Infection
INTERACTIONS
Drugs
3 *Diltiazem:* Increase cilostazol concentrations
3 *Erythromycin, azole antifungals (i.e., ketoconazole et al), fluoxetine, nefazadone, and sertraline:* as CYP3A4 or CYP2C19 inhibitors, may increase cilostazol levels; clinical effects unknown
3 *Omeprazole:* Increase cilostazol concentrations
3 *Foods: Grape fruit juice:* Increases cilostazol levels; *High fat:* increases absorption of cilostazol (80% increase of Cmax, 25% increase of AUC)

SPECIAL CONSIDERATIONS
• Cilostazol has been shown, in a multicenter, randomized, double-blind study (DPPARA 2), to be superior to pentoxifylline for treatment of claudication symptoms
PATIENT/FAMILY EDUCATION
• Take ½ hr before meal or 2 hr after meal
MONITORING PARAMETERS
• Beneficial effects usually seen in 2 to 4 wk, may take up to 12 wk

---

* = non-FDA-approved use

cimetidine

(sye-met'i-deen)
Rx: Tagamet
OTC: Tagamet HB
Chemical Class: Imidazole derivative
Therapeutic Class: Gastrointestinal antiulcer agent

CLINICAL PHARMACOLOGY

Mechanism of Action: Competitive, reversible inhibitor of histamine at gastric H_2-receptors; reduces gastric acid secretion

Pharmacokinetics

IM/IV: Onset 10 min, peak ½ hr, duration 4-5 hr

PO: Peak 1-1½ hr

Well absorbed (PO, IM); 30%-40% metabolized by liver (sulfoxide, major metabolite), excreted in urine (75% unchanged after 24 hr); $t_{1/2}$ 1½-2 hr

INDICATIONS AND USES: Short-term treatment of duodenal and benign gastric ulcers; maintenance therapy for duodenal ulcer; erosive gastroesophageal reflux disease (GERD); prevention of upper gastrointestinal bleeding in critically ill patients; treatment of pathological hypersecretory conditions (i.e., Zollinger-Ellison syndrome, systemic mastocytosis, multiple endocrine adenomas); heartburn, acid indigestion, and sour stomach (OTC only); as part of a multiple-drug regimen to eradicate *Helicobacter pylori* in the treatment of peptic ulcer*; chronic viral warts in children,* chronic idiopathic urticaria (in combination with H_1-receptor antagonists)*

DOSAGE

Adult and Child >16 yr

• *Treatment:* PO 300 mg qid with meals, hs or 400 mg bid or 800 mg hs × 8 wk; after 8 wk give 300-400 mg hs dose only; IV bolus 300 mg/20 ml 0.9% NaC1 over 1-2 min q6h; IV INF 300 mg/50 ml D_5W over 15-20 min q6h; continuous IV INF 37.5 mg/hr (900 mg/day); IM 300 mg q6h, not to exceed 2400 mg/day

• *Prophylaxis of duodenal ulcer:* 400 mg hs

• *GERD:* PO 1600 mg/day (800 mg bid or 400 mg qid) for 12 wk

• *Pathologic hypersecretory states:* PO 300 mg qid; increase prn; do not exceed 2400 mg/day

• *Heartburn, acid indigestion, sour stomach (OTC only):* PO 200 mg (2 tabs) up to bid prn

▧ AVAILABLE FORMS/COST OF THERAPY

• Inj, Sol—IM, IV: 300 mg/2 ml, 8 ml: **$3.31-$21.03**

• Liq—Oral: 300 mg/5 ml, 480 ml: **$111.46-$227.50**

• Tab, Coated—Oral: 200 mg, 12's: **$5.70 (OTC);** 200 mg, 100's: **$13.65-$96.55;** 300 mg, 100's: **$15.53-$101.05;** 400 mg, 100's: **$17.70-$169.70;** 800 mg, 100's: **$41.45-$299.70**

PRECAUTIONS: Organic brain syndrome, hepatic disease, renal disease, elderly

PREGNANCY AND LACTATION: Pregnancy category B; excreted into breast milk and may accumulate; theoretically, adversely affects the nursing infant's gastric acidity, inhibits drug metabolism, and produces CNS stimulation—all not reported; compatible with breast feeding

SIDE EFFECTS/ADVERSE REACTIONS

CNS: Anxiety, confusion, depression, dizziness, headache, psychosis, *seizures,* tremors, weakness

CV: Bradycardia, tachycardia

GI: Abdominal cramps, diarrhea, jaundice, paralytic ileus

---

italic = common side effects   ***bold italic*** = life-threatening reactions

GU: Galactorrhea, gynecomastia, impotence; increase in BUN, creatinine

HEME: **Agranulocytosis, aplastic anemia, neutropenia, thrombocytopenia**

SKIN: Alopecia, **exfoliative dermatitis,** flushing, rash, sweating, urticaria

DRUG INTERACTIONS

Drugs

3 *Amiodarone, benzodiazepines; calcium channel blockers; amiodarone; cyclic antidepressants; carbamazepine; carmustine; chloramphenicol; cisapride; citalopram; clozapine; diltiazem; femoxidine; flecanide; glyburide; glipizide; labetolol; lidocaine; lomustine; melphalan; metoprolol; narcotic analgesics; moricizine; N-acetylprocainamide; nicotine; phenytoin; peridolol; praziquantel; procainamide; propafinone; propranolol; quinidine; tacrine; theophylline; tolbutamide:* Increased concentrations of interacting drugs with potential for toxicity

3 *Ketoconazole, cefpodoxime, cefuroxime:* Reduced concentrations of interacting drugs

2 *Warfarin:* Increased concentrations of interacting drugs with potential for toxicity

Labs

• *False positive:* Hemoccult

SPECIAL CONSIDERATIONS

• Generic formulations offer less costly alternative for patients not at risk for drug interactions

PATIENT/FAMILY EDUCATION

• Stagger doses of cimetidine and antacids

---

cinoxacin
(sin-ox'a-sin)
Rx: Cinobac
Chemical Class: Quinolone derivative
Therapeutic Class: Antibiotic

CLINICAL PHARMACOLOGY

Mechanism of Action: Interferes with the enzyme DNA gyrase needed for the synthesis of bacterial DNA; bactericidal

Pharmacokinetics

PO: Peak 2 hr, duration 6-8 hr, excreted in urine (unchanged/inactive metabolites); $t_{1/2}$ 1½ hr

INDICATIONS AND USES: Infections of the urinary tract caused by susceptible organisms

Antibacterial spectrum usually includes: *E. coli, Klebsiella, Enterobacter, P. mirabilis, P. vulgaris, M. morganii, Serratia, Citrobacter*

DOSAGE

Adult and Child >12 yr

• PO 1 g/day in 2-4 divided doses × 1-2 wk

• *Preventive therapy:* PO 250 mg qhs for up to 5 mo

$ **AVAILABLE FORMS/COST OF THERAPY**

• Cap, Gel—Oral: 250 mg, 40's: **$49.25;** 500 mg, 50's: **$77.60-$111.16**

CONTRAINDICATIONS: Anuria, CNS damage

PRECAUTIONS: Renal disease, hepatic disease

PREGNANCY AND LACTATION: Pregnancy category B

SIDE EFFECTS/ADVERSE REACTIONS

CNS: Agitation, confusion, *dizziness, headache,* insomnia

EENT: Blurred vision, sensitivity to light, tinnitus, visual disturbances

---

GI: Abdominal cramps, anorexia, diarrhea, *nausea, vomiting*
SKIN: Edema, photosensitivity, pruritus, rash, urticaria

---

ciprofloxacin

(sip-ro-floks′a-sin)
Rx: Ciloxan (ophthalmic),
Cipro
Chemical Class: Fluoroquinolone derivative
Therapeutic Class: Antibiotic

CLINICAL PHARMACOLOGY
Mechanism of Action: Interferes with the enzyme DNA gyrase, needed for the synthesis of bacterial DNA; bactericidal
Pharmacokinetics
PO: Peak 1-2 hr; 60%-85% bioavailable PO with minimal 1st pass; widely distributed; 30%-50% excreted in urine as active drug, 20%-40% of dose excreted in feces (biliary excretion); t$_{1/2}$ 4 hr; metabolites less active
INDICATIONS AND USES: Infections of the lower respiratory tract, skin and skin structure, bone and joints, urinary tract, external auditory canal*; uncomplicated gonorrhea; typhoid fever; chronic prostatitis; intra-abdominal infections (in combination with metronidazole); infectious diarrhea; empirical therapy in febrile neutropenia (IV); superficial ocular infections caused by susceptible organisms (ophthalmic)
Antibacterial spectrum usually includes:
• Gram-positive organisms: *Enterococcus faecalis,* (many strains are only moderately susceptible), *Staphylococcus aureus, S. epidermidis, Streptococcus pneumoniae* (minimally)
• Gram-negative organisms: *Campy-*

lobacter jejuni, Citrobacter diversus, C. freundii, Enterobacter cloacae, Escherichia coli, H. influenzae, H. parainfluenzae, Klebsiella pneumoniae, Morganella morganii, Proteus mirabilis, P. vulgaris, Providencia rettgeri, P. stuartii, Pseudomonas aeruginosa, Serratia marcescens, Shigella flexneri, S. sonnei, Neisseria gonorrhoeae
• Most strains of *Pseudomonas cepacia* and some strains of *Pseudomonas maltophilia* are resistant to ciprofloxacin as are most anaerobic bacteria, including *Bacteroides fragilis* and *Clostridium difficile*
DOSAGE
Adult
• *Uncomplicated UTI:* PO 100-250 mg q12h; IV 200 mg q12h × 7 days
• *Complicated/severe urinary tract infections:* PO 500 mg q12h × 14 days; IV 400 mg q12h
• *Respiratory, skin, bone, and joint infections:* (Bone and joint infections may require treatment for 4 to 6 wk or longer) PO 500-750 mg q12h × 7-14 days
• *Infectious diarrhea:* 500 mg q12h × 5-7 days
• *Uncomplicated gonorrhea:* PO 500 mg as a single dose, plus doxycycline 100 mg bid or other agent active against chlamydia
• *Typhoid fever:* PO 500 mg q12h
• *Ocular:* 1 gtt 5-6 times/day
• *Renal impairment:* CrCl 10-50 ml/min 50% of dose; CrCl <10 ml/min 30% of dose
💲 **AVAILABLE FORMS/COST OF THERAPY**
• Inj, Sol—IV: 200 mg/20 ml, 1's: **$14.41;** 400 mg/40 ml, 1's: **$28.81**
• Oint, Ophth—Top: 0.3%, 3.5 g: **$30.00**
• Sol, Ophth—Top: 0.3%, 2, 5 ml: **$13.00**/2 ml
• Sus—Oral: 250 mg/5 ml, 100 ml; **$64.38** 500 mg/5 ml, 100 ml: **$75.40**

---

italic = common side effects   ***bold italic*** = life-threatening reactions

- Tab, Uncoated—Oral: 100 mg, 6's: **$14.40;** 250 mg, 100's: **$303.72;** 500 mg, 100's: **$362.36;** 750 mg, 100's: **$362.36**

PRECAUTIONS: Children (arthropathy in juvenile animals), renal disease, excessive sunlight, caution with known or suspected CNS disorders

PREGNANCY AND LACTATION: Pregnancy category C; appears in breast milk at levels similar to serum; allow 48 hr to elapse after last dose, before resuming breast feeding

SIDE EFFECTS/ADVERSE REACTIONS

CNS: Chills, depression, dizziness, fatigue, fever, hallucinations, headache, insomnia, nightmares, restlessness

EENT: Blurred vision, tinnitus

GI: Abdominal pain/discomfort, nausea, constipation; diarrhea, dysphagia, flatulence, heartburn, increased ALT, AST; oral candidiasis, vomiting

SKIN: Flushing, photosensitivity, pruritus, rash, urticaria

INTERACTIONS

Drugs

3 *Aluminum:* Reduced absorption of ciprofloxacin; do not take within 4 hr of dose

3 *Antacids:* Reduced absorption of ciprofloxacin; do not take within 4 hr of dose

3 *Antipyrine:* Inhibits metabolism of antipyrine; increased plasma antipyrine level

3 *Caffeine:* Inhibits metabolism of caffeine; increased plasma caffeine level

3 *Calcium:* Reduced absorption of ciprofloxacin; do not take within 4 hr of dose

3 *Diazepam:* Inhibits metabolism of diazepam; increased plasma diazepam level

3 *Didanosine:* Markedly reduced absorption of ciprofloxacin; take ciprofloxacin 2 hr before didanosine

3 *Foscarnet:* Coadministration increases seizure risk

3 *Iron:* Reduced absorption of ciprofloxacin; do not take within 4 hr of dose

3 *Magnesium:* Reduced absorption of ciprofloxacin; do not take within 4 hr of dose

3 *Metoprolol:* Inhibits metabolism of metoprolol; increased plasma metoprolol level

3 *Pentoxifylline:* Inhibits metabolism of pentoxifylline; increased plasma pentoxifylline level

3 *Phenytoin:* Inhibits metabolism of phenytoin; increased plasma phenytoin level

3 *Propranolol:* Inhibits metabolism of propranolol; increased plasma propranolol level

3 *Ropinirole:* Inhibits metabolism of ropinirole; increased plasma ropinirole level

3 *Sodium bicarbonate:* Reduced absorption of ciprofloxacin; do not take within 4 hr of dose

3 *Sucralfate:* Reduced absorption of ciprofloxacin; do not take within 4 hr of dose

3 *Theobromine:* Inhibits metabolism of theobromine; increased plasma theobromine level

3 *Theophylline:* Inhibits metabolism of theophylline; cut maintenance theophylline dose in half during therapy with ciprofloxacin

3 *Warfarin:* Inhibits metabolism of warfarin; increases hypoprothrombinemic response to warfarin

3 *Zinc:* Reduced absorption of ciprofloxacin; do not take within 4 hr of dose

Labs

- *False increase:* Urine coproporphyrin I, coproporphyrin III, urine porphyrins

SPECIAL CONSIDERATIONS
• Reserve use for UTI to documented pseudomonal infection or complicated UTI
• Considered 1st-line therapy for otitis externa in diabetic patients

citalopram
(sy-tal'oh-pram)
Rx: Celexa
Chemical Class: Bicyclic phthalane derivative
Therapeutic Class: Selective serotonin reuptake inhibitor antidepressant

CLINICAL PHARMACOLOGY
Mechanism of Action: Inhibitor of CNS neuronal uptake of serotonine (5HT); no significant activity for histaminergic, alpha or beta adrenergic, muscarinic, or dopaminergic
Pharmacokinetics
PO: Peak serum concentrations 2 to 4 hr; bioavailability 80%, unaffected by meals, metabolized by liver enzymes CYP3A4 and CYP2C19. Primary metabolite is desmethylcitalopram, which is active but less selective and less potent than parent drug; 20% (12% unchanged) excreted in urine, significant elimination in feces; $t_{1/2}$ 33 to 37 hr
INDICATIONS AND USES: Major depressive disorder, diabetic neuropathy,* obsessive-compulsive disorder,* panic disorder,* poststroke emotional lability,* premenstrual dysphoria syndrome,* alcohol abuse,* dementia*
DOSAGE
Adult and Child >16 yr
• *Depression:* 20-60 mg qd
• *Alcohol abuse:* 40 mg qd
• *Diabetic neuropathy:* 40 mg qd
• *Poststroke emotional lability:* 20 mg qd if patient <66 yr old

Dosage in renal failure
• No adjustment needed
Dosage in hepatic insufficiency
• 20 mg qd, may increase to 40 mg qd in unresponsive patients
Dosage in geriatric patients
• *Depression:* 20 mg qd, may increase to 40 mg qd in unresponsive patients
• *Dementia:* 20-30 mg qd
• *Poststroke emotional lability:* 10 mg qd in patients >66 yr old
💲 AVAILABLE FORMS/COST OF THERAPY
• Tab, Coated—Oral: 20 mg, 100's: **$193.20**; 40 mg, 100's: **$201.60**
CONTRAINDICATIONS: Concurrent use of MAOIs or use within 2 wk of discontinuation of MAOIs
PRECAUTIONS: Hepatic insufficiency, cardiovascular disease, seizure disorders, suicidal tendencies, mania, children and adolescence (no clinical data)
PREGNANCY AND LACTATION: Pregnancy category C; breastfeeding: unknown, 2 cases of infants experiencing excessive somnolence, decreased feeding, and weight loss have been reported
SIDE EFFECTS/ADVERSE REACTIONS
CNS: Migraine, parethesia, somnolence, impaired concentration, fatigue, drowsiness, sleep disturbance, confusion, restlessness, *amnesia, apathy,* **suicidal attempt, seizures**
CV: Hypotension, postural hypotension, palpitations
EENT: Visual changes
GI: Nausea, vomiting, xerostomia, taste perversion, constipation, dyspepsia, anorexia, increased appetite, flatulence
GU: Polyuria, dysuria, amenorrhea, *abnormal ejaculation* (>5%)
MS: Myalgia
RESP: Cough
SKIN: Increased sweating, rash

---

italic = common side effects   ***bold italic*** = life-threatening reactions

INTERACTIONS
Drugs
❷ *Buspirone:* Increased risk of serotonin syndrome

❸ *Cimetidine:* Increased levels of desmethylcitalopram via inhibition of CYP2D6 by cimetidine

❸ *Imipramine:* Increased bioavailability and half-life of desipramine (the major metabolite of imipramine) via inhibition of CYP2D6 by citalopram

⚠ *MAOIs, dexfenfluramine, sibutramine:* increased risk of sertonin syndrome

❸ *Metoprolol:* May increase levels of metoprolol, but no clinically signfcant changes in blood pressure or heart rate have been observed

❸ *Naratriptan, rizatriptan, sumatriptan, zolmatriptan 4:* Increased risk of weakness, hyperreflexia, and incoordination

SPECIAL CONSIDERATIONS
• No clinical advantage over other SSRIs

PATIENT/FAMILY EDUCATION
• Therapeutic response may take 5 to 6 wk; most commonly taken once daily in the afternoon or evening

---

clarithromycin
(clare-i-thro-mye′sin)
Rx: Biaxin
Chemical Class: Macrolide derivative
Therapeutic Class: Antibiotic

CLINICAL PHARMACOLOGY
Mechanism of Action: Binds to 50S ribosomal subunits of susceptible bacteria and suppresses protein synthesis

Pharmacokinetics
PO: Peak 2-4 hr; 65% bound to plasma proteins; extensively metabolized in liver (14-OH metabolite twice as active as parent compound vs *Haemophilus influenzae*); $t_{1/2}$ 3-7 hr (metabolite 5-7 hr)

INDICATIONS AND USES: Infections of upper and lower respiratory tract, skin and skin structures; disseminated mycobacterial infections due to *Mycoplasma avium* and *M. intracellulare;* eradication of *Helicobacter pylori* associated with active duodenal ulcer disease (in combination with omeprazole and metronidazole)

Antibacterial spectrum usually includes:

Gram-positive organisms: *Staphylococcus aureus, Streptococcus pneumoniae, S. pyogenes, S. agalactiae,* streptococci (Groups C, F, G), Viridans group streptococci, *Listeria monocytogenes*

• Gram-negative organisms: *Haemophilus influenzae, Moraxella catarrhalis, Bordetella pertussis, Campylobacter jejuni, Legionella pneumophila, Neisseria gonorrhoeae, Pasteurella multocida*

• Anaerobes: *Clostridium perfringens, Peptococcus niger, Propionibacterium acnes, Bacteriodes melaninogenicus*

• Other organisms: *Mycoplasma pneumoniae, M. avium* complex (MAC) consisting of *M. avium* and *M. intracellulare; Chlamydia trachomatis, H. pylori*

DOSAGE
Adult
• *Acute maxillary sinusitis:* PO 500 mg bid for 14 days

• *Acute exacerbation of chronic bronchitis:* (due to *Haemophilus influenzae*) PO 500 mg bid for 7-14 days

• *Mycobacterial infections:* PO 500 mg bid

• *Other infections:* PO 250 mg bid for 7-14 days

• *H. pylori:* PO 500 mg bid × 10

---

days (with omeprazole 20 mg bid and amoxicillin 1 g bid)

Dosing adjustment in renal impairment (CrCl <30 ml/min): decrease dose by 50% or double dosing interval

Child

• *Mycobacterial infections:* PO 7.5 mg/kg bid, do not exceed 500 mg bid

AVAILABLE FORMS/COST OF THERAPY

• Powder, Reconst—Oral: 125 mg/5 ml, 100 ml: **$29.85;** 250 mg/5 ml, 100 ml: **$56.85**

• Tab, Coated—Oral: 250, 500 mg, 60's: **$195.59**

PRECAUTIONS: Renal impairment, children

PREGNANCY AND LACTATION: Pregnancy category C; excretion into breast milk unknown; use caution in nursing mothers

SIDE EFFECTS/ADVERSE REACTIONS

CNS: Headache, psychosis

GI: Abdominal pain, abnormal taste, anorexia, *diarrhea,* heartburn, **hepatotoxicity,** *nausea,* stomatitis, *vomiting*

GU: Moniliasis, vaginitis

SKIN: Pruritus, rash, urticaria

INTERACTIONS

Drugs

3 *Alfentanil:* Prolonged anesthesia and respiratory depression

3 *Alprazolam:* Increased plasma alprazolam concentration

3 *Amprenavir:* Plasma concentrations of clarithromycin may be increased by amprenavir; plasma concentrations of amprenavir may be increased by clarithromycin

⚠ *Astemizole:* QT prolongation and life-threatening dysrhythmia

3 *Atorvastatin:* Increased plasma atorvastatin concentration with risk of rhabdomyolysis

3 *Bromocriptine:* Increased bromocriptine concentration with toxicity

3 *Buspirone:* Increased plasma buspirone concentration

3 *Carbamazepine:* Markedly increased plasma carbamazepine concentrations

2 *Cisapride:* QT prolongation and dysrhythmia

2 *Clozapine:* Increased plasma clozapine concentrations

3 *Colchicine:* Potential colchicine toxicity

3 *Cyclosporine:* Increased plasma cyclosporine concentrations

3 *Diazepam:* Increased plasma concentration of diazepam

3 *Digoxin:* Reduced bacterial flora may increase plasma digoxin concentrations

3 *Disopyramide:* Increased plasma disopyramide concentrations

2 *Ergotamine:* Potential for ergotism

3 *Ethanol:* Ethanol reduces plasma clarithromycin concentration

3 *Felodipine:* Increased plasma felodipine concentrations

3 *Food:* Food may increase or decrease the bioavailability of clarithromycin

3 *Indinavir:* Plasma concentrations of clarithromycin may be increased by indinavir; plasma concentrations of indinavir may be increased by clarithromycin

3 *Itraconazole:* Increased plasma itraconazole concentration

3 *Lovastatin:* Increased plasma lovastatin concentration with risk of rhabdomyolysis

3 *Methylprednisolone:* Increased plasma methylprednisolone concentrations

3 *Midazolam:* Increased plasma concentration of midazolam

3 *Nelfinavir:* Plasma concentrations of clarithromycin may be increased by nelfinavir; plasma concentrations of nelfinavir may be increased by clarithromycin

3 *Penicillin:* Decreased activity of penicillin

3 *Quinidine:* Increased plasma concentration of quinidine

3 *Ritonavir:* Plasma concentrations of clarithromycin may be increased by ritonavir, plasma concentrations of ritonavir may be increased by clarithromycin

3 *Saquinavir:* Plasma concentrations of clarithromycin may be increased by saquinavir; plasma concentrations of saquinavir may be increased by clarithromycin

3 *Sildenafil:* Increased plasma sildenafil concentration

2 *Simvastatin:* Increased plasma simvastatin concentration with risk of rhabdomyolysis

3 *Tacrolimus:* Increased plasma tacrolimus concentration

A *Terfenadine:* QT prolongation and life-threatening dysrhythmia

3 *Theophylline:* Increased plasma theophylline concentration

3 *Triazolam:* Increased plasma triazolam concentration

3 *Valproic acid:* Increased plasma valproic acid concentration

3 *Warfarin:* Markedly increased hypoprothrombinemic response to warfarin

3 *Zafirlukast:* Reduced plasma zafirlukast concentration probably by reducing bioavailability

3 *Zopiclone:* Increased plasma zopiclone concentration

clemastine

(klem'as-teen)
Rx: Tavist
OTC: Tavist-1, Antihist-I
Combinations
  OTC: with phenylpropanol-amine (Tavist D)
Chemical Class: Ethanolamine derivative
Therapeutic Class: Antihistamine

CLINICAL PHARMACOLOGY
Mechanism of Action: Decreases allergic response by blocking histamine at H_1-receptors
Pharmacokinetics
PO: Peak 5-7 hr, duration 10-12 hr; metabolized by liver, excreted by kidneys

INDICATIONS AND USES: Perennial and seasonal allergic rhinitis; uncomplicated allergic skin manifestations of urticaria and angioedema
DOSAGE
Adult and Child >12 yr
• PO 1.34-2.68 mg bid-tid, not to exceed 8.04 mg/day
AVAILABLE FORMS/COST OF THERAPY
• Syr—Oral: 0.5 mg/5 ml, 120 ml: **$16.50-$26.22**
• Tab, Uncoated—Oral: 1.34 mg, 16's: **$6.41-$6.55 (OTC)**; 2.68 mg, 100's: **$38.22-$134.74**
CONTRAINDICATIONS: Narrow-angle glaucoma, bladder neck obstruction
PRECAUTIONS: Liver disease, elderly, increased intraocular pressure, hyperthyroidism, cardiovascular disease, hypertension, urinary retention, renal disease, stenosed peptic ulcers
PREGNANCY AND LACTATION: Pregnancy category C; excreted

into breast milk; may cause drowsiness and irritability in nursing infant; use with caution during breast feeding

SIDE EFFECTS/ADVERSE REACTIONS

CNS: Anxiety, confusion, *dizziness, drowsiness,* euphoria, fatigue, neuritis, paresthesia, poor coordination

CV: Hypotension, palpitations, tachycardia

EENT: Blurred vision, dry nose, throat; mydriasis, nasal stuffiness, tinnitus

GI: Anorexia, *constipation,* diarrhea, *dry mouth,* nausea, vomiting

GU: Dysuria, frequency, impotence, retention

HEME: ***Agranulocytosis, hemolytic anemia, thrombocytopenia***

RESP: Chest tightness, increased thick secretions, wheezing

SKIN: Photosensitivity, rash, urticaria

SPECIAL CONSIDERATIONS

• No advantage over loratadine or cetirizine; lower doses associated with less sedation and efficacy

---

clidinium

(kli-din'ee-um)

Rx: Quarzan

Combinations

  Rx: with chlordiazepoxide (Clindex, Librax)

Chemical Class: Synthetic quaternary ammonium derivative

Therapeutic Class: Anticholinergic; gastrointestinal antispasmodic; gastrointestinal antiulcer agent (adjunct)

CLINICAL PHARMACOLOGY

Mechanism of Action: Inhibits gastrointestinal motility and diminishes gastric acid secretion

Pharmacokinetics

PO: Onset 1 hr, duration 3 hr; ionized, excreted in urine

INDICATIONS AND USES: Peptic ulcer disease (in combination with other drugs); functional GI disorders (diarrhea, pylorospasm, hypermotility, neurogenic colon)*; irritable bowel syndrome (spastic colon, mucous colitis)*; acute enterocolitis,* ulcerative colitis,* diverticulitis,* mild dysenteries,* pancreatitis,* splenic flexure syndrome*

DOSAGE

Adult

• PO 2.5-5 mg tid-qid ac, hs (use lower dose for elderly or debilitated patients)

$ **AVAILABLE FORMS/COST OF THERAPY**

• Cap, Gel—Oral: 2.5 mg, 100's: **$20.02;** 5 mg, 100's: **$27.28**

CONTRAINDICATIONS: Narrow-angle glaucoma, obstructive uropathy (e.g., bladder neck obstruction due to prostatic hypertrophy), obstructive disease of the GI tract (e.g., pyloroduodenal stenosis), paralytic ileus, intestinal atony, unstable cardiovascular status in acute hemorrhage, severe ulcerative colitis, toxic megacolon complicating ulcerative colitis, myasthenia gravis

PRECAUTIONS: Hyperthyroidism, coronary artery disease, dysrhythmias, CHF, ulcerative colitis, hypertension, hiatal hernia, hepatic disease, renal disease, urinary retention, prostatic hypertrophy, elderly

PREGNANCY AND LACTATION: Pregnancy category C; excretion into breast milk unknown, although would be expected to be minimal due to quaternary structure (see also atropine)

SIDE EFFECTS/ADVERSE REACTIONS

CNS: Anxiety, confusion, dizziness,

drowsiness, hallucination, headache, insomnia, stimulation (especially in elderly), weakness

CV: Palpitations, tachycardia

EENT: Blurred vision, cycloplegia, increased ocular tension, mydriasis, photophobia

GI: Absence of taste, *constipation, dry mouth,* dysphagia, heartburn, nausea, paralytic ileus, vomiting

GU: Hesitancy, impotence, *retention*

SKIN: Allergic reactions, anhidrosis, fever, pruritus, rash, urticaria

SPECIAL CONSIDERATIONS
• Adjunctive agent; no significant effect on ulcer disease alone

PATIENT/FAMILY EDUCATION
• Avoid driving or other hazardous activities until stabilized on medication
• Avoid alcohol or other CNS depressants; will enhance sedating properties of this drug

---

clindamycin

(klin-da-mye'sin)
Rx: Cleocin, Cleocin T, Cleocin vaginal, Clinda-Derm
Chemical Class: Lincomycin derivative
Therapeutic Class: Antibiotic

CLINICAL PHARMACOLOGY
Mechanism of Action: Inhibits bacterial protein synthesis by preferentially binding to the 50S ribosomal subunit

Pharmacokinetics
PO: Peak 45 min, duration 6 hr
IM: Peak 3 hr, duration 8-12 hr
VAG: Peak 16 hr (total 5% systemic absorption)
90% bound to plasma proteins; metabolized in liver, excreted in urine, bile, feces as active/inactive metabolites; $t_{1/2}$ 2.5 hr

INDICATIONS AND USES: Infec-tions of the respiratory tract (e.g., empyema, anaerobic pneumonitis, lung abscess), skin and soft tissues, female pelvis and genital tract; septicemia; intra-abdominal infections (e.g., peritonitis, abscess); bone and joint infections; CNS toxoplasmosis in AIDS patients (in combination with pyrimethamine)*; *Pneumocystis carinii* pneumonia (in combination with primaquine)*; *Chlamydia trachomatis* infections in women*; acne vulgaris (top formulations); rosacea (top formulations)*; bacterial vaginosis (vag formulation)*

Antibacterial spectrum usually includes:
• Gram-positive organisms: *Staphylococcus aureus, S. epidermidis* (penicillinase and non-penicillinase-producing strains), streptococci (except *Str. faecalis*), pneumococci
• Anaerobes: *Bacteroides* spp. (including *B. fragilis* and *B. melaninogenicus*), *Fusobacterium, Propionibacterium, Eubacterium, Actinomyces* spp., *Peptococcus, Peptostreptococcus, Clostridium perfringens, C. tetani, Veillonella*

DOSAGE
Adult
• PO 150-450 mg q6-8h, not to exceed 1.8 g/day; IM/IV 1.2-1.8 g/day in 2-4 divided doses, not to exceed 4.8 g/day; VAG insert 1 applicatorful qhs for 7 days; TOP apply bid
Child
• PO 10-30 mg/kg/d divided q6h; IM/IV 25-40 mg/kg/d divided q6-8h; TOP apply bid

§ AVAILABLE FORMS/COST OF THERAPY
• Inj, Sol—IM, IV: 150 mg/ml, 2 ml, **$1.51-$11.50**
• Sol—Top: 1%, 30, 60 ml: **$7.17-$29.99**/60 ml
• Gel—Top: 1%, 30, 60 g: **$26.40/** 30 g

- Lotion—Top: 1%, 60 ml: **$36.72**
- Swab, Medicated—Top: 1%, 60's: **$31.97**
- Cre—Vag: 2%, 40 g: **$35.36**
- Cap, Gel—Oral: 75 mg, 100's: **$86.90**; 150 mg, 100's: **$52.01-$160.43**; 300 mg, 100's: **$319.71**
- Granule, Reconst—Oral: 75 mg/5 ml 100 ml: **$13.41**
- Supp—Vag: Not available at publication time

CONTRAINDICATIONS: Regional enteritis, ulcerative colitis, antibiotic-associated colitis

PRECAUTIONS: History of GI disease, liver disease, renal disease, atopic individuals, tartrazine sensitivity (75 and 150 mg caps), elderly, prolonged therapy

PREGNANCY AND LACTATION: Pregnancy category B; excreted into breast milk; compatible with breast feeding

SIDE EFFECTS/ADVERSE REACTIONS

GI: Abdominal pain, anorexia, *diarrhea,* increased AST, ALT, bilirubin, alk phosphatase; jaundice, *nausea,* **pseudomembranous colitis,** *vomiting,* weight loss

GU: Urinary frequency, vaginitis, vulvar irritation

HEME: **Agranulocytosis,** eosinophilia, **leukopenia, thrombocytopenia**

SKIN: Abscess at inj site, erythema, pain, pruritus, rash, urticaria

INTERACTIONS

Drugs

3 *Food:* Decreased clindamycin concentrations with diet foods containing sodium cyclamate

2 *Kaolin-pectin:* Decreased clindamycin concentrations

Labs

- *False increase:* Serum theophylline

SPECIAL CONSIDERATIONS
- Most active antibiotic against anaerobes
- Preferred topical antiacne antibiotic

C

clioquinol (iodochlorhydroxyquin)

(klee-oh-kwee′nole)

Combinations

Rx: with hydrocortisone (Ala-Quin, Corque, Dek-Quin); with hydrocortisone and pramoxine (1 + 1 − F)

Chemical Class: Halogenated hydroxyquinoline

Therapeutic Class: Topical anti-infective

CLINICAL PHARMACOLOGY

Mechanism of Action: Increases cell membrane permeability in susceptible organisms by binding sterols; decreases potassium, sodium, and nutrients in cell; inhibits the growth of various mycotic organisms such as Microsporons, Trichophytons, and *Candida albicans* and gram positive cocci such as staphylococci and enterococci

Pharmacokinetics

Some absorbed through the skin; excreted in urine (conjugated form), the rest excreted slowly

INDICATIONS AND USES: Inflamed conditions of the skin such as eczema, athlete's foot, other fungal infections

DOSAGE

Adult

- Top apply to affected area bid-tid, not for use >1 wk

$ AVAILABLE FORMS/COST OF THERAPY

- Cre—Top: (Clioquinol/Hydrocortisone), 3%/0.5%, 15, 30 g:

$3.00/15 g 3%/1%, 20, 30 g: **$2.01-$6.20**/20 g

• Oint—Top: 3%/1%, 20 g: **$4.28**

CONTRAINDICATIONS: Lesions of the eye, tuberculosis of the skin, most viral skin lesions (including herpes simplex, vaccinia, varicella), children <2 yr of age, diaper rash

PRECAUTIONS: Sensitized skin, deep or puncture wounds, serious burns

PREGNANCY AND LACTATION: Pregnancy category C; excretion into breast milk unknown

SIDE EFFECTS/ADVERSE REACTIONS

CNS: Neurotoxicity with systemic use

SKIN: Burning, contact dermatitis, dry skin, erythema, pruritus, rash, redness, staining of hair and skin, stinging, urticaria

SPECIAL CONSIDERATIONS

• Potential neurotoxicity with absorption (with occlusion); since other agents without this toxicity exist, questionable utility

---

clobetasol
(klo-bet′a-sol)

Rx: Cormax, Embeline E, Temovate, Temovate E

Chemical Class: Synthetic glucocorticoid
Therapeutic Class: Topical corticosteroid, very high potency

CLINICAL PHARMACOLOGY
Mechanism of Action: Depresses formation, release, and activity of endogenous mediators of inflammation, such as prostaglandins, kinins, histamine, liposomal enzymes, and the complement system resulting in decreased edema, erythema, and pruritus

Pharmacokinetics
Absorbed through the skin (increased by inflammation and occlusive dressings); metabolized primarily in the liver

INDICATIONS AND USES: Psoriasis, eczema, contact dermatitis, pruritus (usually reserved for severe dermatoses that have not responded to less potent formulation)

DOSAGE
Adult and Child >12 yr

• TOP apply to affected area bid, rub completely into skin

🚯 **AVAILABLE FORMS/COST OF THERAPY**

• Cre—Top: 0.05%, 15, 30, 45, 60 g: **$29.69-$34.39**/30 g

• Oint—Top: 0.05%, 15, 30, 45, 60 g: **$29.69-$34.39**/30 g

• Gel—Top: 0.05%, 15, 30, 60 g: **$28.56-$34.39**/30 g

• Sol—Top: 0.05%, 25, 50 ml: **$39.60-$54.77**/50 ml

CONTRAINDICATIONS: Fungal infections; use on face, groin, or axilla

PRECAUTIONS: Viral infections, bacterial infections, children, prolonged use

PREGNANCY AND LACTATION: Pregnancy category C; unknown whether top application could result in sufficient systemic absorption to produce detectable amounts in breast milk (systemic corticosteroids are secreted into breast milk in quantities not likely to have detrimental effects on infant)

SIDE EFFECTS/ADVERSE REACTIONS

SKIN: Acne, allergic contact dermatitis, atrophy, burning, dryness, folliculitis, hypertrichosis, hypopigmentation, irritation, itching, miliaria, perioral dermatitis, secondary infection, striae

---

MISC: Potential for systemic absorption and reversible HPA axis suppression (more likely with occlusive dressings, prolonged administration, application to large surface areas, liver failure, and in children)

SPECIAL CONSIDERATIONS
• No demonstrated superiority over other high-potency agents; cost should govern use

PATIENT/FAMILY EDUCATION
• Apply sparingly only to affected area
• Avoid contact with the eyes
• Do not put bandages or dressings over treated area unless directed by clinician
• Do not use on weeping, denuded, or infected areas
• Discontinue drug, notify clinician if local irritation or fever develops

---

clocortolone

(klo-kort′o-lone)
Rx: Cloderm
Chemical Class: Synthetic glucocorticoid
Therapeutic Class: Topical corticosteroid, intermediate potency

CLINICAL PHARMACOLOGY
Mechanism of Action: Depresses formation, release, and activity of endogenous mediators of inflammation, such as prostaglandins, kinins, histamine, liposomal enzymes, and the complement system resulting in decreased edema, erythema, and pruritus

Pharmacokinetics
Absorbed through the skin (increased by inflammation and occlusive dressings); metabolized primarily in the liver

INDICATIONS AND USES:
Psoriasis, eczema, contact dermatitis, pruritus

DOSAGE
Adult and Child
• TOP apply to affected area tid or qid, rub completely into skin

§ AVAILABLE FORMS/COST OF THERAPY
• Cre—Top: 0.1%, 15, 45 g: **$14.60**/15 g

CONTRAINDICATIONS: Fungal infections; use on face, groin, or axilla
PRECAUTIONS: Viral infections, bacterial infections, children
PREGNANCY AND LACTATION: Pregnancy category C; unknown whether top application could result in sufficient systemic absorption to produce detectable amounts in breast milk (systemic corticosteroids are secreted into breast milk in quantities not likely to have detrimental effects on infant)

SIDE EFFECTS/ADVERSE REACTIONS
SKIN: Acne, allergic contact dermatitis, atrophy, burning, dryness, folliculitis, hypertrichosis, hypopigmentation, irritation, itching, miliaria, perioral dermatitis, secondary infection, striae
MISC: Systemic absorption of topical corticosteroids has produced reversible HPA axis suppression (more likely with occlusive dressings, prolonged administration, application to large surface areas, liver failure, and in children)

SPECIAL CONSIDERATIONS
• No demonstrated superiority over other low-potency agents; cost should govern use

PATIENT/FAMILY EDUCATION
• Apply sparingly only to affected area
• Avoid contact with the eyes
• Do not put bandages or dressings over treated area unless directed by clinician

---

- Discontinue drug, notify clinician if local irritation or fever develops
- Do not use on weeping, denuded, or infected areas

---

clofazimine
(kloe-faz'i-meen)
Rx: Lamprene
Chemical Class: Iminophenazine dye
Therapeutic Class: Leprosy, *Mycobacterium avium* complex

CLINICAL PHARMACOLOGY
Mechanism of Action: Binds to mycobacterial DNA and inhibits growth; also exerts anti-inflammatory properties in controlling erythema nodosum leprosum reactions; precise mechanisms of action are unknown
Pharmacokinetics
PO: Deposited in fatty tissue and reticuloendothelial system, $t_{1/2}$ 70 days; small amount excreted in feces, sputum, sweat
INDICATIONS AND USES: Lepromatous leprosy (including dapsone-resistant lepromatous leprosy and lepromatous leprosy complicated by erythema nodosum leprosum); combination therapy with other antiinfectives in *Mycobacterium avium-intracellulare* (MAI) infections*
DOSAGE
Adult
- *Dapsone-resistant leprosy:* PO 100 mg qd in combination with 1 or more other antileprosy drugs for 3 yr, followed by monotherapy with 100 mg clofazamine qd
- *Dapsone-sensitive multibacillary leprosy:* PO 50-100 mg qd in combination with 2 or more other antileprosy drugs for 2 yr, followed by single-drug therapy with an appropriate agent

- *Erythema nodosum leprosum:* PO 100-200 mg qd for up to 3 mo or longer, then taper dose to 100 mg qd when possible
- *MAI infections:* PO 100 mg qd-tid in combination with other mycobacterial agents
Child
- *Leprosy:* PO 1 mg/kg q24h in combination with dapsone and rifampin
$ AVAILABLE FORMS/COST OF THERAPY
- Cap, Elastic—Oral: 50 mg, 100's: **$15.65**
PRECAUTIONS: Children, abdominal pain, diarrhea, depression
PREGNANCY AND LACTATION: Pregnancy category C; excreted into breast milk; do not administer to nursing mother unless clearly indicated
SIDE EFFECTS/ADVERSE REACTIONS
CNS: Dizziness, drowsiness, fatigue, giddiness, headache, neuralgia
EENT: Conjunctival and corneal pigmentation; dry, burning, itching, irritated eyes
GI: Abdominal/epigastric pain, anorexia, constipation, diarrhea, enlarged liver, eosinophilic enteritis, *GI intolerance,* hepatitis, jaundice, nausea, taste disorder, vomiting, weight loss
HEME: Eosinophilia
METAB: Hypokalemia
SKIN: Acneiform eruptions, *dryness,* erythroderma, *ichthyosis,* monilial cheilosis, phototoxicity, *pigmentation (pink to brownish black),* pruritus, rash
INTERACTIONS
Labs
- *Increase:* Albumin, bilirubin, AST
SPECIAL CONSIDERATIONS
- Use in conjunction with other antileprosy agents to prevent development of resistance

---

* = non-FDA-approved use

PATIENT/FAMILY EDUCATION
• May discolor skin from pink to brownish black, as well as discoloring the conjunctivae, lacrimal fluid, sweat, sputum, urine, and feces; skin discoloration may take several mo or yr to disappear after discontinuation of therapy

---

clofibrate
(kloe-fye'brate)
Rx: Atromid-S
Chemical Class: Fibric acid derivative
Therapeutic Class: Antilipemic

CLINICAL PHARMACOLOGY
Mechanism of Action: Acts to lower elevated serum lipids by reducing the very low-density lipoprotein fraction rich in triglycerides; serum cholesterol may be decreased, particularly in those patients whose cholesterol elevation is due to the presence of intermediate-density lipoprotein (IDL) as a result of Type III hyperlipoproteinemia
Pharmacokinetics
PO: Peak 2-6 hr; >90% bound to plasma proteins; metabolized in liver, excreted in urine; $t_{1/2}$ 18-22 hr
INDICATIONS AND USES: Primary dysbetalipoproteinemia (Type III hyperlipidemia); Type IV and V hyperlipidemia (in patients at risk of abdominal pain and pancreatitis)
DOSAGE
Adult
• PO 2 g/day in 4 divided doses
💲 **AVAILABLE FORMS/COST OF THERAPY**
• Cap, Elastic—Oral: 500 mg, 100's: **$84.60-$92.33**
CONTRAINDICATIONS: Severe hepatic or renal disease, primary biliary cirrhosis

PRECAUTIONS: Peptic ulcer
PREGNANCY AND LACTATION: Pregnancy category C; animal data suggest that the drug is excreted into breast milk; use caution in nursing mothers
SIDE EFFECTS/ADVERSE REACTIONS
CNS: Dizziness, drowsiness, fatigue, headache, weakness
CV: Angina, *dysrhythmias,* thrombophlebitis
GI: Abdominal distress, bloating, cholelithiasis, diarrhea, dyspepsia, flatulence, hepatomegaly, increased liver enzymes, *nausea,* stomatitis, vomiting, weight gain
GU: Decreased libido, dysuria, hematuria, impotence, oliguria, proteinuria
HEME: Anemia, bleeding, eosinophilia, *leukopenia*
MS: Arthralgias, myalgias
SKIN: Alopecia, dry hair and skin, pruritus, rash, urticaria
MISC: Polyphagia
INTERACTIONS
Drugs
❸ *Antidiabetics:* Enhanced effect of oral hypoglycemic drugs in some patients
❸ *Furosemide:* Enhanced effects of both drugs in patients with hypoalbuminemia
❷ *Lovastatin:* Increased risk of myopathy
❷ *Oral anticoagulants:* Increased hypoprothrombinemic response to warfarin and possibly other oral anticoagulants; serious bleeding episodes have occurred
SPECIAL CONSIDERATIONS
• No evidence substantiates a beneficial effect from clofibrate on cardiovascular mortality (a 36% increase in incidence of noncardiovascular deaths was reported in one study)
• Fibric acid derivatives only as al-

---

ternative lipid-lowering drugs; clofibrate alternative to gemfibrozil

---

clomiphene
(kloe'mi-feen)
Rx: Clomid, Milophene, Serophene
Chemical Class: Nonsteroidal antiestrogenic
Therapeutic Class: Ovulation stimulant

CLINICAL PHARMACOLOGY
Mechanism of Action: Decreases the number of cytoplasmic estrogenic receptors, stimulating the secretion of luteinizing hormone (LH), follicle-stimulating hormone (FSH), and gonadotropins, which in turn stimulate the maturation and endocrine activity of the ovarian follicle and the subsequent development and function of the corpus luteum
Pharmacokinetics
PO: Metabolized in liver, excreted in feces
INDICATIONS AND USES: Ovulatory dysfunction in patients desiring pregnancy who have normal liver function, good levels of endogenous estrogen (reduced levels are less favorable but do not preclude successful therapy), and whose partners have adequate sperm; male infertility*
DOSAGE
Adult
• *Ovulatory failure:* PO 50 mg qd for 5 days beginning on day 5 of cycle; may be repeated at dosage of 100 mg until conception occurs or 3 cycles of therapy have been completed
• *Male infertility:* PO 25 mg qd for 25 days with 5 days rest, or 100 mg every Monday, Wednesday, and Friday

* = non-FDA-approved use

$ **AVAILABLE FORMS/COST OF THERAPY**
• Tab, Uncoated—Oral: 50 mg, 100's: **$692.00-$883.80**
CONTRAINDICATIONS: Hepatic disease, undiagnosed vaginal bleeding
PRECAUTIONS: Hypertension, depression, seizure disorder, diabetes mellitus, ovarian cyst, polycystic ovary syndrome, uterine fibroids
PREGNANCY AND LACTATION: Pregnancy category X; each new course of drug should be started only after pregnancy has been excluded
SIDE EFFECTS/ADVERSE REACTIONS
CNS: Dizziness, insomnia, lightheadedness, nervousness
CV: Vasomotor flushing
EENT: Blurred vision, diplopia, photophobia
GI: Abdominal pain, bloating, constipation, nausea, vomiting
GU: Abnormal uterine bleeding, breast pain, frequency, multiple ovulation, oliguria, *ovarian enlargement,* polyuria, ***ovarian hyperstimulation syndrome***
SKIN: Alopecia, dermatitis, rash, urticaria
SPECIAL CONSIDERATIONS
• Though gonadotropin therapy is more effective for inducing ovulation, expense and time requirements warrant clomiphene trial
PATIENT/FAMILY EDUCATION
• Risk of multiple births increased—is approx 8% (7% twins, <1% triplets or greater)
• Record basal body temperature to determine whether ovulation has occurred; if ovulation can be determined (there is a slight decrease in temperature, then a sharp increase for ovulation), attempt coitus 3 days before and qod until after ovulation
• Prolonged use may increase the risk of ovarian cancer

clomipramine

(klom-ip'ra-meen)

Rx: Anafranil

Chemical Class: Tertiary amine

Therapeutic Class: Anti-obsessional; tricyclic antidepressant

CLINICAL PHARMACOLOGY

Mechanism of Action: Inhibits the reuptake of serotonin (5-HT) norepinephrine and amine blocking activity, moderate and very high, respectively

Pharmacokinetics

PO: Peak 4.7 hr; extensively bound to tissue and plasma proteins, demethylated in liver; active metabolites excreted in urine; $t_{1/2}$ 32 hr (parent compound), 69 hr (metabolite)

INDICATIONS AND USES: Obsessive-compulsive disorder (OCD), depression,* anxiety disorders*

DOSAGE

Adult

• *OCD:* PO 25 mg hs, increase gradually over 4 wk to a dose of 75-250 mg/day in divided doses; after titration, the entire dose may be given hs

• *Depression:* PO 50-150 mg/day in a single or divided dose

• *Anxiety/agoraphobia:* PO 25-75 mg/day

Child

• PO 25 mg hs, increase gradually over several wk to 3 mg/kg/day or 100 mg, whichever is smaller

💲 AVAILABLE FORMS/COST OF THERAPY

• Cap, Gel—Oral: 25 mg, 100's: **$72.00-$103.41;** 50 mg, 100's: **$97.08-$139.38;** 75 mg, 100's: **$108.79-$183.47**

CONTRAINDICATIONS: Administration within 14 days of MAOI therapy, acute recovery period following MI

PRECAUTIONS: Seizure disorder, suicidal patients, elderly, cardiac disease

PREGNANCY AND LACTATION: Pregnancy category C; withdrawal symptoms, including jitteriness, tremor, and seizures have been reported in neonates whose mothers had taken clomipramine until delivery; has been found in human milk; use caution in nursing mothers

SIDE EFFECTS/ADVERSE REACTIONS

CNS: Abnormal dreaming, agitation, anxiety, confusion, depersonalization, depression, *dizziness,* emotional lability, *headache,* hypertonia, impaired concentration, increased appetite, *insomnia,* irritability, *libido change,* memory impairment, migraine, myoclonus, *nervousness,* panic reaction, paresthesia, psychosomatic disorder, *somnolence,* speech disorder, *tremor,* weight gain, yawning

CV: Bradycardia, **dysrhythmia,** pallor, palpitations, postural hypotension, syncope, tachycardia

EENT: Abnormal vision, tinnitus

GI: Abdominal pain, anorexia, constipation, diarrhea, dry mouth, dyspepsia, dysphagia, esophagitis, flatulence, *nausea,* tooth disorder, ulcerative stomatitis, vomiting

GU: Ejaculation disorder, impotence, urinary retention

MS: Arthralgia, back pain, myalgia

RESP: **Bronchospasm,** coughing, pharyngitis, rhinitis, sinusitis

SKIN: Abnormal skin odor, acne, dermatitis, dry skin, increased sweating, pruritus, rash, urticaria

INTERACTIONS

Drugs

🗓 *Barbiturates:* Reduced serum

concentrations of cyclic antidepressants

2 *Bethanidine:* Reduced antihypertensive effect of bethanidine

3 *Carbamazepine:* Reduced cyclic antidepressant serum concentrations

2 *Clonidine:* Reduced antihypertensive response to clonidine; enhanced hypertensive response with abrupt clonidine withdrawal

3 *Debrisoquin:* Inhibited antihypertensive response of debrisoquin

2 *Epinephrine:* Markedly enhanced pressor response to IV epinephrine

3 *Ethanol:* Additive impairment of motor skills; abstinent alcoholics may eliminate cyclic antidepressants more rapidly than nonalcoholics

3 *Fluoxetine, fluvoxamine, grapefruit juice:* Marked increases in cyclic antidepressant plasma concentrations

3 *Guanethidine:* Inhibited antihypertensive response to guanethidine

A *MAOIs:* Excessive sympathetic response, mania, or hyperpyrexia possible

2 *Moclobemide:* Potential association with fatal or non-fatal serotonin syndrome

3 *Neuroleptics:* Increased therapeutic and toxic effects of both drugs

2 *Norepinephrine:* Markedly enhanced pressor response to norepinephrine

2 *Phenylephrine:* Enhanced pressor response to IV phenylephrine

3 *Propoxyphene:* Enhanced effect of cyclic antidepressants

3 *Quinidine:* Increased cyclic antidepressant serum concentrations

SPECIAL CONSIDERATIONS
PATIENT/FAMILY EDUCATION

• Beneficial effects may take 2-3 wk

• Use caution while driving or during other activities requiring alertness; may cause drowsiness

• Avoid alcohol and other CNS depressants

• Do not discontinue abruptly

---

clonazepam
(kloe-na'zi-pam)
Rx: Klonopin
Chemical Class: Benzodiazepine
Therapeutic Class: Anticonvulsant; anxiolytic
DEA Class: Schedule IV

CLINICAL PHARMACOLOGY
Mechanism of Action: CNS depressants via facilitation of inhibitory GABA at benzodiazepine receptor sites (BZ_1—associated with sleep; BZ_2—associated with memory, motor, sensory, and cognitive function); effects include muscle relaxation (spinal cord), anticonvulsant activity (brain stem), ataxia (cerebellum), emotional behavior (limbic and cortical areas), and anxiolytic effects (separate from general CNS depression); anticonvulsant activity: suppresses the spike and wave discharge in absence seizures (petit mal) and decreases the frequency, amplitude, duration, and spread of discharge in minor motor seizures
Pharmacokinetics
PO: Peak 1-3 hr; 88% bound to plasma proteins; metabolized by liver (principal metabolite is inactive), excreted in urine; $t_{1/2}$ 18-50 hr
INDICATIONS AND USES: Lennox-Gastaut syndrome (petit mal variant), akinetic and myoclonic seizures, absence seizures (petit mal) in patients who have failed to respond to succinimides; anxiety; panic disorder; restless legs,* Parkinsonian dysarthria,* multifocal tic disorders,* acute manic episodes of

* = non-FDA-approved use

bipolar affective disorder,* deafferentation pain syndromes,* schizophrenia (adjunctive therapy)*

DOSAGE

Adult

• PO 1.5 mg/day in 3 divided doses initially, may be increased 0.5-1 mg q3d until desired response or side effects, max 20 mg/day

Child <10 yr or <30 kg

• PO 0.01-0.03 mg/kg/day in 2-3 divided doses, not to exceed 0.05 mg/kg/day, may be increased 0.25-0.5 mg q3d until desired response, not to exceed 0.1-0.2 mg/kg/day

$ AVAILABLE FORMS/COST OF THERAPY

• Tab, Uncoated—Oral: 0.5 mg, 100's: **$66.58-$71.37;** 1 mg, 100's: **$75.95-$90.54;** 2 mg, 100's: **$105.25-$124.05**

CONTRAINDICATIONS: Severe liver disease, acute narrow-angle glaucoma

PRECAUTIONS: COPD, impaired renal function, abrupt discontinuation (may precipitate withdrawal), status epilepticus, elderly

PREGNANCY AND LACTATION: Pregnancy category C; episodes of prolonged apnea in the newborn, apparently related to clonazepam, have been reported; excreted into breast milk; monitor closely for CNS depression or apnea in nursing infant

SIDE EFFECTS/ADVERSE REACTIONS

CNS: Ataxia, behavioral changes, confusion, dizziness, *drowsiness,* headache, insomnia, slurred speech, suicidal tendencies, tremor

CV: Bradycardia, hypotension, palpitations

EENT: Abnormal eye movements, blurred vision, diplopia, nystagmus

GI: Anorexia, constipation, diarrhea, gastritis, nausea, polyphagia, sore gums, xerostomia

GU: Dysuria, enuresis, nocturia, urinary retention

HEME: Anemia, eosinophilia, ***leukocytosis, thrombocytopenia***

RESP: Congestion, dyspnea, respiratory depression

SKIN: Rash

INTERACTIONS

Drugs

3 *Disulfiram:* Increased serum clonazepam concentrations

3 *Valproic acid:* Increased occurrence of absence seizures

SPECIAL CONSIDERATIONS

• Up to 30% of patients have shown a loss of anticonvulsant activity, often within 3 mo of administration; dosage adjustment may reestablish efficacy

PATIENT/FAMILY EDUCATION

• Do not take more than prescribed amount, may be habit-forming

• Avoid driving, activities that require alertness; drowsiness may occur

• Avoid alcohol ingestion or other CNS depressants

• Do not discontinue medication abruptly after long-term use

MONITORING PARAMETERS

• Although relationship between serum concentrations and seizure control is not well established, proposed therapeutic concentrations are 20-80 ng/ml; potentially toxic concentrations >80 ng/ml

• Close attention to seizure frequency is important in order to detect the emergence of tolerance

---

clonidine
(klon'ih-deen)
Rx: Catapres, Catapres-TTS, Duraclon
Combinations
  Rx: with chlorthalidone
    (Chlorpres, Combipress)
Chemical Class: Imidazoline derivative
Therapeutic Class: Antihypertensive, centrally acting sympathoplegic

CLINICAL PHARMACOLOGY
Mechanism of Action: Centrally active antihypertensive: stimulates central α_2-adrenergic receptors resulting in reduced sympathetic outflow from the CNS to the heart, kidneys, and peripheral vasculature; decreases systolic and diastolic blood pressure and pulse; chronic therapy associated with only mild reductions or no change in cardiac output; plasma renin activity is unchanged or mildly reduced
Pharmacokinetics
PO: Bioavailability 65%-95%, peak effect 3-5 hr; duration 6-10 hr
TOP: Therapeutic plasma levels 2-3 days after initial application, drug released at constant rate for approximately 7 days; following removal, plasma levels persist for 8 hr then decline slowly over several days Metabolized in liver, excreted in urine (22% unchanged); $t_{1/2}$ 6-23 hr
INDICATIONS AND USES: Hypertension, alcohol withdrawal,* diabetic diarrhea,* Gilles de la Tourette syndrome,* hypertensive urgencies,* menopausal flushing,* opiate detoxification,* postherpetic neuralgia,* smoking cessation,* ulcerative colitis*; in combination with opiates for severe pain in cancer patients (epidural), surgery,* labor,* hyperhydrosis, spinal cord injury

spasticity, chorea, akathisia, restless leg syndrome, hemodynamic stabilization preoperatively,* postoperative shivering,* atropine/neostigmine tachycardia*
DOSAGE
Adult
• PO 0.1 mg bid initially, increase 0.1-0.2 mg/day if needed, max 2.4 mg/day (minimize sedation by giving majority of daily dose hs); TOP apply patch to hairless area of intact skin on upper arm or torso once q7d, rotate sites, start with TTS-1 (0.1 mg/24 hr) and increase after 1-2 wk if needed (using >2 TTS-3 systems usually does not improve efficacy)
• *Severe cancer pain:* 30 µg/hr via continuous epidural infusion; use caution with infusion rates >40 µg/hr
Child
• PO 5-25 µg/kg/day in divided doses q6h, increase at 5-7 day intervals
💲 AVAILABLE FORMS/COST OF THERAPY
• Tab, Uncoated—Oral: 0.1 mg, 100's: **$3.25-$69.67;** 0.2 mg, 100's: **$4.25-$106.58;** 0.3 mg, 100's: **$4.75-$133.75**
• Film, cont rel—Percutaneous: 0.1 mg/24 hr, 12's: **$113.47** (TTS-1): **$7.73** 0.2 mg/24 hr, 12's: **$191.03** (TTS-2): **$13.02;** 0.3 mg/24 hr, 4's **$88.33** (TTS-3): **$18.07**
• Inj—Epidural: 100 µg/ml, 10 ml: **$51.00**
PRECAUTIONS: Severe coronary insufficiency, recent MI, cerebrovascular disease, chronic renal failure, abrupt discontinuation (PO)
PREGNANCY AND LACTATION: Pregnancy category C; secreted into breast milk; hypotension has not been observed in nursing infants, although clonidine was found in the serum of the infants

* = non-FDA-approved use

SIDE EFFECTS/ADVERSE REACTIONS

Less severe with transdermal systems

CNS: Agitation, anxiety, delirium, depression, *dizziness,* dreams or nightmares, *drowsiness,* hallucinations, headache, insomnia, nervousness, restlessness, *sedation*

CV: Bradycardia, **CHF, dysrhythmias,** orthostatic hypotension, palpitations, Raynaud's phenomenon, rebound hypertension, tachycardia

GI: Anorexia, *constipation, dry mouth,* nausea, parotid pain, transient LFT elevations, vomiting

GU: Impotence, loss of libido, nocturia, urinary retention

METAB: Gynecomastia, transient elevation of blood glucose, weight gain

MS: Cramps of the lower limbs, fatigue, muscle or joint pain, weakness

SKIN: Alopecia, angioedema, hair thinning, pruritus, rash, transient localized skin reactions (TOP), urticaria

INTERACTIONS

Drugs

3 β*-blockers:* Rebound hypertension from clonidine withdrawal exacerbated by noncardioselective β-blockers

2 *Cyclic antidepressants:* Cyclic antidepressants may inhibit the antihypertensive response to clonidine

3 *Cyclosporine, tacrolimus:* Increased cyclosporine or tacrolimus concentrations

3 *Insulin:* Diminished symptoms of hypoglycemia

3 *Neuroleptics, nitroprusside:* Severe hypotension possible

Labs

• Growth hormone-stimulation test

SPECIAL CONSIDERATIONS
PATIENT/FAMILY EDUCATION

• Avoid hazardous activities, since drug may cause drowsiness

• Do not discontinue oral drug abruptly or withdrawal symptoms may occur (anxiety, increased BP, headache, insomnia, increased pulse, tremors, nausea, sweating)

• Response may take 2-3 days if drug is given transdermally

• Do not use OTC (cough, cold, or allergy) products unless directed by clinician

• Rise slowly to sitting or standing position to minimize orthostatic hypotension, especially elderly

• Dizziness, fainting, lightheadedness may occur during 1st few days of therapy

• May cause dry mouth; use hard candy, saliva product, or frequent rinsing of mouth

MONITORING PARAMETERS

• Blood pressure (posturally), blood glucose in patients with diabetes mellitus, confusion, mental depression

clopidogrel
(clo-pid'o-grill)
Rx: Plavix
Chemical Class: Thienopyridine
Therapeutic Class: Platelet aggregation inhibitor

CLINICAL PHARMACOLOGY

Mechanism of Action: Selectively and irreversibly inhibits ADP-induced platelet aggregation by inhibiting the binding of ADP to its receptors on platelets, thereby affecting ADP-dependent activation of the glycoprotein IIb/IIIa complex, the major site of platelet-fibrinogen binding

Pharmacokinetics

PO: Peak 1 hr; (significant antiaggregating activity in 2 hr); steady-state effect on bleeding time (1-2× baseline), 3-7 days; following discontinuation, baseline values return in 5 days; 50% absorbed (PO); clopidogrel is a prodrug that is activated by hepatic metabolism (CYP1A), to the major circulating metabolite, a carboxylic acid derivative, which is a CYP2C9 inhibitor; metabolite excreted in both feces and urine; $t_{1/2}$ of major metabolite, 8 hr

INDICATIONS AND USES: Reduction of atherosclerotic events (myocardial infarction, stroke, and vascular death) in patients with atherosclerosis documented by recent stroke, myocardial infarction, or established peripheral arterial disease; prevention of thrombosis following intracoronary stent placement*

DOSAGE
Adult
• PO 75 mg qd (no dosage adjustments for elderly patients or those with renal impairment)

§ AVAILABLE FORMS/COST OF THERAPY
• Tab, Film-coated—Oral: 75 mg, 90's: **$270.69**

CONTRAINDICATIONS: Active pathological bleeding; coagulation disorders; patients receiving anticoagulants or other antiplatelet agents

PRECAUTIONS: Previous hypersensitivity or other untoward effects related to ticlopidine; hypertension; hepatic or renal impairment; history of bleeding or hemostatic disorders; history of drug-related hematologic disorders; patients scheduled for major surgery; pregnancy

PREGNANCY AND LACTATION: Pregnancy category B; excreted into breast milk in rats

SIDE EFFECTS/ADVERSE REACTIONS
CNS: Dizziness, headache, ***intracranial bleeding***
CV: Hypertension

GI: Abdominal pain, diarrhea, dyspepsia, ***GI ulceration and hemorrhage,*** nausea
GU: Liver enzyme elevation
HEME: Neutropenia (uncommon), prolonged bleeding time, purpura
SKIN: Pruritus, rash, urticaria

INTERACTIONS
Drugs
3 *Fluvastatin:* Inhibition of hepatic metabolism (CYP2C9) of fluvastatin with increased risk of myositis; *in vitro* data
3 *Nonsteroidal antiinflammatory agents:* Increased bleeding risk
3 *Phenytoin:* Inhibition of hepatic metabolism (CYP2C9) of phenytoin and increased risk of toxicity; *in vitro* data
3 *Tamoxifen:* Inhibition of hepatic metabolism (CYP2C9) and increased tamoxifen effects; *in vitro* data
3 *Tolbutamide:* Inhibition of hepatic metabolism (CYP2C9) of tolbutamide with increased risk of hypoglycemia; *in vitro* data
3 *Torsemide:* Inhibition of hepatic metabolism (CYP2C9) of torsemide with enhanced diuretic effects; *in vitro* data; increased bleeding risk
3 *Warfarin:* Inhibition of hepatic metabolism (CYP2C9) of warfarin with enhanced hypoprothrombinemic effects; *in vitro* data; increased bleeding risk

SPECIAL CONSIDERATIONS
• Comparative studies indicate that the drug is at least effective as aspirin; comparisons with ticlopidine lacking, however, no frequent CBC monitoring necessary
• Should probably replace ticlopidine as an aspirin alternative
• 28× the cost of an equivalent supply of aspirin

PATIENT/FAMILY EDUCATION
• Inform clinician of signs and symptoms of bleeding, prior to sur-

---

* = non-FDA-approved use

gery, dental work; inform clinician of sore throat, fever, etc. (consider neutropenia)

---

clorazepate
(klor-az'e-pate)
Rx: Gen-Xene, Tranxene, Tranxene-SD
Chemical Class: Benzodiazepine
Therapeutic Class: Antianxiety agent; anticonvulsant
DEA Class: Schedule IV

CLINICAL PHARMACOLOGY
Mechanism of Action: CNS depressant via facilitation of inhibitory GABA at benzodiazepine receptor sites (BZ_1—associated with sleep; BZ_2—associated with memory, motor, sensory, and cognitive function); effects include muscle relaxation (spinal cord), anticonvulsant activity (brain stem), ataxia (cerebellum), emotional behavior (limbic and cortical areas), and anxiolytic effects (separate from general CNS depression)
Pharmacokinetics
PO: Onset 15 min, peak 1-2 hr, duration 4-6 hr; metabolized by liver to active metabolites, excreted by kidneys; $t_{1/2}$ 30-100 hr
INDICATIONS AND USES: Anxiety disorders, acute alcohol withdrawal, partial seizures (adjunctive therapy)
DOSAGE
Adult
• *Anxiety:* PO 7.5-15 mg bid-qid or as single qhs dose of 15-22.5 mg; lower doses may be indicated for elderly or debilitated patients
• *Alcohol withdrawal:* PO 30 mg initially, then 15 mg bid-qid on 1st day; gradually decrease dose over subsequent days
• *Seizure disorders:* PO 7.5 mg tid;

may increase by 7.5 mg/wk or less; not to exceed 90 mg/day
Child 9-12 yr
• *Seizure disorders:* PO 3.75-7.5 mg bid; increase by 3.75 mg at weekly intervals; max 60 mg/day in 2-3 divided doses

💲 AVAILABLE FORMS/COST OF THERAPY
• Tab, Uncoated—Oral: 3.75 mg, 100's: **$21.95-$158.26;** 7.5 mg, 100's: **$29.95-$196.90;** 15 mg, 100's: **$41.45-$267.14**
• Tab, Uncoated, SUS Action—Oral: 11.25 mg, 100's: **$418.81;** 22.5 mg, 100's: **$536.38**

CONTRAINDICATIONS: Narrow-angle glaucoma, psychosis
PRECAUTIONS: Elderly, debilitated, hepatic disease, renal disease, long-term use, history of drug abuse
PREGNANCY AND LACTATION: Pregnancy category D; excreted into breast milk; drug and metabolites may accumulate to toxic levels in nursing infant
SIDE EFFECTS/ADVERSE REACTIONS
CNS: Anterograde amnesia, anxiety, ataxia, *confusion,* depression, dizziness, *drowsiness,* fatigue, hallucinations, headache, hysteria, insomnia, psychosis, slurred speech, stimulation, tremor
CV: Bradycardia, ***cardiovascular collapse,*** hypertension, hypotension, orthostatic, tachycardia
EENT: Auditory disturbances, blurred vision, mydriasis, nystagmus
GI: Anorexia, constipation, diarrhea, dry mouth, nausea, vomiting
GU: Changes in libido, incontinence, menstrual irregularities, urinary retention
SKIN: Dermatitis, hair loss, hirsutism, itching, rash, urticaria
INTERACTIONS
Drugs
3 *Cimetidine:* Increased plasma

---

italic = common side effects   ***bold italic*** = life-threatening reactions

levels of clorazepate and/or active metabolites

3 *Disulfiram:* Increased serum clorazepate concentrations

3 *Ethanol:* Enhanced adverse psychomotor side effects of benzodiazepines

3 *Rifampin:* Reduced serum clorazepate concentrations

SPECIAL CONSIDERATIONS
• Do not use for everyday stress or for longer than 4 mo
• No advantage over diazepam

PATIENT/FAMILY EDUCATION
Do not discontinue medication abruptly after long-term use

---

clotrimazole

(kloe-trim′a-zole)
Rx: Topical: Lotrimin, Mycelex
Oral: Mycelex
Vaginal: Mycelex-G, Mycelex Twin Pack
OTC: Topical: Gynix Lotrimin AF, Mycelex OTC
Vaginal: Gyne-Lotrimin, Mycelex 7, Femcare
Combinations
  Rx: with betamethasone dipropionate (Lotrisone)
Chemical Class: Imidazole derivative
Therapeutic Class: Topical antifungal

CLINICAL PHARMACOLOGY
Mechanism of Action: Broadspectrum antifungal agent that inhibits growth of pathogenic dermatophytes, yeasts, and *Malassezia furfur;* exhibits fungistatic and fungicidal activity against isolates of *Trichophyton rubrum, T. mentagrophytes, Epidermophyton floccosum, Microsporum canis,* and *Candida* sp., including *C. albicans;* interferes with fungal DNA replication by binding sterols in fungal cell membrane, which increases permeability and causes leaking of cell nutrients

Pharmacokinetics
Well absorbed following oral administration, eliminated mainly as inactive metabolites; minimally absorbed following top and vag administration

INDICATIONS AND USES: Tinea pedis, tinea cruris, tinea corporis, tinea versicolor; *C. albicans* infection of the vagina, vulva, throat, mouth

DOSAGE
Adult and Child >3 yr
• PO 10 mg troche dissolved slowly 5×/day; TOP apply bid
Adult and Child >12 yr
• VAG 100 mg qhs for 7 days or 200 mg qhs for 3 days or 500 mg × 1 or 5 g (1 applicatorful) of 1% VAG cream qhs for 7-14 days

$ AVAILABLE FORMS/COST OF THERAPY
• Cre—Top: 1%, 15, 30, 45 g: **$5.44-$22.70**/30 g
• Cre—Vag: 1%, 45, 90 g: **$5.99-$29.50**/45 g
• Sol—Top: 1%, 10, 30 ml: **$16.20-$24.50**/30 ml
• Lotion—Top: 1%, 30 ml: **$25.65**
• Tab, Uncoated, SUS Action—Vag: 100 mg, 7's: **$5.99-$19.20**; 200 mg, 3's: **$8.65-$9.60**; 500 mg, 1's: **$13.88-$16.91**
• Troche—Buccal: 10 mg, 70's: **$73.26**

PREGNANCY AND LACTATION: Pregnancy category B; excretion in breast milk unknown

SIDE EFFECTS/ADVERSE REACTIONS
GI: Abdominal cramps, bloating
GU: Dyspareunia, urinary frequency
SKIN: Blistering, burning, peeling,

---

* = non-FDA-approved use

rash, skin fissures, stinging, urticaria

INTERACTIONS
Drugs
3 *Cyclosporine, Tacrolimus:* Clotrimazole troche administration may increase cyclosporine or tacrolimus concentrations

---

cloxacillin
(klox-a-sill'in)
Chemical Class: Isoxazolyl penicillin derivative, (penicillinase-resistant)
Therapeutic Class: Antibiotic

CLINICAL PHARMACOLOGY
Mechanism of Action: Inhibits bacterial wall synthesis; bactericidal
Pharmacokinetics
PO: Peak 1 hr, duration 6 hr, $t_{1/2}$ 30-60 min; metabolized in liver, excreted in urine and bile
INDICATIONS AND USES: Infections of the respiratory tract, skin and skin structure, bones and joints
Antibacterial spectrum usually includes:
• Gram-positive organisms: most gram-positive aerobic cocci, *Staphylococcus aureus, S. epidermidis* (except methicillin-resistant strains)
• Gram-negative organisms: Most gram-negative aerobic cocci
DOSAGE
Adult
• PO 250-500 mg q6h
Child
• PO 50-100 mg/kg/day in divided doses q6h, max 4 g/day
$ AVAILABLE FORMS/COST OF THERAPY
• Cap, Gel—Oral: 250 mg, 100's: **$22.95-$37.96**; 500 mg, 100's: **$40.00-$75.65**
• Powder, Reconst—Oral: 125 mg/5 ml, 200 ml: **$7.75**
PRECAUTIONS: Hypersensitivity

to cephalosporins, prolonged or repeated therapy
PREGNANCY AND LACTATION: Pregnancy category B
SIDE EFFECTS/ADVERSE REACTIONS
CNS: Anxiety, depression, fever, hallucinations, headache, twitching
GI: Abdominal pain, colitis, *diarrhea;* glossitis, increased AST, ALT; *nausea, vomiting*
GU: Hematuria, vaginitis
HEME: **Bone marrow depression,** eosinophilia, increased bleeding time
SKIN: Rash, urticaria
INTERACTIONS
Drugs
3 *Tetracyclines:* Possible inhibition of antibacterial activity of penicillins
Labs
• *False increase:* Urine amino acids
• *Interference:* 17-ketosteroids
SPECIAL CONSIDERATIONS
• Sodium content of 250 mg cap = 0.6 mEq; sodium content of 125 mg susp = 0.24 mEq

---

clozapine
(klo'za-peen)
Rx: Clozaril
Chemical Class: Dibenzodiazepine derivative
Therapeutic Class: Antipsychotic

CLINICAL PHARMACOLOGY
Mechanism of Action: Serotonin $5-HT_2$ > dopamine (D_2)-receptor antagonist; activity at several neurotransmitter systems: selective antagonist at limbic dopamine receptors (D_1, D_2, D_4, D_5) and serotonin receptors ($5-HT_2$, $5-HT_6$, $5-HT_7$); antagonism at alpha$_1$-adrenergic receptors; and activity at muscarinic, histamine H_1, or nicotinic recep-

italic = common side effects   ***bold italic*** = life-threatening reactions

tors; high sedation and anticholinergic effects; moderate orthostatic hypotension and weight gain; minimal extrapyramidal symptoms

Pharmacokinetics

PO: Peak 2.5 hr; 95% protein bound; completely metabolized by the liver, excreted in urine and feces (metabolites); $t_{1/2}$ 8-12 hr

INDICATIONS AND USES: Severely ill schizophrenic patients who fail to respond adequately to standard antipsychotic drug treatment

DOSAGE

Adult

• PO 12.5 mg qd-bid initially, increase by 25-50 mg/day to achieve a target range of 300-450 mg/day after 2 wk; increase prn by no more than 100 mg in 2 wk intervals; do not exceed 900 mg/day; use lowest dose to control symptoms

$ **AVAILABLE FORMS/COST OF THERAPY**

• Tab, Uncoated—Oral: 25 mg, 100's: **$121.68;** 100 mg, 100's: **$315.27**

NOTE: Available only through patient management system, combining WBC testing, patient monitoring, pharmacy and drug distribution services, all linked to compliance with required safety monitoring (1-800-448-5938)

CONTRAINDICATIONS: Myeloproliferative disorders, uncontrolled epilepsy, history of clozapine-induced agranulocytosis or severe granulocytopenia, severe CNS depression, comatose states, narrow-angle glaucoma

PRECAUTIONS: Cardiovascular disease, pulmonary disease, elderly, prostatic enlargement, hepatic disease, renal disease, general anesthesia, seizure disorders

PREGNANCY AND LACTATION: Pregnancy category B; may be excreted in breast milk, avoid breast feeding during clozapine therapy

SIDE EFFECTS/ADVERSE REACTIONS

CNS: Agitation, akathisia, akinesia, anxiety, ataxia, confusion, depression, disturbed sleep, *dizziness, drowsiness,* epileptiform movements, fatigue, headache, hyperkinesia, hypokinesia, insomnia, lethargy, myoclonic jerks, nightmares, restlessness, rigidity, *sedation, seizures,* slurred speech, syncope, tremor, *vertigo,* weakness

CV: Angina, cardiac abnormality, chest pain, ECG change, hypertension, hypotension, *tachycardia*

EENT: Blurred vision

GI: Abdominal discomfort, anorexia, constipation, diarrhea, dry mouth, heartburn, LFT abnormality, nausea, *salivation,* vomiting

GU: Abnormal ejaculation; incontinence; urinary urgency, frequency, retention

HEME: **Agranulocytosis,** eosinophilia, **leukopenia, neutropenia**

SKIN: Rash

MISC: Fever, weight gain

INTERACTIONS

Drugs

3 *Carbamazepine, phenytoin, primadone, valproic acid:* Considerable reduction in plasma clozapine concentrations

3 *Cimetidine, clarithromycin, troleandomycin:* Increased serum clozapine concentrations

3 *Diazepam:* Isolated cases of cardiorespiratory collapse have been reported

3 *Epinephrine:* Reversed pressor effects of epinephrine

2 *Erythromycin:* Increased serum clozapine concentrations

2 *Fluvoxamine:* Marked increase in plasma clozapine concentrations and side effects; increased risk of leukocytosis

SPECIAL CONSIDERATIONS

• The risk of agranulocytosis and seizures limits use to patients who have failed to respond or were unable to tolerate treatment with appropriate courses of standard antipsychotics

• Advise patients to report immediately the appearance of lethargy, weakness, fever, sore throat, malaise, mucous membrane ulceration, or other possible signs of infection

MONITORING PARAMETERS

• WBC at baseline and then qwk for the duration of treatment and for 4 wk after discontinuation

• Blood pressure, LFTs

---

codeine

(koe'deen)

Combinations

Rx: with acetaminophen (Tylenol no. 2, Tylenol no. 3, Tylenol no. 4); with aspirin (Empirin no. 3, Empirin no. 4)

OTC: with guaifenesin (Robitussin AC); with APAP (Capital, Aceta); with APAP butalbital, caffeine (Fioricet, Phenaphen); with aspirin (Fiorinal)

Chemical Class: Natural opium alkaloid; phenanthrene derivative
Therapeutic Class: Narcotic analgesic; antitussive
DEA Class: Schedule II (combinations: Schedule III or Schedule V [Elixir])

CLINICAL PHARMACOLOGY

Mechanism of Action: Narcotic agonist with activity at μ-receptors (supraspinal analgesia, euphoria, respiratory and physical depression,

miosis, and reduced GI motility), κ-receptors (pentazocine-like spinal analgesia, sedation, and miosis), and Δ-receptors (dysphoria, psychotomimetic effects [e.g., hallucinations], and respiratory and vasomotor stimulation caused by drugs with antagonist activity); compared to morphine, less analgesia, constipation, respiratory depression, sedation, emesis, and physical dependence; more antitussive effect

Pharmacokinetics
IM: Onset 10-30 min, peak 30-60 min
PO: Onset 30-60 min, peak 60-90 min
Metabolized in liver to morphine, excreted in urine (unchanged and metabolites); $t_{1/2}$ 2½-3½ hr

INDICATIONS AND USES: Mild to moderate pain, antitussive

DOSAGE

Adult
• *Analgesia:* PO/IM/SC 15-60 mg q4h prn
• *Antitussive:* PO 10-20 mg q4-6h; not to exceed 120 mg/day

Child
• *Analgesia:* PO/IM/SC 0.5-1 mg/kg/dose q4-6h prn, max 60 mg/dose
• *Antitussive:* PO 1-1.5 mg/kg/day in divided doses q4-6h prn; max 60 mg/dose

$ **AVAILABLE FORMS/COST OF THERAPY**

• Inj, Sol—IM, SC: 15 mg/ml, 2 ml: **$0.91-$1.26**; 30 mg/ml, 2 ml: **$1.01-$1.38**; 60 mg/ml, 1 ml: **$1.26**
• Sol—Oral: 15 mg/5 ml, 500 ml: **$35.78**
• Tab, Uncoated—Oral: 15 mg, 100's: **$37.41**; 30 mg, 100's: **$40.27-$64.76**; 60 mg, 100's: **$73.77-$119.81**

PRECAUTIONS: Head injury, increased intracranial pressure, acute abdominal conditions, elderly, severe impairment of hepatic or renal

---

function, hypothyroidism, Addison's disease, prostatic hypertrophy, urethral stricture, history of drug abuse

PREGNANCY AND LACTATION: Pregnancy category C (category D if used for prolonged periods or in high doses at term); use during labor produces neonatal respiratory depression; passes into breast milk in very small amounts; compatible with breast feeding

SIDE EFFECTS/ADVERSE REACTIONS

CNS: Agitation, dependency, dizziness, *drowsiness,* lethargy, restlessness, *sedation*

CV: Bradycardia, orthostatic hypotension, palpitations, tachycardia

GI: Anorexia, constipation, nausea, vomiting

GU: Urinary retention

RESP: Respiratory depression

SKIN: Flushing, rash, urticaria

INTERACTIONS

Drugs

3 *Barbiturates:* Additive respiratory and CNS depressant effects

3 *Antihistamines, chloral hydrate, glutethimide, methocarbamol:* Enhanced depressant effects

3 *Cimetidine:* Increased respiratory and CNS depression

3 *Ethanol:* Additive CNS effects

2 *Quinidine:* Inhibited analgesic effect of codeine

Labs

• *Increase:* Urine morphine

• False elevatons of amylase and lipase

SPECIAL CONSIDERATIONS PATIENT/FAMILY EDUCATION

• Minimize nausea by administering with food and remain lying down following dose

• Do not administer agonist/antagonist analgesics (i.e., pentazocine, nalbuphine, butorphanol, dezocine, buprenorphine) to patient who has received a prolonged course of co-deine (a pure agonist). In opioid-dependent patients, mixed agonist/antagonist analgesics may precipitate withdrawal symptoms

---

colchicine

(kol'chi-seen)
Colsalide
Combinations
  Rx: with probenicid
    (Proben-C, Colbenemid)
Chemical Class: Colchicum autumnale alkaloid
Therapeutic Class: Antigout agent

CLINICAL PHARMACOLOGY

Mechanism of Action: Antiinflammatory: decreases leukocyte motility, phagocytosis, and lactate production; binds to microtubular protein; interferes with mitotic spindles in granulocytes; prevents release of glycoprotein that causes joint pain and inflammation

Pharmacokinetics

PO: Peak ½-2 hr, $t_{1/2}$ 20 min $V_d = 2L/kg$; deacetylated in liver; excreted in feces

INDICATIONS AND USES: Gouty arthritis (prevention, treatment), amyloidosis,* aphthous stomatitis,* pseudogout,* Behçet's syndrome,* familial Mediterranean fever,* alcoholic cirrhosis*

DOSAGE

Adult

• *Prevention of gouty arthritis:* PO 0.5-1.8 mg qd depending on severity; IV 0.5-1 mg qd-bid

• *Treatment of gouty arthritis:* PO 0.5-1.2 mg, then 0.5-1.2 mg q1h, until pain decreases or side effects occur; IV 2 mg over 2-5 min, then 0.5 mg q6h, not to exceed 4 mg/day; no colchicine should be given by any route for at least 7 days after a full course of IV therapy (4 mg)

---

* = non-FDA-approved use

AVAILABLE FORMS/COST OF THERAPY

• Inj, Sol—IV: 1 mg/2 ml, 2 ml: **$5.04**
• Tab, Uncoated—Oral: 0.5 mg, 100's: **$32.20-$34.51**; 0.6 mg, 100's: **$3.95-$33.25**

CONTRAINDICATIONS: Serious GI, renal, hepatic, cardiac disorders; blood dyscrasias

PRECAUTIONS: Elderly, lactation, children; may induce ileal vitamin B_{12} malabsorption; extravasation may lead to shock

PREGNANCY AND LACTATION: Pregnancy category D (known teratogen)

SIDE EFFECTS/ADVERSE REACTIONS

CNS: Peripheral neuritis
GI: Anorexia, cramps, *diarrhea, malaise,* metallic taste, *nausea, vomiting*
GU: Azotemia, hematuria, oliguria, reversible azoospermia
HEME: **Agranulocytosis, aplastic anemia, pancytopenia, thrombocytopenia**
MS: Myopathy (more common in persons with renal impairment)
SKIN: Alopecia, dermatitis, erythema, pruritus, purpura

INTERACTIONS

Drugs

3 *Cyclosporine, tacrolimus:* Increased serum level of cyclosporine or tacrolimus

3 *Erythromycin, clarithromycin, troleandomycin:* Potential for severe colchicine toxicity

Labs

• *Interference:* Urinary 17-hydroxycorticosteroids

SPECIAL CONSIDERATIONS
MONITORING PARAMETERS

• CBC, platelets, reticulocytes before and during therapy (q3mo)

---

colestipol

(koe-les´ti-pole)
Rx: Colestid
Chemical Class: Bile acid sequestrant
Therapeutic Class: Antilipemic

CLINICAL PHARMACOLOGY

Mechanism of Action: Combines with bile acids to form insoluble complex that is excreted through feces; increased fecal loss of bile acids leads to increased oxidation of cholesterol to bile acids, increased hepatic uptake of LDLs, and decreased serum LDL levels; serum triglyceride levels may increase or remain unchanged

Pharmacokinetics

PO: Not absorbed; excreted in feces

INDICATIONS AND USES: Primary hypercholesterolemia, xanthomas, pruritus due to biliary obstruction,* diarrhea due to bile acids*

DOSAGE

Adult

• PO 5-30 g qd in 2-4 divided doses, ac and hs; increase dose by 5 g at 1-2 mo intervals

AVAILABLE FORMS/COST OF THERAPY

• Granule—Oral: 5 g/scoop, 500 g: **$99.05**
• Granule—Oral: 5 g/7.5 g flavored, 500 g: **$63.51**
• Packet—Oral: 5 g/pkt, 90's: **$146.66**
• Packet—Oral: 5 g/7.5 g pkt, 60's: **$99.61**
• Tab, Uncoated—Oral: 1 g, 120's: **$46.08**

CONTRAINDICATIONS: Biliary obstruction

PRECAUTIONS: Lactation; children; bleeding disorders; may prevent absorption of fat-soluble vitamins such as A, D, E, and K; pro-

---

longed use may lead to the development of hyperchloremic acidosis;
PREGNANCY AND LACTATION: Pregnancy category B
SIDE EFFECTS/ADVERSE REACTIONS

CNS: Dizziness, headache
GI: Abdominal pain, constipation, fecal impaction, flatulence, hemorrhoids, nausea, peptic ulcer, steatorrhea, vomiting
*HEME: **Bleeding***
METAB: Decreased vitamin A, D, E, K absorption; hyperchloremic acidosis
SKIN: Irritation of perianal area, rash
INTERACTIONS
Drugs
⊟ *Acetaminophen, Amiodarone, Corticosteroids, Diclofenac, Digitalis glycosides, Furosemide, Methotrexate, Metronidazole, Thiazide diuretics, Thyroid hormones, Valproic acid:* Cholestyramine reduces interacting drug concentrations and probably subsequent therapeutic response
⊟ *Oral anticoagulants:* Inhibition of hypoprothrombinemic response; colestipol might be less likely to interact
SPECIAL CONSIDERATIONS
• Bile acid sequestrant choice should be based on cost and patient acceptability
• Give all other medications 1 hr before colestipol or 4 hr after colestipol to avoid poor absorption

---

colfosceril
(kohl-foss'sir-ill)
Rx: Exosurf Neonatal
Chemical Class: Phospholipid
Therapeutic Class: Synthetic lung surfactant

CLINICAL PHARMACOLOGY
Mechanism of Action: Prevents alveoli from collapsing during expiration by lowering surface tension between air and alveolar surfaces
Pharmacokinetics
Administered intratracheally; distributed to all lobes, distal airways, and alveolar spaces; alveolar $t_{1/2}$ 12 hr
INDICATIONS AND USES: Prophylaxis for infants with birth weights of <1350 g who are at risk for developing respiratory distress syndrome (RDS); prophylaxis for infants with birth weights >1350 g who have evidence of pulmonary immaturity; rescue treatment for infants who have developed RDS
DOSAGE
Child
• *Prophylaxis:* Intratracheal 5 ml/kg as soon as possible after birth and q12h for 2 doses to infants remaining on mechanical ventilation
• *Rescue treatment:* Intratracheal administer in two 5 ml/kg doses; give initial dose after diagnosis of RDS, then second dose in 12 hr
• Administered in two 2.5 ml/kg half-doses, instilled over 1 to 2 min in small bursts timed with inspiration; change body position between half-doses
$ AVAILABLE FORMS/COST OF THERAPY
• Inj, Lyphl-Susp—Intratracheal: 108 mg/10 ml vial: **$719.14**
PRECAUTIONS: Colfosceril can rapidly affect pO_2, pCO_2, and lung compliance; pulmonary hemorrhage; mucous plugs; do not suction within 2 hr of dose
SIDE EFFECTS/ADVERSE REACTIONS
*RESP: **Apnea,** congenital pneumonia, interstitial emphysema, **pneumothorax,** pulmonary air leak, pulmonary hemorrhage
SPECIAL CONSIDERATIONS
MONITORING PARAMETERS
• Continuous ECG and transcuta-

neous oxygen saturation monitoring during installation
• Frequent ABG sampling is necessary to prevent postdosing hyperoxia and hypocarbia

---

corticotropin (ACTH)
(kor-ti-koe-troe′pin)
Rx: Acthar Gel, H.P.
Chemical Class: Adrenocorticotropic hormone
Therapeutic Class: Adrenal corticosteroid

CLINICAL PHARMACOLOGY
Mechanism of Action: Stimulates adrenal cortex to produce cortisol, corticosterone, several weakly androgenic steroids, and, to a limited extent, aldosterone
Pharmacokinetics
IV/IM/SC: Onset <1 hr; duration 2-4 hr, repository form has duration up to 3 days; plasma $t_{1/2}$ <20 min; excreted in urine; cortisol response dependent on total dose and total time of administration
INDICATIONS AND USES: Testing adrenocortical function; conditions in which the anti-inflammatory effect of glucocorticoids is desired; ACTH has no advantage over glucocorticoids except perhaps in multiple sclerosis and dermatomyositis/polymyositis
DOSAGE
Adult
• *Testing of adrenocortical function:* IM/SC up to 80 U in divided doses qid; IV 10-25 U in 500 ml D_5W given over 8 hr
• *Anti-inflammatory:* SC/IM 40 U in divided doses qid or 40 U q12-24h (gel/repository form)
• *Acute exacerbations of multiple sclerosis:* IM 80-120 U qd (gel/repository form) for up to 3 wk

Child
• *Anti-inflammatory:* SC/IM 1.6 U/kg in divided doses qid or 0.8 U/kg q12-24h (gel/repository form)
$ AVAILABLE FORMS/COST OF THERAPY
• Inj, Lyphl-Sol—IM, SC: 25 U/vial, 1's: **$21.82;** 40 U/vial, 1's: **$30.60-$32.09**
• Inj, Repos Gel—80 U/ml, 5 ml: **$47.98**
CONTRAINDICATIONS: Systemic fungal infections, smallpox vaccination, ocular herpes simplex, primary adrenocortical insufficiency/hyperfunction
PRECAUTIONS: Latent TB, recent significant intercurrent illness or surgery, scleroderma, osteoporosis, CHF, hypertension, hepatic disease, peptic ulcer disease, hyperthyroidism, childbearing-age women, psychiatric disorders, myasthenia gravis, posterior subcapsular cataracts, systemic infection
PREGNANCY AND LACTATION: Pregnancy category C; monitor infants with significant in utero exposure for hyperadrenalism. Unknown if excreted in breast milk
SIDE EFFECTS/ADVERSE REACTIONS
CNS: Behavioral changes, depression, dizziness, euphoria, headache, insomnia, mood swings, pseudotumor cerebri, psychosis, *seizures*
CV: **CHF,** hyperpertension
EENT: Increased intraocular pressure, posterior subcapsular cataracts
GI: Nausea, **pancreatitis,** peptic ulcer, ulcerative esophagitis, vomiting
METAB: Calcium loss, Cushingoid symptoms, growth retardation in children, hyperglycemia, hypokalemic alkalosis, menstrual irregularities, negative nitrogen balance due

---

italic = common side effects   ***bold italic*** = life-threatening reactions

to protein catabolism, sodium retention

MS: Arthralgia, aseptic necrosis of femoral and humeral heads, compression fractures, muscle atrophy, myalgia, osteoporosis, steroid myopathy, weakness

SKIN: Acne, ecchymoses, hirsutism, hyperpigmentation, *impaired wound healing,* petechiae, rash, suppression of skin test reactions, sweating, urticaria

Labs
• *False increase:* 11-hydroxy-corticosteroids

SPECIAL CONSIDERATIONS
• May mask infections
• Intercurrent illness may require increased corticosteroids
• Drug-induced adrenocorticoid insufficiency may be minimized by gradual systemic dosage reduction; relative insufficiency may exist for up to 1 yr after discontinuation; therefore, be prepared to supplement in situations of stress

---

cortisone
(kor'ti-sone)
Rx: Cortone
Chemical Class: Glucocorticoid
Therapeutic Class: Systemic corticosteroid

CLINICAL PHARMACOLOGY
Mechanism of Action: Decreases inflammation by depressing migration of polymorphonuclear leukocytes and activity of endogenous mediators of inflammation; has many profound metabolic effects, possesses mineralocorticoid activity
Pharmacokinetics
PO: Peak 2 hr, duration 1½ days
IM: Absorbed slowly over 24-48 hr
INDICATIONS AND USES: Antiinflammatory or immunosuppressive agent in the treatment of a variety of diseases of hematologic, allergic, inflammatory, neoplastic and autoimmune origin; in replacement doses for primary or secondary adrenocortical insufficiency

DOSAGE
Adult
• PO 25-300 mg qd or q2d, titrated to patient response

▣ AVAILABLE FORMS/COST OF THERAPY
• Tab, Uncoated—Oral: 5 mg, 50's: **$7.10;** 10 mg, 100's: **$26.23;** 25 mg, 100's: **$7.07-$64.70**

CONTRAINDICATIONS: Systemic fungal infections
PRECAUTIONS: Psychosis, diabetes mellitus, glaucoma, osteoporosis, seizure disorders, ulcerative colitis (intestinal perforation), latent tuberculosis or amebiasis (reactivation of disease), hypertension, CHF, myasthenia gravis (if used with anticholinesterase agents), renal disease, esophagitis, peptic ulcer
PREGNANCY AND LACTATION: Pregnancy category C; excreted in breast milk
SIDE EFFECTS/ADVERSE REACTIONS
CNS: Behavioral changes, depression, dizziness, euphoria, headache, insomnia, mood swings, pseudotumor cerebri, psychosis, *seizures*
CV: CHF, embolism, hypertension, thrombophlebitis
EENT: Fungal infections, increased intraocular pressure, posterior subcapsular cataracts
GI: Intestinal perforation, nausea, *pancreatitis,* peptic ulcer, ulcerative esophagitis, vomiting
HEME: Thrombocytopenia
METAB: Calcium loss, Cushingoid symptoms, growth retardation in children, hyperglycemia, hypokalemic alkalosis, menstrual irregulari-

---

ties, negative nitrogen balance due to protein catabolism, sodium retention

MS: Arthralgia, aseptic necrosis of femoral and humeral heads, compression fractures, muscle atrophy, myalgia, osteoporosis, steroid myopathy, weakness

SKIN: Acne, ecchymoses, hirsutism, hyperpigmentation, *impaired wound healing,* petechiae, rash, suppression of skin test reactions, sweating, urticaria

INTERACTIONS
Drugs

3 *Aminoglutethamide:* Enhanced elimination of corticosteroids; marked reduction in corticosteroid response; increased clearance of prednisone; doubling of dose may be necessary

3 *Antidiabetics:* Increased blood glucose

3 *Barbiturates, carbamazepine:* Reduced serum concentrations of corticosteroids; increased clearance of prednisone

3 *Cholestyramine, colestipol:* Possible reduced absorption of corticosteroids

3 *Cyclosporine:* Possible increased concentration of both drugs, seizures

3 *Erythromycin, troleandomycin, clarithromycin, ketoconazole:* Possible enhanced steroid effect

3 *Estrogens, oral contraceptives:* Enhanced effects of corticosteroids

3 *Isoniazid:* Reduced plasma concentrations of isoniazid

3 *IUDs:* Inhibition of inflammation may decrease contraceptive effect

3 *NSAIDs:* Increased risk GI ulceration

3 *Rifampin:* Reduced therapeutic effect of corticosteroids; may reduce hepatic clearance of prednisone

3 *Salicylates:* Subtherapeutic salicylate concentrations possible

SPECIAL CONSIDERATIONS
• Increased dose of rapidly acting corticosteroids may be necessary in patient subjected to unusual stress
• May mask infections
• Do not give live virus vaccines to patients on prolonged therapy
• Patients on chronic steroid therapy should wear medical bracelet
• Drug-induced adrenocorticoid insufficiency may be minimized by gradual systemic dosage reduction; relative insufficiency may exist for up to 1 yr after discontinuation
• Symptoms of adrenal insufficiency include: nausea, fatigue, anorexia, hypotension, hypoglycemia, fever

MONITORING PARAMETERS
• Serum K and glucose
• Growth in children on prolonged therapy
• Edema, blood pressure, CHF, mental status, weight

cosyntropin
(koe-sin-troe′pin)
Rx: Cortrosyn
Chemical Class: ACTH derivative
Therapeutic Class: Adrenal corticosteroid

CLINICAL PHARMACOLOGY
Mechanism of Action: Stimulates adrenal cortex to produce cortisol; cosyntropin contains the first 24 of the 39 amino acids of natural ACTH; 0.25 mg of cosyntropin stimulates the adrenal cortex maximally and to the same extent as 25 units of natural ACTH

Pharmacokinetics
IV/IM: Onset 5 min, peak 1 hr, duration 2-4 hr

INDICATIONS AND USES: Testing adrenocortical function

DOSAGE

Adult

• IM/IV 0.25 mg

Child

• IM/IV age >2 yr 0.25 mg; age <2 yr 0.125 mg

💲 **AVAILABLE FORMS/COST OF THERAPY**

• Inj, Dry-Sol—IM, IV: 0.25 mg: **$15.40**

PREGNANCY AND LACTATION: Pregnancy category C

SIDE EFFECTS/ADVERSE REACTIONS

SKIN: Flushing, pruritus, rash, urticaria

SPECIAL CONSIDERATIONS

MONITORING PARAMETERS

• Check plasma cortisol levels at baseline and 30-60 min after drug is administered; normal adrenal function indicated by an increase of at least 70 µg/L or a measured level of 20 µg

---

co-trimoxazole (sulfamethoxazole and trimethoprim)

(koe-trye-mox'a-zole)

Rx: Bactrim, Bethaprim, Cotrim, Comoxol, Septra, Sulfatrim, Uroplus

Chemical Class: Sulfonamide derivative (sulfamethoxazole); dihydrofolate reductase inhibitor (trimethoprim)

Therapeutic Class: Antibiotic

CLINICAL PHARMACOLOGY

Mechanism of Action: The combination blocks 2 consecutive steps in the bacterial biosynthesis of essential nucleic acids and proteins

Pharmacokinetics

PO: Rapidly absorbed, peak 1-4 hr;

$t_{1/2}$ (SMX) 10-12 hr, (TMP) 8-11 hr; excreted in urine (metabolites and unchanged); 70% (SMX), 44% (TMP) bound to plasma proteins

INDICATIONS AND USES: Infections of the urinary tract, otitis media, acute exacerbation of chronic bronchitis, enteritis, *Pneumocystis carinii* pneumonia (treatment and prophylaxis), traveler's diarrhea, cholera,* salmonella-type infections,* nocardiosis,* prostatitis*

Antibacterial spectrum usually includes:

• Gram-positive organisms: *Streptococcus pneumoniae, Staphylococcus aureus,* Group A β-hemolytic streptococci (some strains may not respond to co-trimoxazole in tonsillopharyngeal infections), *Nocardia*

• Gram-negative organisms: *Acinetobacter, Enterobacter, Escherichia coli, Klebsiella pneumoniae, Proteus mirabilis, Salmonella, Shigella, H. influenzae, H. ducreyi, N. gonorrhoeae,* indole-positive *Proteus* (70% of isolates), *Providencia* and *Serratia* (50% of isolates)

• Protozoa: *Pneumocystis carinii*

DOSAGE

Adult

• *UTIs, shigellosis, acute exacerbations of chronic bronchitis, acute otitis media:* PO 160 mg TMP/800 mg SMX q12h for 10-14 days (3 days for uncomplicated cystitis in otherwise healthy females, 5 days for shigellosis); IV 8-10 mg TMP/kg/day in 2-4 divided doses q6, 8, or 12h for up to 14 days (5 days for shigellosis)

• *Traveler's diarrhea:* PO 160 mg TMP/800 mg SMX q12h for 5 days

• *Pneumocystis carinii pneumonitis:* PO 20 mg TMP/kg/day divided q6h for 14 days; IV 15-20 mg TMP/kg/day divided q6-8h for 14 days

• *Pneumocystis carinii pneumonia*

---

* = non-FDA-approved use

prophylaxis: PO 160 mg TMP/800 mg SMX qd or 3×/wk

Dosage adjustment for impaired renal function: CrCl >30 ml/min, usual regimen; CrCl 15-30 ml/min, ½ usual regimen; CrCl <15 ml/min, not recommended

Child >2 mo

• *UTIs, shigellosis, and acute otitis media:* PO 8 mg TMP/kg/day divided q12h (1 ml/kg susp divided q12h)

• *Pneumocystis carinii pneumonitis:* PO/IV 15-20 mg TMP/kg/day divided q6h for 14 days

🔋 AVAILABLE FORMS/COST OF THERAPY

• Inj, Conc-Sol—IV: 80 mg SMX/16 mg TMP/5 ml: **$2.79-$6.47**

• Susp—Oral: 200 mg SMX/40 mg TMP/5 ml, 100, 150, 200, 480 ml: **$6.19-$30.89**/200 ml

• Tab, Uncoated—Oral: 400 mg SMX/80 mg TMP, 100's: **$12.46-$102.49;** 800 mg SMX/160 mg TMP, 100's: **$11.00-$76.14**

CONTRAINDICATIONS: Megaloblastic anemia due to folate deficiency, infants <2 mo

PRECAUTIONS: Streptococcal pharyngitis, elderly patients receiving diuretics, renal and hepatic function impairment, possible folate deficiency (elderly, chronic alcoholics, anticonvulsant therapy, malabsorption syndrome, malnutrition), G-6-PD deficiency

PREGNANCY AND LACTATION: Pregnancy category C; **do not use at term,** may cause kernicterus in the neonate; not recommended in the neonatal nursing period because sulfonamides excreted in breast milk may cause kernicterus

SIDE EFFECTS/ADVERSE REACTIONS

CNS: Anxiety, aseptic meningitis, ataxia, chills, depression, fatigue, hallucinations, headache, insomnia, *seizures,* vertigo

GI: Abdominal pain, anorexia, diarrhea, glossitis, hepatitis, *nausea,* pancreatitis, *pseudomembranous enterocolitis,* stomatitis, *vomiting*

GU: Crystalluria, *renal failure, toxic nephrosis*

HEME: Agranulocytosis, eosinophilia, *hemolytic anemia, leukopenia, methemoglobinemia, neutropenia, thrombocytopenia*

RESP: Cough, shortness of breath

SKIN: Dermatitis, erythema, pain and inflammation at inj site; *photosensitivity, rash, Stevens-Johnson syndrome,* urticaria

MISC: Drug fever

INTERACTIONS

Drugs

3 *Dapsone:* Increased dapsone and trimethoprim concentrations

3 *Disulfiram, metronidazole:* Co-trimoxazole contains 10% ethanol, disulfiram reaction possible

3 *Methotrexate:* Elevated methotrexate concentrations and toxicity

3 *Oral anticoagulants:* Enhanced hypoprothrombinemic response to warfarin and possibly other oral anticoagulants

3 *Oral hypoglycemics:* Increased potential for hypoglycemia

3 *Phenytoin:* Increased phenytoin concentrations

Labs

• *False increase:* Creatinine (due to interference with assay), urobilinogen, urine protein, plasma α-aminonitrogen

• *False positive:* Urinary glucose test

• *False decrease:* Serum creatine kinase

SPECIAL CONSIDERATIONS

• Pay special attention to complaints of skin rash, especially those involving mucous membranes (could signify early Stevens-Johnson syndrome), sore throat, mouth sores, fever, or unusual bruising or bleeding

MONITORING PARAMETERS

• Baseline and periodic CBC for patients on long-term or high-dose therapy

---

cromolyn

(kroe'moe-lin)
Inhalation **Rx:** Intal
Opthalmic **Rx:** Crolom, Opticrom
Oral **Rx:** Gastrocrom
Nasal **OTC:** Nasalcrom
Chemical Class: Mast cell stabilizer
Therapeutic Class: Antiasthmatic, inhaled antiinflammatory, nasal anti-inflammatory, ophthalmic antiinflammatory

---

CLINICAL PHARMACOLOGY
Mechanism of Action: Stabilizes membrane of the sensitized mast cell
Pharmacokinetics
Minimal oral absorption, 8% of total cromolyn dose absorbed after inhalation; after inhalation, peak level 15 min, elimination $t_{1/2}$ 80 min; excreted unchanged in feces

INDICATIONS AND USES: Allergic rhinitis; allergic conjunctivitis; bronchial asthma; prevention of acute bronchospasm induced by environmental pollutants or exercise; systemic mastocytosis; prevention of food allergy

DOSAGE
Adult
• *Allergic conjunctivitis:* Ophth sol 1-2 gtt 4-6 times/day
• *Allergic rhinitis:* Nasal sol 1 spray each nostril tid-qid
• *Bronchial asthma:* INH 2 puffs qid via inhaler or 20 mg qid via Spinhaler

• *Exercise-induced bronchospasm:* INH 2 puffs via inhaler or 20 mg via Spinhaler <1 hr before exercise
• *Systemic mastocytosis:* PO 200 mg qid
Child
• *Allergic conjunctivitis:* Age >2 yr ophth sol 1-2 gtt 4-6 times/day
• *Allergic rhinitis:* Age >6 yr nasal sol 1 spray each nostril tid-qid
• *Exercise-induced bronchospasm:* Age 2-5 yr 20 mg qid via nebulized sol; age >5 yr INH 2 puffs qid via inhaler ½ hr before exercise
• *Bronchial asthma:* Age 2-5 yr 20 mg qid via nebulized sol; age >5 yr INH 2 puffs qid via inhaler or 20 mg qid via Spinhaler
• *Systemic mastocytosis:* Age <2 yr PO 5 mg/kg qid; age 2-12 yr PO 100 mg qid

💲 AVAILABLE FORMS/COST OF THERAPY
• Sol—INH: 10 mg/ml, 2 ml 60's: **$42.00-$55.86**
• Aer, Spray—INH: 800 µg/spray, 112 sprays: **$45.30;** 200 sprays: **$72.07**
• Concentrate—Oral: 100 mg/5 ml, 96's: **$139.96**
• Sol—Nasal: 5.2 mg/spray, 100 sprays: **$8.39;** 200 sprays: **$13.91**
• Sol—Ophth: 4%, 10 ml: **$36.47-$44.56**

PRECAUTIONS: Renal disease, hepatic disease, child <5 yr

PREGNANCY AND LACTATION: Pregnancy category B; excretion in breast milk unknown

SIDE EFFECTS/ADVERSE REACTIONS
CNS: Dizziness, headache, neuritis
EENT: Burning eyes, cough, *hoarseness,* nasal burning, nasal congestion, nasal stinging, throat irritation
GI: Anorexia, *bitter taste,* diarrhea, dry mouth, nausea, vomiting
GU: Dysuria, frequency

MS: Joint pain or swelling
RESP: Cough

SPECIAL CONSIDERATIONS
PATIENT/FAMILY EDUCATION
• Therapeutic effect in asthma may take up to 4 wk

---

crotamiton
(kroe-tam'i-ton)
Rx: Eurax
Chemical Class: Synthetic chloroformate salt
Therapeutic Class: Scabicide

CLINICAL PHARMACOLOGY
Mechanism of Action: Toxic to *Sarcoptes scabiei*
Pharmacokinetics
Active topically; systemic absorption after topical use is unknown
INDICATIONS AND USES: Scabies in adults, scabies in children,* pruritic skin
DOSAGE
Adult and Child
• TOP (cre, lotion), massage into skin of entire body from chin down; repeat application 24 hr later

[$] AVAILABLE FORMS/COST OF THERAPY
• Lotion—Top: 10%, 60 ml: **$13.04**
• Cre—Top: 10%, 60 g: **$12.23**
CONTRAINDICATIONS: Inflammation, abrasions, or breaks in skin or mucous membranes
PRECAUTIONS: Children
PREGNANCY AND LACTATION:
Pregnancy category C
SIDE EFFECTS/ADVERSE REACTIONS
SKIN: Contact dermatitis, irritation, itching, rash
SPECIAL CONSIDERATIONS
PATIENT/FAMILY EDUCATION
• 60 g is sufficient for 2 applications/adult
• Reapply locally during 48 hr treatment period after handwashing, etc

• A cleansing bath should be taken 48 hr after the last application
• After treatment, use topical corticosteroids to decrease contact dermatitis, antihistamines for pruritus; pruritus may continue for 4-6 wk

---

cyanocobalamin (vitamin B$_{12}$)
(sye-an-oh-koe-bal'a-min)
Rx: Cyanoject, Cyomin
Chemical Class: Synthetic B complex vitamin
Therapeutic Class: Vitamin supplement; blood modifier

CLINICAL PHARMACOLOGY
Mechanism of Action: Needed for nucleoprotein and myelin synthesis, protein and carbohydrate metabolism, normal growth, normal erythropoiesis
Pharmacokinetics
PO: Irregularly absorbed from the distal small gut; requires intrinsic factor but can be overcome with dosage increases (i.e., mean absorption rate of oral cyanocobalamin by patients with pernicious anemia is 1.2%; daily cobalamin turnover rate is about 2 µg/day, so oral doses of 100-250 µg are sufficient); peak 8-12 hr
IM: Peak 1 hr
Stored in liver, kidneys, stomach; 50%-90% excreted in urine; crosses placenta
INDICATIONS AND USES: Vitamin B$_{12}$ deficiency, pernicious anemia, vitamin B$_{12}$ malabsorption syndrome, Schilling test; increased requirements with pregnancy, thyrotoxicosis, hemolytic anemia, hemorrhage, renal and hepatic disease; prevention and treatment of cyanide toxicity associated with nitroprusside*

---

italic = common side effects   ***bold italic*** = life-threatening reactions

DOSAGE
Adult
• *Deficiency:* PO 250 μg qd × 5-10 days, maintenance 250-500 μg qd; IM/SC 30-100 μg qd 5-10 days, maintenance 100-200 μg IM qmo
• *Pernicious anemia/malabsorption syndrome:* IM 100-1000 μg qd × 2 wk, then 100-1000 μg IM qmo
• *Schilling test:* IM 1000 μg in one dose

Child
• *Deficiency:* Total IM/SC dose is 1-5 mg given in single 100 μg doses qd over 2 or more wk; maintenance 60 μg IM qmo or more
• *Pernicious anemia/malabsorption syndrome:* IM 100-500 μg qd over 2 wk, then 60 μg IM/SC qmo
• *Schilling test:* IM 1000 μg in one dose

💲 AVAILABLE FORMS/COST OF THERAPY
• Inj, Sol—IM, IV, SC: 1,000 μg/ml: **$0.15-$0.52**
• Tab—Oral: 100 μg, 100's: **$1.91**; 250 μg, 100's: **$2.38-$3.90**; 500 μg, 100's: **$3.05**; 1,000 μg, 60's: **$3.05**
• Tab, extended release—Oral: 1,500 μg, 60's: **$3.46-$6.18**
• Loz—Oral: 2,000 μg, 50's: **$3.36**
• Tab—SL: 2,500 μg, 50's: **$4.61**

CONTRAINDICATIONS: Optic nerve atrophy

PREGNANCY AND LACTATION: Pregnancy category C; excreted in breast milk in concentrations that approximate the mother's serum; compatible with breast feeding

SIDE EFFECTS/ADVERSE REACTIONS
CNS: Flushing, optic nerve atrophy
CV: **CHF,** peripheral vascular thrombosis, *pulmonary edema*
GI: *Diarrhea*
METAB: Hypokalemia
SKIN: Itching, pain at injection site, rash

SPECIAL CONSIDERATIONS
• Recommended dietary allowance: 0.5-2.6 μg/day depending on age and status (i.e., more during pregnancy and lactation)
• Nutritional sources: egg yolks, fish, organ meats, dairy products, clams, oysters

MONITORING PARAMETERS
• CBC with reticulocyte count after 1st wk of therapy

---

cyclandelate
(sye-klan'da-late)
Rx: Cyclandelate
Therapeutic Class: Peripheral vasodilator

CLINICAL PHARMACOLOGY
Mechanism of Action: Musculotropic; acts directly to relax vascular smooth muscle; no significant adrenergic-stimulating or adrenergic-blocking actions

Pharmacokinetics
PO: Onset 15 min, peak 1½ hr, duration 4 hr

INDICATIONS AND USES: Possibly effective: intermittent claudication, thrombophlebitis (to control associated vasospasm and muscular ischemia), Raynaud's phenomenon, ischemic cerebrovascular disease, arteriosclerosis obliterans, nocturnal leg cramps, dementia of cerebrovascular origin,* memory disorders,* migraine prophylaxis,* vertigo,* tinnitus and visual disturbances attributable to chronic cerebrovascular insufficiency,* diabetic peripheral polyneuropathy*

DOSAGE
Adult
• PO 200 mg qid, not to exceed 400 mg qid, maintenance dose is 400-800 mg/day in 2-4 divided doses

---

* = non-FDA-approved use

$ AVAILABLE FORMS/COST OF THERAPY
- Cap—Oral: 200 mg, 100's: **$5.25-$31.95;** 400 mg, 100's: **$7.75-$59.95**

PRECAUTIONS: Glaucoma, recent MI, hypertension, severe obliterative coronary artery or cerebrovascular disease ("steal" syndrome, diseased areas compromised by vasodilatory effects elsewhere)

PREGNANCY AND LACTATION: Pregnancy category C

SIDE EFFECTS/ADVERSE REACTIONS

CNS: Dizziness, headache, paresthesias, weakness
CV: Tachycardia
GI: Eructation, heartburn, nausea
HEME: Increased bleeding time (rare)
SKIN: Flushing, sweating

---

cyclobenzaprine
(sye-kloe-ben'za-preen)
Rx: Flexeril
Chemical Class: Tricyclic amine
Therapeutic Class: Skeletal muscle relaxant

CLINICAL PHARMACOLOGY
Mechanism of Action: Reduction of tonic somatic motor activity in the brain stem, producing skeletal muscle relaxant activity without interfering with muscle function; effects similar to tricyclic antidepressants

Pharmacokinetics
PO: Onset 1 hr, peak 3-8 hr, duration 12-24 hr, $t_{1/2}$ 1-3 days; metabolized by liver, excreted in urine

INDICATIONS AND USES: Adjunct to rest and physical therapy for relief of muscle spasm and pain in musculoskeletal conditions; fibrositis syndrome*

DOSAGE
Adult
- PO 10 mg tid × 1 wk (range 20-40 mg/day), max 60 mg/day, use should not exceed 3 wk

$ AVAILABLE FORMS/COST OF THERAPY
- Tab, Coated—Oral: 10 mg, 100's: **$8.91-$106.50**

CONTRAINDICATIONS: Acute recovery phase of MI, dysrhythmias, heart block, CHF, child <12 yr, intermittent porphyria, thyroid disease

PRECAUTIONS: History of urinary retention, angle-closure glaucoma, increased intraocular pressure, patients taking anticholinergic medication, addictive personality, elderly; lowers seizure threshold

PREGNANCY AND LACTATION: Pregnancy category B; no data available, but closely related tricyclic antidepressants are excreted into breast milk

SIDE EFFECTS/ADVERSE REACTIONS

CNS: Asthenia, confusion, depression, *dizziness, drowsiness,* headache, insomnia, nervousness, paresthesia, tremor, *weakness*
CV: **Dysrhythmias,** postural hypotension, tachycardia
EENT: Diplopia, temporary loss of vision
GI: Constipation, *dry mouth,* dyspepsia, hiccups, *nausea,* unpleasant taste, vomiting
GU: Change in libido, frequency, urinary retention
SKIN: Facial flushing, fever, pruritus, rash, sweating

INTERACTIONS
Drugs
3 *Droperidol, fluoxetine:* A patient receiving cyclobenzaprine and fluoxetine developed ventricular

---

italic = common side effects   ***bold italic*** = life-threatening reactions

tachycardia and fibrillation after droperidol was added; relative contribution of each drug to the adverse effect unclear

❷ *MAOIs:* Hyperpyretic crisis, severe convulsions, and deaths have occurred in patients receiving closely related tricyclic antidepressants and MAOIs; separate use by 14 days

Labs

• *Interference:* Serum amitriptyline assay

SPECIAL CONSIDERATIONS

• Avoid use in elderly due to anticholinergic side effects

PATIENT/FAMILY EDUCATION

• Use caution with alcohol, other CNS depressants

• Avoid with hazardous activities if drowsiness or dizziness occur

---

cyclopentolate

(sye-kloe-pen'toe-late)

Rx: AK-Pentolate, Cylate, Cyclogyl, Ocu-Pentolate

Combinations

Rx: with phenylephrine (Cyclomydril)

Chemical Class: Tertiary amine

Therapeutic Class: Mydriatic; cycloplegic; ophthalmic anticholinergic

---

CLINICAL PHARMACOLOGY

Mechanism of Action: Blocks response of iris sphincter muscle and muscle of accommodation of ciliary body to cholinergic stimulation; results in mydriasis and paralysis of accommodation (cycloplegia)

Pharmacokinetics

OPHTH: Peak 30-60 min (mydriasis), 25-74 min (cycloplegia), duration ¼-1 day

INDICATIONS AND USES: Cycloplegic refraction, mydriasis

DOSAGE

Adult

• OPHTH SOL 1 gtt of a 0.5%-2% sol, then 1 gtt in 5 min if necessary

Child >6 yr

• OPHTH SOL 1 gtt of a 0.5%-2% sol, then 1 gtt in 5 min of a 0.5%-1% sol if necessary

💲 **AVAILABLE FORMS/COST OF THERAPY**

• Sol—Opht: 0.5%, 15 ml: **$25.75;** 1%, 2, 15 ml: **$5.63-$8.75**/2 ml; 2%, 2, 15 ml: **$7.44-$11.75**/2 ml

CONTRAINDICATIONS: Infants <3 mo, narrow-angle glaucoma

PRECAUTIONS: Elderly (more risk of increased intraocular pressure), infants, children with spastic paralysis or brain damage

PREGNANCY AND LACTATION: Pregnancy category C

SIDE EFFECTS/ADVERSE REACTIONS

CNS: Ataxia, behavior disturbances, confusion, disorientation, failure to recognize people, *seizures,* hallucinations, irritability, psychotic reaction, restlessness, somnolence

CV: Tachycardia

EENT: Blurred vision, conjunctivitis, eye dryness, increased intraocular pressure, photophobia, temporary burning sensation on instillation

GI: Abdominal discomfort, abdominal distention (in infants), dry mouth, vomiting

MISC: Bladder distension, dry skin, fever, flushing, irregular pulse, respiratory depression

SPECIAL CONSIDERATIONS
PATIENT/FAMILY EDUCATION

• Review method of instillation: no more than one drop; apply pressure to lacrimal sac for 1 min following installation

• Do not touch dropper to eye

---

cyclophosphamide

(sye-kloe-foss'fa-mide)
Rx: Cytoxan, Neosar
Chemical Class: Synthetic
nitrogen mustard
Therapeutic Class: Antineo-
plastic

CLINICAL PHARMACOLOGY

Mechanism of Action: Active metabolites alkylate DNA, RNA, thus
interfering with growth of susceptible, rapidly proliferating malignant cells (mechanism is thought to
involve cross-linking of tumor cell
DNA); activity is not cell cycle phase
specific

Pharmacokinetics

PO: Bioavailability >75%

IV: Peak, 2-3 hr (as metabolites)
Metabolized by liver, excreted in
urine (5%-25% unchanged); $t_{1/2}$ 3-12
hr; 60% bound to plasma proteins

INDICATIONS AND USES:

• Malignant disease: Used concurrently or sequentially with other antineoplastic drugs for lymphomas,
leukemias, and other malignancies

• Nonmalignant disease: Biopsy
proven "minimal change" nephrotic
syndrome in children; severe rheumatic conditions* (Wegener's gran-
ulomatosis, steroid-resistant vascu-
litides, progressive rheumatoid arthritis, systemic lupus erythematosus, polyarteritis nodosa, polymyositis); multiple sclerosis*

DOSAGE

Adult

• *Malignant disease:* PO initially 1-5
mg/kg/day, maintenance is 1-5 mg/
kg/day; IV initially 40-50 mg/kg in
divided doses over 2-5 days, maintenance 10-15 mg/kg q7-10 days, or
3-5 mg/kg q3 days

Child

• *Malignant disease:* PO/IV 2-8

mg/kg or 60-250 mg/m² in divided
doses for 6 or more days; maintenance 10-15 mg/kg q7-10 days or
30 mg/kg q3-4wk; dose should be
reduced by half when bone marrow
depression occurs

• *Nephrotic syndrome:* PO 2.5 to 3
mg/kg/day × 60-90 days

💲 AVAILABLE FORMS/COST OF THERAPY

• Inj, Lyphl-Sol—IV: 1, 2 g/vial:
$51.43/g; 100, 200, 500, mg/vial:
$6.45/100 mg

• Tab, Uncoated—Oral: 25 mg,
100's: **$212.34;** 50 mg, 100's:
$389.68

CONTRAINDICATIONS   Suppressed bone marrow function

PRECAUTIONS: Radiation therapy

PREGNANCY AND LACTATION:
Pregnancy category D; excreted in
breast milk; contraindicated because
of potential for adverse effects re-
lating to immune suppression,
growth, and carcinogenesis

SIDE EFFECTS/ADVERSE REACTIONS

CNS: Dizziness, headache

CV: **Cardiotoxicity** (high doses)

GI: Colitis, *diarrhea,* **hepatotoxicity,** *nausea, vomiting, weight loss*

GU: Amenorrhea, azoospermia, hematuria, hemorrhagic cystitis, neoplasms, *ovarian fibrosis, sterility,*

HEME: **Leukopenia, myelosuppression, pancytopenia, thrombocytopenia**

METAB: Syndrome of inappropriate
antidiuretic hormone (SIADH)

RESP: Fibrosis

SKIN: Alopecia, dermatitis

INTERACTIONS

Drugs

3 *Allopurinol:* Increased cyclophosphamide toxicity

3 *Digoxin:* Decreased digoxin absorption from tablets; Lanoxicaps
and elixir not affected

---

italic = common side effects   ***bold italic*** = life-threatening reactions

3 *Succinylcholine:* Prolonged neuromuscular blockade

3 *Warfarin:* Inhibited hypoprothrombinemic response to warfarin

SPECIAL CONSIDERATIONS
MONITORING PARAMETERS
• CBC, differential, platelet count qwk; withhold drug if WBC is <4000 or platelet count is <75,000
• Renal function studies: BUN, UA, serum uric acid; urine CrCl before, during therapy
• I&O; report fall in urine output ≤30 ml/hr

---

cycloserine
(sye-kloe-ser′een)
Rx: Seromycin
Chemical Class: Streptomyces orchidaceus product
Therapeutic Class: Antituberculosis agent; antibiotic

CLINICAL PHARMACOLOGY
Mechanism of Action: Inhibits cell wall synthesis in susceptible strains of gram-positive and gram-negative bacteria and in *Mycobacterium tuberculosis*
Pharmacokinetics
PO: Peak 4-8 hr, therapeutic levels 25-30 µg/ml, blood levels <30 µg/ml minimizes toxicity; 65% excreted unchanged in urine, remaining metabolized to unknown substances; crosses placenta
INDICATIONS AND USES: Pulmonary and extrapulmonary tuberculosis (like all antituberculosis drugs, cycloserine should be administered in conjunction with other effective chemotherapy and not as the sole therapeutic agent); acute UTI caused by susceptible strains of gram-positive and gram-negative bacteria, especially *Enterobacter* spp. and *E. coli* (when more conventional therapy has failed and when the organism has been demonstrated to be susceptible to the drug)

DOSAGE
Adult
• PO 250 mg q12h × 2 wk, then 250 mg q8h × 2 wk, then 250 mg q6h if there are no signs of toxicity; not to exceed 1 g/day
Child
• PO 10-20 mg/kg/day q12h (max 0.75-1 g); individualize doses

$ AVAILABLE FORMS/COST OF THERAPY
• Cap, Gel—Oral: 250 mg, 40's: **$153.05**

CONTRAINDICATIONS: Seizure disorders, severe renal disease, alcoholism (chronic), depression, severe anxiety, psychosis
PRECAUTIONS: Children, mild renal impairment, anemia
PREGNANCY AND LACTATION: Pregnancy category C; excreted into breast milk (72% of serum levels); compatible with breast feeding

SIDE EFFECTS/ADVERSE REACTIONS
CNS: Aggression, anxiety, confusion, depression, drowsiness, headache, lethargy, psychosis, *seizures,* tremors
CV: CHF
HEME: Leukocytosis, megaloblastic anemia, vitamin B_{12}, folic acid deficiency
SKIN: Dermatitis, photosensitivity

INTERACTIONS
Drugs
3 *Isoniazid:* Increased risk of CNS toxicity

SPECIAL CONSIDERATIONS
• L-enantiomer (1-cycloserine) in Gaucher's disease (Orphan Drug)
• Pyridoxine may prevent neurotoxicity (200-300 mg/day)

PATIENT/FAMILY EDUCATION
• Avoid concurrent alcohol

MONITORING PARAMETERS

• Mental status closely and liver function tests qwk

---

cyclosporine

(sye-kloe-spor'in)

Rx: Neoral, Sandimmune, SangCya

Chemical Class: Cyclic peptide

Therapeutic Class: Immunosuppressant

CLINICAL PHARMACOLOGY

Mechanism of Action: Produces immunosuppression by inhibiting T-lymphocytes (mainly T-helper cells, but T-suppressor cells may also be suppressed); also inhibits lymphokine production and release including interleukin-2; does not cause bone marrow suppression

Pharmacokinetics

PO: Variable bioavailability (4%-89%), peak 3.5 hr; 90% protein bound (lipoproteins); $t_{1/2}$ (terminal) 25 hr; metabolized in liver (mixed function oxidase enzymes) to 17 metabolites, only 0.1% left unchanged; excretion primarily biliary-feces, 0.1% excreted in urine

INDICATIONS AND USES: PO/IV prophylaxis of organ rejection in kidney, liver, and heart allogeneic transplants in conjunction with adrenal corticosteroids; prophylaxis of organ rejection in pancreas, bone marrow, and heart/lung transplantation.* Also used (at dosage 1-10 mg/kg/day) in: severe psoriasis; alopecia areata*; aplastic anemia*; atopic dermatitis*; Behçet's disease*; biliary cirrhosis*; Crohn's disease*; dermatomyositis*; Graves' ophthalmopathy*; insulin-dependent diabetes mellitus*; lupus nephritis*; multiple sclerosis*; myasthenia gravis*; nephrotic syndrome*; pemphigus and pemphigoid*; polymyositis*; psoriatic arthritis*; pulmonary sarcoidosis*; pyoderma gangrenosum*; rheumatoid arthritis*; ulcerative colitis*; uveitis*; Orphan Drug status: ophth keratoconjunctivitis sicca with Sjogren's syndrome; graft rejection following keratoplasty; corneal-melting syndromes (i.e., Mooren's ulcer)

DOSAGE

Adult and Child

• PO 15 mg/kg several hr before surgery, then daily for 2 wk, reduce dosage by 2.5 mg/kg/wk to 5-10 mg/kg/day (adjust based on blood levels); IV 5-6 mg/kg several hr before surgery, then daily, switch to PO form as soon as possible

💲 AVAILABLE FORMS/COST OF THERAPY

Sandimmune dosage forms:

• Cap, Elastic—Oral; 25 mg, 100's; **$165.43;** 100 mg, 100's: **$660.50**

• Inj, Sol—IV: 50 mg/ml, 5 ml: **$291.57**

• Sol—Oral: 100 mg/ml, 50 ml: **$330.04**

Neoral dosage forms:

• Cap (soft gel), for micro emulsion: 25 mg, 100's: **$148.53;** 100 mg, 100's: **$593.50**

• Sol—Oral, for micro emulsion: 100 mg/5 ml, 50 ml: **$322.83**

CONTRAINDICATIONS: Hypersensitivity to Cremophor EL (Sandimmune dosage forms)

PRECAUTIONS: Renal disease, hepatic disease, concurrent nephrotoxic drugs; anaphylaxis possible with 1st IV dose; malabsorption syndromes

PREGNANCY AND LACTATION: Pregnancy category C; excreted into breast milk, avoid nursing.

SIDE EFFECTS/ADVERSE REACTIONS

CNS: Headache, tremors

---

italic = common side effects   ***bold italic*** = life-threatening reactions

CV: Hypertension (50% of renal transplants; most cardiac transplants)
GI: Diarrhea, *gum hyperplasia,* hepatotoxicity, nausea, *oral Candida,* pancreatitis, vomiting
GU: Albuminuria, hematuria, proteinuria, **renal failure**
HEME: **Leukopenia**
METAB: Hypomagnesemia (related to neurotoxicity)
SKIN: Acne, *hirsutism,* rash

INTERACTIONS
Drugs

☒ *Allopurinol, amiodarone, chloroquine, clarithromycin, clonidine, clotrimazole, oral contraceptives, erythromycin, fluconazole, griseofulvin, itraconazole, ketoconazole, miconazole, roxithromycin, ticlopidine:* Increased cyclosporine levels, potential for toxicity

☒ *Aminoglycosides, amphotericin B, colchicine, enalapril, melphalan, sulfonamides:* Additive nephrotoxicity with cyclosporine

❷ *Anabolic steroids:* Increased cyclosporine levels, potential for toxicity

☒ *Barbiturates, carbamazepine, nafcillin, pyrazinamide, phenytoin, sulfonamides:* Reduced cyclosporine levels, potential for therapeutic failure

☒ *Calcium channel blockers:* Diltiazem, verapamil increase cyclosporine levels; isradipine, nifedipine, nitrendipine do not interact

☒ *Cisapride, metoclopramide:* Increased bioavailability and serum levels of single-dose cyclosporine

☒ *Digitalis glycosides:* Cyclosporine in patients stabilized on digitalis leads to increased levels and potential toxicity

☒ *Doxorubicin, imipenem:* CNS toxicity

☒ *HMG-CoA reductase inhibitors:* Increased risk of reversible myopathy

☒ *Methotrexate:* Increased toxicity of both agents

☒ *NSAIDs:* Increased risk of cyclosporine nephrotoxicity

❷ *Rifampin:* Reduced cyclosporine levels, potential for therapeutic failure

SPECIAL CONSIDERATIONS
• Neoral has increased bioavailability compared to Sandimmune (do NOT use interchangeably)

PATIENT/FAMILY EDUCATION
• Oral sol may be mixed with milk, chocolate milk, or orange juice to improve palatability. Do not mix with grapefruit juice (increased cyclosporine levels).

MONITORING PARAMETERS
• Renal function studies: BUN, creatinine q mo during treatment, 3 mo after treatment
• Liver function studies and serum levels during treatment
• Blood level monitoring: maintenance of 24-hr trough levels of 250-800 ng/ml (whole blood, RIA) or 50-300 ng/ml (plasma, RIA) should minimize side effects and rejection events

---

cyclothiazide
(cy-clo-thi'a-zide)
Rx: Anhydron
Chemical Class: Sulfonamide derivative
Therapeutic Class: Antihypertensive; thiazide diuretic

Note: Removed from the market voluntarily by manufacturer

CLINICAL PHARMACOLOGY
Mechanism of Action: Alters renal tubular electrolyte reabsorption; acts on distal tubule, increasing excretion of water, sodium, chloride, potassium, magnesium; renal and extrarenal antihypertensive effects;

---

decreased urinary calcium excretion

Pharmacokinetics

PO: Onset <6 hr, peak effect 7-12 hr, duration of effect 18-24 hr, rapid absorption; eliminated unchanged via kidneys

INDICATIONS AND USES: Edema, hypertension, renal calculi,* diabetes insipidus*

DOSAGE

Adult

• 2 mg qd (max 6 mg qd)

Child

• 20-40 μg/kg/day

$ AVAILABLE FORMS/COST OF THERAPY

• Tab, Plain Coated—Oral: 2 mg, 100's: **$29.28**

CONTRAINDICATIONS: Anuria

PRECAUTIONS: Hypokalemia, renal disease (CrCl <35 ml/min), hepatic disease, gout, diabetes mellitus, elderly

PREGNANCY AND LACTATION: Pregnancy category C; excreted into breast milk

SIDE EFFECTS/ADVERSE REACTIONS

CNS: Dizziness, headache, mood or mental changes, paresthesias, vertigo

CV: Irregular heartbeat, orthostatic hypotension, weak pulse

GI: Anorexia, constipation, cramping, diarrhea, dry mouth, gastric irritation, increased thirst, jaundice, nausea, ***pancreatitis,*** vomiting

GU: Decreased sexual ability

METAB: Gout, hyperglycemia, hyperuricemia, *hypokalemia*

MS: Muscle cramps or pain, tiredness, weakness

SKIN: Hives, skin rash

INTERACTIONS

Drugs

3 *Antidiabetics:* Increased dosage requirements due to increased glucose levels

3 *Calcium:* Increased risk for development of milk-alkali syndrome

3 *Carbenoxolone:* Additive potassium wasting; severe hypokalemia

3 *Cholestyramine, colestipol:* Reduced absorption

3 *Diazoxide:* Hyperglycemia

3 *Digitalis glycosides:* Diuretic-induced hypokalemia increases risk of digitalis toxicity

3 *Lithium:* Increased lithium levels, potential toxicity

3 *Methotrexate:* Increased risk for bone marrow toxicity

SPECIAL CONSIDERATIONS

• Ineffective with decreased renal function (CrCl <40 ml/min)

• No clear clinical advantage over less expensive thiazides (i.e., hydrochlorothiazide)

---

cyproheptadine

(si-proe-hep'ta-deen)

Rx: Periactin

Chemical Class: Piperidine derivative

Therapeutic Class: Antihistamine

CLINICAL PHARMACOLOGY

Mechanism of Action: Decreases allergic response by blocking histamine at H_1-receptors; also a serotonin antagonist

Pharmacokinetics

PO: Duration 4-6 hr; metabolized in liver, excreted by kidneys (40% unchanged)

INDICATIONS AND USES: Perennial and seasonal allergic rhinitis, vasomotor rhinitis, allergic conjunctivitis; allergic skin manifestations of urticaria and angioedema; cold urticaria; dermatographism; adjunctive anaphylactic therapy; appetite stimulant*; cluster headaches*; SSRI-induced sexual dysfunction*

---

italic = common side effects   ***bold italic*** = life-threatening reactions

DOSAGE

Adult

• PO 4 mg tid-qid, not to exceed 0.5 mg/kg/day

Child

• PO (0.25 mg/kg/day); 2-6 yr 2 mg bid-tid, not to exceed 12 mg/day; 7-14 yr 4 mg bid-tid, not to exceed 16 mg/day

⚡ AVAILABLE FORMS/COST OF THERAPY

• Syr—Oral: 2 mg/5 ml, 480 ml: **$6.38-$29.87**
• Tab, Uncoated—Oral: 4 mg, 100's: **$1.59-$45.16**

CONTRAINDICATIONS: Acute asthma attack, lower respiratory tract disease

PRECAUTIONS: Increased intraocular pressure due to closed-angle glaucoma, renal disease, cardiac disease, bronchial asthma, seizure disorder, stenosed peptic ulcers, prostatic hypertrophy, bladder neck obstruction, elderly

PREGNANCY AND LACTATION: Pregnancy category B; excreted in breast milk

SIDE EFFECTS/ADVERSE REACTIONS

CNS: Anxiety, confusion, *dizziness, drowsiness,* euphoria, fatigue, neuritis, paresthesia, poor coordination

CV: Hypotension, palpitations, tachycardia

EENT: Blurred vision, dilated pupils; dry nose, throat, mouth; nasal stuffiness; tinnitus

GI: Anorexia, *constipation,* diarrhea, dry mouth, nausea, vomiting, weight gain

GU: Dysuria, frequency, *retention*

RESP: Chest tightness, increased thick secretions, wheezing

SKIN: Photosensitivity, rash, urticaria

MISC: Increased appetite

INTERACTIONS

Drugs

3 *Fluoxetine:* Potential for worsening of depression when cyproheptodine added to fluoxetine therapy

Labs

• *False positive:* Urine tricyclic antidepressant assay

---

dalteparin

(doll'teh-pare-in)

Rx: Fragmin

Chemical Class: Depolymerized heparin derivative (low molecular weight heparin)

Therapeutic Class: Anticoagulant

CLINICAL PHARMACOLOGY

Mechanism of Action: Enhances the inhibition of Factor Xa and thrombin by binding to and accelerating antithrombin activity; preferentially inhibits Factor Xa; activated partial thromboplastin time (PTT) not affected

Pharmacokinetics

SC: Peak activity 4 hr; renal elimination $t_{1/2}$ 1.47-2.5 hr (prolonged in renal failure)

INDICATIONS AND USES: Prophylaxis against deep vein thrombosis (DVT), which may lead to pulmonary embolism (PE), in patients undergoing abdominal surgery who are at risk for thromboembolic complications and following hip replacement surgery (>40 yr of age, obese, undergoing surgery under general anesthesia lasting longer than 30 min, malignancy, history of DVT or PE); unstable angina/non-Q-wave MI; treatment of venous thromboembolism*

DOSAGE

Adult

• Prevention of DVT, abdominal sur-

---

* = non-FDA-approved use

gery: SC 2,500 IU qd starting 1-2 hr prior to surgery and for 5-10 days postoperatively; high-risk patients (e.g., malignancy) should receive 5,000 IU the evening before surgery, then qd for 5-10 days postoperatively

Prevention of DVT, hip replacement surgery: SC 2,500 IU within 2 hr before surgery, 2nd dose of 2,500 IU in evening of the day of surgery (≥6 hr after 1st dose), omit 2nd dose if surgery performed in evening; on 1st postoperative day begin 5,000 IU SC qd for 5-10 days; alternatively 5,000 IU can be administered evening prior to surgery followed by 5,000 IU qd for 5-10 days starting the evening of surgery

Treatment of DVT: SC 200 IU/kg qd or 100 IU/kg q12h; initiate warfarin therapy concurrently and continue dalteparin for a minimum of 5 days and until therapeutic oral anticoagulant effect has been achieved (INR 2-3)

Unstable angina/non-Q-wave MI: SC 120 IU/kg (max 10,000 IU) q12h with PO ASA (75-165 mg qd); continue until patient clinically stabilized (5-8 days)

§ AVAILABLE FORMS/COST OF THERAPY
• Sol—SC: 2500 anti-Factor Xa/0.2 ml: **$13.95**; 5000 anti-Factor Xa/0.2 ml: **$23.71**; 10,000 anti-Factor Xa/9.5 ml: **$428.00**

CONTRAINDICATIONS: Active major bleeding, thrombocytopenia associated with positive *in vitro* tests for antiplatelet antibody in the presence of dateparin, known hypersensitivity to pork products

PRECAUTIONS: History of heparin-induced thrombocytopenia; severe uncontrolled hypertension, bacterial endocarditis, congenital or acquired bleeding disorders, active ulceration and angiodysplastic gas-

trointestinal disease; hemorrhagic stroke or shortly after brain, spinal, or ophthalmological surgery; bleeding diathesis, thrombocytopenia or platelet defects; severe liver or kidney insufficiency; hypertensive or diabetic retinopathy; recent gastrointestinal bleeding; neuraxial anesthesia

PREGNANCY AND LACTATION: Pregnancy category B

SIDE EFFECTS/ADVERSE REACTIONS
HEME: Hemorrhage, ***thrombocytopenia***
SKIN: Pain at injection site, skin necrosis

DRUG INTERACTIONS
Drug
3 *Aspirin:* Increased risk of hemorrhage
3 *Oral anticoagulants:* Additive anticoagulant effects

SPECIAL CONSIDERATIONS
• Cannot be used interchangeably (unit for unit) with unfractionated heparin or other low molecular weight heparins

MONITORING PARAMETERS
• CBC with platelets, stool occult blood, urinalysis
• Monitoring aPTT is not required

---

danaparoid
(da-nap′ar-oid)
Rx: Orgaran
Chemical Class: Low-molecular weight heparinoid consisting of heparan sulfate, dermatan sulfate and chondroitin sulfate
Therapeutic Class: Anticoagulant

CLINICAL PHARMACOLOGY
Mechanism of Action: Inactivates factor Xa via a catalytic effect on antithrombin activity; factor IIa in-

hibition also occurs, but is substantially less than that seen with unfractionated heparin (anti-Xa/anti-IIa ratio >20:1 compared to 1:1 with unfractionated heparin); has only minor effects on platelet function

Pharmacokinetics

SC: Peak anti-Xa activity 2-5 hr, bioavailability approaches 100%; not metabolized in liver; renal excretion accounts for up to 50% of total plasma clearance of anti-Xa activity; elimination $t_{1/2}$ based on plasma anti-Xa activity 18-28 hr

INDICATIONS AND USES: Prevention of deep vein thrombosis (DVT) in patients undergoing elective total hip replacement surgery; heparin-induced thrombocytopenia*

DOSAGE

Adult

• SC 750 anti-Xa units bid for 7-10 days with the first dose given 1-4 hr prior to surgery; postoperative dose should not be given sooner than 2 hr after surgery

• Heparin-induced thrombocytopenia: IV 2,250 U bolus (1,500 U if <60 kg; 3,000 U if 75-90 kg; 3,750 U if >90 kg), followed by 400 U/hr for 4 hr, then 300 U/hr for 4 hr, then 150-200 U/hr to maintain anti-Xa levels between 0.5-0.8 U/ml; continue until platelet counts recover

$ **AVAILABLE FORMS/COST OF THERAPY**

• Inj, Sol—SC: 750 U./0.6 mL, **$108.00**/amp; **$113.40**/syringe

CONTRAINDICATIONS: Hypersensitivity to sulfites; severe hemorrhagic diathesis (hemophilia and idiopathic thrombocytopenic purpura); cerebrovascular hemorrhage or other active hemorrhagic states (except disseminated intravascular coagulation); positive *in vitro* aggregation test in presence of danaparoid in patients with Type II

thrombocytopenia; hypersensitivity to pork products

PRECAUTIONS: Previous hypersensitivity to unfractionated heparin or low-molecular weight heparins; thrombocytopenia; recent childbirth; peptic ulcer disease; severe uncontrolled hypertension; diabetic retinopathy; acute bacterial endocarditis; renal impairment; liver disease; recent lumbar puncture; vasculitis; neuraxial analgesia

PREGNANCY AND LACTATION: Pregnancy category B

SIDE EFFECTS/ADVERSE REACTIONS

CV: Chest pain, ECG changes, tachycardia

HEME: Hemorrhage, *thrombocytopenia*

SKIN: Injection site hematoma, pain at injection site, rash, wound infection

INTERACTIONS

Drugs

3 *Aspirin:* Increased risk of hemorrhage

3 *Oral anticoagulants:* Additive anticoagulant effects

SPECIAL CONSIDERATIONS

• Offers advantage over low-molecular weight heparins for the management of heparin-induced thrombocytopenia

• Does not offer a significant advantage over unfractionated heparin with respect to bleeding complications for any indication

MONITORING PARAMETERS

• CBC with platelets, stool occult blood, urinalysis

• Monitoring aPTT is not required

---

* = non-FDA-approved use

danazol
(da'na-zole)
Rx: Danocrine
Chemical Class: Ethisterone
derivative
Therapeutic Class: Androgen

CLINICAL PHARMACOLOGY
Mechanism of Action: Suppresses the pituitary-ovarian axis; depresses the output of follicle-stimulating hormone (FSH) and luteinizing hormone (LH); possesses weak androgenic activity; decreases immunoglobulin levels

Pharmacokinetics
PO: Peak 2 hr; extensively metabolized in liver, excreted in urine; $t_{1/2}$ 4½ hr

INDICATIONS AND USES: Endometriosis amenable to hormonal management; reduction of nodularity, pain, and tenderness in fibrocystic breast disease; prevention of attacks of hereditary angioedema (cutaneous, abdominal, laryngeal); precocious puberty*; gynecomastia*; menorrhagia*; idiopathic immune thrombocytopenia*; lupus-associated thrombocytopenia*; autoimmune hemolytic anemia*

DOSAGE
Adult
• *Endometriosis:* PO initially 400 mg bid to achieve rapid response and amenorrhea; decrease to dose sufficient to maintain amenorrhea (100-200 mg bid) for 3-9 mo
• *Fibrocystic breast disease:* PO 100-400 mg/day in 2 divided doses
• *Hereditary angioedema:* PO initially 200 mg bid-tid; decrease dose by 50% or less at 1-3 mo intervals to lowest effective dose; if attack occurs, increase dose by up to 200 mg/day

⑤ AVAILABLE FORMS/COST OF THERAPY
• Cap, Gel—Oral: 50 mg, 100's: **$119.59;** 100 mg, 100's: **$179.42;** 200 mg, 100's: **$208.49-$355.85**

CONTRAINDICATIONS: Undiagnosed abnormal genital bleeding; markedly impaired hepatic, renal, or cardiac function; porphyria, pregnancy

PRECAUTIONS: Breast cancer, long-term use, epilepsy, migraine; cardiac, renal, or hepatic dysfunction

PREGNANCY AND LACTATION: Pregnancy category X may result in androgenic effects in the fetus; initiate therapy during menstruation or rule out pregnancy prior to initiating therapy in women of child-bearing potential; contraindicated during breast feeding

SIDE EFFECTS/ADVERSE REACTIONS
CNS: Dizziness, emotional lability, fatigue, headache, nervousness, sleep disorders, tremor
CV: Elevated blood pressure
GI: Constipation, hepatic dysfunction (doses >400 mg/day), nausea, vomiting, ***pancreatitis***
GU: Clitoral hypertrophy, hematuria, pelvic pain, testicular atrophy, menstrual irregularities (spotting, amenorrhea, cycle disturbances), vaginal dryness
METAB: Decreased HDL, increased LDL
SKIN: Acne, edema, flushing, *mild hirsutism, oily skin or hair,* sweating
MISC: Changes in libido, decrease in breast size, deepening of the voice, glucose intolerance, weight gain

INTERACTIONS
Drugs
❷ *Carbamazepine:* Predictably increases serum carbamazepine concentrations, toxicity possible

---

italic = common side effects   ***bold italic*** = life-threatening reactions

❷ *Cyclosporine:* Increased serum cyclosporine concentrations, toxicity possible

❸ *HMG-CoA reductase inhibitors (lovastatin, pravastatin):* Myositis risk increased

❷ *Oral anticoagulants:* Enhanced hypoprothrombinemic response

❷ *Tacrolimus:* Increased tacrolimus concentrations, toxicity possible

Labs

• *False decrease:* Plasma cortisol, serum testosterone, serum thyroxine

• *False increase:* Plasma cortisol, serum testosterone

SPECIAL CONSIDERATIONS

• Useful for palliative treatment of moderate to severe endometriosis or infertility due to endometriosis and for those whom alternative hormonal therapy is ineffective, intolerable, or contraindicated

• Drug of choice for treating all types of hereditary angioedema except for children or pregnant women where fibrolytic inhibitors (aminocaproic acid) may be preferred

• Breast pain should be treated conservatively (analgesics, supportive bra). Hormonal therapy is not innocuous. Symptoms usually return after discontinuation

• Ovarian function usually returns within 60-90 days after discontinuation

PATIENT/FAMILY EDUCATION

• Use nonhormonal contraceptive measures during therapy; discontinue use if pregnancy is suspected

MONITORING PARAMETERS

• Potassium, blood sugar, urine glucose during long-term therapy

---

dantrolene
(dan'troe-leen)
Rx: Dantrium
Chemical Class: Hydantoin derivative
Therapeutic Class: Skeletal muscle relaxant; malignant hyperthermia antidote

---

CLINICAL PHARMACOLOGY

Mechanism of Action: Reduces contraction of skeletal muscle by a direct action on excitation-contraction coupling, apparently by decreasing the amount of calcium released from the sarcoplasmic reticulum

Pharmacokinetics

PO: Peak 5 hr, highly protein bound, metabolized in liver, excreted in urine (metabolites and unchanged drug); $t_{1/2}$ 8 hr

INDICATIONS AND USES: Control of spasticity resulting from upper motor neuron disorders such as spinal cord injury, stroke, cerebral palsy, or multiple sclerosis; malignant hyperthermia (prevention of initial and recurrent episodes, treatment of crises); exercise-induced muscle pain*; neuroleptic malignant syndrome*; heatstroke*

DOSAGE

Adult

• *Spasticity:* PO 25 mg qd initially; increase to bid-qid, then increase dose by 25 mg q4-7 days; max 400 mg/day

• *Malignant hyperthermia:* PO 4-8 mg/kg/day in 4 divided doses starting 1-2 hr before surgery; the same dose may be used for up to 3 days after a crisis to prevent further hyperthermia; IV 1 mg/kg, may repeat as needed to a cumulative dose of 10 mg/kg then switch to PO

Child
• *Spasticity:* PO 0.5 mg/kg bid initially; increase to tid-qid at 4-7 day intervals then increase dose by 0.5 mg/kg to a max of 3 mg/kg bid-qid; do not exceed 400 mg/day
• *Malignant hyperthermia:* Same as adult

💲 AVAILABLE FORMS/COST OF THERAPY
• Cap, Gel—Oral: 25 mg, 100's: **$82.81;** 50 mg, 100's: **$124.04;** 100 mg, 100's: **$154.31**
• Inj, Sol—IV: 20 mg, 1's: **$65.87**

CONTRAINDICATIONS: Active hepatic disease, muscle spasm resulting from rheumatic disorders
PRECAUTIONS: Age >35 yr (increased risk for hepatotoxicity), long-term use, impaired pulmonary function, severely impaired cardiac function, history of previous liver disease
PREGNANCY AND LACTATION: Pregnancy category C; do not use in nursing women
SIDE EFFECTS/ADVERSE REACTIONS
CNS: Disorientation, *dizziness, drowsiness, fatigue,* headache, insomnia, nervousness, paresthesias, *seizures,* tremors, *weakness*
CV: Chest pain, erratic blood pressure, palpitations
EENT: Blurred vision, mydriasis, nasal congestion
GI: Abdominal pain, anorexia, constipation, *diarrhea,* dry mouth, dysphasia, *GI bleeding, hepatotoxicity,* increased AST and alk phosphatase, *nausea,* vomiting
GU: Crystalluria, hematuria, impotence, nocturia, urinary frequency, urinary incontinence, urinary retention
RESP: Pleural effusion, *pulmonary edema*
SKIN: Acne-like rash, photosensitivity, pruritus, rash, sweating, urticaria

SPECIAL CONSIDERATIONS
• Use carefully where spasticity is utilized to sustain upright posture and balance in locomotion or to obtain or maintain increased function
• Discontinue after 6 wk if improvement does not occur
• Use lowest dose possible (hepatotoxicity dose-related)
PATIENT/FAMILY EDUCATION
• IV therapy may decrease grip strength and increase weakness of leg muscles, especially walking down stairs
MONITORING PARAMETERS
• Baseline and periodic LFTs (AST, ALT, alk phosphatase, total bilirubin)

dapiprazole
(da′pi-prah-zohl)
Rx: Rēv-Eyes
Chemical Class: Pyridine derivative
Therapeutic Class: Miotic

CLINICAL PHARMACOLOGY
Mechanism of Action: Blocks α-adrenergic receptors in smooth muscle producing miosis through an effect on the dilator muscle of the iris; no activity on ciliary muscle contraction or intraocular pressure
Pharmacokinetics
OPHTHAL: Eye color affects the rate of pupillary constriction, individuals with brown irides may have a slightly slower rate of pupillary constriction than those with blue or green irides; eye color does not appear to affect the final pupil size
INDICATIONS AND USES: Reversal of iatrogenically induced mydriasis produced by adrenergic (phenylephrine) or parasympatholytic (tropicamide) agents

italic = common side effects   ***bold italic*** = life-threatening reactions

DOSAGE
Adult
• OPHTH instill 2 gtt, then 2 gtt 5 min later; do not use more than once/wk

💲 AVAILABLE FORMS/COST OF THERAPY
• Sol—Ophth: 0.5%, 5 ml: **$36.43**

CONTRAINDICATIONS: Acute iritis

PRECAUTIONS: Children, severe cardiovascular disease

PREGNANCY AND LACTATION: Pregnancy category B; excretion into breast milk unknown; use caution in nursing mothers

SIDE EFFECTS/ADVERSE REACTIONS
EENT: Blurring vision, browache, *burning, conjunctival injection,* corneal edema, eye dryness, headaches, itching, keratitis, lid edema, lid erythema, photophobia, ptosis, tearing

SPECIAL CONSIDERATIONS
• Use limited to clinician's office following diagnostic mydriasis

---

dapsone
(dap'sone)
Rx: Dapsone
Chemical Class: Sulfone
Therapeutic Class:
Leprostatic; antiprotozoal

CLINICAL PHARMACOLOGY
Mechanism of Action: Competitive antagonist of para-aminobenzoic acid (PABA); prevents normal bacterial utilization of PABA for the synthesis of folic acid

Pharmacokinetics
PO: Rapid, complete absorption; 73% bound to plasma proteins; metabolized in liver, excreted in urine and bile; $t_{1/2}$ 25-31 hr

INDICATIONS AND USES: All forms of leprosy (Hansen's disease) except for cases of proven dapsone resistance; dermatitis herpetiformis; *Pneumocystis carinii* pneumonia (PCP) in HIV-infected patients (in combination with trimethoprim)*; alternative to co-trimoxazole for PCP prophylaxis (alone or in combination with pyrimethamine)*; prevention of the 1st episode of toxoplasmosis in HIV-infected patients (in combination with pyrimethamine)*; treatment of relapsing polychondritis*; prophylaxis of malaria*; brown recluse spider bites*

DOSAGE
Adult
• *Leprosy:* PO 50-100 mg qd for 3-10 yr (addition of rifampin 600 mg qd for the 1st 6 mo is recomended)
• *Dermatitis herpetiformis:* PO 50 mg qd initially; increase to 300 mg qd or higher to achieve full control; reduce dosage to minimum level as soon as possible
• *PCP prophylaxis:* PO 50-100 mg qd

Child
• *Leprosy:* PO 1-2 mg/kg/day; max 100 mg/day

💲 AVAILABLE FORMS/COST OF THERAPY
• Tab, Uncoated—Oral: 25 mg, 100's: **$18.90;** 100 mg, 100's: **$19.75**

PRECAUTIONS: Renal disease, hepatic disease, G-6-PD deficiency, anemia, severe cardiopulmonary disease, methemoglobin reductase deficiency

PREGNANCY AND LACTATION: Pregnancy category C; extensive, but uncontrolled, experience and 2 published surveys in pregnant women have not shown increases in the risk for fetal abnormalities if administered during all trimesters; excreted in breast milk, hemolytic

---

* = non-FDA-approved use

reactions can occur in neonates, discontinue nursing or discontinue drug; alternatively, some authors have suggested infants should be kept with mothers infected with leprosy, and breast feeding during drug therapy encouraged

SIDE EFFECTS/ADVERSE REACTIONS

CNS: Headache, insomnia, paresthesia, peripheral neuropathy, psychosis, vertigo

EENT: Blurred vision, optic neuritis, photophobia, tinnitus

GI: Abdominal pain, anorexia, nausea, vomiting

GU: **Nephrotic syndrome,** proteinuria, **renal papillary necrosis**

HEME: **Agranulocytosis, aplastic anemia, hemolytic anemia** (dose related)

SKIN: Drug-induced systemic lupus erythematosis, photosensitivity

INTERACTIONS

Drugs

3 *Didanosine:* Higher failure rate in pneumocystis infections, possibly due to inhibited dissolution of dapsone in stomach; administer dapsone 2-3 hr before didanosine

3 *Probenecid:* Increased serum dapsone concentrations, clinical importance not established

3 *Rifampin:* Reduced serum dapsone concentrations; increased methemoglobin concentrations

3 *Trimethoprim:* Increased serum dapsone concentrations; increased trimethoprim concentrations

SPECIAL CONSIDERATIONS

• Use in conjunction with either rifampin or clofazimine to prevent development of drug resistance and reduce infectiousness of patient with leprosy more quickly

PATIENT/FAMILY EDUCATION

• Full therapeutic effects on leprosy may not occur for several mo; compliance with dosage schedule, duration is necessary

MONITORING PARAMETERS

• CBC weekly for the 1st mo, qmo for 6 mo, and semiannually thereafter

• Periodic LFTs

---

deferoxamine

(de-fer-ox'a-meen)
Rx: Desferal
Chemical Class: Siderochrome
Therapeutic Class: Heavy metal antidote (aluminum, iron)

CLINICAL PHARMACOLOGY

Mechanism of Action: Chelates iron by forming a stable complex that prevents iron from entering into further chemical reactions; readily chelates free serum iron, iron from ferritin and hemosiderin, but not from transferrin; does not combine with iron from cytochromes and hemoglobin

Pharmacokinetics

Rapidly metabolized by plasma enzymes, excreted in urine; iron chelate excreted renally giving urine a red color, some chelate also excreted in bile; $t_{1/2}$ 1 hr

INDICATIONS AND USES: Acute iron intoxication; promotion of iron excretion in patients who have secondary iron overload from multiple transfusions; aluminum accumulation in bone in renal failure patients,* aluminum-induced dialysis encephalopathy*

DOSAGE

Adult

• *Acute iron intoxication:* IM 1 g stat, then 0.5 g q4h for 2 doses, additional doses of 0.5 g q4-12h prn, max 6 g/day; IV infuse at a rate ≤15 mg/kg/hr, dosage the same as

---

italic = common side effects   **bold italic** = life-threatening reactions

IM max 6 g/day (use only in cardiovascular collapse)

• *Chronic iron overload:* IM 0.5-1 g/day; SC via portable pump INF 1-2 g/day over 8-12 hr; IV give 2 g with, but separate from, each unit of blood at a rate ≤15 mg/kg/hr

Child

• *Acute iron intoxication:* IM 90 mg/kg q8h, max 6 g/day; IV 15 mg/kg/hr, max 6 g/day

• *Chronic iron overload:* IV 15 mg/kg/hr, max 6 g/day; SC via portable pump INF 20-40 mg/kg/day over 8-12 hr

$ AVAILABLE FORMS/COST OF THERAPY

• Inj, Sol—IM, IV, SC: 500 mg: **$11.58**

CONTRAINDICATIONS: Severe renal disease or anuria

PREGNANCY AND LACTATION: Pregnancy category C; excretion into breast milk unknown; use caution in nursing mothers

SIDE EFFECTS/ADVERSE REACTIONS

CV: Hypotension (with rapid IV inj), tachycardia

GI: Abdominal cramps, diarrhea

EENT: Blurred vision, cataracts, ototoxicity

MS: Leg cramps

SKIN: Erythema, pain at inj site, pruritus, urticaria

SPECIAL CONSIDERATIONS

Acute iron intoxication: Deferoxamine indicated if:

• Free serum iron present

• Patient symptomatic

• Serum iron >350 µg/dL

PATIENT/FAMILY EDUCATION

• May turn urine red

MONITORING PARAMETERS

• Visual acuity tests, slit-lamp examinations, funduscopy, and audiometry are recommended periodically in patients treated for prolonged periods of time

• BUN, creatinine, CrCl

• Serum iron levels

---

delavirdine

(deh-la′ver-deen)

Rx: Rescriptor

Chemical Class: Arylpiperazine derivative

Therapeutic Class: Nonnucleoside reverse transcriptase inhibitor

CLINICAL PHARMACOLOGY

Mechanism of Action: Inhibits DNA- and RNA-directed polymerase function of HIV-1 by allosteric inhibition

Pharmacokinetics:

PO: Well-absorbed, peak 1 hr; 99% protein bound; does not penetrate CSF; metabolized by cytochrome P450 3A enzyme system, inhibits its own metabolism causing reduced clearance at higher doses; $t_{1/2}$ 7 hr at daily dose of 1200 mg; 44% of dose excreted in feces, 51% of dose excreted in urine; inhibits CYP3A and CYP2C9

INDICATIONS AND USES: Combination therapy for HIV-1

DOSAGE

Adult and Child >12 yr

• PO: 400 mg tid

• For latest treatment guidelines, see www.hivatis.org

$ AVAILABLE FORMS/COST OF THERAPY

• Tab, Uncoated—Oral: 100 mg, 360's: **$228.58;** 200 mg, 180's: **$282.96**

CONTRAINDICATIONS: Concurrent use of rifampin

PRECAUTIONS: Children, hepatic disease

PREGNANCY AND LACTATION: Pregnancy category C, teratogenic

---

in rats; excreted in breast milk at high concentrations

SIDE EFFECTS/ADVERSE REACTIONS

CNS: Confusion, depression, dizziness, *headache,* insomnia, somnolence

CV: Bradycardia, tachycardia

EENT: Epistaxis, gingivitis, pharyngitis, rhinitis

GI: Diarrhea, dyspepsia, increased alkaline phosphatase, ALT, AST; *nausea (11%)*

GU: Breast enlargement, menorrhagia, nephrolithiasis, proteinuria

HEME: **Anemia (79%), leukopenia (16%), thrombocytopenia (42%)**

METAB: Hyperkalemia

MS: Increased CPK, myalgia

RESP: Cough, dyspnea

SKIN: Rash (45%), pruritus

MISC: Fatigue

INTERACTIONS

Drugs

🔳 *Aluminum:* Antacids reduce GI absorption of delavirdine by 50% if taken at same time; separate doses by at least 1 hr

🔳 *Antacids:* Antacids reduce GI absorption of delavirdine by 50% if taken at same time; separate doses by at least 1 hr

⚠ *Astemizole:* Delavirdine increases astemizole plasma level; coadministration contraindicated

🔳 *Barbiturates:* Barbiturates decrease plasma delavirdine levels

🔳 *Benzodiazepines:* Delavirdine increases benzodiazepine plasma levels by inhibiting hepatic metabolism

🔳 *Calcium:* Antacids reduce GI absorption of delavirdine by 50% if taken at same time; separate doses by at least 1 hr

🔳 *Carbamazepine:* Carbamazepine decreases plasma delavirdine levels

② *Cimetidine:* Cimetidine reduces GI absorption of delavirdine; coadministration not recommended

② *Cisapride:* Delavirdine increases cisapride plasma level; coadministration not recommended

🔳 *Clarithromycin:* Delavirdine increases clarithromycin plasma levels; clarithromycin increases delavirdine plasma levels

🔳 *Dapsone:* Delavirdine increases dapsone plasma level

🔳 *Didanosine:* Delavirdine reduces didanosine absorption; didanosine reduces delavirdine absorption; separate doses by at least 1 hr

② *Ergotamines:* Delavirdine increases ergotamine plasma level; coadministration not recommended

② *Famotidine:* Famotidine reduces GI absorption of delavirdine; coadministration not recommended

🔳 *Fluoxetine:* Fluoxetine increases delavirdine levels by inhibiting hepatic metabolism

🔳 *Indinavir:* Delavirdine increases indinavir AUC by 40%; reduce indinavir dose to 600 mg tid

② *Lansoprazole:* Lansoprazole reduces GI absorption of delavirdine; coadministration not recommended

② *Lovastatin:* Delavirdine increases lovastatin plasma level; coadministration not recommended

🔳 *Magnesium:* Antacids reduce GI absorptioin of delavirdine by 50% if taken at same time; separate doses by at least 1 hr

② *Midazolam:* Delavirdine increases midazolam plasma level; coadministration not recommended

🔳 *Nelfinavir:* Delavirdine increases nelfinavir AUC by 100%; nelfinavir reduces delavirdine AUC by 50%; no data on dose adjustment

② *Nizatidine:* Nizatidine reduces GI absorption of delavirdine; coadministration not recommended

🔳 *Nifedipine:* Delavirdine increases nifedipine plasma level

---

italic = common side effects   ***bold italic*** = life-threatening reactions

❷ *Omeprazole:* Omeprazole reduces GI absorption of delavirdine; coadministration not recommended

❸ *Phenytoin:* Phenytoin decreases plasma delavirdine level

❷ *Quinidine:* Delavirdine increases quinidine plasma level

❷ *Ranitidine:* Ranitidine reduces GI absorption of delavirdine; coadministration not recommended

❷ *Rifabutin:* Rifabutin decreases plasma delavirdine level; coadministration not recommended

⚠ *Rifampin:* Rifampin decreases plasma delavirdine level; coadministration contraindicated

❸ *Ritonavir:* Delavirdine increases ritonavir AUC by 70%; no data on dose adjustment

❷ *Saquinavir:* Delavirdine increases saquinavir AUC by 5-fold; additive hepatic toxicity possible; adjust Fortovase dose to 800 mg tid

❷ *Simvastatin:* Delavirdine increases simvastatin plasma level; coadministration not recommended

❸ *Sodium bicarbonate:* Antacids reduce GI absorption of delavirdine by 50% if taken at same time; separate doses by at least 1 hr

⚠ *Terfenadine:* Delavirdine increases terfenadine plasma level; coadministration contraindicated

❷ *Triazolam:* Delavirdine increases triazolam plasma level; coadministration not recommended

❸ *Warfarin:* Delavirdine increases warfarin effect

SPECIAL CONSIDERATIONS
PATIENT/FAMILY EDUCATION
• May take without regard to food; patients with achlorhydria should take with acidic beverage (orange or cranberry juice); may cause alcohol intolerance

MONITORING PARAMETERS
• CBC, hepatic, and renal function

---

demecarium
(de-mi-kare'ee-um)
Rx: Humorsol Ocumeter
Chemical Class: Quaternary ammonium derivative
Therapeutic Class: Miotic; antiglaucoma agent

CLINICAL PHARMACOLOGY
Mechanism of Action: Produces intense miosis and ciliary muscle contraction due to inhibition of cholinesterase, allowing acetylcholine to accumulate at sites of cholinergic transmission; myopia may be induced or, if present, may be augmented by the increased refractive power of the lens

Pharmacokinetics
• Onset of miosis 15-60 min, duration 3-10 days; peak reduction of intraocular pressure 24 hr, duration 7-28 days

INDICATIONS AND USES: Open-angle glaucoma (should be used only when shorter-acting miotics have proved inadequate); conditions obstructing aqueous outflow, such as synechial formation, that are amenable to miotic therapy; following iridectomy; accommodative esotropia (accommodative convergent strabismus)

DOSAGE
Adult and Child
• *Glaucoma:* Initially instill 1 gtt of 0.125% or 0.25% sol (children) or 1-2 gtt (adults) in the glaucomatous eye, keep the patient under supervision and make tonometric examinations at least for 3 or 4 hr to be sure that no immediate rise in pressure occurs; usual dose 1-2 gtt bid to 1-2 gtt twice/wk; the 0.125% strength used bid usually results in smooth control of the physiologic

---

diurnal variation in intraocular pressure

• *Strabismus:* Essentially equal visual acuity of both eyes is a prerequisite to successful treatment. Diagnosis: 1 gtt ou for 2 wk, then 1 gtt q2d for 2-3 wk, if the eyes become straighter, an accommodative factor is demonstrated. Therapy: In esotropia uncomplicated by amblyopia or anisometropia, instill not more than 1 gtt at a time ou qd for 2-3 wk (too severe a degree of miosis may interfere with vision), reduce to 1 gtt qod for 3-4 wk and reevaluate; may be continued in a dosage of 1 gtt q2d to 1 gtt twice/wk (the latter dosage may be maintained for several mo), evaluate the patient's condition every 4 to 12 wk, if improvement continues, change the schedule to 1 gtt q wk and eventually to a trial without medication; if, after 4 mo, control of the condition still requires 1 gtt q2d, therapy should be stopped

§ AVAILABLE FORMS/COST OF THERAPY

• Sol—Ophth: 0.125%, 5 ml: **$16.28;** 0.25%, 5 ml: **$17.46**

CONTRAINDICATIONS: Active uveal inflammation, glaucoma associated with iridocyclitis

PRECAUTIONS: Myasthenia gravis, narrow-angle glaucoma, asthma, spastic GI disturbances, peptic ulcer, bradycardia, hypotension, recent MI, epilepsy, parkinsonism, children (more frequent occurrence of iris cysts)

PREGNANCY AND LACTATION: Pregnancy category C; ionized at physiologic pH, transplacental passage in significant amounts would not be expected; excretion into breast milk unknown, but would be expected to be low due to ionization at physiologic pH

SIDE EFFECTS/ADVERSE REACTIONS

CNS: Fainting, *headache,* sweating
CV: **Dysrhythmia**
EENT: Accommodative spasm, allergic follicular conjunctivitis, blurred vision, browache, *burning,* conjunctival and ciliary redness, eczematoid lid dermatitis, iris cysts (more frequent in children), *lacrimation,* lens opacities, lid muscle twitching, myopia, paradoxical increase in intraocular pressure, *stinging*
GI: Abdominal cramps, diarrhea, nausea, salivation, vomiting
GU: Urinary incontinence
RESP: Difficulty breathing

SPECIAL CONSIDERATIONS
• Reserved for patients refractory to short-acting miotics secondary to cataractogenic potential

PATIENT/FAMILY EDUCATION
• Use caution while driving at night or performing hazardous tasks in poor light
• Continuous gentle pressure on the lacrimal duct with the index finger for several seconds immediately following instillation of the drops minimizes systemic absorption

MONITORING PARAMETERS
• Frequent evaluations to detect iris cysts, especially in children
• Routine slit-lamp examination during prolonged administration
• Intraocular pressure

---

demeclocycline
(dem-e-kloe-sye'kleen)
Rx: Declomycin
Chemical Class: Tetracycline derivative
Therapeutic Class: Antibiotic

CLINICAL PHARMACOLOGY
Mechanism of Action: Inhibits protein synthesis by binding with the

---

30S and possibly the 50S ribosomal subunit(s) of susceptible bacteria; may also cause alterations in the cytoplasmic membrane; bacteriostatic

Pharmacokinetics

PO: Peak 3-6 hr, t$_{1/2}$ 10-17 hr; excreted in urine; 65%-91% bound to serum protein

INDICATIONS AND USES: Chronic hyponatremia associated with the syndrome of inappropriate antidiuretic hormone (SIADH) secretion*; Rocky Mountain spotted fever, typhus fever, Q fever, rickettsialpox, tick fevers, *Mycoplasma pneumoniae,* psittacosis and ornithosis, lymphogranuloma venereum and granuloma inguinale, relapsing fever, chancroid, infections of the respiratory and urinary tract, syphilis and yaws, Vincent's infection, acute intestinal amebiasis (adjunct to amebicides), trachoma, inclusion conjunctivitis, severe acne

Antibacterial spectrum usually includes:

• Gram-positive organisms: *Bacillus anthracis, Actinomyces israelii, Arachnia propionica, Clostridium perfringens, C. tetani, Listeria monocytogenes, Nocardia, Propionibacterium acnes*

• Gram-negative organisms: *Bartonella bacilliformis, Bordetella pertussis, Brucella, Calymmatobacterium granulomatis, Campylobacter fetus, Francisella tularensis, Haemophilus ducreyi, H. influenzae, Legionella pneumophilia, Leptotrichia buccalis, Neisseria gonorrhoeae, N. meningitidis, Pasteurella multocida, Pseudomonas pseudomallei, P. mallei, Shigella, Spirillum minus, Streptobacillus moniliformis, Vibrio cholerae, V. parahaemolyticus, Yersinia enterocolitica, Y. pestis*

• Other organisms: *Rickettsia akari, R. prowazeki, R. rickettsii, R. tsugamushi, R. typhi, Coxiella burnetii, Chlamydia trachomatis, C. psittaci, Mycoplasma hominis, M. pneumoniae, Ureaplasma urealyticum, Borrelia recurrentis, Leptospira, Treponema pallidum, T. pertenue*

DOSAGE

Adult

• PO 150 mg q6h or 300 mg q12h

• *Gonorrhea:* PO 600 mg, then 300 mg q12h for 4 days; total 3 g

• *SIADH:* PO 600-1200 mg/day in divided doses

Child >8 yr

• PO 6-12 mg/kg/day in divided doses q6-12h

$ AVAILABLE FORMS/COST OF THERAPY

• Cap, Elastic—Oral: 150 mg, 100's: **$285.30**

• Tab, Plain Coated—Oral: 150 mg, 100's: **$438.71;** 300 mg, 48's: **$383.17**

CONTRAINDICATIONS: Children <8 yr

PRECAUTIONS: Renal disease, hepatic disease, nephrogenic diabetes insipidus, exposure to direct sunlight, outdated products

PREGNANCY AND LACTATION: Pregnancy category D; problems associated with use of the tetracyclines during or around pregnancy include adverse effects on fetal teeth and bones, maternal liver toxicity, and congenital defects; excreted into breast milk in low concentrations; use caution in nursing mothers

SIDE EFFECTS/ADVERSE REACTIONS

CNS: Fever, headache, paresthesia

CV: Pericarditis

GI: Abdominal cramps, abdominal pain, anorexia, *diarrhea,* dysphagia, enterocolitis, epigastric burning, flatulence, glossitis, hepatotoxicity, *nausea,* oral candidiasis, *pseudomembranous colitis,* stomatitis, vomiting

GU: Nephrogenic diabetes insipidus, *nephrotoxicity,* polydipsia, polyuria

HEME: Eosinophilia, *hemolytic anemia, neutropenia, thrombocytopenia*

SKIN: Exfoliative dermatitis, photosensitivity, pruritus, rash, urticaria

MISC: Decreased calcification of deciduous teeth, angioedema, pseudotumor cerebri (adults) and bulging fontanels (infants)

INTERACTIONS
Drugs

3 *Antacids:* Reduced serum concentration of demeclocycline; take 2 hr before or 6 hr after antacids containing aluminum, calcium, or magnesium

2 *Bismuth:* Reduced serum concentration of demeclocycline; do not coadminister

3 *Calcium:* See antacids

3 *Cholestyramine:* Reduced serum concentration of demeclocycline; take 2 hr before or 3 hr after cholestyramine

3 *Colestipol:* Reduced serum concentration of demeclocycline; take 2 hr before or 3 hr after colestipol

3 *Digoxin:* Demeclocycline may increase serum digoxin levels

3 *Food:* Reduced serum concentration of demeclocycline; take 2 hr before or 3 hr after food

3 *Iron:* Reduced serum concentration of demeclocycline; take 2 hr before or 3 hr after iron

3 *Magnesium:* See antacids

2 *Methoxyflurane:* Demeclocycline enhances nephrotoxicity of methoxyflurane

3 *Oral contraceptives:* Contraceptive failure may occur rarely; mechanism unknown

3 *Penicillins:* Demeclocycline may reduce penicillin efficacy

3 *Warfarin:* Demeclocycline may increase effect of warfarin

3 *Zinc:* Reduced serum concentration of demeclocycline; take 2 hr before or 3 hr after zinc

Labs
• *False increase:* Urinary catecholamines

SPECIAL CONSIDERATIONS
• No advantages over other tetracyclines as anti-infective; higher incidence of phototoxicity; active against water intoxication and SIADH

PATIENT/FAMILY EDUCATION
• Sunscreen does not seem to decrease photosensitivity
• Avoid milk products; take with full glass of water on an empty stomach 1 hr before meals or 2 hr after meals

MONITORING PARAMETERS
• LFTs during prolonged administration

---

desipramine
(dess-ip'ra-meen)
Rx: Norpramin, Pertofrane
Chemical Class: Dibenzazepine derivative: secondary amine
Therapeutic Class: Tricyclic Antidepressant

CLINICAL PHARMACOLOGY
Mechanism of Action: Inhibits the reuptake of norepinephrine and serotonin (amine blocking activity, very high and moderate, respectively) at the presynaptic neuron, prolonging neuronal activity; inhibits histamine and acetylcholine activity; mild peripheral vasodilator effects and possible "quinidine-like" actions

Pharmacokinetics
PO: Peak 2-4 hr; therapeutic response 2-4 wk; metabolized by liver, excreted by kidneys; $t_{1/2}$ 14-62 hr

---

italic = common side effects   ***bold italic*** = life-threatening reactions

INDICATIONS AND USES: Depression, facilitation of cocaine withdrawal,* eating disorders,* panic attacks*

DOSAGE

Adult

• PO 25 mg/day in single or divided doses initially, increase by 25 mg q3-5 days to 100-200 mg/day, max 300 mg/day

Geriatric/Adolescent

• PO 25-100 mg/day, doses >150 mg/day not recommended

Child 6-12 yr

• PO 10-30 mg/day or 1-5 mg/kg/day in divided doses, max 5 mg/kg/day

AVAILABLE FORMS/COST OF THERAPY

• Tab, Plain Coated—Oral: 10 mg, 100's: **$25.19-$60.12;** 25 mg, 100's: **$23.48-$72.24;** 50 mg, 100's: **$47.02-$135.96;** 75 mg, 100's: **$56.35-$173.10;** 100 mg, 100's: **$100.32-$227.40;** 150 mg, 50's: **$109.50-$164.76**

CONTRAINDICATIONS: Acute recovery phase of MI; concurrent use of MAOIs

PRECAUTIONS: Suicidal patients, convulsive disorders, prostatic hypertrophy, psychiatric disease, severe depression, increased intraocular pressure, narrow-angle glaucoma, urinary retention, cardiac disease, hepatic or renal disease, hyperthyroidism, electroshock therapy, elective surgery, elderly, abrupt discontinuation

PREGNANCY AND LACTATION: Pregnancy category C; excreted into breast milk; effect on the nursing infant unknown, but may be of concern

SIDE EFFECTS/ADVERSE REACTIONS

CNS: Anxiety, confusion (especially in elderly), *dizziness,* EPS (elderly),

fatigue, headache, increased psychiatric symptoms, insomnia, memory impairment, nervousness, nightmares, panic, stimulation, tremors, weakness

*CV: **Dysrhythmias,*** ECG changes, hypertension, *orthostatic hypotension,* palpitations, syncope, tachycardia

EENT: Blurred vision, mydriasis, nasal congestion, ophthalmoplegia, tinnitus

GI: Constipation, cramps, *dry mouth,* epigastric distress, hepatitis, increased appetite, jaundice, nausea, paralytic ileus, stomatitis, vomiting

GU: Urinary retention

*HEME: **Agranulocytosis,*** eosinophilia, ***leukopenia, thrombocytopenia***

METAB: Weight gain

SKIN: Photosensitivity, pruritus, rash, sweating, urticaria

INTERACTIONS

Drugs

3 *Barbiturates:* Reduced serum concentrations of cyclic antidepressants

2 *Bethanidine:* Reduced antihypertensive effect of bethanidine

3 *Carbamazepine:* Reduced serum concentrations of cyclic antidepressants

3 *Cimetidine:* Increased serum concentrations of cyclic antidepressants

2 *Clonidine:* Reduced antihypertensive effect of clonidine; enhanced hypertensive response with abrupt clonidine withdrawal

3 *Debrisoquin:* Reduced antihypertensive effect of debrisoquin

3 *Diltiazem:* Increased serum concentrations of cyclic antidepressants

2 *Epinephrine:* Markedly enhanced pressor response to IV epinephrine

3 *Ethanol:* Additive impairment of motor skills; abstinent alcoholics

---

* = non-FDA-approved use

may eliminate cyclic antidepressants faster than nonalcoholics

3 *Fluoxetine:* Marked increases in serum concentrations of cyclic antidepressants

3 *Fluvoxamine:* Marked increases in serum concentrations of cyclic antidepressants

2 *Guanabenz, guanethidine:* Reduced antihypertensive effect

3 *Guanadrel, guanfacine:* Reduced antihypertensive effect

3 *Indinavir:* Increase in serum concentrations of cyclic antidepressants

3 *Lithium:* Increased risk of neurotoxicity

2 *Moclobemide:* Potential association with fatal or nonfatal serotonin syndrome

2 *MAOIs:* Excessive sympathetic response, manias, or hyperpyrexia possible

3 *Neuroleptics:* Increased therapeutic and toxic effects of both drugs

2 *Norepinephrine:* Markedly enhanced pressor response to IV norepinephrine

3 *Paroxetine:* Marked increases in serum concentrations of cyclic antidepressants

3 *Propoxyphene:* Increased serum concentrations of cyclic antidepressants

3 *Quinidine:* Increased serum concentrations of cyclic antidepressants

3 *Rifampin:* Reduced serum concentrations of cyclic antidepressants

3 *Ritonavir:* Marked increases in serum concentrations of cyclic antidepressants

3 *Sulfonylureas:* Cyclic antidepressants may increase hypoglycemic effect

SPECIAL CONSIDERATIONS
• Equally effective as other tricyclic antidepressants for depression; fewer anticholinergic effects than tertiary amines, less orthostasis, and mild stimulatory property

PATIENT/FAMILY EDUCATION
• Therapeutic effects may take 4-6 wk
• Use caution in driving or other activities requiring alertness
• Avoid alcohol and other CNS depressants
• Do not discontinue abruptly after long-term use

MONITORING PARAMETERS
• Determination of desipramine plasma concentrations is not routinely recommended but may be useful in identifying toxicity, drug interactions, or noncompliance (adjustments in dosage should be made according to clinical response not plasma concentrations); therapeutic level is 50-200 ng/ml

desmopressin
(des-moe-press'in)
Rx: DDAVP, Stimate
Chemical Class: Synthetic arginine vasopressin analog
Therapeutic Class: Antihemophilic; hemostatic; antidiuretic

CLINICAL PHARMACOLOGY
Mechanism of Action: A posterior pituitary hormone analog; has ADH activity (promotes renal tubular reabsorption of water); less vascular or GI smooth muscle constriction than natural vasopressin; causes increase in plasma factor VIII levels, which increases platelet aggregation

Pharmacokinetics
NASAL: Onset 1 hr, peak 1-2 hr, duration 8-20 hr, terminal $t_{1/2}$ 76 min

INDICATIONS AND USES: Primary nocturnal enuresis (intranasal only); neurogenic diabetes insipidus; spontaneous, trauma-induced or prevention of perioperative bleeding in patients with hemophilia A with factor VIII levels >5%; spontaneous, trauma-induced, or prevention of perioperative bleeding in patients with von Willebrand's disease (Type I); determination of the capacity of the kidneys to concentrate urine; chronic autonomic failure (e.g., nocturnal polyuria, overnight weight loss, morning postural hypotension)*

DOSAGE

Adult

• *Neurogenic diabetes insipidus:* Nasal (via rhinal tube) 0.1-0.4 ml qd, as a single or divided dose; most adults require 0.2 ml qd in 2 divided doses; the AM and PM doses should be separately adjusted for an adequate diurnal rhythm of water turnover; PO 0.05 mg bid, titrate to optimum therapeutic dose (range, 0.1-1.2 mg divided 2 or 3× daily; IV/SC 0.5-1 ml/day in 2 divided doses, adjusted separately for an adequate diurnal rhythm of water turnover; when switching from intranasal to IV the comparable antidiuretic dose is 1⁄10 the intranasal dose

• *Hemophilia A and von Willebrand's disease (Type I):* IV 0.3 µg/kg diluted in 50 ml NS infused slowly over 15-30 min, 30 min before procedure; intranasal 300 µg (stimate only; use 2 hr before surgical procedure)

Child

• *Primary nocturnal enuresis:* Nasal (>6yr) initially 20 µg or 0.2 ml sol qhs; may increase up to 40 µg qhs prn; decrease to 10 µg qhs if the patient has shown a response to 20 µg. PO 0.2 mg initially at hs, titrate for response to maximum dose of 0.6 mg

• *Central diabetes insipidus:* Nasal (via rhinal tube) (3 mo-12 yr) 0.05 to 0.3 ml qd, either as single dose or

divided into 2 doses; PO 0.05 mg qd; titrate with fluid restriction

• *Hemophilia A and von Willebrand's disease (Type I):* IV 0.3 mg/kg diluted in 50 ml NS (>10 kg) or 10 ml NS (≤10 kg) infused slowly over 15-30 min, 30 min before procedure; intranasal 300 µg (> 50 kg) or 150 µg (≤50 kg) (stimate only; use 2 hr before surgical procedure)

§ AVAILABLE FORMS/COST OF THERAPY

• Aer, Spray—Nasal: 1.5 mg/ml, 2.5 ml: **$575.00**

• Inj, Sol—IV; SC: 4 µg/ml, 10 ml: **$265.59;** 15 µg/ml, 10 ml: **$972.01**

• Sol—Nasal: 0.1 mg/ml, 2.5 ml: **$61.80-$80.25**

• Tab—Oral: 0.1 mg, 100's: **$174.15;** 0.2 mg, 100's: **$271.03**

CONTRAINDICATIONS: Type IIB von Willebrand's disease

PRECAUTIONS: Coronary artery disease, hypertensive cardiovascular disease, elderly, children: for bleeding disorders, proven safe and effective for age ≥ 3 months (parenteral) or ≥11 months (Stimate intranasal)

PREGNANCY AND LACTATION: Pregnancy category B (no uterotonic action at antidiuretic doses); compatible with breast feeding

SIDE EFFECTS/ADVERSE REACTIONS

CNS: Drowsiness, flushing, headache, lethargy, *seizures*

CV: Increased blood pressure

EENT: Congestion, nasal irritation, rhinitis

GI: Cramps, heartburn, nausea

GU: Vulvar pain

SPECIAL CONSIDERATIONS

• Though useful in the treatment of children with enuresis, relapse following discontinuation is common; conservative therapy preferred long-term; desmopressin best used-intermittently (e.g., overnight with friend)

PATIENT/FAMILY EDUCATION

• Nasal tube delivery system is supplied with a flexible calibrated plastic tube (rhinyle); draw sol into the rhinyle, insert 1 end of tube into nostril, blow on the other end to deposit sol deep into nasal cavity

• Ingest only enough water to satisfy thirst (especially elderly and children)

MONITORING PARAMETERS

• Diabetes insipidus: Urine volume and osmolality, plasma osmolality

• Hemophilia A: Determine factor VIII coagulant activity before injecting desmopressin for hemostasis; if activity is <5% of normal, do not rely on desmopressin

• Von Willebrand's disease: Assess levels of factor VIII coagulant, factor VIII antigen, and ristocetin cofactor; skin bleeding time may also be helpful

---

desonide

(dess'oh-nide)

Rx: Delomide, DesOwen, Tridesilon

Chemical Class: Synthetic glucocorticoid

Therapeutic Class: Topical corticosteroid, low potency

CLINICAL PHARMACOLOGY

Mechanism of Action: Depresses formation, release, and activity of endogenous mediators of inflammation such as prostaglandins, kinins, histamine, liposomal enzymes, and the complement system resulting in decreased edema, erythema, and pruritus

Pharmacokinetics: Absorbed through the skin (increased by inflammation and occlusive dressings); metabolized primarily in the liver

INDICATIONS AND USES: Psoriasis, eczema, contact dermatitis, pruritus, superficial bacterial infections of the external auditory canal (otic preparation)

DOSAGE

Adult and Child

• TOP apply to affected area bid-tid, rub completely into skin; OTIC instill 3-4 gtt tid-qid or insert wick saturated with solution and allow to remain *in situ*

💲 **AVAILABLE FORMS/COST OF THERAPY**

• Cre—Top: 0.05%, 15, 60, 90 g: **$8.19-$15.88**/15 g

• Oint—Top: 0.05%, 15, 60 g: **$9.62-$15.88**/15 g

• Lotion—Top: 0.05%, 60, 120 ml: **$26.94**/60 mL

CONTRAINDICATIONS: Fungal infections

PRECAUTIONS: Viral infections, bacterial infections, children; use on face, genitals, axilla

PREGNANCY AND LACTATION: Pregnancy category C; unknown whether top application could result in sufficient systemic absorption to produce detectable amounts in breast milk (systemic corticosteroids are secreted into breast milk in quantities not likely to have detrimental effects on infant)

SIDE EFFECTS/ADVERSE REACTIONS

SKIN: Acne, allergic contact dermatitis, atrophy, burning, dryness, folliculitis, hypertrichosis, hypopigmentation, irritation, itching, miliaria, perioral dermatitis, secondary infection, striae

MISC: Systemic absorption of topical corticosteroids has produced reversible HPA axis suppression (more likely with occlusive dressings, prolonged administration, application

---

italic = common side effects   ***bold italic*** = life-threatening reactions

to large surface areas, liver failure, and in children)

SPECIAL CONSIDERATIONS
PATIENT/FAMILY EDUCATION
• Apply sparingly only to affected area
• Avoid contact with the eyes
• Do not put bandages or dressings over treated area unless directed by clinician
• Discontinue drug and notify clinician if local irritation or fever develops
• Do not use on weeping, denuded, or infected areas

---

desoximetasone
(des-ox-i-met'a-sone)
Rx: Topicort, Topicort LP
Chemical Class: Synthetic glucocorticoid
Therapeutic Class: Topical corticosteroid, intermediate potency (0.05% cream), high potency (0.05% gel, 0.25% cream, ointment)

CLINICAL PHARMACOLOGY
Mechanism of Action: Depresses formation, release, and activity of endogenous mediators of inflammation such as prostaglandins, kinins, histamine, liposomal enzymes, and the complement system resulting in decreased edema, erythema, and pruritus
Pharmacokinetics: Absorbed through the skin (increased by inflammation and occlusive dressings), metabolized primarily in the liver
INDICATIONS AND USES: Psoriasis, eczema, contact dermatitis, pruritus
DOSAGE
Adult and Child
• Top apply to affected area bid-tid, rub completely into skin

💲 AVAILABLE FORMS/COST OF THERAPY
• Cre—Top: 0.05%, 15, 60 g: **$10.95-$15.12**/15 g; 0.25%, 15, 60 g: **$10.17-$20.04**/15 g
• Gel—Top: 0.05%, 15, 60 g: **$17.40**/15 g
• Oint—Top: 0.25%, 15, 60 g: **$19.86**/15 g
CONTRAINDICATIONS: Fungal infections; use on face, groin, or axilla
PRECAUTIONS: Viral infections, bacterial infections, children
PREGNANCY AND LACTATION: Pregnancy category C; it is unknown whether topical application could result in sufficient systemic absorption to produce detectable amounts in breast milk (systemic corticosteroids are secreted into breast milk in quantities not likely to have any detrimental effects on infant)
SIDE EFFECTS/ADVERSE REACTIONS
HEME: Leukocytosis
METAB: Reduced glucose tolerance
SKIN: Acne, allergic contact dermatitis, atrophy, burning, dryness, folliculitis, hypertrichosis, hypopigmentation, irritation, itching, miliaria, perioral dermatitis, secondary infection, striae
MISC: Reversible HPA axis suppression (more likely with occlusive dressings, prolonged administration, application to large surface areas, liver failure, or use in children)
SPECIAL CONSIDERATIONS
• Potent, fluorinated topical corticosteroid with comparable efficacy to fluocinonide, diflorasone, amcinonide, betamethasone, dipropionate, and halcinonide; cost should govern use
PATIENT/FAMILY EDUCATION
• Apply sparingly only to affected area

---

* = non-FDA-approved use

- Avoid contact with the eyes
- Do not put bandages or dressings over treated area unless directed by clinician
- Discontinue drug, notify clinician if local irritation or fever develops
- Do not use on weeping, denuded, or infected areas

---

desoxyribonuclease
(des-oxy-ribe-o-new'clee-ase)
Rx: Elase
Combinations
  Rx: with chloramphenicol;
    Elase-Chloromycetin
Chemical Class: Lytic enzyme
Therapeutic Class: Debriding agent; irrigating agent

CLINICAL PHARMACOLOGY
Mechanism of Action: Purulent exudates consist largely of fibrinous material and nucleoprotein; desoxyribonuclease attacks the DNA and fibrinolysin attacks principally the fibrin of blood clots and fibrinous exudates
INDICATIONS AND USES:
Top—Debriding agent in general surgical wounds, ulcerative lesions (trophic, decubitus, stasis, arteriosclerotic), 2nd and 3rd degree burns, circumcision, episiotomy; intravaginal—cervicitis (benign, postpartum, and postconization) and vaginitis; irrigating agent—infected wounds (abscesses, fistulae, and sinus tracts), otorhinolaryngologic wounds, superficial hematomas (except when the hematoma is adjacent to or within adipose tissue)
DOSAGE
Adult
- *General topical use:* Apply thin layer of ointment and cover with petrolatum gauze or other nonadherant dressing, change qd-tid; sol may be applied topically as a liquid,

wet dressing, or spray by using a conventional atomizer
- *Wet dressing:* Mix 1 vial of powder with 10-50 ml saline and saturate strips of fine-mesh gauze or unfolded sterile gauze sponge with sol; pack ulcerated area with gauze, allow to dry (approximately 6-8 hr), then remove dried gauze; repeat tid-qid
- *Intravaginal:* Apply 5 g of ointment deep into vagina qhs for 5 applications
- *Abscesses, empyema cavities, fistulae, sinus tracts, or SC hematomas:* Prepare sol by reconstituting contents of each vial of powder with 10 ml isotonic saline; drain and replace sol at 6-10 hr intervals
§ AVAILABLE FORMS/COST OF THERAPY
- Oint—Top: 10, 30 g: **$20.64-$23.99**/10 g
PRECAUTIONS: History of sensitivity to bovine material
SIDE EFFECTS/ADVERSE REACTIONS
SKIN: Local hyperemia
SPECIAL CONSIDERATIONS
Successful enzymatic debridement depends on the following factors: surgical removal of any dense, dry eschar prior to administration; enzyme must be in constant contact with the substrate; periodic removal of accumulated necrotic debris; secondary closure or skin grafting as soon as possible after optimal debridement
PATIENT/FAMILY EDUCATION
- Frequency of application is more important than amount of ointment used
- Do not use sol more than 24 hr after reconstitution

---

italic = common side effects   ***bold italic*** = life-threatening reactions

dexamethasone

(dex-a-meth'a-sone)
Ophthalmic: **Rx:** Ak-Dex
Ophthalmic, Maxidex,
Ocumed *Systemic:*
Rx: Cortastat, Dalalone D.P.,
Decadron, Decaject, Dexa-
sone L.A., Dexone LA,
Solurex, Dalalone, Dexasone,
Dexone
Combinations
  Rx: with neomycin, (Neo-
  Decadron, Ak-Neo-Dex);
  with neomycin and poly-
  mixin B (Dexacidin, Max-
  itrol, Dexasporin); with
  tobramycin (Tobradex);
  with lidocaine (Decadron
  with Xylocaine
Chemical Class: Synthetic
glucocorticoid
Therapeutic Class: Systemic
corticosteroid; ophthalmic
corticosteroid

CLINICAL PHARMACOLOGY
Mechanism of Action: Decreases
inflammation by depressing migration of polymorphonuclear leukocytes and activity of endogenous mediators of inflammation. Has many
profound metabolic effects, does not
possess mineralocorticoid activity
Pharmacokinetics
PO: Peak 1-2 hr
IM: Peak 8 hr
Metabolized in liver, excreted in
urine and bile; biologic $t_{1/2}$ 36-54 hr
INDICATIONS AND USES:
Ophthalmic: Steroid-responsive inflammatory conditions of the pal-
bebral and bulbar conjunctiva, lid,
cornea, and anterior segment of the
globe; corneal injury
Systemic: Anti-inflammatory or immunosuppressant agent in the treatment of a variety of diseases of hematologic, allergic, inflammatory,
neoplastic, and autoimmune origin;
acute mountain sickness*; antiemetic*; bacterial meningitis (to decrease incidence of hearing loss)*;
diagnosis of depression*; hirsutism*; prevention of neonatal respiratory distress syndrome (by administration to mother)*
DOSAGE
Adult
• *Anti-inflammatory:* PO/IM/IV
0.75-9 mg/day in divided doses q6-
12h; IM 8-16 mg q1-3 wk (acetate)
• *Cerebral edema:* IV 10 mg loading dose, then 4 mg IM/IV q6h
• *Shock:* IV 1-6 mg/kg or 40 mg
q2-6h (phosphate)
• *Prophylaxis during premature labor* (to prevent infant respiratory
distress due to immature lungs): 6
mg q12h × 4 doses
• *Intralesional:* 0.8-1.6 mg (acetate)
• *Intra-articular and soft tissue:*
4-16 mg q1-3 wk (acetate); large
joints 2-4 mg (phosphate); small
joints 0.8-1 mg (phosphate); bursae
2-3 mg (phosphate); tendon sheaths
0.4-1 mg (phosphate); soft tissue
infiltration 2-6 mg (phosphate); ganglia 1-2 mg (phosphate)
• *Ophth:* Instill 1 gtt into conjunctival sac q1-4h depending on condition; apply ¼ in ribbon of oint to
lower conjunctival sac tid-qid; reduce frequency of administration
once a favorable response is obtained
Child 6-12 yr
• *Anti-inflammatory:* PO/IM/IV
0.08-0.3 mg/kg/day or 2.5-10 mg/
m^2/day in divided doses q6-12h
• *Bacterial meningitis (>2 mo):* IV
0.6 mg/kg/day divided q6h for 1st
4 days of antibiotic treatment; initiate with 1st dose of antibiotic

---

* = non-FDA-approved use

- *Cerebral edema:* PO/IM/IV 1-2 mg/kg loading dose, then 1-1.5 mg/kg/day (max 16 mg/day) in divided doses q4-6h
- *Physiologic replacement:* PO/IM/IV 0.03-0.15 mg/kg/day or 0.6-0.75 mg/m^2/day in divided doses q6-12h
- *Ophth:* Same as adult

💲 AVAILABLE FORMS/COST OF THERAPY

- Elixir—Oral: 0.5 mg/5ml, 60, 100, 120, 240 ml:**$7.50-$11.08/100 ml**
- Sol—Oral: 1 mg/ml, 30 ml: **$15.73**
- Tab, Uncoated—Oral: 0.25 mg, 100's: **$84.25;** 0.5 mg, 100's: **$6.45-$59.50;** 0.75 mg, 100's: **$7.50-$74.38;** 1 mg, 100's: **$28.37;** 1.5 mg, 100's: **$7.74-$29.08;** 2 mg, 100's: **$54.95;** 4 mg, 100's: **$22.54-$58.41;** 6 mg, 100's: **$63.70-$98.88**
- Inj, Sol (phosphate)—IM, IV: 4 mg/ml, 5 ml: **$2.52-$54.69;** 10 mg/ml, 10 ml: **$4.94-$15.38**
- Inj, Sol (phosphate)—24 mg/ml, 5 ml: **$23.44**
- Inj, Susp—Intra-articular; IM: (acetate) 8 mg/ml, 5 ml: **$11.50-$56.95;** 16 mg/ml, 5 ml: **$25.00**
- Oint—Ophth: 0.05%, 3.5 g: **$1.65-$7.25**
- Sol—Ophth: 0.1%, 5 ml: **$1.95-$17.84**
- Susp—Ophth: 0.1%, 5, 15 ml: **$25.00/5 ml**

CONTRAINDICATIONS: Systemic fungal infections; (ophth): acute superficial herpes simplex keratitis and other viral diseases of the cornea and conjunctiva; fungal diseases of ocular structures; ocular TB; following uncomplicated removal of a superficial corneal foreign body

PRECAUTIONS: Psychosis, cerebral malaria, elderly, AIDS, latent tuberculosis or amebiasis (reactivation of disease), diabetes mellitus, glaucoma, osteoporosis, ulcerative colitis (intestinal perforation), CHF,

myasthenia gravis, renal disease, esophagitis, peptic ulcer, hypertension; (ophth): infections of the eye, glaucoma

PREGNANCY AND LACTATION:
Pregnancy category C; used in patients with premature labor at about 24-36 wk gestation to stimulate fetal lung maturation; excreted in breast milk, could suppress infant's growth and interfere with endogenous corticosteroid production

SIDE EFFECTS/ADVERSE REACTIONS

CNS: Depression, headache, *mood changes, seizures,* vertigo

CV: **CHF,** hypertension, tachycardia, ***thromboembolism,*** thrombophlebitis

EENT: Blurred vision, cataracts, *dryness,* epistaxis, increased intraocular pressure, localized infections of nose and pharynx with *C. albicans, nasal irritation,* nasal septum perforation, rebound congestion, sneezing, sore throat, *stinging* (nasal); cataracts, decreased acuity, glaucoma exacerbation, increased intraocular pressure, increased probability of corneal infection, optic nerve damage, poor corneal wound healing, stinging, transient burning (ophth)

GI: Abdominal distention, diarrhea, **GI hemorrhage,** increased appetite, *nausea,* ***pancreatitis***

GU: Hypercalciuria

METAB: Cushingoid state, decreased glucose tolerance, decreased t$_4$, growth suppression in children, *HPA suppression,* hyperglycemia

MS: Aseptic necrosis of femoral and humeral heads, fractures, myopathy, osteoporosis, weakness

SKIN: Acne, bruising, ecchymosis, petechiae, poor wound healing, striae, suppression of skin test reactions, thin fragile skin

---

italic = common side effects   ***bold italic*** = life-threatening reactions

INTERACTIONS
Drugs
▣ *Aminoglutethamide:* Enhanced elimination of corticosteroids; marked reduction in corticosteroid response; increased clearance of dexamethasone; doubling of dose may be necessary

▣ *Antidiabetics:* Increased blood glucose

▣ *Barbiturates, carbamazepine:* Reduced serum concentrations of corticosteroids; increased clearance of dexamethasone

▣ *Cholestyramine, colestipol:* Possible reduced absorption of corticosteroids

▣ *Cyclosporine:* Possible increased concentration of both drugs, seizures

▣ *Erythromycin, troleandomycin, clarithromycin, ketoconazole:* Possible enhanced steroid effect

▣ *Estrogens, oral contraceptives:* Enhanced effects of corticosteroids

▣ *Isoniazid:* Reduced plasma concentrations of isoniazid

▣ *IUDs:* Inhibition of inflammation may decrease contraceptive effect

▣ *NSAIDs:* Increased risk GI ulceration

▣ *Rifampin:* Reduced therapeutic effect of corticosteroids; may reduce hepatic clearance of prednisone

▣ *Salicylates:* Subtherapeutic salicylate concentrations possible
Labs
• *False negative:* Skin allergy tests
SPECIAL CONSIDERATIONS
• Signs of adrenal insufficiency include fatigue, anorexia, nausea, vomiting, diarrhea, weight loss, weakness, dizziness, and low blood sugar; drug induced secondary adrenocorticoid insufficiency and low blood sugar; drug-induced adrenocorticoid insufficiency may be minimized by gradual systemic dosage reduction; relative insufficiency may exist for up to 1 yr after discontinuation, therefore, be prepared to supplement in situations of stress
• May mask infections
• Do not give live virus vaccines to patients on prolonged therapy
• Patients on chronic steroid therapy should wear medical alert bracelet
MONITORING PARAMETERS
• Potassium and blood sugar during long-term therapy
• Observe growth and development of children on prolonged therapy
• Check lens and intraocular pressure frequently during prolonged use of ophthalmic preparations

---

dexchlorpheniramine
(dex′klor-fen-eer′a-meen)
Rx: Polaramine
Combinations
  Rx: with guaifenesin, pseudoephedrine (Polaramine Expectorant)
Chemical Class: Alkylamine derivative
Therapeutic Class: Antihistamine

CLINICAL PHARMACOLOGY
Mechanism of Action: Decreases allergic response by blocking histamine at H_1 receptors
Pharmacokinetics
PO: Onset 20-60 min, peak 3 hr, duration 8-12 hr; protein binding 60%-70%; detoxified in liver; excreted by kidneys (metabolites/free drug); $t_{1/2}$ 20-24 hr

INDICATIONS AND USES: Perennial and seasonal allergic rhinitis; vasomotor rhinitis, allergic conjunctivitis; allergic skin manifestations of urticaria and angioedema; dermatographism; adjunctive anaphylactic therapy

DOSAGE
Adult
• PO 2-6 mg q6h prn; SUS REL 4-6 mg bid prn
Child
• PO age 6-11 yr 1 mg q6h; age 2-5 yr 0.5 mg q6h

$ AVAILABLE FORMS/COST OF THERAPY
• Syr—Oral: 2 mg/5ml, 480 ml: **$16.49-$51.58**
• Tab, Uncoated—Oral: 2 mg, 100's: **$48.64**
• Tab, Sus-Rel—Oral: 4 mg, 100's: **$34.50-$82.97**; 6 mg, 100's: **$40.95-$115.96**

CONTRAINDICATIONS: Acute asthma attack, lower respiratory tract disease

PRECAUTIONS: History of bronchial asthma, increased intraocular pressure secondary to angle-closure glaucoma; hyperthyroidism, cardiovascular disease, hypertension due to atropine-like actions, elderly

PREGNANCY AND LACTATION: Pregnancy category B

SIDE EFFECTS/ADVERSE REACTIONS
CNS: Anxiety, confusion, *dizziness*, *drowsiness*, euphoria, fatigue, neuritis, paresthesia, poor coordination
EENT: Blurred vision, dilated pupils, dry nose, throat; tinnitus
GI: Anorexia, diarrhea, dry mouth, nausea
GU: Dysuria, frequency, *retention*
HEME: **Agranulocytosis, hemolytic anemia, thrombocytopenia**
RESP: Chest tightness, increased thick secretions, wheezing
SKIN: Photosensitivity

DRUG INTERACTIONS
Labs
• *False negative:* Skin allergy tests

SPECIAL CONSIDERATIONS
• Active dextro-isomer of chlorpheniramine

---

dextroamphetamine
(dex-troe-am-fet′a-meen)
Rx: Dexedrine, Dextrostat
Chemical Class: D-β-phenyl-isopropylamine
Therapeutic Class: CNS stimulant
DEA Class: Schedule II

D

CLINICAL PHARMACOLOGY
Mechanism of Action: Sympathomimetic amines with CNS stimulant activity; increases release of norepinephrine and dopamine in cerebral cortex and reticular activating system; promotes norepinephrine release from peripheral adrenergic nerve terminals; peripheral alpha and beta activity includes elevation of systolic and diastolic blood pressures and weak bronchodilator and respiratory stimulation action; heart rate reflexly slowed at standard doses, arrhythmias with overdose

Pharmacokinetics
PO: Onset 30 min, peak 1-3 hr, duration 4-20 hr; metabolized by liver, urine excretion pH dependent (greater excretion with acidic urine); crosses placenta; $t_{1/2}$ 10-30 hr

INDICATIONS AND USES: Narcolepsy, attention deficit disorder with hyperactivity, exogenous obesity*

DOSAGE
Adult
• *Narcolepsy:* PO 5-60 mg/day in divided doses
• *Obesity:* PO 10-15 mg qd (sus rel) in AM or 5-30 mg/day in divided doses of 5-10 mg, administer 30-60 min ac
Child
• *Narcolepsy:* Age >12 yr PO 10 mg qd increasing by 10 mg qd at weekly intervals; age 6-12 yr PO 5 mg qd increasing by 5 mg/wk (max 60 mg qd)

---

italic = common side effects   ***bold italic*** = life-threatening reactions

• *Obesity:* Age >12 yr PO same as adult

• *Attention deficit disorder:* Age >6 yr PO 5 mg qd-bid increasing by 5 mg qd at weekly intervals; age 3-6 yr PO 2.5 mg qd increasing by 2.5 mg qd at weekly intervals (max dose 40 mg/day)

• Sus rel forms may be used for qd dosage

$ AVAILABLE FORMS/COST OF THERAPY

• Tab, Uncoated—Oral: 5 mg, 100's: **$18.30-$24.55;** 10 mg, 100's: **$35.00**

• Cap, Gel, Sus Action—Oral: 5 mg, 50's: **$26.65;** 10 mg, 50's: **$33.20;** 15 mg, 50's: **$42.45**

CONTRAINDICATIONS: Hyperthyroidism, hypertension, glaucoma, drug abuse, cardiovascular disease, anxiety, within 14 days of taking MAOIs

PRECAUTIONS: Tourette syndrome, child <3 yr; amphetamines have a high abuse potential

PREGNANCY AND LACTATION: Pregnancy category C; excreted in breast milk

SIDE EFFECTS/ADVERSE REACTIONS

CNS: Addiction, aggressiveness, chills, *dependence,* dizziness, dysphoria, headache, *hyperactivity, insomnia,* irritability, *restlessness,* stimulation, *talkativeness,* tremor
CV: Cardiomyopathy, decrease in heart rate, *dysrhythmias,* hypertension, *palpitations, tachycardia*
GI: Anorexia, constipation, diarrhea, dry mouth, metallic taste, weight loss
GU: Change in libido, impotence
SKIN: Urticaria

INTERACTIONS
Drugs
3 *Antacids:* Decreased urinary excretion of dextroamphetamine
3 *Furazolidone:* Hypertensive reactions

3 *Guanadrel, Guanethidine:* Antihypertensive effect inhibited by dextroamphetamine
A *MAOIs:* Severe hypertensive reactions possible
2 *Selegiline:* Severe hypertensive reactions possible
3 *Sodium bicarbonate:* May inhibit dextroamphetamine excretion
Labs
• *False positive:* Urine amino acids
SPECIAL CONSIDERATIONS
• Use for obesity should be reserved for patients failing to respond to alternative therapy; weigh the limited benefit against the substantial risk of addiction and dependence
PATIENT/FAMILY EDUCATION
• Tolerance or dependency is common
• Avoid OTC preparations unless approved by clinician
• Do not crush or chew SUS REL dosage forms

---

dextromethorphan
(dex-troe-meth-or′fan)
OTC: Benylin DM, Children's Hold, Delsym, Hold DM, Pertussin, Robitussin Cough Calmers, Robitussin Pediatric, Scott-Tussin DM Cough Chaser, Sucrets Cough Control, Suppress, Trocal, Vicks Formula 44
Combinations
> **OTC:** with benzocaine (Spec T, Vicks Formula 44 cough control discs, Vicks cough silencers); with guaifenesin (Robitussin DM)

Chemical Class: Levorphanol derivative
Therapeutic Class: Antitussive

CLINICAL PHARMACOLOGY
Mechanism of Action: Depresses cough center in medulla

Pharmacokinetics
PO: Onset 15-30 min, duration 3-6 hr

INDICATIONS AND USES: Nonproductive cough

DOSAGE

Adult

• PO 10-20 mg q4h or 30 mg q6-8h, not to exceed 120 mg/day
• PO EXT REL liq 60 mg bid, not to exceed 120 mg/day

Child

• PO: Age 6-12 yr 5-10 mg q4h, not to exceed 60 mg/day; age 2-6 yr 2.5-5 mg q4h, not to exceed 30 mg/day; EXT REL liq: Age 6-12 yr 30 mg bid, not to exceed 60 mg/day; age 2-5 yr 15 mg bid, not to exceed 30 mg/day

$ **AVAILABLE FORMS/COST OF THERAPY**

• Loz—Oral: 2.5 mg, 20's: **$1.71;** 5 mg, 16's: **$2.45**
• Syr—Oral: 3.5 mg/5 ml, 120 ml: **$2.74;** 7.5 mg/5 ml, 60 ml: **$2.26;** 15 mg/5 ml, 120 ml: **$2.74**
• Liq, EXT REL—Oral: 30 mg/5 ml, 90 ml: **$6.31**

PRECAUTIONS: Chronic, persistent, or productive cough; nausea, vomiting; fever; persistent headache

PREGNANCY AND LACTATION: Pregnancy category C

SIDE EFFECTS/ADVERSE REACTIONS

CNS: Dizziness
GI: Nausea

INTERACTIONS

Drugs

⚠ *Isocarboxazid, MAOIs, Phenelzine:* Increased risk of toxicity due to dextromethorphan

3 *Quinidine, terbinafine:* Reduced hepatic metabolism of dextromethorphan

3 *Fluoxetine:* Case report of a patient on fluoxetine developing visual hallucinations when she began

to take dextromethorphan; causality not established

2 *Sibutramine:* Increased risk of serotonin syndrome

---

dezocine

(dez'o-seen)
Rx: Dalgan
Chemical Class: Synthetic opiate derivative—aminotetralin series
Therapeutic Class: Narcotic agonist-antagonist analgesic

D

CLINICAL PHARMACOLOGY

Mechanism of Action: Analgesia via μ subclass opiate receptor binding in CNS; μ receptors mediate morphine-like supraspinal analgesia, euphoria, and respiratory and physical depression; narcotic antagonist activity is greater than pentazocime

Pharmacokinetics

IM: Onset 30 min, peak 50-90 min, duration 2-4 hr
IV: Onset 10 min, peak 30 min, duration 2-4 hr
Metabolized by liver, excreted by kidneys; may cross placenta

INDICATIONS AND USES: Severe pain

DOSAGE

NOTE: 10 mg parenteral dose equivalent to 10 mg morphine

Adult

• IM 5-20 mg q3-6h, not to exceed 120 mg/day; IV 2.5-10 mg q2-4h

$ **AVAILABLE FORMS/COST OF THERAPY**

• Inj, Sol—IM, IV: 5 mg/ml, 1 ml: **$8.54;** 10 mg/ml, 1 ml: **$9.58;** 15 mg/ml, 1 ml: **$9.56**

PRECAUTIONS: Patients physically dependent on narcotics (may precipitate withdrawal), addictive personality, increased intracranial pressure, respiratory depression, he-

---

italic = common side effects   ***bold italic*** = life-threatening reactions

patic disease, renal disease, child <18 yr, elderly, biliary surgery, COPD, sulfite sensitivity

PREGNANCY AND LACTATION: Pregnancy category C

SIDE EFFECTS/ADVERSE REACTIONS

CNS: Anxiety, confusion, delirium, dependency, depression, dizziness, drowsiness, headache, sedation, sleep disturbances, slurred speech

CV: Chest pain, edema, hypertension, hypotension, pallor, pulse irregularity, thrombophlebitis

EENT: Blurred vision, diplopia

GI: Abdominal pain, anorexia, constipation, cramps, diarrhea, dry mouth, nausea, vomiting

GU: Urinary frequency, hesitancy, retention

RESP: Hiccups, *respiratory depression*

SKIN: Chills, inj site reactions, pruritus, rash, sweating

---

diazepam

(dye-az′e-pam)

Rx: Diastat, Diastat-Pediatric, Valium, Valrelease

Chemical Class: Benzodiazepine

Therapeutic Class: Anxiolytic; sedative/hypnotic; anesthesia adjunct; skeletal muscle relaxant; anticonvulsant

DEA Class: Schedule IV

CLINICAL PHARMACOLOGY

Mechanism of Action: CNS depressants via facilitation of inhibitory GABA at benzodiazepine receptor sites (BZ_1—associated with sleep; BZ_2—associated with memory, motor, sensory, and cognitive function); effects include muscle relaxation (spinal cord), anticonvulsant activity (brain stem), ataxia (cerebellum), emotional behavior (limbic and cortical areas), and anxiolytic effects (separate from general CNS depression); other effects include sedative, appetite-stimulating, and weak analgesic actions

Pharmacokinetics

PO: Rapidly absorbed, onset 15-45 min, peak 0.5-1½ hr, duration 2-3 hr

IM: Absorption slow and erratic (deltoid muscle optimal site), onset 15-30 min, peak 0.5-1½ hr, duration 1-1½ hr

IV: Onset 1-3 min, duration 15 min Metabolized by liver, excreted by kidneys, crosses the blood-brain barrier; $t_{1/2}$ 20-50 hr

PR: Onset 5-15 min, peak 1.5 hr

INDICATIONS AND USES: Anxiety, acute alcohol withdrawal, adjunctive anesthesia; amnesia in cardioversion, endoscopic procedures, etc.; conscious sedation, insomnia, status epilepticus, adjunct in seizure disorders; skeletal muscle spasm relaxation; epilepsy in patients taking stable drug regimens who require intermittent use of diazepam to control episodic increased seizure frequency (rectal viscous solution only); tremor,* tension headache,* panic disorder*

DOSAGE

Adult

• *Anxiety/convulsive disorders:* PO 2-10 mg tid-qid

• *Sedative-hypnotic, alcohol withdrawal:* PO 10 mg tid-qid, tapered prn

• *Skeletal muscle relaxant:* PO 2-10 mg tid-qid

• *Status epilepticus:* IV bolus 5-20 mg infused at a rate of 2 mg/min, may repeat q5-10 min, not to exceed 60 mg; may repeat in 30 min if seizures reappear

• *Adjunct for epilepsy:* PR 0.2 mg/kg prn

Geriatric

• 2-2.5 mg qd-bid, titrated prn

---

* = non-FDA-approved use

Child

• IV bolus 0.1-0.3 mg/kg (over 3 min); may repeat q15 min × 2 doses

• *Tetanic muscle spasms:* Infants >30 days to <5 yr IM/IV 1-2 mg to 5-10 mg q3-4h prn

• *Anxiety/convulsive disorders:* >6 mo PO 1-2.5 mg tid-qid (0.04-0.2 mg/kg tid-qid prn)

• *Adjunct for epilepsy:* PR: age 2-5 yr 0.5 mg/kg prn; age 6-11 yr 0.3 mg/kg prn; age ≥ 12 yr 0.2 mg/kg prn

💲 **AVAILABLE FORMS/COST OF THERAPY**

• Inj, Sol—IM, IV: 5 mg/ml, 2 ml: **$0.42-$6.16**

• Tab, Uncoated—Oral: 2 mg, 100's: **$4.95-$46.56;** 5 mg, 100's: **$6.74-$72.41;** 10 mg, 100's: **$3.85-$121.96**

• Sol—Oral: 5 mg/ml, 30 ml: **$23.52**

• Sol, viscous—Rectal: 5 mg/ml, 2.5 mg, 5 mg, 10 mg, 15 mg, 20 mg, 2's: **$156.00** (with rectal delivery system)

CONTRAINDICATIONS: Narrow-angle glaucoma, psychosis

PRECAUTIONS: Elderly, debilitated, hepatic disease, renal disease, children, low serum albumin

PREGNANCY AND LACTATION: Pregnancy category D; drug and metabolite enter breast milk; lethargy and loss of weight in nursing infant have been reported

SIDE EFFECTS/ADVERSE REACTIONS

CNS: Anxiety, confusion, depression, *dizziness, drowsiness,* fatigue, hallucinations, headache, insomnia, stimulation, tremors, withdrawal syndrome

CV: ECG changes, hypotension; *orthostatic hypotension,* tachycardia, venous thrombosis, phlebitis, local irritation, swelling, and vascular impairment following IV inj into small veins on hand

EENT: Blurred vision, mydriasis, tinnitus

GI: Anorexia, constipation, diarrhea, dry mouth, increased ALT/AST, nausea, vomiting

RESP: **Respiratory depression**

SKIN: Dermatitis, itching, rash

INTERACTIONS

Drugs

❸ *Carbamazepine:* Markedly reduces effect of oral diazepam; parenteral diazepam less affected

❸ *Cimetidine:* Inhibits hepatic metabolism of diazepam

❸ *Ciprofloxacin:* Inhibits hepatic metabolism of diazepam; may also competitively inhibit gamma amino butyric acid receptors

❷ *Clarithromycin:* Inhibits hepatic metabolism of diazepam

❸ *Clozapine:* Additive respiratory and cardiovascular depression

❸ *Delavirdine:* Inhibits hepatic metabolism of diazepam

❸ *Disulfiram:* Inhibits hepatic metabolism of diazepam

❸ *Erythromycin:* Inhibits hepatic metabolism of diazepam

❸ *Ethanol:* Additive CNS effects

❸ *Fluconazole:* Inhibits hepatic metabolism of diazepam

❸ *Fluoxetine:* Inhibits hepatic metabolism of diazepam

❸ *Fluvoxamine:* Inhibits hepatic metabolism of diazepam

❸ *Isoniazid:* Inhibits hepatic metabolism of diazepam

❸ *Itraconazole:* Inhibits hepatic metabolism of diazepam

❸ *Ketoconazole:* Inhibits hepatic metabolism of diazepam

❸ *Levodopa:* May reduce anti-Parkinsonian effect

❸ *Metoprolol:* Inhibits hepatic metabolism of diazepam

❸ *Omeprazole:* Inhibits hepatic metabolism of diazepam

❸ *Phenytoin:* Markedly reduces effect of oral diazepam; parenteral diazepam less affected

3 *Quinolones:* Inhibits hepatic metabolism of diazepam; may also competitively inhibit gamma amino butyric acid receptors

3 *Rifampin:* Markedly reduces effect of diazepam

3 *Troleandomycin:* Inhibits hepatic metabolism of diazepam

Labs
• *Increase:* Urine 5-HIAA

SPECIAL CONSIDERATIONS
• Flumazenil (Mazicon), a benzodiazepine receptor antagonist is indicated for complete or partial reversal of the sedative effects of benzodiazepines

PATIENT/FAMILY EDUCATION
• Avoid driving, activities that require alertness; drowsiness may occur
• Avoid alcohol, other psychotropic medications unless prescribed by clinician

---

diazoxide
(dye-az-ox'ide)
Rx: Hyperstat (IV), Proglycem (PO)
Chemical Class: Benzothiadiazine derivative
Therapeutic Class:
Antihypertensive; antihypoglycemic

CLINICAL PHARMACOLOGY
Mechanism of Action: Vasodilates arteriolar smooth muscle by direct relaxation; reduction in blood pressure with concomitant increases in heart rate, cardiac output; decreases release of insulin from β-cells in pancreas, resulting in an increase in blood glucose

Pharmacokinetics
PO: Onset 1 hr, duration 8 hr

IV: Onset 1-2 min, peak 5 min, duration 3-12 hr

$t_{1/2}$ 20-36 hr; excreted slowly in urine; crosses blood-brain barrier, placenta

INDICATIONS AND USES: Hypertensive crisis when urgent decrease of diastolic pressure required; increase blood glucose levels in hyperinsulinism

DOSAGE
Adult
• *Hypertension:* IV bolus 1-3 mg/kg rapidly up to a max of 150 mg in a single inj; dose may be repeated at 5-15 min intervals until desired response is achieved; give IV in 30 sec or less
• *Hypoglycemia:* PO initial 1 mg/kg q8h, adjusted prn according to response; maintenance 3-8 mg/kg/day given bid-tid (max 15 mg/kg/day)

Child
• *Hypertension:* IV bolus 1-2 mg/kg rapidly; administration same as adult; not to exceed 150 mg
• *Hypoglycemia:* PO initial 3.3 mg/kg q8h, adjusted prn; maintenance 8-15 mg/kg/day given bid-tid

$ AVAILABLE FORMS/COST OF THERAPY
• Inj, Sol—IV: 15 mg/ml, 20 ml: **$114.41**
• Susp—Oral: 50 mg/ml, 30 ml: **$122.25**

CONTRAINDICATIONS: Hypersensitivity to thiazides, sulfonamides; hypertension associated with aortic coarctation or AV shunt; pheochromocytoma; dissecting aortic aneurysm; functional hypoglycemia

PRECAUTIONS: Tachycardia; fluid, electrolyte imbalances; lactation; impaired cerebral or cardiac circulation; gout; diabetes mellitus

PREGNANCY AND LACTATION: Pregnancy category C

SIDE EFFECTS/ADVERSE REACTIONS

CNS: Anxiety, blurred vision, confusion, dizziness, EPS, euphoria, headache, insomnia, malaise, paresthesia, sleepiness, TIAs, weakness

CV: Angina pectoris, edema, hypotension, palpitations, rebound hypertension, *supraventricular tachycardia,* T-wave changes

EENT: Cataracts, diplopia, lacrimation, ring scotoma, subconjunctival hemorrhage, tinnitus

GI: Changes in ability to taste, dry mouth, nausea, vomiting

GU: Decreased urinary output, hematuria, increased BUN, reversible nephrotic syndrome

HEME: Decreased hemoglobin/hematocrit, *thrombocytopenia*

METAB: Hyperglycemia, hyperuricemia

SKIN: Hypertrichosis, rash

MISC: Breast tenderness, allergic reactions

INTERACTIONS

Drugs

🔳 *Carboplatin, cisplatin:* Increased risk of nephrotoxicity

🔳 *Hydralazine:* Severe hypotensive reactions

🔳 *Phenytoin:* Decreased phenytoin levels in children, probably due to enhanced metabolism

🔳 *Thiazide diuretics:* Hyperglycemia

SPECIAL CONSIDERATIONS

• Often administered concurrently with a diuretic to prevent congestive heart failure due to fluid retention

• Oral susp dosage form produces higher concentration than cap form

• Hyperglycemia transient (24-48 hr) after IV administration

• If not effective within 2-3 wk of treatment of hypoglycemia, re- evaluate

---

dibucaine

(dye'byoo-kane)
OTC: Nupercainal
Chemical Class: Amide derivative
Therapeutic Class: Topical anesthetic

D

CLINICAL PHARMACOLOGY

Mechanism of Action: Inhibits nerve impulses from sensory nerves

Pharmacokinetics

TOP: Onset up to 15 min, duration 3-4 hr, readily systemically absorbed through traumatized or abraded skin; hepatic and some renal biotransformation; renally excreted as metabolites

INDICATIONS AND USES: Pruritus, pain, sunburn, toothache, rectal pain and irritation, dermatitis (e.g., poison ivy), minor wounds

DOSAGE

Adult and Child

• TOP apply qid as needed

💲 **AVAILABLE FORMS/COST OF THERAPY**

• Oint—Top: 1%, 30, 60 g: **$4.10/30 g**

• Cre—Top: 0.5%, 45 g: **$3.26;** 1%, 30 g: **$3.70**

CONTRAINDICATIONS: Infants <1 yr, application to large areas

PRECAUTIONS: Child <6 yr, sepsis, denuded skin

PREGNANCY AND LACTATION: Pregnancy category C; excretion into breast milk unknown

SIDE EFFECTS/ADVERSE REACTIONS

SKIN: Irritation, rash, sensitization

SPECIAL CONSIDERATIONS

Cross-sensitivity between amide derivatives and ester anesthetics or pramoxine has not been reported

---

italic = common side effects   ***bold italic*** = life-threatening reactions

dichlorphenamide

(die-klor-fen′a-mide)

Rx: Daranide

Chemical Class: Sulfonamide derivative

Therapeutic Class: Antiglaucoma agent

CLINICAL PHARMACOLOGY

Mechanism of Action: Carbonic anhydrase inhibition reduces rate of aqueous humor formation, decreasing intraocular pressure; inhibits hydrogen ion secretion in renal tubule with increased secretion of sodium, potassium, bicarbonate, water

Pharmacokinetics

PO: Onset 1 hr, peak effect 2-4 hr, duration 6-12 hr

INDICATIONS AND USES: Glaucoma, open-angle and angle-closure

DOSAGE

Adult

• PO 100-200 mg initially, then 100 mg q12h to response; maintenance 25-50 mg qd-tid

** $ AVAILABLE FORMS/COST OF THERAPY**

• Tab, Uncoated—Oral: 50 mg, 100's: **$55.65**

CONTRAINDICATIONS: Hepatic insufficiency, renal failure, adrenocortical insufficiency, hyperchloremic acidosis, hypokalemia, hyponatremia, impaired alveolar ventilation (pulmonary disease, edema, infection, or obstruction)

PRECAUTIONS: Hypokalemia when cirrhosis is present or during concomitant use of steroids or ACTH; respiratory acidosis

PREGNANCY AND LACTATION: Pregnancy category C; safety in lactation not established

SIDE EFFECTS/ADVERSE REACTIONS

CNS: Ataxia, confusion, depression, disorientation, dizziness, drowsiness, *fatigue,* headache, lassitude, *malaise,* nervousness, *paresthesias of the extremities,* **seizures,** tremor, *weakness*

EENT: Myopia, tinnitus

GI: Anorexia, constipation, *diarrhea,* hepatic insufficiency, melena, *nausea, taste alteration, vomiting*

GU: Decreased libido, glycosuria, hematuria, impotence, phosphaturia, renal calculi, renal colic, *urinary frequency*

HEME: **Blood dyscrasias**

METAB: Hyperglycemia, *hypokalemia*

MS: Flaccid paralysis

RESP: Acidosis (shortness of breath, troubled breathing)

SKIN: Photosensitivity, pruritus, rash, **Stevens-Johnson syndrome,** skin eruptions, urticaria

MISC: Fever, hypersensitivity, weight loss

INTERACTIONS

Drugs

 3 *Flecainide:* Increased serum flecainide levels

 3 *Methenamine compounds:* Alkalinization of urine decreases antibacterial effects

 3 *Mexiletine:* Increased serum mexiletine levels

 3 *Phenytoin:* Increased risk of osteomalacia

 3 *Primadone:* Case reports suggest decreased serum primadone levels with a similar drug

 3 *Quinidine:* Alkalinization of urine increases quinidine serum levels

 2 *Salicylates:* Increased serum levels of carbonic anhydrase inhibitors, CNS toxicity

SPECIAL CONSIDERATIONS

• Usually most successful when given in combination with miotics (e.g., pilocarpine)

• If quick relief of angle-closure

---

glaucoma does not occur, surgery may be mandatory

PATIENT/FAMILY EDUCATION
• May cause drowsiness

---

diclofenac
(dye-kloe'fen-ak)
Rx: Potassium (Cataflam) Sodium (Voltaren, Voltaren XR)
Combinations
   Rx: with misoprostol (Arthotec)
Chemical Class: Phenylacetic acid derivative
Therapeutic Class: NSAID with analgesic and antipyretic activity

CLINICAL PHARMACOLOGY
Mechanism of Action: Reversible cyclooxygenase (i.e., prostaglandin synthetase) inhibitor; nonselectively decreases the formation of both prostaglandins and thromboxone A_2; variable effects on lipoxygenase synthesis and subsequent leukotriene production; antiinflammatory, antipyretic, and analgesic activity; inhibits platelet aggregation

Pharmacokinetics
PO: Time to peak, sodium salt 2-3 hr, potassium salt 30 min; $t_{1/2}$ 2 hr, synovial $t_{1/2}$ 3× longer
Completely absorbed, 99.7% bound to plasma proteins; metabolized in liver, 50% bioavailable after 1st pass, excreted in urine and bile
OPHTH: Limited systemic absorption

INDICATIONS AND USES: Actinic keratosis (topically),* ankylosing spondylitis, biliary colic,* cataract removal—inflammation (ophth), cataract removal—mydriasis*(ophth), prevention of cognitive decline,* prevention of colon cancer,* corneal abrasion,* dysmenorrhea, erythermalgia,* fever,* gouty arthritis,* headache,* keratitis,* myalgia,* osteoarthritis, pain—mild to moderate

DOSAGE
Adult
• *Osteoarthritis:* PO 100-150 mg/day in divided doses (50 mg bid-tid or 75 mg bid)
• *Rheumatoid arthritis:* PO 150-200 mg/day in divided doses (50 mg tid-qid or 75 mg bid)
• *Ankylosing spondylitis:* PO 100-125 mg/day; give 25 mg qid and 25 mg hs if needed
• *Pain, dysmenorrhea:* PO 50 mg immediate-release tid; loading dose (100 mg) useful in some patients
• *Postoperative/cataracts:* Ophth 1 gtt qid, starting 24 hr after surgery for 2 wk

⚡ AVAILABLE FORMS/COST OF THERAPY
Diclofenac Sodium
• Tab ER 100 mg 100's: **$300.76**
• Tab, Enteric Coated, Sus Action—Oral: 25 mg, 100's: **$44.30-$63.09;** 50 mg, 100's: **$86.13-$122.57;** 75 mg, 100's: **$104.31-$148.44**
• Sol—Ophth: 0.1%, 5 ml: **$35.75-$42.19** Diclofenac Potassium
• Tab, Uncoated—Oral: 50 mg, 100's: **$149.16-$181.09**

CONTRAINDICATIONS: Bronchospasm, nasal polyps, angioedema precipitated by aspirin or other NSAIDs

PRECAUTIONS: History of GI ulceration, bleeding, or perforation; renal dysfunction, hypertension or cardiac conditions aggravated by fluid retention and edema, history of liver dysfunction, history of coagulation

PREGNANCY AND LACTATION: Pregnancy category B; excreted in breast milk

---

italic = common side effects   ***bold italic*** = life-threatening reactions

SIDE EFFECTS/ADVERSE REACTIONS

CNS: Anxiety, confusion, depression, dizziness, drowsiness, fatigue, insomnia, muscle weakness, nervousness, paresthesia, tremors

CV: **CHF, dysrhythmias,** fluid retention, hypertension, hypotension, palpitations, peripheral edema, tachycardia

EENT: Blurred vision; hearing loss, tinnitus; Ophth: anterior chamber reaction, burning, elevated intraocular pressure, irritation, keratitis, ocular allergy

GI: Anorexia, cholestatic hepatitis, constipation, cramps, diarrhea, dry mouth, flatulence, **GI bleeding,** jaundice, *nausea,* peptic ulcer, *vomiting*

GU: Azotemia, cystitis, dysuria, hematuria, **nephrotoxicity,** oliguria, UTI

HEME: **Blood dyscrasias,** bruising, epistaxis

RESP: **Bronchospasm,** dyspnea, hemoptysis, **laryngeal edema,** pharyngitis, rhinitis, shortness of breath

SKIN: Alopecia, erythema, petechiae, photosensitivity, pruritus, purpura, rash, sweating

INTERACTIONS

Drugs

3 *Aminoglycosides:* Reduced clearance with elevated aminoglycoside levels and potential for toxicity (especially indomethacin in premature infants; other NSAIDs probably)

3 *Anticoagulants:* Excessive hypoprothrombinemia, decreased platelet aggregation with increased risk of GI bleeding

3 *Antihypertensives (alpha blockers, angiotension-converting enzyme inhibitors, angiotensin II receptor blockers, beta blockers, diuretics):* Inhibition of antihypertensive and other favorable hemodynamic effects

3 *Corticosteroids:* Increased risk of GI ulceration

3 *Cyclosporine:* Increased nephrotoxicity risk

3 *Lithium:* Decreased clearance of lithium (mediated via prostaglandins) resulting in elevated serum lithium levels and risk of toxicity

2 *Methotrexate:* Decreased renal secretion of methotrexate resulting in elevated methotrexate levels and risk of toxicity

3 *Phenylpropanolamine:* Possible acute hypertensive reaction

3 *Potassium-sparing diuretics:* Additive hyperkalemia potential

2 *Triamterene:* Acute renal failure reported with addition of indomethacin; caution with other NSAIDs

Labs

• *Increase:* Serum AST, plasma cortisol, plasma glucose (oxidase-peroxidase method)

SPECIAL CONSIDERATIONS

• No significant advantage over other NSAIDs; cost should govern use

MONITORING PARAMETERS

• Initial hemogram and fecal occult blood test within 3 mo of starting regular chronic therapy; repeat every 6-12 mo (more frequently in high-risk patients (>65 years, peptic ulcer disease, concurrent steroids or anticoagulants); electrolytes, creatinine, and BUN within 3 mo of starting regular chronic therapy; repeat every 6-12 mo

---

* = non-FDA-approved use

dicloxacillin

(dye-klox'a-sill-in)
Rx: Dycill, Dynapen
Chemical Class: Penicillin
derivative (penicillinase-
resistant)
Therapeutic Class: Antibiotic

CLINICAL PHARMACOLOGY
Mechanism of Action: Inhibits bacterial wall synthesis, bactericidal
Pharmacokinetics
PO: Peak 1 hr, duration 4-6 hr, $t_{\frac{1}{2}}$ 30-60 min; absorption stable to acid; concurrent food decreases absorption; 98% plasma protein bound; excreted unchanged in urine
INDICATIONS AND USES: Infections of the bone and localized skin and skin structure caused by susceptible organisms
Antibacterial spectrum usually includes:
Gram-positive organisms: *Staphylococcus aureus, Streptococcus pyogenes, S. viridans, S. faecalis, S. bovis, S. pneumoniae,* including those producing penicillinase
DOSAGE
Adult
• PO 125-500 mg q6h
Child
• PO 12.5-25 mg/kg in divided doses q6h, max 4 g/day
💲 AVAILABLE FORMS/COST OF THERAPY
• Cap, Gel—Oral: 250 mg, 100's: **$19.00-$95.46;** 500 mg, 100's: **$36.00-$179.00**
• Powder, Reconst—Oral: 62.5 mg/5 ml, 200 ml: **$16.69**
PRECAUTIONS: Hypersensitivity to cephalosporins; asthma, eczema, mononucleosis (rash)
PREGNANCY AND LACTATION: Pregnancy category B; penicillins are excreted into breast milk in low concentrations; compatible with breast feeding
SIDE EFFECTS/ADVERSE REACTIONS
CNS: Anxiety, coma, depression, hallucinations, lethargy, *seizures,* twitching
GI: Abdominal pain, colitis, *diarrhea,* glossitis, increased AST, ALT; *nausea, **pseudomembranous colitis,** vomiting*
GU: Glomerulonephritis, hematuria, *moniliasis,* oliguria, proteinuria, *vaginitis*
HEME: **Bone marrow depression,** increased bleeding time
INTERACTIONS
Drugs
3 *Macrolide antibiotics, chloramphenicol, tetracyclines:* Possible inhibition of antibacterial activity of penicillins
3 *Methotrexate:* Potentiation of methotrexate toxicity
3 *Oral contraceptives:* Possible impaired contraceptive efficacy
3 *Warfarin:* Reduced hypoprothrombinemic response
Labs
• *False increase:* Nafcillin level
SPECIAL CONSIDERATIONS
PATIENT/FAMILY EDUCATION
• Should be taken with water 1 hr before or 2 hr after meals on an empty stomach

dicumarol

(die-coom'er-all)
Rx: Dicumarol
Chemical Class: Coumarin
derivative
Therapeutic Class: Oral anticoagulant

CLINICAL PHARMACOLOGY
Mechanism of Action: Interferes with hepatic synthesis of vitamin K-dependent clotting factors, caus-

---

italic = common side effects   ***bold italic*** = life-threatening reactions

ing depression in the activity of factors II, VII, IX, X and proteins C and S in a dose-dependent manner; has no direct effect on established thrombus, but prevents further extension of formed clot

Pharmacokinetics

PO: Onset of action 1-5 days; duration of action 2-10 days; slow and incomplete absorption; >99% plasma protein bound, metabolized by hepatic microsomal enzymes; excreted as inactive metabolites in the urine and feces; t½ 1-4 days

INDICATIONS AND USES: Prophylaxis and treatment of deep venous thrombosis and pulmonary thromboembolism; prophylaxis of embolism associated with atrial fibrillation, MI, cardioversion of chronic atrial fibrillation, prosthetic heart valves*; cerebral embolism*

DOSAGE

Adult

• PO 25-200 mg/d, as indicated by INR determinations

💲 **AVAILABLE FORMS/COST OF THERAPY**

• Tab, Uncoated—Oral: 25 mg, 100's: **$10.69**

CONTRAINDICATIONS: Pregnancy; hemorrhagic tendencies; recent or contemplated surgery of the eye or CNS, or surgery resulting in large, open surfaces; bleeding from the GI, respiratory, or GU tract; threatened abortion; aneurysm; ascorbic acid deficiency; polyarthritis; severe uncontrolled or malignant hypertension; severe renal or hepatic disease; pericarditis and pericardial effusion; subacute bacterial endocarditis; visceral carcinoma; following procedures with potential for uncontrollable bleeding; history of warfarin-induced skin necrosis; uncooperative patient

PRECAUTIONS: Trauma, infection, renal insufficiency, hypertension, vasculitis, indwelling catheters, severe diabetes, active tuberculosis, postpartum, protein C deficiency, hepatic insufficiency, elderly, children, hyperthyroidism, hypothyroidism, CHF, polyarteritis, deverticulitis, antibiotic therapy, malnutrition

PREGNANCY AND LACTATION: Pregnancy category D; no adverse effect or any change in PT have been noted in nursing infants; compatible with breast feeding for normal full-term infants

SIDE EFFECTS/ADVERSE REACTIONS

CV: Systemic cholesterol microembolization (purple toe syndrome)

GI: Diarrhea, intestinal obstruction from submucosal or intramural hemorrhage, mouth ulcers, nausea, paralytic ileus, sore mouth

GU: Red-orange urine

HEME: **Hemorrhage**

METAB: Adrenal insufficiency, pyrexia

SKIN: Alopecia, dermatitis, *exfoliative dermatitis, skin necrosis,* urticaria

DRUG INTERACTIONS

Drugs

• Drug interactions involving dicumarol similar to those involving warfarin; refer to warfarin drug interaction section

SPECIAL CONSIDERATIONS

• Warfarin is the coumarin anticoagulant of choice

MONITORING PARAMETERS

• Dosage of anticoagulants must be individualized and adjusted according to INR determinations; it is recommended that INR determinations be performed prior to initiation of therapy, at 24-hr intervals while maintenance dosage is being established, then once or twice weekly for the following 3-4 wks, then at 1-4 wk intervals for the duration of treatment

---

* = non-FDA-approved use

• Maintain INR at 2-3 (2.5-3.5 for mechanical valves, recurrent systemic thromboembolism)

dicyclomine
(dye-sye'kloe-meen)
Rx: Bentyl, Dicyclocot
Chemical Class: Synthetic tertiary amine
Therapeutic Class: Gastrointestinal antispasmodic; anticholinergic

CLINICAL PHARMACOLOGY
Mechanism of Action: Inhibits muscarinic actions of acetylcholine at postganglionic parasympathetic neuroeffector sites
Pharmacokinetics
PO: Onset 1-2 hr, duration 3-4 hr; metabolized by liver; $t_{1/2}$ 9-10 hr; excreted in urine
INDICATIONS AND USES: Functional bowel/irritable bowel syndrome; adjunctive treatment of peptic ulcer disease,* infant colic*
DOSAGE
Adult
• PO 10-40 mg tid-qid prn; IM 20 mg q4-6h prn
Child >2 yr
• PO 10 mg tid-qid prn
Child 6 mo-2 yr
• PO 5 mg tid-qid prn
$ **AVAILABLE FORMS/COST OF THERAPY**
• Cap, Gel—Oral: 10 mg, 100's: **$17.63-$29.58**
• Tab, Uncoated—Oral: 20 mg, 100's: **$9.75-$42.24**
• Syr—Oral: 10 mg/5 ml, 480 ml: **$32.88**
• Inj, Sol—IM: 10 mg/ml, 2 ml: **$1.90-$15.18**
CONTRAINDICATIONS: Narrow-angle glaucoma, GI obstruction, myasthenia gravis, paralytic ileus, GI atony, toxic megacolon

PRECAUTIONS: Hyperthyroidism, coronary artery disease, dysrhythmias, CHF, ulcerative colitis, hypertension, hiatal hernia, hepatic disease, renal disease, urinary retention, prostatic hypertrophy, small children, Down Syndrome
PREGNANCY AND LACTATION: Pregnancy category B; single case report of apnea in nursing infant; avoid in nursing women
SIDE EFFECTS/ADVERSE REACTIONS
CNS: Anxiety, *coma* (child <3 mo), *confusion,* dizziness, drowsiness, hallucination; headache, insomnia, *seizures, stimulation in elderly,* weakness
CV: Palpitations, tachycardia
EENT: Blurred vision, cycloplegia, increased ocular tension, mydriasis, photophobia
GI: Absence of taste, *constipation, dry mouth,* dysphagia, heartburn, nausea, paralytic ileus, vomiting
GU: Hesitancy, impotence, *rentention*
SKIN: Allergic reactions, anhidrosis, fever, pruritus, rash, urticaria
INTERACTIONS
Drugs
3 *Amantadine, Tricyclic antidepressants, MAOIs, H_1-antihistamines:* Increased anticholinergic effects
3 *Phenothiazines, Levodopa, Ketoconazole:* Decreased therapeutic effects
SPECIAL CONSIDERATIONS
• Not for intravenous use

---

italic = common side effects   ***bold italic*** = life-threatening reactions

didanosine (ddI)

(dye-dan′o-seen)
Rx: Videx
Chemical Class: Nucleoside analog
Therapeutic Class: Antiretroviral

CLINICAL PHARMACOLOGY
Mechanism of Action: Nucleoside analog, incorporates into viral DNA, leading to chain termination; interferes with viral replication by inhibiting reverse transcriptase
Pharmacokinetics
PO: Peak 0.5-1 hr, $t_{1/2}$ 1.6 hr; acid labile (administration with meal decreases peak concentrations and AUC); bioavailability variable, average 30%; extensive metabolism; renal elimination accounts for 50%; no accumulation reported
INDICATIONS AND USES: HIV infections in adults and children
DOSAGE
Adult
• PO ≥60 kg, 200 mg bid, or 250 mg buffered powder bid; <60 kg, 125 mg bid, or 167 mg buffered powder bid; 2 tab should be taken at each dose so that adequate buffering is provided to prevent gastric degradation
• For latest treatment guidelines see www.hivatis.org
Child
• PO 1.1-1.4 m², 100 mg tab bid, or 125 mg pedi powder bid; 0.8-1 m², 75 mg tab bid, or 94 mg pedi powder bid; 0.5-0.7 m², 50 mg tab bid, or 62 mg pedi powder bid; <0.4 m², 25 mg tab bid, or 31 mg pedi powder bid
• For latest treatment guidelines see www.hivatis.org

💲 AVAILABLE FORMS/COST OF THERAPY
• Packet—Oral: 100 mg, 30's: **$43.00;** 167 mg, 30's: **$86.00;** 250 mg, 30's: **$126.97**
• Sol—Oral: 20 mg/ml, 100 ml: **$33.86;** 200 ml: **$67.70**
• Tab, Chewable—Oral: 25 mg, 60's: **$25.40;** 50 mg, 60's: **$50.80;** 100 mg, 60's: **$101.56;** 150 mg, 60's: **$152.37**
PRECAUTIONS: Renal, hepatic disease, children, sodium-restricted diets, elevated amylase, hyperuricemia, pre-existing peripheral neuropathy, history of pancreatitis (risk of recurrence 30%; consider stopping ddI permanently for patients with ddI-induced pancreatitis), alcohol consumption; morbid obesity, hypertriglyceridemia, cholelithiasis
PREGNANCY AND LACTATION: Pregnancy category B; unknown if excreted in breast milk; discontinuation of breast feeding recommended
SIDE EFFECTS/ADVERSE REACTIONS
CNS: Abnormal thinking, anxiety, asthenia, chills, CNS depression, confusion, dizziness, fever, hypertonia, insomnia, pain, *peripheral neuropathy (34%),* **seizures**
CV: **CHF, dysrhythmia,** hypertension, palpitation, syncope, vasodilation
EENT: Ear pain, epistaxis, optic neuritis, otitis, photophobia, retinal depigmentation, visual impairment
GI: Abdominal pain, constipation, *diarrhea (34%),* dry mouth, dyspepsia, flatulence, **hepatic failure (rare),** melena, nausea, oral thrush, **pancreatitis (7%),** stomatitis, taste perversion, vomiting
GU: Hyperuricemia
HEME: **Anemia, granulocytopenia, leukopenia, thrombocytopenia**
METAB: Lactic acidosis

MS: Arthritis, muscular atrophy, myalgia, myopathy

RESP: **Bronchospasm,** cough, dyspnea, hypoventilation, pneumonia, sinusitis

SKIN: Alopecia, ecchymosis, hemorrhage, petechiae, pruritus, rash, sweating

INTERACTIONS

Drugs

☒ *Allopurinol:* Increases area under curve for ddI in patients with renal insufficiency

☒ *Dapsone:* Buffering compound may inhibit dissolution of dapsone in the stomach

☒ *Food:* Reduced bioavailability

☒ *Ganciclovir:* Increased ddI concentrations

☒ *Itraconazole, ketoconazole:* Alkalinization of stomach by didanosine reduces the solubility and absorption of antifungal

☒ *Quinolones:* Decreased concentrations after binding to the aluminum and magnesium ions in the didanosine buffering compound

SPECIAL CONSIDERATIONS
MONITORING PARAMETERS

• Amylase, lipase, ophthalmologic examinations

• Suspend use until pancreatitis excluded if patient develops nausea, abdominal pain

• Tablets contain 264.5 mg sodium, packets 1380 mg sodium

• Administer on empty stomach

---

dienestrol

(dye-en-ess'trole)
Rx: Ortho Dienestrol
Chemical Class: Nonsteroidal synthetic estrogen derivative
Therapeutic Class: Estrogen

CLINICAL PHARMACOLOGY
Mechanism of Action: Synthetic estrogen substitute; acts on female GU tract and reproductive system

Pharmacokinetics

TOP: 50% systemic absorption (better than non-vaginal estrogen products); distributed mainly to adipose tissue; primarily hepatic degradation; excreted in urine

INDICATIONS AND USES: Atrophic vaginitis, kraurosis vulvae

DOSAGE

Adult

• VAG CRE 1 applicatorful 1-2×/ day for 2 wk, then ½ dose or every other day for 2 wk, then 1 application 2-3 × weekly as maintenance

💲 AVAILABLE FORMS/COST OF THERAPY

• Cre—Vag: 0.01%, 78 g: **$28.14; $30.00** w/applicator

CONTRAINDICATIONS: Breast cancer, estrogen-dependent neoplasia, thromboembolic disorders, reproductive cancer, genital bleeding (abnormal, undiagnosed)

PRECAUTIONS: Hypertension, asthma, blood dyscrasias, gallbladder disease, CHF, diabetes mellitus, bone disease, depression, migraine headache, convulsive disorders, hepatic disease, renal disease, family history of cancer of the breast or reproductive tract

PREGNANCY AND LACTATION: Pregnancy category X; no reports of adverse effects on nursing infant; may reduce milk volume and decrease nitrogen and protein content

SIDE EFFECTS/ADVERSE REACTIONS

CNS: Depression, dizziness, headache, migraines, **stroke**

CV: Edema, elevated blood pressure, **pulmonary embolism, MI,** thromboembolism, thrombophlebitis

EENT: Contact lens intolerance, increased corneal lens curvature

---

italic = common side effects   **bold italic** = life-threatening reactions

GI: Anorexia, cramps, diarrhea, gallbladder disease, increased appetite, increased weight, *nausea, pancreatitis,* vomiting

GU: Amenorrhea, breakthrough bleeding, breast changes, cervical eversion, dysmenorrhea, **endometrial cancer,** endometrial hyperplasia

SKIN: Chloasma, dermatitis, erythema nodosum/multiforme, melasma, photosensitivity

INTERACTIONS
Drugs

❷ *Anticoagulants:* Possible altered hypoprothrombinemic response

❸ *Corticosteroids:* Estrogen can decrease clearance and increase therapeutic and toxic effects of corticosteroids

❸ *Cyclosporine:* Increased risk of toxicity

---

diethylpropion
(die-ethyl-prop'ion)
Rx: Tenuate
Chemical Class: Phenethylamine derivative
Therapeutic Class: Anorexiant
DEA Class: Schedule IV

CLINICAL PHARMACOLOGY
Mechanism of Action: Alters adrenergic control of nerve impulse transmission in the appetite control center of the hypothalamus; decreases hunger

Pharmacokinetics
PO: Duration 4 hr
PO SUS REL: Duration 10-14 hr
Metabolized by liver; excreted by kidneys; $t_{1/2}$ 1-3½ hr

INDICATIONS AND USES: Treatment adjunct in exogenous obesity

DOSAGE
Adult
• PO 25 mg tid 1 hr ac or 75 mg controlled release qd midmorning

💲 **AVAILABLE FORMS/COST OF THERAPY**
• Tab, Uncoated—Oral: 25 mg, 100's: **$7.13-$45.96**
• Tab, Uncoated, Sus Action—Oral: 75 mg, 100's: **$79.80-$115.44**

CONTRAINDICATIONS: Hyperthyroidism, hypertension, glaucoma, angina pectoris, drug abuse, cardiovascular disease, children <12 yr, severe arteriosclerosis, agitated states

PRECAUTIONS: Convulsive disorders (increased risk of seizures)

PREGNANCY AND LACTATION: Pregnancy category B; excreted in breast milk; no reports of adverse effects

SIDE EFFECTS/ADVERSE REACTIONS
CNS: Anxiety, confusion, depression, dizziness, dysphoria, euphoria, fatigue, headache, *hyperactivity,* incoordination, insomnia, malaise, *restlessness,* tremors

CV: **Dysrhythmias,** ECG changes, hypertension, *palpitations,* pulmonary hypertension, *tachycardia*

EENT: Blurred vision, eye irritation, mydriasis

GI: Anorexia, constipation, diarrhea, dry mouth, nausea, pain, unpleasant taste, vomiting

GU: Change in libido, dysuria, impotence, menstrual irregularities, polyuria, urinary frequency

HEME: **Bone marrow depression**

SKIN: Erythema, rash, urticaria

MISC: Chills, ecchymosis, excessive sweating, fever, flushing, hair loss, muscle/chest pain

DRUG INTERACTIONS
Labs
• *False positive:* Urine cocaine, diazepam, methaqualone, phencyclidine

SPECIAL CONSIDERATIONS
• Tolerance to anorectic effects may

develop within weeks; cross-tolerance is almost universal

• Measure the limited usefulness against the inherent risks (habituation) of this agent

• Most patients will eventually regain weight lost during use of this product

---

diethylstilbestrol (DES)

(dye-eth-il-stil-bess'trole)

Rx: Stilphostrol
(diphosphonate salt)

Chemical Class: Nonsteroidal synthetic estrogen derivative
Therapeutic Class: Antineoplastic

CLINICAL PHARMACOLOGY

Mechanism of Action: Increases cellular synthesis of DNA, RNA, and various proteins in responsive tissues of the female reproductive tract affects release of pituitary gonadotropins

Pharmacokinetics

Primarily hepatic metabolism and renal excretion

INDICATIONS AND USES: Postcoital contraception*; inoperable breast and prostatic cancer

DOSAGE

Adult

• *Postcoital contraception:* PO 25 mg bid × 5 days, starting within 72 hr of intercourse

• *Prostatic cancer:* PO 1-3 mg qd initially, may then be reduced to 1 mg qd; IM 5 mg 2×/wk, then 4 mg 2×/wk; IV 0.25-1 g qd × 5 days, then 1-2×/wk; (diphosphate form) PO 50-200 mg tid, max 1 g/day

• *Breast cancer:* PO 15 mg qd

$ **AVAILABLE FORMS/COST OF THERAPY**

• Tab, Uncoated—Oral: 1 mg, 100's: **$9.14;** 5 mg, 100's: **$24.35**

Diphosphonate Salt:

• Inj, Sol—IV: 250 mg/5 ml, 1's: **$15.17**

CONTRAINDICATIONS: Breast cancer (except in selected patients being treated for metastatic disease), active thromboembolic disorders, known or suspected estrogen-dependent neoplasia, undiagnosed abnormal genital bleeding, pregnancy

PRECAUTIONS: Hypertension, gallbladder disease, CHF, diabetes mellitus, seizure disorders, hepatic disease, uterine fibroids, hypertriglyceridemia, family history of breast or endometrial cancer, hypercalcemia

PREGNANCY AND LACTATION: Pregnancy category X; increased incidence of vaginal and cervical carcinoma in female offspring exposed *in utero;* may reduce quantity and quality of milk

SIDE EFFECTS/ADVERSE REACTIONS

CNS: Depression, migraine headache, emotional lability

CV: **Arterial thromboembolism, pulmonary embolism, CVA, MI,** hypertension, venous thrombosis, edema

EENT: Contact lens intolerance, ***retinal thrombosis***

GI: *Nausea and vomiting,* gallbladder disease, bloating, benign hepatic tumors, ***mesenteric thrombosis***

GU: *Breakthrough bleeding, spotting,* amenorrhea, change in cervical secretions, breast enlargement, breast tenderness, testicular atrophy

METAB: Hyperglycemia, hypertriglyceridemia, hypercalcemia

SKIN: Melasma

INTERACTIONS

Drugs

3 *P450 inducers (e.g., rifampin,*

---

italic = common side effects   ***bold italic*** = life-threatening reactions

barbiturates): Decreased estrogen levels

3 *Corticosteroids:* Increased steroid effect

3 *Phenytoin:* Loss of seizure control, decreased estrogen levels

3 *Warfarin:* Theoretical increased risk thromboembolism

SPECIAL CONSIDERATIONS
PATIENT/FAMILY EDUCATION

• Nausea, especially in the morning is primarily central in origin, but solid food often provides some relief

---

difenoxin and atropine

(dye-fen-ox'in)
Rx: Motofen
Chemical Class: Opiate (phenylpiperidine) derivative
Therapeutic Class: Antidiarrheal
DEA Class: Schedule IV

CLINICAL PHARMACOLOGY
Mechanism of Action: Slows intestinal motility through a local effect on the gastrointestinal wall; atropine is present to discourage deliberate overdosage

Pharmacokinetics
PO: Peak 40-60 min, duration 3-4 hr, terminal $t_{1/2}$ 12-14 hr; metabolized in liver to inactive metabolite, excreted in urine and feces

INDICATIONS AND USES: Acute nonspecific diarrhea; acute exacerbations of chronic functional diarrhea

DOSAGE
Adult

• PO 2 mg stat, then 1 mg after each loose stool or 1 mg q3-4h as needed, not to exceed 8 mg/24 hr

[$] **AVAILABLE FORMS/COST OF THERAPY**

• Tab, Uncoated—Oral: 0.025 mg

atropine/1 mg difenoxin, 100's: **$54.90**

CONTRAINDICATIONS: Diarrhea associated with invasive organisms (toxigenic *E. coli, Salmonella* sp., *Shigella*); pseudomembranous colitis; children <2 yr; jaundice

PRECAUTIONS: Hepatic disease, renal disease, ulcerative colitis, children, fluid and electrolyte imbalances, Down syndrome

PREGNANCY AND LACTATION: Pregnancy category C; excretion into breast milk unknown

SIDE EFFECTS/ADVERSE REACTIONS

CNS: Confusion, *dizziness, drowsiness,* fatigue, headache, insomnia, *lightheadedness,* nervousness

EENT: Blurred vision, burning eyes

GI: Constipation, dry mouth, epigastric distress, *nausea,* vomiting

INTERACTIONS
Drugs

2 *MAOIs:* May cause hypertensive crisis

SPECIAL CONSIDERATIONS
• Meperidine analog
• Equally effective as codeine, diphenoxylate, or loperamide

PATIENT/FAMILY EDUCATION
• Prolonged use not recommended
• Drowsiness or dizziness may occur; use caution when driving or operating dangerous machinery

---

* = non-FDA-approved use

diflorasone

(die-floor'a-sone)
Rx: Florone, Florone E,
Maxiflor, Psorcon, Psorcon E
Chemical Class: Synthetic
glucocorticoid
Therapeutic Class: Topical
corticosteroid, very high potency (0.05% ointment), high
potency (0.05% cream, emo-
lient base ointment)

CLINICAL PHARMACOLOGY
Mechanism of Action: Depresses
formation, release, and activity of
endogenous mediators of inflammation such as prostaglandins, kinins, histamine, liposomal enzymes,
and the complement system resulting in decreased edema, erythema,
and pruritus
Pharmacokinetics: Absorbed
through the skin (increased by inflammation and occlusive dressings);
metabolized primarily in the liver
INDICATIONS AND USES: Psoriasis, eczema, contact dermatitis, pruritus
DOSAGE
Adult and Child
• Apply to affected area bid, rub
completely into skin
💲 **AVAILABLE FORMS/COST
OF THERAPY**
• Cre—Top: 0.05%, 15, 30, 60 g:
$33.66-$48.54/30 g
• Oint—Top: 0.05%, 15, 30, 60 g:
$33.66-$48.54/30 g
CONTRAINDICATIONS: Fungal
infections; use on face, groin, or
axilla
PRECAUTIONS: Viral infections,
bacterial infections, children
PREGNANCY AND LACTATION:
Pregnancy category C; unknown
whether topical application could re-
sult in sufficient systemic absorp-

tion to produce detectable amounts
in breast milk (systemic corticosteroids are secreted into breast milk
in quantities not likely to have detrimental effects on infant)
**SIDE EFFECTS/ADVERSE REAC-
TIONS**
SKIN: Acne, allergic contact dermatitis, atrophy, burning, dryness,
folliculitis, hypertrichosis, hypopigmentation, irritation, itching,
miliaria, perioral dermatitis, secondary infection, striae
MISC: Reversible HPA axis suppression (more likely with occlusive
dressings, prolonged administration,
application to large surface areas,
liver failure, or use in children)
SPECIAL CONSIDERATIONS
• No demonstrated superiority over
other high-potency agents; cost
should govern use
PATIENT/FAMILY EDUCATION
• Apply sparingly only to affected
area
• Avoid contact with the eyes
• Do not put bandages or dressings
over treated area unless directed by
clinician
• Discontinue drug, notify clinician
if local irritation or fever develops
• Do not use on weeping, denuded,
or infected areas

diflunisal

(dye-floo'ni-sal)
Rx: Dolobid
Chemical Class: Salicylate
derivative
Therapeutic Class: NSAID
with analgesic and antipyretic
activity

CLINICAL PHARMACOLOGY
Mechanism of Action: Reversible
cyclooxygenase (i.e., prostaglandin
synthetase) inhibitor; nonselectively
decreases the formation of both pros-

taglandins and thromboxane A_2; variable effects on lipoxygenase synthesis and subsequent leukotriene production; antiinflammatory, antipyretic, and analgesic activity; inhibits platelet aggregation

Pharmacokinetics

PO: Peak 2-3 hr, onset 1 hr, >99% bound to plasma proteins, $t_{1/2}$ 8-12 hr (dose dependent); excreted mainly in urine as glucuronide conjugates

INDICATIONS AND USES: Osteoarthritis, rheumatoid arthritis, ankylosing spondylitis,* prevention of cognitive decline,* pain—mild to moderate, migraine headache,* tendonitis,* dysmenorrhea*

DOSAGE

Adult

• *Mild to moderate pain:* PO 500-1000 mg initially, then 250-500 mg q8-12h

• *Osteoarthritis/rheumatoid arthritis:* PO 500-1000 mg/day in 2 divided doses; max 1500 mg/day

AVAILABLE FORMS/COST OF THERAPY

• Tab, Plain Coated—Oral: 250 mg, 60's: **$46.66-$65.45;** 500 mg, 100's: **$90.29-$101.56**

PRECAUTIONS: History of GI ulceration, bleeding, or perforation; renal dysfunction, hypertension or cardiac conditions aggravated by fluid retention and edema, history of liver dysfunction, history of coagulation, children with fever (potential association with Reye's syndrome)

PREGNANCY AND LACTATION: Pregnancy category C; use during 3rd trimester not recommended due to effects on fetal cardiovascular system (closure of ductus arteriosus); excreted into breast milk in concentrations 2%-7% those in maternal plasma; use caution in nursing mothers

SIDE EFFECTS/ADVERSE REACTIONS

CNS: Confusion, dizziness, flushing, hallucinations, headache, insomnia, paresthesias, somnolence, stimulation, vertigo

CV: Chest pain, palpitations

EENT: Blurred vision, corneal deposits, decreased acuity

GI: Abnormal LFTs, anorexia, constipation, *diarrhea,* flatulance, **GI bleeding,** GI pain, heartburn, hepatitis, *nausea,* vomiting

GU: Uricosuria

HEME: **Agranulocytosis, thrombocytopenia**

RESP: Dyspnea

SKIN: Dry mucous membranes, erythema multiforme, **exfoliative dermatitis,** photosensitivity, pruritus, *rash,* **Stevens-Johnson syndrome,** stomatitis, sweating, **toxic epidermal necrolysis,** urticaria

INTERACTIONS

Drugs

3 *Aminoglycosides:* Reduced clearance with elevated aminoglycoside levels and potential for toxicity (especially indomethacin in premature infants; other NSAIDs probably)

3 *Anticoagulants:* Excessive hypoprothrombinemia, decreased platelet aggregation with increased risk of GI bleeding

3 *Antihypertensives (alpha blockers, angiotensin-converting enzyme inhibitors, angiotensin II receptor blockers, beta blockers, diuretics):* Inhibition of antihypertensive and other favorable hemodynamic effects

3 *Corticosteroids:* Increased risk of GI ulceration

3 *Cyclosporine:* Increased nephrotoxicity risk

3 *Lithium:* Decreased clearance of lithium (mediated via prostaglandins) resulting in elevated serum lithium levels and risk of toxicity

3 *Methotrexate:* Decreased renal secretion of methotrexate resulting in elevated methotrexate levels and risk of toxicity

3 *Phenylpropanolamine:* Possible acute hypertensive reaction

3 *Potassium-sparing diuretics:* Additive hyperkalemia potential

3 *Triamterene:* Acute renal failure reported with addition of indomethacin; caution with other NSAIDs

Labs

• *False increase:* Serum salicylate

• *False decrease:* T_4, T_3 uptake

SPECIAL CONSIDERATIONS

• No significant advantage over other NSAIDs; cost should govern use

MONITORING PARAMETERS

• Initial hemogram and fecal occult blood test within 3 mo of starting regular chronic therapy; repeat every 6-12 mo (more frequently in high-risk patients (> 65 years, peptic ulcer disease, concurrent steroids or anticoagulants); electrolytes, creatinine, and BUN within 3 mo of starting regular chronic therapy; repeat every 6-12 mo

---

digitoxin

(di-ji-tox'in)

Rx: Crystodigin

Chemical Class: Digitalis derivative

Therapeutic Class: Antidysrhythmic; cardiac glycoside

CLINICAL PHARMACOLOGY

Mechanism of Action: Increases influx of calcium ions into intracellular cytoplasm, resulting in increased cardiac muscle contractility (positive inotropic effect); decreases SA and AV node conduction (negative chronotropic effect)

Pharmacokinetics

PO: Onset 1-4 hr, peak 8-12 hr, $t_{1/2}$ 168-192 hr, 90%-97% bound to plasma proteins; metabolized by the liver, excreted via the kidneys (metabolites)

INDICATIONS AND USES: Congestive heart failure (CHF), atrial fibrillation, atrial flutter, paroxysmal atrial tachycardia (PAT), cardiogenic shock

DOSAGE

Adult

• Loading dose PO (rapid) 0.6 mg, followed by 0.4 mg, then 0.2 mg at q4-6h intervals; (slow) 0.2 mg bid for 4 days; maintenance dose PO 0.05-0.3 mg qd. Dosage reduction not needed in renal function impairment

Child

• Loading dose PO <1 yr 0.045 mg/kg, 1-2 yr 0.04 mg/kg, >2 yr 0.03 mg/kg divided into 3, 4, or more portions with >6 hr between doses; maintenance dose PO $\frac{1}{10}$ loading dose

$ **AVAILABLE FORMS/COST OF THERAPY**

• Tab, Uncoated—Oral: 0.05 mg, 100's: **$2.92;** 0.1 mg, 100's: **$5.14**

CONTRAINDICATIONS: Ventricular tachycardia, ventricular fibrillation

PRECAUTIONS: Hypokalemia, hypomagnesemia, hypercalcemia, hypothyroidism, severe pulmonary disease, sick sinus syndrome, hepatic disease, acute MI, AV block, elderly, Wolff-Parkinson-White syndrome

PREGNANCY AND LACTATION: Pregnancy category C; passes readily to fetus; excretion into breast milk unknown; digoxin, a related

---

italic = common side effects   ***bold italic*** = life-threatening reactions

cardiac glycoside, is considered compatible with breast feeding
SIDE EFFECTS/ADVERSE REACTIONS
CNS: Anorexia, apathy, confusion, delirium, disorientation, drowsiness, EEG abnormalities, hallucinations, headache, mental depression, neuralgia, psychosis, restlessness, *seizures,* weakness
CV: Atrial fibrillation, AV block, bradycardia, premature ventricular contractions (PVCs), *ventricular fibrillation, ventricular tachycardia*
EENT: Visual disturbances (blurred, yellow or green vision, halo effect)
GI: Abdominal discomfort, *diarrhea, hemorrhagic necrosis of the intestines,* nausea, *vomiting*
HEME: Eosinophilia, *thrombocytopenia*
SKIN: Rash
INTERACTIONS
Drugs
3 *Alprazolam, amiodarone, diltiazem, verapamil, bepridil, nitrendipine, quinidine, carvedilol, cyclosporine, erythromycin and tetracyclines (change in bacterial flora causing effect may persist for months), hydroxychloroquine, NSAIDs, azole antifungals, omeprazole, lansoprazole, propafenone, quinine, spironolactone, tacrolimus:* Increased digoxin levels
3 *Amphotericin B diuretics:* Enhanced digitalis toxicity secondary to drug-induced hypokalemia
3 *Beta-blockers:* Potentiation of bradycardia
3 *Calcium (IV):* Digitalis toxicity
2 *Charcoal:* Reduced digitalis levels
3 *Cholestyramine, Kaolo-pectin (digoxin tablets only), neomycin, penicillamine, rifampin, sulfasalazine:* Reduced digitalis levels
3 *Metoclopramide, cisapride:* Reduced digitalis levels by slowly dissolving digoxin tablets only (Lanoxin tablets and capsules not affected)
3 *Succinylcholine:* Increased arrhythmias
Labs
• *False increase:* Urine 17-hydroxycorticosteroids
SPECIAL CONSIDERATIONS
• When digitalis indicated digoxin is 1st line drug because of its shorter $t_{1/2}$ and faster clearance in the event toxicity develops
• Rule out digitalis toxicity if nausea, vomiting, arrhythmias develop
• Listed adverse effects are mostly signs of toxicity
MONITORING PARAMETERS
• Heart rate and rhythm, periodic ECGs
• Serum potassium, magnesium, calcium, creatinine
• Serum digitoxin levels when compliance, effectiveness, or systemic availability is questioned or toxicity suspected; therapeutic range 9-25 ng/ml

---

digoxin
(di-jox'in)
Rx: Lanoxicaps, Lanoxin
Chemical Class: Digitalis glycoside
Therapeutic Class: Antidysrhythmic; cardiac glycoside

CLINICAL PHARMACOLOGY
Mechanism of Action: Increases influx of calcium ions into intracellular cytoplasm, resulting in increased cardiac muscle contractility (positive inotropic effect); decreases SA and AV node conduction (negative chronotropic effect)
Pharmacokinetics
IV: Onset 5-30 min, peak 1-5 hr

PO: Onset 30-120 min, peak 2-6 hr, t₁/₂ 30-40 hr, 20%-25% bound to plasma proteins; excreted mainly by kidneys

INDICATIONS AND USES: Congestive heart failure in patients receiving diuretics or diuretics and ACE inhibitors (CHF), control of ventricular response rate in atrial fibrillation, atrial flutter, paroxysmal atrial tachycardia (PAT), cardiogenic shock

DOSAGE

Administer IV slowly over 5 min; IM route not recommended due to local irritation, pain, and tissue damage

Adult

• Loading dose (give ½ total dose initially, then ¼ total dose in each of 2 subsequent doses at 8-12 hr intervals); IV 0.5-1 mg; PO 0.75-1.5 mg; maintenance dose IV 0.1-0.4 mg qd; PO 0.125-0.5 mg qd

Child >10 yr

• Loading dose (administered as for adult); IV 8-12 µg/kg; PO 10-15 µg/kg; maintenance dose IV 2-3 µg/kg qd; PO 2.5-5 µg/kg qd

Child 5-10 yr

• Loading dose (administered as for adult); IV 15-30 µg/kg; PO 20-35 µg/kg; maintenance dose IV 4-8 µg/kg divided q12h; PO 5-10 µg/kg divided q12h

Child 2-5 yr

• Loading dose (administered as for adult); IV 25-35 µg/kg; IV 30-40 µg/kg; maintenance dose IV 6-9 µg/kg divided q12h; PO 7.5-10 µg/kg divided q12h

Child 1-24 mo

• Loading dose (administered as for adult); IV 30-50 µg/kg; PO 35-60 µg/kg; maintenance dose IV 7.5-12 µg/kg divided q12h; PO 10-15 µg/kg divided q12h

Full term infant

• Loading dose (administered as for adult); IV 20-30 µg/kg; PO 25-35 µg/kg; maintenance dose IV 5-8 µg/kg divided q12h; PO 6-10 µg/kg divided q12h

Preterm infant

• Loading dose (administered as for adult); IV 15-25 µg/kg; PO 20-30 µg/kg; maintenance dose: IV 4-6 µg/kg divided q12h; PO 5-7.5 µg/kg divided q12h

AVAILABLE FORMS/COST OF THERAPY

• Inj, Sol—IM, IV: 0.1 mg/ml, 1 ml: **$6.12-$6.48;** 0.25 mg/ml, 2 ml: **$1.45-$2.68**

• Elixir—Oral: 0.05 mg/ml, 60 ml: **$10.40-$30.78**

• Cap, Elastic—Oral: 0.05 mg, 100's: **$24.67;** 0.1 mg, 100's: **$26.93;** 0.2 mg, 100's: **$32.32**

• Tab, Uncoated—Oral: 0.125 mg, 100's: **$7.50-$20.30;** 0.25 mg, 100's: **$7.50-$20.30;** 0.5 mg, 100's: **$14.70-$18.50**

CONTRAINDICATIONS: Ventricular tachycardia, ventricular fibrillation

PRECAUTIONS: Hypokalemia, hypomagnesemia, hypercalcemia, hypothyroidism, severe pulmonary disease, sick sinus syndrome, hepatic disease, acute MI, AV block, elderly, Wolff-Parkinson-White syndrome

PREGNANCY AND LACTATION: Pregnancy category C, passes readily to fetus; excreted into breast milk; considered compatible with breast feeding

SIDE EFFECTS/ADVERSE REACTIONS

CNS: Anorexia, apathy, confusion, delirium, disorientation, drowsiness, EEG abnormalities, hallucinations, headache, mental depression, neuralgia, psychosis, restlessness, *seizures,* weakness

italic = common side effects   ***bold italic*** = life-threatening reactions

CV: **Atrial fibrillation, AV block,** bradycardia, premature ventricular contractions (PVCs), **ventricular fibrillation, ventricular tachycardia**
EENT: Visual disturbances (blurred, yellow or green vision, halo effect)
GI: Abdominal discomfort, *diarrhea,* **hemorrhagic necrosis of the intestines,** nausea, *vomiting*
HEME: Eosinophilia, **thrombocytopenia**
SKIN: Rash

INTERACTIONS
Drugs
■ *Alprazolam, amiodarone, diltiazem, verapamil, bepridil, nitrendipine, quinidine, carvedilol, cyclosporine, erythromycin and tetracyclines (change in bacterial flora causing effect may persist for months), hydroxychloroquine, NSAIDs, azole antifungals, omeprazole, lansoprazole, propafenone, quinine, spironolactone, tacrolimus:* Increased digoxin levels
■ *Amphotericin B diuretics:* Enhanced digitalis toxicity secondary to drug-induced hypokalemia
■ *Beta-blockers:* Potentiation of bradycardia
■ *Calcium (IV):* Digitalis toxicity
❷ *Charcoal:* Reduced digitalis levels
■ *Cholestyramine, Kaolo-pectin (digoxin tablets only) neomycin, penicillamine, rifampin, sulfasalazine:* Reduced digitalis levels
■ *Cyclophosphamide:* Impaired digoxin (especially tablets) absorption; digitoxin not affected
■ *Metoclopramide, cisapride:* Reduced digitalis levels by slowly dissolving digoxin tablets only (Lanoxin tablets and capsules not affected)
■ *Succinylcholine:* Increased arrhythmias

Labs
• *False increase:* Urine 17-hydroxy-corticosteroids

SPECIAL CONSIDERATIONS
• Preferred digitalis glycoside
• Rule out digitalis toxicity if nausea, vomiting, arrhythmias develop
• Listed adverse effects are mostly signs of toxicity

MONITORING PARAMETERS
• Heart rate and rhythm, periodic ECGs
• Serum potassium, magnesium, calcium, creatinine
• Serum digoxin levels when compliance, effectiveness, or systemic availability is questioned or toxicity suspected
• Obtain serum drug concentrations at least 8-12 hr after a dose (preferably prior to next scheduled dose); therapeutic range 0.5-2.0 ng/ml

---

digoxin immune Fab
Rx: Digibind
Chemical Class: Antibody fragment
Therapeutic Class: Digoxin antidote

CLINICAL PHARMACOLOGY
Mechanism of Action: Antibody fragments bind to free digoxin to reverse digoxin toxicity by not allowing digoxin to bind to sites of action; derived from sheep antibodies
Pharmacokinetics
IV: Onset of improvement in signs and symptoms of digoxin toxicity 30 min, $t_{1/2}$ 15-20 hr, antigen binding fragment–digoxin complex accumulates in the blood and is excreted by the kidneys

INDICATIONS AND USES: Potentially life-threatening digoxin intoxication (has also been used successfully to treat life-threatening digitoxin overdose)

DOSAGE

Adult

• IV dose (mg) = dose ingested (mg) × 0.8 × 66.7; if digoxin liq cap or digitoxin used, do not multiply ingested dose by 0.8; if ingested amount is unknown, give 800 mg IV. Alternatively, calculate the equimolar dose required from the total amount of digoxin (or digitoxin) in the patient's body. An estimate of the total body load can be made from a serum level: For digoxin body load in mg = serum digoxin concentration × 0.56 × weight in kg/1000. Each 40 mg vial will bind 0.6 mg of digoxin or digitoxin; calculate the number of vials required by dividing body load in mg by 0.6 mg/vial; dose (in number of vials) = body load (mg)/0.6 mg/vial

§ AVAILABLE FORMS/COST OF THERAPY

• Inj, Conc-Sol—IV: 40 mg/vial, 1's: **$536.88**

PRECAUTIONS: Children, cardiac disease, renal disease, allergy to ovine products

PREGNANCY AND LACTATION: Pregnancy category C; excretion into breast milk unknown; use caution in nursing mothers

SIDE EFFECTS/ADVERSE REACTIONS

METAB: Hypokalemia

MISC: **Hypersensitivity (anaphylaxis, fever)**

DRUG INTERACTIONS

Labs

• *Interference:* Immunoassay digoxin

SPECIAL CONSIDERATIONS MONITORING PARAMETERS

• Potassium, serum digoxin level prior to therapy

• Continuous ECG monitoring

dihydroergotamine

(dye-hye-droe-er-got′a-meen)
Rx: D.H.E. 45, Migranol (nasal)
Chemical Class: Ergot alkaloid
Therapeutic Class: Antimigraine agent

CLINICAL PHARMACOLOGY

Mechanism of Action: Causes vasoconstriction of dilated cranial blood vessels associated with vascular headaches, with a concomitant decrease in the amplitude of pulsations

Pharmacokinetics

IM: Onset 15-30 min

IV: Onset within a few min

NASAL: Onset 60 min

Ninety percent bound to plasma proteins, $t_{1/2}$ (terminal) 21-32 hr; metabolized by liver, excreted in urine and bile

INDICATIONS AND USES: Prevent or abort vascular headaches including migraine and cluster headaches

DOSAGE

Adult

• IM 1 mg at first sign of headache, repeat at 1 hr intervals prn, do not exceed 3 mg/attack or 6 mg/wk; IV 1 mg at first sign of headache, repeat in 1 hr prn, do not exceed 2 mg/attack or 6 mg/wk

• NASAL 1 spray in each nostril at first sign of headache, may repeat in 15 min prn; max 6 sprays/day

§ AVAILABLE FORMS/COSTS OF THERAPY

• Inj, Sol—IM, IV: 1 mg/ml, 1 ml: **$13.18**

• Spray—Nasal: 0.5 mg/inh, 4 ml: **$67.52**

CONTRAINDICATIONS: Pregnancy, peripheral vascular disease, hepatic or renal impairment, coronary artery disease, uncontrolled hypertension, sepsis

PRECAUTIONS: Prolonged administration, excessive dosage

PREGNANCY AND LACTATION: Pregnancy category X; likely excreted into breast milk; ergotamine has caused symptoms of ergotism (e.g., vomiting, diarrhea) in the infant; excessive dosage or prolonged administration may inhibit lactation

SIDE EFFECTS/ADVERSE REACTIONS

CV: Chest pain, coronary vasoconstriction (large doses), increase or decrease in blood pressure, transient tachycardia or bradycardia

GI: Nausea (10%), vomiting

MISC: Itching, localized edema, muscle pain in the extremities, numbness and tingling of fingers and toes, weakness in the legs

INTERACTIONS

Drugs

❷ *Clarithromycin, erythromycin* (not azithromycin or dirithromycin): Increased ergotism (hypertention and ischemia)

❷ *Nitroglycerin:* Enhanced ergot effect, decreased antianginal effects

❷ *Sibutramine:* Increased risk of serotonin syndrome

SPECIAL CONSIDERATIONS

• Considered alternative abortive acute migraine agent; nasal spray less effective than sumatriptan

PATIENT/FAMILY EDUCATION

• Initiate therapy at 1st sign of attack

• Prolonged use may lead to withdrawal headaches

dihydrotachysterol
(dye-hye-droe-tak-iss'ter-ole)
Rx: DHT, Hytakerol
Chemical Class: Sterol derivative
Therapeutic Class: Vitamin D analog; antiosteoporotic

CLINICAL PHARMACOLOGY

Mechanism of Action: Stimulates intestinal calcium absorption and mobilization of bone calcium in the absence of parathyroid hormone and of functioning renal tissue; also increases renal phosphate excretion

Pharmacokinetics

PO: Onset 2 wk; hydroxylated in the liver to 25-hydroxydihydrotachysterol, the major circulating active form of the drug; excreted in bile

INDICATIONS AND USES: Treatment of acute, chronic, and latent forms of postoperative tetany; idiopathic tetany; hypoparathyroidism; pseudohypoparathyroidism*; familial hypophosphatemia*; renal osteodystrophy in chronic renal failure*; osteoporosis (with calcium and flouride)*

DOSAGE

Adult

• PO 0.75-2.5 mg/day for 4 days initially, then 0.2-1.75 mg/day as required for normal serum calcium levels; average dose 0.6 mg qd

Child

• PO 1-5 mg/day for 4 days initially, then 0.5-1.5 mg/day as required for normal serum calcium levels

Neonate

• PO 0.05-0.1 mg/day

$ **AVAILABLE FORMS/COST OF THERAPY**

• Sol—Oral: 0.2 mg/ml, 30 ml: **$38.79**

• Tab, Uncoated—Oral: 0.125 mg,

50's: **$49.36**; 0.2 mg, 100's: **$100.28**; 0.4 mg, 50's: **$90.00**

• Cap, Gel—Oral: 0.125 mg, 50's: **$126.83**

CONTRAINDICATIONS: Hypercalcemia and hypervitaminosis D

PRECAUTIONS: Renal stones, renal failure, heart disease

PREGNANCY AND LACTATION: Pregnancy category A (category D if used in doses above the recommended daily allowance); excretion into breast milk unknown; vitamin D is excreted into breast milk in limited amounts; considered compatible with breast feeding, however, serum calcium levels of the infant should be monitored if the mother is receiving pharmacologic doses

SIDE EFFECTS/ADVERSE REACTIONS

CNS: Amnesia, ataxia, coma, depression, disorientation, drowsiness, fever, hallucinations, headache, lethargy, syncope, vertigo

*CV: **Cardiovascular failure***

EENT: Tinnitus

GI: Anorexia, constipation, cramps, diarrhea, dry mouth, jaundice, metallic taste, nausea, vomiting

GU: Hematuria, hypercalciuria, hyperphosphatemia, polyuria, ***renal failure***

MS: Arthralgia, decreased bone development, hypotonia, myalgia, weakness

SPECIAL CONSIDERATIONS

• Vitamin D analog of choice for prevention and treatment of renal osteodystrophy; less expensive than calcitriol

PATIENT/FAMILY EDUCATION

• Compliance with dosage instructions, diet (evaluate vitamin D ingested in fortified foods, maintain adequate calcium intake) is essential

MONITORING PARAMETERS

• Serum Ca^{++} and phosphate

• If adverse reactions occur rule out hypercalcemia, worsening renal function

D

dihydroxyaluminum sodium carbonate

(dye-hye-drox'ee-a-loom'-a-nim)

OTC: Rolaids

Chemical Class: Aluminum product

Therapeutic Class: Antacid

CLINICAL PHARMACOLOGY

Mechanism of Action: Neutralizes gastric acidity, reduces pepsin

Pharmacokinetics

PO: Onset 20-40 min; excreted in feces

INDICATIONS AND USES: Symptomatic relief of gastroesophageal reflux, acid indigestion; hyperacidity associated with peptic ulcer, gastritis, peptic esophagitis, gastric hyperacidity, hiatal hernia

DOSAGE

Adult

• PO chew 1-2 tab prn

§ AVAILABLE FORMS/COST OF THERAPY

• Tab, Chewable—Oral: 334 mg, 75's: **$4.33**

PRECAUTIONS: Elderly, fluid restriction, decreased GI motility, GI obstruction, dehydration, renal disease, sodium-restricted diets

PREGNANCY AND LACTATION: Pregnancy category C

SIDE EFFECTS/ADVERSE REACTIONS

GI: Anorexia, *constipation,* fecal impaction

METAB: Hypercalciuria, hypophosphatemia

MISC: Aluminum intoxication, osteomalacia

---

italic = common side effects   ***bold italic*** = life-threatening reactions

DRUG INTERACTIONS
Drugs
🔳 *Allopurinol, beta blockers, ateviridine, cefpodoxime and cefuroxime (not cefetamet or cefixime), quinolones, tetracyclines, iron, isoniazid, ketoconazole and itraconazole (not fluconazole), penicillamine:* Decreased absorption

🔳 *Glipizide, glyburide:* Enhanced gastric absorption, monitor for hypoglycemia

🔳 *Lithium:* Lower lithium concentrations

🔳 *Methenamine:* Interference with urinary antibacterial activity if urine pH >5.5

🔳 *Salicylates:* Lower serum concentrations from reduced renal tubular reabsorption

🔳 *Sympathomimetic amines, flecainide, tocainide, mexiletine, quinidine, quinine:* Decreased elimination secondary to increased urine pH, increased drug effects (large doses only)

🔳 *Vitamin C:* Increased aluminum absorption

SPECIAL CONSIDERATIONS
PATIENT/FAMILY EDUCATION
• Thoroughly chew tab before swallowing, follow with a glass of water
• May impair absorption of many drugs; take other drugs 2 hr before or 4-6 hr after antacid
• May cause premature dissolution of enteric coated tablets
• Stools may appear white or speckled

---

diltiazem
(dil-tye'a-zem)
Rx: Cardizem, Cardizem CD, Cardizem SR, Dilacor XR, Diltia XT, Tiamate, Tiazac
Combinations
  Rx: with enalapril (Teczem)
Chemical Class: Benzothiazepine
Therapeutic Class: Calcium channel blocker: Antianginal; antihypertensive; antidysrhythmic (class IV)

CLINICAL PHARMACOLOGY
Mechanism of Action: Inhibits calcium ion influx across cell membrane during cardiac depolarization; produces relaxation of coronary vascular smooth muscle; dilates coronary arteries; slows SA/AV node conduction times, dilates peripheral arteries; hemodynamics: decreases myocardial contractility; no effect or increases cardiac output; decreases peripheral vascular resistance

Pharmacokinetics
PO: Peak serum conc 2-4 hr
PO SUS REL: Peak serum conc 6-11 hr
PO QD CAP: Peak serum conc 10-14 hr
$t_{1/2}$ 4-6 hr, 70%-80% bound to rapid absorption; bioavailability 47%; plasma proteins; Vd 1.7 L/kg metabolized by liver, excreted in urine (96% as metabolites)

INDICATIONS AND USES: *Oral:* Angina pectoris due to coronary artery spasm, chronic stable angina, essential hypertension (SR only); Also prevention of reinfarction of non-Q-wave MI,* tardive dyskinesia,* Raynaud's syndrome,* migraine headache prophylaxis*

---

* = non-FDA-approved use

Parenteral: Atrial fibrillation or flutter (IV), paroxysmal supraventricular tachycardia (IV).

DOSAGE

Adult

• IMMED REL PO 30 mg qid, gradually increase to 180-360 mg/day divided tid-qid until optimal response is obtained; SUS REL (Cardizem SR) PO 60-120 mg bid, adjust at 14 day intervals until optimal response obtained, optimum range 240-350 mg/day; SUS REL (Cardizem CD, Dilacor XR) once daily cap PO 180-240 mg qd, max 540 mg/day; IV 0.25 mg/kg as a bolus over 2 min (a second 0.35 mg/kg bolus dose may be administered after 15 min if response is inadequate), then continuous INF of 5-15 mg/hr for up to 24 hr; conversion from IV to PO, start PO approximately 3 hr after bolus dose; PO (mg/day) = $10 \times \{[\text{rate (mg/hr)} \times 3] + 3\}$; 3 mg/hr = 120 mg/day; 5 mg/hr = 180 mg/day; 7 mg/hr = 240 mg/day; 11 mg/hr = 360 mg/day

💲 AVAILABLE FORMS/COST OF THERAPY

• Cap, Gel, Sus Action—Oral: 60 mg, 100's: **$71.75-$93.48;** 90 mg, 100's: **$82.68-$106.80;** 120 mg, 100's: **$90.01-$139.20;** 180 mg, 100's: **$105.98-$126.83;** 240 mg, 100's: **$112.95-$135.64;** 300 mg, 90's: **$184.79-$241.14;** 360 mg, 90's: **$188.36;** 420 mg, 90's: **$197.42**

• Tab, Plain Coated—Oral: 30 mg, 100's: **$9.87-$50.76;** 60 mg, 100's: **$26.49-$79.68;** 90 mg, 100's: **$78.04-$112.02;** 120 mg, 100's: **$101.67-$146.64**

• Inj, Sol—IV: 5 mg/ml, 5 ml: **$4.80-$14.30**

CONTRAINDICATIONS: Sick sinus syndrome or 2nd or 3rd degree heart block (except with a functioning pacemaker), hypotension <90 mm Hg systolic, acute MI with pulmonary congestion, atrial fibrillation or atrial flutter associated with an accessory bypass tract such as in WPW syndrome or short PR syndrome (IV), ventricular tachycardia (IV)

PRECAUTIONS: CHF, hypotension, hepatic injury, children, impaired renal or hepatic function

PREGNANCY AND LACTATION: Pregnancy category C; excreted into breast milk in concentrations that may approximate those in maternal serum; use caution in nursing mothers

SIDE EFFECTS/ADVERSE REACTIONS

CNS: Abnormal dreams, amnesia, depression, *dizziness,* gait abnormality, hallucinations, *headache,* insomnia, nervousness, paresthesia, personality change, somnolence, tremor

CV: Angina, ***arrhythmia, AV block (1st degree), AV block (2nd or 3rd degree),*** bradycardia, bundle branch block, ***congestive heart failure,*** edema, flushing, hypotension, palpitations, syncope, tachycardia

GI: Anorexia, constipation, diarrhea, dysgeusia, dyspepsia, GERD; mild elevations of LFTs; *nausea,* thirst, vomiting, weight increase

METAB: Metabolic acidosis

SKIN: Petechiae, photosensitivity, pruritus, rash, urticaria

INTERACTIONS

Drugs

🔳 *Alpha blockers:* Additive increased antihypertensive effect

🔳 *Amiodarone:* Cardiotoxicity with bradycardia and decreased cardiac output

🔳 *Antipyrine:* Increased antipyrine concentrations

🔳 *Aspirin:* Enhanced antiplatelet activity

🔳 *Azole antifungals:* Possible in-

---

italic = common side effects   ***bold italic*** = life-threatening reactions

creased calcium channel blocker effects

☒ *Beta-blockers:* Inhibition of metabolism of propranolol and metoprolol (not atenolol); additive effects on cardiac conduction and hypotension

❷ *Carbamazepine:* Increase in carbamazepine toxicity

☒ *Cyclosporine, tacrolimus:* Increased blood concentrations, renal toxicity

☒ *Digitalis glycosides:* Reduced elimination, increased digitalis levels, toxicity

☒ *Ecainide:* Increased ecainide levels

☒ *Erythromycin, troleandomycin:* Increased levels calcium channel blocker

☒ *Fentanyl:* Severe hypotension or increased fluid volume requirements

☒ *H_2-receptor antagonists:* Serum diltiazem concentrations increased

☒ *Lithium:* Neurotoxicity

☒ *Neuromuscular blockers:* Prolonged blockade by vecuronium and pancuronium

☒ *Nitroprusside:* Enhanced hypotension

☒ *Phenobarbital:* Reduced calcium channel blocker concentration

☒ *Phenytoin:* Increased phenytoin levels

☒ *Rifampin:* Decreased diltiazem concentrations

☒ *Tricyclic antidepressants:* Increased TCA levels

Labs
• *False positive:* Urine ketones

---

dimenhydrinate
(dye-men-hye′dri-nate)
Rx: Hydrate
OTC: Calm-X, Dramamine, Triptone
Chemical Class: Ethanolamine derivative
Therapeutic Class: Antihistamine; antivertigo agent

CLINICAL PHARMACOLOGY
Mechanism of Action: Has a depressant action on hyperstimulated labyrinthine function; antiemetic effects may be due to diphenhydramine moiety (dimenhydrinate is a mixture of diphenhydramine and 8-chlorotheophylline)
Pharmacokinetics
PO: Onset 15-30 min
IM: Onset 20-30 min
Duration 3-6 hr; metabolized in liver, excreted in urine
INDICATIONS AND USES: Prevention and treatment of motion sickness; Meniere's disease,* other vestibular disturbances*
DOSAGE
Adult
• PO 50-100 mg q4-6h, do not exceed 400 mg/day; IM/IV 50 mg prn
Child 6-12 yr
• PO 25-50 mg/q6-8h, do not exceed 150 mg/day; IM 1.25 mg/kg or 37.5 mg/m^2 qid, do not exceed 300 mg/day
Child 2-6 yr
• PO 12.5-25 mg q6-8h, do not exceed 75 mg/day
💲 AVAILABLE FORMS/COST OF THERAPY
• Inj, Sol—IM, IV: 50 mg/ml, 10 ml: **$4.00-$12.48**
• Tab, Uncoated—Oral: 50 mg, 100's: **$1.72-$19.50**

---

* = non-FDA-approved use

• Tab, Chewable—Oral: 50 mg, 24's: **$5.86**
• Liq—Oral: 12.5 mg/4 ml, 480 ml: **$10.14-$12.50**

CONTRAINDICATIONS: Neonates (IV products may contain benzyl alcohol)

PRECAUTIONS: Children, prostatic hypertrophy, stenosing peptic ulcer, pyloroduodenal obstruction, bladder neck obstruction, narrow-angle glaucoma, cardiac dysrhythmias, elderly, children <2 yrs

PREGNANCY AND LACTATION: Pregnancy category B; has been used for the treatment of hyperemesis gravidarum; small amounts are excreted into breast milk; use caution in nursing mothers

SIDE EFFECTS/ADVERSE REACTIONS

CNS: Confusion, dizziness, *drowsiness,* excitation, headache, heaviness and weakness of hands, insomnia (especially in children), lassitude, nervousness, restlessness, tingling, vertigo
CV: Palpitations, tachycardia
EENT: Blurring of vision, diplopia, nasal stuffiness
GI: Anorexia, constipation, diarrhea, *dry mouth,* epigastric distress, nausea, vomiting
GU: Difficult or painful urination
HEME: **Hemolytic anemia**
SKIN: Drug rash, photosensitivity, urticaria

SPECIAL CONSIDERATIONS
PATIENT/FAMILY EDUCATION
• For prevention of motion sickness administer at least 30 min before exposure to motion

dimercaprol
(dye-mer-kap'role)
Rx: BAL in Oil, British Anti-Lewisite
Chemical Class: Dithiol derivative
Therapeutic Class: Heavy metal antidote (arsenic, gold, mercury, lead)

CLINICAL PHARMACOLOGY
Mechanism of Action: Promotes excretion of heavy metals by chelation, increasing urinary and fecal elimination of the metals

Pharmacokinetics
IM: Peak 30-60 min; metabolism and excretion are complete within 4 hr, excretion via urine and feces

INDICATIONS AND USES: Treatment of arsenic, gold, and mercury poisoning; acute lead poisoning (in conjunction with calcium edetate disodium)

DOSAGE
Adult and Child
• *Mild arsenic and gold poisoning:* IM 2.5 mg/kg/dose q6h for 2 days, then q12h on 3rd day, then qd thereafter for 10 days
• *Severe arsenic and gold poisoning:* IM 3 mg/kg/dose q4h for 2 days, then q6h on 3rd day, then q12h thereafter for 10 days
• *Mercury poisoning:* IM 5 mg/kg initially followed by 2.5 mg/kg/dose qd-bid for 10 days
• *Lead poisoning:* IM 4 mg/kg alone for first dose, then 3-4 mg/kg/dose with calcium edetate disodium administered at a separate site q4h for 5-7 days

AVAILABLE FORMS/COST OF THERAPY
• Inj, Sol—IM: 100 mg/ml, 3 ml: **$33.00**

---

italic = common side effects   ***bold italic*** = life-threatening reactions

CONTRAINDICATIONS: Hepatic insufficiency (except postarsenical jaundice); iron, cadmium, or selenium poisoning; severe renal disease

PRECAUTIONS: Acute renal insufficiency, G-6-PD deficiency, acidic urine, hypertension

PREGNANCY AND LACTATION: Pregnancy category D; use only in life-threatening poisoning

SIDE EFFECTS/ADVERSE REACTIONS

CNS: Anxiety, headache

CV: Rise in blood pressure, tachycardia

EENT: Burning sensation in the lips, mouth and throat; conjunctivitis, lacrimation, blepharal spasm; feeling of constriction in the throat; rhinorrhea

GI: Abdominal pain, *nausea,* salivation, *vomiting*

GU: Burning sensation in the penis

SKIN: Sweating

SPECIAL CONSIDERATIONS
• Administer by deep IM injection only

MONITORING PARAMETERS
• Blood pressure, pulse
• BUN, Cr, urine pH (alkaline urinary pH decreases renal damage)
• Specific heavy metal levels

---

dinoprostone (PGE$_2$)
(dye-noe-prost'one)
Rx: Cervidil, Prepidil Gel, Prostin E$_2$

Chemical Class: Prostaglandin
Therapeutic Class: Abortifacient; uterine stimulant

CLINICAL PHARMACOLOGY
Mechanism of Action: Stimulates uterine contractions, GI and vascular smooth muscle

Pharmacokinetics
Onset 20 min (more rapid from gel form); metabolized in spleen, kidney, lungs, excreted in urine

INDICATIONS AND USES: Abortion during 2nd trimester, benign hydatidiform mole, expulsion of uterine contents in fetal deaths to 28 wk, missed abortion, cervical ripening, labor induction

DOSAGE
Adult
• *Abortifacient:* Vag supp (Prostin E$_2$)—20 mg high into vagina, repeat q3-5h until abortion occurs, max 240 mg
• *Cervical ripening:* Gel(Prepidil)—administer contents of 1 syringe (0.5 mg) into cervical canal just below the internal os, repeat in 6 hr prn, max 1.5 mg/24 hr; Insert (Cervidil)—Place transversely in posterior fornix of vagina; remove after 12 hr

$ AVAILABLE FORMS/COST OF THERAPY
• Gel—Cervical: 0.5 mg/3 g: **$151.80**
• Supp—Vag: 20 mg/supp: **$439.77**
• Insert—Vag 0.3 mg/hr: **$183.46**

CONTRAINDICATIONS: SUPP: Acute PID; cardiac, pulmonary, renal, or hepatic disease; viable fetus; GEL: History of major uterine surgery (including C-section with vertical uterine scar), cephalopelvic disproportion, grand multiparae (≥6 previous term pregnancies), nonvertex presentation, hyperactive or hypertonic uterine patterns, fetal distress, obstetric emergencies favoring surgical intervention, placenta previa or unexplained vaginal bleeding, vasa previa, active herpes genitalia

PRECAUTIONS: Asthma, glaucoma, hepatic/renal function impairment, hypotension, hypertension, cardiovascular disease, anemia, jaundice, diabetes, epilepsy, chorioamnionitis, cervicitis, infected en-

docervical lesions, acute vaginitis, previous C-section with transverse uterine scar, ruptured membranes
PREGNANCY AND LACTATION: Pregnancy category C; complete any failed attempts at pregnancy termination by some other means
SIDE EFFECTS/ADVERSE REACTIONS

CNS: Chills, dizziness, fever, *headache*

CV: Hypertension (transient)

EENT: Blurred vision

GI: Diarrhea, nausea, vomiting

GU: Vaginal pain, vaginismus, vaginitis, vulvitis

HEME: Transient leukocytosis

MS: Joint swelling, leg cramps, weakness

SKIN: Rash, skin color changes

INTERACTIONS

Drugs

• *Oxytoxin:* Augmented activity, use sequentially not concurrently (6-12 hr after gel, 30 min after removal of insert)

SPECIAL CONSIDERATIONS

• Do not place gel above level of internal os; use 20 mm endocervical catheter if no effacement present; 10 mm catheter if cervix 50% effaced

• May use small amount water soluble lubricant with insert; do not use insert without retrieval system

PATIENT/FAMILY EDUCATION

• Remain supine for 10-15 min (vag supp), 15-30 min (gel), 2h (insert)

MONITORING PARAMETERS

• Blood pressure, fetal monitor (for cervical ripening)

diphenhydramine

(dye-fen-hye'dra-meen)

Rx: Banaril, Benadryl, Dytuss, Hyrexin, Tusstat, Tuxadryl **OTC:** Allermax, Banophen, Banophen Caplets, Belix, Benadryl 25, Benylin Cough, Bydramine Cough, Diphen Cough, Dormarex 2, Genahist, Gen-D-phen, Hydramine Cough, Nidryl, Nordryl Cough, Phendry, Uni-Bent Cough Combinations

　OTC: with acetaminophen (Excedrin PM, Extra Strength Tylenol PM, Sominex Pain Relief, Unisom with Pain Relief); with calamine (Caladryl)

Chemical Class: Ethanolamine derivative

Therapeutic Class: Antihistamine; antivertigo agent; antipruritic; hypnotic; antianaphylactic (adjunct); antiparkinson's agent

CLINICAL PHARMACOLOGY

Mechanism of Action: Decreases allergic response by blocking histamine at H_1-receptors

Pharmacokinetics

PO: Peak 2-4 hr, 78% bound to plasma proteins; metabolized in the liver; $t_{1/2}$ 2-8 hr

INDICATIONS AND USES: Perennial and seasonal allergic rhinitis; vasomotor rhinitis; allergic conjunctivitis; symptomatic relief of common cold; allergic and non-allergic pruritic symptoms; uncomplicated allergic skin manifestations of urticaria and angioedema; adjunctive therapy of anaphylactic reactions; motion sickness; sleep aid; parkinsonism (including drug-induced);

cough suppressant; acute dystonic reactions

DOSAGE

Adult

• PO/IM/IV 15-50 mg q4h, do not exceed 400 mg/day; for sleep PO 50 mg at hs; TOP apply prn

Child

• PO/IM/IV 5 mg/kg/day or 150 mg/m^2/day divided q6-8h, do not exceed 300 mg/day

💲 **AVAILABLE FORMS/COST OF THERAPY**

• Cap, Gel—Oral: 25 mg, 100's: **$1.32-$6.50;** 50 mg, 100's: **$1.91-$6.80**
• Elixir—Oral: 12.5 mg/5 ml, 480 ml: **$2.93-$8.20**
• Syrup—Oral: 12.5 mg/5 ml, 480 ml: **$1.90-$15.84**
• Inj, Sol—IM, IV: 10 mg/ml, 30 ml: **$5.40-$8.25;** 50 mg/ml, 1 ml: **$0.81-$1.54**
• Cream—Top: 2%, 15 g: **$3.16**
• Spray—Top: 2%, 60 ml: **$4.57**

CONTRAINDICATIONS: Narrow-angle glaucoma, bladder neck obstruction

PRECAUTIONS: Liver disease, elderly, increased intraocular pressure, hyperthyroidism, cardiovascular disease, hypertension, urinary retention, renal disease, stenosed peptic ulcers

PREGNANCY AND LACTATION: Pregnancy category C; excreted into breast milk; although levels are not thought to be sufficiently high after therapeutic doses to affect the infant, the manufacturer considers the drug contraindicated in nursing mothers due to the increased sensitivity of newborn or premature infants to antihistamines

SIDE EFFECTS/ADVERSE REACTIONS

CNS: Anxiety, confusion, *dizziness,* *drowsiness,* euphoria, fatigue, neuritis, paresthesia, poor coordination

CV: Palpitations, tachycardia

EENT: Blurred vision, dilated pupils, *dry nose, throat,* nasal stuffiness, tinnitus

GI: Anorexia, *constipation,* diarrhea, *dry mouth,* nausea, vomiting

GU: Dysuria, frequency, impotence, retention

HEME: **Bone marrow suppression, hemolytic anemia**

RESP: Chest tightness, increased thick secretions, wheezing

SKIN: Photosensitivity, rash, urticaria; topical preparations can sensitize the skin

INTERACTIONS

Drugs

❸ *Anticholinergics:* Possible enhanced anticholinergic, CNS effects

Labs

• *False negative:* Skin allergy tests
• *False positive:* Urine methadone, serum and urine tricyclic antidepressant

---

diphenoxylate and atropine

(dye-fen-ox'i-late)
Rx: Lomocot, Lomotil, Lonox. Vi-Atro
Chemical Class: Meperidine analog
Therapeutic Class: Antidiarrheal
DEA Class: Schedule V

CLINICAL PHARMACOLOGY

Mechanism of Action: Direct effect on circular smooth muscle of the bowel that prolongs GI transit time; available only in combination with atropine sulfate; lacks analgesic activity

Pharmacokinetics

PO: Onset 1 hr, peak 2 hr, duration

3-4 hr; metabolized in liver, excreted in bile and urine

INDICATIONS AND USES: Diarrhea, reduction of ileostomy discharge

DOSAGE

Adult

• PO 5 mg (2 tab) qid, then taper dose as tolerated

Child

• PO 0.3-0.4 mg/kg qd in 4 divided doses

$ AVAILABLE FORMS/COST OF THERAPY

• Sol—Oral: 2.5 mg diphenoxylate/ 0.025 mg atropine/5 ml, 60 ml: **$6.28-$15.74**

• Tab, Uncoated—Oral: 2.5 mg diphenoxylate/0.025 mg atropine, 100's: **$4.68-$53.28**

CONTRAINDICATIONS: Obstructive jaundice, diarrhea associated with pseudomembranous enterocolitis or enterotoxin-producing bacteria

PRECAUTIONS: Age <2 yr, acute ulcerative colitis (may induce toxic megacolon), severe hepatorenal disease

PREGNANCY AND LACTATION: Pregnancy category C; excreted in breast milk

INTERACTIONS

Drugs

❷ *MAOIs:* Possible hypertensive crisis

❸ *Barbiturates, tranquilizers, narcotics, alcohol:* Potentiation of effects

SIDE EFFECTS/ADVERSE REACTIONS

CNS: Fatigue, dizziness, drowsiness
EENT: Dry mouth
GI: Abdominal pain or distention, constipation, ileus, nausea, vomiting
SKIN: Rash (hypersensitivity)

---

dipivefrin

(dye-pi've-frin)
Rx: Propine
Chemical Class: Diesterified epinephrine derivative
Therapeutic Class: Antiglaucoma agent

D

CLINICAL PHARMACOLOGY

Mechanism of Action: Converted to epinephrine, which decreases aqueous humor production and increases outflow

Pharmacokinetics

Onset 30 min, peak 1 hr, duration 12 hr

INDICATIONS AND USES: Open-angle glaucoma

DOSAGE

Adult

• 1 gtt in affected eye(s) q12h

$ AVAILABLE FORMS/COST OF THERAPY

• Sol, Top—Ophth: 0.1%, 15 ml: **$30.15-$53.46**

CONTRAINDICATIONS: Narrow-angle glaucoma

PRECAUTIONS: Children, aphakia (may cause reversible macular edema)

PREGNANCY AND LACTATION: Pregnancy category B

SIDE EFFECTS/ADVERSE REACTIONS

CV: **Dysrhythmias,** hypertension, tachycardia
EENT: *Burning,* mydriasis, photophobia, *stinging*

---

dipyridamole
(dye-peer-id'a-mole)
Rx: Persantine
Combinations:
  Rx: with aspirin (Aggrenox)
Chemical Class: Substituted
pyrimidine derivative
Therapeutic Class: Coronary
vasodilator, antiplatelet agent

CLINICAL PHARMACOLOGY
Mechanism of Action: Inhibits
platelet adhesion, likely by inhibiting thromboxane A_2 formation and
inhibiting phosphodiesterase
Pharmacokinetics
PO: Onset 30 min, peak 2-2½ hr,
duration 6 hr
IV: Onset 1 min, peak 7 min, duration 30 min
Protein binding 91%-99%, conjugated in liver to glucuronide, excreted in bile, undergoes enterohepatic recirculation
INDICATIONS AND USES: Adjunct
to warfarin to prevent thromboembolic complications of cardiac valve
replacement; adjunct to aspirin to
prevent coronary bypass graft
occlusion* or transient ischemic
attack*; as diagnostic aid in thallium myocardial perfusion imaging
for the evaluation of CAD; to reduce the risk of stroke in patients
who have had transient ischemia of
the brain or completed ischemic
stroke caused by thrombosis (Aggrenox)
DOSAGE
Adult
• Adjunct to warfarin therapy: PO
75-100 mg qid
• *Diagnostic aid in myocardial perfusion studies:* IV 0.14 mg/kg/min
for 4 min, max dose 60 mg
Child
• *Inhibition of platelet adhesion:* PO
3-6 mg/kg/day in 3 divided doses

**§ AVAILABLE FORMS/COST
  OF THERAPY**
• Tab, Coated—Oral: 25 mg, 100's:
$2.52-$35.82; 50 mg, 100's: **$4.13-
$57.71;** 75 mg, 100's: **$5.93-$77.18**
• Inj, Sol—IV: 5 mg/ml, 10 ml:
$96.00-$142.50
PRECAUTIONS: Ischemic heart
disease, bleeding disorders, hypotension
PREGNANCY AND LACTATION:
Pregnancy category C; excreted in
breast milk
SIDE EFFECTS/ADVERSE REACTIONS
CNS: Dizziness, headache
GI: Abdominal distress, anorexia, diarrhea, nausea, vomiting
SKIN: Flushing, rash
INTERACTIONS
Drugs
3 *Adenosine:* Increased concentrations of adenosine, potentiates adenosine's pharmacologic effects
3 *Beta blockers:* Additive bradycardia
SPECIAL CONSIDERATIONS
• Contributes little to the effect of
aspirin alone

dirithromycin
(die-rith-ro-my'sin)
Rx: Dynabac
Chemical Class: Macrolide
antibiotic
Therapeutic Class: Antibiotic

CLINICAL PHARMACOLOGY
Mechanism of Action: Bacteriostatic via reversible binding to 50S
ribosomal unit, thereby impairing
protein synthesis
Pharmacokinetics
PO: Peak 4 hr; rapidly absorbed and
converted by nonenzymatic hydrolysis to the microbiologically active
compound   erythromycylamine;
15%-32% protein bound; good tis-

* = non-FDA-approved use

sue penetration into upper and lower respiratory tract and prostate; nonenzymatic hydrolysis to inactive metabolites; fecal and renal elimination; $t_{1/2}$ 44 hr

INDICATIONS AND USES: Infections of upper (including otitis media, pharyngitis, tonsillitis) and lower respiratory tract, skin and skin structure caused by susceptible organisms

Antibacterial spectrum usually includes:

- Gram-positive organisms: *Streptococcus pneumonia, Staphylococcus aureus, Str. pyogenes*
- Gram-negative organisms: *Legionella, Moraxella catarrhalis*
- Anerobes: *P. acnes*
- *Other: Mycoplasma pneumonia, Chlamydia trachomatis*

DOSAGE
Adult (Child >12 yrs)
- PO 500 mg qd for 7-14 days

$ AVAILABLE FORMS/COST OF THERAPY
- Tab, Enteric Coated—Oral: 250 mg, 60's: **$112.50**

PRECAUTIONS: Hepatic insufficiency

PREGNANCY AND LACTATION: Pregnancy category C; excreted into rodent breast milk; no human data

SIDE EFFECTS/ADVERSE REACTIONS
CNS: Asthenia, dizziness, headache
GI: Abdominal pain, diarrhea, dyspepsia, gas, *nausea,* vomiting

INTERACTIONS
Drugs
3 *Penicillins:* Dirithromycin may inhibit antibacterial activity of penicillins

SPECIAL CONSIDERATIONS
PATIENT/FAMILY EDUCATION
- Take with food or within 1 hr of having eaten
- Long $t_{1/2}$ and higher tissue concentrations allow qd dosing; however, the improved antimicrobial activity against *H.influenzae* and lower incidence of GI adverse effects have not been realized with this agent; Azithromycin probably best choice pending further comparisons

---

disopyramide
(dye-soe-peer'a-mide)
Rx: Norpace, Norpace CR
Chemical Class: Substituted pyramide derivative
Therapeutic Class: Antidysrhythmic (class IA)

CLINICAL PHARMACOLOGY
Mechanism of Action: Lengthens effective refractory period of the atrium and ventricle; decreases conduction velocity; has minimal effect on effective refractory period of the AV node; decreases the disparity in refractoriness between infarcted and adjacent normal myocardium; anticholinergic actions

Pharmacokinetics
PO: Peak 30 min-3 hr, duration 6-12 hr, $t_{1/2}$ 4-10 hr; metabolized in liver, excreted unchanged in urine (50%) and feces (10%); crosses placenta; protein binding concentration dependent (50%-65% at plasma levels of 2-4 µg/ml)

INDICATIONS AND USES: Life-threatening ventricular dysrhythmias such as sustained ventricular tachycardia; supraventricular tachycardia*

DOSAGE
Adult
- PO 100-200 mg q6h; in renal dysfunction, if CrCl 30-40 ml/min, dose should be 100 mg q8h, if CrCl 15-30 ml/min, dose should be 100 mg q12h, if CrCl <15 ml/min, dose should be 100 mg q24h; may give

loading dose of 300 mg for rapid effect; PO (SUS REL CAP) 200-300 mg q12h; not recommended in renal dysfunction

Child

• PO age 12-18 yr: 6-15 mg/kg/day in divided doses q6h; age 4-12 yr: 10-15 mg/kg/day in divided doses q6h; age 1-4 yr: 10-20 mg/kg/day in divided doses q6h; age <1 yr: 10-30 mg/kg/day in divided doses q6h

$ AVAILABLE FORMS/COST OF THERAPY

• Cap, Gel—Oral: 100 mg, 100's: **$13.50-$68.17;** 150 mg, 100's: **$28.70-$80.52**

• Cap, Gel, Sus Action—Oral: 100 mg, 100's: **$82.09;** 150 mg, 100's: **$97.02**

CONTRAINDICATIONS: 2nd or 3rd degree block, cardiogenic shock, CHF (uncompensated), sick sinus syndrome, QT prolongation

PRECAUTIONS: Children, diabetes mellitus, renal disease, hepatic disease, myasthenia gravis, narrow-angle glaucoma, cardiomyopathy, conduction abnormalities (including accessory pathways)

PREGNANCY AND LACTATION: Pregnancy category C; excreted in breast milk

SIDE EFFECTS/ADVERSE REACTIONS

CNS: Anxiety, depression, *dizziness,* fatigue, *headache,* insomnia, paresthesias, psychosis

CV: Angina, *AV block, bradycardia,* **cardiac arrest, CHF,** chest pain, edema, *hypotension,* increased QRS or QT duration, PVCs, syncope, tachycardia

EENT: Blurred vision; dry nose, throat, eyes; narrow-angle glaucoma

GI: Anorexia, *constipation (11%),* diarrhea, *dry mouth (32%),* flatulence, nausea, vomiting

GU: Hesitancy (14%), impotence, *retention,* urinary frequency, urgency

HEME: **Agranulocytosis,** anemia (rare), **thrombocytopenia**

METAB: Hypoglycemia

MS: Pain in extremities, weakness

SKIN: Pruritus, rash, urticaria

INTERACTIONS

Drugs

3 *Barbiturates, phenytoin, rifampin:* Reduced disopyramide level via induction

3 *Beta blockers:* Enhanced negative inotropy

3 *Clarithromycin, erythromycin, troleandromycin:* Macrolide increased disopyramide-serum concentration resulting in dysrhythmias

3 *Lidocaine:* Arrhythmias or heart failure in predisposed patients

3 *Potassium, potassium-sparing diuretics:* Increased potassium concentration can enhance disopyramide effects on myocardial conduction

Labs

• *Increase:* Liver enzymes, lipids, BUN, creatinine

• *Decrease:* Hgb/hct, blood glucose

SPECIAL CONSIDERATIONS

• Due to potential for prodysrhythmic effects, use for asymptomatic PVCs or lesser dysrhythmias should be avoided

MONITORING PARAMETERS

• Monitor ECG closely; if PR, QRS, or QT interval increase by 25%, stop drug

• Therapeutic plasma levels are 2-4 µg/ml

---

* = non-FDA-approved use

disulfiram

(dye-sul'fi-ram)
Rx: Antabuse
Chemical Class: Thiuram derivative
Therapeutic Class: Alcohol deterrent

CLINICAL PHARMACOLOGY
Mechanism of Action: Blocks oxidation of alcohol at acetaldehyde stage; accumulation of acetaldehyde produces disulfiram–alcohol reaction
Pharmacokinetics
PO: Onset 12 hr, effect lasts up to 2 wk; oxidized by liver; metabolites excreted by kidney, 20% excreted unchanged in feces
INDICATIONS AND USES: Adjunctive treatment of chronic alcoholism
DOSAGE
Adult
• PO 250-500 mg qd for 1-2 wk, then 125-500 mg qd until fully socially recovered
AVAILABLE FORMS/COST OF THERAPY
• Tab, Uncoated—Oral: 250 mg, 100's: **$6.50-$85.58;** 500 mg, 50's: **$7.00-$51.61**
CONTRAINDICATIONS: Alcohol intoxication, psychoses, cardiovascular disease; recent use of metronidazole, isoniazid, paraldehyde, alcohol, or alcohol-containing preparations (e.g., cough syrups, tonics); patients with history of rubber contact dermatitis should be evaluated for hypersensitivity to thiuram derivatives before receiving
PRECAUTIONS: Hypothyroidism, hepatic disease, diabetes mellitus, seizure disorders, nephritis, stroke
PREGNANCY AND LACTATION: Pregnancy category X; excreted in breast milk

SIDE EFFECTS/ADVERSE REACTIONS
CNS: Dizziness, *drowsiness,* fatigue, *headache,* neuritis, peripheral neuropathy, psychosis, restlessness, *seizures,* sweating, tremors
GI: Anorexia, *hepatotoxicity,* metallic or garlic-like taste, nausea, severe thirst, vomiting
METAB: Increased cholesterol
SKIN: Dermatitis, rash, urticaria
MISC: ***Disulfiram–alcohol reaction: flushing, sweating, headache, nausea, vomiting, chest pain, palpitations, dyspnea, tachycardia, confusion, and hypotension (reactions may occur with blood ethanol level as low as 5-10 mg/dl)***
INTERACTIONS
Drugs
❸ *Benzodiazepines (clonazepam, clorazepate, diazepem, flurazepam, halazepam, prazepam, triazolam):* Increased serum concentrations of these drugs
❸ *Cocaine:* Substantial increase in plasma cocaine levels and cardiovascular effects
❸ *Co-trimoxazole:* IV co-trimoxazole contains 10% ethanol; ethanol intolerance possible
🅐 *Ethanol:* Severe ethanol intolerance; warn patients to avoid all forms of ethanol
❷ *Isoniazid:* Use with disulfiram promotes encephalopathy
❸ *Metronidazole:* Use with disulfiram promotes encephalopathy
❷ *Oral anticoagulants:* Increased hypoprothromburemic response to oral anticoagulants
❸ *Phenytoin:* Increased phenytoin levels, toxicity possible
❸ *Theophylline:* Increased theophylline levels, toxicity possible
❸ *Tranylcypromine:* Case report of delirium in one patient

---

italic = common side effects   ***bold italic*** = life-threatening reactions

SPECIAL CONSIDERATIONS
PATIENT/FAMILY EDUCATION
• Disulfiram–alcohol reaction may occur for 2 wk after last dose
• May occur with external use of alcohol-containing products (i.e., liniments)
• Do not administer 1st dose until patient has abstained from alcohol for at least 12 hr

---

dobutamine
(doe-byoo′ta-meen)
Rx: Dobutrex
Chemical Class: Synthetic catecholamine
Therapeutic Class: β-Adrenergic agonist: sypathomimetic

CLINICAL PHARMACOLOGY
Mechanism of Action: Direct acting positive inotropic agent via β-adrenoceptor agonism producing additional mild chronotropic, hypertensive, arrhythmogenic and vasodilative effects; does not release endogenous nonepinepherine; in patients with depressed cardiac function, increases cardiac output, without increased heart rate; systemic vascular resistance is usually decreased

Pharmacokinetics
IV: Onset 1-2 min, peak 10 min, $t_{1/2}$ 2 min; metabolized in liver (inactive metabolites); metabolites excreted in urine

INDICATIONS AND USES: Short-term treatment of adults with cardiac decompensation due to depressed myocardial contractility; diagnostic aid for ischemic heart disease*

DOSAGE
Adult
• IV INF 2.5-15 µg/kg/min, max dose 40 µg/kg/min

* = non-FDA-approved use

💲 AVAILABLE FORMS/COST OF THERAPY
• Inj, Dry-Sol—IV: 12.5 mg/ml, 20 ml: **$1.76-$57.19**
CONTRAINDICATIONS: Hypertrophic cardiomyopathy, uncontrolled atrial fibrillation or flutter (unless a digitalis preparation is used prior to starting therapy with dobutamine)
PRECAUTIONS Children, hypertension, sulfite sensitivity (preparation may contain sulfite)
PREGNANCY AND LACTATION: Pregnancy category C; excreted in breast milk
SIDE EFFECTS/ADVERSE REACTIONS
CNS: Anxiety, dizziness, headache, paresthesia
CV: Angina, *dysrhythmia,* hypertension, palpitations, *PVCs, tachycardia*
GI: Heartburn, nausea, vomiting
METAB: Hypokalemia
MS: Leg cramps
INTERACTIONS
Drugs
• *Sodium bicarbonate:* Alkalinizing substances inactivate dobutamine
SPECIAL CONSIDERATIONS
MONITORING PARAMETERS
• Continuously monitor ECG, BP, and PCWP

docusate

(dok'yoo-sate)
OTC: *Sodium;* Colace, Dioeze, Diocto, DOK, DOSS DSS, Modane Soft, Regulax SS
OTC: *Calcium;* Sulfolax, Surfak Stool Softener
Combinations
   OTC: with senna concentrate (Senokot-S); with phenolphthalein (Doxidan); with casanthranol (Peri-Colace); with cascara sagrada (Nature's Remedy)
Chemical Class: Anionic surfactant
Therapeutic Class: Stool softener; laxative

CLINICAL PHARMACOLOGY
Mechanism of Action: Detergent activity; facilitates admixture of fat and water to soften stool
Pharmacokinetics
PO: Onset 24-72 hr, absorbed to some extent in duodenum and jejunum; excreted in bile
INDICATIONS AND USES: Constipation associated with hard, dry stools; stool softener in patients who should avoid straining during defecation; cerumenolytic*
DOSAGE
Adult
• *Laxative/stool softener:* PO 50-400 mg/day in 1-4 divided doses
• *Cerumenolytic:* Fill ear canal with liquid; produces substantial ear wax disintegration in 15 min, complete disintegration after 24 hr
Child <3 yr
• PO 10-40 mg/day in 1-4 divided doses
Child 3-6 yr
• PO 20-60 mg/day in 1-4 divided doses

Child 6-12 yr
• PO 40-150 mg/day in 1-4 divided doses
💲 **AVAILABLE FORMS/COST OF THERAPY**
• Cap, Softgel—Oral: 50, 100, 250 mg, 100's: **$1.40-$22.88**
• Liq—Oral: 150 mg/15 ml, 480 ml: **$12.00-$88.99**
• Syr—Oral: 60 mg/15 ml, 480 ml: **$3.30-$18.78**
CONTRAINDICATIONS: Obstruction, fecal impaction, nausea/vomiting, acute abdominal pain, concomitant use of mineral oil
PREGNANCY AND LACTATION: Pregnancy category C; no reports linking use of docusate with congenital defects have been located; diarrhea has been reported in 1 infant exposed to docusate while breast feeding, but relationship between symptom and drug is unknown
SIDE EFFECTS/ADVERSE REACTIONS
EENT: Throat irritation
GI: Anorexia, bitter taste, cramps, diarrhea, nausea
SKIN: Rash
SPECIAL CONSIDERATIONS
PATIENT/FAMILY EDUCATION
• Drink plenty of water during administration

dofetilide

(doe-fet'ill-ide)
Rx: Tikosyn
Chemical Class: Methanesulfonanilide derivative
Therapeutic Class: Antiarrhythmic: potassium channel blocker (class III antiarrhythmic)

CLINICAL PHARMACOLOGY
Mechanism of Action: Class III antiarrhythmic (i.e., selective potassium channel blocker); prolongs the

duration of action potential, then, refractoriness by delaying the membrane repolarizatioin; ECG changes include prolongation of the QT and QTc intervals without change in the QRS interval; no effect on cardiac output, stroke volume index, or systemic vascular resistance; dose-dependent negative chronotropic effects but lacks negative inotropic activity

Pharmacokinetics

PO: Peak serum levels within 2-3 hr; bioavailability near 100%, unaffected by food; Vd 3L/kg; 60%-70% protein bound; 50% hepatic metabolism (CYP3A4); 50% unchanged recovered in urine; t½ 10 hr

INDICATIONS AND USES: Maintenance of normal sinus rhythm (delay in time to recurrence of atrial fibrillation/atrial flutter) in patients with atrial fibrillation/atrial flutter of greater than one wk duration who have been converted to normal sinus rhythm; conversion of atrial fibrillation and atrial flutter to normal sinus rhythm

DOSAGE

Adult

NOTE: 1) Dofetilide therapy must be initiated in a setting capable of providing continuous ECG monitoring and management of serious ventricular arrhythmias; 2) Pretherapy anticoagulation should be initiated and continued after conversion according to customary medical practice; 3) Pretherapy ECG for determination of QTc <400 msec (500 msec with ventricular conduction abnormalities); 4) Pretherapy creatinine clearance calculation

• PO: initial dose 125-500 µg bid depending on calculated creatinine clearance; for calculated creatinine clearance >60 ml/min, use initial dose of 500 µg bid; 40-60 ml/min,

250 µg bid; 20-40 ml/min, 125 µg; dofetilide is contraindicated when calculated creatinine clearance is <20 ml/min

• PO continuation dosing 2-3 hr post initial dose, redetermine QTc: 1) if QTc >15% increase from baseline or 2) if QTc >400 msec, adjust dose as follows: if starting dose (based on CrCl) is 500 µg bid, adjusted dose for QTc prolongation is 250 µg bid; if starting dose is 250 µg bid, adjusted dose is 125 µg bid; if starting dose is 125 µg bid, adjusted dose is 125 µg bid

💲 AVAILABLE FORMS/COST OF THERAPY

• Cap—Oral: 125 mcg, 60's; 250 mcg, 60's; 500 mcg, 60's (prices not available)

CONTRAINDICATIONS: Congenital or acquired long QT syndromes; baseline QTc >440 msec (500 msec in patients with ventricular conduction abnormalities); renal impairment (calculated creatinine clearance <20 ml/min)

PRECAUTIONS: Ventricular arrhythmia, renal impairment, hypokalemia

PREGNANCY AND LACTATION: Pregnancy category C; no information on the presence of dofetilide in breast milk; breast feeding while on dofetilide not advised

SIDE EFFECTS/ADVERSE REACTIONS

CNS: Headache, dizziness, insomnia, cerebral ischemia, cerebrovascular accident, facial paralysis, flaccid paralysis, migraine, paresthesia, syncope

*CV: **Ventricular arrhythmias, including torsades de pointes,** ventricular fibrillation, ventricular tachycardia, AV block, bundle branch block, **heart block,** chest pain, bradycardia, edema, myocardial infarction*

---

* = non-FDA-approved use

GI: Nausea, diarrhea, abdominal pain, liver damage
MS: Back pain
RESP: Respiratory tract infection, dyspnea, flu syndrome, angioedema, cough
SKIN: Rash

INTERACTIONS

Drugs

3 *Amiloride:* May compete with dofetilide for renal cationic secretion and subsequently increase dofetilide levels

2 *Cimetidine:* Increases dofetilide levels by 13%-58%, dose dependent

2 *Ketoconazole and other azole antifungals:* Increases dofetilide levels by 53%-97% by inhibition of CYP3A4

3 *Metformin:* May compete with dofetilide for renal cationic secretion and subsequently increase dofetilide levels

2 *Sulfamethoxazole:* Increases dofetilide AUC by 93% and Cmax by 103%

3 *Triamterene:* May compete with dofetilide for renal cationic secretion and subsequently increase dofetilide levels

2 *Trimethoprim:* Increases dofetilide AUC by 93% and Cmax by 103%

2 *Verapamil:* Increases dofetilide levels by 42% and increased risk of torsade de pointes

3 *Other potential drug interactions:* Macrolide antibiotics, protease inhibitors, serotonin reuptake inhibitors, amiodarone, cannabinoids, diltiazem, grapefruit juice, nefazadone, norfloxacin, quinine, zafirlukast: potential to increase dofetilide concentrations via inhibition of CYP3A4

SPECIAL CONSIDERATIONS
MONITORING PARAMETERS
• ECG, QTc intervals, renal function

dolasetron
(doe-lass'eh-tron)
Rx: Anzemat
Chemical Class: Nonbenzamide
Therapeutic Class: Antiemetic

D

CLINICAL PHARMACOLOGY
Mechanism of Action: Selectively blocks the action of serotonin at 5-HT₃ receptors; cytotoxic chemotherapy appears to be associated with release of serotonin from enterochromaffin cells of the small intestine which may stimulate vagal afferents through 5-HT₃ receptors initiating the vomiting reflex

Pharmacokinetics
IV: Peak <1 hr (active metabolite)
PO: Peak 1½ hr, bioavailability 59%
Rapidly metabolized to active metabolite which is 50 times more potent than parent compound; excreted in urine (45%-68%) and feces (25%); $t_{1/2}$ approximately 10 min (parent drug) and 8 hr (active metabolite)

INDICATIONS AND USES: Prevention of nausea and vomiting associated with emetogenic cancer chemotherapy; prevention and treatment of postoperative nausea and vomiting; radiotherapy-induced nausea and vomiting*

DOSAGE
Adult
• Chemotherapy: *IV* 1.8 mg/kg 30 min prior to chemotherapy; PO 100 mg as a single dose administered 1 hr prior to chemotherapy
• Postoperative: IV 12.5 mg as a single dose 15 min before cessation of anesthesia or when nausea and vomiting present; PO 100 mg 2 hr prior to surgery
Child (2-16 yr)
• Chemotherapy: IV 1.8 mg/kg 30

---

italic = common side effects   ***bold italic*** = life-threatening reactions

min prior to chemotherapy (100 mg max); PO 1.8 mg/kg 1 hr prior to chemotherapy (100 mg max)

• Postoperative: IV 0.35 mg/kg as a single dose 15 min before cessation of anesthesia or when nausea and vomiting present; PO 1.2 mg/kg within 2 hr before surgery (100 mg max)

💲 **AVAILABLE FORMS/COST OF THERAPY**

• Inj—IV: 100 mg/vial: **$155.88**
• Tab—Oral: 50 mg, 5's: **$258.96;** 100 mg, 5's: **$343.20**

PRECAUTIONS: Hypertension, CAD, dysrhythmias, cardiac conduction defects, CHF, seizure disorder

PREGNANCY AND LACTATION: Pregnancy category B; excretion in breast milk unknown, use caution in nursing mothers

SIDE EFFECTS/ADVERSE REACTIONS

CNS: Dizziness, headache, lightheadedness
CV: ECG changes, hypertension, hypotension
EENT: Blurred vision
GI: Constipation, diarrhea, elevated transaminases, *increased appetite*
MISC: Chills, fever

SPECIAL CONSIDERATIONS

• No obvious advantage over other agents in this class (ondansetron, granisetron)

---

donepezil

(dah-nep'eh-zil)
Rx: Aricept
Chemical Class: Piperidine derivative
Therapeutic Class: Antidementia agent; cholinergic

CLINICAL PHARMACOLOGY
Mechanism of Action: Enhances cholinergic function by increasing the concentration of acetylcholine through reversible inhibition of its hydrolysis by acetylcholinesterase; does not appear to alter the course of the underlying dementing process

Pharmacokinetics
PO: Peak plasma concentration 3-4 hr; bioavailibility, 100%; 96% bound to plasma proteins; extensively metabolized to 4 major metabolites (2 are active), excreted mainly in urine (unchanged and metabolites); $t_{1/2}$ 70 hr

INDICATIONS AND USES: Mild to moderate dementia of the Alzheimer's type

DOSAGE
Adult

• PO 5 mg hs; may increase to 10 mg hs after 4-6 wk (higher dose has not been shown to provide a significantly greater clinical benefit for most patients and may increase cholinergic adverse events)

💲 **AVAILABLE FORMS/COST OF THERAPY**

• Tab—Film-coated: 5 mg, 30's: **$126.45**
• Tab—Film-coated: 10 mg, 30's: **$126.45**

PRECAUTIONS: Sick sinus syndrome or other supraventricular cardiac conduction conditions, history of peptic ulcer disease, bladder outflow obstruction, seizure disorder, asthma/COPD

PREGNANCY AND LACTATION: Pregnancy category C

SIDE EFFECTS/ADVERSE REACTIONS

CNS: Abnormal dreams, depression, dizziness, *fatigue,* headache, *insomnia,* somnolence
CV: Syncope
GI: Anorexia, *diarrhea, nausea, vomiting*
GU: Frequent urination
HEME: Ecchymosis

METAB: Weight decrease
MS: Arthritis, *muscle cramps*
INTERACTIONS
Drugs
3 *Fluvoxamine:* Possible increase in fluvoxamine levels
SPECIAL CONSIDERATIONS
• Clinicians were unable to notice improvement in the majority of patients in clinical trials; advantages over tacrine include qd dosing and apparent lack of liver toxicity
MONITORING PARAMETERS
• Close monitoring for clinical improvement and periodic reassessment of need for continued therapy

---

dopamine
(doe'pa-meen)
Rx: Intropin
Chemical Class: Synthetic catecholamine
Therapeutic Class: α- and β-adrenergic sympathomimetic; vasosuppressor

---

CLINICAL PHARMACOLOGY
Mechanism of Action: Stimulates both adrenergic and dopaminergic receptors in a dose-dependent manner; low doses (1-5 μg/kg/min) stimulate mainly dopaminergic receptors producing renal and mesenteric vasodilation; intermediate doses (5-15 μg/kg/min) stimulate both dopaminergic and β_1-adrenergic receptors producing cardiac stimulation and renal vasodilation; large doses (>15 μg/kg/min) stimulate α-adrenergic receptors producing vasoconstriction and increases in peripheral vascular resistance and blood pressure
Pharmacokinetics
IV: Onset 5 min, duration <10 min; metabolized in plasma, kidneys, and liver by MAO (75% to inactive metabolites, 25% to norepinephrine); $t_{1/2}$ 2 min

INDICATIONS AND USES: Correction of hemodynamic imbalances in shock syndromes (e.g. MI, trauma, septicemia, renal failure, CHF); COPD*; CHF*; respiratory distress syndrome (RDS) in infants*
DOSAGE
Adult and Child
• IV INF 1-20 μg/kg/min, titrated to desired response; do not exceed 50 μg/kg/min
💲 AVAILABLE FORMS/COST OF THERAPY
• Inj, Conc-Sol—IV: 40 mg/ml, 5 ml: **$1.04-$16.21;** 80 mg/ml, 5 ml: **$1.24-$7.25;** 160 mg/ml, 5 ml: **$1.96-$8.14**
CONTRAINDICATIONS: Pheochromocytoma, uncorrected tachydysrhythmia or ventricular fibrillation
PRECAUTIONS: Hypovolemia, arterial embolism, occlusive vascular disease, abrupt discontinuation, sulfite sensitivity, concurrent use of MAOIs
PREGNANCY AND LACTATION: Pregnancy category C; because dopamine is indicated only in life-threatening situations, chronic use would not be expected; no data available regarding use in breast feeding
SIDE EFFECTS/ADVERSE REACTIONS
CNS: Headache
CV: Aberrant conduction, *anginal pain,* bradycardia, *ectopic beats,* hypertension, *palpitation, tachycardia, vasoconstriction,* widened QRS complex
EENT: Dilated pupils (high doses)
GI: Nausea, vomiting
GU: Azotemia
RESP: Dyspnea
SKIN: **Gangrene** (high doses for prolonged periods of time), **necrosis,**

---

italic = common side effects   ***bold italic*** = life-threatening reactions

piloerection, tissue sloughing with extravasation

INTERACTIONS

Drugs

3️⃣ *Ergot alkaloids:* Gangrene has been reported

3️⃣ *Phenytoin:* Increased risk of hypotension with IV phenytoin administration

Labs

• *False increase:* Urine amino acids; urine catecholamines; serum creatinine

• *False decrease:* Serum creatinine

SPECIAL CONSIDERATIONS

• *Dilute before use if not prediluted;* antidote for extravasation: infiltrate area as soon as possible with 10-15 ml NS containing 5-10 mg phentolamine

MONITORING PARAMETERS

• Urine flow, cardiac output, blood pressure, pulmonary wedge pressure

---

dornase alfa

(door'nace al'fa)

Rx: Pulmozyme

Chemical Class: Recombinant human deoxyribonuclease I

Therapeutic Class: Mucolytic

CLINICAL PHARMACOLOGY

Mechanism of Action: Hydrolyzes DNA in sputum of cystic fibrosis (CF) patients and reduces sputum viscoelasticity

Pharmacokinetics

INH: Does not produce significant elevations in serum DNase concentrations; no accumulation of serum DNase has been noted; following nebulization, enzyme levels are measurable in sputum within 15 min and decline rapidly thereafter

INDICATIONS AND USES: Cystic fibrosis (as an adjunct to standard therapies to reduce the frequency of respiratory infections requiring parenteral antibiotics and to improve pulmonary function)

DOSAGE

Adult and Child ≥5 yr

• NEB 2.5 mg qd; some patients (age >21, forced vital capacity (FVC) >70%) may benefit from bid administration

💲 **AVAILABLE FORMS/COST OF THERAPY**

• Sol—INH: 1 mg/ml, 2.5 ml: **$37.90**

PRECAUTIONS: Safety and efficacy have not been demonstrated in children <5 yr or patients with FVC <40% of predicted

PREGNANCY AND LACTATION: Pregnancy category B; excretion into breast milk unknown; however, since serum levels of DNase have not been shown to increase above endogenous levels, little drug would be expected to be excreted into breast milk

SIDE EFFECTS/ADVERSE REACTIONS

Most events likely reflected sequelae of the underlying lung disease

CNS: Asthenia, fever

CV: Chest pain

EENT: Conjunctivitis, laryngitis, *pharyngitis, voice alteration*

GI: Abdominal pain, gallbladder disease, intestinal obstruction, liver disease, pancreatic disease

METAB: Diabetes mellitus, weight loss

MS: Flu-like syndrome

RESP: Apnea, bronchiectasis, change in sputum, cough increase, dyspnea, hemoptysis, hypoxia, lung function decrease, nasal polyps, rhinitis, sinusitis, sputum increase, wheeze

SKIN: Rash

SPECIAL CONSIDERATIONS

• Safety and efficacy have been demonstrated only with the follow-

---

* = non-FDA-approved use

ing nebulizers and compressors: disposable jet nebulizer *Hudson T Updraft II,* disposable jet nebulizer *Marquest Acorn II* in conjunction with a *Pulmo-Aide* compressor, and reusable *PARI LC Jet+* nebulizer in conjunction with the *PARI PRONEB* compressor

PATIENT/FAMILY EDUCATION

• Must be stored in refrigerator at 2-8°C and protected from strong light (keep refrigerated when transporting and do not leave at room temp for >24 hr)

• Do not dilute or mix with other drugs in nebulizer

---

dorzolamide

(door-zol'a-mide)
Rx: Trusopt Ocumeter
Combinations:
  Rx: with Timolol (Cosopt Ocumeter)
Chemical Class: Sulfonamide derivative
Therapeutic Class: Antiglaucoma agent

CLINICAL PHARMACOLOGY
Mechanism of Action: Inhibition of carbonic anhydrase in ciliary processes of the eye decreases aqueous humor secretion, reducing intraocular pressure
Pharmacokinetics
OPHTH: Systemically absorbed in amounts below that anticipated to be necessary for pharmacological effect on renal function and respiration; 33% plasma protein bound; excreted as *N*-desethyl metabolite and unchanged in urine; $t_{1/2}$ in RBCs 4 mo

INDICATIONS AND USES: Treatment of elevated intraocular pressure in patients with ocular hypertension or open-angle glaucoma

DOSAGE
Adult
• OPHTH 1 gtt in affected eye(s) tid
💲 **AVAILABLE FORMS/COST OF THERAPY**
• Sol—Ophth: 2%, 5, 10 ml: **$24.10/5 ml**
PRECAUTIONS: Renal/hepatic impairment (severe)
PREGNANCY AND LACTATION: Pregnancy category C
SIDE EFFECTS/ADVERSE REACTIONS
EENT: Blurred vision, dryness, ocular allergic reactions, *ocular burning, stinging, or discomfort (25%);* photophobia (1-5%), *superficial punctate keratitis (12.5%)*; tearing, GI: *Bitter taste following administration (25%)*
SPECIAL CONSIDERATIONS
PATIENT/FAMILY EDUCATION
• Can be administered concomitantly with other top ophth products; separate administration by 10 min
• The preservative in dorzolamide sol, benzalkonium chloride, may be absorbed by soft contact lenses

---

doxapram

(dox'a-pram)
Rx: Dopram
Chemical Class: Monohydrated pyrrolidinone derivative
Therapeutic Class: Analeptic

CLINICAL PHARMACOLOGY
Mechanism of Action: Respiratory stimulation through activation of peripheral carotid chemoreceptors; with higher doses medullary respiratory centers are stimulated
Pharmacokinetics
IV: Onset 20-40 sec, peak 1-2 min, duration 5-10 min; metabolized by liver, metabolites excreted by kidneys; $t_{1/2}$ 2.4-4.1 hr

---

italic = common side effects

bold italic = life-threatening reactions

INDICATIONS AND USES: Chronic obstructive pulmonary disease (COPD) associated with acute hypercapnia (temporary measure in hospitalized patients); postanesthesia respiratory stimulation; drug-induced CNS depression; apnea of prematurity resistant to methylxanthines*

DOSAGE

Adult

• *Postanesthetic respiratory stimulation:* IV inj 0.5-1 mg/kg, not to exceed 1.5 mg/kg total as a single inj, or 2 mg/kg total when given as multiple inj at 5 min intervals; IV INF 250 mg in 250 ml sol, initiate at 5 mg/min until response satisfactory, then maintain at 1-3 mg/min to sustain desired effect; recommended total dose 4 mg/kg

• *Drug-induced CNS depression:* IV inj priming dose of 2 mg/kg, repeated in 5 min, repeat q1-2h till patient awakes; IV INF priming dose of 2 mg/kg, if no response continue supportive measures and repeat priming dose in 1-2 hr, if some respiratory stimulation occurs infuse 1 mg/ml sol at 1-3 mg/min, not to exceed 3 g/day

• *COPD:* IV INF 1-2 mg/min, not to exceed 3 mg/min; do not infuse for longer than 2 hr

Child

• *Apnea of prematurity:* IV 2.5-3 mg/kg loading dose, followed by continuous INF of 1 mg/kg/hr; titrate to lowest rate at which apnea is controlled; do not exceed 2.5 mg/kg/hr

$ AVAILABLE FORMS/COST OF THERAPY

• Inj, Sol—IV: 20 mg/ml, 20 ml: **$85.08**

CONTRAINDICATIONS: Seizure disorders; severe hypertension, bronchial asthma, dyspnea, or cardiac disorders; pneumothorax; pulmonary embolism; pulmonary fibrosis, conditions resulting in constriction of chest wall, muscles of respiration, or alveolar expansion; head injury; incompetence of ventilatory mechanism due to muscle paresis; flail chest

PRECAUTIONS: Bronchial asthma, pheochromocytoma, severe tachycardia, dysrhythmias, hypertension, children

PREGNANCY AND LACTATION: Pregnancy category B; excretion into breast milk unknown

SIDE EFFECTS/ADVERSE REACTIONS

CNS: Apprehension, bilateral Babinski, clonus, disorientation, dizziness, *headache,* hyperactivity, increased deep tendon reflexes, involuntary movements, pyrexia, *seizures*

CV: Chest pain, *dysrhythmias,* flushing, lowered T waves, *mild to moderate increase in blood pressure,* phlebitis, tightness in chest, *variations in heart rate*

EENT: **Laryngospasm,** pupillary dilation

GI: Desire to defecate, diarrhea, nausea, vomiting

GU: Proteinuria, spontaneous voiding, urinary retention

HEME: Decreased Hgb, hct, or RBC; decreased WBC in patients with preexisting leukopenia; hemolysis (with rapid infusion)

RESP: **Bronchospasm,** cough, dyspnea, hiccups, rebound hypoventilation, tachypnea

SKIN: Local skin irritation with extravasation

INTERACTIONS

Drugs

3 *Anesthetics, inhalation:* Sensitized myocardium at risk of arrhythmia; delay administration of doxapram 10 min

---

* = non-FDA-approved use

2 *MAO Inhibitors:* Additive pressor effect

SPECIAL CONSIDERATIONS
MONITORING PARAMETERS
• Baseline ABG then q30 min (for use in COPD)

---

doxazosin
(dox-ay′zoe-sin)
Rx: Cardura
Chemical Class: Quinazoline derivative
Therapeutic Class: α_1-adrenergic blocker: antihypertensive; symptomatic benign prostatic hypertrophy

---

CLINICAL PHARMACOLOGY
Mechanism of Action: Selectively blocks postsynaptic α_1-adrenergic receptors; dilates both arterioles and veins, reducing peripheral vascular resistance and blood pressure; no reflex tachycardia or changes in renin release; blockade of α_1-adrenoceptors in bladder neck and prostate relaxes smooth muscle, improving urine flow rates in benign prostatic hypertrophy
Pharmacokinetics
PO: Onset 2 hr, peak 2-3 hr; 98% bound to plasma proteins; extensively metabolized in liver, excreted via bile, feces, and urine; $t_{1/2}$ 22 hr
INDICATIONS AND USES: Hypertension, benign prostatic hyperplasia refractory CHF*
DOSAGE
Adult
• PO 1 mg qd, increasing to 16 mg qd if required; usual range 4-16 mg/day

$ AVAILABLE FORMS/COST OF THERAPY
• Tab, Uncoated—Oral: 1 mg, 100's: **$99.63;** 2 mg, 100's: **$99.63;** 4 mg, 100's: **$104.58;** 8 mg, 100's: **$109.81**

PRECAUTIONS: Children, hepatic disease
PREGNANCY AND LACTATION: Pregnancy category C; may accumulate in breast milk; use caution in nursing mothers
SIDE EFFECTS/ADVERSE REACTIONS
CNS: Anxiety, asthenia, ataxia, depression, *dizziness,* fever, *headache,* hypertonia, insomnia, nervousness, paresthesia, somnolence
CV: Chest pain, **dysrhythmia,** edema, flushing, palpitations, postural hypotension, tachycardia
EENT: Abnormal vision, tinnitus, vertigo
GI: Abdominal discomfort, constipation, diarrhea, dry mouth, flatulence, nausea, vomiting
GU: Incontinence, polyuria
MS: Arthralgia, myalgia
RESP: Dyspnea
SKIN: Pruritus, rash
INTERACTIONS
Drugs
3 *ACE inhibitors:* Increased potential for first dose hypotension
3 *Indomethacin:* Decreased hypotensive effect of doxazosin
3 *Verapamil, nifedipine:* Enhanced hypotensive effects of both drugs
3 β-*adrenergic blockers:* Exaggerated first-dose response
Labs
False positive urinary metabolites of norepinephrine and VMA
No effect on prostate specific antigen (PSA)
SPECIAL CONSIDERATIONS
• Use as a single antihypertensive agent limited by tendency to cause sodium and water retention and increased plasma volume
PATIENT/FAMILY EDUCATION
• Alert patient to the possibility of syncopal and orthostatic symptoms,

---

italic = common side effects   ***bold italic*** = life-threatening reactions

especially with 1st dose ("1st-dose syncope")
• Initial dose should be administered at bedtime in the smallest possible dose

---

doxepin
(dox'eh-pin)
Rx: *Systemic:* Adapin, Sinequan; *Topical:* Zonalon
Chemical Class: Dibenzoxepin derivative: tertiary amine
Therapeutic Class: Tricyclic antidepressant; topical antipruritic

CLINICAL PHARMACOLOGY
Mechanism of Action: Inhibits reuptake of norepinephrine and serotonin (blocking activity slight and moderate, respectively) at the presynaptic neuron prolonging neuronal activity; inhibits histamine and acetylcholine activity; mild peripheral vasodilator effects and possible "quinidine-like" actions on cardiac conduction; moderate anticholinergic and orthostatic hypotensive, high sedative side effects
Pharmacokinetics
PO: Metabolized by liver to desmethyldoxepin (active), excreted by kidneys, $t_{1/2}$ 8-24 hr; 80%-85% bound to plasma proteins
INDICATIONS AND USES: Depression, anxiety, chronic pain,* peptic ulcer disease,* panic disorder,* dermatologic disorders,* pruritus associated with atopic dermatitis and lichen simplex chronicus (top formulation)
DOSAGE
Adult
• PO 50-75 mg/day in divided doses, may increase to 300 mg/day or may give daily dose hs; TOP apply thin film of cream qid for up to 8 days

Adolescents
• PO 25-50 mg/day in single or divided doses, gradually increase to 100 mg/day
[$] AVAILABLE FORMS/COST OF THERAPY
• Cre—Top: 5%, 30, 45 g: **$23.57/30 g**
• Cap, Gel—Oral: 10 mg, 100's: **$10.00-$38.04;** 25 mg, 100's: **$9.10-$49.06;** 50 mg, 100's: **$18.25-$69.06;** 75 mg, 100's: **$29.00-$114.55;** 100 mg, 100's: **$21.00-$124.89;** 150 mg, 100's: **$58.25-$231.71**
• Conc—Oral: 10 mg/ml, 120 ml: **$13.00-$28.59**
CONTRAINDICATIONS: Urinary retention, narrow-angle glaucoma, acute recovery phase of MI, concurrent use of MAOIs
PRECAUTIONS: Suicidal patients, seizure disorders, prostatic hypertrophy, psychiatric disease, severe depression, increased intraocular pressure, cardiac disease, hepatic disease, renal disease, hyperthyroidism, electroshock therapy, elective surgery, elderly, abrupt discontinuation, children
PREGNANCY AND LACTATION: Pregnancy category C (top formulation is category B); paralytic ileus has been observed in an infant exposed to doxepin and chlorpromazine at term; excreted into breast milk (as well as active metabolite); effect on nursing infant unknown, but may be of concern
SIDE EFFECTS/ADVERSE REACTIONS
CNS: Anxiety, confusion (especially in elderly), *dizziness, drowsiness,* extrapyramidal symptoms (elderly), fatigue, headache, increased psychiatric symptoms, insomnia, memory impairment, nervousness, nightmares, panic, stimulation, tremors, weakness

* = non-FDA-approved use

CV: **Dysrhythmias,** ECG changes, hypertension, *orthostatic hypotension,* palpitations, syncope, tachycardia

EENT: *Blurred vision,* mydriasis, nasal congestion, ophthalmoplegia, tinnitus

GI: *Constipation,* cramps, diarrhea, *dry mouth,* epigastric distress, hepatitis, increased appetite, jaundice, nausea, **paralytic ileus,** stomatitis, vomiting

GU: *Urinary retention*

HEME: **Agranulocytosis,** eosinophilia, **leukopenia, thrombocytopenia**

SKIN: *Burning or stinging at application site,* crackling (TOP), *dryness or tightness of skin,* edema, irritation, paresthesias, photosensitivity; pruritus, *pruritus or eczema exacerbation,* rash, scaling, sweating, tingling, urticaria

DRUG INTERACTIONS
Drugs
3 *Barbiturates:* Reduced serum concentrations of cyclic antidepressants

2 *Bethanidine:* Reduced antihypertensive effect of bethanidine

3 *Carbamazepine:* Reduced cyclic antidepressant serum concentrations

2 *Clonidine:* Reduced antihypertensive response to clonidine; enhanced hypertensive response with abrupt clonidine withdrawal

3 *Debrisoquin:* Inhibited antihypertensive response of debrisoquin

2 *Epinephrine:* Markedly enhanced pressor response to IV epinephrine

3 *Ethanol:* Additive impairment of motor skills; abstinent alcoholics may eliminate cyclic antidepressants more rapidly than non-alcoholics

3 *Fluoxetine, flluvoxamine, grapefruit juice:* Marked increases in cyclic antidepressant plasma concentrations

3 *Guanethidine:* Inhibited antihypertensive response to guanethidine

2 *Moclobemide:* Potential association with fatal or non-fatal serotonin syndrome

A *MAOIs:* Excessive sympathetic response, mania, or hyperpyrexia possible

3 *Neuroleptics:* Increased therapeutic and toxic effects of both drugs

2 *Norepinephrine:* Markedly enhanced pressor response to norepinephrine

2 *Phenylephrine:* Enhanced pressor response to IV phenylephrine

3 *Propoxyphene:* Enhanced effect of cyclic antidepressants

3 *Quinidine:* Increased cyclic antidepressant serum concentrations

SPECIAL CONSIDERATIONS
• Equally effective as other tricyclic antidepressants for depression; distinguishing characteristics include: sedative, anxiolytic, antihistaminic properties

PATIENT/FAMILY EDUCATION
• Therapeutic effects may take 4-6 wk
• Do not discontinue abruptly after long-term use
• If drowsiness occurs with top application, decrease surface area being treated or number of daily applications

MONITORING PARAMETERS
• CBC; ECG; mental status: mood, sensorium, affect, suicidal tendencies

---

doxycycline
(dox-i-sye'kleen)
Rx: Atridox, Doryx, Doxy, Doxy Caps, Doxychel Hyclate, Periostat, Vibramycin, Vibra-Tabs
Chemical Class: Tetracycline derivative
Therapeutic Class: Antibiotic

CLINICAL PHARMACOLOGY
Mechanism of Action: Inhibits protein synthesis by binding with the 30S and possibly the 50S ribosomal subunit(s) of susceptible organisms
Pharmacokinetics
PO: Peak 1.5-4 hr, food decreases absorption approximately 20%; 90% bound to plasma proteins; not metabolized in liver, partially inactivated in the GI tract by chelate formation; $t_{1/2}$ 15-26 hr; excreted in urine (23%) and feces (30%)

INDICATIONS AND USES: Rocky Mountain spotted fever; typhus fever and the typhus group; Q fever; rickettsialpox; tick fevers caused by Rickettsiae; respiratory tract infections; lymphogranuloma venereum; psittacosis (ornithosis); trachoma; inclusion conjunctivitis; uncomplicated urethral, endocervical, or rectal infections in adults; nongonococcal urethritis; relapsing fever; chancroid; plague; tularemia; cholera; *Campylobacter fetus* infections; brucellosis; bartonellosis; granuloma inguinale; malaria prophylaxis, acne, periodontitis subgingival scaling and root planing in adults
Antibacterial spectrum usually includes:
• Gram-positive organisms: *Streptococcus pyogenes* (44% of strains found to be resistant), *Str. pneumoniae* (74% of strains found to be resistant), enterococcus group (*Str.*

faecalis and *Str. faecium*), α-hemolytic streptococci (viridans group)
• Gram-negative organisms: *Neisseria gonorrhoeae, Calymmatobacterium granulomatis, Haemophilus ducreyi, H. influenzae, Yersinia pestis, Francisella tularensis, Vibrio cholera, Bartonella bacilliformis, Brucella* spp.
• Other organisms: Rickettsiae, *Clostridium* spp., *Chlamydia psittaci, C. trachomatis, Fusobacterium fusiforme, Actinomyces* spp., *Mycoplasma pneumoniae, Bacillus anthracis, Ureaplasma urealyticum, Propionibacterium acnes, Borrelia recurrentis, Entamoeba* spp., *Treponema pallidum, T. pertenue, Balantidium coli, Plasmodium falciparum*
DOSAGE
Adult
• PO/IV 100-200 mg/day in 1-2 divided doses
Child ≥ 8 yr
• PO/IV 2-5 mg/kg/day in 1-2 divided doses; do not exceed 200 mg/day
🚺 AVAILABLE FORMS/COST OF THERAPY
• Cap, Gel—Oral: 50 mg, 50's: **$6.30-$104.76;** 100 mg, 50's: **$3.93-$188.33**
• Cap, Gel, Coated Pellets—Oral: 100 mg, 50's: **$92.93-$133.81**
• Tab, Plain Coated—Oral: 100 mg, 50's: **$4.45-$188.33**
• Powder, Reconst—Oral: 25 mg/5 ml, 60 ml: **$11.49**
• Syr—Oral: 50 mg/5ml, 480 ml: **$174.26**
• Inj, Sol—IV: 100 mg/vial: **$18.89;** 200 mg/vial: **$37.24**
CONTRAINDICATIONS: Children <8 yr
PRECAUTIONS: Hepatic disease, prolonged or repeated therapy

PREGNANCY AND LACTATION:
Pregnancy category D; excreted into breast milk; theoretical possibility for dental staining seems remote because serum levels in infant undetectable

SIDE EFFECTS/ADVERSE REACTIONS

CNS: Fever, headache, paresthesia

CV: Pericarditis

GI: Abdominal cramps, abdominal pain, anorexia, *diarrhea,* enterocolitis, epigastric burning, flatulence, glossitis, hepatotoxicity, *nausea,* ***pseudomembranous colitis,*** stomatitis, vomiting

GU: Azotemia, increased BUN, polydipsia, polyuria

HEME: Eosinophilia, ***hemolytic anemia, neutropenia, thrombocytopenia***

SKIN: ***Exfoliative dermatitis,*** highly irritating (avoid extravasation), *photosensitivity,* pruritus, rash, urticaria

MISC: Angioedema, bulging fontanels (infants), decreased calcification of deciduous teeth, pseudotumor cerebri (adults)

INTERACTIONS

Drugs

▪ *Antacids:* Reduced serum concentration and efficacy of doxycycline

▪ *Barbiturates:* Reduced serum doxycycline concentrations

▪ *Bismuth:* Reduced bioavailability of doxycycline

▪ *Calcium:* See antacids

▪ *Carbamazepine:* Reduced serum doxycycline concentrations

▪ *Cholestyramine; colestipol:* Reduced serum concentration of doxycycline; take 2 hr before or 3 hr after resin dose

▪ *Ethanol:* Chronic ethanol ingestion may reduce the serum concentrations of doxycycline

▪ *Iron:* Reduced serum concentration and efficacy of doxycycline

▪ *Magnesium:* See antacids

▪ *Oral contraceptives:* Potential for decreased efficacy of oral contraceptives

▪ *Penicillins:* Doxycycline may reduce penicillin efficacy

▪ *Phenytoin:* Reduced serum doxycycline concentrations

▪ *Warfarin:* Potential for enhanced hypoprothrombinenic response to warfarin

▪ *Zinc:* Reduced serum concentration of doxycycline; take 2 hr before or 3 hr after zinc

SPECIAL CONSIDERATIONS
• Tetracycline of choice due to broad spectrum, long $t_{1/2}$, superior tissue penetration, and excellent oral absorption

PATIENT/FAMILY EDUCATION
• Do not take with antacids, iron products
• Take with food

---

dronabinol

(droe-nab´i-nol)

Rx: Marinol

Chemical Class: Synthetic cannabinoid derivative
Therapeutic Class: Antiemetic, appetite stimulant
DEA Class: Schedule II

CLINICAL PHARMACOLOGY

Mechanism of Action: Central sympathomimetic and neural cannabinoid receptor activity mediate effect; tachyphylaxis and tolerance develop to psychological effects but not appetite stimulant effect

Pharmacokinetics

PO: Onset 30-60 min, peak effect 2-4 hr, duration of psychoactive effect 4-6 hr, appetite stimulant effect 24 hr; absorption 90%; highly lipid soluble; 97% protein bound; metabolized in liver; metabolites and drug excreted in bile (85%) and urine

---

italic = common side effects   ***bold italic*** = life-threatening reactions

(15%); metabolites detected in urine for 5 wk after single dose

INDICATIONS AND USES: Nausea related to cancer chemotherapy not responsive to conventional agents; appetite stimulant in AIDS-related anorexia

DOSAGE

Adult

• *Antiemetic:* PO 5 mg/m^2 1-3 hr before chemotherapy, then q2-4h up to 6 doses qd; max dose 15 mg/m^2

• *Appetite stimulant:* PO 2.5 mg bid, 1 hr ac; max dose 20 mg qd

§ AVAILABLE FORMS/COST OF THERAPY

• Cap, Elastic—Oral: 2.5 mg, 100's: **$316.95;** 5 mg, 100's: **$626.99;** 10 mg, 60's: **$781.61**

CONTRAINDICATIONS: Hypersensitivity to any cannabinoid or sesame oil

PRECAUTIONS: Children, history of abuse or dependence

PREGNANCY AND LACTATION: Pregnancy category C; excreted in breast milk

SIDE EFFECTS/ADVERSE REACTIONS

CNS: Abnormal thinking, *anxiety,* ataxia, confusion, depersonalization, *difficulty concentrating, dizziness, euphoria (24%),* hallucination, *mood change,* somnolence

CV: Orthostatic hypotension, palpitations, tachycardia, vasodilation

EENT: Change in vision, dry mouth, rhinitis, sinusitis, tinnitus

GI: Diarrhea, nausea, vomiting

MS: Myalgias

RESP: Cough

SKIN: Sweating

SPECIAL CONSIDERATIONS

• May have additive sedative or behavioral effects with CNS depressants

• Use caution escalating the dose because of increased frequency of adverse reactions at higher doses

---

droperidol

(droe-per'i-dole)

Rx: Inapsine

Combinations

Rx: with fentanyl (Innovar)

Chemical Class: Butyrophenone derivative

Therapeutic Class: Antiemetic; sedative; anesthesia adjunct

CLINICAL PHARMACOLOGY

Mechanism of Action: Alters the action of dopamine at subcortical levels in CNS to produce sedation; produces mild α-adrenergic blockade, peripheral vascular dilation, and reduction of pressor effect of epinephrine

Pharmacokinetics

IV/IM: Onset 3-10 min (full effect may not be apparent for 30 min), duration 2-4 hr; metabolized in liver, excreted in urine and feces; t$_{1/2}$ 2.2 hr

INDICATIONS AND USES: Premedication for surgery; induction, maintenance in general anesthesia; antiemetic in cancer chemotherapy*

DOSAGE

Adult

• *Adjunct to general anesthesia:* IV 2.5 mg/10 kg given with analgesic or general anesthetic

• *Premedication for surgery:* IM 2.5-10 mg 30-60 min preoperatively

• *Maintaining general anesthesia:* IV 1.25-2.5 mg

Child 2-12 yr

• *Adjunct to general anesthesia:* IV 1-1.5 mg/10 kg, titrated to response needed

• *Premedication for surgery:* IM 1-1.5 mg/10 kg 30-60 min preoperatively

---

* = non-FDA-approved use

§ **AVAILABLE FORMS/COST OF THERAPY**

• Inj, Sol—IM, IV: 2.5 mg/ml, 2 ml: **$1.88-$12.21**

PRECAUTIONS: Elderly, cardiovascular disease (hypotension, bradydysrhythmias), renal disease, liver disease, Parkinson's disease, child <2 yr

PREGNANCY AND LACTATION: Pregnancy category C; has been used to promote analgesia for cesarean section patients without affecting respiration of the newborn; excretion into breast milk unknown, use caution in nursing mothers

NOTE: Has been used as a continuous IV infusion for hyperemesis gravidarum during the 2nd and 3rd trimesters without apparent fetal harm

SIDE EFFECTS/ADVERSE REACTIONS

CNS: Akathisia, chills, dizziness, *drowsiness,* dystonia, hallucinations, shivering

CV: Hypertension, *hypotension, tachycardia*

EENT: Oculogyric crisis

MS: Muscular rigidity

RESP: **Apnea, bronchospasm, respiratory arrest, respiratory depression**

SPECIAL CONSIDERATIONS
MONITORING PARAMETERS

• Blood pressure, heart rate, respiratory rate

---

dyclonine
(dye'clo-neen)
Rx: Dyclone
Chemical Class: Pramoxine derivative
Therapeutic Class: Topical anesthetic

CLINICAL PHARMACOLOGY
Mechanism of Action: Blocks nerve impulses at sensory nerve endings in the skin and mucous membranes

Pharmacokinetics

TOP: Onset 2-10 min, duration 30 min

INDICATIONS AND USES: Anesthetizing accessible mucous membranes prior to endoscopic procedures; blocking the gag reflex; relieving pain associated with oral ulcers of stomatitis, postoperative wounds, and ano-genital lesions

DOSAGE

Adult

• Apply to desired area as a rinse, gargle, mouthwash, spray, wet compress, or swab prn; do not exceed 30 ml of 1% sol(300 mg)

§ **AVAILABLE FORMS/COST OF THERAPY**

• Sol—Top: 0.5%, 30 ml: **$32.58;** 1%, 30 ml: **$43.87**

PRECAUTIONS: Traumatized mucosa, sepsis in region intended for application, shock, heart block, child <12 yr

PREGNANCY AND LACTATION: Pregnancy category C; excretion into breast milk unknown

SIDE EFFECTS/ADVERSE REACTIONS

CNS: Depression, dizziness, drowsiness, excitation, nervousness, *seizures,* tremors, unconsciousness

CV: Bradycardia, **cardiac arrest, myocardial depression**

EENT: Blurred vision

GU: Urethritis (when used for urethral anesthesia)

RESP: **Respiratory arrest**

SKIN: Edema, slight irritation, stinging, swelling, urticaria

INTERACTIONS

③ *Tocainide, mexiletine:* Additive or synergistic toxicity

SPECIAL CONSIDERATIONS
PATIENT/FAMILY EDUCATION

• Ingestion of food following use in

---

italic = common side effects **bold italic** = life-threatening reactions

the mouth or throat increases risk of aspiration

• Avoid too frequent dosing to prevent accumulation and systemic side effects

• Drowsiness may be first sign of toxicity

---

dyphylline
(dye'fi-lin)

Rx: Dilor, Dylix, Lufyllin, Neothylline
Combinations
  Rx: with guaifenesin (Dilex-G, Dilor-G, Lufyllin-GG); with ephedrine, guaifenesin, phenobarbital (Lufyllin-EPG)
Chemical Class: Xanthine derivative
Therapeutic Class: Antiasthmatic, bronchodilator; COPD agent

CLINICAL PHARMACOLOGY
Mechanism of Action: Possesses the peripheral vasodilator and bronchodilator actions characteristic of theophylline (approximately 1/10th as potent as theophylline); has diuretic and myocardial stimulant effects
Pharmacokinetics
PO: Bioavailability 68%-82%, peak 1 hr; not metabolized to theophylline; 83% excreted unchanged in urine, $t_{1/2}$ 2 hr
INDICATIONS AND USES: Bronchial asthma, bronchospasm in chronic bronchitis and emphysema
DOSAGE
Adult
• PO up to 15 mg/kg q6h; IM 250-500 mg q6h (administer by slow IM inj; do not administer IV), not to exceed 15 mg/kg/dose

---

$ AVAILABLE FORMS/COST OF THERAPY
• Elixir—Oral: 100 mg/15 ml, 480 ml: **$34.68-$82.34;** 160 mg/5 ml, 480 ml: **$52.37**
• Inj, Sol—IM: 250 mg/ml, 2 ml: **$5.57**
• Tab, Uncoated—Oral: 200 mg, 100's: **$13.78-$131.42** 400 mg, 100's: **$16.86-$193.01**
CONTRAINDICATIONS: Concurrent use with other xanthine preparations
PRECAUTIONS: Severe cardiac disease, hypertension, hyperthyroidism, acute myocardial injury, peptic ulcer, CHF, children
PREGNANCY AND LACTATION: Pregnancy category C; excreted into breast milk, compatible with breast feeding
SIDE EFFECTS/ADVERSE REACTIONS
CNS: Anxiety, dizziness, headache, *insomnia,* light-headedness, muscle twitching, *restlessness,* **seizures**
CV: **Dysrhythmias,** flushing, hypotension, *palpitations, sinus tachycardia*
GI: Anorexia, dyspepsia, epigastric pain, *nausea, vomiting*
RESP: Tachypnea
SKIN: Flushing, urticaria
MISC: Albuminuria, dehydration, fever, hyperglycemia
INTERACTIONS
Drugs
3 *Probenecid:* Increased serum dyphylline concentrations
SPECIAL CONSIDERATIONS
• Though better tolerated, significantly less bronchodilating activity vs theophylline. Serious dosing errors possible if dyphylline monitored with theophylline serum assays
MONITORING PARAMETERS
• Minimal effective serum concentration 12 µg/ml

---

echothiophate iodide

(ek-oh-thye'oh-fate)
Rx: Phospholine Iodide
Chemical Class: Cholinesterase inhibitor
Therapeutic Class: Antiglaucoma agent; miotic

CLINICAL PHARMACOLOGY
Mechanism of Action: Enhances effect of endogenously liberated acetylcholine in iris, ciliary muscle, and other parasympathetically innervated structures of the eye; results in miosis which increases outflow of aqueous humor, fall in intraocular pressure, and potentiation of accommodation

Pharmacokinetics
OPHTH: Onset of miosis 10-30 min, duration of miosis 1-4 wk; onset of intraocular pressure reduction 4-8 hr, peak 24 hr, duration 1-4 wk

INDICATIONS AND USES: Glaucoma (open-angle), accommodative esotropia

DOSAGE
Adult and Child
• OPHTH instill 1 gtt in conjunctival sac, not to exceed 1 gtt qd (accommodative estropia), or 1 gtt bid (glaucoma)

$ **AVAILABLE FORMS/COST OF THERAPY**
• Sol—Ophth: 0.03%, 5 ml: **$27.39;** 0.06%, 5 ml: **$28.70;** 0.125%, 5 ml: **$32.20;** 0.25%, 5 ml: **$36.29**

CONTRAINDICATIONS: Active uveal inflammation, most cases of angle-closure glaucoma (due to the possibility of increasing angle block)

PRECAUTIONS: Asthma, bradycardia, parkinsonism, peptic ulcer, myasthenia gravis, spastic GI disease, recent MI, epilepsy, history of quiescent uveitis

PREGNANCY AND LACTATION: Pregnancy category C; as a quaternary ammonium compound, is ionized at physiologic pH and transplacental passage in significant amounts would not be expected; excretion into breast milk unknown; use caution in nursing mothers

SIDE EFFECTS/ADVERSE REACTIONS
CNS: Headache
CV: Cardiac irregularities
EENT: Activation of latent iritis or uveitis, *browache, burning,* conjunctival and ciliary redness, conjunctival thickening, decreased vision in dim light, destruction of nasolacrimal canals, iris cysts, *lacrimation, lens opacities* (50% over 6 mo); lid muscle twitching, myopia, retinal detachment; *visual blurring*
GI: Abdominal cramps, diarrhea, nausea, salivation, vomiting
GU: Urinary incontinence
RESP: Difficulty breathing
SKIN: Sweating
MISC: Fainting

INTERACTIONS
Drugs
❷ *Succinylcholine:* Prolonged neuromuscular blocking effects of succinylcholine

SPECIAL CONSIDERATIONS
• Reserved for refractory open-angle glaucoma after short-acting miotics, epinephrine, β-blockers, and carbonic anhydrase inhibitors due to cataractogenic properties

PATIENT/FAMILY EDUCATION
• Local irritation and headache may occur at initiation of therapy, then resolve with time
• Use caution while driving at night or performing hazardous tasks in poor light
• Minimize systemic absorption by applying gentle pressure to the lacrimal sac for 3-5 min following administration

---

italic = common side effects   ***bold italic*** = life-threatening reactions

econazole

(e-kone'a-zole)

Rx: Spectazole

Chemical Class: Imidazole
derivative

Therapeutic Class: Antifungal

CLINICAL PHARMACOLOGY

Mechanism of Action: Alteration
of the fungal cell membrane, which
allows leakage of essential intracellular components

Pharmacokinetics

TOP: Systemic absorption extremely
low, inhibitory concentrations have
been found as deep as the middle
region of the dermis, <1% of applied dose recovered in urine and
feces

INDICATIONS AND USES: Tinea
pedis (athlete's foot), tinea cruris
(jock itch), tinea corporis (ringworm), cutaneous candidiasis, tinea
versicolor

Antifungal spectrum usually includes *Trichophyton rubrum, T. mentagrophytes, T. tonsurans, Microsporum canis, M. audouini, M.
gypseum, Epidermophyton floccosum,* the yeasts, *Candida albicans,
Pityrosporum orbiculare*

DOSAGE

Adult and Child

• TOP apply to affected area qd-bid
depending on condition

**$ AVAILABLE FORMS/COST
OF THERAPY**

• Cre—Top: 1%, 15, 30, 85 g:
$25.08/30 g

PREGNANCY AND LACTATION:
Pregnancy category C; excretion
into breast milk unknown; limited
systemic absorption would minimize possibility of exposure to nursing infant

SIDE EFFECTS/ADVERSE REACTIONS

SKIN: Burning, erythema, itching,
pruritic rash, stinging

SPECIAL CONSIDERATIONS

PATIENT/FAMILY EDUCATION

• For external use only; avoid contact with eyes; cleanse skin with
soap and water and dry thoroughly
prior to application

• Use medication for full treatment
time outlined by clinician, even
though symptoms may have improved

• Notify clinician if no improvement after 2 wk (jock itch, ringworm) or 4 wk (athlete's foot)

edetate calcium disodium (calcium EDTA)

(ed'e-tate)

Rx: Calcium Disodium
Versenate

Chemical Class: Chelating
agent

Therapeutic Class: Lead
antidote

CLINICAL PHARMACOLOGY

Mechanism of Action: The calcium in edetate calcium disodium is
readily displaced by heavy metals,
such as lead, to form stable complexes that are excreted in urine

Pharmacokinetics

IV/IM/SC: Not metabolized; distributed primarily in extracellular fluid;
excreted in urine; $t_{1/2}$ 20-60 min

INDICATIONS AND USES: Acute
and chronic lead poisoning, lead encephalopathy

DOSAGE

Adult

• *Acute lead encephalopathy:* IV 1.5
g/m^2/day as either an 8-24 hr INF or
divided into 2 doses q12h for 3-5

days, with dimercaprol; may be given again after 4 days off drug; IM (preferred route) 250 mg/m^2/ dose q4h for 3-5 days, with dimercaprol; may be given again after 4 days off drug

• *Lead poisoning:* IV 1 g/250-500 ml D$_5$W or 0.9% NaCl over 1-2 hr q12h for 3-5 days; may repeat after 2 days; do not exceed 50 mg/kg/day in mildly affected or asymptomatic individuals; IM 35 mg/kg bid, do not exceed 50 mg/kg/day in mildly affected or asymptomatic individuals

Child

• *Acute lead encephalopathy:* Same as adult

• *Lead poisoning:* IM 35 mg/kg/ day in divided doses q8-12h for 3-5 days; off 4 days before next course

💲 **AVAILABLE FORMS/COST OF THERAPY**

• Inj, Sol—IV: 200 mg/ml, 5 ml: **$38.36**

CONTRAINDICATIONS: Anuria, active renal disease, hepatitis

PRECAUTIONS: Vomiting (may lead to dehydration and decreased urine flow), rapid IV INF (especially in lead encephalopathy)

PREGNANCY AND LACTATION: Pregnancy category B; excretion into breast milk unknown; use caution in nursing mothers

SIDE EFFECTS/ADVERSE REACTIONS

CNS: Chills, fever, *headache,* numbness, tingling, tremors

CV: Cardiac rhythm irregularities, hypotension

EENT: Lacrimation, nasal congestion, sneezing

GI: Anorexia, cheilosis, excessive thirst; *mild increases in AST, ALT;* nausea, vomiting

GU: **Acute necrosis of proximal tubules,** glycosuria, infrequent changes in distal tubules and glomeruli, mi-

croscopic hematuria and large epithelial cells in urinary sediment, proteinuria

HEME: Anemia, transient bone marrow suppression

METAB: Hypercalcemia, zinc deficiency

MS: Arthralgia, fatigue, myalgia

SKIN: Rash

MISC: Malaise, pain at inj site

SPECIAL CONSIDERATIONS

PATIENT/FAMILY EDUCATION

• Notify clinician immediately if no urine output in a 12 hr period

MONITORING PARAMETERS

• Urinalysis and urine sediment daily during therapy to detect signs of progressive renal tubular damage

• Renal function tests, liver function tests, and serum electrolytes before and periodically during therapy

• ECG during IV therapy

---

edetate disodium

(ed′e-tate)

Rx: Disotate, Endrate

Chemical Class: Chelating agent

Therapeutic Class: Antihypercalcemic; digitalis antidote

CLINICAL PHARMACOLOGY

Mechanism of Action: Forms chelates with many divalent and trivalent metals that are then excreted in urine

Pharmacokinetics

IV: Not metabolized; t$_{1/2}$ 20-60 min: following chelation 95% excreted in urine as chelates within 24-48 hr

INDICATIONS AND USES: Emergency treatment of hypercalcemia; ventricular dysrhythmias associated with digitalis toxicity

DOSAGE

Adult

• IV INF 50 mg/kg/day (not to exceed 3 g/day), diluted in 500 ml of

---

italic = common side effects   ***bold italic*** = life-threatening reactions

D_5W or 0.9% NaCl and infused over 3-4 hr for 5 consecutive days followed by 2 days without medication
Child

• IV INF 15-50 mg/kg/day (not to exceed 3 g/day), diluted in 500 ml of D_5W or 0.9% NaCl and infused over 3-4 hr for 5 consecutive days followed by 5 days without medication

$ AVAILABLE FORMS/COST OF THERAPY

• Inj, Sol—IV: 150 mg/ml, 20 ml: **$6.35-$32.44**

CONTRAINDICATIONS: Anuria

PRECAUTIONS: Intracranial lesions, seizure disorder, CAD, peripheral vascular disease, tuberculosis, CHF, diabetes

PREGNANCY AND LACTATION: Pregnancy category C; excretion into breast milk unknown; use caution in nursing mothers

SIDE EFFECTS/ADVERSE REACTIONS

CNS: Febrile reactions, *headache,* numbness, *seizures,* transient circumoral paresthesia

CV: **Dysrhythmias,** thrombophlebitis, transient drop in blood pressure

GI: Diarrhea, nausea, vomiting

GU: **Acute tubular necrosis, nephrotoxicity**

HEME: Anemia

METAB: Hyperuricemia, hypocalcemia, hypokalemia, hypomagnesemia

MS: Back pain, muscle cramps

RESP: **Respiratory arrest**

SKIN: **Exfoliative dermatitis,** skin and mucous membrane reactions

SPECIAL CONSIDERATIONS
Have patient remain supine for a short time after INF due to the possibility of orthostatic hypotension

MONITORING PARAMETERS
• ECG, blood pressure during INF
• Renal function before and during therapy
• Serum calcium, magnesium, potassium levels

---

edrophonium
(ed-roe-foe'nee-um)
Rx: Enlon, Reversol, Tensilon
Combinations
  Rx: with atropine (Enlon-Plus)
Chemical Class: Quaternary ammonium derivative
Therapeutic Class: Cholinergic; curare antidote

CLINICAL PHARMACOLOGY
Mechanism of Action: An acetylcholinesterase inhibitor, inhibits destruction of acetylcholine, facilitates transmission of impulses across myoneural junction
Pharmacokinetics
IM: Onset 2-10 min, duration 12-45 min
IV: Onset <1 min, duration 6-24 min
Hydrolyzed by cholinesterase and metabolized by microsomal enzymes of liver, excreted by kidneys; $t_{1/2}$ 1.8 hr

INDICATIONS AND USES: Diagnosis of myasthenia gravis; differentiation of myasthenic crisis from cholinergic crisis; evaluation of treatment requirements in myasthenia gravis; curare antagonist

DOSAGE
Adult

• *Diagnosis of myasthenia gravis:* IV 1-2 mg over 15-30 sec, then 8 mg if no response; IM 10 mg; if cholinergic reaction occurs, retest after ½ hr with 2 mg IM

• *Evaluation of treatment requirements in myasthenia gravis:* IV 1-2 mg 1 hr after PO dose of anticholinesterase; if strength improves, an increase in neostigmine or pyridostigmine dose is indicated

• *Differentiation of myasthenic crisis from cholinergic crisis:* IV 1 mg, if no response in 1 min, may repeat; *myasthenic crisis* clear improvement in respiration, *cholinergic crisis* increased oropharyngeal secretions and further weakening of respiratory muscles (intubation and controlled ventilation may be required)

• *Curare antagonist:* IV 10 mg over 30-45 sec; may repeat; not to exceed 40 mg

Child

• *Diagnosis of myasthenia gravis:* IV 0.04 mg/kg given over 1 min followed by 0.16 mg/kg given within 45 sec if no response; >34 kg IM 2 mg; <34 kg IM 1 mg; infant IV 0.1 mg, followed by 0.4 mg if no response, not to exceed 0.5 mg

• *Evaluation of treatment requirements in myasthenia gravis:* IV 0.04 mg/kg given 1 hr after PO intake of drug being used in treatment; if strength improves, an increase in neostigmine or pyridostigmine is indicated

💲 AVAILABLE FORMS/COST OF THERAPY

• Inj, Sol—IM, IV: 10 mg/ml, 1 ml: **$0.86-$4.08**

CONTRAINDICATIONS: Mechanical, intestinal, and urinary obstructions

PRECAUTIONS: Seizure disorders, bronchial asthma, recent coronary occlusion, hyperthyroidism, dysrhythmias, peptic ulcer, megacolon, poor GI motility, bradycardia, hypotension

PREGNANCY AND LACTATION: Pregnancy category C; because it is ionized at physiologic pH, would not be expected to cross placenta in significant amounts; may cause premature labor; because it is ionized at physiologic pH, would not be expected to be excreted into breast milk

SIDE EFFECTS/ADVERSE REACTIONS

CNS: Dizziness, drowsiness, headache, incoordination, loss of consciousness, paralysis, *seizures,* sweating, weakness

CV: AV block, bradycardia, *cardiac arrest, dysrhythmias,* ECG changes, hypotension, syncope, tachycardia

EENT: Blurred vision, lacrimation, miosis, visual changes

GI: Cramps, diarrhea, dysphagia, increased peristalsis, increased salivary and gastric secretions, nausea, vomiting

GU: Frequency, incontinence, urgency

MS: Arthralgia, fasciculations, muscle cramps and spasms, weakness

RESP: Bronchospasm, dyspnea, increased tracheobronchial secretions, *laryngospasm, respiratory arrest, respiratory depression*

SKIN: Rash, urticaria

INTERACTIONS

Drugs

3 *Procainamide:* Edrophonium tests in patients with myasthenia gravis may be unreliable in procainamide-treated patients

3 *Tacrine:* Increased cholinergic effects of edrophonium

SPECIAL CONSIDERATIONS

MONITORING PARAMETERS

• Preinjection and postinjection strength

• Heart rate, respiratory rate, blood pressure

---

efavirenz

(e-fahv'er-ins)
Rx: Sustiva
Chemical Class: Substituted benzoxazin-one
Therapeutic Class: Non-nucleoside reverse transcriptase inhibitor

CLINICAL PHARMACOLOGY

Mechanism of Action: Noncompetitive inhibitor of reverse transcriptase of HIV-1

Pharmacokinetics

PO: Peak 5 hr; well absorbed PO, bioavailability increased by 50% with high-fat meal; 99% protein bound (mainly albumin); metabolized by hepatic P450 system, primarily CYP3A4 and CYP2B6; induces its own metabolism through the P450 system; excreted unchanged in stool (50%) and urine (1%) and as glucuronidated metabolites in urine (30%); $t_{1/2}$ single dose: 52-76 hr, multiple dose: 40-55 hr; crosses placenta; CSF level 1% of plasma level

INDICATIONS AND USES: Combination therapy for HIV-1

DOSAGE

Adult and Child >40 kg

• 600 mg qd

• For latest treatment guidelines, see www.hivatis.org

Child<40 kg

• 10-<15 kg: 200 mg qd; 15-<20 kg: 250 mg qd; 20-<25 kg: 300 mg qd; 25-<32.5 kg: 350 mg qd; 32.5-<40 kg: 400 mg qd

• For latest treatment guidelines, see www.hivatis.org

$ **AVAILABLE FORMS/COST OF THERAPY**

• Cap—Oral: 50 mg, 100's: **$108.50;** 100 mg, 100's: **$216.81;** 200 mg, 100's: **$438.00**

PRECAUTIONS: Depression, liver disease, pregnancy (fetal malformations observed in monkeys)

PREGNANCY AND LACTATION: Pregnancy category C (fetal malformations observed in monkeys); breast feeding not recommended

SIDE EFFECTS/ADVERSE REACTIONS

CNS: CNS side effects seen in 52% of patients, abnormal dreams, amnesia, anxiety, confusion, depression, *dizziness, impaired concentration, insomnia,* tremor

CV: Flushing, palpitations, tachycardia

EENT: Tinnitus

GI: Diarrhea, elevated transaminases, nausea

METAB: Hyperlipidemia

MS: Arthralgia, myalgia

RESP: Asthma

SKIN: Rash (27%)

INTERACTIONS

Drugs

❷ *Amprenavir:* Efavirenz decreases amprenavir plasma level; amprenavir dose adjustment recommended

⚠ *Astemizole:* Efavirenz increases astemizole plasma level; coadministration contraindicated

❸ *Barbiturates:* Barbiturates decrease plasma efavirenz levels; dose adjustment not recommended

❸ *Carbamazepine:* Carbamazepine decreases plasma efavirenz levels; dose adjustment not recommended

❷ *Cisapride:* Efavirenz increases cisapride plasma level; coadministration not recommended

❸ *Clarithromycin:* Efavirenz decreases clarithromycin plasma levels; coadministration not recommended

❷ *Ergotamines:* Efavirenz increases ergotamine plasma level; coadministration not recommended

3 *Ethinyl estradiol:* Efavirenz increases ethinyl estradiol plasma levels; dose adjustment not recommended

3 *Indinavir:* Efavirenz reduces indinavir AUC by 31%; increase indinavir dose to 1000 mg q8h

3 *Lovastatin:* Efavirenz increases lovastatin plasma level; dose adjustment not recommended

2 *Midazolam:* Efavirenz increases midazolam plasma level; coadministration not recommended

3 *Nelfinavir:* Efavirenz increases nelfinavir AUC by 20%; dose adjustment not recommended

3 *Oral contraceptives:* Efavirenz increases ethinyl estradiol plasma levels; dose adjustment not recommended

3 *Phenytoin:* Phenytoin decreases plasma efavirenz level; dose adjustment not recommended

2 *Rifabutin:* Efavirenz decreases plasma rifabutin level by 35%; no change in plasma efavirenz level; increase rifabutin dose to 450 mg qd

3 *Rifampin:* Rifampin decreases plasma efavirenz level by 25%; dose adjustment not recommended

3 *Ritonavir:* Ritonavir increases efavirenz AUC by 21%; efavirenz increases ritonavir AUC by 18%; dose adjustment not recommended

2 *Saquinavir:* Saquinavir reduces efavirenz AUC by 12%; efavirenz reduces saquinavir AUC by 62%; coadministration not recommended

3 *Simvastatin:* Efavirenz increases simvastatin plasma level; dose adjustment not recommended

A *Terfenadine:* Efavirenz increases terfenadine plasma level; coadministration contraindicated

2 *Triazolam:* Efavirenz increases triazolam plasma level; coadministration not recommended

3 *Warfarin:* Efavirenz increases warfarin effect

Labs

False positive: Cannabinoid screening test by CEDIA DAU Multilevel THC assay

SPECIAL CONSIDERATIONS
PATIENT/FAMILY EDUCATION

• May be taken without regard for meals; absorption increased by a high-fat meal, which should be avoided

• Take at bedtime for first 2-4 wk of therapy; may continue at bedtime if desired

MONITORING PARAMETERS

• ALT, AST, CBC, cholesterol, triglycerides

---

eflornithine
(eh-floor'ni-theen)
Rx: Ornidyl
Chemical Class: Ornithine decarboxylase inhibitor
Therapeutic Class: Antiprotozoal

CLINICAL PHARMACOLOGY
Mechanism of Action: Irreversibly inhibits ornithine decarboxylase; decarboxylation of ornithine by ornithine decarboxylase is an obligatory step in the biosynthesis of polyamines such as putrescine, spermidine, and spermine, which play important roles in cell division and differentiation in all mammalian and many non-mammalian cells

Pharmacokinetics
IV: Not significantly bound to plasma proteins, crosses the blood-brain barrier; 80% excreted unchanged in urine within 24 hr; $t_{1/2}$ 3 hr

INDICATIONS AND USES: Treatment of meningoencephalitic stage of *Trypanosoma brucei gambiense* infection (sleeping sickness); *Pneumocystis carinii* pneumonia*

---

italic = common side effects   ***bold italic*** = life-threatening reactions

DOSAGE
Adult

• IV INF 100 mg/kg/dose infused over a minimum of 45 min q6h for 14 days

• **Note:** Eflornithine for inj concentrate is hypertonic and must be diluted with sterile water for injection, USP, before inf

💲 **AVAILABLE FORMS/COST OF THERAPY**

• Inj, Sol—IV: 200 mg/ml, 100 ml: compassionate use through World Health Organization (WHO)

PRECAUTIONS: Seizure disorder, renal function impairment (reduced doses recommended)

PREGNANCY AND LACTATION: Pregnancy category C; excretion into breast milk unknown; use caution in nursing mothers

SIDE EFFECTS/ADVERSE REACTIONS

CNS: Asthenia, dizziness, headache, *seizures*

EENT: Hearing impairment

GI: Abdominal pain, anorexia, *diarrhea*

HEME: **Anemia (55%),** eosinophilia, **leukopenia (37%), myelosuppression, thrombocytopenia (14%)**

SKIN: Alopecia

MISC: Facial edema

SPECIAL CONSIDERATIONS

The most frequent, serious, toxic effect of eflornithine is myelosuppression, which may be unavoidable if successful treatment is to be completed; decisions to modify dosage or to interrupt or cease treatment depend on the severity of the observed adverse event(s) and the availability of support facilities

MONITORING PARAMETERS

• Serial audiograms if feasible

• CBC with platelets before and twice weekly during therapy and qwk after completion of therapy until hematologic values return to baseline levels

• Follow-up for at least 24 mo is advised to ensure further therapy should relapses occur

---

emedastine
(e-med'a-steen)
Rx: Emadine
Therapeutic Class: Ophthalmic antihistamine

CLINICAL PHARMACOLOGY
Mechanism of Action: Inhibits histamine-stimulated vascular permeability in the conjunctiva; appears to be devoid of effects on adrenergic, dopaminergic and seritonin receptors

Pharmacokinetics
OPHTH: Low systemic bioavailability; metabolized and excreted in urine; $t_{1/2}$ 3-4 hr

INDICATIONS AND USES: Allergic conjunctivitis

DOSAGE
Adult

• Ophth 1 gtt in affected eye(s) up to qid

💲 **AVAILABLE FORMS/COST OF THERAPY**

• Ophth, Sol—0.05%:5 ml: **$32.50**

PRECAUTIONS: Children

PREGNANCY AND LACTATION: Pregnancy category B; use caution in nursing mothers

SIDE EFFECTS/ADVERSE REACTIONS

CNS: Headache, abnormal dreams

EENT: Blurred vision, burning or stinging, corneal infiltrates, corneal staining, dry eyes, foreign body sensation, hyperemia, keratitis, pruritus, rhinitis, sinusitis, tearing

GI: Bad taste

SKIN: Dermatitis

MISC: Asthenia

---

* = non-FDA-approved use

PATIENT/FAMILY EDUCATION
• Do not wear contact lenses if eyes are red; wait at least 10 min after instilling before inserting soft contact lenses

enalapril
(en-al′a-pril)
Rx: Vasotec
Combinations
   Rx: with diltiazem (Teczem); with felodipine (Lexxel); with hydrochlorothiazide (Vaseretic)
Chemical Class: Nonsulfhydryl angiotensin-converting enzyme (ACE) inhibitor
Therapeutic Class: Antihypertensive

CLINICAL PHARMACOLOGY
Mechanism of Action: Antihypertensive, hypoproliferative, and cardioprotective effects attributable to competitive inhibition of angiotensin-converting enzyme (ACE) yielding decreased plasma concentrations of angiotensin II, plasma aldosterone concentrations, systemic vascular resistance, blood pressure, preload, and afterload, not accompanied by changes in heart rate, pressor sensitivity to exogenous norepinephrine, or baroreceptor sensitivity
Pharmacokinetics
PO: Peak ½-1½ hr (enalaprilat 3-4 hr), metabolized by liver to active metabolite (enalaprilat), excreted in urine and feces; $t_{1/2}$ 1½ hr (enalaprilat 11 hr)
IV (enalaprilat): Onset 5-15 min
INDICATIONS AND USES: Hypertension, CHF, MI, erythrocytosis,* nephropathy,* retinopathy,* hyperaldosteronism,* rheumatoid arthritis*

DOSAGE
Adult and Child >16 yr
• *Hypertension:* PO 2.5-5 mg qd, increase prn; usual dose range 10-40 mg/day divided qd-bid; IV 0.625 mg (with concomittant diuretic therapy)—1.25 mg (without concomittant diuretic therapy)/dose given over 5 min q6h
• *Congestive heart failure:* 2.5-10 mg qd-bid, generally given with digitalis and diuretics; maximum daily doses, 40 mg (or until systolic blood pressure 100 mm Hg) greater symptomatic benefits without differences in mortality or tolerability
• *Nephropathy:* 5 mg qd; increasing prn to 20 mg/day
• Dose adjustment for renal impairment: same
Child
• Same

$ AVAILABLE FORMS/COST OF THERAPY
• Tab, Uncoated—Oral: 2.5 mg, 100's: **$82.74;** 5 mg, 100's: **$105.11;** 10 mg, 100's: **$110.36;** 20 mg, 100's: **$157.01**
• Inj, Sol—IV: 1.25 mg/ml, 1 ml: **$14.75**

PRECAUTIONS: History of anaphylaxis, renal insufficiency (<30 ml/min), hypotension (CHF, elderly, volume depletion—diuretics, dialysis, cirrhosis), aortic stenosis, hyperkalemia (potassium supplements, potassium—sparing diuretics, renal disease, diabetes), neutropenia (autoimmune diseases, collagen vascular, febrile illness, immunosuppressant drug therapy), proteinuria, renal artery stenosis, surgery/anesthesia (excessive hypotension, correctable with fluids)

PREGNANCY AND LACTATION: Pregnancy category C (1st trimester), category D (2nd and 3rd trimesters); ACE inhibitors can cause fetal and neonatal morbidity and death when administered to pregnant women; when pregnancy is detected, discontinue ACE inhibitors as soon as possible; detectable in breast milk in trace amounts; effect on nursing infant has not been determined; use with caution in nursing mothers

SIDE EFFECTS/ADVERSE REACTIONS

CNS: Anxiety, dizziness, fatigue, headache, insomnia, paresthesia

CV: Angina, hypotension, palpitations, postural hypotension, syncope (especially with 1st dose)

GI: Abdominal pain, constipation, melena, nausea, vomiting

GU: Decreased libido, impotence, increased BUN/creatinine, UTI

HEME: **Agranulocytosis, neutropenia**

METAB: Hyperkalemia, hyponatremia

MS: Arthralgia, arthritis, myalgia

RESP: Asthma, bronchitis, *cough,* dyspnea, sinusitis

SKIN: **Angioedema,** flushing, rash, sweating

INTERACTIONS

Drugs

❷ *Allopurinol:* Predisposition to hypersensitivity reactions to ACE inhibitors

❸ *Aspirin, NSAIDs:* Inhibition of the antihypertensive response to ACE inhibitors

❸ *Azathioprine:* Increased myelosuppression

❸ *Insulin:* Enhanced insulin sensitivity

❸ *Iron:* Increased risk of anaphylaxis with administration of parenteral (IV) iron

❸ *Lithium:* Increased risk of serious lithium toxicity

❸ *Loop diuretics:* Initiation of ACE inhibitor therapy in the presence of intensive diuretic therapy results in a precipitous fall in blood pressure

in some patients; ACE inhibitors may induce renal insufficiency in the presence of diuretic-induced sodium depletion

❸ *Potassium:* Increased risk for hyperkalemia

❸ *Potassium-sparing diuretics:* Increased risk for hyperkalemia

❸ *Prazosin, terazosin, doxazosin:* Exaggerated first-dose hypotensive response to α-blockers

❸ *Trimethoprim:* Additive risk of hyperkalemia, especially in patient predisposed to renal insufficiency

Labs

ACE inhibition can account for approximately $0.5mEq/L$ rise in serum potassium

SPECIAL CONSIDERATIONS
PATIENT/FAMILY EDUCATION

• Caution with salt substitutes containing potassium chloride

• Rise slowly to sitting/standing position to minimize orthostatic hypotension

• Dizziness, fainting, lightheadedness may occur during 1st few days of therapy

• May cause altered taste perception or cough; persistent dry cough usually does not subside unless medication is stopped; notify clinician if these symptoms persist

MONITORING PARAMETERS

• BUN, creatinine, potassium within 2 wk after initiation of therapy (increased levels may indicate acute renal failure)

---

enoxacin

(en-ox′a-sin)

Rx: Penetrex

Chemical Class: Fluoroquinolone derivative

Therapeutic Class: Antibiotic

CLINICAL PHARMACOLOGY
Mechanism of Action: Interferes

with the enzyme DNA gyrase needed for the synthesis of bacterial DNA; bactericidal

Pharmacokinetics

PO: Peak 1-3 hr, excreted in urine as unchanged drug (80%) and metabolites (20%); $t_{1/2}$ 3-6 hr

INDICATIONS AND USES: Uncomplicated urethral or cervical gonorrhea uncomplicated UTI; complicated UTI

Antibacterial spectrum usually includes: Gram-positive organisms: *Staphylococcus epidermidis, S. saprophyticus*

Gram-negative organisms: *Neisseria gonorrhoeae, E. Coli, Klebsiella pneumoniae, Proteus mirabilis, Pseudomonas, aeruginosa, Enterobacter cloacae*

DOSAGE

Adult

• *Uncomplicated UTI:* PO 200 mg q12h for 3-7 days

• *Complicated UTI:* PO 400 mg q12h for 14 days

• *Uncomplicated gonorrhea:* PO 400 mg as a single dose

• *Renal function impairment* (CrCl <30 ml/min/1.73 m²): PO after a normal initial dose; use 50% recommended dose q12h

⚡ AVAILABLE FORMS/COST OF THERAPY

• Tab, Uncoated—Oral: 200 mg, 50's: **$154.53;** 400 mg, 50's: **$162.25**

PRECAUTIONS: Children <17 yr (potential for arthropathy and osteochondrosis), elderly, renal disease, seizure disorders

PREGNANCY AND LACTATION: Pregnancy category C; excretion into breast milk unknown; due to the potential for arthropathy and osteochondrosis use extreme caution in nursing mothers

SIDE EFFECTS/ADVERSE REACTIONS

CNS: Anxiety, depression, dizziness, fatigue, headache, insomnia, *seizures,* somnolence

EENT: Visual disturbances

GI: Abdominal pain, anorexia, diarrhea, dry mouth; flatulence, heartburn, increased AST, ALT; *nausea, pseudomembranous colitis,* vomiting

SKIN: Photosensitivity, pruritus, rash

INTERACTIONS

Drugs

3 *Aluminum:* Reduced absorption of enoxacin; do not take within 4 hr of dose

3 *Antacids:* Reduced absorption of enoxacin; do not take within 4 hr of dose

3 *Antipyrine:* Inhibits metabolism of antipyrine; increased plasma antipyrine level

3 *Caffeine:* Inhibits metabolism of caffeine; increased plasma caffeine level

3 *Calcium:* Reduced absorption of enoxacin; do not take within 4 hr of dose

3 *Cimetidine:* Reduced absorption of enoxacin

3 *Diazepam:* Inhibits metabolism of diazepam; increased plasma diazepam level

3 *Didanosine:* Markedly reduced absorption of enoxacin; take enoxacin 2 hr before didanosine

3 *Famotidine:* Reduced absorption of enoxacin

3 *Fenbufen:* Coadministration increases seizure risk

3 *Foscarnet:* Coadministration increases seizure risk

3 *Iron:* Reduced absorption of enoxacin; do not take within 4 hr of dose

3 *Lansoprazole:* Reduced absorption of enoxacin

3 *Magnesium:* Reduced absorption of enoxacin; do not take within 4 hr of dose

3 *Metoprolol:* Inhibits metabolism

E

---

italic = common side effects   ***bold italic*** = life-threatening reactions

of metoprolol; increased plasma metoprolol level

▪ *Nizatidine:* Reduced absorption of enoxacin

▪ *Omeprazole:* Reduced absorption of enoxacin

▪ *Pentoxifylline:* Inhibits metabolism of pentoxifylline; increased plasma pentoxifylline level

▪ *Phenytoin:* Inhibits metabolism of phenytoin; increased plasma phenytoin level

▪ *Propranolol:* Inhibits metabolism of propranolol; increased plasma propranolol level

▪ *Ranitidine:* Reduced absorption of enoxacin

▪ *Ropinirole:* Inhibits metabolism of ropinirole; increased plasma ropinirole level

▪ *Sodium bicarbonate:* Reduced absorption of enoxacin; do not take within 4 hr of dose

▪ *Sucralfate:* Reduced absorption of enoxacin; do not take within 4 hr of dose

▪ *Tacrine:* Inhibits metabolism of tacrine; increased plasma tacrine level

❷ *Theobromine:* Inhibits metabolism of theobromine; increased plasma theobromine level

❷ *Theophylline:* Inhibits metabolism of theophylline; cut maintenance theophylline dose in half during therapy with enoxacin

▪ *Warfarin:* Inhibits metabolism of warfarin; increases hypoprothrombinemic response to warfarin

▪ *Zinc:* Reduced absorption of enoxacin; do not take within 4 hr of dose

SPECIAL CONSIDERATIONS

• No demonstrated advantage over other fluoroquinolones for UTI or gonorrhea; choice should be based on availability and cost

PATIENT/FAMILY EDUCATION

• Administer on an empty stomach (1 hr before or 2 hr after meals)
• Drink fluids liberally
• Do not take antacids containing magnesium or aluminum or products containing iron or zinc within 4 hr before or 2 hr after dosing

---

enoxaparin
(e-nox-ah-pair'in)
Rx: Lovenox
Chemical Class: Depolymerized heparin derivative (low-molecular-weight heparin)
Therapeutic Class: Anticoagulant

CLINICAL PHARMACOLOGY

Mechanism of Action: Enhances the inhibition of Factor Xa and thrombin by binding to and accelerating antithrombin activity; preferentially inhibits Factor Xa; activated partial thromboplastin time (aPTT) not affected

Pharmacokinetics

SC: Peak activity 3-5 hr; renal elimination $t_{1/2}$ 4½ hr

INDICATIONS AND USES: Prevention of deep vein thrombosis (DVT), which may lead to pulmonary embolism (PE) following hip or knee replacement surgery or abdominal surgery; in conjunction with warfarin-treatment of DVT with and without PE (inpatient) or treatment of acute DVT without PE (outpatient); unstable angina and non-Q-wave MI (in conjunction with aspirin); prevention of deep vein thrombosis (DVT) long term when other modalities inappropriate*

DOSAGE

Adult

• Prevention of DVT, hip or knee replacement surgery: SC 30 mg

---

q12h; initial dose given 12-24 hr postoperatively provided hemostasis has been established; duration 7-14 days

• Prevention of DVT, abdominal surgery: SC 40 mg qd; initial dose given 2 hr prior to surgery; duration 7-12 days

• Treatment of DVT/PE: SC 1 mg/kg q12h (outpatient or inpatient) or 1.5 mg/kg qd (inpatient); initiate warfarin therapy concurrently and continue enoxaparin for a minimum of 5 days and until therapeutic oral anticoagulant effect has been achieved (INR 2-3)

• Unstable angina/non-Q-wave MI: SC 1 mg/kg q12h in conjunction with aspirin 100-325 mg PO qd; usual duration 2-8 days

[$] AVAILABLE FORMS/COST OF THERAPY

• Inj, Sol—SC: 30 mg/0.3 ml: **$17.64;** 40 mg/0.4 ml: **$23.52;** 60 mg/0.6 ml: **$35.28;** 80 mg/0.8 ml: **$47.04;** 100 mg/1 ml: **$58.80**

CONTRAINDICATIONS: Active major bleeding; thrombocytopenia associated with positive in vitro tests for anti-platelet antibody in the presence of enoxaparin

PRECAUTIONS: Bacterial endocarditis, bleeding disorder, active ulceration, angiodysplastic GI disease, hemorrhagic stroke; recent brain, spinal, or ophthalmological surgery; history of heparin-induced thrombocytopenia; renal function impairment; elderly; children; neuraxial anesthesia

PREGNANCY AND LACTATION: Pregnancy category B; excretion into breast milk unknown; use caution in nursing mothers

SIDE EFFECTS/ADVERSE REACTIONS

CNS: Confusion, fever
CV: Edema
GI: Increased ALT, AST; nausea

HEME: Hemorrhage, hypochromic anemia, ***thrombocytopenia***
SKIN: Ecchymosis, erythema at inj site, hematoma, local irritation, pain

INTERACTIONS

Drugs

[3] *Aspirin:* Increased risk of hemorrhage

[3] *Oral anticoagulants:* Additive anticoagulant effects

SPECIAL CONSIDERATIONS

• Cannot be used interchangeably with unfractionated heparin or other low molecular weight heparins

PATIENT/FAMILY EDUCATION

• Administer by deep SC inj into abdominal wall; alternate inj sites
• Report any unusual bruising or bleeding to clinician

MONITORING PARAMETERS

• CBC with platelets, stool occult blood, urinalysis
• Monitoring aPTT is not required

---

entacapone

(en-tak'a-pone)
Rx: Comtan
Chemical Class: Catechol-O-methyl-tranferase (COMT) inhibitor
Therapeutic Class: Anti-Parkinson's agent

CLINICAL PHARMACOLOGY
Mechanism of Action: Alters the plasma pharmacokinetics of levodopa; when given in combination with levodopa/carbidopa, plasma levels of levodopa are more sustained and result in more constant dopaminergic stimulation in the brain, leading to greater effects on the signs and symptoms of Parkinson's disease; may allow decrease in levodopa dose requirements
Pharmacokinetics
PO: Peak 1 hr, bioavailability 35%; 98% bound to plasma proteins;

99.8% metabolized, main pathway is isomerization to the cis-isomer, followed by glucuronidation (inactive); 0.2% of a dose is found unchanged in the urine; $t_{1/2}$ 2.4 hr

INDICATIONS AND USES: As an adjunct to levodopa/carbidopa for the treatment of signs and symptoms of idiopathic Parkinson's disease in patients who experience "wearing off" symptoms at the end of a dosing interval

DOSAGE

Adult

• PO 200 mg dose, up to a max of 8 ×/day; max daily dose 1600 mg/day; always administer with levodopa/carbidopa; to optimize therapy the levodopa/carbidopa dosage must be reduced, usually by 25%; this reduction is usually necessary when the patient is taking more than 800 mg of levodopa daily

💲 **AVAILABLE FORMS/COST OF THERAPY**

• Tab—PO: 200 mg, 100's: **$168.00**

CONTRAINDICATIONS: Treatment with a nonselective MAO inhibitor (isocarboxide, phenelzine, or tranylcypromine)

PRECAUTIONS: May increase risk of orthostatic hypotension and syncope; may cause diarrhea, hallucinations; may cause or exacerbate dyskinesia; abrupt withdrawal; hepatic impairment, renal impairment

PREGNANCY AND LACTATION: Pregnancy category C; use caution in nursing mothers

SIDE EFFECTS/ADVERSE REACTIONS

CNS: Dyskinesia, dizziness, fatigue, hallucinations, anxiety, somnolence, agitation, hyperpyrexia, confusion
CV: Orthostatic hypotension, syncope
GI: Nausea, diarrhea, abdominal pain, constipation, vomiting, dry mouth, dyspepsia, flatulence, gastritis, taste perversion
GU: Brown-orange urine discoloration
MS: Hyperkinesia, hypokinesia, back pain, weakness
RESP: Dyspnea
SKIN: Purpura
MISC: Increased sweating, rhabdomyolysis, pulmonary fibrosis, retroperitoneal fibrosis

INTERACTIONS

Drugs

❷ *Nonselective MAO inhibitors (phenelzine, tranylcypromine):* Inhibition of the majority of the pathways responsible for normal catecholamine metabolism

❸ *Iron:* Decreased absorption of iron via chelation

❸ *Isoproterenol, epinephrine, norepinephrine, dopamine, dobutamine, alpha-methyldopa, apomorphine, isoetherine, and bitolterol:* Decreased metabolism of these drugs

---

ephedrine

(e-fed′rin)

OTC: Pretz-D, Kondon's Nasal

Combinations

Rx: with potassium iodide, phenobarbital, theophylline (Quadrinal), with hydroxyzine, theophylline (Hydrophed DF, Marax-DF); with guaifenesin (Brancholate, Ephex SR)

Chemical Class: Catecholamine

Therapeutic Class: Bronchodilator; vasopressor; decongestant

CLINICAL PHARMACOLOGY

Mechanism of Action: Stimulates α- and β-adrenergic receptors directly and via norepinepherine release; produces bronchial smooth muscle relaxation, cardiac stimulation, and increased blood pressure; CNS effects similar to amphetamine

Pharmacokinetics

PO: Onset 15-60 min, duration 3-6 hr

IM: Onset 10-20 min

60%-77% of dose excreted as unchanged drug in urine; $t_{1/2}$ 2.5-3.6 hr

INDICATIONS AND USES: Bronchial asthma, nasal congestion (local treatment); vasopressor in shock, enuresis,* myasthenia gravis*

DOSAGE

Adult

• IM/SC 25-50 mg, not to exceed 150 mg/24 hr; IV 10-25 mg, not to exceed 150 mg/24 hr; PO 25-50 mg bid-tid

• *Nasal congestion:* TOP instill 3-4 gtt q4h or small amount of gel in each nostril q4h

Child

• PO/SC/IV 3 mg/kg/day in divided doses q4-6h

• *Nasal congestion:* TOP instill 3-4 gtt q4h or small amount of gel in each nostril q4h

§ AVAILABLE FORMS/COST OF THERAPY

• Cap, Gel—Oral: 25 mg, 100's: **$4.95-$8.48;** 50 mg, 100's: **$5.95**

• Inj, Sol—IM, IV, SC: 50 mg/ml, 1 ml: **$0.56-$2.05**

• Spray—Nasal: 0.25%, 50 ml: **$5.00**

• Sol. 0.48%, 45 ml: **$3.44**

CONTRAINDICATIONS: Narrow-angle glaucoma

PRECAUTIONS: Heart disease, coronary insufficiency, dysrhythmias, angina, hyperthyroidism, diabetes mellitus, prostatic hypertrophy, increased intracranial pressure, hypovolemia

PREGNANCY AND LACTATION: Pregnancy category C; routinely used to treat or prevent maternal hypotension following spinal anesthesia; may cause fetal heart rate changes; excretion into breast milk unknown; one case report of adverse effects (excessive crying, irritability, and disturbed sleeping patterns) in a 3-month-old nursing infant whose mother consumed disoephedrine

SIDE EFFECTS/ADVERSE REACTIONS

CNS: Anxiety, confusion, dizziness, hallucinations, headache, *insomnia, seizures, tremors*

CV: Chest pain, **dysrhythmias,** hypertension, palpitations, tachycardia

EENT: Burning, dryness, irritation, rebound congestion with prolonged use, sneezing, stinging

GI: Anorexia, nausea, vomiting

GU: Dysuria, urinary retention

METAB: Hyperglycemia

RESP: Respiratory difficulty

SKIN: Contact dermatitis, pallor

INTERACTIONS

Drugs

❸ *Antacids:* Increased ephedrine serum concentrations

❸ *Furazolidone:* Hypertensive response possible

❸ *Guanadrel:* Inhibits antihypertensive response

❸ *Guanethidine:* Inhibits antihypertensive response

❷ *MAOIs:* Substantially enhanced pressor response to ephedrine, severe hypertension

❸ *Sodium bicarbonate:* Increased ephedrine serum concentrations

Labs

• *False increase:* Urine amino acids, urine 5-HIAA

SPECIAL CONSIDERATIONS
PATIENT/FAMILY EDUCATION

• May cause wakefulness or nervousness; take last dose 4-6 hr prior to bedtime

---

italic = common side effects   ***bold italic*** = life-threatening reactions

• Do not use nasal products for >3-5 days
MONITORING PARAMETERS
• Heart rate, ECG, blood pressure (when using for vasopressor effect)

---

epinephrine
(ep-i-nef'rin)
Vasopressor: **Rx:** Adrenalin, Sus-Phrine
Bronchodilator: **Rx:** Adrenaline, Ana-Guard, Sus-Phrine; **OTC:** Adrenalin, AsthmaHaler Mist, Asthma-Nefrin, microNefrin, Nephron, Primatene Mist, S-2,
Decongestant: **OTC:** Adrenalin
Antiglaucoma agent: **Rx:** Epifrin, Glaucon
Emergency Kit: **Rx:** Ana-Kit, EpiPen, EpiPen Jr.
Combinations
  Rx: with etidocaine (Duranest with Epinephrine); with prilocaine (Citanest Forte); with lidocaine (Xylocaine with Epinephrine); with pilocarpine (E-Pilo Ophthalmic)
Chemical Class: Catecholamine
Therapeutic Class: Vasopressor; antiglaucoma agent; bronchodilator; decongestant

---

CLINICAL PHARMACOLOGY
Mechanism of Action: Stimulates α-, β_1-, and β_2-adrenergic receptors resulting in bronchodilation, cardiac stimulation, nasal decongestion, and dilation of skeletal muscle vasculature; effects on vasculature are dose dependent, small doses produce vasodilation while large doses produce vasoconstriction; decreases production of aqueous humor and increases aqueous outflow; dilates the pupil by contracting the dilator muscle
Pharmacokinetics
SC: Onset 3-5 min
INH: Onset 1 min
OPHTH: Onset 1 hr
Taken up into the adrenergic neuron and metabolized by monoamine oxidase and catechol-o-methyltransferase; circulating drug metabolized by liver; inactive metabolites excreted in urine
INDICATIONS AND USES: Cardiac arrest, acute asthmatic attacks, nasal congestion, open-angle glaucoma, anaphylactic reactions
DOSAGE
Adult
• *Bronchodilator:* IM/SC (1:1000) 0.1-0.5 mg q12-15 min-4 hr; IV 0.1-0.25 mg (single dose max 1 mg); SC susp (1:200) 0.5-1.5 mg (0.1-0.3 ml); NEB instill 8-15 gtt into nebulizer reservoir, administer 1-3 inhalations 4-6 times/day; MDI 1-2 puffs at 1st sign of bronchospasm
• *Cardiac arrest:* IV/intracardiac 0.1-1 mg (1-10 ml of 1:10,000 dilution) q3-5 min prn; IV intermediate dose 2-5 mg q3-5 min; escalating dose 1 mg-3 mg-5 mg 3 min apart; high dose 0.1 mg/kg q3-5 min; intratracheal 1 mg q3-5 min (higher doses [e.g., 0.1 mg/kg] should be considered only after 1 mg doses have failed)
• *Hypotension:* IV INF 1-4 μg/min
• *Anaphylactic reaction:* IM/SC 0.2-0.5 mg q20 min-4 hr (single dose max 1 mg)
• *Glaucoma:* Ophth 1 gtt qd-bid
• *Nasal congestion:* Intranasal apply prn; do not use for >3-5 days
Child
• *Bronchodilator:* SC 10 μg/kg (0.01 ml/kg of 1:1000), max single dose 0.5 mg; susp (1:200) 0.005 ml/kg/dose (0.025 mg/kg/dose) q6h,

---

* = non-FDA-approved use

max 0.15 ml (0.75 mg)/dose; NEB 0.25-0.5 ml of 2.25% racemic epinephrine solution diluted in 3 ml NS q1-4h

• *Cardiac arrest:* IV/intratracheal 0.01 mg/kg (0.1 ml/kg) of 1:10,000 sol q3-5 min prn, max 5 ml

• *Refractory hypotension:* IV INF 0.1-4 μg/kg/min

• *Anaphylactic reaction:* SC 0.01 mg/kg q15 min for 2 doses then q4h prn, max 0.5 mg/dose

• *Nasal congestion (>6 yr):* Intranasal apply prn

Neonate

• *Cardiac arrest:* IV/intratracheal 0.01-0.03 mg/kg (0.1-0.3 ml/kg) of 1:10,000 sol q3-5 min prn

AVAILABLE FORMS/COST OF THERAPY

• Inj, Sol—IM: 0.15, 0.3 mg/0.3 ml, 1's: **$39.70**

• Inj, Sol—IM, IV, SC: 0.1 mg/ml, 10 ml: **$13.75-$16.47;** 1 mg/ml, 1 ml: **$0.52-$4.22**

• Sol—INH: 1%, 7.5 ml: **$24.88**

• Aer—INH: 0.22 mg/INH, 15 ml: **$6.10-$11.00;** 0.3 mg/INH, 15 ml: **$8.22-$9.35**

• Sol—Ophth: 0.5%, 15 ml: **$37.50**

• Sol—Ophth, Top: 1%, 15 ml: **$40.20**

• Sol—Ophth, Top: 2%, 15 ml: **$43.99**

• Sol—Nasal: 1 mg/ml, 30 ml: **$11.45**

CONTRAINDICATIONS: Cardiac dysrhythmias, angle-closure glaucoma, local anesthesia of fingers and toes, general anesthesia with halogenated hydrocarbons or cyclopropane, organic brain damage, labor, coronary insufficiency

PRECAUTIONS: Elderly, cardiovascular disease, hypertension, diabetes, hyperthyroidism, psychoneurotic individuals, thyrotoxicosis, parkinsonism

PREGNANCY AND LACTATION: Pregnancy category C; excreted into breast milk; use caution in nursing mothers

SIDE EFFECTS/ADVERSE REACTIONS

CNS: Anxiety, dizziness, fear, headache, hemiplegia, restlessness, ***subarachnoid hemorrhage,*** *tremor,* weakness

CV: Anginal pain, ***dysrhythmias,*** hypertension, palpitations

GI: Nausea, vomiting

GU: Urinary retention

RESP: Respiratory difficulty

SKIN: Hemorrhage at inj site, pallor, urticaria, wheal

INTERACTIONS

Drugs

3 β-*blockers:* Noncardioselective β-blockers enhance pressor response to epinephrine resulting in hypertension and bradycardia

3 *Chlorpromazine, clozaril, thioridazine:* Reversal of epinephrine pressor response

2 *Cyclic antidepressants:* Pressor response to IV epinephrine markedly enhanced

SPECIAL CONSIDERATIONS
PATIENT/FAMILY EDUCATION

• Do not exceed recommended doses

• Wait at least 3-5 min between inhalations with MDI

• Notify clinician of dizziness or chest pain

• Do not use nasal preparations for >3-5 days to prevent rebound congestion

• To avoid contamination of ophth preparations, do not touch tip of container to any surface

• Do not use ophth preparations while wearing soft contact lenses

• Transitory stinging may occur on instillation of ophth preparations

---

italic = common side effects   ***bold italic*** = life-threatening reactions

- Report any decrease in visual acuity immediately

MONITORING PARAMETERS
- Blood pressure, heart rate
- Intraocular pressure

---

epoprostenol (prostacyclin)
(e-poe-pros´ten-ol)
Rx: Flolan
Chemical Class: Prostaglandin PGI_2
Therapeutic Class: Vasodilator

CLINICAL PHARMACOLOGY
Mechanism of Action: Direct vasodilator of pulmonary and systemic arterial vascular beds; reduces right and left ventricular afterload, increases cardiac output and stroke volume, decreases pulmonary vascular resistance and mean systemic arterial pressure, inhibits platelet aggregation; may also induce bronchodilation, inhibit gastric acid secretion, and decrease gastric emptying

Pharmacokinetics
IV INF: Steady state reached in 15 min; extensively hydrolyzed in blood, some metabolites have pharmacological activity; excreted (82%) in urine; $t_{1/2}$ 6 min

INDICATIONS AND USES: Long-term IV treatment of primary pulmonary hypertension in New York Heart Association Class III and Class IV patients

DOSAGE
Adult
- IV INF, acute: 2 ng/kg/min, increase by 2 ng/kg/min q15 min until limited by adverse effects, mean maximum-tolerated dose in trials was 8.6 ± 0.3 ng/kg/min
- IV INF, chronic: Initiate at 4 ng/kg/min less than maximum-tolerated rate or at ½ maximum-tolerated rate if maximum rate <5 ng/kg/min; increases in rate can be made by 1-2 ng/kg/min q 15 min, decreases by 2 ng/kg/min q 15 min

AVAILABLE FORMS/COST OF THERAPY
- Inj, dry sol—IV: 0.5 mg/vial: **$17.40**; 1.5 mg/vial: **$34.81**

CONTRAINDICATIONS: CHF secondary to severe left ventricular systolic dysfunction, patients unable to commit to administration and care of indwelling central venous catheter

PRECAUTIONS: Elderly, concurrent vasodilator use

PREGNANCY AND LACTATION: Pregnancy category B; unknown if excreted in breast milk

SIDE EFFECTS/ADVERSE REACTIONS:
CNS: Agitation, anxiety, headache (49%), hyperesthesia, hypoesthesia, nervousness, paresthesia, tremor
CV: Bradycardia (5%), chest pain (11%), dizziness (8%), flushing (58%), hypotension (16%), syncope, tachycardia
GI: Abdominal pain, diarrhea, dyspepsia, nausea/vomiting (32%)
MS: Back pain, jaw pain, musculoskeletal pain, myalgia
RESP: Dyspnea
MISC: Chills, fever, flu-like syndrome, sweating

SPECIAL CONSIDERATIONS
- Clinically shown to improve exercise capacity, dyspnea, and fatigue as early as 1st week of therapy
- Drug is administered chronically on an ambulatory basis with a portable infusion pump through a permanent central venous catheter; peripheral IV infusions may be used temporarily until central venous access obtained

---

* = non-FDA-approved use

- Patients must be taught sterile technique, drug reconstitution, and care of catheter
- Do not interrupt infusion or decrease rate abruptly, may cause rebound symptoms (dyspnea, dizziness, asthenia, death)
- Unless contraindicated, patients should be anticoagulated to reduce risk of pulmonary thromboembolism or systemic embolism through a patent foramen ovale

MONITORING PARAMETERS
- Postural BP and heart rate for several hr following dosage adjustments

---

eprosartan
(eh-pro-sar'tan)
Rx: Teveten
Chemical Class: Angiotensin II receptor antagonist
Therapeutic Class: Antihypertensive

CLINICAL PHARMACOLOGY
Mechanism of Action: Antihypertensive (inhibition of vasoconstrictor and aldosterone secretion), smooth muscle hypoproliferative, and cardioprotective effects are attributable to selective blockade of angiotensin II (AT1) receptors found throughout the cardiovascular and renal systems; effects independent of angiotension II synthesis
Pharmacokinetics
PO: Peak 4 hr (range 2-6 hr)
PO bioavailability, 13%, possibly delayed or enhanced by concurrent food; 98% protein bound, 20% metabolized by liver (no active metabolites), 70% excreted in feces, 7% in urine; elimination $t_{1/2}$ 5-9 hr
INDICATIONS AND USES: Hypertension, congestive heart failure (left

ventricular dysfunction),* chronic renal failure,* diabetic nephropathy*
DOSAGE
Adult and Child >16 yr
- Initially, 400 mg qd or 200 mg bid, with titration to 800 mg per day (36%-50% response in reaching goal reductions in sitting diastolic blood pressure)
Dosage in Renal Failure
Dose reduction necessary; peak plasma levels approximately 50% higher in moderate to severe renal failure

AVAILABLE FORMS/COST OF THERAPY
- Tab—Oral: 400 mg, 100's: **$94.00;** 600 mg, 100's: **$125.00**

PRECAUTIONS: Angioedema (associated with aspirin and/or penicillin allergy), aortic or mitral valve stenosis, biliary cirrhosis or biliary obstruction, breast feeding period, coronary artery disease, elderly patients, hepatic dysfunction (adjust dose), hypertrophic cardiomyopathy, hypotension (sodium- or volume-depleted patients), pregnancy, renal artery stenosis, solitary kidney, or congestive heart failure
PREGNANCY AND LACTATION: Pregnancy category C, first trimester—category D, second and third trimesters; drugs acting directly on the renin-angiotensin-aldosterone system are documented to cause fetal harm (hypotension, oligohydramnios, neonatal anemia, hyperkalemia, neonatal skull hypoplasia, anuria, and renal failure; neonatal limb contractures, craniofacial deformities, and hypoplastic lung development)
SIDE EFFECTS/ADVERSE REACTIONS
CNS: Dizziness (2.4%), fatigue (1.4%), headache (3.8%)
MS: Myalgia (1.9%)
RESP: Cough (1.8%-6.5%)

---

italic = common side effects   ***bold italic*** = life-threatening reactions

SKIN: Facial edema, angioedema, diaphoresis

MISC: Angioedema

SPECIAL CONSIDERATIONS

• Potentially as or more effective than angiotensin-converting enzyme inhibitors, without cough; no evidence for reduction in morbidity and mortality as first line agents in hypertension, yet; whether they provide the same cardiac and renal protection also still tentative; like ACE inhibitors, less effective in black patients

PATIENT/FAMILY EDUCATION

• Call your clinician immediately if note following side effects: wheezing, lip, throat, or face swelling; hives or rash

MONITORING PARAMETERS

• Baseline electrolytes, urinalysis, blood urea nitrogen and creatinine with recheck at 2-4 wk after initiation (sooner in volume-depleted patients); monitor sitting blood pressure; watch for symptomatic hypotension, particulary in volume-depleted patients

---

eptifibatide

(ep-tih-fib'ah-tide)

Rx: Integrilin

Chemical Class: Glycoprotein (GP) IIb/IIIa inhibitor

Therapeutic Class: Antiplatelet agent

CLINICAL PHARMACOLOGY

Mechanism of Action: Reversibly prevents fibrinogen, von Willebrand's factor, and other adhesion ligands from binding to platelet GP IIb/IIIa receptors, thereby inhibiting platelet aggregation

Pharmacokinetics

Steady state achieved within 4-6 hr; 25% bound in human plasma; 50% cleared by renal excretion; t½ 2.5 hr

INDICATIONS AND USES: Acute coronary syndromes (unstable angina and non Q-wave MI), including patients who are to be managed medically and those undergoing percutaneous coronary intervention (PCI)

DOSAGE

Adult

• Acute coronary syndrome: IV bolus of 180 mcg/kg as soon as possible following diagnosis, followed by a continuous INF of 2 mcg/kg/min until hospital discharge or initiation of CABG surgery, up to 72 hr; if patient is to undergo PCI during INF, consider decreasing INF rate to 0.5 mcg/kg/min at the time of procedure, continue INF additional 20-24 hr after procedure, allowing up to 96 hr of therapy; patients weighing >121 kg have received max bolus of 22.6 mg followed by max INF rate of 15 mg/hr

• Nonemergent PCI: IV bolus of 135 mcg/kg immediately prior to procedure, followed by continuous INF of 0.5 mcg/kg/min for 20-24 hr

$ AVAILABLE FORMS/COST OF THERAPY

• Inj, Sol—IV: 0.75 mg/ml, 100 ml: **$157.50**; 2 mg/ml, 10 ml: **$50.40**

CONTRAINDICATIONS: Active internal bleeding or history of bleeding diathesis within previous 30 days; history of stroke within 30 days; history of hemorrhagic stroke; major surgical procedure or severe physical trauma within previous month; systolic blood pressure >200 mm Hg or diastolic blood pressure >110 mm Hg; history of intracranial hemorrhage, intracranial neoplasm, arteriovenous malformation or aneurysm; history, symptoms or findings of aortic dissection, acute pericarditis; platelet count <100,000/mm^3, serum creatinine ≥2 mg/dL (for the 180 mcg/kg bolus and the

---

2 mcg/kg/min INF) or ≥4 mg/dL (for the 135 mcg/kg bolus and the 0.5 mcg/kg/min INF), dependency on renal dialysis

PRECAUTIONS: Platelet count <150,000/mm^3; hemorrhagic retinopathy; IM injections, urinary catheters, nasotracheal intubation, nasogastric tubes; elderly

PREGNANCY AND LACTATION: Pregnancy category B; use caution in nursing mothers

SIDE EFFECTS/ADVERSE REACTIONS

CV: Hypotension

HEME: **Bleeding** (major bleeding 4.4%-10.8%, minor bleeding 10.5%-14.2%)

INTERACTIONS

Drugs

3 *Antithrombotics (aspirin, heparin, warfarin, ticlopidine, clopidogrel):* Increased risk of bleeding

SPECIAL CONSIDERATIONS

• When bleeding cannot be controlled with pressure, discontinue INF

• Most major bleeding occurs at arterial access site for cardiac catheterization; prior to pulling femoral artery sheath, discontinue heparin for 3-4 hr and document activated clotting time (ACT) <180 sec or aPTT <45 sec; achieve sheath hemostasis ≥4 hr before discharge

• In patients who undergo CABG, discontinue eptifibatide INF prior to surgery

• Eptifibatide, tirofiban, and abciximab can all decrease the incidence of cardiac events associated with acute coronary syndromes; direct comparisons are needed to establish which, if any, is superior; for angioplasty, until more data become available, abciximab appears to be the drug of choice

MONITORING PARAMETERS

• Platelet count, hemoglobin, hematocrit, PT/aPTT (baseline, within 6 hr following bolus dose, then daily thereafter)

• In patients undergoing PCI, also measure ACT; maintain aPTT between 50 and 70 sec unless PCI is to be performed; during PCI, maintain ACT between 300 and 350 sec

E

---

ergocalciferol

(er-goe-kal-sif'e-role)

Rx: Calciferol, Drisdol, Deltalin

OTC: Calciferol Drops, Drisdol Drops

Chemical Class: Sterol derivative

Therapeutic Class: Vitamin D analog

CLINICAL PHARMACOLOGY

Mechanism of Action: Regulates calcium homeostasis; promotes active absorption of calcium and phosphorus by the small intestine; increases rate of accretion and resorption of bone minerals; promotes resorption of phosphate by renal tubules; also involved in magnesium metabolism

Pharmacokinetics

PO: Peak effect in approximately 1 mo following daily dosing, readily absorbed from GI tract, absorption requires intestinal presence of bile; inactive until hydroxylated in the liver and kidney to calcifediol and then to calcitriol (most active form)

INDICATIONS AND USES: Refractory rickets, osteoporosis, familial hypophosphatemia and hypoparathyroidism

DOSAGE

Adult

• *Dietary supplementation* (including prevention of osteoporosis): PO 400-800 IU qd

---

italic = common side effects   ***bold italic*** = life-threatening reactions

• *Hypoparathyroidism:* PO 25,000-200,000 IU qd (with calcium supplements)

• *Refractory rickets:* PO 12,000-500,000 IU qd (with phosphate supplements)

• *Familial hypophosphatemia:* PO 10,000-80,000 IU qd (with 1-2 g/day elemental phosphorus)

• IM therapy reserved for patients with GI, liver, or biliary disease associated with vitamin D malabsorption

Child

• *Dietary supplementation:* PO 400 IU qd

• *Hypoparathyroidism:* PO 50,000-200,000 IU qd (with calcium supplements)

• *Refractory rickets:* PO 400,000-800,000 IU qd (with phosphate supplements)

$ AVAILABLE FORMS/COST OF THERAPY

• Sol—Oral: 8,000 IU/ml, 60 ml: **$20.59** (OTC)

• Cap, Elastic—Oral: 50,000 IU, 100's: **$5.78-$102.44**

• Tab, Plain Coated—Oral: 50,000 IU, 100's: **$5.99-$46.95**

• Inj, Sol—IM: 50,000 IU/ml, 1 ml: **$19.67**

CONTRAINDICATIONS: Hypercalcemia, malabsorption syndrome, hypervitaminosis D, decreased renal function

PRECAUTIONS: Renal stones, coronary disease, arteriosclerosis, elderly

PREGNANCY AND LACTATION: Pregnancy category A (category D if used in doses above the recommended daily allowance); excreted into breast milk in limited amounts; compatible with breast feeding, however, serum calcium levels of the infant should be monitored if mother is receiving pharmacologic doses

SIDE EFFECTS/ADVERSE REACTIONS

CNS: Anorexia, headache, hyperthermia, irritability, overt psychosis, somnolence

CV: **Dysrhythmia,** generalized vascular calcification, hypertension

EENT: Conjunctivitis (calcific), rhinorrhea

GI: Constipation, dry mouth, elevated AST and ALT, metallic taste, nausea, **pancreatitis,** polydipsia, vomiting

GU: Albuminuria, decreased libido, elevated BUN, nephrocalcinosis, nocturia, polyuria, reversible azotemia

METAB: Hypercholesterolemia, mild acidosis

MS: Bone pain, muscle pain, weakness

SKIN: Photophobia, pruritis

MISC: Weight loss

SPECIAL CONSIDERATIONS
MONITORING PARAMETERS

The following monitoring suggestions are recommended for pharmacologic dosing, not dietary supplementation

• Serum and urinary calcium, phosphorus, and BUN

• X-ray bones monthly until condition is corrected and stabilized

• Ensure adequate calcium intake; maintain serum calcium concentration between 9-10 mg/dl

• Periodically determine magnesium and alk phosphatase

• 24 hr urinary calcium and phosphate (hypoparathyroid patients)

• Serum calcium times phosphorus should not exceed 70 mg/dl to avoid ectopic calcification

ergoloid mesylates

(er'goe-loid)
Rx: Gerimal, Hydergine
Chemical Class: Ergot alkaloid
Therapeutic Class: Cerebral metabolic enhancer

CLINICAL PHARMACOLOGY
Mechanism of Action: May increase brain metabolism, possibly increasing cerebral blood flow
Pharmacokinetics
PO: Rapidly absorbed, peak 0.6-3 hr; extensive 1st-pass metabolism by the liver; $t_{1/2}$ 2.6-5.1 hr
INDICATIONS AND USES: Age-related mental capacity decline
DOSAGE
Adult
• PO 1 mg tid initially, increase to 4.5-12 mg/day in divided doses
§ AVAILABLE FORMS/COST OF THERAPY
• Tab—SL: 1 mg, 100's: **$16.45**
• Tab, Uncoated—Oral: 1 mg, 100's: **$21.40-$88.35**
• Cap, Elastic—Oral: 1 mg, 100's: **$92.97**
• Liq—Oral: 1 mg/ml, 100 ml: **$72.72**
CONTRAINDICATIONS: Acute or chronic psychosis
PRECAUTIONS: Acute intermittent porphyria
SIDE EFFECTS/ADVERSE REACTIONS
GI: Nausea, sublingual irritation, vomiting
SPECIAL CONSIDERATIONS
PATIENT/FAMILY EDUCATION
• Results may not be observed for 3-4 wk
• May cause transient GI disturbances; allow sublingual tablets to completely dissolve under tongue; do not chew or crush sublingual tablets
MONITORING PARAMETERS
• Before prescribing, exclude the possibility that the patient's signs and symptoms arise from a potentially reversible and treatable condition
• Periodically reassess the diagnosis and the benefit of current therapy to the patient; discontinue if no benefit

ergonovine

(er-gone-o'veen)
Rx: Ergotrate Maleate
Chemical Class: Ergot alkaloid
Therapeutic Class: Oxytocic

CLINICAL PHARMACOLOGY
Mechanism of Action: Partial agonist or antagonist at α-adrenergic, dopaminergic, and tryptaminergic receptors; increases the strength, duration, and frequency of uterine contractions and decreases uterine bleeding when used after placental delivery
Pharmacokinetics
IM: Onset 7-8 min, duration 45 min
IV: Onset 40 sec, duration 3 hr
Principally eliminated by nonrenal mechanisms (metabolism in liver, excretion in feces); $t_{1/2}$ ½-2 hr
INDICATIONS AND USES: Postpartum/postabortal hemorrhage due to uterine atony; adjunct to coronary arteriography to diagnose coronary artery spasm*; migraine headache*
DOSAGE
Adult
• IM/IV 0.2 mg, severe uterine bleeding may require repeated doses, but rarely more than 0.2 mg per 2-4

---

italic = common side effects   ***bold italic*** = life-threatening reactions

hr (confine IV route to emergencies)

💲 AVAILABLE FORMS/COST OF THERAPY

• Inj, Sol—IV: 0.2 mg/ml, 1 ml: **$4.75**

CONTRAINDICATIONS: Augmentation of labor; administration before delivery of placenta; threatened spontaneous abortion

PRECAUTIONS: Calcium deficiency, prolonged use, hypertension, heart disease, venoarterial shunts, mitral valve stenosis, obliterative vascular disease, sepsis, hepatic or renal impairment

PREGNANCY AND LACTATION: Not recommended for routine use prior to delivery of the placenta; may lower prolactin levels, which may decrease lactation

SIDE EFFECTS/ADVERSE REACTIONS

CNS: Dizziness, fainting, headache
CV: Chest pain, hypertension, *MI*
EENT: Tinnitus
GI: Nausea, vomiting
GU: Cramping
RESP: Dyspnea
SKIN: Sweating

INTERACTIONS

Drugs

3 *Dopamine:* Excessive vasoconstriction

SPECIAL CONSIDERATIONS

• Symptoms of ergotism occur with overdosage (nausea, vomiting, diarrhea, seizure, hallucinations delirium, numb/gangrenous extremities)

MONITORING PARAMETERS

• Blood pressure, pulse, and uterine response

---

ergotamine
(er-got′a-meen)
Rx: Ergomar
Combinations
  Rx: with caffeine (Cafergot, Ercaf, Wigraine); with belladonna alkaloids, phenobarbital (Bellergal-S)
Chemical Class: Ergot alkaloid
Therapeutic Class: Antimigraine agent

CLINICAL PHARMACOLOGY

Mechanism of Action: Partial agonist and/or antagonist activity against tryptaminergic, dopaminergic, and α-adrenergic receptors depending upon their site; uterine stimulant; causes constriction of peripheral and cranial blood vessels

Pharmacokinetics

PO: Peak 2 hr; metabolized in liver, excreted as metabolites in bile; plasma $t_{1/2}$ 2 hr

INDICATIONS AND USES: Abortive therapy for vascular headaches including migraine and cluster headaches

DOSAGE

Adult

• PO, SL or PR 2 mg stat, then 1-2 mg q½h prn until relief, not to exceed 6 mg/day or 10 mg/wk; PR 1 supp stat, then ½ supp q1h prn until relief, not to exceed 2 mg per attack

Older Child and Adolescent

• PO or SL 1 mg stat, then 1 mg q½h prn until relief, not to exceed 3 mg/attack

💲 AVAILABLE FORMS/COST OF THERAPY

• Supp—PR: (caffeine/ergotamine) 100 mg/2 mg, 100's: **$729.84**
• Tab—Oral: 2 mg, 100's: **$442.25**
• Tab—Oral: (caffeine/ergotamine) 100 mg/1 mg, 100's: **$66.26-$73.70**

---

* = non-FDA-approved use

CONTRAINDICATIONS: Pregnancy (or women at risk for pregnancy), peripheral vascular disease, hepatic or renal impairment, CAD, uncontrolled hypertension, sepsis

PRECAUTIONS: Prolonged administration, excessive dosage

PREGNANCY AND LACTATION: Pregnancy category X; excreted into breast milk; has caused symptoms of ergotism (e.g., vomiting, diarrhea) in the infant; excessive dosage or prolonged administration may inhibit lactation

SIDE EFFECTS/ADVERSE REACTIONS

CV: Chest pain, coronary vasoconstriction (large doses), increase or decrease in blood pressure, transient tachycardia or bradycardia

GI: Nausea, vomiting

MISC: Itching, localized edema, muscle pain in extremities, numbness and tingling of fingers and toes, weakness in legs

INTERACTIONS

Drugs

❷ *Azithromycin, dirithromycin, erythromycin:* Coadministration may result in ergotism

❷ *Nitroglycerin:* Decreased antianginal effects of nitroglycerin

SPECIAL CONSIDERATIONS

PATIENT/FAMILY EDUCATION

• Initiate therapy at 1st sign of attack

• DO NOT exceed recommended dosage

• Notify clinician of irregular heart beat, nausea, vomiting, numbness or tingling of fingers or toes, pain or weakness of extremities

• Regular use may lead to withdrawal headaches

---

erythromycin

(er-ith-roe-mye′sin)

Systemic: **Rx:** E-Mycin, Eryc, Ery-Tab, PCE Dispertab, Ilosone, E.E.S., Eryped, Ilotycin

Topical: **Rx:** A/T/S, Akne-Mycin, C-Solve 2, Emgel, Erycette, Eryderm, Erygel, Erymax, E-Solve 2, ETS-2%, Staticin, Theramycin Z, T-Stat

Ophth: **Rx:** AK-Mycin, Ilotycin

Combinations

Rx: with sulfisoxazole (Pediazole); with benzoyl peroxide (Benzamycin)

Chemical Class: Macrolide derivative

Therapeutic Class: Antibiotic

CLINICAL PHARMACOLOGY

Mechanism of Action: Binds to 50S ribosomal subunits of susceptible bacteria and suppresses protein synthesis

Pharmacokinetics

PO: Peak 4 hr, duration 6 hr; 70% bound to plasma proteins; $t_{1/2}$ 1-3 hr; metabolized in liver, excreted in bile, feces

INDICATIONS AND USES: Systemic: treatment of infections caused by susceptible strains of the designated microorganisms; upper and lower respiratory tract infections caused by *Streptococcus pyogenes* and *Str. pneumoniae;* respiratory tract infections due to *Mycoplasma pneumoniae;* pertussis (whooping cough) caused by *Bordatella pertussis;* diphtheria, as an adjunct to antitoxin in infections due to *Corynebacterium diphtheriae;* erythrasma due to *Corynebacterium minutissimum;* intestinal amebiasis caused by *Entamoeba histolytica* (PO only); acute pelvic inflamma-

---

tory disease caused by *Neisseria gonorrhoeae;* infections due to *Listeria monocytogenes;* skin and soft tissue infections caused by *Str. pyogenes* and *Staphylococcus aureus;* infections caused by *Chlamydia trachomatis* (conjunctivitis of the newborn, pneumonia of infancy, urogenital infections during pregnancy, uncomplicated urethral, endocervical, or rectal infections in adults); nongonococcal urethritis caused by *Ureaplasma urealyticum;* Legionnaires' disease caused by *Legionella pneumophila;* prevention of initial/recurrent attacks of rheumatic fever; prevention of bacterial endocarditis

Topical: acne vulgaris

Ophthalmic: superficial ocular infections involving the conjunctiva or cornea; prophylaxis of ophthalmia neonatorum due to *Neisseria gonorrhoeae* or *Chlamydia trachomatis*

Systemic: diabetic gastroparesis*; as an alternative to penicillins in anthrax*; Vincent's gingivitis*; actinomycosis*; *Nocardia* infections (with a sulfonamide)*; *Eikenella corrodens* infections*; *Borrelia* infections (including early Lyme disease)*; campylobacter enteritis*; *Lymphogranuloma venereum*; chancroid*

DOSAGE

Adult

• PO base 333 mg q8h; estolate, stearate, or base 250-500 mg q6-12h; ethyl succinate 400-800 mg q6-12h; IV 15-20 mg/kg/day divided q6h; TOP apply to affected area bid; OPHTH apply ¼ in ribbon of ointment qd-qid as needed

• *Endocarditis prophylaxis:* PO ethyl succinate 800 mg 1 hr prior to procedure and 400 mg 6 hr after

Child

• PO base, ethyl succinate 30-50 mg/kg/day divided q6-8h; estolate: 30-50 mg/kg/day divided q8-12h; stearate 20-40 mg/kg/day divided q6h; IV lactobionate 20-40 mg/kg/day divided q6h, do not exceed 4 g/day; gluceptate: 20-50 mg/kg/day divided q6h; TOP apply to affected area bid; OPHTH apply ¼ in ribbon of ointment qd-qid as needed

$ **AVAILABLE FORMS/COST OF THERAPY**

• Oint—Ophth: 5 mg/g, 3.5 g: **$2.25-$5.58**

• Gel—Top: 2%, 5, 30, 50, 60 g: **$16.48-$26.20/30 g**

• Sol—Top: 1.5%, 60 ml: **$5.25-$24.29;** 2%, 60, 120 ml: **$3.42-$20.96/60 ml**

• Swab, Medicated—Top: 2%, 60's: **$16.93-$23.00**

• Oint—Top: 2%, 25 g: **$19.94**

• Cap, Gel, SUS Action (base)—Oral: 250 mg, 100's: **$17.93-$46.81**

• Cap, Gel (estolate)—Oral: 250 mg, 100's: **$22.92-$56.91**

• Tab, Chewable (ethyl succinate)—Oral: 200 mg, 40's: **$21.02**

• Tab, Plain Coated (base)—Oral: 250 mg, 100's: **$13.95-$16.33;** 333 mg, 60's: **$83.38;** 500 mg, 100's: **$25.60-$164.33**

• Tab, Plain Coated (stearate)—Oral: 250 mg, 100's: **$9.00-$18.16;** 500 mg, 100's: **$24.18-$40.84**

• Tab, Plain Coated (ethyl succinate)—Oral: 400 mg, 100's: **$20.75-$27.75**

• Tab, Coated (estolate)—Oral: 500 mg, 50's: **$49.56**

• Tab, Enteric Coated, SUS Action (base)—Oral: 250 mg, 100's: **$24.44-$30.65;** 333 mg, 100's: **$31.04-$50.85;** 500 mg, 100's: **$41.27**

• Susp (estolate)—Oral: 125 mg/5 ml, 480 ml: **$23.90-$31.95;** 250 mg/5 ml: 480 ml: **$35.00-$84.58**

• Susp (ethyl succinate)—Oral: 200 mg/5 ml, 100, 480 ml: **$12.14-**

$23.50/480 ml; 400 mg/5 ml, 100, 480 ml: **$20.92-$42.50**/480 ml

• Powder, Granules, Reconst (ethyl succinate)—Oral: 200 mg/5 ml, 100, 200 ml: **$14.08-$16.30**/200 ml; 400 mg/5 ml, 100, 200 ml: **$23.14**/200 ml

• Drops (ethyl succinate)—Oral: 200 mg/5 ml, 50 ml: **$6.65**

• Inj, Lyphl-Sol (lactobionate)—IV: 500 mg/vial, 1's: **$6.25-$11.25**; 1 g/vial, 1's: **$11.58-$19.89**

• Inj, Dry Sol (gluceptate)—IV: 1 g/ampule, 50 ml: **$25.07**

CONTRAINDICATIONS: Systemic: pre-existing liver disease (estolate); ophthalmic: epithelial herpes simplex keratitis; vaccinia, varicella, mycobacterial, fungal infections

PRECAUTIONS: Systemic: hepatic disease, prolonged or repeated therapy; ophthalmic: antibiotic hypersensitivity; topical: child <12 yr

PREGNANCY AND LACTATION: Pregnancy category B; excreted into breast milk; compatible with breast feeding

SIDE EFFECTS/ADVERSE REACTIONS

CV: ***Ventricular dysrhythmias*** (rare)
EENT: Hearing loss, overgrowth of nonsusceptible organisms (ophth), poor corneal wound healing, temporary visual haze, tinnitus
GI: Abdominal cramping and discomfort, anorexia, cholestatic hepatitis (most common with estolate), *diarrhea,* heartburn, *nausea,* pruritus ani, stomatitis, *vomiting*
GU: Moniliasis, vaginitis
SKIN: Pruritus, rash, thrombophlebitis, urticaria (IV site), burning; dry, scaly, oily skin; pruritus, rash, stinging; urticaria (top)

INTERACTIONS
Drugs
🅱 *Alfentanil:* Prolonged anesthesia and respiratory depression

🅱 *Alprazolam:* Increased plasma alprazolam concentration

🅱 *Amprenavir:* Plasma concentrations of erythromycin may be increased by amprenavir; plasma concentrations of amprenavir may be increased by erythromycin

🅰 *Astemizole:* QT prolongation and life-threatening dysrhythmia

🅱 *Atorvastatin:* Increased plasma atorvastatin concentration with risk of rhabdomyolysis

🅱 *Bromocriptine:* Increased bromocriptine concentration with toxicity

🅱 *Buspirone:* Increased plasma buspirone concentration

🅱 *Carbamazepine:* Markedly increased plasma carbamazepine concentrations

❷ *Cisapride:* QT prolongation and dysrhythmia

❷ *Clozapine:* Increased plasma clozapine concentrations

🅱 *Colchicine:* Potential colchicine toxicity

🅱 *Cyclosporine:* Increased plasma cyclosporine concentrations

🅱 *Diazepam:* Increased plasma concentration of diazepam

🅱 *Digoxin:* Reduced bacterial flora may increase plasma digoxin concentrations

🅱 *Disopyramide:* Increased plasma disopyramide concentrations

❷ *Ergotamine:* Potential for ergotism

🅱 *Ethanol:* Ethanol reduces plasma erythromycin concentration

🅱 *Felodipine:* Increased plasma felodipine concentrations

🅱 *Food:* Food may increase or decrease the bioavailability of erythromycin

🅱 *Indinavir:* Plasma concentrations of erythromycin may be increased by indinavir; plasma concentrations of indinavir may be increased by erythromycin

🔳 *Itraconazole:* Increased plasma itraconazole concentration

🔳 *Lovastatin:* Increased plasma lovastatin concentration with risk of rhabdomyolysis

🔳 *Methylprednisolone:* Increased plasma methylprednisolone concentrations

🔳 *Midazolam:* Increased plasma concentration of midazolam

🔳 *Nelfinavir:* Plasma concentrations of erythromycin may be increased by nelfinavir; plasma concentrations of nelfinavir may be increased by erythromycin

🔳 *Penicillin:* Decreased activity of penicillin

🔳 *Quinidine:* Increased plasma concentration of quinidine

🔳 *Ritonavir:* Plasma concentrations of erythromycin may be increased by ritonavir; plasma concentrations of ritonavir may be increased by erythromycin

🔳 *Saquinavir:* Plasma concentrations of erythromycin may be increased by saquinavir; plasma concentrations of saquinavir may be increased by erythromycin

🔳 *Sildenafil:* Increased plasma sildenafil concentration

2️⃣ *Simvastatin:* Increased plasma simvastatin concentration with risk of rhabdomyolysis

🔳 *Tacrolimus:* Increased plasma tacrolimus concentration

⚠ *Terfenadine:* QT prolongation and life-threatening dysrhythmia

🔳 *Theophylline:* Increased plasma theophylline concentration

🔳 *Triazolam:* Increased plasma triazolam concentration

🔳 *Valproic acid:* Increased plasma valproic acid concentration

🔳 *Warfarin:* Markedly increased hypoprothrombinemic response to warfarin

🔳 *Zafirlukast:* Reduced plasma zafirlukast concentration probably by reducing bioavailability

🔳 *Zopiclone:* Increased plasma zopiclone concentration

Labs
- *False decrease:* Folate assay
- *False increase:* Urine 17-ketosteroids, AST, urine amino acids

SPECIAL CONSIDERATIONS
PATIENT/FAMILY EDUCATION
- Take with food to minimize GI discomfort
- Take each dose with 180-240 ml of water
- Wash, rinse, and dry affected area prior to top application
- Keep top preparations away from eyes, nose, and mouth
- Ophth ointments may cause temporary blurring of vision following administration

MONITORING PARAMETERS
- LFTs if hepatotoxicity suspected
- Check daily for vein irritation and phlebitis in patients receiving IV forms

---

erythropoietin (epoetin alfa)
(er-ith-row-poe'ee-tin)
Rx: Epogen, Procrit
Chemical Class: Amino acid glycoprotein
Therapeutic Class: Hematopoietic agent

CLINICAL PHARMACOLOGY
Mechanism of Action: Induces red blood cell production by stimulating the division and differentiation of committed erythroid progenitor cells; induces release of reticulocytes from bone marrow into the bloodstream, where they mature to erythrocytes

Pharmacokinetics
SC: Peak 5-24 hr, onset takes several days; elimination poorly under-

stood; some metabolism in liver and bone marrow, 10% excreted unchanged in urine; $t_{1/2}$ 4-13 hr in patients with chronic renal failure (20% shorter in patients with normal renal function)

INDICATIONS AND USES: Anemia in patients with chronic renal failure; anemia related to zidovudine therapy in HIV-infected patients; anemia in cancer patients on chemotherapy and other patients requiring elective surgery (attempt to reduce the need for blood transfusions); anemia of prematurity*; pruritus associated with renal failure*

DOSAGE

Adult

• *Chronic renal failure:* IV (dialysis patients)/IV or SC (non-dialysis chronic renal failure patients) 50-100 U/kg 3 times/wk initially; increase dose if hct increases by <5-6 points after 8 wk and is below target range; decrease dose when target hct is reached or hct increases >4 points in any 2 wk period; maintenance dose should be individualized, but is generally about 25 U/kg 3 times/wk

• *Zidovudine-treated HIV-infected patients:* IV/SC 100 U/kg 3 times/wk initially; after 8 wk adjust dose by 50-100 U/kg to a max of 300 U/kg 3 times/wk

• *Cancer patients on chemotherapy:* SC 150 U/kg 3 times/wk initially; after 8 wk adjust dose by 50-100 U/kg to a max of 300 U/kg 3 times/wk

• *Prior to elective surgery:* SC 300 U/kg/d for 10 days prior to surgery, the day of surgery and for 4 days after surgery

Neonate

• *Anemia of prematurity:* SC 150-250 U/kg 3 times/wk

💲 AVAILABLE FORMS/COST OF THERAPY

• Inj, Sol—IV, SC: 2000 U/ml, 1 ml: **$24.00;** 3000 U/ml, 1 ml: **$36.00;** 4000 U/ml, 1 ml: **$48.00;** 10,000 U/ml, 1 ml: **$120.00;** 20,000 U/ml, 1 ml: **$240.00-$253.20**

CONTRAINDICATIONS: Uncontrolled hypertension; hypersensitivity to mammalian cell-derived products or to human albumin; use to enhance athletic performance

PRECAUTIONS: Severe anemia, seizure disorder, vascular disease, history of thrombosis, children, porphyria

PREGNANCY AND LACTATION: Pregnancy category C; excretion into breast milk unknown; use caution in nursing mothers

SIDE EFFECTS/ADVERSE REACTIONS

CNS: Headache, **seizures**
CV: Hypertension, tachycardia
GI: Diarrhea, *nausea,* vomiting
HEME: Clotted vascular access
METAB: Hyperkalemia
MS: Arthralgia, myalgia
RESP: Shortness of breath
SKIN: Inj site stinging

SPECIAL CONSIDERATIONS

• Iron supplementation (325 mg bid-tid) should be given during therapy to provide for increased requirements during expansion of red cell mass secondary to marrow stimulation by erythropoietin

• Use prior to elective surgery should be limited to patients with presurgery hemoglobin of >10 but ≤13 g/dl undergoing noncardiac, nonvascular procedures

PATIENT/FAMILY EDUCATION

• Do not shake vials as this may denature the glycoprotein rendering the drug inactive

• Notify clinician if severe headache develops

E

---

italic = common side effects   ***bold italic*** = life-threatening reactions

• Frequent blood tests required to determine optimal dose

MONITORING PARAMETERS

• Hct (target range 30%-33%, max 36%), serum iron, ferritin (keep >100 ng/dl)

• Baseline erythropoietin level (treatment of patients with erythropoietin levels >200 mU/ml is not recommended)

• Blood pressure

• BUN, uric acid, creatinine, phosphorus, potassium on a regular basis

---

esmolol
(ess'moe-lol)

Rx: Brevibloc

Chemical Class: β₁-selective (cardioselective) adrenoceptor blocker

Therapeutic Class: Antidysrhythmic (Class II)

CLINICAL PHARMACOLOGY

Mechanism of Action: Competitive β-adrenergic antagonist; produces negative inotropic and chronotropic responses; slows AV nodal conduction; decreases heart rate; decreases myocardial oxygen consumption; antiarrhythmic effects (class II); reduction in platelet aggregation and blood viscosity; suppression of renin release; inhibition of central sympathetic outflow; decreases presynaptic receptor neurotransmitter release; no intrinsic sympathomimetic or membrane stabilizing activity; low lipid solubility

Pharmacokinetics

IV: Onset very rapid, duration short; 55% bound to plasma proteins; metabolized by hydrolysis of the ester linkage by esterases in the cytosol of red blood cells, excreted via kidneys; $t_{1/2}$ 9 min

INDICATIONS AND USES: Supraventricular arrhythmias (atrial fibrillation, atrial flutter, paroxysmal supraventricular tachycardia), aggressive behavior,* angina pectoris,* anxiety,* hyperthyroidism,* neuroleptic-induced akathisia,* aortic dissection,* cardiac surgery (myocardial protection),* electroconvulsive therapy,* pheochromocytoma,* tetanus,* neuroleptic-induced akathisia, angina pectoris,* anxiety,* postmyocardial infarction*

DOSAGE

Adult and Child >16 yr

• *Acute myocardial ischemia:* IV loading INF 500 µg/kg, followed by 50-150 mcg/kg/min INF

• *Arrhythmias:* IV 50-200 µg/kg/min

Child

• *Arrhythmias:* IV 300 µg/kg/min INF initially; titrate upward in 50-100 µg/kg/min increments every 10 minutes; mean effective doses much higher than adults

⚡ AVAILABLE FORMS/COST OF THERAPY

• Inj, Sol—IV: 10 mg/ml, 10 ml: **$18.03;** 250 mg/ml, 10 ml: **$85.21**

CONTRAINDICATIONS: Bronchial asthma, cardiogenic shock, overt cardiac failure, 2nd and 3rd degree AV block, severe sinus bradycardia

PRECAUTIONS: Anesthesia/surgery (myocardial depression), avoid abrupt withdrawal, bronchospastic airways, congestive heart failure, diabetes mellitus, hyperthyroidism/thyrotoxicosis (atenolol, unlike propranolol, does not decrease T_3 levels), concurrent clonidine (discontinue atenolol several days prior to withdrawal of clonidine), peripheral vascular disease, renal disease

PREGNANCY AND LACTATION: Pregnancy category C; potential for hypotension and subsequent decreased uterine blood flow and fetal hypoxia should be considered; ex-

---

* = non-FDA-approved use

cretion into breast milk unknown; use caution in nursing mothers

SIDE EFFECTS/ADVERSE REACTIONS

CNS: Depression, *dizziness,* drowsiness, *fatigue,* hallucinations, insomnia, *lethargy,* memory loss, mental changes, strange dreams

CV: Bradycardia, **CHF,** cold extremities, *hypotension,* **2nd or 3rd degree heart block**

EENT: Dry, burning eyes; sore throat; visual disturbances

GI: Diarrhea, dry mouth, **ischemic colitis, mesenteric arterial thrombosis,** *nausea,* vomiting

GU: Impotence, sexual dysfunction

HEME: **Agranulocytosis, thrombocytopenia**

METAB: Masked hypoglycemic response to insulin (sweating excepted)

RESP: **Bronchospasm,** dyspnea, wheezing

SKIN: Alopecia, pruritis, rash

INTERACTIONS

Drugs

3 *Alpha-1 adrenergic blockers:* Potential enhanced first dose response (marked initial drop in blood pressure, particularly on standing (especially prazocin)

3 *Amiodarone:* Symptomatic bradycardia and sinus arrest; AV node refractory period is prolonged and sinus node automaticity is decreased by amiodarone. The sinus rate can be further slowed or AV block worsened in patients with bradycardia, sick sinus syndrome, or partial AV

3 *Dihydropyridine calcium channel blockers:* Severe hypotension or impaired cardiac performance; most prevalent with impaired left ventricular function, cardiac arrhythmias, or aortic stenosis

3 *Digoxin:* Additive prolongation of atrioventricular (AV) conduction time

3 *Diltiazem:* Potentiates β-adrenergic effects; hypotension, left ventricular failure, and AV conduction disturbances problematic in elderly, patients with left ventricular dysfunction, aortic stenosis, or with large doses of either drug

3 *Hypoglycemic agents:* Masked hypoglycemia, hyperglycemia

3 *Verapamil:* Potentiates β-adrenergic effects; hypotension, left ventricular failure, and AV conduction disturbances problematic in elderly, patients with left ventricular dysfunction, aortic stenosis, or with large doses of either drug

SPECIAL CONSIDERATIONS

• Transfer to alternative agent (e.g., propranolol, digoxin, verapamil): ½ hr after 1st dose of alternative agent, reduce esmolol INF rate by 50%; following 2nd dose of alternative agent, monitor patient's response and, if satisfactory control is maintained for the 1st hr, discontinue esmolol INF

MONITORING PARAMETERS

• Angina: Reduction in nitroglycerin usage; frequency, severity, onset, and duration of angina pain; heart rate

• Arrhythmias: Heart rate

• Hypertension: Blood pressure

• Postmyocardial infarction: Left ventricular function, lower resting heart rate

• Toxicity: Blood glucose, bronchospasm, hypotension, bradycardia, depression, confusion, hallucination, sexual dysfunction

PATIENT/FAMILY EDUCATION

• Do not discontinue abruptly; may require taper; rapid withdrawal may produce rebound hypertension or angina

---

italic = common side effects   **bold italic** = life-threatening reactions

estazolam

(ess-ta'zoe-lam)
Rx: ProSom
Chemical Class: Benzodiazepine
Therapeutic Class: Sedative-hypnotic
DEA Class: Schedule IV

CLINICAL PHARMACOLOGY
Mechanism of Action: CNS depressants via facilitation of inhibitory GABA at benzodiazepine receptor sites (BZ_1—associated with sleep; BZ_2—associated with memory, motor, sensory, and cognitive function); effects include muscle relaxation (spinal cord), anticonvulsant activity (brain stem), ataxia (cerebellum), emotional behavior (limbic and cortical areas), and anxiolytic effects (separate from general CNS depression); decreases sleep latency, the number of awakenings, and the time spent in stage 0 (awake) sleep; stage 2 (unequivocal sleep) is increased; in sum, sleep time increased

Pharmacokinetics
PO: Onset 15-45 min, peak 2 hr, duration 7-8 hr; 93% bound to plasma proteins; metabolized by liver, excreted by kidneys (inactive/active metabolites); $t_{1/2}$ 8-28 hr
INDICATIONS AND USES: Insomnia
DOSAGE
Adult
• PO 1-2 mg qhs; 0.5 mg in elderly or debilitated patients
💲 AVAILABLE FORMS/COST OF THERAPY
• Tab, Uncoated—Oral: 1 mg, 100's: **$88.70-$114.33;** 2 mg, 100's: **$98.80-$127.36**
PRECAUTIONS: Renal or hepatic function impairment, elderly, depression, history of drug abuse, abrupt withdrawal, respiratory depression, sleep apnea
PREGNANCY AND LACTATION: Pregnancy category X; may cause fetal damage when administered during pregnancy; excreted into breast milk; may accumulate in breast-fed infants and is therefore not recommended
SIDE EFFECTS/ADVERSE REACTIONS

CNS: Abnormal thinking, agitation, amnesia, anxiety, apathy, *asthenia,* ataxia, decreased libido, decreased reflexes, emotional lability, hangover, hostility, *hypokinesia,* neuritis, *seizures,* sleep disorder, *somnolence,* stupor, twitch
CV: **Dysrhythmia,** syncope
EENT: Ear pain; epistaxis, eye irritation, pain, pharyngitis, photophobia, rhinitis, sinusitis, swelling
GI: Abdominal pain, appetite changes; dyspepsia; enterocolitis, flatulence, gastritis, increased AST, melena, mouth ulceration
GU: Frequent urination, hematuria, menstrual cramps; nocturia, oliguria, penile discharge, urinary hesitancy, urgency; urinary incontinence, vaginal discharge, itching
HEME: **Agranulocytosis**
MS: Back pain, lower extremity pain
RESP: Asthma, cold symptoms, cough, dyspnea, hyperventilation
SKIN: Acne, dry skin, photosensitivity, urticaria
INTERACTIONS
Drugs
3 *Cimetidine:* Increased serum benzodiazepine concentrations
3 *Disulfiram:* May increase benzodiazepine serum concentrations
3 *Erythromycin:* Increased estazolam sedative effects
3 *Ethanol:* Enhanced adverse psychomotor effects of benzodiazepines

3 *Rifampin:* Reduced serum benzodiazepine concentrations

SPECIAL CONSIDERATIONS
PATIENT/FAMILY EDUCATION
• Do not discontinue abruptly after prolonged therapy
• May experience disturbed sleep for the 1st or 2nd night after discontinuing the drug

---

esterified estrogens
Rx: Estratab, Menest
Combinations
  Rx: with methyltestosterone (Estratest, Menogen)
Chemical Class: Estrogen derivative
Therapeutic Class: Estrogen; antineoplastic; antiosteoporotic

CLINICAL PHARMACOLOGY
Mechanism of Action: Necessary for adequate functioning of female reproductive system; affects release of pituitary gonadotropins, inhibits ovulation, inhibits bone resorption
Pharmacokinetics
PO: Well absorbed; metabolized and inactivated in the liver, excreted in urine

INDICATIONS AND USES: Symptoms associated with menopause (vasomotor symptoms, atrophic vaginitis, kraurosis vulvae), female hypogonadism, female castration, primary ovarian failure, breast cancer (palliation), prostatic carcinoma (palliation), postpartum breast engorgement,* osteoporosis,* prevention of cardiovascular disease*

DOSAGE
Adult
• *Menopause:* PO 0.3-1.25 mg qd or days 1-25 of mo (combined with progestin in women with intact uterus)
• *Female hypogonadism:* PO 2.5 to 7.5 mg/day in divided doses for 20 days, followed by 10 day rest period, repeat if bleeding does not occur by the end of this period; if bleeding occurs before the end of the 10 day period, begin 2.5-7.5 mg/day in divided doses days 1-20 of mo (administer oral progestin during last 5 days of estrogen cycle)
• *Female castration and primary ovarian failure:* PO 1.25 mg qd, 3 wk on, 1 wk off
• *Prostate cancer (inoperable, progressing):* 1.25-2.5 mg tid
• *Breast cancer (inoperable, progressing):* 10 mg tid for 3 mo or longer

$ AVAILABLE FORMS/COST OF THERAPY
• Tab, Sugar Coated—Oral: 0.3 mg, 100's: **$16.44-$39.19;** 0.625 mg, 100's: **$23.31-$52.72;** 1.25 mg, 100's: **$39.20;** 2.5 mg, 100's: **$73.02**
• Tab—Oral: 0.625 mg/2.5 mg methyltestostane, 100's: **$87.55;** 1.25 mg/2.5 mg methyltestosterone, 100's: **$107.64**

CONTRAINDICATIONS: Breast cancer (except in selected patients being treated for metastatic disease), active thromboembolic disorders, known or suspected estrogen-dependent neoplasia, undiagnosed abnormal genital bleeding

PRECAUTIONS: Hypertension, gallbladder disease, CHF, diabetes mellitus, depression, migraine headache, seizure disorders, hepatic disease, family history of breast or endometrial cancer, history of thromboembolic disorders, uterine fibroids, hyperglyceridemia, hypercalcemia

PREGNANCY AND LACTATION: Pregnancy category X; may decrease quantity and quality of breast milk

---

italic = common side effects   ***bold italic*** = life-threatening reactions

SIDE EFFECTS/ADVERSE REACTIONS

CNS: Depression, migraine headache, emotional lability

*CV: **Arterial thromboembolism, pulmonary embolism, CVA, MI,** hy*pertension, venous thrombosis, edema

EENT: Contact lens intolerance, ***retinal thrombosis***

GI: Nausea and vomiting, gallbladder disease, bloating, benign hepatic tumors, ***mesenteric thrombosis***

GU: Breakthrough bleeding, spotting, amenorrhea, change in cervical secretions, breast enlargement, breast tenderness, ***testicular atrophy, endometrial cancer***

METAB: Hyperglycemia, hypertriglyceridemia, hypercalcemia

SKIN: Melasma

INTERACTIONS

Drugs

🔳 *P450 inducers (e.g., rifampin, barbiturates):* Decreased estrogen levels

🔳 *Corticosteroids:* Increased steroid effect

🔳 *Phenytoin:* Loss of seizure control, decreased estrogen levels

🔳 *Warfarin:* Theoretical increased risk thromboembolism

SPECIAL CONSIDERATIONS

• Progestins recommended in non-hysterectomized women

estradiol

(ess-tra-dye′ole)

Oral: **Rx:** Estrace, Vagifem
Estradiol Cypionate Inj:
Rx: Depo-Estradiol, DepoGen, Estro-Cyp
Estradiol Valerate Inj:
Rx: Delestrogen, Valergen
Transdermal: **Rx:** Estraderm, Climara, Vivelle, E$_2$ III
Vaginal insert: **Rx:** Estring
Combinations
  Rx: with testosterone cypionate (Depo-Testadiol)
  Rx: with testosterone enanthate (Deladumone)
  Rx: Transdermal with norethindrone (CombiPatch)
  Rx: with norgestimate (Ortho-Prefest)
Chemical Class: Estrogen derivative
Therapeutic Class: Estrogen; antineoplastic; antiosteoporotic

CLINICAL PHARMACOLOGY

Mechanism of Action: Necessary for adequate functioning of female reproductive system; affects release of pituitary gonadotropins, inhibits bone resorption

Pharmacokinetics

PO/IM/TRANSDERM: Degraded in liver; excreted in urine; crosses placenta; excreted in breast milk

INDICATIONS AND USES: Symptoms associated with menopause (vasomotor symptoms, atrophic vaginitis, kraurosis vulvae), breast cancer, prostatic cancer, atrophic vaginitis, hypogonadism, castration, primary ovarian failure, prevention of osteoporosis, prevention of cardiovascular disease*

DOSAGE

Adult

• *Menopause/hypogonadism/cas-*

---

* = non-FDA-approved use

tration/ovarian failure: PO 1-2 mg qd 3wk on, 1 wk off or 5 days on, 2 days off; IM 1-5 mg q3-4wk (cypionate); 10-20 mg q4wk (valerate); TRANSDERM 0.05-0.1 mg worn continuously, change once (Climara, E₂III) or twice (Estraderm, Vivelle, CombiPatch) per week; VAG RING insert ring into vagina, change rings q3mo

• *Prostatic cancer:* IM 30 mg q1-2 wk (valerate); PO 1-2 mg tid (oral estradiol)

• *Breast cancer:* PO 10 mg tid for 3 mo or longer

• *Atrophic vaginitis:* Vag cre 2-4 g (marked on applicator) qd for 1-2 wk, then 1 g 1-3 times/wk

§ AVAILABLE FORMS/COST OF THERAPY

• Tab, Uncoated—Oral: 0.5 mg, 100's: **$22.78-$36.52;** 1 mg, 100's: **$31.33-$48.66;** 2 mg, 100's: **$45.74-$49.50**

• Cre—Vag: 0.01%, 42.5 g: **$38.57**

• Insert, CONT REL—Vag: 0.0075 mg/24 hr, 1's: **$69.46**

• Film, CONT REL—Percutaneous: 0.025 mg/24 hr 4's: **$24.25** (Climara) 0.0375 mg/24 hr, 8's: **$22.87** (Vivelle); 0.05 mg/24 hr, 8's: **$23.34** (Vivelle); 8's: **$22.57** (Estraderm); 4's: **$27.98** (Climara); 0.075 mg/24 hr, 8's: **$26.72** (Vivelle); 0.1 mg/24 hr, 8's: **$27.28** (Vivelle); 8's: **$23.88** (Estraderm), 4's: **$26.31** (Climara)

• Film, CONT REL-Percutaneous: .05/.14 norethindrone/24 hr (9 sq cm); 8's: **$26.69;** .05/.25 norethindrone/24 hr (16 sq cm), 8's: **$26.69**

• Inj (Valerate)—IM: 10 mg/ml: **$43.93/5 ml;** 20 mg/ml: **$12.29/10 ml;** 40 mg/ml: **$16.95-$29.95/10 ml**

• Inj (Cypionate)—IM: 5 mg/ml, 5, 10 ml: **$5.50-$14.00/10 ml**

CONTRAINDICATIONS: Breast cancer (except in selected patients being treated for metastatic disease), active thromboembolic disorders, known or suspected estrogen-dependent neoplasia, undiagnosed abnormal genital bleeding

PRECAUTIONS: Hypertension, gallbladder disease, CHF, diabetes mellitus, depression, migraine headache, seizure disorders, hepatic disease, family history of breast or endometrial cancer, history of thromboembolic disorders, uterine fibroids, hypertriglyceridemia, hypercalcemia

PREGNANCY AND LACTATION: Pregnancy category X; may reduce quantity and quality of breast milk

SIDE EFFECTS/ADVERSE REACTIONS

CNS: Depression, migraine headache, emotional lability

*CV: **Arterial thromboembolism, pulmonary embolism, CVA, MI,** hy*pertension, venous thrombosis, edema

EENT: Contact lens intolerance, ***retinal thrombosis***

GI: Nausea and vomiting, gallbladder disease, bloating, benign hepatic tumors, ***mesenteric thrombosis***

GU: Breakthrough bleeding, spotting, amenorrhea, change in cervical secretions, breast enlargement, breast tenderness, ***testicular atrophy, endometrial cancer***

METAB: Hyperglycemia, hypertriglyceridemia, hypercalcemia

SKIN: Melasma

INTERACTIONS

Drugs

3 *P450 inducers* (e.g., rifampin, barbiturates): Decreased estrogen levels

3 *Corticosteroids:* Increased steroid effect

3 *Phenytoin:* Loss of seizure control, decreased estrogen levels

3 *Warfarin:* Theoretical increased risk thromboembolism

---

italic = common side effects   ***bold italic*** = life-threatening reactions

SPECIAL CONSIDERATIONS
• Progestins recommended in non-hysterectomized women. Estring may have minimal systemic absorption

---

estrogens, conjugated

Rx: Premarin, Cenestin

Combinations

   Rx: with medroxyprogesterone (Prempro [daily product]), Premphase [cycled product]; with meprobamate (PMB); with methyltestosterone (Premarin with methyltestosterone)

Chemical Class: Estrogen derivative

Therapeutic Class: Estrogen; antineoplastic; antiosteoporotic

CLINICAL PHARMACOLOGY

Mechanism of Action: Necessary for adequate functioning of female reproductive system; affects release of pituitary gonadotropins, inhibits bone resorption

Pharmacokinetics

PO/IV/IM: Degraded in liver, excreted in urine, crosses placenta, excreted in breast milk

INDICATIONS AND USES: Menopause, breast cancer (inoperable, in postmenopausal women and men), prostatic cancer, dysfunctional uterine bleeding, hypogonadism, castration, primary ovarian failure, atrophic vaginitis, prevention of osteoporosis, prevention of cardiovascular disease*

DOSAGE

Adult

• *Menopause/atrophic vaginitis:* PO 0.3-1.25 mg qd cyclically or continuously, with medroxyprogesterone in women with an intact uterus

• *Atrophic vaginitis:* Vag cre 2-4 g qd cyclically, reduce dosage as tolerated (typically, 2-4 g once or twice weekly for maintenance)

• *Osteoporosis prevention:* PO 0.625 mg qd cyclically or continuously, with medroxyprogesterone in women with an intact uterus

• *Prostatic cancer:* PO 1.25-2.5 mg tid

• *Breast cancer:* PO 10 mg tid for 3 mo or longer

• *Dysfunctional uterine bleeding:* IV/IM 25 mg, repeat in 6-12 hr

• *Castration/primary ovarian failure:* PO 1.25 mg qd cyclically or continuously, with medroxyprogesterone in women with an intact uterus

• *Hypogonadism:* PO 2.5 mg qd-tid cyclically, with medroxyprogesterone in women with an intact uterus

§ AVAILABLE FORMS/COST OF THERAPY

• Cre, Top—Vag: 0.625 mg/g, 42.5 g: **$39.19-$43.66**

• Inj, Lyphl-Sol—IM, IV: 25 mg/5 ml, 5 ml: **$48.64**

• Tab, Sugar Coated—Oral: 0.3 mg, 100's: **$25.48;** 0.625 mg, 100's: **$39.45;** 0.9 mg, 100's: **$46.73-$64.05;** 1.25 mg, 100's: **$53.98-$73.99;** 2.5 mg, 100's: **$126.01**

Combination Products

• Tab, Uncoated—Oral: 0.625 mg/2.5 mg medroxyprogesterone (both dosed qd), 28's: **$22.60;** 0.625 mg/5.0 mg medroxyprogesterone (both dosed qd), 28's: **$22.60**

• Tab, Uncoated—Oral: 0.625 mg/5 mg medroxyprogesterone (estrogen dosed qd day 1-28, medroxyprogesterone dosed day 15-28), 28's: **$20.71**

CONTRAINDICATIONS: Breast cancer (except in selected patients being treated for metastatic disease), active thromboembolic disorders, known or suspected estrogen-dependent neoplasia, undiagnosed abnormal genital bleeding

---

* = non-FDA-approved use

PRECAUTIONS: Hypertension, gallbladder disease, CHF, diabetes mellitus, depression, migraine headache, seizure disorders, hepatic disease, family history of breast or endometrial cancer, history of thromboembolic disorders, uterine fibroids, hypertriglyceridemia, hypercalcemia

PREGNANCY AND LACTATION: Pregnancy category X; may decrease quantity and quality of breast milk

SIDE EFFECTS/ADVERSE REACTIONS

CNS: Depression, migraine headache, emotional lability

*CV: **Arterial thromboembolism, pulmonary embolism, CVA, MI,** hypertension, venous thrombosis, edema*

EENT: Contact lens intolerance, ***retinal thrombosis***

*GI: Nausea and vomiting, gallbladder disease, bloating, benign hepatic tumors, **mesenteric thrombosis***

*GU: Breakthrough bleeding, spotting, amenorrhea, change in cervical secretions, breast enlargement, breast tenderness, **endometrial cancer***

METAB: Hyperglycemia, hypertriglyceridemia, hypercalcemia

SKIN: Melasma

INTERACTIONS

Drugs

3 *P450 inducers* (e.g., rifampin, barbiturates): Decreased estrogen levels

3 *Corticosteroids:* Increased steroid effect

3 *Phenytoin:* Loss of seizure control, decreased estrogen levels

3 *Warfarin:* Theoretical increased risk thromboembolism

SPECIAL CONSIDERATIONS
• Progestins recommended in non-hysterectomized women

• Premarin is derived from pregnant mare's urine; Cenestin from yams and soy. Although probably therapeutically equivalent, they are not substitutable by the pharmacist.

---

estrone
(ess'trone)

Rx: Estragyn-5, Estro-A, Kestrone-5, Primestrin

Chemical Class: Estrogen derivative

Therapeutic Class: Estrogen; antineoplastic

CLINICAL PHARMACOLOGY

Mechanism of Action: Necessary for adequate functioning of female reproductive system; affects release of pituitary gonadotropins, inhibits ovulation, inhibits bone resorption

Pharmacokinetics

IM: Degraded in liver, excreted in urine, crosses placenta, excreted in breast milk

INDICATIONS AND USES: Menopause, inoperable prostatic cancer, atrophic vaginitis, hypogonadism, primary ovarian failure, dysfunctional uterine bleeding

DOSAGE

Adult

• *Dysfunctional uterine bleeding:* IM 2-5 mg qd for several days

• *Menopause/atrophic vaginitis:* IM 0.1-0.5 mg 2-3 times/wk, cyclically or continuously

• *Female hypogonadism/primary ovarian failure:* IM 0.1-2 mg q wk in 1 dose or divided doses, cyclically or continuously

• *Prostatic cancer:* IM 2-4 mg 2-3 times/wk

$ AVAILABLE FORMS/COST OF THERAPY

• Inj, Susp—IM: 2 mg/ml, 10 ml: **$9.75-$14.95;** 5 mg/ml, 10 ml: **$9.75-$14.75**

---

italic = common side effects   ***bold italic*** = life-threatening reactions

CONTRAINDICATIONS: Breast cancer, active thromboembolic disorders, known or suspected estrogen-dependent neoplasia, undiagnosed abnormal genital bleeding

PRECAUTIONS: Hypertension, gallbladder disease, CHF, diabetes mellitus, migraine headache, hepatic disease, family history of breast or endometrial cancer, uterine fibroids, history of thromboembolic disorders, hypertriglyceridemia, hypercalcemia

PREGNANCY AND LACTATION: Pregnancy category X; may reduce quantity and quality of breast milk

SIDE EFFECTS/ADVERSE REACTIONS

CNS: Depression, migraine headache, emotional lability

CV: Arterial thromboembolism, pulmonary embolism, CVA, MI, hypertension, venous thrombosis, edema

EENT: Contact lens intolerance, *retinal thrombosis*

GI: Nausea and vomiting, gallbladder disease, bloating, benign hepatic tumors, *mesenteric thrombosis*

GU: Breakthrough bleeding, spotting, amenorrhea, change in cervical secretions, breast enlargement, breast tenderness, *testicular atrophy, endometrial cancer*

METAB: Hyperglycemia, hypertriglyceridemia, hypercalcemia

SKIN: Melasma

INTERACTIONS

Drugs

3 *P450 inducers* (e.g., rifampin, barbiturates): Decreased estrogen levels

3 *Corticosteroids:* Increased steroid effect

3 *Phenytoin:* Loss of seizure control, decreased estrogen levels

3 *Warfarin:* Theoretical increased risk thromboembolism

SPECIAL CONSIDERATIONS
• Progestins recommended in non-hysterectomized women

---

estropipate
(es-tro-pip′ate)
Rx: Ogen, Ortho-Est
Chemical Class: Estrogen derivative
Therapeutic Class: Estrogen; antiosteoporotic

CLINICAL PHARMACOLOGY

Mechanism of Action: Necessary for adequate functioning of female reproductive system; affects release of pituitary gonadotropins, inhibits bone resorption

Pharmacokinetics

PO: Metabolized in liver (significant 1st-pass effect) primarily to estrone, excreted in urine

INDICATIONS AND USES: Vasomotor symptoms, atrophic vaginitis or kraurosis vulvae associated with menopause; female hypogonadism, female castration, or primary ovarian failure; osteoporosis prevention; prevention of cardiovascular disease*

DOSAGE

Adult

• *Vasomotor symptoms:* PO 0.75-3 mg qd for 25-31 days monthly

• *Atrophic vaginitis:* PO 0.75-3 mg qd for 25-31 days monthly; vag 2-4 g qd initially, then weekly or twice weekly

• *Female hypogonadism, female castration, or primary ovarian failure:* PO 1.5-9 mg/day × 3 wk, followed by a rest period of 8-10 days, repeated cyclically

• *Osteoporosis prevention:* PO 0.75 mg qd for 25-31 days monthly

---

* = non-FDA-approved use

§ AVAILABLE FORMS/COST OF THERAPY

• Tab, Uncoated—Oral: 0.75 mg, 100's: **$40.06-$70.30;** 1.5 mg, 100's: **$54.90-$98.56;** 3 mg, 100's: **$100.39-$157.59**

• Cre—Vag: 1.5 mg/g, 45 g: **$47.68**

CONTRAINDICATIONS: Breast cancer (except in selected patients being treated for metastatic disease), active thromboembolic disorders, known or suspected estrogen-dependent neoplasia, undiagnosed abnormal genital bleeding

PRECAUTIONS: Hypertension, gallbladder disease, CHF, diabetes mellitus, depression, migraine headache, seizure disorders, hepatic disease, family history of breast or endometrial cancer, history of thromboembolic disorders, uterine fibroids, hypertriglyceridemia, hypercalcemia

PREGNANCY AND LACTATION: Pregnancy category X; may reduce quantity and quality of breast milk

SIDE EFFECTS/ADVERSE REACTIONS

CNS: Depression, migraine headache, emotional lability

CV: Arterial thromboembolism, pulmonary embolism, CVA, MI, hypertension, venous thrombosis, edema

EENT: Contact lens intolerance, *retinal thrombosis*

GI: Nausea and vomiting, gallbladder disease, bloating, benign hepatic tumors, *mesenteric thrombosis*

GU: Breakthrough bleeding, spotting, amenorrhea, change in cervical secretions, breast enlargement, breast tenderness, *endometrial cancer*

METAB: Hyperglycemia, hypertriglyceridemia, hypercalcemia

SKIN: Melasma

INTERACTIONS

Drugs

§ *P450 inducers* (e.g., rifampin, barbiturates): Decreased estrogen levels

§ *Corticosteroids:* Increased steroid effect

§ *Phenytoin:* Loss of seizure control, decreased estrogen levels

§ *Warfarin:* Theoretical increased risk thromboembolism

SPECIAL CONSIDERATIONS

Unopposed estrogen increases risk of endometrial cancer; recommended administration of concurrent progestational agents for non-hysterectomized women

---

etanercept
(e-tan′er-cept)
Rx: Enbrel
Chemical Class: Recombinant human fusion protein
Therapeutic Class: Immuno-modulatory agent; disease-modifying antirheumatic drug (DMARD)*

CLINICAL PHARMACOLOGY

Mechanism of Action: Tumor necrosis factor receptor p75 Fc fusion protein (TNFR:Fc); binds specifically with human TNF and blocks its interaction with cell surface TNF receptors, preventing TNF's contribution to the normal inflammatory and immune responses of rheumatoid arthritis

Pharmacokinetics

SQ: Cmax 72 hr; 2-5 fold increases in serum level with repeated dosing; 60% bioavailability; Vd 17 L; cleared via the reticuloendothelial system (liver, spleen); $t_{1/2}$ 115 hr

INDICATIONS AND USES: Rheumatoid arthritis, juvenile rheumatoid arthritis

DOSAGE

Adult and Child >16 yr

• SQ 25 mg twice weekly

Children 4-17 yr

• SQ 0.4 mg/kg (max 25 mg) twice weekly

$ AVAILABLE FORMS/COST OF THERAPY

• Inj, Pow—SQ: 25 mg; 1's: **$141.49**

CONTRAINDICATIONS: Sepsis

PRECAUTIONS: Immunogenicity, potential declines in host defenses against malignancies and infections; immunization-related infections; latex allergies

PREGNANCY AND LACTATION: Pregnancy category B; information on breast milk excretion is unknown; breast feeding not advised

SIDE EFFECTS/ADVERSE REACTIONS

CNS: Headache, dizziness, asthenia, *cerebral ischemia, depression, dyspnea*

CV: Heart failure, *MI,* hypertension, hypotension

EENT: Rhinitis, pharyngitis, sinusitis

GI: Abdominal pain, dyspepsia, cholycystitis, *pancreatitis, GI hemorrhage*

MS: Bursitis

RESP: Respiratory tract infections, cough

SKIN: Rash

MISC: Injection site reactions; infections (varicella), aseptic meningitis

SPECIAL CONSIDERATIONS

• Immunizations should be up to date, especially in children prior to starting therapy

PATIENT/FAMILY EDUCATION

• Review injection techniques to ensure safe self-administration

MONITORING PARAMETERS

• Efficacy: ESR, C-reactive protein, rheumatoid factor, improvement in tender/painful swollen joints, quality of life

---

ethacrynic acid

(eth-a-kri'nik)

Rx: Edecrin

Chemical Class: Ketone derivative of aryloxyacetic acid

Therapeutic Class: Loop diuretic

CLINICAL PHARMACOLOGY

Mechanism of Action: Inhibits absorption of sodium and chloride at proximal and distal tubule sites and in the loop of Henle

Pharmacokinetics

PO: Onset ½ hr, peak 2 hr, duration 6-8 hr

IV: Onset 5 min, peak 15-30 min, duration 2 hr

Hepatic metabolism; excreted in urine and feces, crosses placenta; $t_{1/2}$ 30-70 min

INDICATIONS AND USES: Pulmonary edema; edema (CHF, hepatic cirrhosis nephrotic syndrome, ascites); glaucoma*; hypertension (in combination with other agents),* hypercalcemia*

DOSAGE

Adult

• PO 50-200 mg/day; may give up to 200 mg bid, adjust dose in 25-50 mg increments; IV 50 mg or 0.5-1.0 mg/kg given over several min

Child

• PO 25 mg, increased by 25 mg/day until desired effect occurs; not established for infants or parenterally

$ AVAILABLE FORMS/COST OF THERAPY

• Inj, Sol—IV: 50 mg/vial: **$21.84**

• Tab, Uncoated—Oral: 25 mg, 100's: **$34.25;** 50 mg, 100's: **$48.81**

CONTRAINDICATIONS: Anuria,

hypovolemia, electrolyte depletion, infants, hepatic coma

PRECAUTIONS: Fluid and electrolyte imbalance (including sodium, chloride, potassium, magnesium, calcium), renal disease, hepatic disease (may precipitate hepatic encephalopathy), gout, COPD, lupus erythematosus, diabetes mellitus, hyperparathyroidism, vomiting, diarrhea, elevated cholesterol/triglycerides

PREGNANCY AND LACTATION: Pregnancy category B; cardiovascular disorders such as pulmonary edema, severe hypertension, or CHF are probably the only valid indications for loop diuretics during pregnancy; no data on nursing; contraindicated per manufacturer

SIDE EFFECTS/ADVERSE REACTIONS

CNS: Encephalopathy in hepatic disease, fatigue, headache, vertigo, weakness

CV: Chest pain, ***circulatory collapse,*** ECG changes, hypotension

EENT: Blurred vision, ear pain, hearing loss, tinnitus

GI: Abdominal distension, abdominal pain, ***acute pancreatitis,*** anorexia, cramps, dry mouth, ***GI bleeding,*** jaundice, nausea, severe diarrhea, upset stomach, vomiting

GU: Glycosuria, polyuria, ***renal failure,*** sexual dysfunction

HEME: ***Agranulocytosis, leukopenia, neutropenia, thrombocytopenia***

METAB: Decreased glucose tolerance, hyperglycemia, hyperuricemia, hypocalcemia, hypochloremic alkalosis, *hypokalemia,* hypomagnesemia, hyponatremia

MS: Arthritis, cramps, stiffness

SKIN: Photosensitivity, pruritis, purpura, rash, ***Stevens-Johnson syndrome,*** sweating

INTERACTIONS
Drugs

❷ *Aminoglycosides (gentamicin, kanamycin, neomycin, streptomycin):* Additive ototoxicity (ethacrynic acid > furosemide, torsemide, bumetanide)

❸ *Angiotensin converting enzyme inhibitors:* Initiation of ACEI with intensive diuretic therapy may result in precipitous fall in blood pressure; ACEIs may induce renal insufficiency in the presence of diuretic-induced sodium depletion

❸ *Barbiturates (phenobarbital):* Reduced diuretic response

❸ *Bile acid-binding resins (cholestyramine, colestipol):* Resins markedly reduce the bioavailability and diuretic response

❸ *Carbenoxolone:* Severe hypokalemia from coadministration

❸ *Cephalosporins (cephaloridine, cephalothin):* Enhanced nephrotoxicity with coadministration

❷ *Cisplatin:* Additive ototoxicity (ethacrynic acid > furosemide, torsemide, bumetanide)

❸ *Clofibrate:* Enhanced effects of both drugs, especially in hypoalbuminemic patients

❸ *Corticosteroids:* Concomitant loop diuretic and corticosteroid therapy can result in excessive potassium loss

❸ *Digitalis glycosides (digoxin, digitoxin):* Diuretic-induced hypokalemia may increase risk of digitalis toxicity

❸ *Nonsteroidal antiinflammatory drugs (flurbiprofen, ibuprofen, indomethacin, naproxen, piroxicam, sulindac):* Reduced diuretic and antihypertensive effects

❸ *Phenytoin:* Reduced diuretic response

❸ *Serotonin-reuptake inhibitors (fluoxetine, paroxetine, sertraline):* Case reports of sudden death; en-

---

italic = common side effects   ***bold italic*** = life-threatening reactions

hanced hyponatremia proposed; causal relationships not established

🔳 *Terbutaline:* Additive hypokalemia

🔳 *Tubocurarine:* Prolonged neuromuscular blockade

SPECIAL CONSIDERATIONS

• Inhibits reabsorption of filtered sodium more than other loop diuretics, therefore, may be effective in patients with significant degrees of renal insufficiency

• Reserve for patients not responding to or intolerant of furosemide or bumetanide

MONITORING PARAMETERS

• Urine volume, creatinine clearance, BUN, electrolytes, reduction in edema, increased diuresis, decrease in body weight, reduction in blood pressure, glucose, uric acid, serum calcium (tetany), tinnitus, vertigo, hearing loss (especially in those at risk for ototoxicity—IV doses > 120 mg; concomitant ototoxic drugs; renal disease)

---

ethambutol

(e-tham′byoo-tole)
Rx: Myambutol
Chemical Class: Diisopropyl-ethylene diamide derivative
Therapeutic Class: Antituberculosis agent

CLINICAL PHARMACOLOGY
Mechanism of Action: Inhibits RNA synthesis, decreases tubercle bacilli replication
Pharmacokinetics
PO: Peak 2-4 hr, metabolized in liver; excreted in urine (unchanged drug/inactive metabolites), and feces, crosses placenta; $t_{1/2}$ 3-4 hr
INDICATIONS AND USES: Adjunct in treatment of pulmonary tuberculosis; mycobacterium avium complex (MAC) in AIDS (2nd line)*

DOSAGE
Adult and Child >13 yr
Tuberculosis
• *Initial treatment:* PO 15 mg/kg/day as a single daily dose
• *Retreatment:* PO 25 mg/kg/day as single dose for 2 mo with at least 1 other drug, then decrease to 15 mg/kg/day as single daily dose
Mycobacterium avium complex in AIDS
• PO: 15 mg/kg with 3 or 4 other antimycobacterial agents

💲 **AVAILABLE FORMS/COST OF THERAPY**

• Tab, Uncoated—Oral: 100 mg, 100's: **$55.18;** 400 mg, 100's: **$184.63**

CONTRAINDICATIONS: Optic neuritis, child <13 yr

PRECAUTIONS: Renal disease, diabetic retinopathy, cataracts, ocular defects, hepatic and hematopoietic disorders, gout

PREGNANCY AND LACTATION: Pregnancy category B; compatible with breast feeding

SIDE EFFECTS/ADVERSE REACTIONS

CNS: Confusion, disorientation, dizziness, fever, hallucinations, headache, malaise

EENT: Bloody sputum, blurred vision, changes in color perception, decreased visual acuity, optic neuritis, photophobia

GI: Abdominal distress, anorexia, nausea, vomiting

HEME: **Thrombocytopenia**

METAB: Acute gout, elevated uric acid, liver function impairment

MS: Joint pain

SKIN: Dermatitis, pruritis

SPECIAL CONSIDERATIONS

• Initial therapy in tuberculosis should include 4 drugs: isoniazid, rifampin, pyrazinamide, and etham-

---

* = non-FDA-approved use

butol, until drug susceptibility results available

PATIENT/FAMILY EDUCATION

• Administer with meals to decrease GI symptoms

MONITORING PARAMETERS

• Perform visual acuity testing before beginning therapy and periodically during drug administration (qmo if dose >15 mg/kg/day)

---

ethanolamine oleate
(eth-an-ole′a-meen ol′ee-ate)

Rx: Ethamolin

Chemical Class: Fatty acid ester

Therapeutic Class: Sclerosing agent

CLINICAL PHARMACOLOGY

Mechanism of Action: Following IV inj, irritates intimal endothelium of the vein and produces a sterile dose-related inflammatory response, leading to fibrosis and occlusion of the vein; oleic acid component of compound is responsible for the inflammatory response

Pharmacokinetics

IV: Disappears from inj site within 5 min via portal vein; sclerosis of varices lasts 2½ mo

INDICATIONS AND USES: Esophageal varices that have recently bled, to prevent rebleeding

DOSAGE

Adult

• IV 1.5-5 ml per varix, max total dose per treatment should not exceed 20 ml; to obliterate the varix, inj should be made at time of acute bleeding, then after 1 wk, 6 wk, 3 mo, and 6 mo as indicated

Child

• IV 2-5 ml per varix to a max of 20 ml

💲 AVAILABLE FORMS/COST OF THERAPY

• Inj, Sol—IV: 50 mg/ml, 2 ml: **$28.65**

CONTRAINDICATIONS: Esophageal varices that have not bled

PRECAUTIONS: Severe inj necrosis possible; concomitant cardiorespiratory disease; elderly, critically ill patients; severe liver dysfunction

PREGNANCY AND LACTATION: Pregnancy category C

SIDE EFFECTS/ADVERSE REACTIONS

GI: Esophageal ulcer, stricture

METAB: Pyrexia

RESP: Pleural effusion/infiltration, pneumonia

MISC: Retrosternal pain

INTERACTIONS

Labs

• *False decrease:* Serum ionized calcium

SPECIAL CONSIDERATIONS

• Orphan drug

---

ethchlorvynol
(eth-klor-vi′nole)

Rx: Placidyl

Chemical Class: Tertiary acetylenic alcohol

Therapeutic Class: Sedative-hypnotic

DEA Class: Schedule IV

CLINICAL PHARMACOLOGY

Mechanism of Action: Produces cerebral depression; mechanism unknown

Pharmacokinetics

PO: Onset 15-60 min, peak 2 hr, duration 5 hr, extensive distribution to adipose tissue; metabolized by liver (90%), renal elimination; $t_{1/2}$ 10-20 hr

INDICATIONS AND USES: Insomnia (short-term therapy); sedation*

DOSAGE
Adult
• *Insomnia:* PO 500 mg-1 g ½ hr before hs, may repeat 200 mg if needed
• *Sedation:* PO 200 mg bid or tid
Child
• PO 25 mg/kg in 1 dose, not to exceed 1 g

$ AVAILABLE FORMS/COST OF THERAPY
• Cap, Gel—Oral: 200 mg, 100's: **$112.99**; 500 mg, 100's: **$139.20**; 750 mg, 100's: **$184.73**

CONTRAINDICATIONS: Porphyria
PRECAUTIONS: Depression, hepatic disease, renal disease, suicidal tendencies, elderly, history of drug abuse, tartrazine sensitivity
PREGNANCY AND LACTATION: Pregnancy category C
SIDE EFFECTS/ADVERSE REACTIONS
CNS: Ataxia, dizziness, facial numbness, fatigue, giddiness, hangover, hysteria, nightmares, weakness
CV: Hypotension
EENT: Blurred vision
GI: Bitter aftertaste, cholestatic jaundice, nausea, vomiting
HEME: **Thrombocytopenia**
SKIN: Rash, urticaria
INTERACTIONS
Drugs
3 *Warfarin:* Decreased hypoprothrombinemic response to oral anticoagulents
SPECIAL CONSIDERATIONS
• Geriatric patients may be more sensitive to usual adult dose
• Do not prescribe for periods >1 wk

---

ethinyl estradiol
(eth-in'il ess-tra-dye'ole)
Rx: Estinyl
Combinations
  See oral contraceptives monograph for combined oral contraceptives containing ethinyl estradiol
Chemical Class: Synthetic estrogen derivative
Therapeutic Class: Estrogen; contraceptive

CLINICAL PHARMACOLOGY
Mechanism of Action: Necessary for adequate functioning of female reproductive system; affects release of pituitary gonadotropins; inhibits bone resorption
Pharmacokinetics
PO: Peak 2-3 hr; addition of 17-α-ethinyl group to estradiol enhances potency and oral activity; degraded in liver; excreted in urine
INDICATIONS AND USES: Vasomotor symptoms associated with menopause; atrophic vaginitis, kraurosis vulvae*; breast engorgement*; female hypogonadism; osteoporosis*; contraceptive (combined with progestins, see oral contraceptives monograph); female breast cancer (inoperable, progressing); prostatic carcinoma (inoperable)
DOSAGE
Adult
• *Menopause:* PO 0.02-0.05 mg qd 3 wk on, 1 wk off (may add progestational agent during latter part of the cycle)
• *Prostatic cancer:* PO 0.15-2 mg qd
• *Hypogonadism:* PO 0.05 mg qd-tid × 2 wk/mo, then 2 wk progesterone; repeat cycle for 3-6 mo, then 2 mo off
• *Breast cancer:* PO 1 mg tid

---

* = non-FDA-approved use

• *Breast engorgement:* PO 0.5-1 mg qd × 3 days, then tapered off over 7 days

• *Combined oral contraceptive:* Combined with progestins, 20-80 μg qd cycled 21 days, off 7 days

$ AVAILABLE FORMS/COST OF THERAPY

• Tab, Coated—Oral: 0.02 mg, 100's: **$37.28**; 0.05 mg, 100's: **$62.81**

CONTRAINDICATIONS: Breast cancer (except in selected patients being treated for metastatic disease), active thromboembolic disorders, known or suspected estrogen-dependent neoplasia, undiagnosed abnormal genital bleeding

PRECAUTIONS: Hypertension, gallbladder disease, CHF, diabetes mellitus, depression, migraine headache, seizure disorders, hepatic disease, family history of breast or endometrial cancer, history of thromboembolic disorders, uterine fibroids, hypertriglyceridemia, hypercalcemia

PREGNANCY AND LACTATION: Pregnancy category X; may reduce quantity and quality of breast milk

SIDE EFFECTS/ADVERSE REACTIONS

CNS: Depression, migraine headache, emotional lability

CV: Arterial thromboembolism, pulmonary embolism, CVA, MI, hypertension, venous thrombosis, edema

EENT: Contact lens intolerance, *retinal thrombosis*

GI: Nausea and vomiting, gallbladder disease, bloating, benign hepatic tumors, *mesenteric thrombosis*

GU: Breakthrough bleeding, spotting, amenorrhea, change in cervical secretions, breast enlargement, breast tenderness, *testicular atrophy, endometrial cancer*

METAB: Hyperglycemia, hypertriglyceridemia, hypercalcemia

SKIN: Melasma

MISC: Changes in libido, weight gain

INTERACTIONS

Drugs

3 *P450 inducers* (e.g., *rifampin, barbiturates*): Decreased estrogen levels

3 *Corticosteroids:* Increased steroid effect

3 *Phenytoin:* Loss of seizure control, decreased estrogen levels

3 *Warfarin:* Theoretical increased risk of thromboembolism

SPECIAL CONSIDERATIONS

• Unopposed estrogen increases risk of endometrial cancer; recommended administration of concurrent progestational agents for non-hysterectomized women

---

ethionamide

(e-thye-on'am-ide)

Rx: Trecator-SC

Chemical Class: Thiomine derivative

Therapeutic Class: Antituberculosis agent

CLINICAL PHARMACOLOGY

Mechanism of Action: Bacteriostatic against *Mycobacterium tuberculosis* via inhibition of peptide synthesis

Pharmacokinetics

PO: Peak 3 hr, metabolized in liver, renal excretion (primarily inactive metabolites); $t_{1/2}$ 3 hr

INDICATIONS AND USES: Pulmonary, extrapulmonary TB when other antitubercular drugs have failed

DOSAGE

Adult

• PO 500 mg-1 g qd in divided doses with another antitubercular drug and pyridoxine

---

italic = common side effects   ***bold italic*** = life-threatening reactions

Child

• PO 15-20 mg/kg/day in 3-4 doses, not to exceed 1 g; concomitant pyridoxine recommended

💲 **AVAILABLE FORMS/COST OF THERAPY**

• Tab, Sugar Coated—Oral: 250 mg, 100's: **$212.75**

CONTRAINDICATIONS: Severe hepatic disease

PRECAUTIONS: Renal disease, diabetes, hepatic impairment, children

PREGNANCY AND LACTATION: Pregnancy category D

SIDE EFFECTS/ADVERSE REACTIONS

CNS: Depression, dizziness, drowsiness, headache, peripheral neuritis, psychosis, *seizures,* tremors

CV: Postural hypotension

EENT: Blurred vision, olfactory disturbances, optic neuritis

GI: Anorexia, diarrhea (50% can't tolerate >500 mg), hepatitis (5%), jaundice, metallic taste, *nausea, vomiting*

GU: Impotence, menorrhagia

HEME: Purpura, *thrombocytopenia*

METAB: Difficulty managing diabetes mellitus

SKIN: Acne, alopecia, dermatitis

MISC: Gynecomastia

INTERACTIONS

Labs

• *False decrease:* Urine alkaline phosphatase, urine lactate dehydrogenase

SPECIAL CONSIDERATIONS

• Use only with at least 1 other effective antituberculous agent

MONITORING PARAMETERS

• Serum transaminases (AST, ALT) biweekly during therapy

ethosuximide

(eth-oh-sux′i-mide)
Rx: Zarontin
Chemical Class: Succinimide derivative
Therapeutic Class: Anticonvulsant

CLINICAL PHARMACOLOGY

Mechanism of Action: Increases seizure threshold and inhibits spike-and-wave formation in absence (petit mal) seizures; decreases amplitude, frequency, duration, spread of discharge in minor motor seizures

Pharmacokinetics

PO: Peak 3-7 hr; steady state 4-7 days; rapid and complete absorption; freely distributed, except to fat; insignificant protein binding; metabolized by liver, excreted in urine (20% unchanged); $t_{1/2}$ 56-60 hr (adults), 26-30 hr (children)

INDICATIONS AND USES: Absence seizures, partial seizures*

DOSAGE

Adult and Child >6 yr

• PO 250 mg bid initially; may increase by 250 mg q4-7 days, not to exceed 1.5 g/day

Child 3-6 yr

• PO 250 mg/day or 125 mg bid initially; may increase by 250 mg q4-7 days, not to exceed 1 g/day (20 mg/kg/day)

💲 **AVAILABLE FORMS/COST OF THERAPY**

• Syr—Oral: 250 mg/5 ml, 480 ml: **$80.95-$92.66**

• Cap, Gel—Oral: 250 mg, 100's: **$88.09**

PRECAUTIONS: Hepatic function impairment; renal dysfunction; acute intermittent porphyria; monotherapy with mixed types of epilepsy (may increase frequency of grand-mal seizures)

---

* = non-FDA-approved use

PREGNANCY AND LACTATION:
Pregnancy category C; freely enters breast milk; no adverse effects on infants reported; compatible with breast feeding

SIDE EFFECTS/ADVERSE REACTIONS

CNS: Aggressiveness, anxiety, depression, *dizziness, drowsiness, euphoria, fatigue,* headache, insomnia, irritability, *lethargy*

EENT: Blurred vision, myopia

GI: Abdominal pain, *anorexia,* constipation, cramps, diarrhea, gum hypertrophy, *heartburn,* hiccups, *nausea,* tongue swelling, *vomiting,* weight loss

GU: Hematuria, **renal damage,** vaginal bleeding

HEME: **Agranulocytosis, aplastic anemia,** eosinophilia, **leukocytosis, pancytopenia, thrombocytopenia**

SKIN: Hirsutism, pruritic erythema, **Stevens-Johnson syndrome,** urticaria

MISC: Systemic lupus erythematosis

SPECIAL CONSIDERATIONS

PATIENT/FAMILY EDUCATION

• Take doses at regularly spaced intervals

• OK with food or milk

MONITORING PARAMETERS

• Blood counts, renal function tests, liver function tests, urinalysis periodically

• Therapeutic serum concentrations 40-100 µg/ml

---

ethotoin

(eth-oh-to′in)

Rx: Peganone

Chemical Class: Hydantoin derivative

Therapeutic Class: Anticonvulsant

E

CLINICAL PHARMACOLOGY

Mechanism of Action: Stabilizes neuronal membranes decreasing seizure activity by increasing efflux or decreasing influx of sodium ions across cell membranes the motor cortex during generation of impulses

Pharmacokinetics

PO: Therapeutic serum concentration 15-50 µg/ml; rapid absorption; metabolized by liver (substantial nonlinear kinetics), excreted in urine; $t_{1/2}$ 3-9 hr

INDICATIONS AND USES: Generalized tonic-clonic or complex-partial seizures (2nd-line agent)

DOSAGE

Adult

• PO 250 mg qid initially; may increase over several days to 3 g/day in divided doses (<2 g/day ineffective in most adults)

Child

• PO initial dose should not exceed 750 mg/day in divided doses; usual maintenance dose 500 mg-1 g/day in 4-6 divided doses

💲 AVAILABLE FORMS/COST OF THERAPY

• Tab, Uncoated—Oral: 250 mg, 100's: **$44.39**

CONTRAINDICATIONS: Hematologic disease, hepatic disease

PRECAUTIONS: Geriatric patients metabolize hydantoins slowly

PREGNANCY AND LACTATION: Pregnancy category C (fetal hydan-

---

toin syndrome); excreted in breast milk

SIDE EFFECTS/ADVERSE REACTIONS

CNS: Ataxia, dizziness, *drowsiness,* fatigue, fever, headache, insomnia, numbness, slurred speech

CV: Chest pain

EENT: Diplopia, nystagmus

GI: Diarrhea, gingival hypertrophy, liver damage, nausea, toxic hepatitis, vomiting

HEME: **Agranulocytosis, leukopenia,** lymphadenopathy, **megaloblastic anemia, pancytopenia, thrombocytopenia**

SKIN: Rash

INTERACTIONS

Drugs

3 *Alcohol or CNS depression-producing drugs:* Enhanced CNS depression

3 *Amiodarone:* Increased plasma concentration of ethotoin

3 *Antacids:* Decrease bioavailability of ethotoin

3 *Chloramphenicol, Cimetidine, Disulfiram, Isoniazid, Phenylbutazone, Sulfonamides:* All inhibit metabolism and increase concentration of ethotoin

3 *Estrogen contraceptives, Corticosteroids, Corticotropin:* All may have effects decreased because of increased metabolism

3 *Fluconazole:* Decreases the metabolism of ethotoin

3 *Lidocaine:* Concurrent IV use may produce additive cardiac depressant effects

3 *Methadone:* Increased methadone metabolism, decreased activity

3 *Oral anticoagulants:* Increased serum concentration of ethotoin; increased anticoagulant effect initially, then decreased with continued use

3 *Oral diazoxide:* Decreased efficacy of both agents

3 *Rifampin:* Increased metabolism of ethotoin, decreased effect

3 *Streptozocin:* Ethotoin may protect pancreatic β-cells from the toxic effects of streptozocin

3 *Sucralfate:* Decreased ethotoin absorption

3 *Valproic acid:* Displaces ethotoin from binding sites, inhibits ethotoin metabolism, increased or additive liver toxicity

3 *Xanthines:* Increased hepatic xanthine metabolism, decreased serum concentration; xanthines inhibit ethotoin absorption with decreased serum ethotoin levels

SPECIAL CONSIDERATIONS
PATIENT/FAMILY EDUCATION

• Strictly enforced program of teeth cleaning and plaque control to prevent gingival hyperplasia is necessary

• Take doses at regularly spaced intervals

MONITORING PARAMETERS

• Therapeutic serum level: 40-100 µg/ml

etidocaine
(eh-tee'doe-kane)
Rx: Duranest-MPI
Combinations
   Rx: with epinephrine
      (Duranest-MPF with Epinephrine)
Chemical Class: Amide derivative
Therapeutic Class: Local anesthetic

CLINICAL PHARMACOLOGY
Mechanism of Action: Blocks generation and conduction of nerve impulses; the order of loss of nerve function is: (1) pain, (2) temperature, (3) touch, (4) proprioception, and (5) skeletal muscle tone

Pharmacokinetics
Inj: Onset 2-8 min, duration 3-6 hr; metabolized by liver; high lipid solubility; $t_{1/2}$ 2.7 hr (adult), 4-8 hr (neonate); metabolites excreted in urine
INDICATIONS AND USES: Infiltration anesthesia, peripheral nerve blocks, central neural blocks (lumbar or caudal, epidural)
DOSAGE
Dose varies with procedure, depth of anesthesia, vascularity of tissues, duration of anesthesia, and condition of patient
• Peripheral nerve block (5-40 ml), central nerve block or lumbar peridural, caudal (10-30 ml): 1%
• Intra-abdominal or pelvic surgery, lower limb surgery or cesarean section (10-20 ml): 1% or 1.5%
• Maxillary infiltration or inferior alveolar nerve block (1-5 ml): 1.5%
💲 **AVAILABLE FORMS/COST OF THERAPY**
• Inj—Sol: 1%, 30 ml: **$21.58**
• Inj—Sol (w/epinephrine): 1%, 30 ml: **$23.47**; 1.5%, 20 ml: **$25.90**
PRECAUTIONS: Severe drug allergies, sulfite sensitivity (preparations containing epinephrine), severe shock, heart block, children, elderly, hepatic disease, peripheral vascular disease (preparations containing epinephrine)
PREGNANCY AND LACTATION: Pregnancy category B; although no breast milk excretion data, problems in humans have not been documented
SIDE EFFECTS/ADVERSE REACTIONS
CNS: Anxiety, disorientation, drowsiness, loss of consciousness, restlessness, *seizures,* shivering, tremors
CV: Bradycardia, ***cardiac arrest, dysrhythmias,*** fetal bradycardia, hypertension, hypotension, myocardial depression

EENT: Blurred vision, pupil constriction, tinnitus
GI: Nausea, vomiting
RESP: ***Respiratory arrest, status asthmaticus***
SKIN: Allergic reactions, burning, edema, rash, skin discoloration at inj site, tissue necrosis, urticaria
INTERACTIONS
Drugs
3 *Beta-blockers:* Hypertensive reactions possible, especially with local anesthetics containing epinephrine; acute discontinuation of β-blockers before local anesthesia may increase the risk of side effects due to anesthetic
SPECIAL CONSIDERATIONS
• Amide-type local anesthetic

---

etidronate
(ee-tid'roe-nate)
Rx: Didronel
Chemical Class: Synthetic analog of pyrophosphate
Therapeutic Class: Bisphosphonate

CLINICAL PHARMACOLOGY
Mechanism of Action: Binds to hydroxyapatite at sites of bone resorption, inhibiting normal and abnormal bone resorption ("crystal poison"); minimal secondary reduction in bone formation (resorption coupled to formation)
Pharmacokinetics
Therapeutic response, Paget's Disease, and osteoporosis 1-3 mo; hypercalcemia 24 hr; duration of effect, Paget's Disease 1 yr after discontinuing therapy; hypercalcemia 14 days of normocalcemia; poorly absorbed orally (1%-6%); chemically adsorbed to bone; not metabolized, excreted in urine/feces; $t_{1/2}$ 1-6 hr

italic = common side effects   ***bold italic*** = life-threatening reactions

INDICATIONS AND USES: Paget's disease, heterotropic ossification caused by spinal cord injury or complicating total hip replacement, hyperparathyroidism, bone pain in prostatic carcinoma and metastatic breast cancer, prevention of glucocorticoid-induced osteoporosis, hypercalcemia of malignancy (IV), osteoporosis*

DOSAGE

Adult

• *Paget's disease:* PO 5-10 mg/kg/day 2 hr ac with H_2O; not to exceed 20 mg/kg/day; max course 6 mo

• *Heterotropic ossification:* PO (due to spinal cord injury) 20 mg/kg qd × 2 wk, then 10 mg/kg/day for 10 wk, total 12 wk; (complicating total hip replacement) 20 mg/kg qd × 1 mo preoperatively, then 20 mg/kg qd for 3 mo postoperatively

• *Hypercalcemia:* IV 7.5 mg/kg/day for 3 successive days (diluted in at least 250 ml normal saline) over at least 2 hr; retreatment interval at least 7 days

• *Osteoporosis:* PO 400 mg qd 2 hr ac with H_2O × 2 wk, repeat every 3 mo

AVAILABLE FORMS/COST OF THERAPY

• Inj, Sol—IV: 300 mg/6 ml, 6 ml: **$67.00**

• Tab, Uncoated—Oral: 200 mg, 60's: **$148.43;** 400 mg, 60's: **$296.80**

CONTRAINDICATIONS: Severe renal disease, overt osteomalacia

PRECAUTIONS: Renal disease, restricted vitamin D and calcium intake, enterocolitis

PREGNANCY AND LACTATION: Pregnancy category B; breast milk excretion not known; problems in humans have not been documented

SIDE EFFECTS/ADVERSE REACTIONS

GI: Diarrhea, metallic taste, nausea

GU: Mild to moderate abnormalities in renal function

MS: Bone pain, decreased mineralization of nonaffected bones, hypocalcemia

SPECIAL CONSIDERATIONS

PATIENT/FAMILY EDUCATION

• Administer on empty stomach with H_2O, 2 hr ac

• Exceeding the 2 wk treatment periods for osteoporosis may lead to bone demineralization and osteomalacia

---

etodolac

(e-toe-doe'lak)
Rx: Lodine
Chemical Class: Acetic acid derivative
Therapeutic Class: NSAID with analgesic and antipyretic activity

---

CLINICAL PHARMACOLOGY

Mechanism of Action: Reversible cyclooxygenase (i.e., prostaglandin synthetase) inhibitor; non-selectively decreases the formation of both prostaglandins and thromboxane A_2; variable effects on lipoxygenase synthesis and subsequent leukotriene production; antiinflammatory, antipyretic, and analgesic activity; inhibits platelet aggregation

Pharmacokinetics

PO: Peak serum levels 1-2 hr; analgesic onset 30 min, analgesic duration 4-12 hr; rapidly and completely absorbed; serum protein binding >99%; metabolized by liver, metabolites excreted in urine and feces; $t_{1/2}$ 7.3 hr

INDICATIONS AND USES: Prevention of cognitive decline,* osteoarthritis, pain—mild to moderate, rheumatoid arthritis, soft tissue injuries*

DOSAGE

Adult

• *Osteoarthritis:* PO 800-1200 mg/day in divided doses initially, then adjust dose to 600-1200 mg/day in divided doses; do not exceed 1200 mg/day; patients <60 kg, not to exceed 20 mg/kg; SUS REL PO 400-1000 mg qd

• *Analgesia:* PO 200-400 mg q6-8h prn for acute pain, do not exceed 1200 mg/day; patients <60 kg, not to exceed 20 mg/kg

🔋 AVAILABLE FORMS/COST OF THERAPY

• Cap, Gel—Oral: 200 mg, 100's: **$106.18-$132.63;** 300 mg, 100's: **$120.23-$150.20**

• Tab, Uncoated—Oral: 400 mg, 100's: **$117.66-$158.78;** 500 mg, 100's: **$139.05-$159.80**

• Tab, SUS REL—Oral: 400 mg, 100's: **$144.28;** 500 mg 100's: **$150.78;** 600 mg, 100's: **$272.98**

CONTRAINDICATIONS: Bronchospasm, nasal polyps, angioedema precipitated by aspirin or other NSAIDs

PRECAUTIONS: History of GI ulceration, bleeding, or perforation; renal dysfunction, hypertension or cardiac conditions aggravated by fluid retention and edema, history of liver dysfunction

PREGNANCY AND LACTATION: Pregnancy category C (category D if used near term); breast milk excretion unknown; problems in humans have not been documented

SIDE EFFECTS/ADVERSE REACTIONS

CNS: Anxiety, confusion, depression, *dizziness,* drowsiness, fatigue, *headache,* insomnia, lightheadedness, tremors, vertigo

CV: **CHF, dysrhythmias,** fluid retention, palpitations, peripheral edema, tachycardia

EENT: Blurred vision, hearing loss, tinnitus

GI: Anorexia, cholestatic hepatitis, constipation, cramps, diarrhea, dry mouth, dyspepsia, flatulence, *GI bleeding,* jaundice, *nausea,* peptic ulcer, vomiting

GU: Azotemia, cystitis, dysuria, hematuria, oliguria, UTI

HEME: **Blood dyscrasias**

SKIN: Erythema, pruritus, purpura, rash, sweating, urticaria

INTERACTIONS

Drugs

3 *Aminoglycosides:* Reduced clearance with elevated aminoglycoside levels and potential for toxicity (especially indomethacin in premature infants; other NSAIDs probably)

3 *Antihypertensives (α-blockers, angiotensin-converting enzyme inhibitors, angiotensin II receptor blockers, β-blockers, diuretics):* Inhibition of antihypertensive and other favorable hemodynamic effects

3 *Corticosteroids:* Increased risk of GI ulceration

3 *Anticoagulants:* Excessive hypoprothrombinemia, decreased platelet aggregation with increased risk of GI bleeding

3 *Cyclosporine:* Increased nephrotoxicity risk

3 *Lithium:* Decreased clearance of lithium (mediated via prostaglandins) resulting in elevated serum lithium levels and risk of toxicity

3 *Methotrexate:* Decreased renal secretion of methotrexate resulting in elevated methotrexate levels and risk of toxicity

3 *Phenylpropanolamine:* Possible acute hypertensive reaction

3 *Potassium-sparing diuretics:* Additive hyperkalemia potential

---

italic = common side effects **bold italic** = life-threatening reactions

3 *Triamterene:* Acute renal failure reported with addition of indomethacin; caution with other NSAIDs

SPECIAL CONSIDERATIONS
• No significant advantage over other NSAIDs; cost should govern use

MONITORING PARAMETERS
• Initial hemogram and fecal occult blood test within 3 mo of starting regular chronic therapy; repeat every 6-12 mo (more frequently in high-risk patients (>65 years, peptic ulcer disease, concurrent steroids or anticoagulants); electrolytes, creatinine, and BUN within 3 mo of starting regular chronic therapy; repeat every 6-12 mo

---

etretinate
(e-tret'in-ate)
Rx: Tegison
Chemical Class: Retinoic acid derivative
Therapeutic Class: Antipsoriatic

CLINICAL PHARMACOLOGY
Mechanism of Action: Unknown; might reduce cell proliferation by inhibiting ornithine decarboxylase, a rate-limiting enzyme in regulation of cell growth, proliferation, and differentiation

Pharmacokinetics
PO: Peak 2-6 hr during chronic therapy; absorbed in small intestine; accumulates in adipose tissue, especially the liver and subcutaneous fat; significant 1st-pass hepatic metabolism to active acid form; primarily biliary excretion; $t_{1/2}$ 120 days

INDICATIONS AND USES: Severe recalcitrant psoriasis, including erythrodermic and generalized pustular types; bronchial metaplasia,*

mycosis fungoides,* actinic keratoses,* arsenical keratoses,* basal cell carcinomas,* genodermatosis,* pustular bacterids,* hyperkeratotic eczema of palms and soles,* cutaneous lupus erythematosus*

DOSAGE
Adult
• Psoriasis: PO 0.75-1 mg/kg/day in divided doses, not to exceed 1.5 mg/kg/day; maintenance dose 0.5-0.75 mg/kg/day generally beginning after 8-16 wk of therapy; terminate therapy in patients whose lesions have sufficiently resolved

$ **AVAILABLE FORMS/COST OF THERAPY**
• Cap, Gel—Oral: 10 mg, 30's: **$61.46;** 25 mg, 30's: **$96.11**

PRECAUTIONS: Children, hepatic disease, diabetes, obesity, increased alcohol intake, hypertriglyceridemia

PREGNANCY AND LACTATION: Pregnancy category X (effective contraception must be used at least 1 mo before, during, and following discontinuation of therapy for an indefinite period of time); excreted into milk of lactating rats; human breast milk data not available; not recommended during lactation

SIDE EFFECTS/ADVERSE REACTIONS
CNS: Amnesia, anxiety, depression, *dizziness, fatigue, fever, headache, pain,* pseudotumor cerebri
CV: Atrial fibrillation, chest pain, coagulation disorders, CV obstruction, edema
EENT: Change in lacrimation, cheilitis, *double vision, dry nose, eyes; earache, eye irritation,* nosebleed, *otitis externa; pain,* sore tongue
GI: Abdominal pain, anorexia, constipation, diarrhea, flatulence, hepatitis, increased transaminases, *nausea,* weight loss
GU: Acetonuria, casts, dysuria, gly-

---

* = non-FDA-approved use

cosuria; hematuria, hemoglobinuria, *increased BUN, creatinine;* proteinuria, *WBC in urine*

METAB: Decrease in HDL cholesterol; elevation of plasma triglycerides, total cholesterol; increased or decreased fasting blood sugar, increase or decrease K, Ca, P, Na, Cl

MS: Bone pain, cramps, gout, *hyperostosis,* hypertonia, *myalgia*

RESP: Cough, dyspnea

SKIN: Alopecia; bruising, dryness; itching, nail changes, onycholysis, paronychia, *peeling of palms, soles, fingertips; rash,* perspiration change, pyogenic granuloma, rash, red scaling face; sunburn

INTERACTIONS

Drugs

❷ *Methotrexate:* Increased potential for hepatotoxicity

❸ *Vitamin A:* Additive toxicity possible

SPECIAL CONSIDERATIONS

PATIENT/FAMILY EDUCATION

• Take with food or milk

• Contact lens intolerance is common

• Transient exacerbation of psoriasis common during initiation of therapy

• Do not take vitamin A supplements

MONITORING PARAMETERS

• Fasting lipid panels

---

famciclovir

(fam-si′klo-veer)

Rx: Famvir

Chemical Class: Acyclic purine nucleoside analog

Therapeutic Class: Antiviral

CLINICAL PHARMACOLOGY

Mechanism of Action: Converted to penciclovir in intestinal and hepatic tissue, then phosphorylated intracellularly to penciclovir triphosphate which inhibits viral DNA synthesis

Pharmacokinetics

PO: Onset 15 min, peak 45-55 min, duration 6 hr; bioavailability 80%, not affected by food; protein binding 20%; metabolized to penciclovir, which is excreted in urine (60%) and stool; $t_{1/2}$ 2 hr (longer in renal insufficiency), intracellular $t_{1/2}$ 10-20 hr

INDICATIONS AND USES: Acute herpes zoster infection, acute treatment of initial* and recurrent episodes of genital herpes simplex, suppression of recurrent genital herpes

DOSAGE

Adult

• *Herpes zoster:* 500 mg q8h for 7 days, initiated as soon as possible after diagnosis; if CrCl 40-59 ml/min, use 500 mg q12h for 7 days; if CrCl 20-39 ml/min, use 500 mg q24h for 7 days; if CrCl <20 ml/min, use 500 mg q48h

• *Genital herpes simplex:* 125 mg q12h for 5 days; if CrCl 20-39 ml/min, use 125 mg q24h for 5 days; if CrCl <20 ml/min, use 125 mg q48h for 5 days

• *Suppression of genital herpes:* 250 mg bid; if CrCl 20-39 ml/min, use 125 mg q12h; if CrCl <20 ml/min, use 125 mg q24h

💲 **AVAILABLE FORMS/COST OF THERAPY**

• Tab—Oral: 125 mg, 30's: **$92.25;** 250 mg, 30's: **$105.10**; 500 mg, 30's: **$210.95**

PRECAUTIONS: Renal insufficiency, children

PREGNANCY AND LACTATION: Pregnancy category B; excreted in breast milk

SIDE EFFECTS/ADVERSE REACTIONS

CNS: Bradykinesia, confusion, dizziness, *headache,* somnolence

---

italic = common side effects   ***bold italic*** = life-threatening reactions

GI: Anorexia, constipation, *diarrhea (8%), nausea (13%)*
MS: Arthralgia
SKIN: Pruritus, purpura

SPECIAL CONSIDERATIONS
• Reserve chronic suppressive therapy for patients without prodromal symptoms who have frequent recurrences

---

famotidine
(fam-o'tah-deen)
Rx: Pepcid, Pepcid RPD
OTC: Mylanta AR, Pepcid AC
Chemical Class: Thiazole derivative
Therapeutic Class: Gastrointestinal antiulcer agent

CLINICAL PHARMACOLOGY
Mechanism of Action: Competitive, reversible inhibitor of histamine at gastric H_2-receptors; reduces gastric acid secretion
Pharmacokinetics
PO: Onset 30-60 min, duration 6-12 hr, peak 1-3 hr
IV: Onset immediate, peak 30-60 min, duration 6-12 hr
Oral absorption 50%; plasma protein binding 15%-20%; metabolized in liver 30%; 70% excreted by kidneys unchanged; $t_{1/2}$ 2½-3½ hr (>20 hr with CrCl <10 ml/min)

INDICATIONS AND USES: Short-term treatment of duodenal and benign gastric ulcers; maintenance therapy for duodenal ulcer; pathological hypersecretory conditions (e.g., Zollinger-Ellison syndrome, multiple endocrine adenomas); gastroesophageal reflux disease (GERD) and esophagitis due to GERD; heartburn, acid indigestion, and sour stomach (OTC), GI bleeding,* prophylaxis for aspiration pneumonitis*

DOSAGE
Adult
• *Duodenal ulcer:* PO 40 mg qd hs × 4-8 wk, then 20 mg qd hs if needed (maintenance); IV 20 mg q12h if unable to take PO
• *Gastric ulcer:* PO 40 mg qhs
• *GERD:* PO 20 mg bid for up to 6 wk; for esophagitis due to GERD, 20-40 mg bid for up to 12 wk
• *Hypersecretory conditions:* PO 20 mg q6h; may give 160 mg q6h if needed; IV 20 mg q12h if unable to take PO
• *Heartburn, acid indigestion, and sour stomach (OTC):* PO 10 mg bid prn; for prevention of heartburn, take 1 hr ac
• *Renal failure (CrCl <10 ml/min):* PO 20 mg qhs or increase dosing interval to 36-48 hr

💲 AVAILABLE FORMS/COST OF THERAPY
• Granule, Reconst—Oral Susp: 40 mg/5 ml, 50 ml: **$90.53**
• Tab, Plain Coated—Oral (OTC): 10 mg, 18's: **$6.30-$6.71**
• Tab, Chewable—Oral (OTC): 10 mg, 18's: **$6.71**
• Tab, Plain Coated—Oral: 20 mg, 100's: **$170.45;** 40 mg, 100's: **$329.41**
• Tab, Oral Disintegrating—Oral: 20 mg, 100's: **$187.50;** 40 mg, 100's: **$362.50**
• Inj, Sol—IV: 10 mg/ml, 2 ml: **$3.98**

PRECAUTIONS: Severe renal disease, severe hepatic function

PREGNANCY AND LACTATION: Pregnancy category B; concentrated in breast milk (less than cimetidine or ranitidine); no problems reported with other H_2-histamine receptor antagonists; compatible with breast feeding

SIDE EFFECTS/ADVERSE REACTIONS
CNS: Anxiety, depression, dizziness,

---

* = non-FDA-approved use

fever, headache, insomnia, paresthesia, *seizures,* somnolence
EENT: Orbital edema, taste change, tinnitus
GI: Abnormal liver enzymes, anorexia, constipation, cramps, nausea, vomiting
*HEME: **Thrombocytopenia***
MS: Arthralgia, myalgia
*RESP: **Bronchospasm***
SKIN: Rash

INTERACTIONS
Drugs
🔢 *Cefpodoxime, cefuroxime, enoxacin, ketoconazole:* Reduction in gastric acidity reduces absorption, decreased plasma levels, potential for therapeutic failure
🔢 *Glipizide; glyburide; tolbutamide:* Increased absorption of these drugs, potential for hypoglycemia
🔢 *Nifedipine; nitrendipine; nisoldipine:* Increased concentrations of these drugs

SPECIAL CONSIDERATIONS
• No advantage over other agents in this class, base selection on cost
PATIENT/FAMILY EDUCATION
• Stagger doses of famotidine and antacids

---

felodipine
(fell-o'da-peen)
Rx: Plendil
Combinations
  Rx: with enalapril (Lexxel)
Chemical Class: Dihydropyridine
Therapeutic Class: Calcium channel blocker: antihypertensive; antianginal

CLINICAL PHARMACOLOGY
Mechanism of Action: Inhibits calcium ion influx across cell membrane in vascular smooth muscle and cardiac muscle; produces relaxation of coronary and peripheral vascular smooth muscle; hemodynamics: increases myocardial contractility and cardiac output; significantly decreases peripheral vascular resistance
Pharmacokinetics
PO: Onset 2-5 hr, peak 2.5-5 hr, rapid and complete absorption; extensive 1st pass metabolism; 15% systemic bioavailability; 99% protein bound; metabolized in liver, 0.5% excreted unchanged in urine; t₁/₂ 11-16 hr

INDICATIONS AND USES: Hypertension, vasospastic angina,* effort-associated angina,* primary pulmonary hypertension,* Raynaud's disease,* CHF*
DOSAGE
Adult
• *Hypertension:* PO 5 mg qd initially (2.5 mg in elderly and impaired liver function), usual range 5-10 mg qd; do not exceed 20 mg qd; do not adjust dosage at intervals of <2 wk
💲 **AVAILABLE FORMS/COST OF THERAPY**
• Tab, Uncoated, SUS Action—Oral: 2.5, 5 mg, 100's: **$99.37;** 10 mg, 100's: **$178.56**
PRECAUTIONS: Hypotension (<90 mm Hg systolic), hepatic injury, children, renal disease, elderly
PREGNANCY AND LACTATION: Pregnancy category C
SIDE EFFECTS/ADVERSE REACTIONS
CNS: Anxiety, depression, dizziness, fatigue, headache, insomnia, light headedness, tinnitus
CV: Edema, hypotension, *MI,* palpitations, pulmonary edema, tachycardia, syncope
EENT: Cough, epistaxis, nasal congestion
GI: Gastric upset, gingival hyperplasia
GU: Nocturia, polyuria

italic = common side effects   ***bold italic*** = life-threatening reactions

HEME: Anemia

RESP: Shortness of breath, wheezing

SKIN: Pruritus, rash

MISC: Flushing, sexual difficulties

INTERACTIONS

Drugs

3 *Barbiturates:* Decreased felodipine bioavailability

3 *Digitalis glycosides:* Increased digitalis levels; increased risk of toxicity

3 *Erythromycin:* Increased felodipine concentrations

3 *Fentanyl:* Severe hypotension or increased fluid volume requirements

3 *Grapefruit juice:* Inhibits felodipine metabolism, 200% increase in AUC

3 *Histamine H_2 antagonists:* Increased bioavailability of felodipine

3 *Hydantoins:* Serum felodipine level may be decreased

3 *Propranolol:* Enhanced hypotension, increased propranolol concentrations

SPECIAL CONSIDERATIONS

• Results of V-HeFT III indicate felodipine may be used safely in patients with left ventricular dysfunction

PATIENT/FAMILY EDUCATION

• Administer as whole tablet (do not crush or chew)

• Avoid grapefruit juice (see drug interactions)

---

fenoldopam

(fen-ole'doe-pam)

Rx: Corlopam

Chemical Class: Benzazepine derivative

Therapeutic Class: Antihypertensive

CLINICAL PHARMACOLOGY

Mechanism of Action: Selective agonist at dopamine (DA_1) receptors; exerts hypotensive effects via decrease in peripheral vascular resistance, with increased renal blood flow, diuresis, and natriuresis

Pharmacokinetics

IV: Steady state plasma concentration in 15-20 min; duration 1 hr following discontinuation of infusion; metabolized in liver to a variety of sulfate, glucuronide and methoxy metabolites; 80% excreted in urine (metabolites), 20% excreted in feces; elimination $t_{1/2}$ 5 min

INDICATIONS AND USES: In-hospital, short-term (≤48 hr) management of severe hypertension when rapid, but quickly reversible, emergency reduction of blood pressure is needed

DOSAGE

Adult

• IV INF 0.1 µg/kg/min initially with upward titration q15min; average required maintenance dose in clinical studies was 0.5 µg/kg/min; in severe CHF, doses of 0.1-1.5 µg/kg/min have been studied

$ **AVAILABLE FORMS/COST OF THERAPY**

• Inj—Conc: 10 mg/mL, 5 mL: **$1155.00;** 1 ml: **$240.00**

PRECAUTIONS: History of portal hypertension or previous variceal bleeding; history of dysrhythmia; CAD; angle-closure glaucoma

PREGNANCY AND LACTATION: Pregnancy category B; breast milk excretion unknown; use caution

SIDE EFFECTS/ADVERSE REACTIONS

CNS: Dizziness, *headache*

CV: Angina, *dysrhythmia,* ECG changes, hypotension, peripheral edema, *tachycardia,* ischemic heart disease

EENT: Blurred vision, increased intraocular pressure

GI: Diarrhea, dry mouth, nausea, vomiting

---

* = non-FDA-approved use

HEME: Leukocytosis, bleeding
METAB: Elevated BUN, glucose, transaminase, LDH
RESP: Dyspnea, URT
SKIN: Flushing

SPECIAL CONSIDERATIONS
• Equivalent to nitroprusside in head-to-head comparison in patients with severe hypertension; renal function was improved in patients with hypertension and renal dysfunction
• Use should probably be limited to those patients with severe hypertension

MONITORING PARAMETERS
• Blood pressure, heart rate, urine volume, urinary sodium, serum creatinine, serum potassium, and BUN

---

fenoprofen
(fen-oh-proe′fen)
Rx: Nalfon
Chemical Class: Propionic acid derivative
Therapeutic Class: NSAID with analgesic and antipyretic activity

CLINICAL PHARMACOLOGY
Mechanism of Action: Reversible cyclooxygenase (i.e., prostaglandin synthetase) inhibitor; non-selectively decreases the formation of both prostaglandins and thromboxane A_2; variable effects on lipoxygenase synthesis and subsequent leukotriene production; antiinflammatory, antipyretic, and analgesic activity; inhibits platelet aggregation
Pharmacokinetics
PO: Rapid absorption, peak level 2 hr, metabolized in liver, metabolites excreted in urine; 99% protein binding to albumin; $t_{1/2}$ 3 hr

INDICATIONS AND USES: Osteoarthritis, rheumatoid arthritis, ankylosing spondylitis,* prevention of cognitive decline,* pain—mild to moderate, migraine headache,* tendonitis*

DOSAGE
Adult
• *Pain:* PO 200 mg q4-6h prn
• *Arthritis:* PO 300-600 mg tid-qid, not to exceed 3.2 g/day

$ AVAILABLE FORMS/COST OF THERAPY
• Cap, Gel—Oral: 200 mg, 100's: **$56.04;** 300 mg, 100's: **$43.89**
• Tab, Uncoated—Oral: 600 mg, 100's: **$47.19-$67.95**

CONTRAINDICATIONS: Bronchospasm, nasal polyps, angioedema precipitated by aspirin or other NSAIDs

PRECAUTIONS: History of GI ulceration, bleeding, or perforation; renal dysfunction, hypertension or cardiac conditions aggravated by fluid retention and edema, history of liver dysfunction, history of coagulation deficits

PREGNANCY AND LACTATION: Pregnancy category B (D, 3rd trimester); excreted in breast milk

SIDE EFFECTS/ADVERSE REACTIONS
CNS: Anxiety, confusion, depression, dizziness, drowsiness, fatigue, headache, insomnia, tremors
CV: **Dysrhythmias,** palpitations, peripheral edema, tachycardia
EENT: Blurred vision, hearing loss, tinnitus
GI: Anorexia, cholestatic hepatitis, *constipation,* cramps, diarrhea, dry mouth, *dyspepsia, nausea,* **peptic ulcer,** vomiting
GU: Azotemia, dysuria, hematuria, *interstitial nephritis*
HEME: **Agranulocytosis, aplastic anemia, hemolytic anemia, thrombocytopenia**
METAB: Hyperkalemia

---

italic = common side effects **bold italic** = life-threatening reactions

SKIN: Pruritus, purpura, rash, sweating

INTERACTIONS
Drugs

3 *Aminoglycosides:* Reduced clearance with elevated aminoglycoside levels and potential for toxicity (especially indomethacin in premature infants; other NSAIDs probably)

3 *Antihypertensives (α-blockers, angiotensin-converting enzyme inhibitors, angiotensin II receptor blockers, β-blockers, diuretics):* Inhibition of antihypertensive and other favorable hemodynamic effects

3 *Corticosteroids:* Increased risk of GI ulceration

3 *Anticoagulants:* Excessive hypoprothrombinemia, decreased platelet aggregation with increased risk of GI bleeding

3 *Cyclosporine:* Increased nephrotoxicity risk

3 *Lithium:* Decreased clearance of lithium (mediated via prostaglandins) resulting in elevated serum lithium levels and risk of toxicity

3 *Methotrexate:* Decreased renal secretion of methotrexate resulting in elevated methotrexate levels and risk of toxicity

3 *Phenylpropranolamine:* Possible acute hypertensive reaction

3 *Potassium-sparing diuretics:* Additive hyperkalemia potential

3 *Triamterene:* Acute renal failure reported with addition of indomethacin; caution with other NSAIDs

Labs
• *False increase:* Free and total triiodothyronine levels, plasma cortisol
• *False positive:* Urine barbiturate, urine benzodiazepine

SPECIAL CONSIDERATIONS
• No significant advantage over other NSAIDs; cost should govern use

MONITORING PARAMETERS
• Initial hemogram and fecal occult blood test within 3 mo of starting regular chronic therapy; repeat every 6-12 mo (more frequently in high-risk patients (>65 years, peptic ulcer disease, concurrent steroids or anticoagulants); electrolytes, creatinine, and BUN within 3 mo of starting regular chronic therapy; repeat every 6-12 mo

---

fentanyl
(fen'ta-nill)
Rx: *Injection:* Sublimaze
Transdermal: Duragesic
Lozenge: Fentanyl Oralet, Actiq
Combinations
  Rx: with droperidol (Innovar)
Chemical Class: Synthetic opium alkaloid; phenylpiperidine derivative
Therapeutic Class: Narcotic analgesic
DEA Class: Schedule II

CLINICAL PHARMACOLOGY
Mechanism of Action: Narcotic agonist with activity at μ-receptors (supraspinal analgesia, euphoria, respiratory and physical depression, miosis, and reduced GI motility), Kappa receptors (pentazocine-like spinal analgesia, sedation, and miosis), and Delta receptors (dysphoria, psychotomimetic effects [e.g., hallucinations], and respiratory and vasomotor stimulation caused by drugs with antagonist activity); compared to morphine, equal analgesia, less respiratory depression and emesis

Pharmacokinetics

IM: Onset 7-15 min, peak 30 min, duration 1-2 hr

IV: Onset 1-2 min, peak 3-5 min, duration ½-1 hr

LOZ: Onset 5-15 min, peak 20-30 min; 50% bioavailability with rapid transmucosal and slower GI absorption

TRANS: Steady state plasma level 24 hr after application, 6 days after change of dose; plasma level $t_{1/2}$ 17 hr after patch removal due to some continued absorption

Metabolized by liver, excreted by kidneys, excretion $t_{1/2}$ 2½-4 hr; highly lipophilic, 80% bound to plasma proteins, crosses placenta, stored in fat and muscle (may lead to prolonged effect with repeated administration)

INDICATIONS AND USES: Perioperative analgesia; adjunct to general anesthesia (alone or combined with droperidol); general anesthesia; chronic pain (transdermal)

DOSAGE

Adult and Child >12 yr

• *Chronic pain:* Trans 25 µg/hr system initially; initial dose may be increased after 3 days, thereafter a minimum of 6 days should elapse between dosage increases; to convert patients already receiving other narcotics, refer to manufacturer product information; change system q72h

• *Sedation for minor procedure:* Buccal 5 µg/kg (max 400 µg) 20-40 min prior to procedure

• *Preoperatively:* IM 50-100 µg 30-60 min before surgery

• *Adjunct to general anesthesia:* IV 2-50 µg/kg

• *Adjunct to regional anesthesia:* IM/IV 50-100 µg when additional analgesia required

• *General anesthesia:* IV 50-100 µg/kg with oxygen and a muscle relaxant

• *Postoperatively:* IM 50-100 µg q1-2h prn

Child 2-12 yr

• *Sedation for minor procedure:* Buccal 5-10 µg/kg (max 400 µg) 20-40 min prior to procedure; children <40 kg may require doses of 10-15 µg/kg (max 400 µg); do not use in child <2 yr

• *Adjunct to anesthesia:* IV 2-3 µg/kg

Notes:

1. IV/IM dose of 0.1 mg fentanyl equianalgesic to 10 mg of morphine, 75 mg of meperidine

2. Transdermal fentanyl dose of 100 µg/hr equianalgesic to 60 mg morphine IM or 360 mg morphine PO per 24 hr

3. Buccal dose of 5 µg fentanyl equianalgesic to 1 µg IM fentanyl

💲 **AVAILABLE FORMS/COST OF THERAPY**

• Inj, Sol—IM, IV: 0.05 mg/ml, 2 ml: **$0.36-$9.31**

• Loz, Top—Oral: 200, 300, 400 µg, 1's: **$137.50**

• Loz, Top—on a stick: 0.2 mg, **$166.23;** 0.4 mg, **$214.32;** 0.6 mg, **$261.92;** 0.8 mg, **$309.51;** 1.2 mg, **$404.99;** 1.6 mg, **$499.89**

• Film, CON REL—Percutaneous: 25 µg/hr, 5's: **$58.79;** 50 µg/hr, 5's: **$92.46;** 75 µg/hr, 5's: **$148.14;** 100 µg/hr, 5's: **$184.56**

CONTRAINDICATIONS: Lozenge for child <15 kg, transdermal for child <12 yr

PRECAUTIONS: Elderly, respiratory depression, increased intracranial pressure, seizure disorders, severe respiratory disorders, cardiac dysrhythmias

PREGNANCY AND LACTATION: Pregnancy category C; excreted in breast milk

---

italic = common side effects   ***bold italic*** = life-threatening reactions

**SIDE EFFECTS/ADVERSE REAC-
TIONS**

CNS: Asthenia, *confusion,* delirium,
dizziness, euphoria, *somnolence*

CV: Bradycardia, hypotension or hypertension

EENT: Blurred vision, *dry mouth,*
miosis

GI: Constipation, nausea, vomiting

GU: Urinary retention

MS: Muscle rigidity

RESP: Laryngospasm, **respiratory
depression**

SKIN: Pruritis, sweating

INTERACTIONS

Drugs

3 *Antihistamines, chloral hydrate,
glutethimide, methocarbamol:* Enhanced depressant effects

3 *Barbiturates:* Additive respiratory and CNS-depressant effects

3 *Cimetidine:* Increased respiratory and CNS depression

3 *Diazepam:* Cardiovascular depression

3 *Ethanol:* Additive CNS effects

3 *Nitrous oxide:* Cardiovascular
depression

Labs

False elevations of serum amylase
and lipase

SPECIAL CONSIDERATIONS

• Increased skin temperature increases absorption rate of transdermal preparation

• Lozenge should be used only in a
monitored anesthesia care setting

• Following removal of transdermal system, 17 hr are required for
50% decrease in serum fentanyl concentrations

• Do not administer agonist/antagonist analgesics (i.e., pentazocine,
nalbuphine, butorphanol, dezocine,
buprenorphine) to patient who has
received a prolonged course of fentanyl (a pure agonist). In opioid-

dependent patients, mixed agonist/
antagonist analgesics may precipitate withdrawal symptoms

---

ferrous salts

OTC: *Sulfate:* Feosol,
Feratab, Fer-in-sol, Fer-Iron,
Fero-Gradumet, Mol-Iron
Sulfate exsiccated: Feosol,
Fer-in-Sol, Ferra-TD, Slow Fe
Gluconate: Fergon, Simron
Fumarate: Femiron, Feostat,
Hemocyte, Ircon, Nephro-Fer
Polysaccharide-Iron complex:
Hytinic, Niferex, Nu-Iron
Combinations

OTC: with magnesium and
aluminum hydroxide
(Fermalox); with docusate
(Ferocyl, Ferro-Sequels,
Ferro-Docusate, Ferro-dok
TR, Ferro-DSS SR); with
vitamin C (Mol-Iron with
Vitamin C, Ferancee-HP,
Vitron-C Plus, Cevi-Fer,
Irospan, Fero-Grad,
Hemaspan); with folate
(Palafer CF); with multivitamins (Flintstones Plus
Iron, Stresstabs with Iron)

Chemical Class: Iron preparation

Therapeutic Class: Hematinic

CLINICAL PHARMACOLOGY

Mechanism of Action: Replaces
iron stores; hematologic response
begins in 3 days

Pharmacokinetics

PO: Absorbed in duodenum and upper jejunum, absorption decreased
by food and achlorhydria; bound to
transferrin; crosses placenta; excreted in feces, urine

INDICATIONS AND USES: Prevention and treatment of iron deficiency anemia; adjunct to epoetin
therapy*

---

* = non-FDA-approved use

DOSAGE (all expressed in elemental iron)

Adult

• *Iron deficiency:* PO 100-200 mg/day divided tid

• *Pregnancy:* PO 30 mg/day

Child

• *Iron deficiency:* (2-12 yr) PO 3 mg/kg/day divided tid-qid; (6 mo-2 yr) PO up to 6 mg/kg/day divided tid-qid; (infants) PO 10-25 mg/day divided tid-qid

• *Prophylaxis:* 1-2 mg/kg/day in 3 divided doses

NOTE: Ferrous fumarate is 33% elemental iron (325 mg has 106 mg); gluconate 12% elemental iron (325 mg has 38 mg); sulfate 20% elemental iron (325 mg has 65 mg)

$ AVAILABLE FORMS/COST OF THERAPY

Ferrous fumarate

• Tab—Oral: 63 mg, 40's: **$5.38**

• Tab—Oral: 200 mg, 100's: **$8.00**

• Tab—Oral: 325 mg, 100's: **$1.87-$20.00**

• Tab—Oral: 350 mg, 30's: **$7.14**

• Tab, Chewable—Oral: 100 mg, 100s: **$18.73**

• Liq—Oral: 45 mg/0.6 ml, 60 ml: **$18.20**

• Susp—Oral: 100 mg/5 ml, 240 ml: **$21.00**

Ferrous gluconate

• Tab—Oral: 300 mg, 100's: **$3.18-$4.43**

• Tab—Oral: 320 mg, 100's: **$6.52**

• Tab, Enteric Coated—Oral: 325 mg, 100's: **$3.50**

• Cap, soft Gel—Oral: 86 mg, 100's: **$35.65**

• Tab—Oral: 325 mg, 100s: **$1.45-$6.08**

• Elixir—Oral: 300 mg/5 ml, 480 ml: **$19.25**

Ferrous sulfate

• Tab—Oral: 50 mg, 100's: **$23.41;** 195 mg, 100's: **$5.42;** 200 mg, 100's: **$7.72;** 300 mg, 100's: **$3.96;** 325 mg, 100's: **$0.85-$5.85**

• Tab, Enteric Coated—Oral: 325 mg, 100's: **$1.95-$2.95**

• Tab, SUS REL—Oral: 160 mg, 90's: **$17.33;** 525 mg, 100's: **$27.65**

• Cap—Oral: 325 mg, 100's: **$4.43**

• Cap, SUS REL—Oral: 150 mg, 100's: **$2.25;** 250 mg, 100's: **$2.25-$5.00**

• Elixir—Oral: 220 mg/5 ml, 480 ml: **$3.75-$9.95**

• Liq—Oral: 75 mg/0.6 ml, 50 ml: **$1.60-$9.69**

• Syr—Oral: 90 mg/5 ml, 480 ml: **$14.76**

CONTRAINDICATIONS: Ulcerative colitis; regional enteritis, hemosiderosis; hemochromatosis, hemolytic anemia

PREGNANCY AND LACTATION: Pregnancy category A; excreted in breast milk

SIDE EFFECTS/ADVERSE REACTIONS

GI: Black stools, *constipation,* diarrhea, *epigastric pain, nausea,* vomiting

SKIN: Temporarily discolored tooth enamel (liq) and eyes

INTERACTIONS

Drugs

3 *Antacids:* Reduce iron absorption

3 *Ciprofloxacin, levodopa, levofloxacin, methyldopa, norfloxacin, penicillamine, tetracyclines, vitamin E:* Absorption reduced by iron

3 *Enalapril:* Three patients on enalapril developed systemic reactions following IV iron; causal relationship not established

Labs

• Urine discoloration black, brown, or dark color

• *Glucose:* Decreased with clinistix, diastix; no effect observed with testape

---

italic = common side effects   ***bold italic*** = life-threatening reactions

• *Occult blood:* 25-65% false positives

SPECIAL CONSIDERATIONS PATIENT/FAMILY EDUCATION

• Best absorbed on empty stomach, may take with food if GI upset occurs

• Drink liquid iron preparations in water or juice and through a straw to prevent tooth stains

• 4-6 mo of therapy generally required

• Iron changes stools black or dark green

MONITORING PARAMETERS

• Hemoglobin, hematocrit

---

fexofenadine

(fex-oh-fen'eh-deen)
Rx: Allegra
Chemical Class: Piperidine derivative
Therapeutic Class: Antihistamine

CLINICAL PHARMACOLOGY

Mechanism of Action: Decreases allergic response by blocking histamine at H_1-receptors; no QT prolongation even at very high plasma concentrations

Pharmacokinetics

PO: Active metabolite of terfenadine; onset 1 hr, peak 2.6 hr, duration 12 hr; absorption 90%, protein binding 70%, minimal metabolism; $t_{1/2}$ 14.4 hr; excreted in stool (80%) and urine (11%)

INDICATIONS AND USES: Seasonal allergic rhinitis

DOSAGE

Adult

• PO: 60 mg bid; if CrCl <40 ml/min, reduce dose to 60 mg qd

Child >12 yr

• PO: 60 mg bid; if CrCl <40 ml/min, reduce dose to 60 mg qd

AVAILABLE FORMS/COST OF THERAPY

• Tab—Oral: 60 mg, 100's: **$99.42**; 180 mg, 100's: **$206.00**

PRECAUTIONS: Concurrent use of macrolide antibiotics, azole antifungals, or agents that inhibit cytochrome P450 3A4 isozyme

PREGNANCY AND LACTATION: Pregnancy category C; breast milk excretion unknown

SIDE EFFECTS/ADVERSE REACTIONS

CNS: Drowsiness (1%), fatigue, headache
GI: Dyspepsia, nausea
GU: Dysmenorrhea

SPECIAL CONSIDERATIONS

• Essentially the same as terfenadine without the potential for QT prolongation; relatively weak antihistamine with minimal sedation

• Consider alternating q hs chlorpeniramine with qam fexofenadine 60 mg to minimize cost

---

finasteride

(feen-as'ter-ide)
Rx: Proscar, Propecia
Chemical Class: 5α-reductase inhibitor
Therapeutic Class: Benign prostatic hypertrophy agent, hair growth stimulant

CLINICAL PHARMACOLOGY

Mechanism of Action: Inhibits the enzyme responsible for converting testosterone to 5α-dihydrotestosterone (DHT) reducing the levels of DHT available for development of the prostate gland and other DHT-dependent organs

Pharmacokinetics

PO: Bioavailability 63%, peak 1-2 hr, plasma protein binding 90%; metabolized in the liver, 39% excreted in urine (metabolites), 57%

---

in feces; $t_{1/2}$ 6 hr; crosses blood-brain barrier

INDICATIONS AND USES: Symptomatic benign prostatic hypertrophy (<50% of patients experience an increase in urinary flow and improvement in symptoms), male pattern hair loss (vertex and anterior midscalp), prostate cancer*

DOSAGE

Adult

• *BPH:* PO 5 mg qd

• Hair loss: PO 1 mg qd; ≥3 mos necessary for benefit to be noted

💲 **AVAILABLE FORMS/COST OF THERAPY**

• Tab, Plain Coated—Oral: 5 mg, 100's: **$227.95-$232.09**; 1 mg, 100's: **$156.25**

CONTRAINDICATIONS: Children, women

PRECAUTIONS: Hepatic function impairment, obstructive uropathy

PREGNANCY AND LACTATION: Pregnancy category X; not indicated for use in women; pregnant women should not handle crushed tablets

SIDE EFFECTS/ADVERSE REACTIONS

GU: Decreased libido, decreased volume of ejaculate, impotence

SPECIAL CONSIDERATIONS

• Minimal benefit for benign prostatic hypertrophy if the prostate is not very large; response is not immediate

• Combination therapy with α-blocker may be optimal

• Whether long-term treatment can reduce prostate cancer risk is unknown; decreases prostate specific antigen (PSA)

PATIENT/FAMILY EDUCATION

• Condoms should be used if the female partner is at risk of pregnancy

• Withdrawal of drug for hair loss leads to reversal within 12 mo

MONITORING PARAMETERS

• 6-12 mo of therapy may be necessary in some patients to assess effectiveness (BPH), 3 or more mo for hair loss

---

flavoxate

(fla-vox'ate)

Rx: Urispas

Chemical Class: Flavone derivative

Therapeutic Class: Genitourinary muscle relaxant

CLINICAL PHARMACOLOGY

Mechanism of Action: Relaxes the detrusor and other smooth muscle by cholinergic blockade, also exerts a direct effect on the muscle

Pharmacokinetics

PO: Onset 55 min, peak 112 min; 57% excreted in urine within 24 hr

INDICATIONS AND USES: Relief of nocturia, incontinence, suprapubic pain, dysuria, frequency associated with urologic conditions (symptomatic only)

DOSAGE

Adult and Child >12 yr

• PO 100-200 mg tid-qid, reduce dose when symptoms improve

💲 **AVAILABLE FORMS/COST OF THERAPY**

• Tab, Plain Coated—Oral: 100 mg, 100's: **$85.80**

CONTRAINDICATIONS: Pyloric or duodenal obstruction, obstructive intestinal lesions or ileus, achalasia, GI hemorrhage, obstructive uropathies of the lower urinary tract

PRECAUTIONS: Glaucoma, children <12 yr

PREGNANCY AND LACTATION: Pregnancy category B; excretion

italic = common side effects   ***bold italic*** = life-threatening reactions

into breast milk unknown; use caution in nursing mothers

SIDE EFFECTS/ADVERSE REACTIONS

CNS: Drowsiness, headache, mental confusion (especially in the elderly), nervousness, vertigo

CV: Tachycardia and palpitation

EENT: Blurred vision, disturbance in eye accommodation, increased ocular tension

GI: Dry mouth, *nausea,* vomiting

GU: Dysuria

*HEME: **Leukopenia*** (rare)

SKIN: Urticaria and other dermatoses

SPECIAL CONSIDERATIONS
• Urinary antispasmodic that is no more effective than propantheline or other similar agents

---

flecainide

(fle′kah-nide)

Rx: Tambocor

Chemical Class: Benzamide derivative

Therapeutic Class: Antidysrhythmic (Class IC)

CLINICAL PHARMACOLOGY

Mechanism of Action: Produces a dose-related decrease in intracardiac conduction in all parts of the heart with the greatest effect on the His-Purkinje system; causes slight prolongation of refractory periods; decreases the rate of rise of the action potential without affecting its duration

Pharmacokinetics

PO: Peak 3 hr, 40%-50% bound to plasma proteins (α_1-glycoprotein), $t_{1/2}$ 12-27 hr; metabolized by liver, excreted by kidneys

INDICATIONS AND USES: Paroxysmal atrial fibrillation (PAF) and paroxysmal supraventricular tachycardias (PSVT) associated with disabling symptoms; documented life-threatening ventricular dysrhythmias

DOSAGE

Adult

• *PSVT and PAF:* PO 50 mg q12h; may increase q4d by 50 mg q12h to desired response; not to exceed 300 mg/day

• *Sustained ventricular tahcycardia:* PO 100 mg q12h; may increase q4d by 50 mg q12h to desired response; not to exceed 400 mg/day

Child

• PO 3 mg/kg/day divided tid; may increase up to 11 mg/kg/day for uncontrolled patients with subtherapeutic levels

§ AVAILABLE FORMS/COST OF THERAPY

• Tab, Uncoated—Oral: 50 mg, 100's: **$128.46;** 100 mg, 100's: **$206.76;** 150 mg, 100's: **$284.58**

CONTRAINDICATIONS: Severe heart block, cardiogenic shock, nonsustained ventricular dysrhythmias, frequent PVCs, non-life-threatening dysrhythmias (due to proarrhythmic effects), recent MI

PRECAUTIONS: Children, renal disease, liver disease, CHF, respiratory depression, myasthenia gravis, sick sinus syndrome, electrolyte disturbances

PREGNANCY AND LACTATION: Pregnancy category C; excreted into breast milk with milk-plasma ratios 1.6:3.7, but considered compatible with breast feeding

SIDE EFFECTS/ADVERSE REACTIONS

CNS: Amnesia, anxiety, ataxia, confusion, depression, *dizziness,* euphoria, *faintness, fatigue, headache,* hypoesthesia, insomnia, *lightheadedness,* malaise, neuropathy, paresis, paresthesia, ***seizures,*** somnolence, stupor, syncope, tremor, twitching, unsteadiness, vertigo, weakness

CV: Angina pectoris, *AV block, bradycardia,* chest pain, *CHF, dysrhythmia,* edema, hypertension, hypotension, palpitation, *sinus arrest, sinus pause,* tachycardia

EENT: Blurred vision, diplopia; eye pain, irritation; nystagmus, photophobia, visual disturbances

GI: Abdominal pain, anorexia, change in taste, *constipation,* dry mouth, dyspepsia, flatulence, *nausea,* vomiting

GU: Decreased libido, impotence, polyuria, urinary retention

HEME: Leukopenia, thrombocytopenia

MS: Arthralgia, myalgia

RESP: Bronchospasm

SKIN: Alopecia, *exfoliative dermatitis,* pruritus, rash, urticaria

INTERACTIONS

Drugs

3 *Acetazolamide, ammonium chloride, antacids, sodium bicarbonate:* Increases in urine pH decreases flecanide urinary clearance

3 *Amiodarone:* Reduced flecainide dosage requirements

3 *Cimetidine:* Inhibits metabolism of flecainide

3 *Propranolol:* Inhibitors of each other's metabolism; additive negative inotropic effects

3 *Sotolol:* Additive myocardial conduction depression; cardiac arrest reported

SPECIAL CONSIDERATIONS

• Not 1st line therapy

• Reserve for resistant arrhythmias due to proarrhythmic effects

• Initiate therapy in facilities capable of providing continuous ECG monitoring and managing life-threatening dysrhythmias

MONITORING PARAMETERS

• Monitor trough plasma levels periodically, especially in patients with moderate to severe chronic renal failure or severe hepatic disease and CHF; therapeutic range 0.2-1 µg/ml

---

fluconazole
(floo-con'a-zole)
Rx: Diflucan
Chemical Class: Triazole derivative
Therapeutic Class: Antifungal

CLINICAL PHARMACOLOGY

Mechanism of Action: Interferes with cytochrome P450 activity, decreasing ergosterol synthesis (principal sterol in fungal cell membrane) and inhibiting cell membrane formation

Pharmacokinetics

IV/PO: Peak 1-2 hr (PO), 11%-12% bound to plasma proteins, extensive distribution into all studied body fluids, $t_{1/2}$ 20-50 hr; cleared primarily by renal excretion

INDICATIONS AND USES: Oropharyngeal and esophageal candidiasis; candidal UTI, peritonitis and systemic candidal infections; vaginal candidiasis; prophylaxis of candidiasis in patients undergoing bone marrow transplant who receive cytotoxic chemotherapy or radiation therapy; cryptococcal meningitis

DOSAGE

Adult

• *Cryptococcal meningitis:* PO/IV 400 mg on 1st day, then 200 mg qd for 10-12 wk after CSF becomes culture negative; increase up to 400 mg/day based on response

• *Esophageal candidiasis:* PO/IV 200 mg on 1st day, then 100 mg qd for at least 3 wk and for 2 wk following resolution of symptoms; doses up to 400 mg/day may be used based on response

---

italic = common side effects   ***bold italic*** = life-threatening reactions

• *Oropharyngeal candidiasis:* PO/IV 200 mg on 1st day, then 100 mg qd for at least 2 wk

• *Other candidiasis:* PO/IV 50-200 mg/day, doses up to 400 mg/day may be used based on response

• *Prevention of candidiasis in bone marrow transplant:* PO/IV 400 mg qd, initiate several days before anticipated onset of neutropenia, continue 7 days after neutrophil count rises above 1000 cells/mm^3

• *Vaginal candidiasis:* PO 150 mg as a single dose

• *Renal function impairment:* PO/IV reduce dose by 50% in patients with CrCl <50 ml/min

Child

• Equivalent doses for children are 3 mg/kg for adult dose of 100 mg; 6 mg/kg for adult dose of 200 mg; 12 mg/kg for adult dose of 400 mg; do not exceed 600 mg dose

⚡ AVAILABLE FORMS/COST OF THERAPY

• Inj, Sol—IV: 2 mg/ml, 100 ml: **$83.44**

• Powder—Oral: 50 mg/5 ml, 60 ml: **$28.88;** 200 mg/5 ml, 60 ml: **$104.88**

• Tab, Plain Coated—Oral: 50 mg, 30's: **$134.79;** 100 mg, 30's: **$211.81;** 150 mg, 12's: **$134.88;** 200 mg, 30's: **$346.61**

PRECAUTIONS: Hypersensitivity to other azoles, children, renal disease

PREGNANCY AND LACTATION: Pregnancy category C; excreted into breast milk in concentrations similar to plasma; not recommended in nursing mothers

SIDE EFFECTS/ADVERSE REACTIONS

CNS: Headache, *seizures*

GI: Cramping, diarrhea, flatus, *hepatic injury,* nausea, vomiting

*HEME: **Leukopenia, thrombocytopenia***

METAB: Hypercholesterolemia, hypertriglyceridemia, hypokalemia

*SKIN: **Exfoliative skin disorders***

INTERACTIONS

Drugs

3 *Alprazolam:* Increased plasma alprazolam concentration

⚠ *Astemizole:* QT prolongation and life-threatening dysrhythmia

3 *Atevirdine:* Increased plasma atevirdine concentration

3 *Atorvastatin:* Increased plasma atorvastatin concentration with risk of rhabdomyolysis

3 *Buspirone:* Increased plasma buspirone concentration

3 *Caffeine:* Increased plasma caffeine concentration

3 *Chlordiazepoxide:* Increased plasma chlordiazepoxide concentration

2 *Cisapride:* QT prolongation and dysrhythmia

3 *Cyclosporine:* Increased plasma cyclosporine concentration

3 *Diazepam:* Increased plasma diazepam concentration

3 *Felodipine:* Increased plasma felodipine concentration

3 *Fluvastatin:* Increased plasma fluvastatin concentration with risk of rhabdomyolysis

3 *Losartan:* Reduced concentration of losartan's active metabolite may reduce efficacy of losartan

2 *Lovastatin:* Increased plasma lovastatin concentration with risk of rhabdomyolysis

3 *Methadone:* Increased plasma methadone concentration

3 *Midazolam:* Increased plasma midazolam concentration

3 *Oral anticoagulants:* Increased hypoprothrombinemic response

2 *Phenytoin:* Markedly reduced plasma fluconazole concentration

3 *Pravastatin:* Increased plasma pravastatin concentration with risk of rhabdomyolysis

3 *Quinidine:* Increased plasma quinidine concentration

3 *Rifampin:* Decreased plasma fluconazole concentration; decreased plasma rifampin concentration

2 *Simvastatin:* Increased plasma simvastatin concentration with risk of rhabdomyolysis

3 *Tacrolimus:* Increased plasma tacrolimus concentration

3 *Terfenadine:* Increased plasma terfenadine concentration; QT prolongation and life-threatening dysrhythmia possible

2 *Triazolam:* Increased plasma triazolam concentration

3 *Tolbutamide:* Increased plasma tolbutamide concentration

3 *Warfarin:* Increased hypoprothrombinemic response

Labs:

• *Benzoylecgonine:* False negative urine results

SPECIAL CONSIDERATIONS
MONITORING PARAMETERS

• Periodic liver function tests with prolonged therapy

---

flucytosine

(floo-sye'toe-seen)
Rx: Ancobon

Chemical Class: Fluorinated pyrimidine derivative
Therapeutic Class: Antifungal

CLINICAL PHARMACOLOGY
Mechanism of Action: Acts directly on fungal organisms by competitive inhibition of purine and pyrimidine uptake and indirectly by metabolism within the fungal organism to 5-fluorouracil, which inhibits synthesis of both DNA and RNA
Pharmacokinetics
PO: Peak 2 hr, $t_{1/2}$ 2-5 hr; excreted in urine (unchanged); well-distributed to peritoneal fluid, aqueous humor, joints, and other body fluids and tissues; CSF concentrations approximately 65%-90% of serum levels

INDICATIONS AND USES: Serious infections caused by susceptible strains of *Candida* (septicemia, endocarditis, UTIs) or *Cryptococcus* (meningitis, pulmonary, urinary tract infections, septicemia); treatment of chromomycosis*

DOSAGE
Adult and Child >50 kg

• PO 50-150 mg/kg/day divided q6h; initiate dose at the lower level if renal impairment is present

Adult and Child <50 kg

• PO 1.5-4.5 g/m^2/day in 4 divided doses

$ **AVAILABLE FORMS/COST OF THERAPY**

• Cap, Gel—Oral: 250 mg, 100's: **$277.50;** 500 mg, 100's: **$552.00**

PRECAUTIONS: Renal disease, impaired hepatic function, bone marrow depression, blood dyscrasias, radiation/chemotherapy

PREGNANCY AND LACTATION: Pregnancy category C; 4% of drug metabolized to 5-fluorouracil, an antineoplastic suspected of producing congenital defects in humans; excretion into breast milk unknown; use caution in nursing mothers

SIDE EFFECTS/ADVERSE REACTIONS

CNS: Ataxia, confusion, hallucinations, headache, hearing loss, paresthesia, parkinsonism, peripheral neuropathy, psychosis, pyrexia, sedation, vertigo

CV: **Cardiac arrest,** chest pain

GI: Abdominal pain, *anorexia,* bilirubin elevation, diarrhea, dry mouth, duodenal ulcer, elevation of hepatic enzymes, **GI hemorrhage,** hepatic dysfunction, jaundice, *nausea,* ulcerative colitis, *vomiting*

GU: Azotemia, creatinine and BUN elevation, crystalluria, **renal failure**

HEME: **Agranulocytosis,** anemia,

---

italic = common side effects   ***bold italic*** = life-threatening reactions

aplastic anemia, eosinophilia, *leukopenia, pancytopenia, thrombocytopenia*

METAB: Hypoglycemia, hypokalemia

RESP: Dyspnea, *respiratory arrest*

SKIN: Photosensitivity, pruritus, rash, urticaria

INTERACTIONS

Drugs

3 *Cytosine arabinoside:* Inactivates antifungal activity by competitive inhibition

Labs

• *False increase:* Serum creatinine (when Ektachem analyzer is used)

SPECIAL CONSIDERATIONS

Rarely used as monotherapy; generally used in combination with amphotericin B

PATIENT/FAMILY EDUCATION

• Reduce or avoid GI upset by taking caps a few at a time over a 15 min period

MONITORING PARAMETERS

• Creatinine, BUN, alk phosphatase, AST, ALT, CBC

• Serum flucytosine concentrations (therapeutic range 25-100 μg/ml)

---

fludrocortisone

(floo-droe-kor'ti-sone)

Rx: Florinef

Chemical Class: Synthetic mineralocorticoid

Therapeutic Class: Mineralocorticoid

CLINICAL PHARMACOLOGY

Mechanism of Action: Acts on the distal tubules of the kidney to enhance reabsorption of sodium from tubular fluid into the plasma; increases urinary excretion of both potassium and hydrogen

Pharmacokinetics

PO: Peak 1.7 hr, plasma $t_{1/2}$ 3½ hr, biological $t_{1/2}$ 18-36 hr; metabolized by liver, excreted in urine

INDICATIONS AND USES: Adrenocortical insufficiency in Addison's disease; salt-losing adrenogenital syndrome; severe orthostatic hypotension*

DOSAGE

Adult

• PO 0.05-0.2 mg qd

Child

• PO 0.05-0.1 mg qd

$ **AVAILABLE FORMS/COST OF THERAPY**

• Tab, Uncoated—Oral: 0.1 mg, 100's: **$66.58**

CONTRAINDICATIONS: Systemic fungal infections

PRECAUTIONS: Trauma, surgery, severe illness (supportive dosage may be required), abrupt discontinuation

PREGNANCY AND LACTATION: Pregnancy category C; observe newborn for signs and symptoms of adrenocortical insufficiency; corticosteroids are found in breast milk; use caution in nursing mothers

SIDE EFFECTS/ADVERSE REACTIONS

CNS: Headache

CV: **CHF,** *edema,* enlargement of the heart, flushing, hypertension

METAB: Hypernatremia, hypokalemic alkalosis

MS: Fractures, osteoporosis, weakness

SKIN: Allergic rash, bruising, hives, increased sweating

INTERACTIONS

Drugs

3 *Amphotericin:* Excessive potassium depletion

3 *Diuretics, loop:* Opposite therapeutic effect; excessive potassium loss

3 *Diuretics, thiazide:* Opposite therapeutic effect; excessive potassium loss

---

3 *Digitalis:* Increased potential for digitalis toxicity associated with hypokalemia

SPECIAL CONSIDERATIONS
PATIENT/FAMILY EDUCATION
• Notify clinician of dizziness, severe headache, swelling of feet or lower legs, unusual weight gain
• Do not discontinue abruptly

MONITORING PARAMETERS
• Serum electrolytes, blood pressure, serum renin

---

flumazenil
(floo-maz'en-ill)
Rx: Romazicon
Chemical Class: Imidazobenzodiazepine derivative
Therapeutic Class: Benzodiazepine antagonist

CLINICAL PHARMACOLOGY
Mechanism of Action: Antagonizes the actions of benzodiazepines in the CNS; competitively inhibits activity at the benzodiazepine recognition site on the GABA/benzodiazepine receptor

Pharmacokinetics
IV: 50% bound to plasma proteins, metabolized in the liver, primarily excreted in urine; terminal $t_{1/2}$ 41-79 min

INDICATIONS AND USES: Complete or partial reversal of sedative effects of benzodiazepines

DOSAGE
Adult
• *Reversal of conscious sedation*: IV 0.2 mg (2 ml) initially over 15 sec, repeat at 60 sec intervals prn to a max total dose of 1 mg (10 ml)
• *Suspected benzodiazepine overdose:* IV 0.2 mg (2 ml) given over 30 sec; wait 30 sec, then give 0.3 mg (3 ml) over 30 sec if consciousness does not occur; further doses of 0.5 mg (5 ml) can be given over 30 sec

at intervals of 1 min up to cumulative dose of 3 mg; patients with a partial response at 3 mg may require additional titration up to a total dose of 5 mg (administered slowly in the same manner)

AVAILABLE FORMS/COST OF THERAPY
• Inj, Sol—IV: 0.1 mg/ml, 5, 10 ml: **$35.46**/5 ml

CONTRAINDICATIONS: Serious cyclic antidepressant overdose, patients given benzodiazepine for control of life-threatening condition

PRECAUTIONS: Children, elderly, renal disease, seizure disorders, head injury, labor and delivery, hepatic disease, hypoventilation, panic disorder, drug and alcohol dependency, ambulatory patients (resedation may occur)

PREGNANCY AND LACTATION: Pregnancy category C; excretion into breast milk unknown; use caution in nursing mothers

SIDE EFFECTS/ADVERSE REACTIONS
CNS: Agitation, confusion, *dizziness,* emotional lability, headache, **seizures,** somnolence
CV: Bradycardia, **dysrhythmias,** chest pain, cutaneous vasodilation, hypertension, palpitations, tachycardia
EENT: Abnormal vision, blurred vision, tinnitus
GI: Hiccups, *nausea, vomiting*
SKIN: Increased sweating
MISC: Inj site pain, fatigue

SPECIAL CONSIDERATIONS
PATIENT/FAMILY EDUCATION
• Resedation may occur; do not engage in any activities requiring complete alertness or operate hazardous machinery or a motor vehicle until at least 18 to 24 hr after discharge
• Do not use any alcohol or non-

italic = common side effects   ***bold italic*** = life-threatening reactions

prescription drugs for 18 to 24 hr after flumazenil administration

MONITORING PARAMETERS

• Monitor for seizures, sedation, respiratory depression, or other residual benzodiazepine effects for an appropriate period (up to 120 min) based on dose and duration of effect of the benzodiazepine employed; pharmacokinetics of benzodiazepines are not altered in the presence of flumazenil

---

flunisolide
(floo-niss'oh-lide)
Rx: *Aerosol INH:* AeroBid, *Nasal:* Nasalide, Nasarel
Chemical Class: Synthetic glucocorticoid
Therapeutic Class: Antiasthmatic; inhaled corticosteroid; nasal corticosteroid

---

CLINICAL PHARMACOLOGY
Mechanism of Action: Decreases inflammation by suppression of migration of polymorphonuclear leukocytes, fibroblasts, reversal of increased capillary permeability, and lysosomal stabilization

Pharmacokinetics
INH: Systemic availability 40%
NASAL: 50% absorption after nasal inhalation
Rapidly metabolized in liver to inactive metabolites; $t_{1/2}$ 1.8 hr; excreted in urine and feces

INDICATIONS AND USES: Seasonal or perennial rhinitis; (nasal sol); chronic asthma (oral inhaler)

DOSAGE
Adult
• NASAL SOL 2 sprays (50 µg) in each nostril bid-tid, max 8 sprays/nostril/day (400 µg/day); ORAL INHALER 2 inhalations (500 µg) bid, not to exceed 4 inhalations bid (2000 µg)

Child
• NASAL SOL 1 spray (25 µg) in each nostril tid or 2 sprays (50 µg) in each nostril bid, max 4 sprays/nostril/day (200 µg/day); ORAL INHALER (age 6-15 yr) 2 inhalations bid (1000 µg/day)

AVAILABLE FORMS/COST OF THERAPY
• Aer—Inhaler: 250 µg/inh, 100 doses: **$59.64**
• Sol—Nasal: 25 µg/inh, 200 doses: **$39.83**
• Aer, Spray—Nasal: 25 µg/inh, 200 doses: **$38.36**

CONTRAINDICATIONS: Fungal, bacterial infection of nose (nasal sol); status asthmaticus (oral inhaler)

PRECAUTIONS: Quiescent tuberculosis; nasal septal ulcers, recurrent epistaxis, nasal surgery or trauma; untreated fungal, bacterial, or viral infections

PREGNANCY AND LACTATION: Pregnancy category C; excretion into breast milk unknown, use caution in nursing mothers

SIDE EFFECTS/ADVERSE REACTIONS
CNS: Dizziness, headache, nervousness, restlessness
EENT: Candida infection of oral cavity, hoarseness, hoarseness/dysphonia, *sore throat* (oral sol); dryness, epistaxis, nasal irritation and stinging, rebound congestion, sneezing (nasal sol)
GI: Dry mouth, nausea, vomiting
SKIN: Urticaria

SPECIAL CONSIDERATIONS
PATIENT/FAMILY EDUCATION
• To be used on a regular basis, not for acute symptoms
• Use bronchodilators before oral inhaler (for patients using both)
• Nasal sol may cause drying and irritation of nasal mucosa

---

* = non-FDA-approved use

• Clear nasal passages prior to use of nasal sol

MONITORING PARAMETERS

• Monitor children for growth as well as for effects on the HPA axis during chronic therapy

• Monitor patients switched from chronic systemic corticosteroids to avoid acute adrenal insufficiency in response to stress

---

fluocinolone
(floo-oh-sin'oh-lone)

Rx: Derma-Smoothe/FS, FS Shampoo, Synalar, Synemol

Chemical Class: Synthetic glucocorticoid
Therapeutic Class: Topical corticosteroid, low potency (0.01% cream, solution, oil, shampoo), intermediate potency (0.025% cream, ointment)

CLINICAL PHARMACOLOGY

Mechanism of Action: Depresses formation, release, and activity of endogenous mediators of inflammation such as prostaglandins, kinins, histamine, liposomal enzymes, and the complement system resulting in decreased edema, erythema, and pruritus

Pharmacokinetics

Absorbed through the skin (increased by inflammation and occlusive dressings); metabolized primarily in the liver

INDICATIONS AND USES: Psoriasis, eczema, contact dermatitis, pruritus of corticosteroid responsive dermatoses; moderate to severe stable atopic dermatitis (0.01% oil) in patients ≥6 yr

DOSAGE

Adult and Child

• TOP apply to affected area bid-tid, rub completely into skin

§ AVAILABLE FORMS/COST OF THERAPY

• Cre—Top: 0.01%, 15, 30, 60, 425 g: **$2.48-$5.48**/60 g; 0.025%, 15, 30, 60, 425 g: **$3.45-$41.80**/60 g

• Oint—Top: 0.025%, 15, 30, 60 g: **$8.67-$40.19**/60 gm

• Sol—Top: 0.01%, 20, 60 ml: **$5.62-$42.42**/60 ml

• Oil—Top: 0.01%, 120, 360 ml: **$18.28**/120 ml

• Shampoo—Top: 0.01%, 120 ml: **$14.62**

CONTRAINDICATIONS: Fungal infections; use on face, groin, or axilla

PRECAUTIONS: Viral infections, bacterial infections, children

PREGNANCY AND LACTATION: Pregnancy category C; unknown whether topical application could result in sufficient systemic absorption to produce detectable amounts in breast milk (systemic corticosteroids are secreted into breast milk in quantities not likely to have detrimental effects on infant)

SIDE EFFECTS/ADVERSE REACTIONS

SKIN: Acne, allergic contact dermatitis, atrophy, burning, dryness, folliculitis, hypertrichosis, hypopigmentation, irritation, itching, miliaria, perioral dermatitis, secondary infection, striae

MISC: Systemic absorption of topical corticosteroids has produced reversible HPA axis suppression (more likely with occlusive dressings, prolonged administration, application to large surface areas, liver failure, and in children)

SPECIAL CONSIDERATIONS
PATIENT/FAMILY EDUCATION

• Apply sparingly only to affected area

• Avoid contact with eyes

• Do not put bandages or dressings

---

italic = common side effects   ***bold italic*** = life-threatening reactions

over treated area unless directed by clinician

• Do not use on weeping, denuded, or infected areas

• Discontinue drug, notify clinician if local irritation or fever develops

---

fluocinonide
(floo-oh-sin'oh-nide)
Rx: Lidex, Lidex-E
Chemical Class: Synthetic glucocorticoid
Therapeutic Class: Topical corticosteroid, high potency

CLINICAL PHARMACOLOGY
Mechanism of Action: Depresses formation, release, and activity of endogenous mediators of inflammation such as prostaglandins, kinins, histamine, liposomal enzymes, and the complement system resulting in decreased edema, erythema, and pruritus
Pharmacokinetics
Absorbed through the skin (increased by inflammation and occlusive dressings); metabolized primarily in the liver
INDICATIONS AND USES: Psoriasis, eczema, contact dermatitis, pruritus of corticosteroid responsive dermatoses
DOSAGE
Adult and Child
• TOP apply to affected area bid-tid, rub completely into skin
§   AVAILABLE FORMS/COST OF THERAPY
• Cre—Top: 0.05%, 15, 30, 60, 120 g: **$3.77-$29.87**/30 g
• Gel—Top: 0.05%, 15, 30, 60, 120 g: **$35.87-$50.07**/60 g
• Oint—Top: 0.05%, 1, 15, 30, 60, 120 g: **$16.39-$29.87**/30 g
• Sol—Top: 0.05%, 20, 60 ml: **$14.52-$48.53**/60 ml
CONTRAINDICATIONS: Fungal

infections; use on face, groin, or axilla
PRECAUTIONS: Viral infections, bacterial infections, children
PREGNANCY AND LACTATION: Pregnancy category C; unknown whether topical application could result in sufficient systemic absorption to produce detectable amounts in breast milk (systemic corticosteroids are secreted into breast milk in quantities not likely to have detrimental effects on infant)
SIDE EFFECTS/ADVERSE REACTIONS
SKIN: Acne, allergic contact dermatitis, atrophy, burning, dryness, folliculitis, hypertrichosis, hypopigmentation, irritation, itching, miliaria, perioral dermatitis, secondary infection, striae
MISC: Systemic absorption of topical corticosteroids has produced reversible HPA axis suppression (more likely with occlusive dressings, prolonged administration, application to large surface areas, liver failure, and in children)
SPECIAL CONSIDERATIONS
PATIENT/FAMILY EDUCATION
• Apply sparingly only to affected area
• Avoid contact with eyes
• Do not put bandages or dressings over treated area unless directed by clinician
• Do not use on weeping, denuded, or infected areas
• Discontinue drug, notify clinician if local irritation or fever develops

---

* = non-FDA-approved use

fluorescein

(flure'e-seen)
Rx: AK-Fluor, Angioscein,
Fluorescite, Fluorets, Fluor-I-
Strip, Fluor-I-Strip-A.T., Ful-
Glo, Ocu-Flur 10
Combinations
  Rx: with proparacaine (Fluo-
racaine)
Chemical Class: Xanthine dye
Therapeutic Class: Ophthal-
mic diagnostic agent

CLINICAL PHARMACOLOGY
Mechanism of Action: Breaks in
corneal tissue absorb dye and appear bright green under cobalt blue
light

INDICATIONS AND USES: Diagnostic aid in identifying foreign bodies, hard fitting contact lenses, fundus photography, tonometry, identifying corneal abrasions, retinal angiography

DOSAGE
Adult
• *Detection of foreign bodies/
corneal abrasions:* Ophth 1 gtt 2%
sol, allow a few sec for staining,
wash out excess with sterile irrigating solution; strips moisten strip with
sterile water, place moistened strip
at the fornix in lower cul-de-sac close
to the punctum, have patient close
lid tightly over strip until desired
amount of staining obtained
• *Retinal angiography:* IV 500-750
mg inj rapidly in antecubital vein
Child
• *Retinal angiography:* IV 7.5 mg/
kg inj rapidly in antecubital vein

**$ AVAILABLE FORMS/COST
OF THERAPY**
• Inj, Sol—IV; 10% 5 ml: **$3.90-
$14.25**
• Inj, Sol—IV; 25%, 2 ml: **$3.90-
$17.00**

• Sol—Ophth: 2%, 15 ml: **$14.19-
$23.99**; 10%, 5 ml: **$0.25**
• Strip—Ophth: 0.6 mg, 300's:
$36.88; 1 mg, 300's: **$72.68**; 9 mg,
300's: **$72.68**

CONTRAINDICATIONS: Soft contact lenses (lenses may become discolored)

PRECAUTIONS: History of allergies, asthma

PREGNANCY AND LACTATION:
Pregnancy category C; avoid parenteral use, especially in 1st trimester; excreted into breast milk; use
caution in nursing mothers

**SIDE EFFECTS/ADVERSE REAC-
TIONS**
CNS: Seizures, dizziness, headache,
paresthesia
CV: Bradycardia, *cardiac arrest,* hypotension, *shock,* syncope
EENT: Burning, conjunctival redness, pruritis, stinging, urticaria
GI: GI distress, nausea, strong taste,
vomiting
GU: Bright yellow discoloration of
urine
*RESP: Acute pulmonary edema,
bronchospasm, dyspnea*
SKIN: Severe local tissue damage
with extravasation, yellowish discoloration of skin

SPECIAL CONSIDERATIONS
PATIENT/FAMILY EDUCATION
• May cause temporary yellowish
discoloration of skin (fades in
6-12 hr)
• Urine will appear bright yellow
(fades in 24-36 hr)
• Soft contact lenses may become
stained, wait at least 1 hr after thorough rinsing of eye before replacing
lenses

MONITORING PARAMETERS
• Luminescence appears in the retina and choroidal vessels 9-15 min
following IV inj; can be observed
by standard viewing equipment

F

---

italic = common side effects   ***bold italic*** = life-threatening reactions

fluoride, sodium

Rx: Fluorinse, Fluoritab, Flura, Gel-Kam, Karidium, Karigel, Listermint with Fluoride, Luride, Minute-Gel, Pediaflor, Pharmaflur, Phos-Flur, Prevident, Stop, Thera-Flur
Sodium fluoride, slow release: Slow Fluoride
OTC: Fluorigard, Gel-Tin
Chemical Class: Fluoride ion
Therapeutic Class: Antiosteoporotic; anti-dental caries agent

CLINICAL PHARMACOLOGY
Mechanism of Action: Needed for hard tooth enamel and for resistance to periodontal disease; reduces acid production by dental bacteria; potent stimulator of bone formation—increases bone mass in intermediate doses

Pharmacokinetics
PO: Absorption related to solubility; sodium fluoride almost completely absorbed; calcium or magnesium delays absorption; 50% deposited in bone and teeth; excreted in urine, feces, and breast milk; crosses placenta
INDICATIONS AND USES: Prevention of dental caries; osteoporosis*
DOSAGE
NOTE: 2.2 mg sodium fluoride equivalent to 1 mg of fluoride ion
Adult and Child >12 yr
• *Dental rinse:* Top apply 10 ml 0.2% sol qd after brushing teeth, rinse mouth for >1 min with sol then expectorate
• *Osteoporosis: PO 8-80 mg/day* (slow release formulation pending FDA approval)
Child
• *Brush-on gel:* After brushing with toothpaste, >6 yr apply thin ribbon of gel to teeth with toothbrush for at least 1 min hs, expectorate gel and rinse mouth thoroughly
• *Dental rinse:* Top 5 ml 0.2% sol qd after brushing teeth, rinse mouth for >1 min with sol then expectorate
• *Gel Drops >6 yr:* Use applicators supplied by dentist; apply 4-8 gtt to inner surface of applicator, spread evenly with tip of bottle; place applicator over upper and lower teeth and bite down gently for 6 min; remove and rinse mouth
• *Systemic protection from periodontal disease:* PO in areas where fluoride content of drinking water < 0.3 ppm, <2 yr 0.25 mg fluoride qd; 2-3 yr 0.5 mg qd; 3-12 yr 1 mg qd; in areas where fluoride content of drinking water is 0.3-0.7 ppm, <2 yr 0.125 mg fluoride qd; 2-3 yr 0.25 mg qd, 3-14 yr 0.25-0.75 mg qd

$ **AVAILABLE FORMS/COST OF THERAPY**
• Gel, Swab—Dental: 0.1% (0.4% sodium fluoride), 122 g, 12's: **$11.40;** 0.5% (1.1% sodium fluoride), 120 g: **$3.97**
• Gel, Drops—Dental: 0.5% (1.1% sodium fluoride), 24 ml: **$5.63**
• Rinse—Dental: 0.01% (0.02% sodium fluoride), 360 ml: **$3.07;** 0.02% (0.05% sodium fluoride), 480 ml: **$3.49;** 0.09% (0.2% sodium fluoride); 480 ml: **$7.49**
• Tab, Chewable—Oral: 0.25 mg (0.55 mg sodium fluoride), 1000's: **$11.45;** 0.5 mg (1.1 mg sodium fluoride), 1000's: **$9.75-$11.45;** 1 mg (2.2 mg sodium fluoride), 1000's: **$9.75-$19.95**
• Drops—Oral: 0.125 mg/gtt (0.275 mg sodium fluoride), 30 ml: **$3.30;** 0.25 mg/gtt (0.55 mg sodium fluoride), 23 ml: **$1.90;** 0.5 mg/ml (1.1 mg sodium fluoride), 50 ml: **$14.11**
CONTRAINDICATIONS: Hypersensitivity

---

* = non-FDA-approved use

PRECAUTIONS: Drinking water with >0.7 ppm fluoride
PREGNANCY AND LACTATION: Administration from 3rd-9th mo of gestation safe (no information on teratogenicity); small amounts excreted into breast milk, inadequate therapeutically due to small amount of excretion and complexation with calcium
SIDE EFFECTS/ADVERSE REACTIONS
EENT: Watery eyes
GI: Black tarry stools, constipation, diarrhea, discoloration of teeth, *hematemesis,* increased salivation, loss of appetite, nausea, stomatitis, weight loss
METAB: Hypocalcemia
MS: Articular and juxta-articular pain, osteomalacia, stress fractures, tetany
RESP: Decreased respiration, *respiratory arrest*
SPECIAL CONSIDERATIONS
• Therapy begun prenatally and continued through age 16 is effective in reducing the number of decayed, missing, or filled surfaces and teeth; especially beneficial in areas where fluoride content of drinking water is below 0.7 ppm
• Treatment of osteoporosis, combined with 1 or more of the following—calcium, estrogen, or vitamin D—increases bone density, reduces rate of new vertebral fractures, if correct dose and in slow-release preparation; role in steroid-induced osteoporosis being investigated, reports to date indicate a poor response rate
PATIENT/FAMILY EDUCATION
• Avoid use with dairy products

fluorometholone
(flure-oh-meth'oh-lone)
Rx: Eflone, Flarex, Fluor-Op, FML Liquifilm, FML Forte Liquifilm
Combinations
  Rx: with sulfacetamide (FML-S Liquifilm)
Chemical Class: Synthetic glucocorticoid
Therapeutic Class: Ophthalmic corticosteroid

CLINICAL PHARMACOLOGY
Mechanism of Action: Suppresses aspects of the inflammatory process such as hyperemia, cellular infiltration, vascularization, and fibroblastic proliferation
Pharmacokinetics
OPHTHAL: Absorbed into aqueous humor with slight systemic absorption
INDICATIONS AND USES: Steroid-responsive inflammatory conditions of the palpebral and bulbar conjunctiva, lid, cornea, and anterior segment of the globe; corneal injury; graft rejection after keratoplasty
DOSAGE
Adult and Child
• SUSP instill 1 gtt in conjunctival sac q1h during the day and q2h during night, reduce to tid-qid when a favorable response is observed; OINT apply ¼ inch ribbon in lower conjunctival sac tid-qid, taper when favorable response is observed
AVAILABLE FORMS/COST OF THERAPY
• Sol—Ophth: 0.1%, 10 ml: **$19.88**
• Susp—Ophth: 0.1%, 2, 5, 10, 15 ml: **$12.53-$19.75**/5 ml; 0.25%, 2, 5, 10, 15 ml: **$28.16**/10 ml
CONTRAINDICATIONS: Acute superficial herpes simplex; fungal, vi-

ral diseases of the eye or conjunctiva; ocular TB

PRECAUTIONS: Corneal abrasions, glaucoma, children, eye infections

PREGNANCY AND LACTATION: Pregnancy category C

SIDE EFFECTS/ADVERSE REACTIONS

EENT: Cataracts, decreased acuity, glaucoma exacerbation, increased possibility of corneal infections, *optic nerve damage,* poor corneal wound healing, transient stinging or burning, visual field defects

SPECIAL CONSIDERATIONS
PATIENT/FAMILY EDUCATION

• Do not discontinue use without consulting clinician

• Notify clinician if condition worsens or persists or if pain, itching, or swelling of the eye occurs

---

fluoxetine

(floo-ox′e-teen)
Rx: Prozac
Chemical Class: Trifluoro propylamine derivative
Therapeutic Class: Selective serotonin reuptake inhibitor (SSRI), antidepressant

CLINICAL PHARMACOLOGY
Mechanism of Action: Selective, potent inhibition of CNS neuronal uptake of serotonin (5HT); no significant affinity for histaminergic, α- or β-adrenergic, muscarinic, or dopaminergic receptors

Pharmacokinetics
PO: Peak 4-8 hr; 94.5% bound to plasma proteins; metabolized to norfluoxetine (active); $t_{1/2}$ 48-216 hr (including active metabolite)

INDICATIONS AND USES: Depression, obsessive-compulsive disorder, obesity,* bulimia nervosa

DOSAGE
Adult

• PO 20 mg qAM, increase after 4-6 wks prn, max 80 mg/day; doses >20 mg can be divided into morning and noon doses

$ **AVAILABLE FORMS/COST OF THERAPY**

• Cap, Gel—Oral: 10 mg, 100's: **$252.41;** 20 mg, 100's: **$258.89;** 40 mg, 30's: **$155.34**

• Sol—Oral: 20 mg/5 ml, 120 ml: **$114.97**

• Tab 10 mg, 30's **$75.72**

CONTRAINDICATIONS: Concurrent use with MAOI, or within 14 days of discontinuing MAOI

PRECAUTIONS: Renal or hepatic function impairment, elderly, children, bipolar affective disorder, seizure disorder, suicidal ideation, diabetes

PREGNANCY AND LACTATION: Pregnancy category B; excreted into breast milk; use caution in nursing mothers

SIDE EFFECTS/ADVERSE REACTIONS

CNS: Anxiety, apathy, decreased libido, delusions, *dizziness, drowsiness, euphoria, fatigue,* hallucinations, *headache, insomnia, nervousness,* psychosis, *seizures,* serotonergic syndrome (anxiety, hyperreflexia, confusion), *tremor*

CV: Hot flushes, palpitations

EENT: Blurred vision, visual disturbance

GI: Anorexia, constipation, *diarrhea,* dry mouth, *dyspepsia,* hyperbilirubinemia, *loose stools, nausea,* taste changes

GU: Painful menstruation, sexual dysfunction

METAB: Altered glycemic control, hypoglycemia

MS: Joint or muscle pain

SKIN: Pruritus, rash, sweating

---

* = non-FDA-approved use

MISC: Weight loss
INTERACTIONS
Drugs

🟥 *Benzodiazepines (alprazolam, diazepam):* Probable inhibition of metabolism (CYP3A4) leading to accumulation of diazepam and alprazolam

🟥 *Beta-blockers (metroprolol, propranolol, sotalol):* Inhibition of metabolism (CYP2D6) leads to increased plasma concentrations of selective beta blockers and potential cardiac toxicity; atenolol may be safer choice

🟥 *Buspirone:* Reduced therapeutic effect of both drugs; possible seizures

🟥 *Carbamazepine:* Inhibition of hepatic metabolism of carbamazepine, but the formation of carbamazepine epoxide is not inhibited, contributing to increased toxicity

🟥 *Cyproheptadine:* Serotonin antagonist may partially reverse antidepressant and other effects

❷ *Dexfenfluramine:* Duplicate effects on inhibition of serotonin reuptake; inhibition of dexfenfluramine metabolism (CYP2D6) exaggerates effect; both mechanisms increase risk of serotonin syndrome

🟥 *Dextromethorphan:* Inhibition of dextromethorphan's metabolism (CYP2D6) by fluoxetine and additive serotonergic effects

🟥 *Diuretics, loop (bumetanide, furosemide, torsemide):* Possible additive hyponatremia; 2 fatal case reports with furosemide and fluoxetine

❷ *Fenfluramine:* Duplicate effects on inhibition of serotonin reuptake; inhibition of dexfenfluramine metabolism (CYP2D6) exaggerates effect; both mechanisms increase risk of serotonin syndrome

🟥 *Haloperidol:* Inhibition of haloperidol's metabolism (CYP2D6) may increase risks of extrapyramidal symptoms

❷ *HMG-Co A reductase inhibitors (atorvastatin, lovastatin, simvastatin):* Inhibition of statin metabolism (CYP3A4), by fluoxetine, may lead to rhabdomyolysis

🟥 *Lithium:* Neurotoxicity (tremor, confusion, ataxia, dizziness, dysarthria, and absence seizures) reported in patients receiving this combination; mechanism unknown

⚠ *MAOI's (isocarboxazid, phenelzine, tranylcypromine):* Increased CNS serotonergic effect has been associated with severe or fatal reactions with this combination

❷ *Non-sedating antihistamines (astemizole, terfenadine):* Metabolite, norfluoxetine, may inhibit metabolism (CYP3A4) for detoxifying these antihistamines; cardiac rhythm disturbance

🟥 *Phenytoin:* Inhibition of metabolism and phenytoin toxicity

🟥 *Selegiline:* Sporadic cases of mania and hypertension

🟥 *Tricyclic antidepressants (clomipramine, desipramine, doxepin, imipramine, nortriptylline, trazodone):* Marked increases in tricyclic antidepressant levels due to inhibition of metabolism (CYP2D6)

❷ *Tryptophan:* Additive serotonergic effects

SPECIAL CONSIDERATIONS
PATIENT/FAMILY EDUCATION
• Therapeutic response may take 4-6 wk
• May cause insomnia, administer in AM; sedating antidepressants, in small doses (i.e. trazodone 50 mg), frequently administered H.S., concurrently

---

italic = common side effects   **bold italic** = life-threatening reactions

fluoxymesterone

(floo-ox-ee-mess'te-rone)
Rx: Halotestin
Chemical Class: Testosterone derivative
Therapeutic Class: Androgen; antineoplastic
DEA Class: Schedule III

CLINICAL PHARMACOLOGY

Mechanism of Action: Promotes weight gain via retention of nitrogen, potassium, and phosphorus, increased protein anabolism, and decreased catabolism; endogenous androgens are essential for normal growth and development of male sex organs and maintenance of secondary sex characteristics; androgenic activity is minor, effects are predominantly anabolic

Pharmacokinetics

PO: Metabolized in liver, excreted in urine; $t_{1/2}$ 9.2 hr

INDICATIONS AND USES: Males: primary hypogonadism (congenital or acquired), hypogonadotropic hypogonadism (congenital or acquired), delayed puberty; females: palliative therapy of metastatic breast cancer, postpartum breast pain/engorgement

DOSAGE

Adult Males

• *Hypogonadism:* PO 5-20 mg qd
• *Delayed puberty:* 2.5-20 mg qd for 4-6 mo

Adult Females

• *Breast cancer:* PO 10-40 mg/day in divided doses
• *Breast engorgement:* PO 2.5 mg after delivery, 5-10 mg/day in divided doses for 4-5 days

💲 **AVAILABLE FORMS/COST OF THERAPY**

• Tab, Uncoated—Oral: 2 mg, 100's:

$63.44; 5 mg, 100's: **$155.63;** 10 mg, 100's: **$141.47-$231.40**

CONTRAINDICATIONS: Serious cardiac, hepatic, or renal disease; carcinoma of breast or prostate (males); pregnancy, enhancement of athletic performance

PRECAUTIONS: Diabetes mellitus, cardiovascular disease, risk factors for atherosclerosis, hepatic disease, seizure disorder, renal disease, BPH (urethral obstruction), acute intermittent porphyria

PREGNANCY AND LACTATION: Pregnancy category X; causes virilization of external genitalia of female fetus; excretion into breast milk unknown; use extreme caution in nursing mothers

SIDE EFFECTS/ADVERSE REACTIONS

CNS: Anxiety, decreased or increased libido, dizziness, fatigue, flushing, headache, insomnia, lability, paresthesias, sweating, tremors

CV: Increased blood pressure, *CHF,* edema

EENT: Conjunctival edema, nasal congestion, deepening of voice

GI: Cholestatic jaundice, constipation, nausea, vomiting, weight gain, *hepatocellular neoplasm*

GU: Decreased breast size, gynecomastia, priapism, menstrual irregularities, oligospermia, testicular atrophy, vaginitis, virilization in females

HEME: Polycythemia, suppression of clotting factors

METAB: Hypercalcemia (in breast cancer), hypercholesterolemia, hyperglycemia, hyperkalemia

SKIN: Acneiform lesions, acne vulgaris, alopecia, flushing, hirsutism, oily hair, skin, rash, sweating

INTERACTIONS

Drugs

❷ *Cyclosporine, tacrolimus:* Increased cyclosporin and tacrolimus levels with potential toxicity

❷ *Oral anticoagulants:* Enhanced hypoprothrombinemic response to oral anticoagulants

SPECIAL CONSIDERATIONS
MONITORING PARAMETERS
• Frequent urine and serum calcium determinations (breast cancer)
• Periodic LFTs, Hct
• X-ray examinations of bone age q6mo during treatment of prepubertal males

---

fluphenazine

(floo-fen'a-zeen)
Rx: Permitil, Prolixin
Chemical Class: Piperazine; phenothiazine derivative
Therapeutic Class: Antipsychotic

CLINICAL PHARMACOLOGY
Mechanism of Action: Dopamine receptor antagonist, with higher affinity for D_2- over D_1-receptors, and variable selectivity among the cortical dopamine tracts; also activity on nondopaminergic sites, i.e., cholinergic, α_1-adrenergic, and histaminic receptors (explaining side effects); high risk extrapyramidal reactions; minimal orthostatic hypotension, sedation, and anticholinergic effects

Pharmacokinetics
PO: Peak 2-4 hr, onset 1 hr, duration 6-8 hr
IM/SC (depends on salt): (HCl) peak 1.5-2 hr, onset 1 day; (enanthate) peak 2-3 days, onset 1-3 days, duration 1-3 wk; (decanoate) peak 1-2 days, onset 1-3 days, duration ≥4 wk, 6.8-14.3 hr
Widely distributed in tissues, 91%-99% bound to plasma proteins; metabolized in liver, excreted in urine and bile; $t_{1/2}$ 33 hr (salt

delays absorption but does not alter $t_{1/2}$)

INDICATIONS AND USES: Management of psychotic disorders, Huntington's chorea,* control of acute agitation,* dementia*

DOSAGE
NOTE: 2 mg equivalent to chlorpromazine 100 mg
Adult and Child >16 yr
• PO 0.5-10 mg/day divided q6-8h initially, reduce dosage gradually to daily maintenance doses of 1-5 mg (may give as single daily dose); IM (HCl) 1.25-10 mg/day divided q6-8h; IM/SC (enanthate and decanoate) 12.5-25 mg q1-4 wk based on patient response, do not exceed 100 mg
Child <16 yr
• PO 0.25-3.5 mg/day in divided doses q 4-6 hr, max 10 mg/day

💲 **AVAILABLE FORMS/COST**
OF THERAPY
• Conc—Oral: 5 mg/ml, 120 ml: **$134.03**/120 ml
• Eli—Oral: 2.5 mg/5 ml, 60 ml: **$15.90-$21.31**; 480 ml: **$142.75-$169.86**
• Inj, Sol—IM, SC: 2.5 mg/ml, 10 ml: **$42.57-$61.46**
• Tab, Plain Coated—Oral: 1 mg, 100's: **$18.81-$97.86**; 2.5 mg, 100's: **$26.91-$138.78**; 5 mg, 100's: **$35.21-$179.00**; 10 mg 100's: **$42.24-$232.99**
• Inj, Sol (decanoate)—IM, SC: 25 mg/ml, 5 ml: **$52.56-$89.37**
• Inj, Sol (enanthate)—SC: 25 mg/ml, 5 ml: **$114.76**

CONTRAINDICATIONS: Liver damage, cerebral arteriosclerosis, CAD, severe hypertension/hypotension, blood dyscrasias, coma, subcortical brain damage, bone marrow depression

PRECAUTIONS: Depression, acute pulmonary infection, chronic respi-

---

italic = common side effects   ***bold italic*** = life-threatening reactions

ratory disorders, cardiovascular disease, glaucoma, seizure disorder; impaired hepatic/renal function; elderly, children <12 yr, alcohol withdrawal, electroconvulsive therapy

PREGNANCY AND LACTATION: Pregnancy category C; EPS in the newborn have been attributed to *in utero* exposure; other reports have indicated that phenothiazines are relatively safe during pregnancy; excretion into breast milk unknown; use caution in nursing mothers

SIDE EFFECTS/ADVERSE REACTIONS

CNS: Drowsiness, *EPS: pseudoparkinsonism, akathisia, dystonia, tardive dyskinesia;* fatigue, headache, insomnia, *neuroleptic malignant syndrome, seizures,* vertigo

CV: Cardiac arrest, ECG changes, hypertension, *orthostatic hypotension,* tachycardia

EENT: Blurred vision, dry eyes, glaucoma

GI: Anorexia, constipation, diarrhea, *dry mouth, hepatitis,* jaundice, *nausea, paralytic ileus, vomiting,* weight gain

GU: Bladder paralysis, ejaculation inhibition, enuresis, male impotence, polyuria, priapism, urinary retention, frequency or incontinence

HEME: Agranulocytosis, anemia, *aplastic anemia, hemolytic anemia, leukocytosis, leukopenia, thrombocytopenia*

METAB: Amenorrhea, elevated prolactin levels, galactorrhea, hyperglycemia or hypoglycemia, hyponatremia, lactation, menstrual irregularities, moderate breast engorgement (females), SIADH

RESP: Bronchospasm, dyspnea, laryngospasm

SKIN: Dermatitis, photosensitivity, *rash*

MISC: Heat intolerance

INTERACTIONS
Drugs

3 *Anticholinergics:* Inhibition of therapeutic response to neuroleptics, additive anticholinergic effects

3 *Antimalarials (amodiaquine, chloroquine, sulfadoxine-pyrimethamine):* Increased neuroleptic concentrations

3 *Barbiturates:* Reduced serum neuroleptic concentrations

3 *Beta-blockers:* Potential increases in serum concentrations of both drugs

3 *Bromocriptine:* Reduced effects of both drugs

3 *Clonidine:* Acute organic brain syndrome

3 *Cyclic antidepressants:* Increased serum concentrations of both drugs

3 *Epinephrine:* Reversal of pressor response to epinephrine

3 *Guanadrel:* Inhibits antihypertensive response

2 *Levodopa:* Inhibition of the antiparkinsonian effect of levodopa

3 *Lithium:* Rare cases of severe neurotoxicity have been reported in acute manic patients

3 *Meperidine:* Hypotension, excessive CNS depression

3 *Orphenadrine:* Reduced serum neuroleptic concentrations

Labs

• Urine pregnancy test: false positive

SPECIAL CONSIDERATIONS

Concentrate must be diluted prior to administration; use only the following diluents: water, saline, 7-Up, homogenized milk, carbonated orange beverage, and pineapple, apricot, prune, orange, V-8, tomato, and grapefruit juices; do not mix with beverages containing caffeine, tannics (tea), or pectinates (apple juice), as physical incompatibility may result

---

* = non-FDA-approved use

PATIENT/FAMILY EDUCATION
• May cause drowsiness; use caution while driving or performing other tasks requiring alertness
• Avoid contact with skin when using concentrates
• Avoid prolonged exposure to sunlight
• May discolor urine pink or reddish-brown
• Use caution in hot weather, heatstroke may result
• Arise slowly from a reclining position

MONITORING PARAMETERS
• Monitor closely for the appearance of tardive dyskinesia

---

flurandrenolide
(flure-an-dren'oh-lide)
Rx: Cordran, Cordran SP, Cordran Tape
Chemical Class: Synthetic glucocorticoid
Therapeutic Class: Topical corticosteroid, intermediate potency

CLINICAL PHARMACOLOGY
Mechanism of Action: Depresses formation, release, and activity of endogenous mediators of inflammation such as prostaglandins, kinins, histamine, liposomal enzymes, and the complement system resulting in decreased edema, erythema, and pruritus of corticosteroid responsive dermatoses
Pharmacokinetics
Absorbed through the skin (increased by inflammation and occlusive dressings); metabolized primarily in the liver

INDICATIONS AND USES: Psoriasis, eczema, contact dermatitis, pruritus of corticosteroid responsive dermatoses

DOSAGE
Adult and Child
• TOP apply to affected area bid-tid; rub completely into skin; apply tape q12-24h

💲 AVAILABLE FORMS/COST OF THERAPY
• Lotion—Top: 0.05%, 15, 60 ml: **$35.43/60 ml**
• Cre—Top: 0.025%, 30, 60 g: **$16.42/30 g**; 0.05%, 15, 30, 60 g: **$20.95/30 g**
• Oint—Top: 0.025%, 30, 60 g: **$16.42/30 g**; 0.05%, 15, 30, 60 g: **$20.95/30 g**
• Tape, Medicated—Top: 4 µg/cm³, 24″ × 3″: **$15.38**

CONTRAINDICATIONS: Fungal infections, use on face, groin, or axilla
PRECAUTIONS: Viral infections, bacterial infections, children
PREGNANCY AND LACTATION: Pregnancy category C; unknown whether topical application could result in sufficient systemic absorption to produce detectable amounts in breast milk (systemic corticosteroids are secreted into breast milk in quantities not likely to have detrimental effects on infant)

SIDE EFFECTS/ADVERSE REACTIONS
SKIN: Acne, allergic contact dermatitis, atrophy, burning, dryness, folliculitis, hypertrichosis, hypopigmentation, irritation, itching, miliaria, perioral dermatitis, secondary infection, striae
MISC: Systemic absorption of topical corticosteroids has produced reversible HPA axis suppression (more likely with occlusive dressings, prolonged administration, application to large surface areas, liver failure, and in children)

SPECIAL CONSIDERATIONS
PATIENT/FAMILY EDUCATION
• Apply sparingly only to affected area

- Avoid contact with the eyes
- Do not put bandages or dressings over treated area unless directed by clinician
- Do not use on weeping, denuded, or infected areas
- Discontinue drug, notify clinician if local irritation or fever develops

---

flurazepam

(flure-az′e-pam)
Rx: Dalmane
Chemical Class: Benzodiazepine
Therapeutic Class: Sedative-hypnotic
DEA Class: Schedule IV

CLINICAL PHARMACOLOGY

Mechanism of Action: CNS depressants via facilitation of inhibitory GABA at benzodiazepine receptor sites (BZ_1—associated with sleep; BZ_2—associated with memory, motor, sensory, and cognitive function); effects include muscle relaxation (spinal cord), anticonvulsant activity (brain stem), ataxia (cerebellum), emotional behavior (limbic and cortical areas), and anxiolytic effects (separate from general CNS depression; decreases sleep latency, the number of awakenings, and the time spent in stage 0 (awake) sleep; stage 2 (unequivocal sleep) is increased; in sum, sleep time increased

Pharmacokinetics
PO: Onset 15-45 min, peak ½-1 hr; 97% bound to plasma proteins; metabolized by liver to an active metabolite (N-desalkylflurazepam); $t_{1/2}$ of active metabolite 47-100 hr

INDICATIONS AND USES: Insomnia

DOSAGE

Adult
- PO 15-30 mg qhs

Elderly and Child >15 yr
- PO 15 mg qhs

💲 AVAILABLE FORMS/COST OF THERAPY

- Cap, Gel—Oral: 15 mg, 100's: **$21.50-$112.38**; 30 mg, 100's: **$23.85-$122.25**

CONTRAINDICATIONS: Pregnancy
PRECAUTIONS: Renal or hepatic function impairment, elderly, depression, history of drug abuse, abrupt withdrawal, respiratory depression, sleep apnea
PREGNANCY AND LACTATION: Pregnancy category X; administration to nursing mothers is not recommended

SIDE EFFECTS/ADVERSE REACTIONS

CNS: Anxiety, confusion, *daytime sedation,* dizziness, *drowsiness,* headache, irritability, *lethargy,* lightheadedness
CV: Chest pain, hypotension (rare), palpitations, pulse changes
GI: Abdominal pain, constipation, diarrhea, heartburn, increased liver function tests, nausea, vomiting
HEME: **Granulocytopenia** (rare), **leukopenia**
SKIN: Dermatitis or allergy, flushes, pruritus, rash, sweating

INTERACTIONS

Drugs
❷ *Azole antifungals (fluconazole, itraconazole, ketoconazole):* Increased serum concentrations of flurazepam via inhibition of oxidative metabolism (CYP3A4)
❸ *Beta blockers (labetalol, metoprolol, propranolol):* Reduces the metabolism of benzodiazepines and may increase the pharmacodynamic effects
❸ *Cimetidine:* Increased plasma levels of flurazepam and metabolites via inhibition of hepatic oxidative metabolism

---

* = non-FDA-approved use

3 *Clozapine:* Isolated cases of cardiorespiratory collapse, but a causal relationship not established

3 *Disulfiram:* May increase serum concentrations of flurazepam via inhibition of oxidative metabolism (CYP3A4)

3 *Isoniazid:* May increase flurazepam serum concentrations via inhibition of metabolism

3 *Loxapine:* Isolated cases of respiratory depression, stupor, and hypotension reported; role of drug interaction not established

3 *Macrolide antibiotics (clarithromycin, erythromycin, troleandomycin):* Macrolides increase flurazepam plasma concentrations via inhibition of metabolism (CYP3A4)

3 *Omeprazole:* Increases plasma concentrations of flurazepam via inhibition of hepatic metabolism

3 *Rifampin:* Reduced serum concentrations of flurazepam via enhanced hepatic metabolism (CYP3A4)

3 *Serotonin reuptake inhibitors (fluoxetine, fluvoxamine):* May increase serum concentrations of flurazepam via inhibition of oxidative metabolism (CYP3A4)

SPECIAL CONSIDERATIONS
PATIENT/FAMILY EDUCATION
• Avoid alcohol and other CNS depressants
• Do not discontinue abruptly after prolonged therapy
• May experience disturbed sleep for the 1st or 2nd night after discontinuing the drug
• May cause drowsiness or dizziness; use caution while driving or performing other tasks requiring alertness; hangover daytime drowsiness possible secondary to long duration of action
• Inform clinician if you are planning to become pregnant, you are

pregnant, or if you become pregnant while taking this medicine

***

flurbiprofen
(flure-bi′proe-fen)
Rx: Ansaid, Ocufen (ophthalmic)
Chemical Class: Propionic acid derivative
Therapeutic Class: NSAID with analgesic and antipyretic activity

CLINICAL PHARMACOLOGY
Mechanism of Action: Reversible cyclooxygenase (i.e., prostaglandin synthetase) inhibitor; non-selectively decreases the formation of both prostaglandins and thromboxane A_2; variable effects on lipoxygenase synthesis and subsequent leukotriene production; antiinflammatory, antipyretic, and analgesic activity; inhibits platelet aggregation; OPHTH: antiinflammatory and antimiotic
Pharmacokinetics
PO: Peak 1.5 hr, >99% bound to plasma proteins; extensively metabolized, excreted primarily in urine; $t_{1/2}$ 5.7 hr

INDICATIONS AND USES: Intraoperative miosis, ocular inflammation, ankylosing spondylitis,* prevention of cognitive decline,* prevention of colon cancer,* dysmenorrhea,* acute gout,* migraine headache, mild-moderate pain* (bursitis, dental, cancer, episiotomy, osteoarthritis, postoperative sickle cell disease), peridontal disease, rheumatoid arthritis, tendonitis, soft tissue injury,* sunburn

DOSAGE
Adult
• *Rheumatoid and osteoarthritis:* PO 200-300 mg/day divided bid-qid
• *Dysmenorrhea:* PO 50 mg qid
• *Inhibition of intraoperative mio-*

sis: Ophth 1 gtt q30 min beginning 2 hr before surgery (total 4 gtt)

$ **AVAILABLE FORMS/COST OF THERAPY**

• Tab, Coated—Oral: 50 mg, 100's: **$68.02-$111.10;** 100 mg, 100's: **$39.85-$171.79**

• Sol—Ophth: 0.03%, 2.5 ml: **$8.73-$16.56**

CONTRAINDICATIONS: Bronchospasm, nasal polyps, angioedema precipitated by aspirin or other NSAIDs, dendritic keratitis (ophth)

PRECAUTIONS: History of GI ulceration, bleeding, or perforation; renal dysfunction, hypertension or cardiac conditions aggravated by fluid retention and edema, history of liver dysfunction, history of coagulation deficits

PREGNANCY AND LACTATION: Pregnancy category C; excreted into breast milk; use caution in nursing mothers

SIDE EFFECTS/ADVERSE REACTIONS

CNS: Dizziness, headache, lightheadedness

CV: Chest pain, ***CHF,*** dysrhythmias, edema, hypertension, hypotension, palpitation, tachycardia

EENT: Burning or stinging upon instillation, dry eyes, hearing disturbances, photophobia, tinnitus, visual disturbances

GI: Abdominal cramps, constipation, diarrhea, *dyspepsia,* flatulence, **gastric or duodenal ulcer with bleeding or perforation, hepatitis, nausea,** occult blood in stool, pancreatitis, vomiting

GU: **Acute renal failure**

HEME: **Agranulocytosis, eosinophilia, leukopenia, neutropenia, pancytopenia, thrombocytopenia**

METAB: Hyperglycemia, hyperkalemia, hypoglycemia, hyponatremia

RESP: Bronchospasm, dyspnea

SKIN: Photosensitivity, rash, urticaria

INTERACTIONS

Drugs

3 *Aminoglycosides:* Reduced clearance with elevated aminoglycoside levels and potential for toxicity (especially indomethacin in premature infants; other NSAIDs probably)

3 *Antihypertensives (α-blockers, angiotensin-converting enzyme inhibitors, angiotensin II receptor blockers, β-blockers, diuretics):* Inhibition of antihypertensive and other favorable hemodynamic effects

3 *Corticosteroids:* Increased risk of GI ulceration

3 *Anticoagulants:* Excessive hypoprothrombinemia, decreased platelet aggregation with increased risk of GI bleeding

3 *Cyclosporine:* Increased nephrotoxicity risk

3 *Lithium:* Decreased clearance of lithium (mediated via prostaglandins) resulting in elevated serum lithium levels and risk of toxicity

3 *Methotrexate:* Decreased renal secretion of methotrexate resulting in elevated methotrexate levels and risk of toxicity

3 *Phenylpropanolamine:* Possible acute hypertensive reaction

3 *Potassium-sparing diuretics:* Additive hyperkalemia potential

3 *Triamterene:* Acute renal failure reported with addition of indomethacin; caution with other NSAIDs

Labs

• *Cortisol:* Increased at high flurbiprofen levels

SPECIAL CONSIDERATIONS

PATIENT/FAMILY EDUCATION

• Avoid aspirin and alcoholic beverages

• Take with food, milk, or antacids to decrease GI upset

• Notify clinician if edema, black stools, or persistent headache occurs

MONITORING PARAMETERS

• Initial hemogram and fecal occult blood test within 3 mo of starting regular chronic therapy; repeat every 6-12 mo (more frequently in high-risk patients (>65 years, peptic ulcer disease, concurrent steroids or anticoagulants); elecrolytes, creatinine, and BUN within 3 mo of starting regular chronic therapy; repeat every 6-12 mo

---

flutamide

(floo′ta-mide)
Rx: Eulexin
Chemical Class: Acetanilid derivative
Therapeutic Class: Androgen inhibitor; antineoplastic

CLINICAL PHARMACOLOGY

Mechanism of Action: Inhibits androgen uptake or inhibits nuclear binding of androgen in target tissues; arrests tumor growth in androgen-sensitive tissue, e.g., prostate gland

Pharmacokinetics

PO: Rapidly and completely absorbed, 94% bound to plasma proteins; excreted in urine and feces as metabolites; $t_{1/2}$ 6 hr, geriatric $t_{1/2}$ 8 hr

INDICATIONS AND USES: In combination with LHRH agonists (e.g., leuprolide) for management of locally confined stage B_2-C and Stage D_2 metastatic prostate carcinoma

DOSAGE

Adult

• PO 250 mg (125 mg × 2) q8h

💲 AVAILABLE FORMS/COST OF THERAPY

• Cap, Gel—Oral: 125 mg, 100's: **$215.05**

PREGNANCY AND LACTATION:

Pregnancy category D

SIDE EFFECTS/ADVERSE REACTIONS

CNS: Anxiety, confusion, depression, drowsiness, *hot flashes*
CV: Edema, hypertension
GI: Anorexia, *diarrhea,* **hepatitis,** increased liver function studies, *nausea, vomiting*
GU: Decreased libido, impotence
HEME: **Anemia, leukopenia, thrombocytopenia**
SKIN: Photosensitivity, rash
MISC: Gynecomastia

INTERACTIONS

Drugs

3 *Warfarin:* Increased hypoprothrombinemic effect

SPECIAL CONSIDERATIONS

• Begin 8 wk before radiation therapy in Stage B_2-C carcinoma, continue during radiation
• In metastatic carcinoma continue until progression noted

PATIENT/FAMILY EDUCATION

• Feminization may occur during therapy
• Do not discontinue therapy without discussion with clinician

MONITORING PARAMETERS

• Periodic LFTs during long-term treatment

---

fluticasone

(flu-tic′a-zone)
Rx: Cutivate, Flonase, Flovent, Flovent Rotadisk
Chemical Class: Glucocorticoid
Therapeutic Class: Inhaled corticosteroid; nasal corticosteroid; topical corticosteroid, intermediate potency

---

CLINICAL PHARMACOLOGY

Mechanism of Action: Inhibits inflammatory cells and production or

---

italic = common side effects   ***bold italic*** = life-threatening reactions

secretion of cell mediators of inflammation

Pharmacokinetics

INH: Peak (following 880 µg) 0.1-1 ng/ml

Systemic bioavailability, 30% of dose delivered from the actuator; high total clearance due to efficient 1st-pass hepatic metabolism and minimally active metabolites

INDICATIONS AND USES: Asthma, chronic maintenance treatment; allergic rhinitis; corticosteroid-responsive dermatoses

DOSAGE

Adult

• *Asthma, chronic:* Previous asthma therapy (bronchodilators alone): 88-440 µg bid; previous asthma therapy (including inhaled corticosteroids): 88-440 µg bid; previous asthma therapy (including chronic systemic corticosteroids): 880 µg bid

• *Allergic rhinitis:* 1-2 sprays in each nostril qd or 1 spray in each nostril bid; do not exceed 2 sprays/nostril/day

• TOP apply to affected area qd-bid

Child

• Use not recommended in children <12 yr

Children ≥12 yr

• *Asthma:* Previous asthma therapy (bronchodilators alone): 88-440 µg bid; previous asthma therapy (including inhaled corticosteroids): 88-440 µg bid; previous asthma therapy (including chronic systemic corticosteroids): 880 µg bid

• *Allergic rhinitis:* 1 spray in each nostril qd; may increase to 2 sprays in each nostril qd

🚺 AVAILABLE FORMS/COST OF THERAPY

• Cre—Top: 0.05%, 15, 30, 60 g: **$24.18**/30 g

• Oint—Top: 0.005%, 15, 30, 60 g: **$24.18**/30 g

• Aer, metered—Nasal inh: 0.05 mg/inh, 16 g: **$49.87-$52.56**

• Aer, metered—Inh: 44 µg/inh, 7.9 g (60 puffs): **$33.86;** 13 g (120 puffs): **$45.14;** 110 µg/inh, 7.9 g (60 puffs): **$33.97;** 13 g (120 puffs): **$57.55;** 220 µg/inh, 7.9 g (60 puffs): **$62.64;** 13 g (120 puffs): **$88.54**

• Disk—Inh: 44 µg/inh, 60's: **$33.71;** 88 mcg/inh, 60's: **$45.14;** 220 mcg/inh, 60's: **$60.43**

CONTRAINDICATIONS: Relief of acute bronchospasm

PREGNANCY AND LACTATION: Pregnancy category C; no information on excretion into human breast milk

SIDE EFFECTS/ADVERSE REACTIONS

CNS: Fatigue, headache

EENT: Dysphonia, nasal congestion or discharge, *oropharyngeal candidiasis,* sinusitis, upper respiratory tract infections

MS: Muscle soreness

RESP: **Bronchospasm**

SKIN: Urticaria

MISC: Angioedema, *hypersensitivity reactions* (shortness of breath, tightness in chest, wheezing)

INTERACTIONS

Labs

• Cholesterol: Increased

SPECIAL CONSIDERATIONS

• Improvement following inhalation, 24 hr to 1-2 wk

• Systemic corticosteroid effects from inhaled and nasal steroids inadequate to prevent adrenal insufficiency in most patients withdrawn abruptly from corticosteroids

• Observe for evidence of inadequate adrenal response following periods of stress; use caution with extended use in children and adolescents as reduction in growth velocity may occur

---

* = non-FDA-approved use

PATIENT/FAMILY EDUCATION
• Rinsing the mouth following INH and using a spacer device reduces common EENT adverse effects
• Review proper MDI administration technique regularly

---

fluvastatin
(floo′va-sta-tin)
Rx: Lescol
Chemical Class: Substituted hexahydronaphthalene
Therapeutic Class: Antilipemic (HMG-CoA reductase inhibitor); "statin"

CLINICAL PHARMACOLOGY
Mechanism of Action: Competitively inhibits 3-hydroxy-3-methylglutaryl-coenzyme A (HMG-CoA) reductase, an early rate-limiting step in cholesterol biosynthesis; increases HDL cholesterol minimally [2.5%-7.8%], moderately decreases total and LDL cholesterol [15%-20%, 19%-35%, respectively, minimal lowering effect on triglycerides [3%-11%]
Pharmacokinetics
PO: Onset 15 min, peak 30-60 min, duration 3-4 hr; fully absorbed if taken without food; food slows absorption and reduces peak plasma level by 50%-70%; protein binding 98%; $t_{1/2}$ 0.5-1 hr; metabolized in liver (CYP2C9), excreted in bile
INDICATIONS AND USES: Primary hypercholesterolemia (heterozygous familial and nonfamilial hypercholesterolemia) and secondary prevention of cardiovascular events
DOSAGE
Adult
• PO: 20-40 mg hs, increase to 40 mg bid if necessary

AVAILABLE FORMS/COST OF THERAPY
• Cap—Oral: 20 mg, 100's: **$125.45**; 40 mg, 100's: **$125.45**
CONTRAINDICATIONS: Pregnancy, lactation, active liver disease, unexplained transaminase elevations
PRECAUTIONS: History of liver disease, heavy ethanol use, patients at risk for rhabdomyolysis (acute infection, hypotension, major surgery, or trauma)
PREGNANCY AND LACTATION: Pregnancy category X; contraindicated in breast feeding—present in breast milk (2 : 1 milk: plasma ratio)
SIDE EFFECTS/ADVERSE REACTIONS
CNS: Headache, insomnia
GI: Diarrhea, dyspepsia, elevated transaminase levels (1%), ***hepatotoxicity,*** nausea
EENT: Posterior subcapsular abnormalities
MS: Myalgia, myopathy, ***rhabdomyolysis***
INTERACTIONS
Drugs
🔳 *Alcohol:* 20 g of alcohol within 1 hr of dosing, increased fluvastatin AUC by 30%
❷ *Azole antifungals (fluconazole, itraconazole, ketoconazole, miconazole):* Increased fluvastatin levels via inhibition of metabolism with increased risk of rhabdomyolysis
🔳 *Cholestyramine, colestipol:* Reduced bioavailability of fluvastatin
🔳 *Cimetidine, ranitidine, omeprazole:* Coadministration increases fluvastatin Cmax 43%-70% with 18%-23% decrease in plasma clearance
🔳 *Cyclosporine:* Concomitant administration increases risk of severe myopathy or rhabdomyolysis
🔳 *Danazol:* Inhibition of metabolism (CYP3A4) thought to yield in-

---

italic = common side effects   ***bold italic*** = life-threatening reactions

creased fluvastatin levels with increased risk of rhabdomyolysis

3 *Fluoxetine:* Less likely to inhibit CYP3A4 hepatic metabolism (vs lovastatin) with less risk of rhabdomyolysis

2 *Gemfibrazil:* Small increased risk of myopathy with combination, especially at high doses of statin

3 *Isradipine:* Isradipine probably decreases fluvastatin plasma concentrations minimally

3 *Macrolide antibiotics (clarithromycin, erythromycin, troleandomycin):* Increased fluvastatin levels via inhibition of metabolism with increased risk of rhabdomyolysis

3 *Niacin:* Concomitant administration increases risk of severe hepatotoxicity

3 *Nefazadone:* Less likely to inhibit CYP3A4 hepatic metabolism (vs lovastatin) with less risk of rhabdomyolysis

3 *Rifampin:* Coadministration decreases fluvastatin Cmax and AUC

3 *Terbinafine:* Minimal effect on the metabolism of fluvastatin

3 *Warfarin:* Addition of fluvastatin may increase hypoprothrombinemic response to warfarin via inhibition of metabolism (CYP2C9)

SPECIAL CONSIDERATIONS
• Statin selection based on lipid-lowering prowess, cost, and availability

PATIENT/FAMILY EDUCATION
• Report symptoms of myalgia, muscle tenderness, or weakness
• Take daily doses in the evening for increased effect

MONITORING PARAMETERS
• Cholesterol (max therapeutic response 4-6 wk)
• LFT's (AST, ALT) at baseline and at 12 wk of therapy; if no change, nor further monitoring necessary (discontinue if elevations persists at >3 times upper limit of normal)

• CPK in patients complaining of diffuse myalgia, muscle tenderness, or weakness

---

fluvoxamine
(floo-vox′a-meen)
Rx: Luvox
Chemical Class: Aralkylketone derivative
Therapeutic Class: Selective serotonin reuptake inhibitor (SSRI), antidepressant

CLINICAL PHARMACOLOGY
Mechanism of Action: Selectively inhibits CNS neuronal uptake of serotonin (5HT); no significant activity for histaminergic, α- or β- adrenergic, muscarinic, or dopaminergic receptors

Pharmacokinetics
PO: Peak 3-8 hr; 77%-80% bound to plasma proteins; primarily eliminated by kidneys; $t_{1/2}$ 13.6-15.6 hr

INDICATIONS AND USES:
Obsessive-compulsive disorder (adults and children), depression

DOSAGE
Adult
• PO 50 mg qhs initially, increase in 50 mg increments q4-7d, as tolerated, until max therapeutic benefit is achieved; do not exceed 300 mg/day; doses >100 mg should be divided bid

Child
• PO 25 mg qhs initially, increase in 25 mg increments q4-6d, as tolerated, therapeutic benefit is achieved, or maximum daily dose of 200 mg; doses >100 mg should be divided bid

8 **AVAILABLE FORMS/COST OF THERAPY**
• Tab, Uncoated—Oral: 25 mg, 100's: **$255.89;** 50 mg, 100's: **$252.41;** 100 mg, 100's: **$258.90**

CONTRAINDICATIONS: Administration within 14 days of discontinuing MAOI therapy

PRECAUTIONS: History of mania, seizure disorder, liver dysfunction, suicidal ideation, children

PREGNANCY AND LACTATION: Pregnancy category C; excreted into breast milk; use caution in nursing mothers

SIDE EFFECTS/ADVERSE REACTIONS

CNS: Agitation, anxiety, decreased libido, depression, dizziness, *headache, insomnia,* nervousness, *somnolence,* tremor

CV: Hypertension, hypotension, orthostatic, palpitations, syncope, tachycardia

EENT: Amblyopia, taste perversion/change

GI: Anorexia, constipation, *diarrhea, dry mouth, dyspepsia,* flatulence, *nausea,* vomiting

GU: Abnormal ejaculation, sexual dysfunction, urinary frequency

RESP: Dyspnea

SKIN: Sweating

INTERACTIONS

Drugs

⚠ *Antihistamines, nonsedating (astemizole, terfenadine):* Fluvoxamine inhibits metabolism (CYP3A4) for detoxifying these antihistamines; cardiac rhythm disturbances

❸ *Benzodiazepines (alprazolam, diazepam):* Probable inhibition of metabolism (CYP3A4) leading to accumulation of diazepam and alprazolam

❸ *Beta-blockers (metoprolol, propranolol, sotalol):* Inhibition of metabolism (CYP2D6) leads to increased plasma concentrations of selective beta blockers and potential cardiac toxicity; atenolol may be safer choice

❸ *Buspirone:* Reduced therapeutic effect of both drugs; possible seizures

❸ *Carbamazepine:* Inhibition of hepatic metabolism of carbamazepine, but the formation of carbamazepine epoxide is not inhibited, contributing to increased toxicity

❷ *Clozapine:* Fluvoxamine markedly increases clozapine concentrations as a potent inhibitor of CYP1A2

❸ *Cyclic antidepressants (clomipramine, desipramine, doxepin, imipramine, nortriptylline, trazadone):* Inhibition of metabolism (CYP1A2 and CYP3A4) leading to accumulation of cyclic antidepressants; dosage adjustments necessary

❸ *Cyproheptadine:* Serotonin antagonist may partially reverse antidepressant and other effects

❷ *Dexfenfluramine:* Duplicate effects on inhibition of serotonin reuptake; inhibition of dexfenfluramine metabolism (CYP2D6) exaggerates effect; both mechanisms increase risk of serotonin syndrome

❷ *Fenfluramine:* Duplicate effects on inhibition of serotonin reuptake; inhibition of dexfenfluramine metabolism (CYP2D6) exaggerates effect; both mechanisms increase risk of serotonin syndrome

❷ *HMG-Co A reductase inhibitors (atorvastatin, lovastatin, simvastatin):* Inhibition of statin metabolism (CYP3A4), by fluoxetine, may lead to rhabdomyolysis

❸ *Lithium:* Neurotoxicity (tremor, confusion, ataxia, dizziness, dysarthria, and absence seizures) reported in patients receiving this combination; mechanism unknown

⚠ *MAOIs (isocarboxazid, phenelzine, tranylcypromine):* Increased CNS serotonergic effects have been associated with severe or fatal reactions with this combination

---

italic = common side effects   ***bold italic*** = life-threatening reactions

3 *Phenytoin:* Inhibition of metabolism and phenytoin toxicity

2 *Selegiline:* Sporadic cases of mania and hypertension

2 *Theophylline:* Theophylline toxicity increased via accumulation due to inhibition of metabolism (CYP1A2) by fluvoxamine

2 *Tryptophan:* Additive serotonergic effects

3 *Warfarin:* Increased hypothrombinemic response

SPECIAL CONSIDERATIONS
PATIENT/FAMILY EDUCATION
• May cause dizziness or drowsiness; use caution driving or performing tasks requiring alertness

---

folic acid
(foe'lik)
Rx: Folic acid
OTC: Folic acid
Chemical Class: B complex vitamin
Therapeutic Class: Hematinic; vitamin

CLINICAL PHARMACOLOGY
Mechanism of Action: Required for nucleoprotein synthesis and maintenance of normal erythropoiesis; stimulates production of RBC, WBC, and platelets in certain megaloblastic anemias
Pharmacokinetics
PO: Peak 1 hr, metabolized in liver to 7,8-dihydrofolic acid and eventually to 5,6,7,8-tetrahydrofolic acid, excreted in urine (percentage dependent on dose)
INDICATIONS AND USES: Treatment of megaloblastic anemias due to folic acid deficiency; prophylaxis of fetal neural tube defects; hyperhomocysteinemia*
DOSAGE
Adult and Child >11 yr
• *Folic acid deficiency:* PO/IV/ IM/SC 1 mg/day initially; maintenance dose 0.5 mg/day
• *Prophylaxis of fetal neural tube defects:* Low risk: PO at least 0.4 mg/day beginning at least 1 mo prior to conception and increasing to 0.8 mg/day during pregnancy; high risk: PO 4 mg/day at least 1 mo prior to conception and for 2 mo after conception
• Hyperhomocysteinemia: PO 0.4 mg qd
Child
• *Folic acid deficiency:* PO/IV/ IM/SC 1 mg/day initially; maintenance dose 0.1-0.4 mg/day
Infants
• *Folic acid deficiency:* PO/IV/ IM/SC 15 µg/kg/dose daily or 50 µg/day

$ **AVAILABLE FORMS/COST OF THERAPY**
• Inj, Sol—IM, IV, SC: 5 mg/ml, 10 ml: **$12.50-$13.27**
• Tab, Uncoated—Oral: 1 mg, 100's: **$1.95-$12.00**
• Tab—Oral: 0.4 mg, 100's (OTC): **$2.50-$3.00**; 0.8 mg, 100's (OTC): **$2.50-$3.00**
• Cap—Oral: 0.8 mg, 120's (OTC): **$4.95**
CONTRAINDICATIONS: Anemias other than megaloblastic/macrocytic anemia, vitamin B_{12} deficiency anemia
PREGNANCY AND LACTATION: Pregnancy category A; folic acid deficiency during pregnancy is a common problem in undernourished women and in women not receiving supplements; evidence has accumulated that folic acid deficiency, or abnormal folate metabolism, may be related to the occurrence of neural tube defects; actively excreted in human breast milk; compatible with breast feeding; recommended daily allowance during lactation is 0.5 mg/ day

---

* = non-FDA-approved use

SIDE EFFECTS/ADVERSE REACTIONS

RESP: Bronchospasm (rare)
SKIN: Allergic reactions have been reported, itching, rash

INTERACTIONS

Drugs

3 *Phenytoin:* Decreased serum phenytoin concentrations; long-term phenytoin frequently leads to subnormal folate levels

2 *Pyrimethamine:* Inhibition of antimicrobial effect of pyrimethamine

SPECIAL CONSIDERATIONS

• Recent evidence supports the premise that lowering elevated plasma homocysteine levels may reduce the risk of coronary heart disease

PATIENT/FAMILY EDUCATION

• Take only under medical supervision

MONITORING PARAMETERS

• CBC; serum folate concentrations <0.005 µg/ml indicate folic acid deficiency and concentrations <0.002 µg/ml usually result in megaloblastic anemia

---

fomepizole

(foe-mep′i-zoll)
Rx: Antizol
Chemical Class: Pyrzole derivative
Therapeutic Class: Ethylene glycol (antifreeze) antidote

CLINICAL PHARMACOLOGY

Mechanism of Action: Competitively inhibits alcohol dehydrogenase; alcohol dehydrogenase catalyzes the oxidation of ethanol to acetaldehyde and the initial steps of ethylene glycol and methanol metabolism, which yields toxic metabolites

Pharmacokinetics

IV: Metabolized by the liver (autoinduction of metabolism occurs with multiple dosing); excreted primarily in urine; $t_{1/2}$ varies with dose and has not been calculated

INDICATIONS AND USES: As an antidote for ethylene glycol (antifreeze) poisoning or for use in suspected ethylene glycol ingestion

DOSAGE

Adult

• *Treatment:* IV 15 mg/kg loading dose, followed by doses of 10 mg/kg q12h for 4 doses, then 15 mg/kg q12h thereafter until ethylene glycol levels have been reduced to <20 mg/dl; administer all doses as a slow IV infusion over 30 min

• *Dialysis:* Administer next scheduled dose at the beginning of dialysis if ≥6 hr since last dose; administer q4h during dialysis; at the end of dialysis, administer ½ of next scheduled dose if it has been 1-3 hr since last dose, or administer next scheduled dose if it has been >3 hr since last dose; for maintenance dosing of hemodialysis, administer next scheduled dose 12 hr from the last dose

$ **AVAILABLE FORMS/COST OF THERAPY**

• Conc—IV, 1 g/ml, 1.5 ml: **$1150.00**

PRECAUTIONS: Elderly, children

PREGNANCY AND LACTATION: Pregnancy category C; use caution in nursing mothers

SIDE EFFECTS/ADVERSE REACTIONS

CNS: Headache, dizziness, *seizures,* vertigo, lightheadedness, nystagmus, feeling of drunkenness, strange feeling, slurred speech, decreased environmental awareness

CV: Bradycardia, tachycardia, hypotension, phlebosclerosis

GI: Nausea, vomiting, diarrhea, anorexia, heartburn

HEME: Lymphangitis, eosinophilia, anemia

---

italic = common side effects   *bold italic* = life-threatening reactions

RESP: Hiccups, pharyngitis
MISC: Abdominal pain, fever, somnolence, lumbalgia, hangover, rash, injection site reaction

INTERACTIONS
Drugs

3 *Ethanol:* Reduced elimination rate of ethanol; reduced elimination rate of fomepizole

MONITORING PARAMETERS
• Frequently monitor both ethylene glycol levels and acid-base balance, as determined by serum electrolyte (anion gap) or arterial blood gas analysis
• In patients with high ethylene glycol levels ($\geq$50 mg/dl), significant metabolic acidosis or renal failure, consider hemodialysis to remove ethylene glycol and its toxic metabolites
• Treatment with fomepizole may be discontinued when ethylene glycol levels have been reduced to <20 mg/dl

---

fomvirsen
(fom-veer'-sen)
Rx: Vitravene
Chemical Class: Synthetic antisense oligonucleotide
Therapeutic Class: Antiviral

CLINICAL PHARMACOLOGY
Mechanism of Action: As an antisense oligonucleotide, fomvirsen is complementary to messenger RNA of the immediate-early transcriptional unit (IE2) of human CMV. Fomvirsen binding to this messenger RNA results in selective inhibition of IE2 proteins necessary for CMV replication
Pharmacokinetics
INTRAVITREAL: No systemic absorption documented; metabolized intravitreally by exonucleases yielding shortened oligonucleotides and mononucleotides, which are further catabolized and excreted as low-molecular-weight metabolites

INDICATIONS AND USES: CMV retinitis in AIDS patients

DOSAGE
Adult
• *Intravitreal:* 330 µg day 1 and day 15, then 330 µg qmo

§ AVAILABLE FORMS/COST OF THERAPY
• Inj, Sol—Intravitreal: 330 µg/0.25 ml, **$800**

PRECAUTIONS: Ocular infection other than retinitis, ocular diseases/conditions (e.g., glaucoma), recent treatment with cidofovir (potential exacerbation of ocular inflammation)

PREGNANCY AND LACTATION: Pregnancy category C; breast milk excretion unlikely

SIDE EFFECTS/ADVERSE REACTIONS
EENT: Abnormal vision, cataract, eye pain, conjunctival hemorrhage, *increased intraocular pressure (19%), intaocular inflammation (e.g., iritis, vitreitis; 20%),* retinal hemorrhage

SPECIAL CONSIDERATIONS
PATIENT/FAMILY EDUCATION
• Does not treat systemic aspects of CMV infection
MONITORING PARAMETERS
• Ophthalmologic examination

---

foscarnet
(foss-car'net)
Rx: Foscavir
Chemical Class: Pyrophosphate analog
Therapeutic Class: Antiviral

CLINICAL PHARMACOLOGY
Mechanism of Action: Selective inhibition at the pyrophosphate binding site on virus-specific DNA polymerases and reverse transcriptases;

does not require activation by thymidine kinase or other kinases

Pharmacokinetics

IV: 14%-17% bound to plasma proteins; 80%-90% excreted unchanged in urine; $t_{1/2}$ 2-8 hr in normal renal function

INDICATIONS AND USES: CMV retinitis in patients with AIDS; acyclovir-resistant HSV and herpes zoster infections; with ganciclovir for CMV retinitis after relapse with either agent alone

DOSAGE

Adult and Adolescent

• *Induction:* IV INF 60 mg/kg via infusion pump over 1 hr q8h for 2-3 wk depending on clinical response
• *Maintenance:* IV INF 90-120 mg/kg/day via infusion pump over 2 hr
• *Dose adjustment in renal impairment (based on CrCl ml/min/kg):* Induction for CrCl ≥1.6, 60 mg/kg/8 hr; CrCl 1.3, 50 mg/kg/8 hr; CrCl 1.0, 40 mg/kg/8 hr; CrCl 0.7, 30 mg/kg/8 hr; CrCl 0.4, 20 mg/kg/8 hr; maintenance for CrCl ≥1.4, 100 mg/kg/day; CrCl 0.7, 70 mg/kg/day; CrCl 0.5, 60 mg/kg/day

$ AVAILABLE FORMS/COST OF THERAPY

• Sol—IV: 24 mg/ml, 250 ml: **$74.95;** 500 ml: **$145.93**

PRECAUTIONS: Renal function impairment, electrolyte disturbances, neurologic abnormalities, cardiac abnormalities, seizure disorder, elderly, children, severe anemia

PREGNANCY AND LACTATION: Pregnancy category C; excretion into breast milk unknown; use caution in nursing mothers

SIDE EFFECTS/ADVERSE REACTIONS

CNS: Fever, headache, *seizures*
CV: Bradycardia, *cardiac failure, arrest;* cardiomyopathy; dysrhythmias, ECG abnormalities (sinus tachycardia, 1st degree AV block, non-specific ST-T segment changes), extrasystole, flushing, hypertension, hypotension, palpitations, phlebitis
EENT: Conjunctivitis, eye abnormalities, eye pain, taste perversions, vision abnormalities
GI: Abdominal pain, anorexia, constipation, *diarrhea,* dry mouth, dyspepsia, dysphagia, flatulence, melena, *nausea,* **pancreatitis,** rectal hemorrhage, ulcerative stomatitis, *vomiting*
GU: **Abnormal renal function (acute renal failure, decreased CrCl and increased serum creatinine),** albuminuria, dysuria, nocturia, polyuria, urethral disorder, urinary retention, UTI
HEME: **Anemia, granulocytopenia, leukopenia,** lymphadenopathy, platelet abnormalities, **thrombocytopenia,** thrombosis, WBC abnormalities
METAB: Acidosis, cachexia, decreased weight, hypercalcemia, hypocalcemia, hypokalemia, hypomagnesemia, hyponatremia, hypophosphatemia or hyperphosphatemia, increased alkaline phosphatase, increased LDH and BUN, thirst
MS: Arthralgia, back pain, chest pain, myalgia
RESP: Bronchospasm, coughing, dyspnea, hemoptysis, pharyngitis, pneumonia, pneumothorax, pulmonary infiltration, respiratory disorders, rhinitis, sinusitis, stridor
SKIN: Erythematous rash, facial edema, maculopapular rash, pruritus, rash, seborrhea, skin discoloration, skin ulceration, sweating

INTERACTIONS

Drugs

3 *Quinolones:* **Increased seizure risk (rare)**

SPECIAL CONSIDERATIONS
• Hydration to establish diuresis both prior to and during administration is recommended to minimize renal tox-

icity; the standard 24 mg/ml sol may be used undiluted via a central venous catheter, dilute to 12 mg/ml with D$_5$W or NS when a peripheral vein catheter is used

PATIENT/FAMILY EDUCATION

• Foscarnet is not a cure for CMV retinitis

• Notify clinician of perioral tingling, numbness in the extremities, or paresthesias (could signify electrolyte imbalances)

MONITORING PARAMETERS

• Serum creatinine, calcium, phosphorus, potassium, magnesium at baseline and 2-3 times/wk during induction and at least every 1-2 wk during maintenance

• Hemoglobin

• Regular ophthalmologic examinations

---

fosfomycin

(foss-fo-mye'sin)

Rx: Monurol

Chemical Class: Phosphoric acid derivative

Therapeutic Class: Antibiotic

CLINICAL PHARMACOLOGY

Mechanism of Action: Inactivates the enzyme enolpyruvul transferase; irreversibly blocks condensation of uridine diphosphate-N-acetylglucosamine with p-enolpyruvate which is one of the first steps in bacterial cell wall synthesis; bactericidal

Pharmacokinetics

PO: Peak 2 hr, absolute bioavailability 37% (reduced to 30% with food); not bound to plasma proteins, crosses the placenta; excreted unchanged in urine (38% of 3 g dose) and feces (18% of 3 g dose); t$_{1/2}$ 5.7 hr (11-50 hr in renal function impairment)

INDICATIONS AND USES: Uncomplicated acute cystitis in women Antibacterial spectrum usually includes:

• Gram-positive organisms: *Enterococcus faecalis, E. faecalis*

• Gram-negative organisms: *Escherichia coli, Citrobacter diversus, C. freundii, Enterobacter aerogenes, Klebsiella oxytoca, K. pneumoniae, Proteus mirabilis, P. vulgaris, Serratia marcenscens*

DOSAGE

Adult ≥18 yr

• PO 3 g packet mixed with 90-120 ml of water as a single dose

$ AVAILABLE FORMS/COST OF THERAPY

• Granule—Oral: 3 g/packet, 3's: **$83.56**

PRECAUTIONS: Children

PREGNANCY AND LACTATION: Pregnancy category B; excretion into breast milk unknown

SIDE EFFECTS/ADVERSE REACTIONS

CNS: Dizziness, headache

EENT: Pharyngitis, rhinitis

GI: Abdominal pain, *diarrhea*, dyspepsia, nausea

GU: Dysmenorrhea, vaginitis

HEME: **Aplastic anemia (rare)**

MS: Back pain

SKIN: Rash

MISC: Asthenia

INTERACTIONS

Drugs

3 *Metoclopramide:* Decreased serum concentration and urinary excretion of fosfomycin

SPECIAL CONSIDERATIONS

• Inferior 5-11 day posttherapy microbiologic eradication rates compared to ciprofloxacin and cotrimoxazole for acute cystitis; eradication rates comparable to nitrofurantoin

• Reserve for women unable to tolerate or unlikely to comply with

---

* = non-FDA-approved use

3-day courses of cotrimoxazole or trimethoprim

PATIENT/FAMILY EDUCATION

• Always mix with water before ingesting

---

fosinopril
(fo-sin'o-pril)
Rx: Monopril
Chemical Class: Nonsulfhydryl angiotensin-converting enzyme (ACE) inhibitor
Therapeutic Class: Antihypertensive

CLINICAL PHARMACOLOGY

Mechanism of Action: Antihypertensive, hypoproliferative, and cardioprotective effects attributable to competitive inhibition of angiotensin-converting enzyme (ACE) yielding decreased plasma concentrations of angiotensin II and plasma aldosterone concentrations, systemic vascular resistance, blood pressure, preload and afterload, not accompanied by changes in heart rate, pressor sensitivity to exogenous norepinephrine, or baroreceptor sensitivity

Pharmacokinetics

PO: Onset 1 hr, duration 24 hr, peak 3 hr; metabolized to active metabolite (fosinoprilat), $t_{1/2}$ (fosinoprilat) 12 hr; excreted in urine (50%) and feces (50%)

INDICATIONS AND USES: Hypertension, CHF (left ventricular dysfunction), MI, erythrocytosis,* nephropathy,* retinopathy*

DOSAGE

Adult and Child >16 yr

• *Hypertension:* PO 10 mg qd; usual dose range, 20-40 mg qd; maximal dose 80 mg qd, though dose-response curve usually flat after 40 mg qd

• *Congestive heart failure:* PO 5 (for volume-depleted, moderate to severe renal failure) = 10 mg qd; usual dose range 20-40 mg qd or titrate to systolic blood pressure of 100 mm Hg

• *Myocardial infarction:* PO 5 mg initial dose, repeated in 24 hr, with progressive doubling to a maximum dose of 20 mg qd, if systolic blood pressure remains over 100 mm Hg (fosinopril in acute myocardial infarction study, FAMIS)

• *Dosage in renal failure:* PO ≤7.5 mg qd if CrCl <10 ml/min

$ AVAILABLE FORMS/COST OF THERAPY

• Tab, Uncoated—Oral: 10 mg, 90's: **$77.58;** 20 mg, 90's: **$77.58;** 40 mg, 90's: **$77.58**

PRECAUTIONS: History of anaphylaxis, renal insufficiency (<30 ml/min), hypotension (CHF, elderly, volume depletion—diuretics, dialysis, cirrhosis), aortic stenosis, hyperkalemia (potassium supplements, potassium-sparing diuretics, renal disease, diabetes), neutropenia (autoimmune diseases, collagen vascular, febrile illness, immunosuppressant drug therapy), proteinuria, renal artery stenosis, surgery/anesthesia (excessive hypotension, correctable with fluids)

PREGNANCY AND LACTATION: Pregnancy category C (1st trimester), category D (2nd and 3rd trimesters); ACE inhibitors can cause fetal and neonatal morbidity and death when administered to pregnant women; when pregnancy is detected, discontinue ACE inhibitors as soon as possible; detectable in breast milk in trace amounts, a newborn would receive <0.1% of the mg/kg maternal dose; effect on nursing infant has not been determined; use with caution in nursing mothers

---

italic = common side effects   ***bold italic*** = life-threatening reactions

SIDE EFFECTS/ADVERSE REACTIONS

CNS: Anxiety, *dizziness, fatigue, headache,* insomnia, paresthesia

CV: Angina, hypotension, palpitations, postural hypotension, syncope (especially with 1st dose)

GI: Abdominal pain, constipation, melena, nausea, vomiting

GU: Decreased libido, impotence, increased BUN, creatinine, UTI

HEME: **Agranulocytosis, neutropenia**

METAB: Hyperkalemia, hyponatremia

MS: Arthralgia, arthritis, myalgia

RESP: Asthma, bronchitis, *cough,* dyspnea, sinusitis

SKIN: **Angioedema,** flushing, rash, sweating

INTERACTIONS

Drugs

❷ *Allopurinol:* Combination may predispose to hypersensitivity reactions

❸ *Alpha adrenergic blockers:* Exaggerated first dose hypotensive response when added to fosinopril

❸ *Aspirin:* May reduce hemodynamic effects of fosinopril; less likely at doses under 236 mg; less likely with nonacetylated salicylates

❸ *Azathioprine:* Increased myelosuppression

❸ *Cyclosporine:* Combination may cause renal insufficiency

❸ *Insulin:* Fosinopril may enhance insulin sensitivity

❸ *Iron:* Fosinopril may increase chance of systemic reaction to IV iron

❸ *Lithium:* Reduced lithium clearance

❸ *Loop diuretics:* Initiation of fosinopril may cause hypotension and renal insufficiency in patients taking loop diuretics

❸ *NSAIDs:* May reduce hemodynamic effects of fosinopril

❸ *Potassium-sparing diuretics:* Increased risk of hyperkalemia

❸ *Trimethoprim:* Additive risk of hyperkalemia, especially in patient predisposed to renal insufficiency

Labs

ACE inhibition can account for approximately 05. mEq/L rise in serum potassium

SPECIAL CONSIDERATIONS

PATIENT/FAMILY EDUCATION

• Caution with salt substitutes containing potassium chloride

• Rise slowly to sitting/standing position to minimize orthostatic hypotension

• Dizziness, fainting, lightheadedness may occur during 1st few days of therapy

• May cause altered taste perception or cough; persistent dry cough usually does not subside unless medication is stopped; notify clinician if these symptoms persist

MONITORING PARAMETERS

• BUN, creatinine, potassium within 2 wk after initiation of therapy (increased levels may indicate acute renal failure)

---

furazolidone

(fyur-a-zoh'li-done)

Rx: Furoxone

Chemical Class: Synthetic nitrofuran derivative

Therapeutic Class: Antibiotic; antiprotozoal

CLINICAL PHARMACOLOGY

Mechanism of Action: Exerts bactericidal action via interference with several bacterial enzyme systems; MAOI

Pharmacokinetics

PO: Systemically absorbed; extensively metabolized (possibly in the

---

intestine), colored metabolites excreted in urine

INDICATIONS AND USES: Bacterial or protozoal diarrhea and enteritis caused by susceptible organisms

Antimicrobial spectrum usually includes:

• Gram-positive organisms: Staphylococci

• Gram-negative organisms: *E. coli, Salmonella, Shigella, Proteus, Enterobacter aerogenes, Vibrio cholerae;* protozoan organisms: *Giardia lamblia*

DOSAGE
Adult
• PO 100 mg qid
Child
• PO 25-50 mg qid (≥5 yr); 17-25 mg qid (1-4 yr); 8-17 mg qid (1 mo-1 yr)

$ AVAILABLE FORMS/COST OF THERAPY
• Liq—Oral: 50 mg/15 ml, 60, 473 ml: **$16.06**/60 ml
• Tab, Coated—Oral: 100 mg, 100's: **$257.68**

CONTRAINDICATIONS: Infants <1 mo

PRECAUTIONS: Hypertension, diabetes, G-6-PD deficiency

PREGNANCY AND LACTATION: Pregnancy category C; could theoretically produce hemolytic anemia in a G-6-PD deficient newborn if given at term; excretion into breast milk unknown; use caution in nursing mothers

SIDE EFFECTS/ADVERSE REACTIONS
CNS: Fever, headache, malaise
*CV: **Hypertensive crisis,** orthostatic hypotension*
GI: Anal pruritus, colitis, nausea, proctitis, staphylococcic enteritis, vomiting
HEME: Hemolysis in G-6-PD deficiency
METAB: Hypoglycemia
MS: Arthralgia
SKIN: Vesicular morbilliform rash

DRUG INTERACTIONS
Drugs
3 *Amphetamines:* Hypertensive crisis
3 *Ephedrine:* Hypertensive response
3 *Ethanol:* Disulfiram-like reaction
3 *Foods high in amine content:* Hypertensive crisis
3 *Phenylpropanolamine:* Hypertensive response
Labs
• *Urine discoloration:* Metabolites may produce brown color
• *Glucose:* Metabolites give false positive with Benedict's reagent

SPECIAL CONSIDERATIONS
PATIENT/FAMILY EDUCATION
• Avoid ingestion of alcohol during and within 4 days after furazolidone therapy
• Avoid foods containing tyramine, especially if therapy extends beyond 5 days
• Avoid OTC drugs containing sympathomimetic drugs
• May color the urine brown

furosemide
(fur-oh'se-mide)
Rx: Furocot, Fumide, Lasix, Lo-Aqua, Myrosemide, Terbolan
Chemical Class: Anthranilic acid
Therapeutic Class: Loop diuretic

CLINICAL PHARMACOLOGY
Mechanism of Action: Inhibits the absorption of sodium and chloride at proximal and distal tubule sites and in the loop of Henle

italic = common side effects   ***bold italic*** = life-threatening reactions

Pharmacokinetics

PO: Onset 1 hr, peak 1-2 hr, duration 6-8 hr, 60% bioavailability; oral absorption is slower and less complete in patients with decompensated CHF; IV administration or increased oral dosing overcomes this deficit

IV/IM: Onset 5 min (slightly delayed with IM), peak ½ hr (IM), duration 2 hr; 98% bound to plasma proteins; 50% of PO dose and 80% of IV dose excreted in the urine within 24 hr, remainder eliminated by non-renal pathways (liver metabolism, excreted unchanged in feces); $t_{1/2}$ 30 min (9 hr in renal failure)

INDICATIONS AND USES: Edema (CHF, hepatic cirrhosis, renal disease, nephrotic syndrome); hypertension, pulmonary edema, hypercalcemia*

DOSAGE

Adult

• PO 20-80 mg/day in AM; may give another dose in 6 hr; increase in increments of 20-40 mg up to 400 mg/day if response is not satisfactory

• IM/IV 20-40 mg, increased by 20 mg q2h until desired response (rule of thumb: IV dose = ½ PO dose)

• *Pulmonary edema:* IV 40 mg given over several min, repeated in 1 hr; increase to 80 mg if needed

Child

• PO/IM/IV 1-2 mg/kg/dose up to 6 mg/kg/day in divided doses q6-12h

💲 AVAILABLE FORMS/COST OF THERAPY

• Inj, Sol—IM, IV: 10 mg/ml, 2, 4, 8, 10 ml: **$1.63-$14.96**/10 ml

• Sol—Oral: 10 mg/ml, 60, 120 ml: **$9.10-$10.50**/60 ml; 40 mg/5 ml, 500 ml: **$29.04**

• Tab, Uncoated—Oral: 20 mg, 100's: **$2.00-$19.14;** 40 mg, 100's:

$2.50-$26.82; 80 mg, 100's: **$7.75-$41.60**

CONTRAINDICATIONS: Anuria, hepatic coma

PRECAUTIONS: Fluid and electrolyte imbalance (including sodium, chloride, potassium, magnesium, calcium), renal disease, hepatic disease (may precipitate hepatic encephalopathy), gout, COPD, lupus erythematosus, diabetes mellitus, hyperparathyroidism, vomiting, diarrhea, elevated cholesterol/triglycerides

PREGNANCY AND LACTATION: Pregnancy category C; cardiovascular disorders such as pulmonary edema, severe hypertension, or CHF are probably the only valid indications for this drug during pregnancy; furosemide has been used after the first trimester without causing fetal or newborn adverse effects; does not appear to significantly alter amniotic fluid volume; maternal use during pregnancy has not been associated with toxic or teratogenic effects, although metabolic complications have been observed (hyponatremia, hyperuricemia); reduces placental and/or maternal hepatic perfusion; excreted into breast milk; no reports of adverse effects in nursing infants

SIDE EFFECTS/ADVERSE REACTIONS

CNS: Dizziness, fever, headache, paresthesia, restlessness, vertigo

CV: Chest pain, *circulatory collapse,* ECG changes, orthostatic hypotension

EENT: Blurred vision, ototoxicity

GI: Anorexia, constipation, cramping, diarrhea, dry mouth, *ischemic hepatitis,* jaundice, *nausea,* oral and gastric irritation, pancreatitis, vomiting

---

* = non-FDA-approved use

GU: Glycosuria, hyperuricemia, urinary bladder spasm

HEME: **Agranulocytosis, anemia, aplastic anemia, leukopenia,** purpura, **thrombocytopenia**

METAB: Hyperglycemia

SKIN: Erythema multiforme, **exfoliative dermatitis,** interstitial nephritis, necrotizing angiitis, photosensitivity, pruritus, *rash,* urticaria

INTERACTIONS
Drugs

2 *Aminoglycosides (gentamicin, kanamycin, neomycin, streptomycin):* Additive ototoxicity (ethacrynic acid > furosemide, torsemide, bumetanide)

3 *Angiotensin converting enzyme inhibitors:* Initiation of ACEI with intensive diuretic therapy may result in precipitous fall in blood pressure; ACEIs may induce renal insufficiency in the presence of diuretic-induced sodium depletion

3 *Barbiturates (phenobarbital):* Reduced diuretic response

3 *Bile acid-binding resins (cholestyramine, colestipol):* Resins markedly reduce the bioavailability and diuretic response of furosemide

3 *Carbenoxolone:* Severe hypokalemia from coadministration

3 *Cephalosporins (cephaloridine, cephalothin):* Enhanced nephrotoxicity with coadministration

2 *Cisplatin:* Additive ototoxicity (ethacrynic acid > furosemide, torsemide, bumetanide)

3 *Clofibrate:* Enhanced effects of both drugs, especially in hypoalbuminemic patients

3 *Corticosteroids:* Concomitant loop diuretic and corticosteroid therapy can result in excessive potassium loss

3 *Digitalis glycosides (digoxin, digitoxin):* Diuretic-induced hypokalemia may increase risk of digitalis toxicity

3 *Nonsteroidal antiinflammatory drugs (flurbiprofen, ibuprofen, indomethacin, naproxen, piroxicam, aspirin, sulindac):* Reduced diuretic and antihypertensive effects

3 *Phenytoin:* Reduced diuretic response

3 *Serotonin-reuptake inhibitors (fluoxetine, paroxetine, sertraline):* Case reports of sudden death; enhanced hyponatremia proposed; causal relationships not established

3 *Terbutaline:* Additive hypokalemia

3 *Tubocurarine:* Prolonged neuromuscular blockade

Labs

• *Cortisol:* False increases

• *Glucose:* Falsely low urine tests with clinistix and diastix

• *Thyroxine:* Increased serum concentration

• T_3 *uptake:* Interference causes increased serum values

SPECIAL CONSIDERATIONS
PATIENT/FAMILY EDUCATION

• May cause GI upset, take with food or milk

• Take early in the day

• Avoid prolonged exposure to sunlight

MONITORING PARAMETERS

• Urine volume, creatinine clearance, BUN electrolytes, reduction in edema, increased diuresis, decrease in body weight, reduction in blood pressure, glucose, uric acid, serum calcium (tetany), tinnitus, vertigo, hearing loss (especially in those at risk for ototoxicity—IV doses >120 mg; concomitant ototoxic drugs; renal disease)

---

gabapentin

(ga'ba-pen-tin)
Rx: Neurontin
Chemical Class: Cyclohexan-acetic acid derivative
Therapeutic Class: Anticonvulsant

CLINICAL PHARMACOLOGY
Mechanism of Action: Structurally related to gamma-aminobutyric acid (GABA) but does not interact with GABA receptors; binds to receptors in neocortex and hippocampus; identity and function remain to be elucidated
Pharmacokinetics
PO: Over dosage range of 300 to 600 mg tid, bioavailability drops 60%; not protein bound; not metabolized; elimination $t_{1/2}$ 5-7 hr if CrCl normal, 52 hr if CrCl <30 ml/min; removed by hemodialysis
INDICATIONS AND USES: Anticonvulsant adjunctive therapy for partial seizures with or without secondary generalization; adjunctive pain management*
DOSAGE
Adult and Child >12 yr
• PO 900 to 2400 mg/day given in 3 divided doses; start with 300 mg on day 1, 300 mg bid on day 2, and 300 mg tid on day 3
• *Adjustment for renal dysfunction:* CrCl >60 ml/min, daily dose 1200 mg; CrCl 30-60 ml/min, daily dose 600 mg; CrCl 15-30 ml/min, daily dose 300 mg; CrCl <15 ml/min, daily dose 150 mg; hemodialysis, 200-300 mg after dialysis
$ **AVAILABLE FORMS/COST OF THERAPY**
• Cap, Gel—Oral: 100 mg, 100's: **$46.43;** 300 mg, 100's: **$116.08;** 400 mg, 100's: **$139.28**

• Tab—Oral, 600 mg, 100's: **$210.03;** 800 mg, 100's: **$252.03**
PRECAUTIONS: Severe renal dysfunction, age <12 yr, tumorigenic in rats (pancreatic adenomas and carcinomas); significance to humans unknown
PREGNANCY AND LACTATION: Pregnancy category C; excretion into breast milk unknown
SIDE EFFECTS/ADVERSE REACTIONS
CNS: Abnormal thinking, amnesia, *ataxia (13%),* depression, *dizziness (17%),* dysarthria, *fatigue (11%),* nervousness, *nystagmus (8%),* somnolence *(19%),* tremor *(7%)*
EENT: Diplopia, rhinitis
GI: Dry mouth, dyspepsia
GU: Impotence
HEME: **Leukopenia (1%)**
MS: Myalgia, twitching
SKIN: Flushing, pruritus
INTERACTIONS
Drugs
3 *Antacids:* Reduce bioavailability of gabapentin by 20%
SPECIAL CONSIDERATIONS
PATIENT/FAMILY EDUCATION
Do not stop abruptly; taper over 1 wk
MONITORING PARAMETERS
• Drug level monitoring not necessary

gallium nitrate

(gal'ee-yum)
Rx: Ganite
Chemical Class: Hydrated nitrate salt of gallium
Therapeutic Class: Hypocalcemic agent

CLINICAL PHARMACOLOGY
Mechanism of Action: Inhibits calcium resorption from bone, reducing increased bone turnover

---

* = non-FDA-approved use

Pharmacokinetics
IV: Steady state achieved in 24-48 hr, not metabolized, excreted by the kidneys

INDICATIONS AND USES: Symptomatic cancer-related hypercalcemia unresponsive to adequate hydration

DOSAGE
Adult
• IV INF 200 mg/m^2/day for 5 consecutive days; dilute in 1 L NS or D$_5$W and infuse over 24 hr

⚡ AVAILABLE FORMS/COST OF THERAPY
• Inj, Sol—IV: 25 mg/ml, 20 ml: **$152.46**

CONTRAINDICATIONS: Severe renal disease (serum creatinine >2.5 mg/dl)

PRECAUTIONS: Concurrent use of potentially nephrotoxic drugs, children, renal disease

PREGNANCY AND LACTATION: Pregnancy category C; excretion into breast milk unknown, use caution in nursing mothers

SIDE EFFECTS/ADVERSE REACTIONS
CNS: Confusion, fever, hypothermia, lethargy, paresthesia
CV: Edema, hypotension, tachycardia
EENT: Acute optic neuritis, decreased hearing, visual impairment
GI: Constipation, diarrhea, nausea, vomiting
GU: **Acute renal failure, nephrotoxicity**
HEME: **Anemia** (very high doses), **leukopenia**
METAB: *Decreased serum bicarbonate,* hypocalcemia, *transient hypophosphatemia*
RESP: Dyspnea, pleural effusion, pulmonary infiltrates, rales, rhonchi
SKIN: Rash

INTERACTIONS
Drugs
3 *Aminoglycosides:* Increased risk of nephrotoxicity
3 *Amphotericin B:* Increased risk of nephrotoxicity

SPECIAL CONSIDERATIONS
Maintain adequate hydration throughout the treatment period; avoid overhydration in patients with compromised cardiovascular status

MONITORING PARAMETERS
• Serum creatinine daily (discontinue if exceeds 2.5 mg/dl)
• Urine output (≥2 L/day is recommended)
• Serum calcium and phosphorus

---

ganciclovir
(gan-sy'clo-ver)
Rx: Cytovene
Chemical Class: Synthetic nucleoside analog
Therapeutic Class: Antiviral

CLINICAL PHARMACOLOGY
Mechanism of Action: Preferentially phosphorylated in virus-infected cells to ganciclovir-triphosphate, which inhibits viral DNA synthesis

Pharmacokinetics
IV: t$_{1/2}$ 3.5 hr (prolonged in renal failure); excreted unchanged by the kidneys; crosses blood-brain barrier; 1%-2% bound to plasma proteins
PO: Bioavailability 5% fasting, 6-9% with food; elimination t$_{1/2}$ 4.8 hr

INDICATIONS AND USES: CMV retinitis in immunocompromised patients; prevention of CMV disease in transplant patients at risk; prevention of CMV in patients with advanced HIV infection; other CMV disease (e.g., pneumonitis, gastroenteritis, hepatitis)*

---

italic = common side effects   ***bold italic*** = life-threatening reactions

DOSAGE
Adult and Child >3 mo

• *CMV retinitis:* Induction IV 5 mg/kg q12h as a 1-2 hr INF for 14-21 days; maintenance IV 5 mg/kg/day as a single daily dose for 7 days/wk or 6 mg/kg/day for 5 days/wk; PO 1 g tid with food

• *CMV prevention in transplant recipients:* Induction IV 5 mg/kg q12h as a 1-2 hr INF for 7-14 days; maintenance IV 5 mg/kg/day as a single daily dose for 7 days/wk or 6 mg/kg/day for 5 days/wk

• *CMV prevention in AIDS patients:* PO 1 g tid with food

• *Renal function impairment (dosage for CrCl in ml/min):*
CrCl 50-69 IV 2.5 mg/kg q12h (induction) and 2.5 mg/kg q24h (maintenance); PO 500 mg tid
CrCl 25-49 IV 2.5 mg/kg q24h (induction) and 1.25 mg/kg q24h (maintenance); PO 500 mg bid
CrCl 10-24 IV 1.25 mg/kg q24h (induction) and 0.625 mg/kg q24h (maintenance); PO 500 mg qd
CrCl <10 IV 1.25 mg/kg 3×/wk after hemodialysis (induction) and 0.625 mg/kg 3×/wk after hemodialysis (maintenance); PO 500 mg 3×/wk after hemodialysis

💲 **AVAILABLE FORMS/COST OF THERAPY**

• Cap, Gel—Oral: 250 mg, 180's: **$719.55**
• Cap, Gel—Oral: 500 mg, 180's: **$1439.11**
• Inj, Lyphl-Sol—IV: 500 mg/vial: **$35.66**

PRECAUTIONS: Pre-existing cytopenias, renal function impairment, children <6 mo, elderly, platelet count <25,000/mm^3

PREGNANCY AND LACTATION: Pregnancy category C; excretion into breast milk unknown, not recommended in nursing mothers due to potential for serious adverse reactions in the nursing infant; do not resume nursing for at least 72 hr after last dose of ganciclovir

SIDE EFFECTS/ADVERSE REACTIONS

CNS: Abnormal thoughts or dreams, ataxia, chills, *coma,* confusion, dizziness, fever, *headache,* malaise, nervousness, paresthesia, psychosis, somnolence, tremor

CV: Dysrhythmia, hypertension, hypotension

EENT: Retinal detachment in CMV retinitis

GI: Abdominal pain, abnormal LFTs, anorexia, diarrhea, *hemorrhage,* nausea, vomiting

GU: Hematuria; increased serum creatinine, BUN

HEME: Anemia, eosinophilia, *granulocytopenia, thrombocytopenia*

METAB: Decrease in blood glucose

RESP: Dyspnea

SKIN: Alopecia, pruritus, rash, urticaria

MISC: Sepsis, infections

INTERACTIONS
Drugs

❸ *Didanosine:* Increased hematological toxicity

🅰 *Zidovudine:* Increased hematological toxicity

SPECIAL CONSIDERATIONS
PATIENT/FAMILY EDUCATION

• Compliance with laboratory monitoring is essential

MONITORING PARAMETERS

• CBC with differential and platelets q2 days during induction and weekly thereafter

• Serum creatinine q2 wk

---

* = non-FDA-approved use

gemfibrozil
(gem-fi'broe-zil)
Rx: Lopid
Chemical Class: Fibric acid derivative
Therapeutic Class: Antilipemic

CLINICAL PHARMACOLOGY
Mechanism of Action: Inhibits peripheral lipolysis and decreases hepatic extraction of free fatty acids, thus reducing hepatic triglyceride production; inhibits synthesis of VLDL carrier apolipoprotein B, leading to a decrease in VLDL production; in the process of decreasing triglyceride production, accelerates turnover and removal of cholesterol from the liver and increases excretion of cholesterol in the feces
Pharmacokinetics
PO: Peak 1-2 hr, >90% bound to plasma proteins, $t_{1/2}$ 1½ hr (biologic $t_{1/2}$ considerably longer due to enterohepatic recycling); metabolized in liver, excreted in urine (glucuronide conjugates)
INDICATIONS AND USES: Hypertriglyceridemia (Types IV and V hyperlipidemia); Type IIb hyperlipidemia; reduction of coronary heart disease risk in patients with low HDL cholesterol in addition to elevated LDL cholesterol and triglyceride levels that haven't responded to weight loss, dietary therapy, and other pharmacologic agents
DOSAGE
Adult
• PO 600 mg bid, 30 min before morning and evening meals
$ AVAILABLE FORMS/COST OF THERAPY
• Tab, Plain Coated—Oral: 600 mg, 60's: **$25.20-$84.22**
CONTRAINDICATIONS: Severe hepatic disease, pre-existing gallbladder disease, severe renal disease, primary biliary cirrhosis
PRECAUTIONS: Children, cholelithiasis
PREGNANCY AND LACTATION: Pregnancy category C; excretion into breast milk unknown; use caution in nursing mothers
SIDE EFFECTS/ADVERSE REACTIONS
CNS: Fatigue, headache, hypesthesia, paresthesia, vertigo
CV: Atrial fibrillation
EENT: Blurred vision, cataracts, retinal edema
GI: *Abdominal pain,* constipation, diarrhea, *dyspepsia,* nausea, taste perversion, vomiting, cholelithiasis
GU: Impotence
HEME: ***Anemia, bone marrow hypoplasia,*** eosinophilia, ***leukopenia, thrombocytopenia***
METAB: Increased blood glucose
MS: Arthralgia, myalgia, myasthenia, myopathy, painful extremities, ***rhabdomyolysis,*** synovitis
SKIN: Alopecia, dermatitis, ***exfoliative dermatitis,*** pruritus
MISC: Weight loss, carcinogenesis
INTERACTIONS
Drugs
3 *Binding resins:* Reduced bioavailability of gemfibrozil, separate doses by >2 hr
3 *Glyburide:* Increased risk of hypoglycemia
2 *HMG CoA reductase inhibitors (lovastatin, simvastatin, atorvastatin):* Increased likelihood of drug-induced myopathy
3 *Pravastatin:* Increased likelihood of drug-induced myopathy
2 *Warfarin:* Increased hypoprothrombinemic, response to warfarin
SPECIAL CONSIDERATIONS
PATIENT/FAMILY EDUCATION
• May cause dizziness or blurred vision; use caution while driving or

G

---

performing other tasks requiring alertness
• Notify clinician if GI side effects become pronounced
MONITORING PARAMETERS
• Serum CK level in patients complaining of muscle pain, tenderness, or weakness
• Periodic CBC during first 12 mo of therapy
• Periodic LFTs; discontinue therapy if abnormalities persist
• Blood glucose

---

gentamicin

(jen-ta-mye′sin)
Rx: *Cre/oint:* Ed-Mycin, G-Myticin, Garamycin *Ophth:* Ed-Mycin, Garamycin, Genoptic, Gent-AK, Gentrasul, Infa-Gen, Spectro Genta *Systemic:* G Mycin, Garamycin, Combinations
  Rx: with prednisolone (Pred-G)
Chemical Class: Aminoglycoside
Therapeutic Class: Antibiotic

CLINICAL PHARMACOLOGY
Mechanism of Action: Interferes with protein synthesis in bacterial cell by binding to 30S ribosomal subunit, which causes misreading of genetic code; inaccurate peptide sequence forms in protein chain, causing bacterial death
Pharmacokinetics
IM: Onset rapid, peak 30-90 min
IV: Onset immediate, peak 30 min after a 30 min INF
<30% bound to plasma proteins, plasma $t_{1/2}$ 1-2 hr, duration 6-8 hr; not metabolized, eliminated unchanged in urine via glomerular filtration
INDICATIONS AND USES: Bacterial neonatal sepsis; bacterial septicemia; serious bacterial infections of the CNS (meningitis), urinary tract, respiratory tract, GI tract, skin, bone, and soft tissue; superficial ocular infections involving the conjunctiva or cornea; infection prophylaxis in minor cuts, wounds, burns, and skin abrasions; superficial infections of the skin; alternative regimen for PID (in combination with clindamycin)*
Antibacterial spectrum usually includes:
• Gram-positive organisms: *Staphylococcus* spp. (including penicillin- and methicillin-resistant strains), *Streptococcus faecalis* (in combination with cell wall synthesis inhibitor)
• Gram-negative organisms: *Escherichia coli*, *Proteus* spp. (indole-positive and indole-negative), *Pseudomonas aeruginosa*, *Klebsiella* spp., *Enterobacter* spp., *Serratia* spp., *Citrobacter* spp., *Providencia* spp., *Salmonella* spp. and *Shigella* spp., *Yersinia pestis*
DOSAGE
• Use ideal body weight for dosage calculations
Adult
• *Severe systemic infections:* IV INF 3-5 mg/kg/day diluted in 50-100 ml NS or D_5W and infused over 30-60 min in divided doses q8h, adjust dosage based on results of gentamicin peak and trough levels (once-daily dosage*: 7 mg/kg q24h; not for pediatrics, pregnant, burns, ascites, dialysis, enterococcal endocarditis); IM 3 mg/kg/day in divided doses q8h, adjust dosage based on results of gentamicin peak and trough levels; intrathecal 4-8 mg/day
• *Conjunctivitis:* INSTILL 1 gtt q2-4h; OPHTH apply 1/4 in ribbon of ointment to conjunctival sac bid-tid

---

- TOP rub into affected area qd-qid, cover with sterile bandage if needed

Infants and Children <5 yr

- IV/IM 2.5 mg/kg/dose q8h, adjust dosage based on results of gentamicin peak and trough levels; INTRATHECAL (>3 mo) 1-2 mg/day

Child ≥5 yr

- IV/IM 1.5-2.5 mg/kg/dose q8h, adjust dosage based on results of gentamicin peak and trough levels

§ AVAILABLE FORMS/COST OF THERAPY

- Inj, Sol—IM; IV: 10 mg/ml, 2 ml: **$1.75-$2.24**; 40 mg/ml, 2 ml: **$2.15-$4.37**
- Inj, Sol—Intrathecal: 2 mg/ml, 2 ml: **$2.70**
- Sol—Ophth: 0.3%, 5, 15 ml: **$2.40-$18.02**/5 ml
- Oint—Ophth: 0.3% , 3.5 g: **$9.55-$18.02**
- Oint—Top: 0.1%, 15, 30, 45 g: **$1.80-$19.92**/15 g
- Cre—Top: 0.1%, 15, 30 g: **$1.80-$19.92**/15 g

PRECAUTIONS: Neonates, renal disease, myasthenia gravis, hearing deficits, Parkinson's disease, elderly, dehydration, hypokalemia, prolonged use

PREGNANCY AND LACTATION: Pregnancy category C; ototoxicity has not been reported as an effect of *in utero* exposure; 8th cranial nerve toxicity in the fetus is well known following exposure to other aminoglycosides and could potentially occur with gentamicin; potentiation of magnesium sulfate-induced neuromuscular weakness in neonates has been reported, use caution during the last 32 hr of pregnancy; data on excretion into breast milk are lacking

SIDE EFFECTS/ADVERSE REACTIONS

CNS: Confusion, *convulsions,* depression, dizziness, muscle twitching, myasthenia gravis-like syndrome, *neurotoxicity,* numbness, tremors, vertigo

CV: Hypertension, hypotension, palpitations

EENT: Deafness, ototoxicity, tinnitus, visual disturbances; Ophth, burning, conjunctival erythema, conjunctival paresthesia, inflammation, itching, lid itching, lid swelling, mydriasis, overgrowth of nonsusceptible organisms, poor corneal wound healing, stinging, temporary visual haze (ointment), transient irritation

GI: Anorexia, hepatomegaly, increased ALT, AST, bilirubin; *nausea,* splenomegaly, *vomiting*

GU: Azotemia, hematuria, nephrotoxicity, oliguria, renal damage, renal failure

HEME: Agranulocytosis, anemia, *eosinophilia, leukopenia, thrombocytopenia*

METAB: Decreased serum calcium, sodium, potassium, magnesium

RESP: Respiratory depression

SKIN: Alopecia, burning, dermatitis, photosensitivity, pruritis, *rash,* urticaria

INTERACTIONS

Drugs

§ *Amphotericin B:* Synergistic nephrotoxicity

❷ *Atracurium:* Gentamicin potentiates respiratory depression by atracurium

§ *Carbenicillin:* Potential for inactivation of gentamicin in patients with renal failure

§ *Carboplatin:* Additive nephrotoxicity or ototoxicity

§ *Cephalosporins:* Increased potential for nephrotoxicity in patients with preexisting renal disease

§ *Cisplatin:* Additive nephrotoxicity or ototoxicity

§ *Cyclosporine:* Additive nephrotoxicity

---

italic = common side effects   ***bold italic*** = life-threatening reactions

❷ *Ethacrynic acid:* Additive ototoxicity

❸ *Indomethacin:* Reduced renal clearance of gentamicin in premature infants

❸ *Methoxyflurane:* Additive nephrotoxicity

❷ *Neuromuscular blocking agents:* Gentamicin potentiates respiratory depression by neuromuscular blocking agents

❸ *NSAIDs:* May reduce renal clearance of gentamicin

❸ *Penicillins (extended spectrum):* Potential for inactivation of gentamicin in patients with renal failure

❸ *Piperacillin:* Potential for inactivation of gentamicin in patients with renal failure

❷ *Succinylcholine:* Gentamicin potentiates respiratory depression by succinylcholine

❸ *Ticarcillin:* Potential for inactivation of gentamicin in patients with renal failure

❸ *Vancomycin:* Additive nephrotoxicity or ototoxicity

❷ *Vecuronium:* Gentamicin potentiates respiratory depression by vecuronium

Labs
• *Amino acids:* Increase in urine amino acids
• *AST:* False elevations
• *Protein:* False urine elevations

SPECIAL CONSIDERATIONS
PATIENT/FAMILY EDUCATION
• Report headache, dizziness, loss of hearing, ringing, roaring in ears, or feeling of fullness in head
• Tilt head back, place medication in conjunctival sac, and close eyes
• Apply light finger pressure on lacrimal sac for 1 min following instill (gtt)
• May cause temporary blurring of vision following administration
• Notify clinician if stinging, burning, or itching becomes pronounced or if redness, irritation, swelling, decreasing vision, or pain persists or worsens
• Do not touch tip of container to any surface
• For external use only
• Cleanse affected area of skin prior to application
• Notify clinician if condition worsens or if rash or irritation develops

MONITORING PARAMETERS
• Urinalysis for proteinuria, cells, casts
• Urine output
• Serum peak, drawn at 30-60 min after IV INF or 60 min after IM inj, trough level drawn just before next dose; adjust dosage per levels (usual therapeutic plasma levels, peak 4-8 μg/ml, trough ≤ 2 μg/ml)
• Serum creatinine for CrCl calculation
• Serum calcium, magnesium, sodium
• Audiometric testing, assess hearing before, during, after treatment

glatiramer
(gla-teer'a-mer)
Rx: Copaxone
Chemical Class: Synthetic polypeptide
Therapeutic Class: Multiple sclerosis agent

CLINICAL PHARMACOLOGY
Mechanism of Action: Inhibits the immune response to myelin basic protein and possibly other myelin antigens that are thought to be involved in the pathogenesis of multiple sclerosis

Pharmacokinetics
SC: Substantial fraction hydrolyzed locally; some fraction enters lymphatic circulation; some may enter systemic circulation intact

INDICATIONS AND USES: Relapsing-remitting multiple sclerosis
DOSAGE
Adult
• SC 20 mg qd
💲 **AVAILABLE FORMS/COST OF THERAPY**
• Inj—SC:20 mg/vial, 32's: **$922.98**
PRECAUTIONS: Advanced relapsing-remitting multiple sclerosis, chronic-progressive multiple sclerosis
PREGNANCY AND LACTATION: Pregnancy category B; excretion into breast milk unknown, use caution in nursing mothers
SIDE EFFECTS/ADVERSE REACTIONS
CNS: Dizziness, faintness
CV: Transient chest pain
GI: Anorexia, constipation, nausea, vomiting
HEME: Transient eosinophilia
MS: Joint pain, muscle cramps
SKIN: Pain at injection site, rash, urticaria
MISC: Systemic reaction (combination of flushing, palpitations, chest tightness, diaphoresis, dyspnea, and/or anxiety)
SPECIAL CONSIDERATIONS
• May be useful for relapsing-remitting multiple sclerosis in patients who are not benefiting from, or are intolerant of, interferon β-1 a/b; less effective in patients with advanced disease or chronic-progressive multiple sclerosis; not a cure for multiple sclerosis and benefits achieved are relatively modest
• Sites for injection include arms, abdomen, hips, and thighs

---

glimepiride
(gly-mep′er-ide)
Rx: Amaryl
Chemical Class: Sulfonylurea (2nd generation)
Therapeutic Class: Oral hypoglycemic

G

CLINICAL PHARMACOLOGY
Mechanism of Action: Decreases blood sugar via stimulation of insulin secretion and increased tissue responsiveness to insulin; initial hypoglycemic effects due to stimulation of pancreatic islets (dependent upon functioning β-cells); extrapancreatic effect predominantly due to inhibition of hepatic glucose production, but may also facilitate improved insulin-insulin receptor binding
Pharmacokinetics
PO: Peak 2-3 hr, duration 24 hr; >99.5% bound to plasma proteins; completely metabolized by liver, metabolites excreted in urine (60%) and feces (40%)
INDICATIONS AND USES: Diabetes mellitus, type 2
DOSAGE
Adult
• PO 1-2 mg qd with breakfast or the 1st main meal; usual maintenance dose 1-4 mg qd; mfg. maximum dose 8 mg/day (NOTE: Daily doses >4 mg provide little added benefit.)
💲 **AVAILABLE FORMS/COST OF THERAPY**
• Tab—Oral: 1 mg, 100's: **$24.48;** 2 mg, 100's: **$39.66;** 4 mg, 100's: **$74.76**
CONTRAINDICATIONS: Diabetes mellitus, type 1; ketoacidosis
PRECAUTIONS: Elderly, cardiac disease, severe renal disease, severe hepatic disease, thyroid disease, ad-

---

renal or pituitary insufficiency, debilitated or malnourished patients

PREGNANCY AND LACTATION: Pregnancy category C; inappropriate for use during pregnancy due to inadequacy for blood glucose control, potential for prolonged neonatal hypoglycemia, and risk of congenital abnormalities; insulin is the drug of choice for control of blood sugars during pregnancy; breast milk secretion, unknown; the potential for neonatal hypoglycemia dictates caution in nursing mothers

SIDE EFFECTS/ADVERSE REACTIONS

CNS: Dizziness, drowsiness, headache, paresthesia

EENT: Blurred vision, tinnitus, vertigo

GI: Cholestatic jaundice, constipation, diarrhea, elevated liver function tests, gastralgia, nausea

HEME: **Agranulocytosis, aplastic anemia, hemolytic anemia,** hepatic porphyria, **leukopenia, pancytopenia, thrombocytopenia**

METAB: Hypoglycemia, hyponatremia, SIADH

MS: Fatigue, weakness

SKIN: Eczema, erythema, morbilliform or maculopapular eruptions, pruritus, urticaria

INTERACTIONS

Drugs

❸ *Anabolic steroids:* Enhanced hypoglycemic response

❸ *Angiotensin converting enzyme inhibitors*: Increased risk of hypolycemia

❸ *Antacids:* Enhanced rate of absorption

❸ *Aspirin:* Enhanced hypoglycemic effect

❸ β-*Adrenergic blockers:* Altered response to hypoglycemia; prolonged recovery of normoglycemia, hypertension, blockade of tachycardia; may increase blood glucose concentration

❸ *Clofibrate:* Enhanced effects of oral hypoglycemic drugs

❸ *Corticosteroids:* Increased blood glucose in diabetic patients

❸ *Cyclosporine:* Increased cyclosporine levels

⚠ *Ethanol:* Excessive intake may lead to altered glycemic control; "Antabuse"-like reaction may occur

❸ *Gemfibrozil:* Increased risk of hypoglycemia

❸ *H$_2$-receptor antagonists:* Enhanced rate of absorption

❸ *MAOIs:* Excessive hypoglycemia may occur in patients with diabetes

❷ *Phenylbutazole:* Increases serum concentrations of oral hypoglycemic drugs

❸ *Proton pump blockers:* Enhanced rate of absorption

❸ *Rifampin:* Reduced sulfonylurea concentrations

❸ *Sulfonamides:* Enhanced hypoglycemic effects of sulfonylureas

❸ *Thiazide diuretics:* Potential increased dosage requirement of antidiabetic drugs

SPECIAL CONSIDERATIONS

• No demonstrated advantage over existing 2nd generation sulfonylureas

PATIENT/FAMILY EDUCATION

• Multiple drug interactions, including alcohol and salicylates

• Symptoms of hypoglycemia: tingling lips/tongue, nausea, confusion, fatigue, sweating, hunger, visual changes (spots)

MONITORING PARAMETERS

• Self-monitored blood glucoses; glycosolated hemoglobin q 3-6 mo

---

* = non-FDA-approved use

glipizide
(glip'i-zide)
Rx: Glucotrol, Glucotrol XL
Chemical Class: Sulfonylurea
(2nd generation)
Therapeutic Class: Oral hypoglycemic

CLINICAL PHARMACOLOGY
Mechanism of Action: Decreases blood sugar via stimulation of insulin secretion and increased tissue responsiveness to insulin; initial hypoglycemic effects due to stimulation of pancreatic islets (dependent upon functioning β-cells); extrapancreatic effect predominantly due to inhibition of hepatic glucose production, but may also facilitate improved insulin-insulin receptor binding

Pharmacokinetics
PO: Completely absorbed by GI route, onset 1-1½ hr, duration 10-24 hr, $t_{1/2}$ 2-4 hr; metabolized in liver to inactive metabolites, excreted in urine; 90%-95% bound to plasma proteins

INDICATIONS AND USES: Type 2 diabetes mellitus

DOSAGE
Adult and Child >16 yr
• PO 2.5-5 mg 30 min before breakfast; adjust dose in 2.5-5 mg increments; manufacturer recommended max dose 40 mg/day; best to divide dose if daily dose exceeds 10 mg (i.e., 10 mg bid); (NOTE: little if any benefit from daily doses >20 mg)

💲 AVAILABLE FORMS/COST OF THERAPY
• Tab, Uncoated—Oral: 5 mg, 100's: **$6.75-$45.01;** 10 mg, 100's: **$12.05-$81.64**
• Tab, Coated, SUS Action—Oral: 5 mg, 100's: **$27.56;** 10 mg, 100's: **$54.54**

CONTRAINDICATIONS: Diabetes mellitus, type 1; ketoacidosis

PRECAUTIONS: Elderly, cardiac disease, severe renal disease, severe hepatic disease, thyroid disease, adrenal or pituitary insufficiency, debilitated or malnourished patients

PREGNANCY AND LACTATION: Pregnancy category C; inappropriate for use during pregnancy due to inadequate for blood glucose control, potential for prolonged neonatal hypoglycemia, and risk of congenital abnormalities; insulin is the drug of choice for control of blood sugars during pregnancy; breast milk secretion unknown; the potential for neonatal hypoglycemia dictates caution in nursing mothers

SIDE EFFECTS/ADVERSE REACTIONS
CNS: Dizziness, drowsiness, headache, paresthesia
EENT: Tinnitus, vertigo
GI: Cholestatic jaundice, constipation, diarrhea, elevated liver function tests, gastralgia, nausea
GU: Mild to moderate elevations in BUN and creatinine
*HEME: **Agranulocytosis, aplastic anemia, hemolytic anemia,** hepatic porphyria, **leukopenia, pancytopenia, thrombocytopenia***
*METAB: **Hypoglycemia,** SIADH*
MS: Fatigue, weakness
SKIN: Eczema, erythema, morbilliform or maculopapular eruptions, pruritus, urticaria

INTERACTIONS
Drugs
🔳 *Anabolic steroids:* Enhanced hypoglycemic response
🔳 *Angiotensin converting enzyme inhibitor:* Increased risk of hypoglycemia
🔳 *Antacids:* Enhanced rate of absorption

---

italic = common side effects   ***bold italic*** = life-threatening reactions

3 *Aspirin:* Enhanced hypoglycemic effects

3 β-*Adrenergic blockers:* Altered response to hypoglycemia; prolonged recovery of normoglycemia, hypertension, blockade of tachycardia; may increase blood glucose concentration

3 *Clofibrate:* Enhanced effects of oral hypoglycemic drugs

3 *Corticosteroids:* Increased blood glucose in diabetic patients

⚠ *Ethanol:* Excessive intake may lead to altered glycemic control; Antabuse-like reaction may occur

3 *Gemfibrozil:* Increased risk of hypoglycemia

3 *H₂-receptor antagonists (cimetidine, ranitidine, etc.):* Enhanced rate of absorption

3 *MAOIs:* Excessive hypoglycemia may occur in patient with diabetes

3 *Phenylbutazone:* Increases serum concentrations of oral hypoglycemics

3 *Rifampin:* Reduced sulfonylurea concentrations

3 *Sulfonamides:* Enhanced hypoglycemic effects of sulfonylureas

3 *Thiazide diuretics:* Potential increased dosage requirement of antidiabetic drugs

SPECIAL CONSIDERATIONS
PATIENT/FAMILY EDUCATION
• Administer 30 min ac
• Notify clinician of fever, sore throat, rash, unusual bruising, or bleeding
• Multiple drug interactions, including alcohol and salicylates
• Symptoms of hypoglycemia: tingling lips/tongue, nausea, confusion, fatigue, sweating, hunger, visual changes (spots)
• Notify clinician of fever, sore throat, rash, unusual bruising, or bleeding

MONITORING PARAMETERS
• Self-monitored blood glucose; glycosylated hemoglobin q 3-6 mo

---

glucagon
(gloo′ka-gon)
Rx: Glucagon
Chemical Class: Polypeptide hormone (pancreas)
Therapeutic Class: Antihypoglycemic agent

CLINICAL PHARMACOLOGY
Mechanism of Action: Accelerates liver glycogenolysis and inhibits glycogen synthetase resulting in blood glucose elevation; stimulates hepatic gluconeogenesis; relaxes smooth muscle of the GI tract
Pharmacokinetics
IV/IM/SC: Onset within 15 min; degraded in liver, kidney and plasma; $t_{1/2}$ 3-6 min

INDICATIONS AND USES: Hypoglycemia; diagnostic aid in radiologic examination of GI tract when hypotonic state is advantageous
DOSAGE
Adult
• *Hypoglycemia:* IV/IM/SC 0.5-1 mg, may repeat in 20 min prn
• *Diagnostic aid:* IV/IM/SC 0.25-2.0 mg 10 min prior to procedure
Child
• *Hypoglycemia:* IV/IM/SC 30 μg/kg/dose, not to exceed 1 mg/dose, repeat in 20 min prn
Neonate
• *Hypoglycemia:* IV/IM/SC 30 μg/kg/dose, max 1 mg/dose

💲 AVAILABLE FORMS/COST OF THERAPY
• Inj, Powder for inj—IM, IV, SC: 1 mg: **$66.00**
• Inj, Sol—IM, IV, SC: 1 mg/vial: (Glucagon emergency kit): **$66.00**

PRECAUTIONS: Insulinoma, pheochromocytoma

PREGNANCY AND LACTATION: Pregnancy category B; excretion into breast milk unknown; use caution in nursing mothers

SIDE EFFECTS/ADVERSE REACTIONS

CV: Hypotension

GI: Nausea, vomiting

*RESP: **Respiratory distress***

SKIN: Urticaria

INTERACTIONS

Drugs

3 *Oral anticoagulants:* Enhanced hypoprothrombinemic response to warfarin and possibly other oral anticoagulants

SPECIAL CONSIDERATIONS

PATIENT/FAMILY EDUCATION

• Notify clinician when hypoglycemic reactions occur so that antidiabetic therapy can be adjusted

MONITORING PARAMETERS

• Blood sugar, level of consciousness

---

glutethimide

(gloo-teth'i-mide)

Chemical Class: Piperidine derivative

Therapeutic Class: Sedative-hypnotic

DEA Class: Schedule II

CLINICAL PHARMACOLOGY

Mechanism of Action: CNS depressant: depresses the sensory cortex, decreases motor activity, alters cerebellar function, produce drowsiness, sedation, and hypnosis; dose-dependent respiratory depression; exhibits pronounced anticholinergic activity; suppresses REM sleep and is associated with REM rebound

Pharmacokinetics

PO: Erratically absorbed from GI tract, peak 1-6 hr, $t_{1/2}$ 10-12 hr, 50% bound to plasma proteins; metabolized in liver to an active metabolite; significant enterohepatic recirculation

INDICATIONS AND USES: Short-term relief of insomnia

DOSAGE

Adult

• PO 250-500 mg hs

💲 AVAILABLE FORMS/COST OF THERAPY

• Tab, Uncoated—Oral: 500 mg, 100's: **$10.50-$16.95**

CONTRAINDICATIONS: Porphyria

PRECAUTIONS: History of drug abuse, children, elderly

PREGNANCY AND LACTATION: Pregnancy category C; newborn infants of mothers dependent on glutethimide may exhibit withdrawal symptoms; excretion into breast milk unknown; use caution in nursing mothers

SIDE EFFECTS/ADVERSE REACTIONS

CNS: Ataxia, *dizziness,* hangover, headache, *residual sedation,* stimulation

EENT: Blurred vision

GI: Diarrhea, dry mouth, hiccups, jaundice, nausea, vomiting

*HEME: **Aplastic anemia, leukopenia, megaloblastic anemia,*** porphyria, ***thrombocytopenia***

*SKIN: **Exfoliative dermatitis (rare),*** purpura, *rash,* urticaria

INTERACTIONS

Drugs

3 *Ethanol:* Excessive CNS depression and impaired psychomotor performance

2 *Oral anticoagulants:* Decreased hypoprothrombinemic response to warfarin and probably other oral anticoagulants

3 *Tacrolimus:* Glutethimide increases gut metabolism (CYP3A4)

---

italic = common side effects **bold italic** = life-threatening reactions

of tacrolimus, decreasing levels and effect

Labs

• *Ethosuximide:* Cross-reacts to cause false increases

SPECIAL CONSIDERATIONS
Has generally been replaced with safer and more effective agents

PATIENT/FAMILY EDUCATION

• Use caution when driving or performing tasks requiring alertness
• Avoid alcohol and other CNS depressants

MONITORING PARAMETERS

• Toxic serum glutethimide concentrations are >6 µg/ml

---

glyburide
(glye′byoor-ide)
Rx: Diaβeta, Glynase Prestab, Micronase
Chemical Class: Sulfonylurea (2nd generation)
Therapeutic Class: Oral hypoglycemic

CLINICAL PHARMACOLOGY
Mechanism of Action: Decreases blood sugar via stimulation of insulin secretion and increased tissue responsiveness to insulin; initial hypoglycemic effects due to stimulation of pancreatic islets (dependent upon functioning β cells); extrapancreatic effect predominantly due to inhibition of hepatic glucose production, but may also facilitate improved insulin-insulin receptor binding

Pharmacokinetics

PO: Completely absorbed by GI route, onset 2-4 hr, peak 2-8 hr, duration 24 hr, $t_{1/2}$ 10 hr (4 hr for micronized formulation); metabolized in liver to weakly active metabolites; excreted in urine, feces (metabolites); 90%-95% bound to plasma proteins

INDICATIONS AND USES: Diabetes mellitus, type 2

DOSAGE

Adult and Child >16 yr

• PO 1.25-5 mg qd (0.75-3 mg for micronized formulation) with breakfast or 1st main meal; manufacturer max dose 20 mg/day (2 mg/day for micronized formulation); best to divide dose bid for doses >5 mg (i.e., 5 mg bid) (NOTE: Daily doses >10 mg [6 mg for micronized] provide little added benefit)

$ **AVAILABLE FORMS/COST OF THERAPY**

• Tab, Uncoated—Oral: 1.25 mg, 100's: **$9.38-$28.79;** 2.5 mg, 100's: **$13.13-$47.96;** 5 mg, 100's: **$13.15-$81.09**
• Tab, Uncoated, Micronized—Oral: 1.5 mg, 100's: **$29.52-$43.00;** 3 mg, 100's: **$37.67-$72.00;** 6 mg, 100's: **$84.09-$113.50**

CONTRAINDICATIONS: Diabetes mellitus, type 1; ketoacidosis

PRECAUTIONS: Elderly, cardiac disease, severe renal disease, severe hepatic disease, thyroid disease, adrenal or pituitary insufficiency, debilitated or malnourished patients

PREGNANCY AND LACTATION: Pregnancy category B; inappropriate for use during pregnancy due to inadequacy for blood glucose control, potential for prolonged neonatal hypoglycemia, and risk of congenital abnormalities; insulin is the drug of choice for control of blood sugars during pregnancy; breast milk secretion unknown; the potential for neonatal hypoglycemia dictates caution in nursing mothers

SIDE EFFECTS/ADVERSE REACTIONS

CNS: Dizziness, drowsiness, headache, paresthesia

EENT: Tinnitus, vertigo

GI: Cholestatic jaundice, constipation, diarrhea, elevated liver function tests, gastralgia, nausea

GU: Mild to moderate elevations in BUN and creatinine

HEME: **Agranulocytosis, aplastic anemia, hemolytic anemia,** hepatic porphyria, **leukopenia, pancytopenia, thrombocytopenia**

METAB: **Hypoglycemia,** SIADH

MS: Fatigue, weakness

SKIN: Eczema, erythema, morbilliform or maculopapular eruptions, pruritus, urticaria

INTERACTIONS

Drugs

▨ *Anabolic steroids:* Enhanced hypoglycemic response

▨ *Angiotensin converting enzyme inhibitor:* Increased risk of hypoglycemia

▨ *Antacids:* Enhanced rate of absorption

▨ *Aspirin:* Enhanced hypoglycemic effects

▨ *β-Adrenergic blockers:* Altered response to hypoglycemia; prolonged recovery of normoglycemia, hypertension, blockade of tachycardia; may increase blood glucose concentration

▨ *Clofibrate:* Enhanced effects of oral hypoglycemic drugs

▨ *Corticosteroids:* Increased blood glucose in diabetic patients

⚠ *Ethanol:* Excessive intake may lead to altered glycemic control; Antabuse-like reaction may occur

▨ *Gemfibrozil:* Increased risk of hypoglycemia

▨ *H₂-receptor antagonists (cimetidine, ranitidine, etc.):* Enhanced rate of absorption

▨ *MAOIs:* Excessive hypoglycemia may occur in patient with diabetes

▨ *Phenylbutazone:* Increases serum concentrations of oral hypoglycemics

▨ *Rifampin:* Reduced sulfonylurea concentrations

▨ *Sulfonamides:* Enhanced hypoglycemic effects of sulfonylureas

▨ *Thiazide diuretics:* Potential increased dosage requirement of antidiabetic drugs

Labs

• *Protein:* False-urine increases with Ponceaus dye method

SPECIAL CONSIDERATIONS

• Micronized formulations do not provide bioequivalent serum concentrations to non-micronized formulations; retitrate patients when transferring from any hypoglycemic to micronized glyburide

PATIENT/FAMILY EDUCATION

• Multiple drug interactions including alcohol and salicylates

• Notify clinician of fever, sore throat, rash, unusual bruising, or bleeding

MONITORING PARAMETERS

• Self-monitored blood glucose; glycosylated Hgb q3-6 mo

---

glycerin
(gli'ser-in)

OTC: *Laxative: Fleets Babylax, Glycerol, Sani-Supp*

Rx: *Ophth: Ophthalgan*
Oral: Osmoglyn

Chemical Class: Trihydric alcohol

Therapeutic Class: Laxative; antiglaucoma agent; osmotic diuretic

---

CLINICAL PHARMACOLOGY

Mechanism of Action: (Laxative) Osmotic shifts stimulate defecation; (Ophth) Osmotic agent reduces intraocular pressure transiently

Pharmacokinetics

PO: Well absorbed, onset 10-60 min, duration 5 hr

---

italic = common side effects   ***bold italic*** = life-threatening reactions

OPHTH: Onset 10 min, peak 20 min, duration 4-8 hr

PR: Poorly absorbed, onset 15-30 min

Metabolized and eliminated by kidney

INDICATIONS AND USES: (Rect) constipation; (Ophth) edematous cornea; (Oral) interruption of acute glaucoma attack, reduction of intraocular pressure preocular and postocular surgery, lowering intracranial pressure*

DOSAGE

Adult

• *Constipation:* PR 1 adult supp 1-2 times/day prn or 5-15 ml as an enema

• *Reduction of corneal edema:* OPHTH instill 1 gtt q3-4h

• *Reduction of intraocular pressure:* PO 1-1.8 g/kg 1-1½ hr preoperatively; additional doses may be administered at 5 hr intervals

• *Reduction of intracranial pressure:* PO 1.5 g/kg/day divided q4h or 1 g/kg/dose q6h

Child

• *Constipation:* PR (<6 yr) 1 infant supp 1-2 times/day prn or 2-5 ml as an enema; (>6 yr) same as adult

• *Reduction of corneal edema:* Same as adult

• *Reduction of intraocular pressure:* Same as adult

• *Reduction of intracranial pressure:* Same as adult

Neonate

• *Constipation:* PR 0.5 ml/kg/dose

🚫 AVAILABLE FORMS/COST OF THERAPY

• Sol—Ophth: 99.5%, 7.5 ml: **$25.75**

• Sol—Oral: 50%, 220 ml: **$24.79**

• Supp—Rect: Pediatric 12's: **$0.93-$4.82;** Adult 12's: **$0.93-$4.82**

• Liq—Rect: Ped 4 ml, 6's: **$2.48**

CONTRAINDICATIONS: (Laxative) Symptoms of appendicitis,

acute surgical abdomen, fecal impaction, intestinal obstruction, undiagnosed abdominal pain; (Oral) well-established anuria, severe dehydration, pulmonary edema, cardiac decompensation

PRECAUTIONS: (Laxative) fluid and electrolyte imbalance, chronic use, rectal bleeding; (Oral) hypervolemia, confused mental status, CHF, diabetes, severe dehydration; cardiac, renal, hepatic disease

PREGNANCY AND LACTATION: Pregnancy category C; data regarding use in breast feeding are unavailable

SIDE EFFECTS/ADVERSE REACTIONS

CNS: Confusion, disorientation, headache (oral); dizziness, fainting (laxative)

CV: **Dysrhythmias** (oral); palpitations (laxative)

EENT: Pain or irritation upon instillation (ophth)

GI: Abdominal pain, bloating, excessive bowel activity, flatulence, perianal irritation (laxative); nausea, vomiting (oral)

METAB: **Hyperosmolar nonketotic coma**

INTERACTIONS

Labs

• *Increase:* Amniotic fluid phosphatidylglycerol, serum triglycerides

• *Decrease:* Serum ionized calcium

SPECIAL CONSIDERATIONS

PATIENT/FAMILY EDUCATION

• Do not use laxative in the presence of abdominal pain, nausea, or vomiting

• Do not use longer than 1 wk

• Prolonged or frequent use may result in dependency or electrolyte imbalance

• Notify clinician if unrelieved constipation, rectal bleeding, muscle cramps, weakness, or dizziness occurs

MONITORING PARAMETERS
• Blood glucose, intraocular pressure

---

glycopyrrolate
(glye-koe-pye'roe-late)
Rx: Robinul, Robinul Forte
Chemical Class: Quaternary ammonium derivative
Therapeutic Class: Anticholinergic; gastrointestinal antiulcer agent (adjunct)

CLINICAL PHARMACOLOGY
Mechanism of Action: Inhibits action of acetylcholine on structures innervated by postganglionic cholinergic nerves and on smooth muscles that respond to acetylcholine but lack cholinergic innervation; diminishes volume and free acidity of gastric secretions and controls excessive pharyngeal, tracheal, and bronchial secretions; antagonizes muscarinic symptoms (e.g., bronchorrhea, bronchospasm, bradycardia, and intestinal hypermotility) induced by cholinergic drugs such as the anticholinesterases
Pharmacokinetics
PO: Onset 1 hr, duration 6 hr
IM: Onset 15-30 min, duration 7 hr
IV: Onset 1-10 min, duration 7 hr
Does not penetrate CNS; excreted primarily unchanged via bile, feces
INDICATIONS AND USES: Peptic ulcer (adjunctive therapy); decreases secretions prior to induction of anesthesia, intubation, and surgery; interoperatively to counteract drug-induced or vagal traction reflexes with the associated dysrhythmias; protection against peripheral muscarinic effects of cholinergic agents such as neostigmine and pyridostigmine used to reverse neuromuscular

blockade due to non-depolarizing muscle relaxants
DOSAGE
Adult
• *Preoperatively:* IM 0.004 mg/kg 0.5-1 hr before surgery
• *Intraoperative:* IV 0.1 mg repeat prn at 2-3 min intervals
• *Peptic ulcer:* PO 1-2 mg bid-tid; IM/IV 0.1-0.2 mg tid-qid
• *Reversal of neuromuscular blockade:* IV 0.2 mg for each 1 mg of neostigmine or 5 mg of pyridostigmine administered
Child
• *Preoperatively:* IM (<2 yr) 4.4-8.8 µg/kg 0.5-1 hr before surgery; (>2 yr) 4.4 µg/kg 0.5-1 hr before surgery
• *Intraoperative:* IV 4 µg/kg (max 0.1 mg), repeat prn at 2-3 min intervals
• *Reversal of neuromuscular blockade:* Same as adult
💲 AVAILABLE FORMS/COST OF THERAPY
• Inj, Sol—IM, IV: 0.2 mg/ml, 1, 2, 5, 20 ml: **$1.07-$1.44**/2 ml
• Tab, Uncoated—Oral: 1 mg, 100's: **$21.89;** 2 mg, 100's: **$34.85**
CONTRAINDICATIONS: Narrow-angle glaucoma, obstructive uropathy, GI tract obstruction, paralytic ileus, intestinal atony, acute hemorrhage, severe ulcerative colitis, toxic megacolon, myasthenia gravis
PRECAUTIONS: Glaucoma, asthma, elderly, prostatic hypertrophy, renal disease, CHF, pulmonary disease, hyperthyroidism, CAD, hypertension
PREGNANCY AND LACTATION: Pregnancy category B; has been used prior to cesarean section to decrease gastric secretions; quaternary structure results in limited placental transfer; excretion into breast

G

---

milk is unknown, but should be minimal due to quaternary structure

SIDE EFFECTS/ADVERSE REACTIONS

CNS: Anxiety, confusion, delusions, depression, dizziness, flushing, hallucinations, headache, incoherence, irritability, lethargy, restlessness, sedation, weakness

CV: Palpitations, paradoxical bradycardia, postural hypotension, tachycardia

EENT: Blurred vision, cycloplegia, difficulty swallowing, dilated pupils, increased intraocular pressure, mydriasis, nasal congestion, photophobia

GI: Abdominal distress, altered taste perception, *constipation, dry mouth,* nausea, paralytic ileus, vomiting

GU: Hesitancy, impotence, retention

SKIN: Allergic reactions, decreased sweating, urticaria

---

gonadorelin
(goe-nad-oh-rell'in)
Rx: Factrel
Chemical Class: Synthetic gonadotropin-releasing hormone (GnRH or LHRH)
Therapeutic Class: Diagnostic agent; ovulation stimulant

CLINICAL PHARMACOLOGY
Mechanism of Action: Stimulates release of lutenizing hormone (LH) from the anterior pituitary
Pharmacokinetics
IV: Rapidly metabolized to various biologically inactive peptide fragments, which are readily excreted in urine; $t_{1/2}$ 2-10 min (initial), 10-40 min (terminal)

INDICATIONS AND USES: Evaluating gonadotropic function of the anterior pituitary

DOSAGE
Adult
• *Evaluating functional capacity and response of gonadotropes of the anterior pituitary:* IV/SC: 100 µg; in females, perform the test in the early follicular phase (days 1-7) of menstrual cycle
Child
• *Evaluating functional capacity and response of gonadotropes of the anterior pituitary:* IV: 100 µg

$ AVAILABLE FORMS/COST OF THERAPY
• Inj, Sol—IV, SC: 50 µg/ml, 2 ml: **$155.76;** 250 µg/ml, 2 ml: **$206.90**

CONTRAINDICATIONS: Reproductive hormone-dependent tumor; ovarian cysts

PRECAUTIONS: Ovarian hyperstimulation is possible

PREGNANCY AND LACTATION: Pregnancy category B; possibility of fetal harm appears remote if used during pregnancy

SIDE EFFECTS/ADVERSE REACTIONS

CNS: Flushing, headache, lightheadedness

GI: Abdominal discomfort, nausea

GU: Multiple pregnancy, *ovarian hyperstimulation* (sudden ovarian enlargement, ascites, pleural effusion)

RESP: **Anaphylaxis**

INTERACTIONS
Drugs
3 *Androgen, Estrogen, Glucocorticoid, Progestin-containing preparations:* May reduce LH release from anterior pituitary
Labs
• Do not conduct diagnostic tests during administration of these agents

---

goserelin

(go'seh-rel-in)

Rx: Zoladex

Chemical Class: Synthetic gonadotropin-releasing hormone (GnRH or LHRH)

Therapeutic Class: Antineoplastic; antiendometriosis agent

CLINICAL PHARMACOLOGY

Mechanism of Action: Causes initial increase in serum luteinizing hormone (LH) and follicle stimulating hormone (FSH); chronic administration leads to sustained suppression of pituitary gonadotropins with subsequent reductions in serum testosterone (males) and estradiol (females)

Pharmacokinetics

SC: Peak 12-15 days; released from depot at slower rate for 1st 8 days, and then more rapidly during the remainder of the 28-day dosing period; $t_{1/2}$ 4.2 hr; cleared via a combination of hepatic metabolism and urinary excretion

INDICATIONS AND USES: Advanced prostate carcinoma, endometriosis, breast cancer,* endometrial thinning agent for dysfunctional uterine bleeding*

DOSAGE

Adult

• SC 3.6 mg into upper abdominal wall 4 wk; recommended duration in endometriosis is 6 mo

• Prostate carcinoma: SC 10.8 mg into upper abdominal wall q12 wk

💲 AVAILABLE FORMS/COST OF THERAPY

• Implant, CONT REL—SC: 3.6 mg: **$469.99;** 10.8 mg: **$1409.98**

CONTRAINDICATIONS: Pregnancy

PRECAUTIONS: Patients at risk for osteoporosis (alcoholism, tobacco abuse, family history, chronic anticonvulsant therapy, chronic corticosteroid use)

PREGNANCY AND LACTATION: Pregnancy category X; excretion into breast milk unknown; use caution in nursing mothers

SIDE EFFECTS/ADVERSE REACTIONS

CNS: Anxiety, *depression, emotional lability, headaches,* insomnia, nervousness, **spinal cord compression**

CV: **Cerebrovascular accident,** chest pain, **dysrhythmia,** hot flashes, hypertension, **MI**

GI: Constipation, diarrhea, nausea, ulcer, vomiting

GU: Breakthrough bleeding, decreased libido, renal insufficiency, *spotting,* urinary obstruction, UTI, vaginal dryness

METAB: Gout, hyperglycemia

MS: Decreased bone mineral density, osteoneuralgia

SKIN: Alopecia, dry skin, pain on inj, rash, skin discoloration, *sweating*

MISC: Breast tenderness, *change in breast size,* gynecomastia

INTERACTIONS

Labs

• *Increase:* Alk phosphatase, estradiol, FSH, LH, testosterone levels (1st week)

• *Decrease:* Testosterone levels (after 1st week), progesterone

SPECIAL CONSIDERATIONS

PATIENT/FAMILY EDUCATION

• Notify clinician if regular menstruation persists (females)

• An initial flare in bone pain may occur (prostate cancer therapy)

MONITORING PARAMETERS

• Prostate-specific antigen, acid phosphatase, alk phosphatase

• Testosterone level (<25 ng/dl)

• Bone density if therapy prolonged

---

italic = common side effects   ***bold italic*** = life-threatening reactions

granisetron
(gra-ni'se-tron)
Rx: Kytril
Chemical Class: Carbazole derivative
Therapeutic Class: Antiemetic

CLINICAL PHARMACOLOGY
Mechanism of Action: Selectively blocks the action of serotonin at $5\text{-}HT_3$ receptors; cytotoxic chemotherapy appears to be associated with release of serotonin from enterochromaffin cells of the small intestine, which may stimulate vagal afferents through $5\text{-}HT_3$ receptors, initiating the vomiting reflex
Pharmacokinetics
PO: Onset 15-30 min
IV: Onset 1-3 min
Mean $t_{1/2}$ 9 hr in cancer patients (range 1-31 hr); mean 5 hr in normals (range 1-15 hr); 65% protein bound; metabolized by cytochrome P-450 3A, some metabolites active; 12% of drug excreted unchanged in urine; metabolites excreted in urine and feces

INDICATIONS AND USES: Prevention and treatment of emesis due to cancer chemotherapy; radiation; postsurgical nausea and vomiting*
DOSAGE
Adult
• IV 10 µg/kg infused over ½-5 min, beginning 30 min before initiation of chemotherapy, no adjustment for renal or hepatic disease; PO 1 mg q12h, or 2 mg × 1, 1st dose given 1 hr before chemotherapy, only on the day(s) chemotherapy is given
Child 2-16 yr
• IV 10 µg/kg INF over 5 min, beginning 30 min before initiation of chemotherapy, no adjustment for renal or hepatic disease

💲 AVAILABLE FORMS/COST OF THERAPY
• Inj, Sol—IV: 1 mg/ml, 1 ml: **$186.10**
• Tab, Uncoated—Oral: 1 mg, 2's: **$89.70**
PRECAUTIONS: Child <2 yr
PREGNANCY AND LACTATION: Pregnancy category B; breast milk excretion unknown
SIDE EFFECTS/ADVERSE REACTIONS
CNS: Anxiety, *headache,* somnolence, weakness
CV: Atrioventricular block, hypertension, hypotension, ventricular ectopy
EENT: Dysgeusia
GI: Constipation, diarrhea, elevated transaminase
MISC: Fever

grepafloxacin
(gree-pah-floks'a-sin)
Rx: Raxar
Chemical Class: Fluoroquinolone derivative
Therapeutic Class: Antibiotic

NOTE: Removed from market October, 1999 due to ECG QT interval prolongation
CLINICAL PHARMACOLOGY
Mechanism of Action: Interferes with the enzyme DNA gyrase, needed for the synthesis of bacterial DNA
Pharmacokinetics
PO: Peak 2-3 hr; 70% bioavailable PO not affected by food; widely distributed, 50% protein bound; metabolized in liver by cytochrome P450 1A2 and 3A4 to inactive metabolites; $t_{1/2}$ 16 hr; 50% excreted in feces, 38% in urine as metabolites; clearance impaired in patients with hepatic insufficiency but not with renal insufficiency; clearance in-

creased by 40% in cigarette smokers due to cytochrome P450 1A2 induction

INDICATIONS AND USES: Acute bacterial exacerbations of chronic bronchitis, community-acquired pneumonia, uncomplicated gonorrhea (urethral in males; endocervical and rectal in females), nongonococcal urethritis and cervicitis

Antibacterial spectrum usually includes:

• Gram-positive organisms: *Staphylococcus aureus* (methicillin-susceptible strains), *S. epidermidis*, *Streptococcus pneumoniae, S. pyogenes*

• Gram-negative organisms: *Citrobacter freundii, C. diversus, Enterobacter aerogenes, E. cloacae, Escherichia coli, H. influenza, H. parainfluenza, Klebsiella pneumoniae, Moraxella catarrhalis, Morganella morganii, N. gonorrhoeae, Proteus mirabilis, P. vulgaris*

• Other: *Chlamydia trachomatis, Mycoplasma pneumoniae;* not active against anaerobic bacteria

DOSAGE

Adult

• *Bronchitis:* PO 400-600 mg qd × 10 days

• *Community-acquired pneumonia:* PO 600 mg qd × 10 days

• *Non-gonococcal urethritis and cervicitis:* PO 400 mg qd × 7 days

• *Uncomplicated gonorrhea:* PO 400 mg as single dose (plus treatment for *chlamydia trachomatis*)

💲 AVAILABLE FORMS/COST OF THERAPY

• Tab, Uncoated—Oral: 200 mg, 20's: **$41.20**

CONTRAINDICATIONS: Hepatic failure, patients with QT interval prolongation or taking other medications known to prolong the QT interval

PRECAUTIONS: Patients with hepatic insufficiency, seizure disorder, history of proarrhythmic conditions (e.g., hypokalemia, significant bradycardia, CHF, myocardial ischemia, atrial fibrillation), taking NSAIDs (increased risk of CNS side effects)

PREGNANCY AND LACTATION: Pregnancy category C; excreted in breast milk at levels similar to serum; do not breast feed within 48 hours after a dose

SIDE EFFECTS/ADVERSE REACTIONS

CNS: Anxiety, *dizziness,* headache, hyperkinesia, insomnia, somnolence, ***toxic psychosis***

CV: Arrhythmia, QT prolongation

EENT: Dry mouth, *dysgeusia (18%)*, tinnitus

GI: Abdominal pain, anorexia, constipation, dyspepsia, *nausea (16%), vomiting*

GU: Vaginitis

MS: Arthralgia, tendon rupture

SKIN: Alopecia, photosensitivity, pruritus, rash, sweating

INTERACTIONS

Drugs

③ *Antacids:* Reduced absorption of grepafloxacin; do not take within 4 hr of dose

③ *Benzodiazepines:* May increase serum concentrations of benzodiazepines

③ β-*Adrenergic blockers:* May increase serum concentrations of hepatically metabolized β-adrenergic blockers

③ *Caffeine:* Inhibits metabolism of caffeine

③ *Cyclosporine:* Inhibits metabolism of cyclosporine

③ *Iron:* Reduced absorption of grepafloxacin; do not take within 4 hr of dose

③ *Sucralfate:* Reduced absorption of grepafloxacin; do not take within 4 hr of dose

3 *Theobromine:* Inhibits metabolism of theobromine

3 *Theophylline:* Inhibits metabolism of theophylline; cut maintenance theophylline dose in half during therapy with grepafloxacin

3 *Warfarin:* May increase hypoprothrombinemic response to warfarin

3 *Zinc:* Reduced absorption of grepafloxacin; do not take within 4 hr of dose

Labs

• *Interference:* Urine coproporphyrin, urine uroporphyrin

PATIENT/FAMILY EDUCATION

• Do not take antacids or iron within 4 hr of taking grepafloxacin

---

griseofulvin
(gri-see-oh-ful'vin)

Rx: Fulvicin P/G, Fulvicin-U/F, Grifulvin V, Grisactin, Grisactin 500, Grisactin-Ultra, Gris-PEG

Chemical Class: Penicillium griseofulvum derivative
Therapeutic Class: Antifungal

CLINICAL PHARMACOLOGY
Mechanism of Action: Deposited in the keratin precursor cells, which are gradually exfoliated and replaced by non-infected tissue; has a greater affinity for diseased tissue; tightly bound to the new keratin, which becomes highly resistant to fungal invasions

Pharmacokinetics
PO: GI absorption exhibits high interindividual variability; absorption increased by meals with high fat content; ultramicrosize absorbed 1.5 times more efficiently than conventional microsized formulation; peak 4 hr, $t_{1/2}$ 9-24 hr; metabolized in liver; excreted in urine (inactive metabolites), feces, perspiration

INDICATIONS AND USES: Fungal infections of the skin, hair, and nails (i.e., tinea corporis, tinea pedis, tinea cruris, tinea barbae, tinea capitis, and tinea unguium) caused by susceptible organisms

Antifungal spectrum usually includes: *Trichophyton rubrum, T. tonsurans, T. mentagrophytes, T. interdigitalis, T. verrucosum, T. megnii, T. gallinae, T. crateriform, T. sulphureum, T. schoenleinii, Microsporum audouinii, M. canis, M. gypseum, Epidermophyton floccosum*

DOSAGE
Adult

• PO (microsize) 500-1000 mg/day in single or divided doses; (ultramicrosize) 330-375 mg/day in single or divided doses, max 750 mg/day

Child ≥2 yr

• PO (microsize) 10-15 mg/kg/day in single or divided doses; (ultramicrosize) 5.5-7.3 mg/kg/day in single or divided doses

Duration

• *Tinea corporis:* 2-4 wk
• *Tinea capitis:* At least 4-6 wk
• *Tinea pedis:* 4-8 wk
• *Tinea unguium:* 3-6 mo

$ **AVAILABLE FORMS/COST OF THERAPY**
Microsize:

• Tab, Uncoated—Oral: 250 mg, 100's: **$91.81-$94.70;** 500 mg, 100's: **$88.94-$135.48**

• Cap, Gel—Oral: 125 mg, 100's: **$27.98;** 250 mg, 100's: **$59.25-$87.68**

• Susp—Oral: 125 mg/5 ml, 120 ml: **$28.26**

Ultramicrosize:

• Tab, Uncoated—Oral: 125 mg, 100's: **$38.93-$57.53;** 165 mg, 100's: **$53.15-$77.57;** 250 mg, 100's: **$50.93-$108.33;** 330 mg, 100's: **$40.32-$133.85**

---

* = non-FDA-approved use

CONTRAINDICATIONS: Porphyria, hepatocellular failure

PRECAUTIONS: Penicillin allergy (possible cross-sensitivity), lupus erythematosus

PREGNANCY AND LACTATION: Pregnancy category C; since the use of an antifungal is seldom essential during pregnancy, avoid use during this time; excretion into breast milk unknown; use caution in nursing mothers

SIDE EFFECTS/ADVERSE REACTIONS

CNS: Dizziness, fatigue, headache, insomnia, mental confusion, paresthesias (chronic use)

GI: Diarrhea, epigastric distress, *GI bleeding, hepatic toxicity,* nausea, oral thrush, vomiting

GU: Menstrual irregularities, proteinuria

HEME: **Granulocytopenia, leukopenia**

SKIN: Angioneurotic edema, photosensitivity, *rash, urticaria*

INTERACTIONS

Drugs

3 *Aspirin:* Reduces plasma salicylate level

3 *Cyclosporine:* Reduces plasma cyclosporine level

3 *Oral contraceptives:* Menstrual irregularities, increased risk of pregnancy possible

3 *Phenobarbital:* Reduces plasma griseofulvin level

3 *Tacrolimus:* Reduces plasma tacrolimus level

3 *Warfarin:* Reduces anticoagulant response

SPECIAL CONSIDERATIONS

Prior to therapy, the type of fungus responsible for the infection should be identified

PATIENT/FAMILY EDUCATION

• Response to therapy may not be apparent for some time; complete entire course of therapy

• Avoid prolonged exposure to sunlight or sunlamps

• Notify clinician if sore throat or skin rash occurs

• Store oral suspensions at room temp in light-resistant container

MONITORING PARAMETERS

• Periodic assessments of renal, hepatic, and hematopoietic function during prolonged therapy

G

guaifenesin

(gwye-fen′e-sin)

Rx: Allfen, Amibid LA, Aquamist, Bidex, Duratuss G, Fenesin, GG-200 NR, Ganidin NR, Gua-SR, Guaibid-LA, Guaifenesin Expectorant, Guaifenesin LA, Guaifenesin-SR, Guaifenex G, Guaifenex LA, Humavent LA, Humibid LA, Humibid Pediatric, Iofen-NR, Iophen- NR, Liquibid, Monafed, Muco-Fen 800, Muco-Fen 1200, Muco-Fen LA, Orgadin, Organ-1 NEF, Organidin NR, Pneumomist, Q-Bid LA, Respa-GF, Simumist-SR, Touro EX

OTC: Anti-Tuss, Breonesin, Genatuss, Glytuss, Guiatuss, Hytuss, Hytuss 2X, Mytussin, Naldecon Senior EX, Robitussin

Combinations

  Rx: with codeine (Guiatussin AC); with dextromethorphan (Guaibid-DM); with hydrocodone (Hycotuss); with phenylpropanolamine (Entex LA)

Chemical Class: Glyceryl derivative

Therapeutic Class: Expectorant; mucolytic

CLINICAL PHARMACOLOGY

Mechanism of Action: Supposedly

---

italic = common side effects   ***bold italic*** = life-threatening reactions

increases the output of respiratory tract fluid by reducing adhesiveness and surface tension; promotes ciliary action and facilitates removal of viscous mucus; lack of convincing studies to document efficacy

Pharmacokinetics

PO: Readily absorbed from GI tract; rapidly metabolized, excreted in urine; $t_{1/2}$ 1 hr

INDICATIONS AND USES: Dry, non-productive cough; sinusitis*

DOSAGE

Adult

• PO 100-400 mg q4-6h or 600 mg sustained release q12h, not to exceed 2.4 g/day

Child

• PO (6-12 yr) 100-200 mg q4h, not to exceed 1.2 g/day; (2-6 yr) 50-100 mg q4h, not to exceed 600 mg/day

💲 **AVAILABLE FORMS/COST OF THERAPY**

• Syrup—Oral: 100 mg/5 ml, 480 ml: **$4.10-$36.95**

• Liq—Oral: 100 mg/5 ml, 480 ml: **$36.95-$93.40;** 200 mg/5 ml, 120 ml: **$5.00**

• Cap—Oral: 200 mg, 100's: **$45.29**

• Cap, SUS Action—Oral: 300 mg, 100's: **$48.44**

• Tab—Oral: 100 mg, 100's: **$10.12;** 200 mg, 100's: **$15.70-$35.70**

• Tab, SUS Action—Oral: 575 mg, 100's: **$43.16;** 600 mg 100's: **$8.87-$75.01;** 800 mg, 100's: **$24.48-$28.54;** 1000 mg, 100's: **$49.80;** 1200 mg, 100's: **$32.25-$54.36**

PRECAUTIONS: Recurrent cough; cough associated with fever, rash, persistant headache, excessive secretions

PREGNANCY AND LACTATION: Pregnancy category C; excretion into breast milk unknown

SIDE EFFECTS/ADVERSE REACTIONS

CNS: Dizziness, drowsiness, headache

GI: Nausea, stomach pain, *vomiting*

SKIN: Rash

INTERACTIONS

Labs

• *Interference:* Urine 5-HIAA, VMA

SPECIAL CONSIDERATIONS

PATIENT/FAMILY EDUCATION

• Drink a full glass of water with each dose to help further loosen mucus

• Notify clinician if cough persists after medication has been used for 7 days or cough is associated with headache, high fever, skin rash, or sore throat

---

guanabenz

(gwan'a-benz)

Rx: Wytensin

Chemical Class: Dichlorobenzene derivative

Therapeutic Class: Antihypertensive, centrally acting sympathoplegic

CLINICAL PHARMACOLOGY

Mechanism of Action: Stimulates central α_2-adrenergic receptors resulting in reduced sympathetic outflow from the CNS to the heart, kidneys, and peripheral vasculature; decreases systolic and diastolic blood pressure, and pulse

Pharmacokinetics

PO: 75% bioavailable; onset 1 hr, duration 12 hr; 90% bound to plasma proteins; extensive metabolism excreted in urine (1% unchanged); $t_{1/2}$ approximately 7-10 hr

INDICATIONS AND USES: Hypertension

DOSAGE

Adult

• PO 4 mg bid initially, increase in 4-8 mg/day increments q1-2 wk prn, not to exceed 32 mg bid

---

* = non-FDA-approved use

AVAILABLE FORMS/COST OF THERAPY

• Tab, Uncoated—Oral: 4 mg, 100's: **$53.20-$90.43**; 8 mg, 100's: **$79.80-$135.75**

PRECAUTIONS: Severe coronary insufficiency, recent MI, cerebrovascular disease; severe renal, hepatic dysfunction; sudden discontinuation

PREGNANCY AND LACTATION: Pregnancy category C; excretion into breast milk unknown; use caution in nursing mothers

SIDE EFFECTS/ADVERSE REACTIONS

CNS: Anxiety, ataxia, depression, *dizziness, drowsiness, headache, sedation,* sleep disturbance, *weakness*

CV: Chest pain, dysrhythmias, edema, palpitations, ***rebound hypertension with abrupt cessation***

EENT: Blurred vision, nasal congestion

GI: Abdominal discomfort, constipation, diarrhea, *dry mouth,* epigastric pain, nausea, taste disorder, vomiting

GU: Disturbances of sexual function, urinary frequency

METAB: Gynecomastia

MS: Myalgias

RESP: Dyspnea

SKIN: Pruritis, rash

INTERACTIONS

Drugs

3 β-*blockers:* Rebound hypertension from guanabenz withdrawal exacerbated by noncardioselective β-blockers

3 *Tricyclic antidepressants:* Inhibit the antihypertensive response

SPECIAL CONSIDERATIONS

PATIENT/FAMILY EDUCATION

• Avoid hazardous activities, since drug may cause drowsiness

• Do not discontinue oral drug abruptly, or withdrawal symptoms may occur (anxiety, increased BP, headache, insomnia, increased pulse, tremors, nausea, sweating)

• Do not use OTC (cough, cold, or allergy) products unless directed by clinician

• Rise slowly to sitting or standing position to minimize orthostatic hypotension, especially elderly

• May cause dizziness, fainting, lightheadedness during 1st few days of therapy

• May cause dry mouth; use hard candy, saliva product, or frequent rinsing of mouth

MONITORING PARAMETERS

• Blood pressure (posturally), mental depression

---

guanadrel

(gwahn'a-drel)

Rx: Hylorel

Chemical Class: Guanidine derivative

Therapeutic Class: Antihypertensive, postganglionic adrenergic neuron inhibitor

---

CLINICAL PHARMACOLOGY

Mechanism of Action: Adrenergic neuron inhibitor: lowers arterial pressure secondary to decreased peripheral vascular resistance and cardiac output by depletion of catecholamines from adrenergic nerve endings, the myocardium, and vascular walls; hypotensive effects most pronounced in the erect position; approximately one-third as potent as guanethidine

Pharmacokinetics

PO: Peak levels 1½-2 hr, onset 2 hr, duration 4-14 hr; <20% bound to plasma proteins; metabolized in liver, excreted in urine (40% as unchanged drug); $t_{1/2}$ approximately 10 hr (high interindividual variation)

---

italic = common side effects   ***bold italic*** = life-threatening reactions

INDICATIONS AND USES: Hypertension (not 1st-line) thyrotoxicosis*

DOSAGE

Adult

• PO 10 mg/day as a single dose or divided bid; usual range 20-75 mg/day generally divided bid-qid

• *Renal function impairment:* CrCl 30-60 ml/min, 5 mg qd; CrCl <30 ml/min, 5 mg qod

§ AVAILABLE FORMS/COST OF THERAPY

• Tab, Uncoated—Oral: 10 mg, 100's: **$165.07;**

CONTRAINDICATIONS: Pheochromocytoma, CHF, concurrent use with or within 1 wk of MAOI

PRECAUTIONS: Cerebral vascular disease, CAD, elective surgery, orthostatic hypotension, asthma, renal function impairment, children, peptic ulcer, elderly, diabetes (causes hypoglycemia unawareness)

PREGNANCY AND LACTATION: Pregnancy category B; excretion into breast milk unknown; use caution in nursing mothers

SIDE EFFECTS/ADVERSE REACTIONS

CNS: *Confusion, depression, drowsiness, faintness, fatigue, headache, paresthesias,* psychological problems, sleep disorder

CV: Bradycardia, chest pain, **CHF,** *orthostatic hypotension,* palpitations, *peripheral edema,* syncope

EENT: Double vision, dry burning eyes, *nasal stuffiness,* sore throat, *tinnitus,* visual changes

GI: Abdominal pain, anorexia, *constipation,* dry throat; glossitis, *increased bowel movements,* nausea, vomiting

GU: Ejaculation disturbances, impotence, hematuria, *nocturia; urinary frequency,* urgency

MS: Aching limbs, joint pain, leg cramps

RESP: **Bronchospasm**

SKIN: Alopecia, purpura, rash

MISC: Weight gain, loss

INTERACTIONS

Drugs

❷ *Amitriptyline:* Inhibits antihypertensive effect

❸ *Dextroamphetamine:* Inhibits antihypertensive effect

❸ *Ephedrine:* Inhibits antihypertensive effect

❸ *MAOIs:* Inhibits antihypertensive effect

❸ *Methylphenidate:* Inhibits antihypertensive effect

❸ *Norepinephrine:* Exaggerated pressor response to norepinephrine

❸ *Phenothiazines:* Inhibits antihypertensive effect

❸ *Tricyclic antidepressants:* Inhibit antihypertensive effect

Labs

Increase: BUN

Decrease: Urinary VMA excretion

SPECIAL CONSIDERATIONS

PATIENT/FAMILY EDUCATION

• Arise slowly from a reclining position, especially in the morning

• Avoid OTC medications except as directed by clinician

• Avoid driving, hazardous activities if drowsiness occurs

• Use alcohol with caution

• Use caution when standing for prolonged periods, exercising, and during hot weather (enhanced orthostatic hypotension)

• Do not discontinue abruptly

MONITORING PARAMETERS

• Sitting and standing blood pressure, pulse, weight, edema

---

* = non-FDA-approved use

guanethidine
(gwahn-eth'i-deen)
Rx: Ismelin
Chemical Class: Guanidine derivative
Therapeutic Class: Antihypertensive, postganglionic adrenergic neuron inhibitor

CLINICAL PHARMACOLOGY
Mechanism of Action: Adrenergic neuron inhibitor: lowers arterial pressure secondary to decreased peripheral vascular resistance and cardiac output by depletion of catecholamines from adrenergic nerve endings, the myocardium, and vascular walls; hypotensive effects most pronounced in the erect position

Pharmacokinetics
PO: Oral absorption highly variable (3%-50%), maximum hypotensive response in 14 days; metabolized in liver, excreted in urine (25%-50% as unchanged drug); $t_{1/2}$ 5-10 days

INDICATIONS AND USES: Hypertension (not 1st-line), angina (add on),* bladder instability,* exophthalmos,* glaucoma

DOSAGE
Adult
• *Ambulatory patients:* PO 10 mg qd, increase at 5-7 day intervals to a max of 25-50 mg/day
• *Hospitalized patients:* PO 25-50 mg qd; increase by 25-50 mg/day to desired therapeutic response
Child
• PO 0.2 mg/kg/day; increase by 0.2 mg/kg/day at 7-10 day intervals to a max of 3 mg/kg/day

⚡ AVAILABLE FORMS/COST OF THERAPY
• Tab, Uncoated—Oral: 25 mg, 100's: **$102.66**

CONTRAINDICATIONS: Pheochromocytoma, CHF, concurrent use with or within 1 wk of MAOI

PRECAUTIONS: Elective surgery (discontinue 2 wk prior to procedure), fever (reduced dosage requirements), asthma, recent MI, CAD, peptic ulcer, elderly, orthostatic hypotension, renal dysfunction, sexual dysfunction

PREGNANCY AND LACTATION: Pregnancy category C; breast milk excretion unknown

SIDE EFFECTS/ADVERSE REACTIONS
CNS: Dizziness, fatigue, *lassitude,* mental depression, tremor, *weakness*
CV: Angina, *bradycardia,* **CHF,** edema, fluid retention, *orthostatic hypotension,* syncope
EENT: Blurred vision, *nasal congestion,* ptosis, unpleasant taste
GI: Diarrhea, dry mouth, nausea, parotid tenderness, vomiting
GU: Impotence, *inhibition of ejaculation,* nocturia, priapism, rise in BUN, urinary incontinence, urinary retention
HEME: Anemia, **leukopenia, thrombocytopenia**
METAB: Weight gain, hyperglycemia
MS: Myalgia, myopathy
RESP: Asthma, dyspnea
SKIN: Alopecia, dermatitis

INTERACTIONS
Drugs
❷ *Amitriptyline:* Inhibits antihypertensive effect
❸ *Dextroamphetamine:* Inhibits antihypertensive effect
❸ *Ephedrine:* Inhibits antihypertensive effect
❸ *Haloperidol:* Inhibits antihypertensive effect
❸ *MAOIs:* Inhibits antihypertensive effect
❸ *Methylphenidate:* Inhibits antihypertensive effect

---

italic = common side effects   ***bold italic*** = life-threatening reactions

3 *Norepinephrine:* Exaggerated pressor response to norepinephrine

3 *Phenothiazines:* Inhibits antihypertensive effect

3 *Phenylephrine:* Guanethidine enhances pupillary response to phenylephrine

3 *Thiothixene:* Inhibits antihypertensive effect

3 *Tricyclic antidepressants:* Inhibits antihypertensive effect

Labs

• *Increase:* BUN

• *Decrease:* Urinary VMA excretion

SPECIAL CONSIDERATIONS
PATIENT/FAMILY EDUCATION

• Arise slowly from a reclining position, especially in the morning

• Use alcohol with caution

• Use caution when standing for prolonged periods of time, exercising, and during hot weather (enhanced orthostatic hypotension)

• Avoid OTC medications unless discussed with clinician

• Avoid driving; hazardous activities if drowsiness occurs

• Do not discontinue abruptly

MONITORING PARAMETERS

• Sitting and standing blood pressure, pulse, weight, edema

---

guanfacine

(gwan'fa-seen)

Rx: Tenex

Chemical Class: Phenylacyl guanidine

Therapeutic Class: Antihypertensive, centrally acting sympathoplegic

CLINICAL PHARMACOLOGY
Mechanism of Action: Centrally acting antihypertensive stimulates central α_2-adrenergic receptors resulting in reduced sympathetic outflow from the CNS to the heart, kidneys, and peripheral vasculature; decreases systolic and diastolic blood pressure and pulse; considered more selective α-2 receptor agonist than clonidine; no dopamine inhibition; does not activate opiate receptors

Pharmacokinetics

PO: Bioavailability 80%; peak concentration 1-4 hr, onset (multiple doses) 1 wk, 70% bound to plasma proteins, 50% bound to erythrocytes; metabolized in liver, excreted in urine (40%-75% as unchanged drug); $t_{1/2}$ 17 hr

INDICATIONS AND USES: Hypertension, heroin withdrawal syndrome,* migraine headache*

DOSAGE

Adult

• PO 1 mg qd, increase to 2 mg qd after 3-4 wk prn

$ **AVAILABLE FORMS/COST**
OF THERAPY

• Tab, Uncoated—Oral: 1 mg, 100's: **$70.58-$110.65;** 2 mg, 100's: **$96.75-$151.69**

PRECAUTIONS: Chronic renal or hepatic failure, severe coronary insufficiency, recent MI, cerebrovascular disease

PREGNANCY AND LACTATION: Pregnancy category B; excretion into human breast milk unknown

SIDE EFFECTS/ADVERSE REACTIONS

CNS: Dizziness, fatigue, headache, somnolence, amnesia, depression

CV: Bradycardia, chest pain, palpitations, orthostatic hypotension/withdrawal symptoms—rebound phenomenon (hypertension and sympathetic overactivity)

EENT: Nasal congestion, rhinitis, taste change, tinnitus, vision change

GI: Constipation, cramps, diarrhea, *dry mouth,* nausea

GU: Impotence, urinary incontinence

MS: Leg cramps

---

* = non-FDA-approved use

RESP: Dyspnea
SKIN: Dermatitis, pruritus, purpura
INTERACTIONS
Drugs

■ β*-blockers:* Rebound hypertension from guanfacine withdrawal exacerbated by noncardioselective β-blockers

■ *Cyclosporine, tacrolimus:* Increased immunosuppressant plasma levels

■ *Insulin, sulfonylureas hypoglycemics:* Diminished symptoms of hypoglycemia

■ *Neuroleptics, nitroprusside:* Severe hypotension possible

■ *Tricyclic antidepressants:* Inhibit the antihypertensive response

SPECIAL CONSIDERATIONS
PATIENT/FAMILY EDUCATION

• Avoid hazardous activities, since drug may cause drowsiness

• Do not discontinue oral drug abruptly, or withdrawal symptoms may occur after 3-4 days (anxiety, increased BP, headache, insomnia, increased pulse, tremors, nausea, sweating)

• Do not use OTC (cough, cold, or allergy) products unless directed by clinician

• Rise slowly to sitting or standing position to minimize orthostatic hypotension, especially elderly

• Dizziness, fainting, lightheadedness may occur during 1st few days of therapy

• May cause dry mouth; use hard candy, saliva product, or frequent rinsing of mouth

MONITORING PARAMETERS

• Blood pressure (posturally), blood glucose in patients with diabetes mellitus; confusion, mental depression

halazepam
(hal-az′e-pam)
Rx: Paxipam
Chemical Class: Benzodiazepine
Therapeutic Class: Anxiolytic
DEA Class: Schedule IV

CLINICAL PHARMACOLOGY
Mechanism of Action: CNS depressants via facilitation of inhibitory GABA at benzodiazepine receptor sites (BZ_1—associated with sleep; BZ_2—associated with memory, motor, sensory, and cognitive function); effects include muscle relaxation (spinal cord), anticonvulsant activity (brain stem), ataxia (cerebellum), emotional behavior (limbic and cortical areas), and anxiolytic effects (separate from general CNS depression)
Pharmacokinetics
PO: Peak 1-3 hr; metabolized by the liver to active metabolites, eliminated in urine; $t_{1/2}$ 14 hr
INDICATIONS AND USES: Anxiety
DOSAGE
Adult
• PO 20-40 mg tid-qid
Geriatric
• PO 20 mg qd-bid
■ **AVAILABLE FORMS/COST OF THERAPY**
• Tab, Uncoated—Oral: 20 mg, 100's: **$58.14;** 40 mg, 100's: **$80.81**
CONTRAINDICATIONS: Narrow angle glaucoma, psychosis, pregnancy
PRECAUTIONS: Elderly, debilitated, hepatic disease, renal disease, history of drug abuse, abrupt withdrawal, respiratory depression
PREGNANCY AND LACTATION: Pregnancy category D; may cause fetal damage when administered dur-

H

italic = common side effects   ***bold italic*** = life-threatening reactions

ing pregnancy; excreted into breast milk; may accumulate in breast-fed infants and is therefore not recommended

SIDE EFFECTS/ADVERSE REACTIONS

CNS: Abnormal thinking, agitation, amnesia, anxiety, apathy, *asthenia,* ataxia, decreased libido, decreased reflexes, emotional lability, hangover, hostility, *hypokinesia,* neuritis, seizures, sleep disorder, *somnolence,* stupor, twitch

CV: Dysrhythmia, syncope

EENT: Ear pain, epistaxis, eye irritation, pain, swelling; pharyngitis, photophobia, rhinitis, sinusitis

GI: Abdominal pain, decreased, increased appetite; dyspepsia, enterocolitis, flatulence, gastritis, increased serum transaminase levels, melena, mouth ulceration

GU: Frequent urination, hematuria, itching, menstrual cramps, nocturia, oliguria, penile discharge, urinary hesitancy, urgency; urinary incontinence, vaginal discharge

HEME: **Agranulocytosis**

MS: Back pain, lower extremity pain

RESP: Asthma, cold symptoms, cough, dyspnea, hyperventilation

SKIN: Acne, dry skin, photosensitivity, urticaria

INTERACTIONS

Drugs

🔳 *Carbamazepine:* Markedly reduces effect of halazepam

🔳 *Cimetidine:* Inhibits hepatic metabolism of halazepam

🔳 *Ciprofloxacin:* Inhibits hepatic metabolism of halazepam; may also competitively inhibit gamma amino butyric acid receptors

❷ *Clarithromycin:* Inhibits hepatic metabolism of halazepam

🔳 *Clozapine:* Additive respiratory and cardiovascular depression

🔳 *Delavirdine:* Inhibits hepatic metabolism of halazepam

🔳 *Disulfiram:* Inhibits hepatic metabolism of halazepam

🔳 *Erythromycin:* Inhibits hepatic metabolism of halazepam

🔳 *Ethanol:* Additive CNS effects

🔳 *Fluconazole:* Inhibits hepatic metabolism of halazepam

🔳 *Fluoxetine:* Inhibits hepatic metabolism of halazepam

🔳 *Fluvoxamine:* Inhibits hepatic metabolism of halazepam

🔳 *Isoniazid:* Inhibits hepatic metabolism of halazepam

🔳 *Itraconazole:* Inhibits hepatic metabolism of halazepam

🔳 *Ketoconazole:* Inhibits hepatic metabolism of halazepam

🔳 *Levodopa:* May reduce anti-Parkinsonian effect

🔳 *Metoprolol:* Inhibits hepatic metabolism of halazepam

🔳 *Omeprazole:* Inhibits hepatic metabolism of halazepam

🔳 *Phenytoin:* Markedly reduces effect of halazepam

🔳 *Quinolones:* Inhibits hepatic metabolism of halazepam; may also competitively inhibit gamma amino butyric acid receptors

🔳 *Rifampin:* Markedly reduces effect of halazepam

🔳 *Troleandomycin:* Inhibits hepatic metabolism of halazepam

SPECIAL CONSIDERATIONS

PATIENT/FAMILY EDUCATION

• Avoid alcohol and other CNS depressants

• Do not discontinue abruptly after prolonged therapy

• May cause drowsiness or dizziness, use caution while driving or performing other tasks requiring alertness

• Inform clinician if you are planning to become pregnant, you are pregnant, or if you become pregnant while taking this medicine

• May be habit forming

MONITORING PARAMETERS
• Periodic CBC, UA, blood chemistry analyses during prolonged therapy

halcinonide
(hal-sin'o-nide)
Rx: Halog, Halog-E
Chemical Class: Synthetic glucocorticoid
Therapeutic Class: Topical corticosteroid, high potency

CLINICAL PHARMACOLOGY
Mechanism of Action: Depresses formation, release, and activity of endogenous mediators of inflammation such as prostaglandins, kinins, histamine, liposomal enzymes, and the complement system resulting in decreased edema, erythema, and pruritus
Pharmacokinetics
Absorbed through the skin (increased by inflammation and occlusive dressings); metabolized primarily in the liver
INDICATIONS AND USES: Psoriasis, eczema, contact dermatitis, pruritus
DOSAGE
Adult and Child
• Top apply to affected area bid-tid, rub completely into skin
💲 **AVAILABLE FORMS/COST OF THERAPY**
• Cre—Top: 0.1%, 15, 30, 60, 240 g: **$35.35**/30 g
• Oint—Top: 0.1%, 15, 30, 60, 240 g: **$35.35**/30 g
• Sol—Top: 0.1%, 20, 60 ml: **$26.05**/20 ml
CONTRAINDICATIONS: Fungal infections; use on face, groin, or axilla
PRECAUTIONS: Viral infections, bacterial infections, children

PREGNANCY AND LACTATION:
Pregnancy category C; unknown whether top application could result in sufficient systemic absorption to produce detectable amounts in breast milk (systemic corticosteroids are secreted into breast milk in quantities not likely to have detrimental effects on infant)
SIDE EFFECTS/ADVERSE REACTIONS
SKIN: Acne, allergic contact dermatitis, atrophy, burning, dryness, folliculitis, hypertrichosis, hypopigmentation, irritation, itching, miliaria, perioral dermatitis, secondary infection, striae
MISC: Systemic absorption of topical corticosteroids has produced reversible HPA axis suppression (more likely with occlusive dressings, prolonged administration, application to large surface areas, liver failure, and in children)
SPECIAL CONSIDERATIONS
PATIENT/FAMILY EDUCATION
• Apply sparingly only to affected area
• Avoid contact with the eyes
• Do not put bandages or dressings over treated area unless directed by clinician
• Do not use on weeping, denuded, or infected areas
• Discontinue drug, notify clinician if local irritation or fever develops

halobetasol
(hal-oh-be'ta-sol)
Rx: Ultravate
Chemical Class: Synthetic glucocorticoid
Therapeutic Class: Topical corticosteroid, very high potency

CLINICAL PHARMACOLOGY
Mechanism of Action: Depresses

formation, release, and activity of endogenous mediators of inflammation such as prostaglandins, kinins, histamine, liposomal enzymes, and the complement system resulting in decreased edema, erythema, and pruritus

Pharmacokinetics

Absorbed through the skin (increased by inflammation and occlusive dressings); metabolized primarily in the liver

INDICATIONS AND USES: Psoriasis, eczema, contact dermatitis, pruritus

DOSAGE

Adult and Child

• Top apply to affected area bid-tid, rub completely into skin; total dosage should not exceed 50 g/wk because of the drug's potential to suppress the hypothalamic-pituitary-adrenal (HPA) axis; treatment beyond 2 consecutive wk not recommended

§ AVAILABLE FORMS/COST OF THERAPY

• Cre—Top: 0.05%, 15, 50 g: **$25.49**/15 g
• Oint—Top: 0.05%, 15, 50 g: **$25.49**/15 g

CONTRAINDICATIONS: Fungal infections; use on face, groin, or axilla; occlusive dressings

PRECAUTIONS: Viral infections, bacterial infections, children

PREGNANCY AND LACTATION: Pregnancy category C; unknown whether top application could result in sufficient systemic absorption to produce detectable amounts in breast milk (systemic corticosteroids are secreted into breast milk in quantities not likely to have detrimental effects on infant)

SIDE EFFECTS/ADVERSE REACTIONS

SKIN: Acne, allergic contact dermatitis, atrophy, burning, dryness, fol-liculitis, hypertrichosis, hypopigmentation, irritation, itching, miliaria, perioral dermatitis, secondary infection, striae

MISC: Systemic absorption of topical corticosteroids has produced reversible HPA axis suppression (more likely with occlusive dressings, prolonged administration, application to large surface areas, liver failure, and in children)

SPECIAL CONSIDERATIONS
PATIENT/FAMILY EDUCATION

• Apply sparingly only to affected area
• Avoid contact with the eyes
• Do not put bandages or dressings over treated area
• Do not use on weeping, denuded, or infected areas
• Discontinue drug, notify clinician if local irritation or fever develops
• Treatment should be limited to 2 wk, and amounts greater than 50 g/wk should not be used

---

haloperidol

(ha-loe-per′idole)
Rx: Haldol
Chemical Class: Butyrophenone derivative
Therapeutic Class: Antipsychotic

CLINICAL PHARMACOLOGY

Mechanism of Action: Dopamine receptor antagonist, with higher affinity for D_2- over D_1-receptors, and variable selectivity among the cortical dopamine tracts; also activity on nondopaminergic sites, i.e., cholinergic, α_1-adrenergic and histaminic receptors (explaining side effects); high risk extrapyramidal reactions; minimal orthostatic hypotension, sedation, and anticholinergic effects

---

* = non-FDA-approved use

Pharmacokinetics

PO: Peak 3-6 hr, $t_{1/2}$ 17 hr

IM: Peak 10-20 min, $t_{1/2}$ 17 hr

IM (decanoate): Peak 3-9 days, $t_{1/2}$ approximately 3 wk

>90% bound to plasma proteins, metabolized by the liver, excreted in urine and feces

INDICATIONS AND USES: Psychosis, Gilles de la Tourette syndrome, severe behavioral problems, hyperactive children (short-term), prolonged parenteral neuroleptic therapy for chronic schizophrenia (decanoate), antiemetic* (small doses)

DOSAGE

NOTE: 2 mg equivalent to chlorpromazine 100 mg

Adult and Child >16 yr

• *Psychosis/Tourette's syndrome:* PO 0.5-5 mg bid or tid initially depending on severity of condition, dose is increased to desired dose, max 100 mg/day; IM 2-5 mg q1-8h

• *Chronic schizophrenia:* IM 10-15 times the individual patient's stabilized PO dose q4 wk (decanoate)

Child 3-12 yr

• *Psychosis:* PO/IM 0.05-0.15 mg/kg/day in 2-3 divided doses

• *Tourette's syndrome:* PO 0.05-0.075 mg/kg/day in 2-3 divided doses

• *Hyperactivity:* PO 0.05-0.075 mg/kg/day in 2-3 divided doses

$ AVAILABLE FORMS/COST OF THERAPY

• Conc—Oral: 2 mg/ml, 120 ml: **$14.16-$54.32**

• Inj, Sol—IM: 5 mg/ml, 1, 10 ml: **$1.17-$7.50**/1 ml

• Inj, Sol—IM (decanoate): 50 mg/ml, 1 ml: **$28.80;** 100 mg/ml, 1 ml: **$52.80**

• Tab, Uncoated—Oral: 0.5 mg, 100's: **$1.88-$19.75;** 1 mg, 100's: **$2.25-$28.26;** 2 mg, 100's: **$2.40-$38.86;** 5 mg, 100's: **$2.93-$66.09;**

10 mg, 100's: **$4.94-$69.55;** 20 mg, 100's: **$17.88-$112.49**

CONTRAINDICATIONS: Severe toxic CNS depression, comatose states from any cause, Parkinson's disease

PRECAUTIONS: Elderly, severe cardiac disorders, seizure disorder, hepatic dysfunction, child <3 yr, alcohol withdrawal, electroconvulsive therapy, abrupt withdrawal, glaucoma, COPD

PREGNANCY AND LACTATION: Pregnancy category C; has been used for hyperemesis gravidarum, chorea gravidarum, and manic-depressive illness during pregnancy; excreted into breast milk; effect on nursing infant unknown, but may be of concern

SIDE EFFECTS/ADVERSE REACTIONS

CNS: Agitation, anxiety, catatonic-like behavioral states, confusion, depression, *drowsiness, EPS (pseudoparkinsonism, akathisia, dystonia, tardive dyskinesia),* euphoria, exacerbation of psychotic symptoms including hallucinations, *headache,* insomnia, lethargy, **neuroleptic malignant syndrome,** restlessness, **seizures,** vertigo

CV: ECG changes, hypertension, hypotension, **tachycardia**

EENT: Blurred vision, cataracts, dry eyes, glaucoma, retinopathy

GI: Anorexia, constipation, diarrhea, *dry mouth,* dyspepsia, hypersalivation, *nausea,* vomiting

GU: Priapism, urinary retention

HEME: **Agranulocytosis,** anemia, leukocytosis, minimal decreases in red blood cell counts, transient leukopenia

METAB: Breast engorgement, gynecomastia, hyperglycemia, hyperprolactinemia, hypoglycemia, hyponatremia, impotence, increased libido,

---

italic = common side effects   ***bold italic*** = life-threatening reactions

lactation, mastalgia, menstrual irregularities

RESP: Bronchospasm, increased depth of respiration, laryngospasm

SKIN: Diaphoresis, isolated cases of photosensitivity, loss of hair, maculopapular and acneiform skin reactions

INTERACTIONS

Drugs

3 *Anticholinergics:* Inhibition of therapeutic effect of neuroleptics

3 *Barbiturates:* Potential reduction of serum neuroleptic concentrations

3 *Bromocriptine:* Inhibition of bromocriptine's ability to lower serum prolactin concentrations in patients with pituitary adenoma; theoretical inhibition of antipsychotic effects of neuroleptics

3 *Carbamazepine:* Decreased serum haloperidol concentrations

3 *Guanethidine:* Inhibition of antihypertensive effect of guanethidine

2 *Levodopa:* Inhibition of antiparkinsonian effects of levodopa

3 *Lithium:* Rare reports of severe neurotoxicity in patients receiving lithium and neuroleptics

3 *Quinidine:* Increases haldol concentrations; increased risk of toxicity

SPECIAL CONSIDERATIONS
PATIENT/FAMILY EDUCATION

• Do not mix liquid formulation with coffee or tea
• Use calibrated dropper
• Take with food or milk
• Arise slowly from reclining position
• Do not discontinue abruptly
• Use a sunscreen during sun exposure to prevent burns
• Take special precautions to stay cool in hot weather

MONITORING PARAMETERS

• Observe closely for signs of tardive dyskinesia

---

haloprogin
(ha-loe-proe'jin)
Rx: Halotex
Chemical Class: Iodinated phenolic ester
Therapeutic Class: Antifungal

CLINICAL PHARMACOLOGY

Mechanism of Action: Interferes with fungal cell membrane permeability

Pharmacokinetics

TOP: Absorbed poorly through the skin

INDICATIONS AND USES: Tinea pedis (athlete's foot), tinea cruris (jock itch), tinea corporis (ringworm), tinea manuum, tinea versicolor

Antifungal spectrum usually includes: *Trichophyton rubrum, T. tonsurans, T. mentagrophytes, Microsporum canis, Epidermophyton floccosum, Malassezia furfur*

DOSAGE

Adult and Child

• TOP apply to affected area bid for 14-21 days, intertriginous lesions may require up to 28 days of therapy

$ **AVAILABLE FORMS/COST OF THERAPY**

• Cre, Sol—Top: 1%, 15, 30 g: **$12.24-$22.98**

PREGNANCY AND LACTATION: Pregnancy category B; excretion into breast milk unknown; problems have not been documented

SIDE EFFECTS/ADVERSE REACTIONS

SKIN: Burning sensation, erythema, folliculitis, itching, local irritation, pruritus, scaling, vesicle formation

---

* = non-FDA-approved use

SPECIAL CONSIDERATIONS
PATIENT/FAMILY EDUCATION
• For external use only
• Avoid contact with eyes
• Complete full course of therapy
• Notify clinician if condition worsens or if irritation, redness, swelling, stinging, or burning persists

---

heparin
(hep′a-rin)
Rx: Heparin
Chemical Class: Sulfated glycosaminoglycan
Therapeutic Class: Anticoagulant

CLINICAL PHARMACOLOGY
Mechanism of Action: Potentiates inhibitory action of antithrombin III (heparin cofactor) on several activated coagulation factors, including thrombin (factor IIa) and factors IXa, Xa, XIa, and XIIa, by forming a complex with and inducing a conformational change in the antithrombin III molecule

Pharmacokinetics
IV: Onset immediate (if no loading dose is given, onset may depend on rate of INF)
SC: Onset 20-60 min
Highly bound to plasma proteins; primary route of removal from circulation via uptake by the reticuloendothelial system; also metabolized by liver, eliminated in urine usually as metabolites (50% of IV dose may be excreted unchanged); $t_{1/2}$ 90 min

INDICATIONS AND USES: Deep vein thrombosis (DVT), pulmonary embolism (PE), peripheral arterial embolism; coagulopathies (e.g., disseminated intravascular coagulation); DVT/PE prophylaxis; clotting prevention in arterial and heart surgery, blood transfusions, extracorporeal circulation, dialysis and blood samples; prophylaxis of LV thrombi and CVA after MI*; evolving stroke*; adjunctive therapy of coronary occlusion with acute MI*

DOSAGE
Adult
• *DVT/PE:* IV INF 80 U/kg bolus, then 18 U/kg/hr, adjust based on aPTT results; intermittent IV 10,000 U initially, then 75-125 U/kg q4-6h adjust based on aPTT results; SC 10,000-20,000 units initially, then 8000-10,000 U q8h, or 15,000-20,000 U q12h, adjust based on aPTT results drawn at mid-dosing interval
• *Prevention of DVT/PE:* SC 5000-7500 U q8-12h until patient is ambulatory
Child
• IV INF 50 U/kg initially, then 15-25 U/kg/hr, increase dose by 2-4 U/kg/hr q6-8h based on aPTT results; intermittent IV 50-100 U/kg initially, then 50-100 U/kg q4h adjust based on aPTT results

💲 AVAILABLE FORMS/COST OF THERAPY
• Inj, Sol—IV, SC: 1000 U/ml, 1, 2, 10, 30 ml: **$0.73-$1.11**/ml; 2500 U/ml, 0.25, 1, 10 ml: **$1.34**/ml; 5000 U/ml, 1, 10 ml: **$1.03-$1.61;** 10,000 U/ml, 0.5, 1, 2, 4, 5, 10 ml: **$1.71-$4.05**/ml; 20,000 U/ml, 1, 2, 5 ml: **$1.44-$7.61**/ml

CONTRAINDICATIONS: Severe thrombocytopenia, uncontrolled bleeding (except when due to DIC), suspected intracranial hemorrhage, shock, severe hypotension

PRECAUTIONS: IM inj (avoid due to risk for hematoma), elderly, children, diabetes, renal insufficiency, severe hypertension, subacute bacterial endocarditis, acute nephritis, peptic ulcer disease, severe renal disease

---

italic = common side effects   ***bold italic*** = life-threatening reactions

PREGNANCY AND LACTATION:
Pregnancy category C; does not cross the placenta, has major advantages over oral anticoagulants as the treatment of choice during pregnancy; is not excreted into breast milk due to its high molecular weight

SIDE EFFECTS/ADVERSE REACTIONS

CNS: Fever, headache

CV: Allergic vasospastic reactions, shock

EENT: Lacrimation, rhinitis

GI: Nausea, vomiting

GU: Hematuria, priapism

HEME: Hemorrhage, heparin-induced thrombocytopenia (HIT), white clot syndrome (new thrombus formation associated with heparin administration)

METAB: Rebound hyperlipidemia, suppressed aldosterone synthesis,

MS: Osteoporosis (after long-term, high doses)

RESP: Anaphylactoid reactions, asthma

SKIN: Chills, *cutaneous necrosis,* delayed transient alopecia, erythema, hematoma/ulceration, histamine-like reactions, local irritation, urticaria

INTERACTIONS

Drugs

3 *Aspirin:* Increased risk of hemorrhage

3 *Warfarin:* Warfarin may prolong the aPTT in patients receiving heparin; heparin may prolong the PT in patients receiving warfarin

SPECIAL CONSIDERATIONS

PATIENT/FAMILY EDUCATION

• Report any signs of bleeding: gums, under skin, urine, stools

MONITORING PARAMETERS

• aPTT (usual goal is to prolong aPTT to a value that corresponds to a plasma heparin level of 0.2 to 0.4 U/ml by protamine titration or to an antifactor Xa level of about 0.3 to 0.6 U/ml; this range must be deter-

mined for each individual laboratory), usually measure 6-8 hr after initiation of IV and 6-8 hr after INF rate changes; increase or decrease INF by 2-4 U/kg/hr dependent on aPTT

• For intermittent inj, measure aPTT 3.5-4 hr after IV inj

• Platelet counts, signs of bleeding, Hgb, hct

---

homatropine
(hoe-mat′ro-peen)
Rx: Isopto Homatropine
Chemical Class: Belladonna alkaloid
Therapeutic Class: Mydriatic; cycloplegic

CLINICAL PHARMACOLOGY

Mechanism of Action: Blocks responses of the sphincter muscle of the iris and the accommodative muscle of the ciliary body to stimulation by acetylcholine; dilation of the pupil (mydriasis) and paralysis of accommodation (cycloplegia) result

Pharmacokinetics

OPHTH: Peak ½-1 hr, duration 1-3 days

INDICATIONS AND USES: Uveitis, iritis, mydriasis, cycloplegic refraction

DOSAGE

Adult and Child

• INSTILL 1 gtt; repeat in 5-10 min for refraction or q3-4h for uveitis; patients with heavily pigmented irides may require larger doses; use only 2% strength in children

$ **AVAILABLE FORMS/COST OF THERAPY**

• Sol—Ophth: 2%, 5, ml: **$14.00;** 5%, 5, 15 ml: **$11.35-$16.00/5 ml**

CONTRAINDICATIONS: Adhesions between the iris and the lens, primary glaucoma, narrow anterior chamber angle

---

* = non-FDA-approved use

PRECAUTIONS: Elderly, small children, and infants

PREGNANCY AND LACTATION: Pregnancy category C; may be detectable in very small amounts in breast milk; compatible with breastfeeding

SIDE EFFECTS/ADVERSE REACTIONS

CNS: Confusion, fever, headache, somnolence, visual hallucinations

CV: Tachycardia, vasodilation

EENT: Blurred vision, edema, increased intraocular pressure, irritation, *photophobia*

GI: Abdominal distension in infants, decreased GI motility, dry mouth

GU: Urinary retention

SKIN: Dry skin, rash

SPECIAL CONSIDERATIONS

PATIENT/FAMILY EDUCATION

• Do not touch tip of dropper to any surface

• May cause blurred vision; do not drive or engage in any hazardous activities while pupils are dilated

• May cause sensitivity to light; protect eyes from bright light

• Wash hands immediately following instillation

• Discontinue immediately if eye pain occurs

• To minimize systemic effects, compress the lacrimal sac for several minutes following instillation

---

hyaluronidase

(hye-al-yoor-on′ĭ-dase)

Rx: Wydase

Chemical Class: Protein enzyme

Therapeutic Class: Adjuvant for injectables

CLINICAL PHARMACOLOGY

Mechanism of Action: Modifies permeability of connective tissue through hydrolysis of hyaluronic acid; enhances diffusion of substances injected SC

INDICATIONS AND USES: Hypodermoclysis; adjunct in subcutaneous urography for improving resorption of radiopaque agents; adjunct to increase the absorption and dispersion of other drugs; enhances diffusion of locally irritating or toxic drugs in management of IV extravasation*

DOSAGE

Adult and Child

• *Adjunct to dispersion of other drugs:* Inj 150 U with other drug; consult appropriate references regarding physical or chemical incompatibilities before adding hyaluronidase to sol containing other drug

• *Hypodermolysis:* SC 150 U/1000 ml of clysis sol; for child <3 yr, limit volume of single clysis to 200 ml

• *SC urography:* SC 75 U over each scapula, then contrast medium injected at same sites

💲 **AVAILABLE FORMS/COST OF THERAPY**

• Inj, Lyphl-Sol—SC: 150 U/ml: **$8.26**

CONTRAINDICATIONS: Inj into infected, acutely inflamed, or cancerous area

PREGNANCY AND LACTATION: Pregnancy category C; excretion into breast milk unknown, use caution in nursing mothers

SIDE EFFECTS/ADVERSE REACTIONS

SKIN: Itching, rash, urticaria

SPECIAL CONSIDERATIONS

Prior to administration, conduct a preliminary test for sensitivity: 0.02 ml of 150 U/ml sol is injected intradermally; if wheal with pseudopods develops within 5 min and persists for 20-30 min, test is positive

---

italic = common side effects   ***bold italic*** = life-threatening reactions

hydralazine

(hye-dral'a-zeen)
Rx: Apresoline
Combinations
  Rx: with hydrochlorothiazide
  (Apresazide); with hydro-
  chlorothiazide, reserpine
  (Ser-Ap-Es)
Chemical Class: Phthalazine
derivative
Therapeutic Class: Direct
vasodilator antihyper-
tensive; congestive heart
failure

CLINICAL PHARMACOLOGY
Mechanism of Action: Preferentially dilates arterioles with little effect on veins; interferes with calcium movement within vascular
smooth muscle responsible for initiating or maintaining the contractile state; increases cardiac output,
decreases systemic resistance, reduces afterload
Pharmacokinetics
PO: Well absorbed; undergoes 1st-
pass metabolism; bioavailability
50% (slow acetylators) or 30% (fast
acetylators); peak 60 min, onset 45
min, duration 3-8 hr
IM: Onset 5-10 min, peak 1 hr, duration 2-4 hr
IV: Onset 10-20 min, duration 3-8 hr
Metabolized by liver (genetic variation among individuals in rate of
acetylation), excreted in urine; $t_{1/2}$
0.44-0.47 hr (metabolite 2-4 hr)
INDICATIONS AND USES: Hypertension, CHF,* afterload reduction
in severe aortic insufficiency and
after valve replacement,* eclampsia*
DOSAGE
Adult
• PO 10 mg qid, increase by 10-25
mg/dose q2-5 days as needed to max

of 300 mg/day; IM/IV 10-20 mg
q4-6h, may increase to 40 mg/dose
Child
• PO 0.75-1 mg/kg/day divided bid-
qid, increase over 3-4 wk to 7.5
mg/kg/day divided bid-qid if necessary, do not exceed 200 mg/day;
IM/IV 0.1-0.2 mg/kg/dose q4-6h,
do not exceed 20 mg/dose
💲 **AVAILABLE FORMS/COST**
  OF THERAPY
• Inj, Sol—IM, IV: 20 mg/ml, 1 ml:
$8.75-$9.75
• Tab, Uncoated—Oral: 10 mg,
100's: **$2.75-$26.07;** 25 mg, 100's:
$3.25-$29.44; 50 mg, 100's: **$3.50-
$55.54;** 100 mg, 100's: **$8.29-$78.13**
CONTRAINDICATIONS: CAD, mitral valvular rheumatic heart disease
PRECAUTIONS: Advanced renal
disease, children, pulmonary hypertension
PREGNANCY AND LACTATION:
Pregnancy category C; commonly
used in pregnant women; excreted
into breast milk; compatible with
breast feeding
**SIDE EFFECTS/ADVERSE REAC-
  TIONS**
CNS: Anxiety, depression, *dizziness,
headache,* peripheral neuritis, psychotic reactions, *tremor*
CV: Angina, flushing, hypotension,
palpitations, reflex tachycardia
EENT: Nasal congestion
GI: Anorexia, constipation, *diar-
rhea,* hepatitis, *nausea,* paralytic il-
eus, *vomiting, pancreatitis*
GU: Frequency, glucosuria, poly-
uria, uremia incresed creatinine BUN
HEME: **Agranulocytosis, aplastic
anemia,** hemolytic anemia, neutro-
penia, thrombocytopenia, eosino-
philia, *leukopenia*
MS: Arthralgia, muscle cramps
RESP: Dyspnea
SKIN: Pruritus, rash, urticaria
MISC: Lupus-like syndrome (arthral-

gia, dermatoses, fever, splenomegaly, glomerulonephritis)

INTERACTIONS

Drugs

3 *Diazoxide:* Severe hypotension

3 *NSAIDs:* Inhibited antihypertensive response to hydralazine

Labs

• *False increase:* Ca^{++} (slight); urine 17-ketogenic steroids; glucose, uric acid

• *False decrease:* Glucose, uric acid

SPECIAL CONSIDERATIONS

Lupus-like syndrome more common in "slow acetylators" and following higher doses for prolonged periods

PATIENT/FAMILY EDUCATION

• Take with meals

• Notify clinician of any unexplained prolonged general tiredness or fever, muscle or joint aching, or chest pain

• Stools may turn black

MONITORING PARAMETERS

• CBC and ANA titer before and during prolonged therapy

---

hydrochlorothiazide
(hye-droe-klor-oh-thye'a-zide)

Rx: Aquazide-H, Diaqua, Esidrix, Ezide, HydroDiuril, Hydro-Par, Lexor, Microzide, Oretic, Zide

Combinations

with angiotensin-converting inhibitors: quinapril (Accuretic); captopril (Acediur, Capozide); lisinopril (Prinzide, Zestoretic); benazepril (Lotensin HCT); moexipril (Uniretic); enalapril (Vaseretic); with spironolactone (Aldactazide, Spirozide) with methyldopa (Aldoril), with hydralazine (Apresazide) with reserpine (Aqwesine, Hydropres, Hydroserpine, Hydrotensin, Mallopres, Marpres, Unipres) with angiotensin II receptor blockers: irbesartan (Avalide), valsartan (Diovan HCT), losartan (Hyzaar), with hydralazine and reserpine (Cam-ap-es, H.H.R., Hyserp, Lo-Ten, Ser-A-Gen, Seralazide, Ser-Ap-Es, Serpex, Uni-Serp), with triamterene: (Dyazide, Maxzide) with potassium (Esidrix-K) with guanethidine (Esimil), with betablockers: propranolol: (Inderide); metoprolol: (Lopressor HCT); labetolol (Normazide, Trandate-HCT); timolol: (Timolide); bisoprolol (Ziac) with amiloride (Moduretic)

Chemical Class: Sulfonamide derivative

Therapeutic Class: Thiazide diuretic, antihypertensive

H

---

italic = common side effects   ***bold italic*** = life-threatening reactions

CLINICAL PHARMACOLOGY

Mechanism of Action: Inhibits reabsorption of sodium and chloride in cortical thick ascending limb of the loop of Henle and the early distal tubules, increasing the urinary excretion of sodium and chloride; sulfonamide moiety provides some carbonic anhydrase inhibition activity; other actions: increased potassium and bicarbonate excretion; decreased calcium excretion; uric acid retention; antihypertensive action dependent on sodium depletion, drop in peripheral vascular resistance, and reduction in extracellular volume

Pharmacokinetics

PO: Readily absorbed (60%-80% of dose) peak 4 hr, onset 2 hr, duration 6-12 hr; excreted unchanged in urine; $t_{1/2}$ 5.6-14.8 hr

INDICATIONS AND USES: Edema (CHF, hepatic cirrhosis, corticosteroid and estrogen therapy, nephrotic syndrome, acute glomerulonephritis); hypertension; calcium nephrolithiasis*; prevention of osteoporosis*; diabetes insipidus*

DOSAGE

Adult

• PO 12.5-50 mg qd, max 200 mg/day; doses >50 mg/day generally not recommended due to increased incidence of hypokalemia and other metabolic disturbances

Child

• PO (<6 mo) 1-3.3 mg/kg/day divided bid; (>6 mo) 2 mg/kg/day divided bid

💲 AVAILABLE FORMS/COST OF THERAPY

• Sol—Oral: 50 mg/5ml, 500 ml: **$16.91**
• Tab, Uncoated—Oral: 12.5 mg, 100's: **$44.50;** 25 mg, 100's: **$1.75-$15.43;** 50 mg, 100's: **$2.49-$57.95;** 100 mg, 100's: **$2.75-$6.87**

CONTRAINDICATIONS: Anuria, renal decompensation

PRECAUTIONS: Fluid and electrolyte imbalance (including sodium, potassium, magnesium, calcium), renal disease, hepatic disease, gout, COPD, lupus erythematosus, diabetes mellitus, hyperparathyroidism, vomiting, diarrhea, elevated cholesterol/triglycerides

PREGNANCY AND LACTATION: Pregnancy category B; 1st trimester use may increase risk of congenital defects, use in later trimesters does not seem to carry this risk; therapy for preexisting hypertension can be continued throughout pregnancy with minimal risk; initiating for simple edema not recommended; few unequivocal indications for diuretic therapy in pregnancy except for pulmonary edema or congestive heart failure, excreted into breast milk in small amounts; considered compatible with breast feeding

SIDE EFFECTS/ADVERSE REACTIONS

CNS: Depression, *dizziness,* drowsiness, *fatigue,* headache, paresthesia, *weakness*

CV: **Arrhythmias,** irregular pulse, orthostatic hypotension, palpitations, volume depletion

EENT: Blurred vision

GI: Anorexia, constipation, cramps, diarrhea, *nausea,* pancreatitis, *vomiting*

GU: Frequency, decreased libido, impotence

*HEME: **Agranulocytosis, aplastic anemia, hemolytic anemia, leukopenia, neutropenia, thrombocytopenia***

METAB: Hypercalcemia, *hyperglycemia, hyperuricemia,* hypochloremia, *hypokalemia,* hypomagnesemia, hyponatremia, increased creatinine, BUN, lipid abnormalities (increased total triglycerides, LDL cholesterol)

SKIN: Fever, photosensitivity, purpura, *rash,* urticaria

INTERACTIONS

Drugs

❷ *Angiotensin-converting enzyme inhibitors:* Risk of postural hypotension when added to ongoing diuretic therapy; more common with loop diuretics; first dose hypotension possible in patients with sodium depletion or hypovolemia due to diuretics or sodium restriction; hypotensive response is usually transient; hold diuretic day of first dose

❸ *Calcium* (high doses): Risk of milk-alkali syndrome; monitor for hypercalcemia

❸ *Carbenoxolone:* Additive potassium wasting; severe hypokalemia

❸ *Cholestyramine/colestipol:* Reduced serum concentrations of thiazide diuretics

❸ *Corticosteroids:* Concomitant therapy may result in excessive potassium loss

❸ *Diazoxide:* Hyperglycemia

❸ *Digitalis glycosides:* Diuretic-induced hypokalemia may increase the risk of digitalis toxicity

❸ *Hypoglycemic agents:* Thiazide diuretics tend to increase blood glucose, may increase dosage requirements of antidiabetic drugs

❸ *Lithium:* Increased serum lithium concentrations, toxicity may occur

❸ *Methotrexate:* Increased bone marrow suppression

❸ *Nonsteroidal antiinflammatory drugs:* Concurrent use may reduce diuretic and antihypertensive effects

Labs

• *False decrease:* Urine estriol

SPECIAL CONSIDERATIONS

• May protect against osteoporotic hip fractures

• Loop diuretics or metolazone more effective if CrCl <40-50 ml/min

• Combinations with triamterene, lisinopril have potassium sparing effect

• Doses above 25 mg provide no further blood pressure reduction, but are more likely to induce metabolic disturbance (i.e., hypokalemia, hyperuricemia, etc.)

PATIENT/FAMILY EDUCATION

• Will increase urination temporarily (for about 3 wk); take early in the day

• May cause sensitivity to sunlight; avoid prolonged exposure to the sun and other ultraviolet light

• May cause gout attacks; notify clinician if sudden joint pain occurs

MONITORING PARAMETERS

• Weight, urine output, serum electrolytes, BUN, creatinine, CBC, uric acid, glucose, lipids

H

hydrocodone
(hye-droe-koe'done)
Rx: Hycodan
Combinations
  Rx: with acetaminophen
(Anexsia, Bancap-HC,
Ceta-plus, Co-gesic, Duo-
cet, Hydrocet, Hydrogesic,
Hy-Phen, Lorcet, Lortab,
Margesic-H, Norco, Pana-
cet, Stagesic, T-Gesic,
Vidocin, Zydone); with
aspirin (Alor, Azdone,
Damason-P, Lortab with
ibuprofen (Vicoprofen);
with pseudoephedrine,
guaifenesin (Entuss-D for
Duratuss, Pizotuss-D,
Deconamine CX,
Entuss-D, Cophene XP,
SRC Liquid, Tussafin),
with pseudoephedrine,
chlorpheniramine, guaifenesin (Ztuss); with phenylpropanolamine, pyrilamine,
guaifenesin (Triaminic
Expectorant DH, S-T
Forte, Vetuss HC, Statuss);
with phenindamine,
guaifenesin (P-V-Tussin);
with phenylpropanolamine,
guaifenesin (Tussanil);
with phenylephrine, chlorpheniramine (Atuss-HD);
with phenylephrine,
guaifenesin (Donatussin
DC, Tussafed HC,
Atuss-G)
  Chemical Class: Semisynthetic opium alkaloid; phenanthrene derivative
  Therapeutic Class: Narcotic
analgesic; antitussive
  DEA Class: Schedule III

CLINICAL PHARMACOLOGY
Mechanism of Action: Narcotic agonist with activity at Mu receptors
(supraspinal analgesia, euphoria, respiratory and physical depression,
miosis, and reduced GI motility),
Kappa receptors (pentazocine-like
spinal analgesia, sedation, and miosis), and Delta receptors (dysphoria, psychotomimetic effects [e.g.,
hallucinations], and respiratory and
vasomotor stimulation caused by
drugs with antagonist activity); compared to morphine, less analgesia,
equal antitussive, less respiratory depression and less physical dependence

Pharmacokinetics
Peak 1.3 hr, duration 4.6 hr, $t_{1/2}$ 3.8
hr; metabolized in liver, excreted
mainly in urine

INDICATIONS AND USES: Moder-
ate to moderately severe pain, non-
productive cough
DOSAGE
• NOTE: Only available commercially in combination (USA)
Adult
• PO 5-10 mg q4-6h prn
Child
• PO 0.6 mg/kg/day in 3-4 divided
doses; do not exceed 1.25 mg/dose
(<2 yr), 5 mg/dose (2-12 yr), 10
mg/dose (>12 yr)
**💲 AVAILABLE FORMS/COST
OF THERAPY**
• Cap, Gel—Oral: 500 mg (acetaminophen)/5 mg, 100's: **$18.69-
$103.91**
• Elixir—Oral: 100 mg (guaife-
nisen) 5 mg/5 ml, 480 ml: **$39.95-
$70.06**
• Tab, Uncoated—Oral: 500 mg
(acetaminophen)/2.5 mg, 100's:
$24.98-$46.62; 500 mg (acetaminophen)/5 mg, 100's: **$4.91-
$45.59;** 500 mg (acetaminophen)/
7.5 mg, 100's: **$18.37-$51.41;** 556
mg (acetaminophen)/5 mg, 100's:
$23.88; 650 mg (acetaminophen)/
7.5, 100's: **$34.25-$56.15;** 650 mg

(acetaminophen)/10 mg, 100's: **$35.14-$71.96;** 750 mg (acetaminophen)/7.5 mg, 100's: **$21.83-$51.59;** 200 mg (ibuprofen)/7.5 mg, 100's: **$92.87**

PRECAUTIONS: Head injury, increased intracranial pressure, acute abdominal conditions, elderly, severe impairment of hepatic or renal function, hypothyroidism, Addison's disease, prostatic hypertrophy, urethral stricture, history of drug abuse

PREGNANCY AND LACTATION: Pregnancy category B (category D if used for prolonged periods or in high doses at term); withdrawal could theoretically occur in infants exposed *in utero* to prolonged maternal ingestion; excretion into breast milk unknown; use caution in nursing mothers

SIDE EFFECTS/ADVERSE REACTIONS

CNS: Agitation, dependency, dizziness, *drowsiness,* lethargy, restlessness, *sedation*

CV: Bradycardia, orthostatic hypotension, palpitations, tachycardia

GI: Anorexia, constipation, nausea, vomiting

GU: Urinary retention

RESP: **Respiratory depression, respiratory paralysis**

SKIN: Flushing, rash, urticaria

INTERACTIONS

Drugs

3 *Antihistamines, chloral hydrate, glutethimide, methocarbamol:* Enhanced depressant effects

3 *Barbiturates:* Additive respiratory and CNS depressant effects

3 *Cimetidine:* Increased respiratory and CNS depression

3 *Ethanol:* Additive CNS effects

3 *Protease inhibitors:* Enhanced CNS and respiratory depression

Labs

False elevations of amylase and lipase

SPECIAL CONSIDERATIONS
PATIENT/FAMILY EDUCATION

• Report any symptoms of CNS changes, allergic reactions

• Physical dependency may result when used for extended periods

• Change position slowly, orthostatic hypotension may occur

• Avoid hazardous activities if drowsiness or dizziness occurs

• Avoid alcohol, other CNS depressants

• Minimize nausea by administering with food and remain lying down following dose

• Do not administer agonist/antagonist analgesics (i.e., pentazocine, nalbuphine, butorphanol, dezocine, buprenorphine) to patient who has received a prolonged course of hydrocodone (a pure agonist). In opioid-dependent patients, mixed agonist/antagonist analgesics may precipitate withdrawal symptoms

H

---

italic = common side effects   ***bold italic*** = life-threatening reactions

hydrocortisone

(hye-dro-kor'ti-sone)

Rx: *Ano-Rectals:* Proctocort, Anusol-HC, Proctofoam-HC, Anucort-HC, Cortenema
Systemic: Cortef, Hydrocortone, Hydrocortone Phosphate, Hydrocortone Acetate, Solu-Cortef
Topical: Cetacort, Cort-Dome, Dermacort, Hytone, Locoid, Synacort, Westcort
OTC: Cortizone, Cortaid, Lanacort-5, Gynecort Female Creme, Dermolate, Tegrin-HC

Combinations

> **Rx:** with choloramphenicol (Chloromycetin/HC suspension—ophthalmic); with neomycin and polymyxin B (Cortisporin Otic, Drotic, Otocort—otic); with neomycin, polymyxin B, and bacitracin (Cortisporin Ointment, Neotricin HC—ophthalmic); with oxytetracycline (Terra-Cortril—ophthalmic); with urea (Carmol HC)

Chemical Class: Glucocorticoid
Therapeutic Class: Systemic and topical corticosteroid, low potency

CLINICAL PHARMACOLOGY
Mechanism of Action: Decreases inflammation by depressing migration of polymorphonuclear leukocytes and activity of endogenous mediators of inflammation, has many profound metabolic effects, possesses mineralocorticoid activity
Pharmacokinetics
PO: Onset 1-2 hr, peak 1 hr, duration 1-1½ days
PR: Onset 3-5 days

TOP: Absorbed through the skin (increased by inflammation and occlusive dressings); metabolized by liver, excreted in urine (17-OHCS, 17-KS)

INDICATIONS AND USES: Anti-inflammatory or immunosuppressant agent in the treatment of a variety of diseases of hematologic, allergic, inflammatory, neoplastic, and autoimmune origin; in replacement doses for primary or secondary adrenocortical insufficiency

DOSAGE
Adult and Child
• *Otitis externa:* With head tilted for 2 min instill 4 gtt 3-4 ×/day
• *Inflammatory ocular conditions:* Instill 1 gtt or ointment q3-4h
Adult
• *Acute adrenal insufficiency:* PO 5-30 mg bid-qid; IM/IV/SC 15-240 mg q12h
• *Anti-inflammatory:* PO 5-30 mg bid-qid; IM/IV/SC 15-240 mg q12h
• *Shock:* IM/IV 500-2000 mg q2-6h
• *Rect:* Enema 100 mg nightly for 21 days; suppository 25 mg bid-qid prn
• *Intra-articular and soft tissue (acetate):* Large joints 25 mg; small joints 10-25 mg; bursae 25-37.5 mg; tendon sheaths 5-12.5 mg; soft tissue infiltration 25-50 mg; ganglia 12.5-25 mg
Child
• *Acute adrenal insufficiency:* IM/IV/SC 1-2 mg/kg bolus, then 25-150 mg/day in divided doses (infants and younger children); 1-2 mg/kg bolus, then 150-250 mg/day in divided doses (older children)
• *Physiologic replacement:* PO 0.5-0.75 mg/kg/day or 20-25 mg/m^2/day divided q8h; IM 0.25-0.35 mg/kg/day or 12-15 mg/m^2/day qd
• *Shock:* IM/IV 50 mg/kg initially,

then repeated in 4 hr and/or q24h prn

Adult and Child

• TOP apply to affected area bid-qid, rub completely into skin

$ AVAILABLE FORMS/COSTS OF THERAPY

• Supp (acetate)—Rect: 25 mg, 12's: **$5.93-$33.91**

• Aerosol, Foam (acetate)—Rect: 10%, 15 g: **$68.10**

• Enema—Rect: 100 mg/60 ml: **$9.28**

• Tab, Uncoated—Oral: 5 mg, 100's: **$14.91;** 10 mg, 100's: **$27.85;** 20 mg, 100's: **$11.25-$52.80**

• Susp (cypionate)—Oral: 10 mg/5 ml, 120 ml: **$23.61**

• Inj, Sol (sodium phosphate)—IM, IV, SC: 50 mg/ml, 2, 10 ml: **$10.75**/12 ml

• Inj, Lyph-Sol (sodium succinate)—IM, IV: 100 mg/vial: **$3.26;** 250 mg/2 ml: **$7.56;** 500 mg/4 ml: **$14.71;** 1000 mg/8 ml: **$29.29**

• Inj, Susp (acetate)—Intra-Articular, IM: 25 mg/ml, 5, 10 ml: **$3.60**/10 ml

• Cre, Oint (butyrate)—Top: 0.1%, 15, 45 g: **$17.10-$21.20**/15 g

• Sol (butyrate)—Top: 0.1%, 20, 60 ml: **$24.70**/20 ml

• Aer—Top: 1%, 52.5 ml: **$2.94**

• Cre—Top: 0.5%, 15, 30, 45, 60, 120, 454 g: **$1.20-$5.39**/30 g; 1%, 15, 30, 45, 60, 120, 454 g: **$1.25-$28.68**/30 g; 2.5%, 15, 30, 45, 60, 120, 454 g: **$5.55-$42.45**/30 g

• Cre—Rect: 2.5%, 30 g: **$30.48**

• Lotion—Top: 0.25%, 120 ml: **$5.40-$6.75;** 0.5%, 30, 60, 120 ml: **$3.25**/60 ml; 1%, 30, 60, 75, 120 ml: **$4.48-$29.85**/60 ml; 2.5%, 60, 120 ml: **$25.23-$41.17**/60 ml

• Oint—Top: 0.5%, 15, 30 g: **$1.20-$2.79**/30 g; 1%: **$1.25-$4.25**/30 g; 2.5%: **$8.84-$27.59**/30 g

• Sol—Top: 1%, 30, 60 ml: **$9.93**/30 ml; 2.5%, 30, 60 ml: **$16.33**/30 ml

CONTRAINDICATIONS: Systemic fungal infections

PRECAUTIONS: Psychosis, diabetes mellitus, glaucoma, osteoporosis, seizure disorders, ulcerative colitis (intestinal perforation), CHF, hypertension, myesthenia gravis (if used with anticholinesterase agents), renal disease, esophagitis, peptic ulcer, latent tuberculosis or amebiasis (reactivation of disease). Topical: use on face, groin, or axilla, ocular herpes simplex

PREGNANCY AND LACTATION: Pregnancy category C; excreted in breast milk, could interfere with infant's growth and endogenous corticosteroid production

SIDE EFFECTS/ADVERSE REACTIONS

CNS: Depression, *mood changes, seizures*

CV: CHF, hypertension, tachycardia, ***thromboembolism,*** thrombophlebitis

EENT: Blurred vision, cataract, increased intraocular pressure

*GI: Abdominal distension, diarrhea, **GI hemorrhage,** increased appetite, nausea, pancreatitis*

GU: Menstrual irregularities

HEME: Increased neutrophils

METAB: Alkalosis, Cushingoid state, decreased glucose tolerance, growth suppression in children, HPA suppression

MS: Aseptic necrosis of femoral and humeral heads, fractures, muscle mass loss, osteoporosis, tendon rupture, weakness

SKIN: Acne, allergic contact dermatitis, atrophy, bruising, burning, dryness, ecchymosis, folliculitis, hypertrichosis, hypopigmentation, irritation, itching, miliaria, perioral dermatitis, petechiae, poor wound healing, secondary infection, striae,

---

italic = common side effects   ***bold italic*** = life-threatening reactions

suppression of skin test reactions, thin fragile skin

INTERACTIONS

Drugs

■ *Aminoglutethamide:* Enhanced elimination of hydrocortisone; reduction in corticosteroid response

■ *Antidiabetics:* Increased blood glucose in patients with diabetes

■ *Barbiturates:* Reduction in the serum concentrations of corticosteroids

■ *Cholestyramine, colestipol:* Possible reduced absorption of corticosteroids

■ *Cyclosporine:* Increased levels of both drugs increases the risk of seizures

■ *Estrogens:* Enhanced effects of corticosteroids

■ *Isoniazid (INH):* Reduced INH levels, enhanced corticosteroid effect

■ *IUDs:* Inhibition of inflammation may decrease contraceptive effect

■ *NSAIDs:* Increased risk GI ulceration

■ *Phenytoin:* Reduced therapeutic effect of corticosteroids

■ *Rifampin:* Reduced therapeutic effect of corticosteroids

■ *Salicylates:* Enhanced elimination of salicylates; subtherapeutic salicylate concentrations possible

Labs

• *False negative:* Skin allergy tests

SPECIAL CONSIDERATIONS
PATIENT/FAMILY EDUCATION

• May cause GI upset; take with meals or snacks

• Take single daily doses in AM

• Increased dose of rapidly acting corticosteroids may be necessary in patients subjected to unusual stress

• Signs of adrenal insufficiency include fatigue, anorexia, nausea, vomiting, diarrhea, weight loss, weakness, dizziness, and low blood sugar

• Avoid abrupt withdrawal of therapy following high-dose or long-term therapy

• May mask infections

• Do not give live virus vaccines to patients on prolonged therapy

• Patients on chronic steroid therapy should wear medical alert bracelet

MONITORING PARAMETERS

• Serum K and glucose

• Edema, blood pressure, CHF, mental status, weight

• Growth in children on prolonged therapy

---

hydroflumethiazide
(hye-droe-flu-me-thye'a-zide)
Rx: Diucardin, Saluron
Combinations
  reserpine (Salutensin, Salutensin-Demi)
Chemical Class: Sulfonamide derivative
Therapeutic Class: Thiazide diuretic; antihypertensive

CLINICAL PHARMACOLOGY

Mechanism of Action: Inhibits reabsorption of sodium and chloride in cortical thick ascending limb of the loop of Henle and the early distal tubules, increasing the urinary excretion of sodium and chloride; sulfonamide moiety provides some carbonic anhydrase inhibition activity; other actions: increased potassium and bicarbonate excretion; decreased calcium excretion; uric acid retention; antihypertensive action dependent on sodium depletion, drop in peripheral vascular resistance, and reduction in extracellular volume

Pharmacokinetics

PO: Onset 2 hr, peak 4 hr, duration 12-24 hr; metabolized and biphasic excreted in the urine; $t_{1/2}$ approximately 17 hr

INDICATIONS AND USES: Edema (CHF, hepatic cirrhosis, corticosteroid and estrogen therapy, nephrotic syndrome, acute glomerulonephritis); hypertension; calcium nephrolithiasis*; prevention of osteoporosis*; diabetes insipidus*

DOSAGE

NOTE: Equivalent hydrochlorothiazide dose: 50 mg-50 mg

Adult

• *Edema:* PO 50 mg qd-bid initially; maintenance 25-200 mg/day; administer in divided doses when dosage >100 mg/day

• *Hypertension:* PO 50 mg bid initially; maintenance 50-100 mg/day, do not exceed 200 mg/day

§ AVAILABLE FORMS/COST OF THERAPY

• Tab, Uncoated—Oral: 50 mg, 100's: **$59.05-$72.94**

CONTRAINDICATIONS: Anuria, renal decompensation

PRECAUTIONS: Fluid and electrolyte imbalance (including sodium, potassium, magnesium, calcium), renal disease, hepatic disease, gout, COPD, lupus erythematosus, diabetes mellitus, hyperparathyroidism, vomiting, diarrhea, elevated cholesterol/triglycerides, tartrazine sensitivity

PREGNANCY AND LACTATION: Pregnancy category C; therapy for preexisting hypertension can be continued throughout pregnancy with minimal risk; initiating for simple edema not recommended; few unequivocal indications for diuretic therapy in pregnancy except for pulmonary edema or congestive heart failure, excreted into breast milk in small amounts; considered compatible with breast feeding

SIDE EFFECTS/ADVERSE REACTIONS

CNS: Depression, *dizziness,* drowsiness, *fatigue,* headache, paresthesia

CV: **Arrhythmias** Orthostatic hypotension, palpitations, volume depletion

EENT: Blurred vision

GI: Anorexia, constipation, cramps, diarrhea, hepatitis, *nausea,* **pancreatitis,** *vomiting*

GU: Frequency, impotence, reduced libido, glucosuria, polyuria, increased creatinine, BUN

HEME: **Agranulocytosis, aplastic anemia, hemolytic anemia, leukopenia, neutropenia, thrombocytopenia**

METAB: Lipid abnormalities (incr total, LDL cholesterol, triglycerides); hypercalcemia, *hyperglycemia, hyperuricemia, hypokalemia,* hypomagnesemia, hyponatremia

SKIN: Photosensitivity, purpura, *rash,* urticaria

INTERACTIONS

Drugs

❷ *Angiotensin-converting enzyme inhibitors:* Risk of postural hypotension when added to ongoing diuretic therapy; more common with loop diuretics; first dose hypotension possible in patients with sodium depletion or hypovolemia due to diuretics or sodium restriction; hypotensive response is usually transient; hold diuretic day of first dose

❸ *Calcium (high dose):* Risk of milk-alkali syndrome. Monitor for hypoglycemia

❸ *Cholestyramine, Colestipol:* Reduced serum concentrations of thiazide diuretics

❸ *Corticosteroids:* Concomitant therapy may result in excessive potassium loss

❸ *Diazoxide:* Hyperglycemia

H

---

italic = common side effects   ***bold italic*** = life-threatening reactions

3 *Digitalis glycosides:* Diuretic-induced hypokalemia may increase the risk of digitalis toxicity

3 *Hypoglycemic agents:* Thiazide diuretics tend to increase blood glucose; may increase dosage requirements of hypoglycemic agents

3 *Lithium:* Increased serum lithium concentrations, toxicity may occur

3 *Methotrexate:* Increased bone marrow suppression

3 *Nonsteroidal antiinflammatory drugs:* Concurrent may reduce diuretic and antihypertensive effects

Labs

• *False decrease:* Urine estriol

SPECIAL CONSIDERATIONS

• Doses above 2.5 mg provide no further blood pressure reduction, but are more likely to induce metabolic disturbance (i.e., hypokalemia, hyperuricemia, etc.)

• May protect against osteoporotic hip fractures

• Loop diuretics or metolazone more effective if CrCl <40-50 ml/min

PATIENT/FAMILY EDUCATION

• Will increase urination temporarily (approximately 3 wk); take early in the day to prevent sleep disturbance

• May cause sensitivity to sunlight; avoid prolonged exposure to the sun and other ultraviolet light

• May cause gout attacks; notify clinician if sudden joint pain occurs

MONITORING PARAMETERS

• Weight, urine output, serum electrolytes, BUN, creatinine, CBC, uric acid, glucose, lipids

hydromorphone

(hye-droe-mor′fone)

Rx: Dilaudid

Chemical Class: Synthetic opium alkaloid; phenanthrene derivative

Therapeutic Class: Narcotic analgesic; antitussive

DEA Class: Schedule II

CLINICAL PHARMACOLOGY

Mechanism of Action: Narcotic agonist with activity at Mu receptors (supraspinal analgesia, euphoria, respiratory and physical depression, miosis, and reduced GI motility), Kappa receptors (pentazocine-like spinal analgesia, sedation, and miosis), and Delta receptors (dysphoria, psychotomimetic effects [e.g., hallucinations], and respiratory and vasomotor stimulation caused by drugs with antagonist activity); compared to morphine, equal analgesia, constipation, respiratory depression, and sedation; less emesis

Pharmacokinetics

PO: Peak 45 min

IM: Onset 15-30 min, peak 0.5-1½ hr, duration 4-5 hr

Metabolized by liver, excreted by kidneys

INDICATIONS AND USES: Moderate to severe pain, non-productive cough

DOSAGE

Adult

• *Pain:* PO/IM/IV/SC 1-4 mg q4-6h prn; PR 3 mg q6-8h

• *Antitussive:* PO 1 mg q3-4h prn

Child

• *Pain:* PO 0.03-0.08 mg/kg/dose q4-6h prn, max 5 mg/dose; IV 0.015 mg/kg/dose q4-6h prn

• *Antitussive:* (6-12 yr) 0.5 mg q3-4h prn

---

* = non-FDA-approved use

$ **AVAILABLE FORMS/COST OF THERAPY**

• Inj, Sol—IM, IV, SC: 1, 2, 4, 10 mg/ml, 1 ml: **$0.95-$4.49**
• Sol—Oral: 1 mg/ml, 480 ml: **$104.03**
• Supp—Rect: 3 mg, 6's: **$23.05**
• Tab, Uncoated—Oral: 2 mg, 100's: **$28.12-$47.44;** 4 mg, 100's: **$45.45-$77.44;** 8 mg, 100's: **$121.98-$140.95**

CONTRAINDICATIONS: Acute bronchial asthma, obstetrical anesthesia (parenteral)

PRECAUTIONS: Head injury, increased intracranial pressure, acute abdominal conditions, elderly, severe impairment of hepatic or renal function, hypothyroidism, Addison's disease, prostatic hypertrophy, urethral stricture, history of drug abuse, hypotension

PREGNANCY AND LACTATION: Pregnancy category C (category D if used for prolonged periods or in high doses at term); use during labor produces neonatal respiratory depression; excretion into breast milk unknown; use caution in nursing mothers

SIDE EFFECTS/ADVERSE REACTIONS

CNS: Agitation, dependency, dizziness, *drowsiness, sedation*
CV: Bradycardia, orthostatic hypotension, palpitations, tachycardia
GI: Anorexia, constipation, nausea, vomiting
GU: Urinary retention
*RESP: **Respiratory depression***
SKIN: Flushing, rash, urticaria
METAB: Transient hyperglycemia

INTERACTIONS
Drugs
3 *Antihistamines, chloral hydrate, glutethimide, methocarbamol:* Enhanced depressant effects
3 *Barbiturates:* Additive respiratory and CNS depressant effects
3 *Cimetidine:* Increased respiratory and CNS depression
3 *Ethanol:* Additive CNS effects
Labs
• *False increase:* Amylase and lipase

SPECIAL CONSIDERATIONS
• Do not administer agonist/antagonist analgesics (i.e., pentazocine, nalbuphine, butorphanol, dezocine, buprenorphine) to patient who has received a prolonged course of hydromorphone (a pure agonist). In opioid-dependent patients, mixed agonist/antagonist analgesics may precipitate withdrawal symptoms.

PATIENT/FAMILY EDUCATION
• Physical dependency may result when used for extended periods
• Avoid hazardous activities if drowsiness or dizziness occurs
• Avoid alcohol, other CNS depressants unless directed by clinician
• Minimize nausea by administering with food and remain lying down following dose

H

---

hydroquinone
(hye-droe-kwin'own)
Rx: Alphaquin HP, Eldopaque-Forte, Eldoquin-Forte, Lustra, Solaquin Forte, Melpaque HP, Melquin HP, Melquin 3, NuQuin HP, Melanex, Viquin Forte
OTC: Esoterica Sensitive Skin Formula, Eldopaque, Solaquin
Chemical Class: Monobenzone derivative
Therapeutic Class: Depigmenting agent

CLINICAL PHARMACOLOGY
Mechanism of Action: Depigments hyperpigmented skin by inhibiting the enzymatic oxidation of tyrosine and suppressing other melanocyte

---

italic = common side effects   ***bold italic*** = life-threatening reactions

metabolic processes, thereby inhibiting melanin formation

INDICATIONS AND USES: Temporary bleaching of hyperpigmented skin conditions (e.g., freckles, senile lentigines, chloasma and melasma, other forms of melanin hyperpigmentation)

DOSAGE

Adult and Child ≥12 yr

• *TOP:* apply to affected skin bid

💲 **AVAILABLE FORMS/COST OF THERAPY**

• Cre—Top: 1.5%, 90 g: **$5.44** (OTC)
• Cre—Top: 2%, 30 g: **$22.26** (OTC)
• Cre—Top: 4%, 15, 30, 60 g: **$29.00-$41.45/30 g**
• Gel—Top: 4%, 15, 30, 60 g: **$29.00-$35.94//30 g**
• Sol—Top: 3%, 30 ml: **$10.30-$13.13**

PRECAUTIONS: Sulfite sensitivity

PREGNANCY AND LACTATION: Pregnancy category C; degree of systemic absorption unknown; excretion into breast milk unknown

SIDE EFFECTS/ADVERSE REACTIONS

SKIN: Contact dermatitis, dryness and fissuring of paranasal and infraorbital areas, erythema, irritation, sensitization, stinging

INTERACTIONS

Labs

• *False decrease:* Urine glucose

SPECIAL CONSIDERATIONS

PATIENT/FAMILY EDUCATION

• Apply small amount to an unbroken patch of skin and check in 24 hr; if vesicle formation, itching, or excessive inflammation occurs, further treatment not advised
• Positive response may require 3 wk to 6 mo
• Protect the treated area from UV light by using a sunscreen, sun block, or protective clothing

• Avoid application to lips or near eyes

---

hydroxocobalamin (vitamin B$_{12}$)

(hye-drox'oh-co-bal'a-min)

Rx: Hydroxy-Cobal, LA-12

Chemical Class: B complex vitamin

Therapeutic Class: Vitamin supplement; blood modifier; nitroprusside antidote

---

CLINICAL PHARMACOLOGY

Mechanism of Action: Physiologic role is associated with methylation, participating in nucleic acid and protein synthesis; participates in red blood cell formation through activation of folic acid coenzymes

Pharmacokinetics

IM: Slowly absorbed from inj site; distributed into liver, bone marrow, and other tissue; available for urinary excretion when administered parenterally in doses that exceed binding capacity of plasma, liver, and other tissues

INDICATIONS AND USES: Vitamin B$_{12}$ deficiency (pernicious anemia, GI pathology, fish tapeworm infestation, malignancy of pancreas or bowel, gluten enteropathy, sprue, gastrectomy); increased vitamin B$_{12}$ requirement (pregnancy, thyrotoxicosis, hemolytic anemia, hemorrhage, malignancy, hepatic or renal disease); Schilling test for vitamin B$_{12}$ absorption; cyanide toxicity associated with sodium nitroprusside*

DOSAGE

Adult

• IM 30-100 µg/day for 5-10 days, followed by 100 µg q mo

Child

• IM 1-5 mg over 2 or more wk in

---

* = non-FDA-approved use

doses of 100 µg, then 30-100 µg q mo for maintenance

💰 AVAILABLE FORMS/COST OF THERAPY

• Inj, Sol—IM: 1000 µg/ml, 30 ml: **$9.75-$11.85**

CONTRAINDICATIONS: Hypersensitivity to cobalt

PRECAUTIONS: IV route, infection, uremia, concurrent iron or folic acid deficiency, severe megaloblastic anemia, hypokalemia

PREGNANCY AND LACTATION: Pregnancy category A (C if dose exceeds recommended daily allowance); vitamin B_{12} is an essential vitamin and needs are increased during pregnancy; excreted into breast milk; 2.6 µg/day should be consumed during pregnancy and lactation

SIDE EFFECTS/ADVERSE REACTIONS

CV: **CHF,** peripheral vascular thrombosis
GI: Diarrhea
METAB: Hypokalemia
SKIN: Pain at inj site

INTERACTIONS
Labs
• *False positive:* Intrinsic factor
• *Interference:* Methotrexate, pyrimethamine and most antibiotics interfere with vitamin B_{12} assay

SPECIAL CONSIDERATIONS
PATIENT/FAMILY EDUCATION
• Therapy may require life-long monthly injections

MONITORING PARAMETERS
• Serum potassium for 1st 48 hr during treatment of severe megaloblastic anemia
• Reticulocyte counts, Hct, vitamin B_{12}, iron, and folic acid plasma levels prior to treatment, between days 5 and 7 of treatment, then frequently until Hct is normal

hydroxychloroquine
(hye-drox-ee-klor'oh-kwin)
Rx: Plaquenil, Quineprox
Chemical Class: 4-aminoquinoline derivative
Therapeutic Class: Antimalarial; disease-modifying antirheumatic drug (DMARD)

CLINICAL PHARMACOLOGY
Mechanism of Action: Antimalarial: Inhibits DNA/RNA synthesis (mammalian and protozoal cells); within parasite: raises pH of organelles causing interference with utilization of host erythrocyte hemoglobin; interference with phospholipid metabolism
Inflammation: Suppress responsiveness of T cells to mitogens; decreases leukocyte chemotaxis; stabilizes lysosomal membranes; inhibits DNA/RNA synthesis; traps free radicals

Pharmacokinetics
PO: Rapidly and completely absorbed, peak 1-6 hr; protein-binding 55%; partially metabolized, slowly excreted by kidneys (parent drug and metabolites)

INDICATIONS AND USES: Prophylaxis and treatment of acute attacks of malaria due to *Plasmodium vivax, P. malariae, P. ovale,* and susceptible strains of *P. falciparum;* discoid and systemic lupus erythematosus; rheumatoid arthritis, juvenile rheumatoid arthritis,* sarcoid associated hypercalcemia,* polymorphous light eruption,* prophyria cutanea tarda,* urticaria solar,* chronic cutaneous vasculitis*

DOSAGE
NOTE: hydroxychloroquine sulfate 200 mg = 155 mg hydroxychloroquine base
Adult
• *Prophylaxis of malaria:* PO 400

mg q wk on same day each wk; begin 1-2 wk before exposure, continue 6-8 wk after leaving endemic area

• *Acute malaria attack:* PO 800 mg initial dose, followed by 400 mg in 6 hr on day 1, then 400 mg as single dose on days 2 and 3

• *Rheumatoid arthritis:* PO 400-600 mg qd initially, increase dose until optimal response achieved (usually 4-12 wk); maintenance dose 200-400 mg qd

• *Lupus erythematosus:* PO 400 mg qd-bid for several wk depending on response; maintenance 200-400 mg/day

Child

• *Prophylaxis of malaria:* PO 5 mg/kg (base) q wk on same day each wk; begin 1-2 wk before exposure, continue 6-8 wk after leaving endemic area; do not exceed recommended adult dose

• *Acute malaria attack:* PO 10 mg/kg (base) initial dose, followed by 5 mg/kg (base) in 6 hr on day 1, then 5 mg/kg (base) as a single dose on days 2 and 3

• *Juvenile rheumatoid arthritis/ lupus erythematosus:* PO 3-5 mg/ kg/day divided 1-2 times/day, max 400 mg/day

$ AVAILABLE FORMS/COST OF THERAPY

• Tab, Uncoated—Oral: 200 mg, 100's: **$100.00-$141.05**

CONTRAINDICATIONS: Retinal or visual field changes, children (long-term therapy)

PRECAUTIONS: Psoriasis, porphyria, children (NOTE: Children especially sensitive to the effects of the 4-aminoquinolones), hepatic function impairment, G-6-PD deficiency, alcoholism

PREGNANCY AND LACTATION: Pregnancy category C; excreted in breast milk; safe use during nursing has not been established

SIDE EFFECTS/ADVERSE REACTIONS

CNS: Headache, neuropathy, psychic stimulation, psychosis, *seizures*

CV: ECG changes (inversion or depression of T-wave, widening of QRS complex), hypotension

*EENT: **Irreversible retinal damage*** (prolonged high doses), nerve-type deafness (prolonged high doses), nyctalopia, reduced hearing, scotomatous vision, tinnitus, visual disturbances

GI: Abdominal cramps, *anorexia,* diarrhea, *nausea, vomiting*

*HEME: **Agranulocytosis, blood dyscrasias, hemolytic anemia***

MS: Muscular weakness

SKIN: Lichen planus-like eruptions, pleomorphic skin eruptions (prolonged therapy), pruritus, skin and mucosal pigmentary changes

INTERACTIONS

Drugs

3 *Digitalis glycosides:* Increased serum digoxin concentrations

3 *Praziquantel:* Reduced praziquantel concentration

SPECIAL CONSIDERATIONS
PATIENT/FAMILY EDUCATION

• Report any muscle weakness, visual disturbances, difficulty hearing, or ringing in ears to clinician

MONITORING PARAMETERS

• Baseline and periodic ophthalmologic examinations (visual acuity, slit lamp, funduscopic, and visual field tests); periodic tests of knee and ankle reflexes to detect muscular weakness

• Periodic CBCs during prolonged therapy

hydroxyprogesterone
(hye-drox-ee-proe-jess'te-rone)
Rx: Hylutin, Prodrox
Chemical Class: Progestin derivative
Therapeutic Class: Progestin; antineoplastic

CLINICAL PHARMACOLOGY
Mechanism of Action: Exerts a progestational effect on the endometrium, alters cervical mucus, suppresses evaluation in some patients
Pharmacokinetics
IM: Duration 9-17 days; metabolized primarily in the liver, excreted by the kidney
INDICATIONS AND USES: Amenorrhea (primary and secondary), dysfunctional uterine bleeding, metrorrhagia, metastatic endometrial carcinoma (palliative therapy)
DOSAGE
Adult
• *Amenorrhea and uterine bleeding:* IM 375 mg, repeated q4 wk prn
• *Endometrial carcinoma:* IM 1-7 g/wk
$ AVAILABLE FORMS/COST OF THERAPY
• Inj, Sol—IM: 250 mg/ml, 5 ml: **$13.50-$24.95**
CONTRAINDICATIONS: Active thromboembolic disorders or thrombophlebitis, cerebral hemorrhage, impaired liver function or disease, breast cancer, undiagnosed vaginal bleeding, missed abortion, use as a diagnostic test for pregnancy
PRECAUTIONS: Epilepsy, migraine, asthma, cardiac or renal dysfunction, depression, diabetes
PREGNANCY AND LACTATION: Pregnancy category D; an increased risk of hypospadias in the male fetus and mild virilization of the female fetus have been reported with progestin use; progestins compatible with breast feeding
SIDE EFFECTS/ADVERSE REACTIONS
CNS: Depression, dizziness, fatigue, headache
CV: Edema
GI: Anorexia, *cholestatic jaundice,* increased weight, *nausea,* vomiting
GU: Amenorrhea, breakthrough bleeding, breast changes, dysmenorrhea, *gynecomastia*
METAB: Hyperglycemia
SKIN: Acne, alopecia, hirsutism, melasma, rash
INTERACTIONS
Drugs
3 *Aminoglutethimide:* Decreases progestin concentration
SPECIAL CONSIDERATIONS
PATIENT/FAMILY EDUCATION
• Take protective measures against exposure to UV light or sunlight

hydroxyzine
(hye-drox'i-zeen)
Rx: Atarax, Vistaril, Vistazine
Chemical Class: Piperazine derivative
Therapeutic Class: Antihistamine; sedative/hypnotic; anxiolytic; antiemetic (parenteral)

CLINICAL PHARMACOLOGY
Mechanism of Action: Antianxiety: depresses subcortical levels of CNS; other: primary skeletal muscle relaxation, bronchodilator activity, antihistaminic and analgesic effects, antispasmodic and antiemetic effects
Pharmacokinetics
Onset 15-30 min, duration 4-6 hr, $t_{1/2}$ 3 hr

INDICATIONS AND USES: Anxiety, nausea, vomiting, to potentiate narcotic analgesics; sedation; pruritus

DOSAGE

Adult

• PO 10-100 mg q4-6h; IM 25-100 mg q4-6h

Child

• PO (>6 yr) 50-100 mg/day in divided doses; PO (<6 yr) 50 mg/day in divided doses; IM 1.1 mg/kg q4-6h

§ AVAILABLE FORMS/COST OF THERAPY

• Inj—IM: 25 mg/ml, 10 ml: **$3.00;** 50 mg/ml, 10 ml: **$2.59-$18.73**

• Cap—Oral: 25 mg, 100's: **$7.95-$93.25;** 50 mg, 100's: **$11.25-$113.66;** 100 mg, 100's: **$18.95-$139.66**

• Tab—Oral: 10 mg, 100's: **$5.25-$63.58;** 25 mg, 100's: **$6.95-$93.25;** 50 mg, 100's: **$8.75-$113.66;** 100 mg, 100's: **$22.50-$139.66**

• Sus—Oral: 25 mg/5 ml, 120 ml: **$28.00-$35.57**

• Syr—Oral: 10 mg/5 ml, 120 ml: **$4.64-$13.01**

PRECAUTIONS: Elderly, debilitated, hepatic disease, renal disease, pregnancy, IM only (avoid IV, SC, or intraarterial administration)

PREGNANCY AND LACTATION: Pregnancy category C (but no excess in birth defects documented); safe during labor for relief of anxiety; no data on breast feeding

SIDE EFFECTS/ADVERSE REACTIONS

CNS: Confusion, depression, dizziness, *drowsiness,* fatigue, headache, *seizures,* tremor

GI: Dry mouth

GU: Urinary retention

Labs

• *False increase:* Urine 17-hydroxycorticosteroids and 17-ketogenic steroids

---

hyoscyamine

(hye-oh-sye'a-meen)

Rx: A-Spas S/L, Anaspaz, Cystospaz, Cystospaz-M, Donnamar, ED-SPAZ, Gastrosed, Hyco Drops, Hyosol/SL, Hyospaz, Levbid, Levsin, Levsin/SL, Levsinex, Liqui-Sooth, Medispaz, Spacol, Spasdel, Symax-SL, Symax-SR

Combinations

Rx: with phenobarbital (Levsin PB)

Chemical Class: Belladonna alkaloid

Therapeutic Class: Anticholinergic, gastrointestinal

CLINICAL PHARMACOLOGY

Mechanism of Action: Inhibits muscarinic actions of acetylcholine at postganglionic parasympathetic neuroeffector sites

Pharmacokinetics

PO: Duration 4-6 hr; metabolized by liver, excreted in urine; $t_{1/2}$ 3.5 hr

INDICATIONS AND USES: Irritable bowel syndrome, biliary colic, hypermotility in cystitis, adjunctive treatment of peptic ulcer disease, renal colic, sinus bradycardia (parenteral), acute rhinitis; sialorrhea*; hyperhidrosis*

DOSAGE

Adult

• PO/SL 0.125-0.25 mg tid-qid ac, hs; TIME REL 0.375 mg q12h; IM/SC/IV 0.25-0.5 mg q6h

Child

• 2-12 yr ¼ – ½ adult dose; <2 yr ⅛ – ¼ adult dose

§ AVAILABLE FORMS/COST OF THERAPY

• Cap, Gel, SUS Action—Oral: 0.375 mg, 100's: **$44.06-$88.56**

• Tab, Uncoated—SL: 0.125 mg, 100's: **$13.66-$51.70**

---

* = non-FDA-approved use

• Tab—Oral: 0.125 mg, 100's: **$11.25-$46.10;** 0.15 mg, 100's: **$21.25-$43.13**
• Tab, SUS Action—Oral: 0.375 mg, 100's: **$39.95-$78.74**
• Elixir—Oral: 0.125 mg/5 ml, 480 ml: **$20.00-$61.11**
• Sol—Oral: 0.125 mg/ml, 15, 120 ml: **$9.70-$23.61**
• Inj, Sol—IM, IV, SC: 0.5 mg/ml, 1 ml: **$10.67**

CONTRAINDICATIONS: Narrow-angle glaucoma, GI obstruction, myasthenia gravis, paralytic ileus, GI atony, toxic megacolon, prostatic hypertrophy

PRECAUTIONS: Hyperthyroidism, CAD, dysrhythmias, CHF, ulcerative colitis, hypertension, hiatal hernia, hepatic disease, renal disease, urinary retention

PREGNANCY AND LACTATION: Pregnancy category C; excreted in breast milk; infants sensitive to anticholinergics

SIDE EFFECTS/ADVERSE REACTIONS

CNS: Anxiety, *confusion,* dizziness, drowsiness, hallucination, headache, insomnia, *stimulation in elderly,* weakness
CV: Palpitations, tachycardia
EENT: Blurred vision, cycloplegia, increased intraocular pressure, mydriasis, photophobia
GI: Absence of taste, *constipation, dry mouth,* dysphagia, heartburn, ileus, nausea, vomiting
GU: Hesitancy, impotence, *retention*
SKIN: Anhidrosis, fever, pruritus, rash, urticaria

ibuprofen
(eye-byoo'pro-fen)
Rx: Motrin, Ibuprohm, IBU, Rufen, Saleto
OTC: Arthritis Foundation Pain Reliever, Advil, Ibuprin, Motrin IB, Nuprin
Combinations
  Rx: with Hydrocodone (Vicoprofen)
  OTC: With pseudoephedrine (Sine-Aid IB, Motrin IB Sinus)
Chemical Class: Propionic acid derivative
Therapeutic Class: NSAID with analgesic and antipyretic activity

CLINICAL PHARMACOLOGY
Mechanism of Action: Reversible cyclooxygenase (i.e., prostaglandin synthetase) inhibitor; nonselectively decreases the formation of both prostaglandins and thromboxane A2; variable effects on lipoxygenase synthesis and subsequent leukotriene production; antiinflammatory, antipyretic, and analgesic activity; inhibits platelet aggregation
Pharmacokinetics
PO: Onset ½ hour, peak 1-2 hr, $t_{1/2}$ 2-4 hr; metabolized in liver (inactive metabolites), excreted in urine (inactive metabolites) within 24 hr; does not enter breast milk; food decreases rate but not extent of absorption
INDICATIONS AND USES: Rheumatoid arthritis, osteoarthritis, primary dysmenorrhea, gout,* pain, fever, tocolysis in preterm labor*; prevention of cognitive decline,* colon cancer,* cystic fibrosis,* headache*
DOSAGE
Adult
• PO 200-800 mg qid, not to exceed

italic = common side effects   ***bold italic*** = life-threatening reactions

3200 mg/day (NOTE: Doses <1600 mg/day analgesic only; >1600 mg/day needed for antiinflammatory activity)

Child

• PO 20-40 mg/kg/day divided tid or qid

💲 AVAILABLE FORMS/COST OF THERAPY

• Cap—Oral: 200 mg 50's: **$2.19**
• Tab, Chewable—Oral: 50 mg, 24's: **$2.95;** 100 mg, 100's: **$25.33**
• Tab—Oral: 200 mg, 100's: **$1.60-$19.10;** 400 mg, 100's: **$3.95-$41.00;** 600 mg, 100's: **$4.45-$44.14;** 800 mg, 100's: **$7.13-$45.34**
• Susp—Oral: 100 mg/5 ml, 120 ml: **$3.38-$8.16;** 50 mg/1.5 mL 15 mL **$4.12-$4.97**

CONTRAINDICATIONS: Hypersensitivity to NSAIDs (including symptoms of asthma, nasal polyps, angioedema)

PRECAUTIONS: History of GI ulceration, bleeding, or perforation; renal dysfunction, hypertension or cardiac conditions aggravated by fluid retention and edema, history of liver dysfunction, history of coagulation

PREGNANCY AND LACTATION: Pregnancy category B; reduces amniotic fluid volume, constriction of the ductus arteriosus in 3rd trimester; compatible with breast feeding

SIDE EFFECTS/ADVERSE REACTIONS

CNS: Anxiety, confusion, depression, *dizziness,* drowsiness, fatigue, insomnia, tremors

CV: **CHF,** dysrhythmias, hypertension, palpitations, peripheral edema, tachycardia

EENT: Blurred vision, hearing loss, tinnitus

GI: Anorexia, cholestatic hepatitis, constipation, cramps, diarrhea, dry mouth, flatulence, *GI bleeding,* jaundice, nausea, peptic ulcer, vomiting

GU: Azotemia, hematuria, ***nephrotoxicity,*** oliguria

HEME: **Blood dyscrasias,** increased bleeding time

SKIN: Pruritus, purpura, rash, sweating

INTERACTIONS

Drugs

🔳 *Aminoglycosides:* Reduced clearance with elevated aminoglycoside levels and potential for toxicity (especially indomethacin in premature infants; other NSAIDs probably)

🔳 *Anticoagulants:* Excessive hypoprothrombinemia, decreased platelet aggregation with increased risk of GI bleeding

🔳 *Antihypertensives (α-blockers, angiotensin-converting enzyme inhibitors, angiotensin II receptor blockers, β-blockers, diuretics):* Inhibition of antihypertensive and other favorable hemodynamic effects

🔳 *Corticosteroids:* Increased risk of GI ulceration

🔳 *Cyclosporine:* Increased nephrotoxicity risk

🔳 *Lithium:* Decreased clearance of lithium (mediated via prostaglandins) resulting in elevated serum lithium levels and risk of toxicity

🔳 *Methotrexate:* Decreased renal secretion of methotrexate resulting in elevated methotrexate levels and risk of toxicity

🔳 *Phenylpropanolamine:* Possible acute hypertensive reaction

🔳 *Potassium-sparing diuretics:* Additive hyperkalemia potential

🔳 *Triamterene:* Acute renal failure reported with addition of indomethacin; caution with other NSAIDs

Labs

• *False decrease:* ALT, AST

SPECIAL CONSIDERATIONS
• Administer with food or antacids if GI symptoms occur

MONITORING PARAMETERS
• Initial hemogram and fecal occult blood test within 3 mo of starting regular chronic therapy; repeat every 6-12 mo (more frequently in high-risk patients, >65 years, peptic ulcer disease, concurrent steroids or anticoagulants); electrolytes, creatinine, and BUN within 3 mo of starting regular chronic therapy; repeat every 6-12 mo

---

ibutilide
(eye-byoo'ti-lide)
Rx: Corvert
Chemical Class: Methanesulfonamide derivative
Therapeutic Class: Antidysrhythmic (Class III)

CLINICAL PHARMACOLOGY
Mechanism of Action: Delays repolarization by activation of a slow, inward current (predominantly sodium); prolongs atrial and ventricular action potential duration and refractoriness; produces mild slowing of the sinus rate and AV conduction; produces dose-related prolongation of QT interval

Pharmacokinetics
IV: 40% bound to plasma proteins; metabolized to 8 metabolites (1 active), excreted in urine (~80%) and feces (~19%); $t_{1/2}$ 6 hr

INDICATIONS AND USES: Rapid conversion of atrial fibrillation or atrial flutter of recent onset to sinus rhythm (atrial arrhythmias of longer duration less likely to respond)

DOSAGE
Adult
• IV (≥60 kg) 1 mg (1 vial) infused over 10 min; (<60 kg) 0.01 mg/kg (0.1 ml/kg); if arrhythmia does not terminate within 10 min after end of initial infusion, a 2nd 10 min infusion of equal strength may be administered

$ **AVAILABLE FORMS/COST OF THERAPY**
• Sol—IV: 0.1 mg/ml, 10 ml: **$206.86**

PRECAUTIONS: Heart block; can worsen or induce ventricular dysrhythmias (including torsades de pointes)

PREGNANCY AND LACTATION: Pregnancy category C

SIDE EFFECTS/ADVERSE REACTIONS
CNS: Headache
CV: Bradycardia, bundle branch block, ***CHF,*** hypertension, hypotension, palpitation, postural hypotension, QT segment prolongation, syncope, tachycardia, ***ventricular dysrhythmias***
GI: Nausea

INTERACTIONS
Drugs
3 *Disopyramide, quinidine, procainamide, amiodarone, sotalol:* Potential to prolong refractoriness
2 *Phenothiazines, tricyclic antidepressants, terfenadine, astemizole:* Increased potential for prodysrhythmia due to prolongation of QT interval

SPECIAL CONSIDERATIONS
MONITORING PARAMETERS
• Continuous ECG monitoring for at least 4 hr following infusion or until QTc returns to baseline (longer monitoring if dysrhythmic activity noted). Defibrillator must be available

---

italic = common side effects **bold italic** = life-threatening reactions

idoxuridine (IDU)
(eye-dox-your'ih-deen)
Rx: Herplex
Chemical Class: Pyrimidine nucleoside
Therapeutic Class: Ophthalmic antiviral

CLINICAL PHARMACOLOGY
Mechanism of Action: Inhibits viral replication by interfering with viral DNA synthesis
Pharmacokinetics
Deactivated by deaminases and nucleotidases, penetrates cornea poorly

INDICATIONS AND USES: Herpes simplex keratitis, CMV, and varicella zoster keratitis*

DOSAGE
Adult and Child
• INSTILL 1 gtt q1h during day and q2h during night

💲 AVAILABLE FORMS/COST OF THERAPY
• Sol, Ophth—Top: 0.1%, 15 ml: **$13.21**

PRECAUTIONS: Sensitivity to iodine

PREGNANCY AND LACTATION: Pregnancy category C; crosses placenta, teratogenic in rabbits and mice; no data available for breast feeding but shown to have tumorgenicity in animal studies

SIDE EFFECTS/ADVERSE REACTIONS
EENT: Overgrowth of non-susceptible organisms, photosensitivity, poor corneal wound healing, temporary visual haze

DRUG INTERACTIONS
❷ *Boric acid:* Precipitate formation

PATIENT/FAMILY EDUCATION
• Wearing sunglasses decreases sensitivity to bright light. Notify clinician if no improvement in 14 days

imipenem-cilastin
(i-me-pen'em)
Rx: Primaxin
Chemical Class: Thienamycin antibiotic; renal dipeptidase inhibitor
Therapeutic Class: Antibiotic

CLINICAL PHARMACOLOGY
Mechanism of Action: Inhibits bacterial wall synthesis, results in cell lysis; formulated with cilastin, which prevents renal metabolism of imipenem; bactericidal
Pharmacokinetics
IV: Onset immediate, peak ½-1 hr, $t_{1/2}$ 1 hr
IM: Peak 2 hr, $t_{1/2}$ 6-8 hr
Excreted by kidney (75%) and unknown non-renal mechanism (25%); rapidly cleared by hemodialysis; $t_{1/2}$ longer in children (2 hr in neonates, 1.2 hr in older children)

INDICATIONS AND USES: Serious infections of the lower respiratory tract, urinary tract, skin; intra-abdominal infections, gynecologic infections, septicemia, endocarditis
Antibacterial spectrum usually includes:
Gram-positive organisms: *Streptococcus pneumoniae,* group A β-hemolytic streptococci, *Staphylococcus aureus,* enterococci
Gram-negative organisms: *Acinetobacter, Citrobacter, Enterobacter, E. Coli, Hemophilus, Klebsiella, Proteus, Pseudomonas aeruginosa, Salmonella, Serratia, Shigella*
• *Anaerobes: Bacteroides* including *B. fragilis, Peptococcus, Peptostreptococcus*

DOSAGE
Adult
• IV 250-500 mg q6h; severe in-

fections may require 1 g q6h; max 50 mg/kg/day or 4 g/day (whichever is lower)

• IM 500 or 750 mg q12h to max 1500 mg qd

• *Dosage adjustment in impaired renal function:* CrCl 40-70 ml/sec, 250-500 mg q6-8h; CrCl 20-40 ml/sec, 250 mg q6-8h-500 mg q8h; CrCl 6-20 ml/sec, 250-500 mg q12h

• *Hemodialysis patients:* Supplemental dose after hemodialysis, unless scheduled dose within 4 hr

Child

• IV >40 kg, adult dose

• IV <40 kg, 60 mg/kg/day in divided doses

§ AVAILABLE FORMS/COST OF THERAPY

• Inj, Dry-Sol—IV: 250 mg: **$15.89;** 500 mg: **$30.32**

• Inj, Dry-Sol—IM: 500 mg: **$28.80;** 750 mg: **$43.20**

CONTRAINDICATIONS: IM: hypersensitivity to local anesthetics of the amide type (contains lidocaine)

PRECAUTIONS: Elderly, hypersensitivity to penicillins, seizure disorders, renal disease, children <12 yr

PREGNANCY AND LACTATION: Pregnancy category C; unknown if excreted in breast milk

SIDE EFFECTS/ADVERSE REACTIONS

CNS: Dizziness, fever, myoclonus, **seizures,** somnolence, weakness

CV: Hypotension, palpitations

GI: Diarrhea, glossitis, hepatitis, nausea, **pseudomembranous colitis,** vomiting

GU: Proteinuria, increased BUN/creatinine

HEME: Eosinophilia, **neutropenia**

RESP: Chest discomfort, dyspnea, hyperventilation

SKIN: Erythema at inj site, pain at inj site, phlebitis, pruritus, rash, urticaria

INTERACTIONS

Drugs

🔳 *Cyclosporine, tacrolimus:* Risk of CNS toxicity

🔳 *Theophylline:* Increased seizure risk without elevated theophylline levels

Labs

• *Interference:* Clindamycin, erythromycin, metronidazole, polymyxin, tetracycline, trimethoprim colistin levels

---

imipramine
(im-ip'ra-meen)

Rx: Tofranil, Tofranil PM

Chemical Class: Dibenzazepine derivative; tertiary amine, tertiary amine dibenzazepine derivative

Therapeutic Class: Tricyclic antidepressant; antiincontinence agent

---

CLINICAL PHARMACOLOGY

Mechanism of Action: Inhibits reuptake of norepinephrine and serotonin (blocking activity moderate and very high, respectively) at the presynaptic neuron, prolonging neuronal activity; inhibits histamine and acetylcholine activity; mild peripheral vasodilator effects and possible quinidine-like action on cardiac conduction; moderate anticholinergic and sedative, high orthostatic hypotensive side effects

Pharmacokinetics

PO: Steady state 2-5 days; metabolized by liver, excreted in urine, feces; crosses placenta; excreted in breast milk; $t_{1/2}$ 6-20 hr

INDICATIONS AND USES: Depression, enuresis in children, headache*

DOSAGE

Adult

• PO/IM 75-100 mg/day in divided doses, may increase by 25-50 mg to

---

italic = common side effects   ***bold italic*** = life-threatening reactions

200 mg, not to exceed 300 mg/day; may give daily dose hs

Child

• *Depression: PO:* 1.5 mg/kg/d, increasing by 1-1.5 mg/kg/d q 3-5 days to maximum 5 mg/kg/d

• *Eneuresis:* (≥5 yrs): *PO:* 25 mg qhs, increase to 50 mg in 1 wk Maximum dose 2.5 mg/kg/d or 75 mg

§ AVAILABLE FORMS/COST OF THERAPY

• Tab, Sugar Coated—Oral: 10 mg, 100's: **$3.25-$32.88;** 25 mg, 100's: **$4.50-$54.94;** 50 mg, 100's: **$4.14-$93.30**

• Inj—IM: 25 mg/2 ml: **$2.25**

• Cap, Gel—Oral (pamoate): 75 mg, 100's: **$130.46;** 100 mg, 100's: **$171.56;** 125 mg, 100's: **$213.94;** 150 mg, 100's: **$243.81**

CONTRAINDICATIONS: Hypersensitivity to tricyclic antidepressants, recovery phase of MI, convulsive disorders, prostatic hypertrophy

PRECAUTIONS: Suicidal patients, severe depression, increased intraocular pressure, narrow-angle glaucoma, urinary retention, cardiac disease, hepatic disease, hyperthyroidism, electroshock therapy, elective surgery, elderly

PREGNANCY AND LACTATION: Pregnancy category C

SIDE EFFECTS/ADVERSE REACTIONS

CNS: Anxiety, confusion, *dizziness, drowsiness,* EPS (elderly), headache, increased psychiatric symptoms, insomnia, nightmares, paresthesia, stimulation, tremors, weakness

CV: ECG changes, hypertension, *orthostatic hypotension,* palpitations, *tachycardia*

EENT: Blurred vision, mydriasis, tinnitus

GI: Cramps, *diarrhea, dry mouth,* epigastric distress, hepatitis, increased appetite, jaundice, nausea, paralytic ileus, stomatitis, vomiting

GU: Acute renal failure, impotence, *retention*

HEME: Bone marrow depression, eosinophilia

METAB: Hyperprolactinemia

SKIN: Photosensitivity, pruritus, rash, sweating, urticaria

INTERACTIONS

Drugs

3 *Altretamine:* Orthostatic hypotension

3 *Amphetamines:* Theoretical increase in amphetamine effect

3 *Antidiabetics:* Possible enhanced hypoglycemic effects

2 *Bethanidine, clonidine:* Inhibition of antihypertensive effect, possible hypertensive crisis

3 *Carbamazepine, cholestyramine, colestipol, barbiturates:* Reduces imipramine levels

2 *Epinephrine, norepinephrine:* Hypertension and dysrhythmias

3 *Ethanol:* Enhanced motor skill impairment

3 *Guanethidine, guanfacine:* Inhibition of antihypertensive effect

3 *Isoproterenol and possibly other* β-*agonists:* Increased risk of arrhythmias

3 *Lithium:* Possible increased CNS toxicity, especially in elderly

A *MAOIs:* Serotonin syndrome, some fatal

2 *Moclobemide:* Risk serotonin syndrome

3 *Phenothiazines, cimetidine,* calcium channel blockers, selective serotonin reuptake inhibitors, quinidine, ritonavir, indinavir* (not other H₂-blockers):* Increased imipramine levels

3 *Phenylephrine:* Enhanced pressor response

3 *Propantheline:* Excessive anticholinergic effects

Labs
• *False increase:* Carbamazepine levels
• *False decrease:* Urine 5-HIAA, VMA

SPECIAL CONSIDERATIONS
PATIENT/FAMILY EDUCATION
• Withdrawal symptoms (headache, nausea, vomiting, muscle pain, weakness) may occur if drug discontinued abruptly
• At doses of 20 mg/kg ventricular arrhythmias occur

---

imiquimod
(im-ick'wih-mod)
Rx: Aldara
Chemical Class: Immune response modifier
Therapeutic Class: Antiviral

CLINICAL PHARMACOLOGY
Mechanism of Action: Unknown, but may involve the induction of cytokines, including interferon-α and others
Pharmacokinetics
TOP: Minimal systemic absorption; <0.9% of dose excreted in urine and feces

INDICATIONS AND USES: External genital and perianal warts (condyloma acuminata)

DOSAGE
Adult
• TOP apply to warts 3 times weekly prior to normal sleeping hours; leave on for 6-10 hr then wash off with mild soap and water; continue until warts are completely cleared or 16 wk, whichever comes first

§ AVAILABLE FORMS/COST OF THERAPY
• Cre—Topical: 5%, 250 mg/single-use packet, 12's: **$116.64**

PRECAUTIONS: Urethral, intra-

vaginal, cervical, rectal, or intra-anal warts; children <18 yr

PREGNANCY AND LACTATION: Pregnancy category B; excretion into breast milk unknown but would be expected to be small given minimal systemic absorption

SIDE EFFECTS/ADVERSE REACTIONS
CNS: Headache
MS: Myalgia
SKIN: Itching, erythema, erosion, burning, excoriation, flaking, edema, local pain, induration, ulceration, scabbing, vesicles, soreness
MISC: Flu-like symptoms

SPECIAL CONSIDERATIONS
• New option for treatment of genital and perianal warts which can be applied by patient at home and appears to have low toxicity compared to podofilox
• Response rates approximately 50% and relapses are common

PATIENT/FAMILY EDUCATION
• Apply thin layer to wart(s) and rub in until cream is no longer visible
• Do not occlude application site
• Should severe local reaction occur, remove cream by washing with soap and water; treatment may be resumed once skin reaction has subsided

---

indapamide
(in-dap'a-mide)
Rx: Lozol
Chemical Class: Indoline derivative
Therapeutic Class: Thiazide-like diuretic; antihypertensive

CLINICAL PHARMACOLOGY
Mechanism of Action: Structural and pharmacological similarities to thiazide diuretics; inhibits reabsorption of sodium and chloride in cor-

---

italic = common side effects   ***bold italic*** = life-threatening reactions

tical thick ascending limb of the loop of Henle and the early distal tubules—minimal effect on glomerular filtration rate or renal plasma flow, unlike other thiazide diuretics; decreases peripheral resistance (perhaps via calcium channel blockade) with little or no effect on cardiac output, rate or rhythm. Antihypertensive effects decrease in patients with decreasing renal function; less effect on electrolyte excretion

Pharmacokinetics

PO: Onset 1-2 hr, peak 2 hr, duration up to 36 hr; excreted in urine, feces; $t_{1/2}$ 14-18 hr

INDICATIONS AND USES: Edema (CHF, cirrhosis, corticosteroid and estrogen therapy); hypercalciuria; hypertension, Raynaud's disease*

DOSAGE

Adult

• PO 2.5-5 mg qd in AM NOTE: Equivalent hydrochlorothiazide dose: 2.5 mg-50 mg

💲 **AVAILABLE FORMS/COST OF THERAPY**

• Tab, Plain Coated—Oral: 1.25 mg, 100's: **$59.18-$88.25;** 2.5 mg, 100's: **$65.97-$109.16**

CONTRAINDICATIONS: Renal decompensation; anuria

PRECAUTIONS: Fluid and electrolyte imbalance (including sodium, potassium, chloride, magnesium, calcium), renal disease, hepatic disease, gout, COPD, lupus erythematosus, diabetes mellitus, hyperparathyroidism, vomiting, diarrhea

PREGNANCY AND LACTATION: Pregnancy category B; therapy for preexisting hypertension can be continued throughout pregnancy with minimal risk; initiating for edema not recommended; few unequivocal indications for diuretic therapy in pregnancy except for pulmonary edema or congestive heart failure; not known if excreted in breast milk

SIDE EFFECTS/ADVERSE REACTIONS

CNS: Vertigo, *dizziness,* fatigue, *headache,* paresthesias, *weakness*
CV: Dysrhythmias, orthostatic hypotension, palpitations
EENT: Blurred vision, increased intraocular pressure, loss of hearing, nasal congestion, tinnitus
GI: Abdominal pain, anorexia, constipation, cramps, diarrhea, dry mouth, hepatitis, jaundice, *nausea,* pancreatitis, vomiting
GU: Decreased libido, frequency, impotence, increased creatinine, BUN
HEME: Inhibits platelet aggregation
METAB: Hypercalcemia, hyperglycemia, *hyperuricemia, hypochloremic alkalosis,* hypokalemia, *hypomagnesemia, hyponatremia*
MS: Cramps
SKIN: Photosensitivity, pruritus, rash, urticaria

INTERACTIONS

Drugs

❷ *Angiotensin-converting enzyme inhibitors:* Risk of postural hypotension when added to ongoing diuretic therapy; more common with loop diuretics; first dose hypotension possible in patients with sodium depletion or hypovolemia due to diuretics or sodium restriction; hypotensive response is usually transient; hold diuretic day of first dose

❸ *Corticosteroids:* Concomitant therapy may result in excessive potassium loss

❸ *Diazoxide* Blunt insulin secretion; results in hyperglycemia

❸ *Lithium:* Concurrent use may result in elevated serum levels of lithium; monitor carefully

❸ *Nonsteroidal antiinflammatory*

drugs: Concurrent may reduce diuretic and antihypertensive effects

SPECIAL CONSIDERATIONS

PATIENT/FAMILY EDUCATION

• May cause sensitivity to sunlight; avoid prolonged exposure to the sun and other ultraviolet light
• May cause gout attacks; notify clinician if sudden joint pain occurs
• May worsen control or increase requirements of hypoglycemic agents

MONITORING PARAMETERS

• Weight, urine output, serum electrolytes, BUN, creatinine, CBC, uric acid, glucose, lipids

---

indinavir

(in-din'ah-veer)
Rx: Crixivan
Chemical Class: HIV protease inhibitor
Therapeutic Class: HIV infection

CLINICAL PHARMACOLOGY

Mechanism of Action: Inhibits HIV protease preventing cleavage of viral polyproteins resulting in the formation of immature non-infectious viral particles

Pharmacokinetics

PO: Peak 0.8 hr; AUC decreased by high-calorie, fat and protein meals; 60% bound to plasma proteins; metabolized in liver to 7 metabolites, excreted in feces (83%) and urine; $t_{1/2}$ 1.8 hr

INDICATIONS AND USES: HIV infection when antiretroviral treatment is warranted

DOSAGE

Adult

• PO 800 mg (two 400 mg caps) q8h on an empty stomach; reduce dose to 600 mg q8h in mild-to-moderate hepatic insufficiency
• Adjust dose when used with ke-

toconazole, nelfinavir, rifabutin, ritonavir

• For latest treatment guidelines, see www.hivatis.org

💲 AVAILABLE FORMS/COST OF THERAPY

• Cap—Oral: 200 mg, 270's: **$347.63**
• Cap—Oral: 333 mg, 135's: **$289.40**
• Cap—Oral: 400 mg, 180's: **$463.50**

CONTRAINDICATIONS: Concurrent use of rifampin

PRECAUTIONS: Renal and hepatic function impairment, dehydration, children

PREGNANCY AND LACTATION: Pregnancy category C; not recommended for breast-feeding mothers

SIDE EFFECTS/ADVERSE REACTIONS

CNS: Dizziness, headache, insomnia, somnolence
EENT: Taste perversion
GI: Acid regurgitation, anorexia, diarrhea, dry mouth, *hyperbilirubinemia, nausea,* vomiting
GU: Flank pain, hematuria, nephrolithiasis (4%)
METAB: Hyperbilirubinemia
MS: Back pain

INTERACTIONS

Drugs

⚠ *Astemizole:* Increased plasma levels of astemizole
3 *Barbiturates:* Increased clearance of indinavir; reduced clearance of barbiturates
❷ *Carbamazepine:* Increased clearance of indinavir; reduced clearance of carbamazepine
⚠ *Cisapride:* Increased plasma levels of cisapride
3 *Clarithromycin:* Indinavir reduces clearance of clarithromycin
3 *Delavirdine:* Decreased clear-

ance of indinavir; reduce dose of indinavir to 600 mg q8h

❷ *Efavirenz:* Reduced saquinavir level; increase indinavir dose to 1000 mg q8h

▲ *Ergot alkaloids:* Increased plasma levels of ergot alkaloids

❸ *Erythromycin:* Reduced clearance of indinavir; indinavir reduces clearance of erythromycin

❸ *Ketoconazole:* Decreased clearance of indinavir; decrease indinavir dose to 600 mg tid

▲ *Lovastatin:* Indinavir reduces clearance of lovastatin

▲ *Midazolam:* Increased plasma levels of midazolam and prolonged effect

❸ *Nelfinavir:* Decreased clearance of indinavir; reduce dose of indinavir to 1200 mg bid

❸ *Nevirapine:* Reduces plasma indinavir levels; no dose adjustment needed

❸ *Oral contraceptives:* Indinavir may reduce efficacy

❸ *Phenytoin:* Increased clearance of indinavir; reduced clearance of phenytoin

❷ *Rifabutin:* Increased clearance of indinavir; reduced clearance of rifabutin—reduce rifabutin dose to 150 mg qd and increase indinavir dose to 1000 mg tid

▲ *Rifampin:* Increased clearance of indinavir

❸ *Ritonavir:* Decreased clearance of indinavir; decrease indinavir dose to 400 mg bid

❸ *Saquinavir:* Decreased clearance of saquinavir; reduce dose of Fortovase (saquinavir soft gel capsule) to 800 mg tid

▲ *Simvastatin:* Indinavir reduces clearance of simvastatin

▲ *Terfenadine:* Increased plasma levels of terfenadine

▲ *Triazolam:* Increased plasma levels of triazolam and prolonged effect

❸ *Troleandomycin:* Reduced clearance of indinavir; indinavir reduces clearance of troleandomycin

SPECIAL CONSIDERATIONS
• Antiretroviral activity of indinavir may be increased when used in combination with reverse transcriptase inhibitors

PATIENT/FAMILY EDUCATION
• Drink plenty of water, at least 48 oz/day
• Take with water or light, low-fat meals (dry toast, apple juice, corn flakes, skim milk). High fat meals and grapefruit juice reduce absorption
• Capsules sensitive to moisture. Keep dessicant in bottle
• If dose is missed take next dose on schedule; do not double this dose
• Separate dosing with didanosine by 1 hour
• Take 1 hr before or 2 hr after meals; may take with skim milk or low-fat meal

---

indomethacin
(in-doe-meth´a-sin)
Rx: Indocin, Indocin IV, Indocin SR, Indochron, Indo-Lemmon
Chemical Class: Indole acetic acid derivative
Therapeutic Class: NSAID with analgesic and antipyretic activity

---

CLINICAL PHARMACOLOGY
Mechanism of Action: Reversible cyclooxygenase (i.e., prostaglandin synthetase) inhibitor; nonselectively decreases the formation of both prostaglandins and thromboxane A2; variable effects on lipoxygenase synthesis and subsequent leukotriene production; antiinflammatory, anti-

pyretic, and analgesic activity; inhibits platelet aggregation

Pharmacokinetics

PO: Completely absorbed; onset 1-2 hr, peak 3 hr, duration 4-6 hr; metabolized in liver, kidneys; excreted in urine, bile, feces; 99% plasma protein binding

PR: 80%-90% absorbed

IV: $t_{1/2}$ $4\frac{1}{2}$ in adults; in infants, inversely related to gestational age and wt (<7 days age, <1000 g, $t_{1/2}$ 20-21 hr; >7 days age, >1000 g, $t_{1/2}$ 12-15 hr)

INDICATIONS AND USES: Ankylosing spondylitis, apnea of prematurity,* cholecystitis,* cognitive decline—prevention,* colon cancer—prevention,* dysmenorrhea,* erythema nodosum,* fever,* gouty arthritis, headache,* heterotopic bone ossification—prevention,* hypotension,* interferon intrathecal toxicity,* male infertility,* muromonab (OKT3) toxicity,* neonatal intraventricular hemorrhage,* nephrotic syndrome,* neurogenic, osteoarthritis, pain,* patent ductus arteriosus (PDA), pericarditis,* polyhydramnios,* premature labor,* Reiter's syndrome,* renal tubular dysfunction,* rheumatoid arthritis,* shoulder—acute pain,* Sweet's syndrome,* systemic lupus erythematosus,* ureteral colic*

DOSAGE

Adult

• *Antirheumatic/anti-inflammatory:* PO 25-50 mg bid-qid, may increase by 25 mg/day q wk, not to exceed 200 mg/day; SUS REL 75 mg qd, may increase to 75 mg bid; PR 50 mg bid-qid

• *Gout:* PO 100 mg initially then 50 mg tid until pain relieved, then reduce dose; PR 50 mg bid-qid

Child

• *Antirheumatic/anti-inflammatory:* PO/PR 1.5-2.5 mg/kg/day divided

doses tid-qid to max 4 mg/kg/day or 150-200 mg qd

• *Patent ductus arteriosus:* IV (preferred)/PO/PR 200 μg/kg initial dose; may follow with 100 μg/kg (infants ≤48 hr age), 200 μg/kg (infants 2-7 days age), 250 μg/kg (infants >7 days age) q12-24 hr for 2 doses

💲 AVAILABLE FORMS/COST OF THERAPY

• Inj, Lyphl-Sol—IV: 1 mg/vial: **$29.70**

• Cap, Gel—Oral: 25 mg, 100's: **$6.50-$61.85;** 50 mg, 100's: **$7.50-$100.96**

• Cap, Gel, Sus Rel—Oral: 75 mg, 100's: **$92.60-$151.33**

• Supp—Rect: 50 mg, 30's: **$49.90-$53.26**

• Susp—Oral: 25 mg/5 ml, 237 ml: **$46.44**

CONTRAINDICATIONS: Bronchospasm, nasal polyps, angioedema precipitated by aspirin or other NSAIDs

PRECAUTIONS: History of GI ulceration, bleeding, or perforation; renal dysfunction, hypertension or cardiac conditions aggravated by fluid retention and edema, history of liver dysfunction, history of coagulation

PREGNANCY AND LACTATION: Pregnancy category B; crosses placenta; excreted in breast milk

SIDE EFFECTS/ADVERSE REACTIONS

CNS: Anxiety, confusion, depression, dizziness, drowsiness, fatigue, *headache,* insomnia, tremors

CV: **CHF,** dysrhythmias, hypertension, palpitations, peripheral edema, tachycardia

EENT: Blurred vision, hearing loss, tinnitus

GI: Anorexia, cholestatic hepatitis, constipation, cramps, diarrhea, *dyspepsia,* flatulence, **GI bleeding,**

---

italic = common side effects   ***bold italic*** = life-threatening reactions

green stools, jaundice, *nausea,* peptic ulcer

GU: Azotemia, hematuria, **nephrotoxicity,** oliguria

HEME: **Blood dyscrasias**

RESP: Asthma

SKIN: Pruritus, purpura, rash, sweating

MISC: Fever

INTERACTIONS

Drugs

3 *Aminoglycosides:* Reduced clearance with elevated aminoglycoside levels and potential for toxicity (especially indomethacin in premature infants; other NSAIDs probably)

3 *Anticoagulants:* Excessive hypoprothrombinemia, decreased platelet aggregation with increased risk of GI bleeding

3 *Antihypertensives (alpha blockers, angiotensin-converting enzyme inihibitors, angiotensin II receptor blockers, beta blockers, diuretics:* Inhibition of antihypertensive and other favorable hemodynamic effects

3 *Corticosteroids:* Increased risk of GI ulceration

3 *Cyclosporine:* Increased nephrotoxicity risk

3 *Lithium:* Decreased clearance of lithium (mediated via prostaglandins) resulting in elevated serum lithium levels and risk of toxicity

3 *Methotrexate:* Decreased renal secretion of methotrexate resulting in elevated methotrexate levels and risk of toxicity

3 *Phenylpropanolamine:* Possible acute hypertensive reaction

3 *Potassium-sparing diuretics:* Additive hyperkalemia potential

3 *Triamterene:* Acute renal failure reported with addition of indomethacin; caution with other NSAIDs

SPECIAL CONSIDERATIONS

PATIENT/FAMILY EDUCATION

• Take with food

• No significant advantage over other oral NSAIDs; cost and clinical situation should govern use

MONITORING PARAMETERS

• Renal and hepatic function with prolonged use: check after 3 months, then q6-12 months

• Initial CBC and fecal occult blood test within 3 months of starting regular chronic therapy; repeat q6-12 months (more frequently in high-risk patients)

---

* = non-FDA-approved use

insulin

(in'su-lin)

Rx: *RAPID-ACTING INSULIN ANALOG:* (Lispro): Humalog
OTC: *RAPID ACTING:*
REGULAR INSULIN: Humulin R, Regular Iletin II (Beef), Regular Iletin II (Pork), Regular Iletin I (Beef-Pork), Novolin R, Velosulin
PROMPT INSULIN-ZINC SUSPENSION: Semilente Iletin I/(Beef-Pork)
INTERMEDIATE ACTING:
INSULIN-ZINC SUSPENSION: Humulin L, Lente Iletin I (Beef-Pork), Lente Iletin II (Pork), Iletin II (Pork), Novolin-L
ISOPHANE-INSULIN SUSPEN-SION (NPH): Humulin N, NPH Iletin III (Beef), NPH Iletin II (Pork), NPH Iletin I (Beef-Pork), Novolin N
LONG ACTING:
EXTENDED INSULIN-ZINC SUSPENSION: Humulin-U, Ultralente Iletin I (Beef-Pork), *PROTAMINE ZINC-INSULIN SUSPENSION (PZI):* PZI III (Beef), PZI II (Pork), PZI I (Beef-Pork)
INSULIN MIXTURES:
Isophane Insulin and Regular Insulin: Humulin 50/50, Humulin 70/30, Novolin 70/30
CONCENTRATED INSULIN:
Regular Concentrated Insulin: Humulin RU-500, Regular Iletin II U-500 (Pork)
Chemical Class: Exogenous insulin
Therapeutic Class: Antidiabetic

CLINICAL PHARMACOLOGY

Mechanism of Action: Stimulates carbohydrate metabolism; facilitates transfer of glucose into muscle and adipose tissue (lowers blood glucose); converts glucose to glycogen; stimulates both lipogenesis and protein synthesis; shifts potassium and magnesium intracellularly

Pharmacokinetics

See Insulins Table, p. 1069 SC and IM absorption not significantly different

Metabolized by liver, muscle, kidneys; excreted in urine; $T_{1/2}$ elimination: 5-15 minutes (IV administration); range: 1.6-5.2 hr (SQ or IM administration) with $T_{1/2}$ increasing with increased dose

INDICATIONS AND USES: Diabetes mellitus types 1 and 2, ketoacidosis, hyperkalemia, nonketotic hyperosmolar syndrome; human insulin is insulin of choice in insulin allergy, insulin resistance, pregnancy

DOSAGE

Adult and Child

• *Ketoacidosis:* IV bolus or IM 0.1-0.25 U/kg regular insulin, then 0.1 U/kg/hr IV INF/IM q1h until blood glucose 250 mg/dl, then give SC replacement dose

• *Type I diabetes mellitus (DM) replacement:* SC dosage individualized by blood glucose levels; initial total daily dose based on presence of urine ketones; if ketones negative—moderate 0.5 U/kg; if ketones large 0.7 U/kg; give ⅔ total dose in AM, ⅓ in PM; use mixture regular/NPH insulin (ratio 1:2 for AM dose, 1:1 for PM dose)

• *Type II DM replacement:* SC dosage individualized by blood glucose levels; initial total daily dose 0.3 U/kg; give ⅔ total dose in AM, ⅓ in PM; use mixed insulin 70/30 or 50/50 or mixture of regular/NPH (ratio 1:2 for AM dose, 1:1 for PM dose)

---

italic = common side effects   ***bold italic*** = life-threatening reactions

• *Type II DM combination with oral agent* (unable to achieve targets on max dose oral agent, AM hyperglycemia): Decrease oral agent to ½ max dose, give as single AM dose; add insulin with evening snack SC 0.1 U/kg NPH

• *Nonketotic hyperosmolar syndrome:* IV 10-20 U regular insulin, then IV/IM 5-15 U/hr until glucose 250 mg/dl, then give SC replacement dose

• *Gestational DM:* SC dosage individualized by blood glucose levels; initial total daily dose 0.4 U/kg current wt given as mixture regular/NPH distributed as for Type I DM

• *Hyperkalemia:* Adult IV 5-10 U regular insulin with 25 g dextrose (1 ampule D₅₀); child: 0.5g/kg dextrose with 0.3 U regular insulin/g dextrose over 2 hr

$ AVAILABLE FORMS/COST OF THERAPY

Rapid-acting insulin analog:
• Inj, Sol—SC: 100 U/ml, 1.5 ml, 5's: **$39.96;** 10 ml: **$33.08**
Rapid-acting insulin:
• Inj, Sol—IM, IV, SC: 100 U/ml, (human) 1.5 ml, 5's: **$27.50-$29.65;** 10 ml: (human): **$22.94-$29.65;** (beef/pork) **$28.25;** (pork) **$46.13**
Intermediate-acting insulin:
• Inj, Susp—SC: 100 U/ml, (human) 1.5 ml, 5's: **$27.50-$29.65;** 10 ml: (human) **$22.94;** (beef/pork) **$28.25;** (pork) **$46.13**
Long-acting insulin:
• Inj, Vsp—SC: 100 U/ml, 10 ml: **$22.94**
Mixed insulin 70/30:
• Inj, Sol—SC: 100 U/ml, 1.5 ml, 5's: **$27.50-$29.65;** 10 ml: **$22.94**
Mixed insulin 50/50:
• Inj, Susp—SC: 100 U/ml, 10 ml: **$22.94**
Concentrated insulin:
• Inj, Sol—SC: 500 U/ml, 20 ml: **$165.07**

PREGNANCY AND LACTATION:
Pregnancy category B; insulin requirements of pregnant diabetic patients often decreased in 1st half and increased in the latter half of pregnancy; elevated blood glucose levels associated with congenital abnormalities; does not pass into breast milk

SIDE EFFECTS/ADVERSE REACTIONS
SKIN: Flushing, rash, urticaria, warmth, lipodystrophy, lipohypertrophy
META: Hypoglycemia, decreased K, Ca, PO₄, Mg

INTERACTIONS
Drugs
▣ *Beta-blockers:* Increased glucose levels, hypoglycemia symptoms masked (except sweating)
▣ *Cigarette smoking, marijuana, corticosteroids, thiazides:* Increased glucose levels
▣ *Clonidine, Guanfacine, Guanabenz:* Hypoglycemia symptoms masked
▲ *Ethanol (excessive):* Hypoglycemia
▣ *Salicylates, ACE inhibitors, anabolic steroids, MAO inhibitors:* Enhanced hypoglycemic response

SPECIAL CONSIDERATIONS
PATIENT/FAMILY EDUCATION
• Symptoms of hypoglycemia include: fatigue, weakness, confusion, headache, convulsions, hunger, nausea, pallor, sweating, rapid breathing
• For hypoglycemia, give 1 mg glucagon, glucose 25 g IV (via dextrose 50% sol, 50 ml) or oral glucose if tolerated
• When mixing insulins, draw up regular first
• Dosage adjustment may be necessary when changing insulin products
• Human insulin considered insulin

of choice secondary to antigenicity of animal insulins

---

interferon alfa-2a/2b
(in-ter-feer'on)
Rx: Roferon-A (alfa-2a), Intron-A (alfa-2b)
Combinations
  Rx: Interferon alfa 2b with ribavirin (Rebetron Combination Therapy)
Chemical Class: Recombinant interferon
Therapeutic Class: Antineoplastic, antiviral

CLINICAL PHARMACOLOGY
Mechanism of Action: Altered synthesis of RNA, DNA, cellular proteins
Pharmacokinetics
SC: Absorption >80%; $t_{1/2}$ (alfa-2a) 6-8 hr, peak 7.3 hr; $t_{1/2}$ (alfa-2b) 2-3 hr, peak 3-12 hr
IV: $t_{1/2}$ 4-8 hr
IM: Absorption >80%; $t_{1/2}$ (alfa-2a) 6-8 hr, peak 3.8 hr; $t_{1/2}$ (alfa-2b) 2-3 hr, peak 3-12 hr
INTRALESIONAL: Minimal systemic absorption
Excreted by kidney; unknown if excreted in human breast milk
INDICATIONS AND USES: Hairy cell leukemia, condylomata acuminata, chronic hepatitis C, chronic hepatitis B, malignant melanoma, AIDS-associated Kaposi's sarcoma, renal carcinoma,* chronic myelocytic leukemia, laryngeal papillomatosis,* non-Hodgkin's lymphoma,* multiple myeloma,* mycosis fungoides,* other cancers*
DOSAGE
• A variety of dosage schedules have been used; consult medical literature prior to choosing specific dosage

---

Interferon alfa-2a
Adult
• *Hairy cell leukemia:* IM/SC 3 million U qd for 16-24 wk then 3 million U 3 times/wk
• *Kaposi's sarcoma:* IM/SC 36 million U qd for 10-12 wk or 3 million U qd days 1-3 then 9 million U qd days 4-6, then 18 million U days 7-9, then 36 million U qd for remainder of 10-12 wk; maintenance with 36 million U 3 times/wk
• *Hepatitis C:* IM/SC 3 million U 3 times/wk × 12 months
For relapse 3-6 million U 3 times/wk for 6-12 additional months
Child
• Not established; caution in adolescent females because interferes with serum estradiol and progesterone concentration
Interferon alfa-2b
Adult
• *Hairy cell leukemia:* IM/SC 2 million U/m² body surface area 3 times/wk
• *Condylomata acuminata:* Intralesional 1 million U (0.1 ml) per wart (up to five warts) 3 times/wk for 3 wk; 2nd course may be given 12-16 wk after 1st course; treat more warts sequentially in groups of 5
• *Kaposi's sarcoma:* IM/SC 30 million U/m² body surface area 3 times/wk
• *Chronic active hepatitis:* IM/SC 3 million U 3 times/wk
Child
• Not established

$ AVAILABLE FORMS/COST OF THERAPY
Interferon alfa-2a
• Inj, Dry-Sol—IM, SC: 3 million IU/vial: **$34.97**; 6 million IU/vial: **$69.91**; 9 million IU/vial: **$98.44**; 36 million IU/vial: **$419.26**
Interferon alfa-2b
• Inj, Dry-Sol,—IM, SC, ID: 3 million IU/vial: **$34.93**; 5 million IU/

---

vial: **$58.21;** 10 million IU/vial: **$116.44;** 18 million IU/vial: **$209.58;** 25 million IU/vial: **$291.11;** 50 million IU/vial: **$582.17**

PRECAUTIONS: Severe hypotension, dysrhythmia, tachycardia, severe renal or hepatic disease, seizure disorder

PREGNANCY AND LACTATION: Pregnancy category C; abortifacient in animal models; avoid breast feeding

SIDE EFFECTS/ADVERSE REACTIONS

CNS: Amnesia, anxiety, *coma, confusion, dizziness,* hallucinations, mood changes, *numbness, paresthesias, seizures*

CV: Chest pain, *CHF,* dysrhythmias, hypertension, hypotension, palpitations

EENT: Blurred vision, *dry mouth*

GI: Anorexia, diarrhea (15-45%), *nausea (20-50%), taste changes, vomiting, weight loss*

GU: Impotence

HEME: **Anemia, leukopenia, thrombocytopenia**

SKIN: Alopecia, dry skin, flushing, *itching, rash*

MISC: Chills, fatigue, fever (40-80%), flu-like syndrome, headache, myalgias

INTERACTIONS

Drugs

3 *Theophylline:* Increased theophylline levels

SPECIAL CONSIDERATIONS

• Rebetron Combination Therapy (kit containing interferon alfa-2b inj plus ribavirin capsules) more effective than interferon alfa-2b monotherapy for chronic hepatitis C infection

PATIENT/FAMILY EDUCATION

• Drink plenty of fluids

• Flu-like symptoms decrease during treatment. Acetaminophen (do not exceed recommended dose) may alleviate fever and headache

---

interferon alfa-n3

(in-ter-feer'on)
Rx: Alferon N
Chemical Class: Human leukocyte interferon
Therapeutic Class: Antiviral

CLINICAL PHARMACOLOGY

Mechanism of Action: Altered synthesis of RNA, DNA, and cellular proteins

Pharmacokinetics

INJ: Unable to detect by assay although some systemic effects noted

INDICATIONS AND USES: Condylomata acuminata

DOSAGE

Adult ≥18 yr

• INTRALESIONAL (into base of wart): 0.05 ml (250,000 IU) per wart, given 2 times/wk for max 8 wk; max 0.5 ml/treatment session

$ **AVAILABLE FORMS/COST OF THERAPY**

• Inj, Sol—ID, SC: 5 million U/ml: **$159.11**

CONTRAINDICATIONS: Anaphylaxis to egg protein, neomycin, mouse IgG

PRECAUTIONS: CHF, angina (unstable), COPD, diabetes mellitus with ketoacidosis, hemophilia, pulmonary embolism, thrombophlebitis, bone marrow depression, seizure disorder

PREGNANCY AND LACTATION: Pregnancy category C: Abortifacient in animal models; unknown if excreted into breast milk

SIDE EFFECTS/ADVERSE REACTIONS

CNS: Dizziness, insomnia, sleepiness

GI: Diarrhea, heartburn, *nausea,* vomiting

SKIN: Pain at inj site, pruritis
MISC: Chills, fatigue, fever (40%), flu-like syndrome, myalgias
INTERACTIONS
Drugs
■ *Theophylline:* Increased theophylline levels

---

interferon alfacon-1
(in-ter-feer'on)
Rx: Infergen
Chemical Class: Recombinant interferon
Therapeutic Class: Antiviral

CLINICAL PHARMACOLOGY
Mechanism of Action: Binds to cell surfaces, has antiviral, immunoregulatory, antiproliferative effects
Pharmacokinetics
SC: Unable to detect serum levels; metabolism mainly by kidney
INDICATIONS AND USES: Chronic hepatitis C infection in adults with compensated liver disease
DOSAGE
Adult ≥18 yrs
• No previous interferon therapy: SC 9 μg 3 times/wk for 24 wk
• Previous interferon therapy/relapse: SC 15 μg 3 times/wk for 6 months
§ **AVAILABLE FORMS/COST OF THERAPY**
• Inj, sol—SC: 9 μg/0.3 cc vial: **$35.28**
• Inj, sol—SC: 15 μg/0.5 cc vial: **$58.80**
CONTRAINDICATIONS: Hypersensitivity to *E. coli*-derived products
PRECAUTIONS: Cardiovascular disease, myelodepression or myelodepressive drugs, thyroid disorders, severe psychiatric disorders, transplant patients, immunosuppression

PREGNANCY AND LACTATION: Pregnancy category C; unknown if excreted in breast milk
SIDE EFFECTS/ADVERSE REACTIONS
CNS: Amnesia, confusion, dizziness, insomnia, mild to moderate depression (26%), paresthesia, somnolence, **suicide,** suicidal ideation (1%)
CV: Hypertension, palpitations, tachycardia
EENT: Cotton wool spots *URI,* retinal hemorrhages
GI: Abdominal pain, anorexia, constipation, diarrhea, dyspepsia, nausea, vomiting
GU: Dysmenorrhea
HEME: **Granulocytopenia** *(25%),* lymphadenopathy, **thrombocytopenia** *(18%)*
METAB: Abnormal thyroid test (5-9%), hypertriglyceridemia (6%)
MISC: Flu-like symptoms: arthralgia (45%), fatigue (65%), fever (50-60%), headache (80%), myalgia (55%); injection site erythema (20%)
INTERACTIONS
Drugs
■ *Theophylline:* Increased theophylline levels
SPECIAL CONSIDERATIONS
• Response rates (normal ALT, HCV RNA negative) of 9 μg dose approx 35%, about half those have sustained response 24 wk after treatment
• Withold dosage temporarily if severe adverse reaction occurs, consider decreasing dose to 7.5 μg
PATIENT/FAMILY EDUCATION
• Needs to be refrigerated (36-46° F), may allow to reach room temp before injection; call manufacturer for advice if left out
MONITORING PARAMETERS
• CBC, plts, TSH, triglycerides, LFTs initially, repeat after 2 wk treatment and periodically thereafter

---

italic = common side effects   ***bold italic*** = life-threatening reactions

• Withold for ANC <0.5×10^9/L or platelets <50×10^9/L

interferon beta

(in-ter-feer´on)
Rx: Betaseron
Chemical Class: Recombinant interferon
Therapeutic Class: Multiple sclerosis agent

See next monograph for updated information on interferon beta-1b (Betaseron)

CLINICAL PHARMACOLOGY
Mechanism of Action: Antiviral, immunoregulatory; action not clearly understood

Pharmacokinetics
SC: Serum levels very low or not detectable at recommended dose; at higher doses 50% bioavailable, peak 1-8 hr

INDICATIONS AND USES: Ambulatory patients with relapsing or remitting multiple sclerosis, treatment of AIDS,* AIDS-related Kaposi's sarcoma,* malignant melanoma,* metastatic renal cell carcinoma,* cutaneous T-cell lymphoma,* acute non-A, non-B hepatitis*

DOSAGE
Adult
• *Relapsing/remitting multiple sclerosis:* SC 0.25 mg (8 IU) qod
Child
• Not established

$ AVAILABLE FORMS/COST OF THERAPY
• Inj, Lyphl-Sol—SC: 0.3 mg/vial: **$72.00**

CONTRAINDICATIONS: Hypersensitivity to human albumin

PRECAUTIONS: Children under 18 yr, chronic progressive MS, depression, mental disorders, seizure disorder, heart disease

PREGNANCY AND LACTATION: Pregnancy category C; possible abortifacient; not known if excreted in breast milk; avoid in nursing mothers

SIDE EFFECTS/ADVERSE REACTIONS
CNS: Dizziness, mental changes
CV: Hypertension, palpitations, peripheral vascular disorders, tachycardia
EENT: Conjunctivitis
GI: Abdominal pain, constipation, diarrhea, vomiting
GU: Breast pain, cystitis, *dysmenorrhea, irregular menses, metrorrhagia*
HEME: Lymphadenopathy, lymphopenia, ***neutropenia***
RESP: Dyspnea, *sinusitis*
SKIN: Inj site reaction (85%), sweating
MISC: Flu-like syndrome (76%): chills, fever, headache, myalgias

DRUG INTERACTIONS
Drugs
• *Zidovudine, theophylline:* Increased levels

SPECIAL CONSIDERATIONS
• 31% reduction in annual exacerbation rate (1.31 in placebo group, 0.9 in treatment group)

PATIENT/FAMILY EDUCATION
• Use acetaminophen for relief of flu-like symptoms
• Avoid prolonged sun exposure (photosensitivity)

MONITORING PARAMETERS
• Follow CBC, platelets, LFTs q3mo
• D/C for ANC <750/mm³, ALT/AST >10× upper limits normal, bilirubin >5× upper limits normal; when labs return to these levels restart at 50% reduction dose

* = non-FDA-approved use

interferon beta-1a/b
(in-ter-feer'on)
Rx: Avonex (beta-1a),
Betaseron (beta-1b)
Chemical Class: Purified
protein product
Therapeutic Class: Multiple
sclerosis agent

CLINICAL PHARMACOLOGY
Mechanism of Action: Binds to cell surfaces; has antiviral, immunoregulatory, antiproliferative effects
Pharmacokinetics
SC: Serum levels very low or not detectable at recommended dose; at higher doses 50% bioavailable; peak 1-8 hr
IM: Peak 9.8 hr; biologic response within 12 hr, maximal at 48 hr; duration at least 4 days, $t_{1/2}$ 10 hr
INDICATIONS AND USES: Relapsing forms of multiple sclerosis (slows the accumulation of physical disability and decreases frequency of clinical exacerbations); treatment of AIDS-related Kaposi's sarcoma,* metastatic renal cell carcinoma*; herpes of the lips, genitals*; malignant melanoma,* cutaneous T-cell lymphoma*; acute non-A, non-B hepatitis*

DOSAGE
Adult
• *Relapsing multiple sclerosis:* IM 30 µg IM q wk (Avonex); SC 0.25 mg (8 IU) qod (Betaseron)

$ **AVAILABLE FORMS/COST OF THERAPY**
• Inj—IM: 33 µg/vial, 4's: **$852.00**
• Inj, Lyphl-Sol—SC: 0.3 mg/vial: **$72.00**
CONTRAINDICATIONS: Hypersensitivity to human albumin
PRECAUTIONS: Depression, seizure disorder, heart disease, chil-

dren <18 yr, chronic progressive ms, mental disorders
PREGNANCY AND LACTATION: Pregnancy category C; possible abortifacient; not known if excreted into breast milk; avoid in nursing mothers
SIDE EFFECTS/ADVERSE REACTIONS
CNS: Dizziness, insomnia, **seizures,** *mental changes*
CV: Syncope, vasodilation, hypertension, palpitations, peripheral vascular disorders, tachycardia
EENT: Decreased hearing, conjunctivitis
GI: Abdominal pain, anorexia, diarrhea, dyspepsia, nausea
GU: Dysmenorrhea, irregular menses, metrorrhagia
HEME: Anemia, eosinophilia, **neutropenia**
RESP: Dyspnea, sinusitis, upper respiratory tract infection
SKIN: Alopecia, inj site reaction, urticaria, sweating
MISC: Flu-like symptoms (61%-76%): chills, fever, headache, myalgias
INTERACTIONS
Drugs
3 *Zidovudine, theophylline:* Increased levels of these drugs
SPECIAL CONSIDERATIONS
PATIENT/FAMILY EDUCATION
• Use acetaminophen for relief of flu-like symptoms
• Avoid prolonged sun exposure (photosensitivity)
• Benefit in chronic progressive multiple sclerosis has not been evaluated
• Patients treated × 2 yr had significantly longer time to progression of disability compared with placebo group
MONITORING PARAMETERS
• CBC, platelets, liver function tests, and blood chemistries q3 mo

---

italic = common side effects   ***bold italic*** = life-threatening reactions

• DC for ANC <750/m^3, ALT/AST >10× upper normal limits; when labs return to these levels, restart at 50% of dose

---

interferon gamma-1b
(in-ter-feer'on)
Rx: Actimmune
Chemical Class: Recombinant interferon
Therapeutic Class: Biologic response modifier

CLINICAL PHARMACOLOGY
Mechanism of Action: Interacts with other lymphokines (e.g., interleukin-2); activates macrophages, enhancing phagocytic function; enhances cellular cytotoxicity
Pharmacokinetics
SC: 89% dose absorbed, $t_{1/2}$ 5.9 hr, peak 7 hr
INDICATIONS AND USES: Reduction of frequency and severity of serious infections associated with chronic granulomatous disease
DOSAGE
Adult and Child
• SC 50 μg/m^2 (1.5 million U/m^2) for patients with surface area of >0.5 m^2; 1.5 μg/kg/dose for patient with a surface area of <0.5/m^2; given 3 ×/wk
• Reduce dose 50% for adverse reactions
[$] **AVAILABLE FORMS/COST OF THERAPY**
• Inj, Sol—SC: 100 μg (3 million U)/0.5 ml: **$140.00**
CONTRAINDICATIONS: Hypersensitivity to *E. coli*-derived products
PRECAUTIONS: Cardiac disease, seizure disorders, CNS disorders, myelosuppression, safety not established in children <1 yr
PREGNANCY AND LACTATION: Pregnancy category C; possible abor-

tifacient; not known if excreted in breast milk; not recommended in breast feeding
SIDE EFFECTS/ADVERSE REACTIONS
CNS: Chills, fatigue (14%), fever (52%), headache (33%)
GI: Abdominal pain, *diarrhea, nausea (10%), vomiting, weight loss*
HEME: **Neutropenia, thrombocytopenia**
MS: Myalgia
SKIN: Pain at inj site, rash
INTERACTIONS
Drugs
3 *Theophylline, zidovudine:* Increased levels of these drugs
SPECIAL CONSIDERATIONS
• Optimal sites for inj are the right and left deltoid and anterior thigh
PATIENT/FAMILY EDUCATION
• Use acetaminophen to relieve fever, headache

---

iodinated glycerol
Rx: Iophen, Organidin, Par Glycerol, R-Gen
Combinations
  Rx: with theophylline (Theo-Oridol, Theo-R-Gen); with codeine (Iophen-C Liquid, Tussi-Organidin Liquid)
Chemical Class: Iodopropylidene glycerol isomer
Therapeutic Class: Expectorant

CLINICAL PHARMACOLOGY
Mechanism of Action: Increases respiratory tract fluid by decreasing surface tension, increases removal of mucus
Pharmacokinetics
PO: Readily absorbed, concentrated in respiratory secretions; excreted by kidneys
INDICATIONS AND USES: Mucolytic expectorant in asthma, emphy-

---

* = non-FDA-approved use

sema, bronchitis, cystic fibrosis, chronic sinusitis; **efficacy not proven**

DOSAGE

Adult

• PO tab 60 mg qid; ELI 5 ml qid; SOL 20 gtt qid

Child

• PO up to half adult dose depending on weight

$ AVAILABLE FORMS/COST OF THERAPY

• Eli—Oral: 60 mg/5 ml, 120 ml: **$1.25-$6.93**

• Sol—Oral: 50 mg/ml, 30 ml: **$5.50-$27.62**

• Tab, Uncoated—Oral: 30 mg, 100's: **$10.66-$18.07**

CONTRAINDICATIONS: Hypersensitivity to iodides, pulmonary TB, hyperthyroidism, hyperkalemia, newborns, lactation, acute bronchitis

PRECAUTIONS: Thyroid disease, cystic fibrosis (increased goitrogenic effect in children with cystic fibrosis)

PREGNANCY AND LACTATION: Contraindicated in pregnancy, category X; not recommended in nursing mothers (rash and thyroid suppression in infant)

SIDE EFFECTS/ADVERSE REACTIONS

CNS: CNS depression, fever, frontal headache, parkinsonism

EENT: Burning mouth, throat, eye irritation, swelling of eyelids

GI: Gastric irritation

METAB: Iodism, goiter, myxedema

RESP: Pulmonary edema

*SKIN: **Angioedema,*** rash

INTERACTIONS

Drugs

3 *Lithium, antithyroid drugs:* Increased hypothyroid effects

iodoquinol

(eye-oh-do-kwin′ole)

Rx: Yodoxin

Chemical Class: 8-hydroxyquinolone derivative

Therapeutic Class: Amebicide

CLINICAL PHARMACOLOGY

Mechanism of Action: Direct-acting amebicide; action occurs in intestinal lumen

Pharmacokinetics

PO: Poorly absorbed, excreted in feces

INDICATIONS AND USES: Intestinal amebiasis

DOSAGE

Adult

• PO 650 mg tid after meals for 20 days, not to exceed 2 g/day

Child

• PO 30-40 mg/kg/day in 3 divided doses for 20 days, not to exceed 1.95 g/24 hr for 20 days; do not repeat treatment before 2-3 wk

$ AVAILABLE FORMS/COST OF THERAPY

• Tab, Uncoated—Oral: 210 mg, 100's: **$43.38;** 650 mg, 100's: **$19.50-$53.29**

CONTRAINDICATIONS: Hypersensitivity to iodine; renal disease, hepatic disease, severe thyroid disease, pre-existing optic neuropathy

PRECAUTIONS: Thyroid disease

PREGNANCY AND LACTATION: Pregnancy category C; excretion into breast milk unknown

SIDE EFFECTS/ADVERSE REACTIONS

CNS: Agitation, headache, malaise, peripheral neuropathy

EENT: Blurred vision, optic atrophy, optic neuritis, retinal edema, sore throat

GI: Abdominal cramps, anal itching, *anorexia,* constipation, diar-

---

italic = common side effects   ***bold italic*** = life-threatening reactions

rhea, epigastric distress, gastritis, *nausea,* rectal irritation, vomiting
HEME: **Agranulocytosis** (rare)
SKIN: Alopecia, discolored skin, hair, nails; pruritus; rash
MISC: Chills, fever, thyroid enlargement, vertigo

---

ipecac
(ip'e-kak)
OTC: Ipecac
Chemical Class: Cephaelis ipecacuanha derivative
Therapeutic Class: Emetic

CLINICAL PHARMACOLOGY
Mechanism of Action: Acts on chemoreceptor trigger zone to induce vomiting; irritates gastric mucosa
Pharmacokinetics
PO: Onset 15-30 min; minimal systemic absorption
INDICATIONS AND USES: In poisoning to induce vomiting
DOSAGE
Adult
• PO 15-30 ml, then 3-4 glasses water
Child 1-12 yr
• PO 15 ml, then 1-2 glasses water
Child <1 yr
• PO 5-10 ml, then ½-1 glass water, may repeat dose if needed
$ AVAILABLE FORMS/COST OF THERAPY
• Liq—Oral (1.5%-2.0% in ethanol): 30 ml: **$1.41-$5.25**
CONTRAINDICATIONS: Unconsciousness, semiconsciousness; depressed gag reflex, poisoning with petroleum products or caustic substances, seizures
PREGNANCY AND LACTATION: Pregnancy category C; not known if excreted in breast milk
SIDE EFFECTS/ADVERSE REACTIONS
CNS: **Coma, seizures**

CV: **Atrial fibrillation, dysrhythmias, fatal myocarditis, hypotension**
GI: Bloody diarrhea, nausea, vomiting
INTERACTIONS
Drugs
3 *Activated charcoal:* Decreased effect of ipecac; if both drugs used, give activated charcoal after emesis induced
SPECIAL CONSIDERATIONS
• May not work on empty stomach
• Do not confuse with ipecac fluid extract (14 times stronger)

---

ipratropium
(eye-pra-troep'ee-um)
Rx: Atrovent
Combinations
  Rx: with albuterol (Combivent)
Chemical Class: Quaternary ammonium compound
Therapeutic Class: Bronchodilator

CLINICAL PHARMACOLOGY
Mechanism of Action: Inhibits action of acetylcholine at receptor sites on bronchial smooth muscle, resulting in bronchodilation; has antisecretory properties when applied locally
Pharmacokinetics
INH: Onset 5-15 min; peak effect 1-2 hr, duration of action 3-6 hr; absorption minimal; does not cross blood-brain barrier; 90% excreted in feces
INDICATIONS AND USES: Maintenance treatment of bronchospasm in COPD; perennial rhinitis, rhinorrhea associated with the common cold; bronchial asthma,* cough after respiratory infection* (not indicated for acute bronchospasm)

---

* = non-FDA-approved use

DOSAGE
Adult
• INH 1-2 puffs qid, not to exceed 12 puffs/24 hr
• SOL 500 µg via nebulizer q6-8 hr, can be mixed with albuterol
• *Perennial rhinitis:* Nasal 2 sprays of 0.03% sol bid-tid
• *Rhinitis associated with common cold:* Nasal 2 sprays of 0.06% sol tid-qid for 4 days
Child <12 yr
• *Perennial rhinitis:* Nasal 2 sprays of 0.03% sol bid-tid
• *Rhinitis associated with common cold:* Nasal 2 sprays of 0.06% sol tid-qid for 4 days

$ **AVAILABLE FORMS/COST OF THERAPY**
• Aer—INH: 18 µg/inh, 14 g: **$35.93**
• Sol—INH: 0.2 mg/ml, 2.5 ml: **$1.62-$2.34**
• Sol—Nasal: 0.03%, 30 ml: **$38.74; 0.06%, 15 ml: $33.19**

CONTRAINDICATIONS: Hypersensitivity to atropine
PRECAUTIONS: Angle-closure glaucoma, prostatic hypertrophy, bladder neck obstruction, urinary retention
PREGNANCY AND LACTATION: Pregnancy category B; not known if excreted in breast milk, but little systemic absorption when administered by INH
SIDE EFFECTS/ADVERSE REACTIONS
CNS: Anxiety, dizziness, headache, nervousness
CV: Palpitations
EENT: Blurred vision, dry mouth, metallic taste, stomatitis
GI: Cramps, *nausea,* vomiting
RESP: **Bronchospasm,** *cough, worsening of symptoms*
SKIN: Rash

SPECIAL CONSIDERATIONS
• Bronchodilator of choice for COPD

---

irbesartan
(erb'ba-sar-tan)
Rx: Avapro
Chemical Class: Angiotensin II receptor antagonist
Therapeutic Class: Antihypertensive

CLINICAL PHARMACOLOGY
Mechanism of Action: Antihypertensive (inhibition of vasoconstriction and aldosterone secretion), smooth muscle hypoproliferative, and cardioprotective effects are attributable to selective blockade of angiotensin II (AT_1) receptors found throughout the cardiovascular and renal systems; effects independent of angiotensin II synthesis
Pharmacokinetics
PO: Peak, 1-2 hrs; peak response, 2 hrs (blood pressure reduction, increased plasma renin activity), 4-8 hrs (reductions in plasma aldosterone)
PO bioavailability, 60%-80%, no food effect; 90% protein bound; extensively metabolized by liver (CYP2C9) to inactive metabolite, 65% fecal, 20% renal excretion; elimination $t_{1/2}$, 11-15 hrs
INDICATIONS AND USES: Hypertension; congestive heart failure (left ventricular dysfunction),* myocardial infarction,* diabetic nephropathy*
DOSAGE
Adult
• PO 150-300 mg qd
$ **AVAILABLE FORMS/COST OF THERAPY**
• Capsule—Oral: 75 mg, 90's: **$107.15;** 150 mg, 90's: **$112.79;** 300 mg, 90's: **$135.56**

---

italic = common side effects   ***bold italic*** = life-threatening reactions

PRECAUTIONS: Angioedema (associated with aspirin and/or penicillin allergy), aortic or mitral valve stenosis, biliary cirrhosis or biliary obstruction, breast feeding period, coronary artery disease, elderly patients, hepatic dysfunction (adjust dose), hypertrophic cardiomyopathy, hypotension (sodium or volume depleted patients), pregnancy, renal artery stenosis, solitary kidney, or congestive heart failure

PREGNANCY AND LACTATION: Pregnancy category C (first trimester—category D, second and third trimesters; drugs acting directly on the renin-angiotensin-aldosterone system are documented to cause fetal harm (hypotension, oligohydramnios, neonatal anemia, hyperkalemia, neonatal skull hypoplasia, anuria, and renal failure; neonatal limb contractures, craniofacial deformities, and hypoplastic lung development

SIDE EFFECTS/ADVERSE REACTIONS

CNS: Dizziness, headache, weakness or tiredness

CV: First dose hypotension, fluid retention, orthostatic effects, syncope

GI: Diarrhea, dyspepsia/heartburn

MS: Trauma

RESP: Cough, upper respiratory infection

MISC: Angioedema

SPECIAL CONSIDERATIONS
• Potentially as or more effective than angiotensin-converting enzyme inhibitors, without cough; no evidence for reduction in morbidity and mortality as first line agents in hypertension, yet; whether they provide the same cardiac and renal protection also still tentative; Like ACE inhibitors, less effective in black patients

PATIENT/FAMILY EDUCATION
• Call your clinician immediately if

note following side effects: wheezing; lip, throat or face swelling; hives or rash

MONITORING PARAMETERS
• Baseline electrolytes, urinalysis, blood urea nitrogen and creatinine with recheck at 2-4 weeks after initiation (sooner in volume depleted patients); monitor sitting blood pressure; watch for symptomatic hypotension, particularly in volume depleted patients

---

iron dextran
Rx: InFeD, Dexferrum
Chemical Class: Ferric hydroxide complexed with dextran
Therapeutic Class: Hematinic

CLINICAL PHARMACOLOGY
Mechanism of Action: Iron is carried by transferrin to bone marrow and incorporated into hemoglobin

Pharmacokinetics
IM: Excreted in feces, urine, bile, breast milk; crosses placenta; most absorbed through lymphatics; can be gradually absorbed over weeks/months from fixed locations

INDICATIONS AND USES: Iron deficiency anemia when oral administration not satisfactory; patients receiving epoetin therapy*

DOSAGE
• To calculate total amount of iron (in mg) required to restore hemoglobin to normal levels and replenish iron stores in iron deficient anemia: $(0.3) \times$ (weight in lb) $\times$ [100-(Hgb in g/dl $\times$ 100/14.8)]
• Divide this result by 50 to obtain dose in ml

Adult
• IM 0.5 ml as a test dose by Z-track (pull skin laterally prior to injection); wait ≥1 hr before giving re-

mainder of therapeutic dose; max dose 2 ml (100 μg) qd
• IV 0.5 ml as test dose; give slowly, ≤1 ml/min; follow same protocol and dose as for IM; alternatively the entire dose may be diluted in 500 ml of normal saline and infused over 4-6 hr if the test dose is tolerated

Child
• If <30 lb, total dose is 80% of dose as calculated by above formula
• IM/IV 0.5 ml as a test dose as above, then no more than the following per day: <10 lb 0.5 ml (25 mg); <20 lb 1 ml (50 mg)

$ AVAILABLE FORMS/COST OF THERAPY
• Inj, Sol—IM, IV: 50 mg/ml, 2 ml: **$37.71**

CONTRAINDICATIONS: Anemias other than iron deficiency anemia, hepatic disease

PRECAUTIONS: Acute renal disease, asthma, rheumatoid arthritis (IV), severe liver disease, infants <4 mo

PREGNANCY AND LACTATION: Pregnancy category C; excreted in breast milk

SIDE EFFECTS/ADVERSE REACTIONS

CNS: Dizziness, headache, paresthesia, *seizures,* shivering, weakness
CV: Chest pain, hypotension, *shock,* tachycardia
GI: Abdominal pain, dark stools, metallic taste, *nausea,* vomiting
HEME: Leukocytosis
RESP: Dyspnea
SKIN: Brown skin discoloration, chills, fever, necrosis, pain at inj site, phlebitis, pruritus, rash, sterile abscesses, sweating, urticaria

INTERACTIONS
Drugs
3 *Enalapril:* Three patients on enalapril receiving IV iron developed systemic reactions (GI symp-

toms, hypotension); causality not established
3 *Vitamin E:* Decreased reticulocyte response in anemic children
Labs
• *False increase:* Serum calcium, serum glucose, serum iron
• *False positive:* Stool guaiac

SPECIAL CONSIDERATIONS
• Discontinue oral iron before giving
• Delayed reaction (fever, myalgias, arthralgias, nausea) may occur 1-2 days after administration
• When giving IM, give only in gluteal muscle

---

isocarboxazid
(eye-soe-kar-box'a-zid)
Rx: Marplan
Chemical Class: Hydrazine derivative
Therapeutic Class: MAOI

CLINICAL PHARMACOLOGY
Mechanism of Action: Increases concentrations of endogenous epinephrine, norepinephrine, serotonin, dopamine in storage sites in CNS by inhibition of monoamine oxidase; increased concentrations reduce depression
Pharmacokinetics
PO: Duration up to 2 wk; metabolized by liver; excreted by kidneys

INDICATIONS AND USES: Depression uncontrolled by other means

DOSAGE
Adult
• PO 30 mg/day in single or divided doses; reduce dose to lowest effective dose (10-20 mg qd) when condition improves; full effect may take 3-4 wk

$ AVAILABLE FORMS/COST OF THERAPY
• Tab, Uncoated—Oral: 10 mg, 100's: **$70.66**

CONTRAINDICATIONS: Elderly, hypertension, CHF, severe hepatic disease, pheochromocytoma, severe renal disease, severe cardiac disease

PRECAUTIONS: Suicidal patients, seizure disorders, severe depression, schizophrenia, hyperactivity, diabetes mellitus

PREGNANCY AND LACTATION: Pregnancy category C; breast feeding data not available

SIDE EFFECTS/ADVERSE REACTIONS

CNS: Anxiety, confusion, *dizziness, drowsiness,* fatigue, headache, hyperreflexia, insomnia, mania, stimulation, tremors, weakness

CV: **Dysrhythmias,** hypertension, **hypertensive crisis,** orthostatic hypotension

EENT: Blurred vision

GI: *Anorexia,* constipation, diarrhea, dry mouth, nausea, vomiting, weight gain

GU: Change in libido, frequency

HEME: Anemia

METAB: Hypoglycemia, syndrome of inappropriate antidiuretic hormone-like syndrome

SKIN: Flushing, increased perspiration, jaundice, rash

INTERACTIONS

Drugs

❸ *Barbiturates:* Prolonged action of barbiturate

⚠ *Dextromethorphan:* Agitation, seizure, increased BP, hyperpyrexia

⚠ *Ephedrine, amphetamines, phenylephrine, phenylpropanolamine, pseudoephedrine:* Hypertension, severe

⚠ *Ethanol:* Alcoholic beverages containing tyramine may cause severe hypertensive reaction

❸ *Guanethidine:* Decreased antihypertensive response to guanethidine

❸ *Levodopa:* Hypertension, severe

❷ *Lithium:* Hyperpyrexia possible

⚠ *Meperidine:* Sweating, rigidity, hypertension

⚠ *Methotrimeprazine:* Case report of fatality in patient taking these drugs, causality not established

❸ *Norepinephrine:* Increased pressor response to norepinephrine

⚠ *Reserpine:* Potential for hypertensive reaction, clinical evidence lacking

⚠ *Sertraline, fluoxetine, fluvoxamine, paroxetine, venlafaxine:* Increased CNS effects (serotonergic)

⚠ *Tricyclic antidepressants:* Excessive sympathetic response, mania, hyperpyrexia

SPECIAL CONSIDERATIONS

• Phentolamine for severe hypertension

PATIENT/FAMILY EDUCATION

• Avoid high-tyramine foods: cheese (aged), sour cream, beer, wine, pickled products, liver, raisins, bananas, figs, avocados, meat tenderizers, chocolate, yogurt; soy sauce, caffeine

• Do not discontinue medication quickly after long-term use

---

isoetharine

(eye-soe-eth′a-reen)
Rx: Isoetharine
Chemical Class: Sympathomimetic amine; B_2-adrenergic agonist
Therapeutic Class: Antiasthmatic, bronchodilator

CLINICAL PHARMACOLOGY
Mechanism of Action: Causes bronchodilation by β-$_2$ stimulation, resulting in relaxation of bronchial smooth muscle; inhibits mast cell degranulation; stimulates cilia to remove secretions

Pharmacokinetics
INH: Onset rapid, peak 5-15 min, duration 1-4 hr; metabolized in liver, GI tract, lungs; excreted in urine
INDICATIONS AND USES: Bronchial asthma; reversible bronchospasm that occurs with bronchitis and emphysema
DOSAGE
Adult
• NEB 1%, 0.25-0.5 ml, q4h prn
💲 AVAILABLE FORMS/COST OF THERAPY
• Sol—INH: 1%, 30 ml: **$54.75-$96.11**
PRECAUTIONS: Ischemic heart disease, cardiac dysrhythmias, hyperthyroidism, diabetes mellitus, prostatic hypertrophy, hypertension
PREGNANCY AND LACTATION: Pregnancy category C; no breast feeding data available
SIDE EFFECTS/ADVERSE REACTIONS
CNS: Anxiety, dizziness, headache, insomnia, stimulation, *tremors*
*CV: **Cardiac arrest, dysrhythmias,*** hypertension, palpitations, tachycardia
GI: Nausea
METAB: Hyperglycemia
INTERACTIONS
Drugs
❷ *Beta-blockers:* Decreased action of isoetharine, cardioselective beta-blockers preferable if concurrent use necessary
❸ *Furosemide:* Potential for additive hypokalemia
SPECIAL CONSIDERATIONS
• Inhalation technique critical
• Re-educate routinely

isoflurophate
(eye-soe-flure'oh-fate)
Rx: Floropryl
Chemical Class: Cholinesterase inhibitor
Therapeutic Class: Antiglaucoma agent; miotic

CLINICAL PHARMACOLOGY
Mechanism of Action: Irreversibly inhibits acetylcholinesterase, which prevents breakdown of neurotransmitter acetylcholine, which then accumulates, causing intense miosis and ciliary muscle contraction
Pharmacokinetics
OPHTH: Onset of miosis 5-10 min, duration 1-4 wk; peak reduction in intraocular pressure in 24 hr, duration 1 wk
INDICATIONS AND USES: Open-angle glaucoma (when shorter-acting miotics have proved inadequate), accommodative esotropia, conditions obstructing aqueous outflow; following iridectomy
DOSAGE
Adult and Child
• *Glaucoma:* Instill ¼ inch strip in conjunctival sac q8-72 hr hs
• *Esotropia:* Instill ¼ inch strip in conjunctival sac qhs for 2 wk, then qod hs, and finally q wk for 1 mo, then reevaluate
💲 AVAILABLE FORMS/COST OF THERAPY
• Oint—Ophth: 0.025%, 3.5 g: **$8.14**
CONTRAINDICATIONS: Uveal inflammation, glaucoma associated with iridocyclitis
PRECAUTIONS: History of retinal detachment, asthma, bradycardia, parkinsonism, peptic ulcer, spastic GI disease, recent MI, epilepsy, myasthenia gravis, angle-closure glaucoma

PREGNANCY AND LACTATION: Pregnancy category X; no data available on breast feeding

SIDE EFFECTS/ADVERSE REACTIONS

CNS: Headache

CV: Bradycardia, hypotension, paradoxic tachycardia

EENT: Blurred vision, brow ache, conjunctival congestion, lacrimation, lid muscle twitching, stinging, burning

GU: Urinary incontinence

GI: Abdominal cramps, diarrhea, increased salivation, nausea, vomiting

RESP: Bronchoconstriction, ***bronchospasm,*** dyspnea, wheezing

SPECIAL CONSIDERATIONS

PATIENT/FAMILY EDUCATION

• Wash hands immediately after application

MONITORING PARAMETERS

• Routine slit-lamp exam during prolonged therapy

---

isometheptene

(i-so-meh-thep′tene)

Only available in combination with dichloralphenazone and acetaminophen:

Rx: Amidrine Duradin, I.D.A., Iso-Acetazone, Midchlor, Midrin, Migrapap, Migratine, Migrazone, Migquin, Migrex, VA-Zone

Chemical Class: Sympathomimetic amine

Therapeutic Class: Vasoconstrictor (in combination with analgesic and sedative)

CLINICAL PHARMACOLOGY

Mechanism of Action: Indirect-acting sympathomimetic agent with vasoconstricting activity; vasoconstriction of cerebral blood vessels may reduce pulsation of cerebral arteries; dichloralphenazone is a mild sedative; acetaminophen an analgesic

INDICATIONS AND USES: Tension headache; possibly effective for relief of vascular headaches

DOSAGE

Adult

• *Tension headache:* PO 1-2 caps q4h prn to max 8 caps qd

• *Vascular headache:* PO 2 caps at once, then 1 cap qhr prn to max 5 caps/12 hr

$ AVAILABLE FORMS/COST OF THERAPY

• Cap, Gel—Oral: acetaminophen 325 mg/dichloralphenazone 100 mg/isometheptene 65 mg, 100's: **$4.50-$48.75**

CONTRAINDICATIONS: Glaucoma, severe renal disease, severe hepatic disease (acetaminophen), organic heart disease, MAOI therapy

PRECAUTIONS: Hypertension, peripheral vascular disease, recent CVA

PREGNANCY AND LACTATION: Data not available

SIDE EFFECTS/ADVERSE REACTIONS

CNS: Dizziness

SKIN: Rash

INTERACTIONS

Drugs

⚠ *Bromocriptine:* Potential for hypertension and ventricular tachycardia

Labs

• *False positive:* Urine amphetamine

---

isoniazid (INH)

(eye-soe-nye'a-zid)
Rx: INH, Nydrazid
Combinations
  Rx: with rifampin
    (Rifamate); with rifampin,
    pyrazinamide (Rifater)
Chemical Class: Synthetic
isonicotinic acid derivative
Therapeutic Class: Antituber-
culosis agent

CLINICAL PHARMACOLOGY
Mechanism of Action: Interferes
with lipid and nucleic acid biosynthesis in growing tubercle bacilli;
active only against mycobacteria,
primarily those that are actively dividing
Pharmacokinetics
PO: Peak 1-2 hr, duration 6-8 hr;
Widely distributed to all fluids and
tissues; low protein binding; metabolized in liver, primarily by acetylation; rate of metabolism geneti-
cally determined; eliminated in
urine; $t_{1/2}$ 0.5-1.6 hr (fast acetylators), 2-5 hr (slow acetylators)
INDICATIONS AND USES: Treatment and prophylaxis of tuberculosis; severe tremor in patients with
multiple sclerosis*
DOSAGE
Adult
• *Treatment:* PO or IM 5 mg/kg/
day (up to 300 mg total) in a single
dose; use in conjunction with other
effective antituberculosis agents; duration of treatment 6 mo-2 yr
• *Disseminated disease:* PO 10 mg/
kg/day in 1-2 divided doses
• *Prophylaxis:* PO or IM 300 mg qd
Child
• *Treatment:* PO or IM 10-20 mg/
kg/day (up to 300 mg total) in 1-2
divided doses

• *Prophylaxis:* PO or IM 10 mg/
kg/day qd, do not exceed 300 mg/
day
$ AVAILABLE FORMS/COST OF THERAPY
• Inj, Sol—IM: 100 mg/ml, 10 ml:
$16.00
• Syr—Oral: 50 mg/ml, 480 ml:
$16.90-$20.00
• Tab, Uncoated—Oral: 100 mg,
100's: **$0.68-$5.61;** 300 mg, 100's:
$4.47-$5.25
CONTRAINDICATIONS: Previous
isoniazid-associated hepatic injury,
acute liver disease
PRECAUTIONS: Active chronic
liver disease, severe renal dysfunction, malnutrition, slow acetylators,
elderly, diabetes, alcoholics (increased
risk of peripheral neuropathy)
PREGNANCY AND LACTATION:
Pregnancy category C; the American Thoracic Society recommends
use of isoniazid for tuberculosis during pregnancy; excreted in breast
milk; women can safely breast feed
their infants while taking isoniazid
if the infant is periodically exam-
ined for signs and symptoms of peripheral neuritis or hepatitis
SIDE EFFECTS/ADVERSE REACTIONS
CNS: Fever, memory impairment, *pe-*
ripheral neuropathy, **seizures, toxic**
encephalopathy, toxic psychosis
EENT: Optic neuritis and atrophy
GI: Epigastric distress, **hepatotox-**
icity (mild and transient elevation of
serum transaminases in 10%-20%
does not require discontinuation;
progressive liver damage rare in patients <20 yr, but is seen in as many
as 2.3% of those >50 yr), nausea,
vomiting
HEME: **Agranulocytosis;** eosinophilia, **hemolytic, sideroblastic, or**
aplastic anemia; thrombocytope-
nia

---

italic = common side effects   ***bold italic*** = life-threatening reactions

METAB: Gynecomastia, hyperglycemia, hypocalcemia, hypophosphatemia, metabolic acidosis, pellagra, pyridoxine deficiency

SKIN: Skin eruptions, vasculitis

MISC: Rheumatic syndrome, systemic lupus erythematosis-like syndrome

INTERACTIONS

Drugs

◼ *Acetaminophen:* Increased acetaminophen concentrations, potential for hepatotoxicity

◼ *Antacids:* Reduced plasma isoniazid concentrations

◼ *Carbamazepine:* Increased serum carbamazepine concentrations, toxicity may occur

◼ *Corticosteroids:* Reduced plasma concentrations of isoniazid

◼ *Cycloserine:* Increased potential for CNS toxicity

◼ *Diazepam, triazolam:* Increased concentrations of these drugs

❷ *Disulfiram:* Adverse mental changes and coordination problems

◼ *Ethanol:* Higher incidence of isoniazid-induced hepatitis in alcoholics

◼ *Phenytoin:* Predictable increases in serum phenytoin concentrations, toxicity possible

◼ *Rifampin:* Increased hepatotoxicity of isoniazid in some patients; more common with slow acetylators of isoniazid, and/or pre-existing liver disease

◼ *Theophylline:* Increased theophylline concentrations, toxicity possible

◼ *Valproic acid:* Increased valproic acid concentration possible

◼ *Warfarin:* Potential for enhanced hypoprothrombinemic response to warfarin

Labs

• *False increase:* Serum AST, serum uric acid

• *False decrease:* Serum glucose

• *False positive:* Urine sugar

SPECIAL CONSIDERATIONS
PATIENT/FAMILY EDUCATION

• Take on empty stomach if possible; however, may be taken with food to decrease GI upset

• Minimize daily alcohol consumption to lessen the risk of hepatitis

• Notify clinician of weakness, fatigue, loss of appetite, nausea and vomiting, yellowing of skin or eyes, darkening of urine, numbness or tingling of hands and feet

MONITORING PARAMETERS

• Periodic ophthalmologic examinations even when visual symptoms do not occur

• Periodic liver function tests

---

isoproterenol

(eye-soe-proe-ter'e-nole)

Rx: Isuprel, Medihaler-Iso

Combinations

Rx: with phenylephrine (Duo-Medihaler)

Chemical Class: Synthetic catecholamine

Therapeutic Class: β-adrenergic agonist: antiasthmatic, bronchodilator; vasopressor; sympathomimetic

---

CLINICAL PHARMACOLOGY

Mechanism of Action: Stimulates β_1- and β_2-adrenergic receptors resulting in relaxation of bronchial, GI, and uterine smooth muscle, increased heart rate and contractility, vasodilation of peripheral vasculature; increases renal perfusion, cardiac output, decreases total peripheral resistance, and increasing blood pressure in cardiogenic or septicemic shock

Pharmacokinetics

IV: Onset rapid, duration 10 min

INH: Onset immediate

SC: Onset 30 min, duration up to 2 hr

Metabolized by conjugation in many tissues including the liver and lungs; $t_{1/2}$ 2½-5 min; excreted in urine (principally as sulfate conjugates)

INDICATIONS AND USES: Mild or transient episodes of heart block; serious episodes of heart block and Stokes-Adams attacks (except when caused by ventricular tachycardia or fibrillation); cardiac arrest (until electric shock or pacemaker is available); bronchospasm occurring during anesthesia, asthma, chronic bronchitis, or emphysema; hypovolemic and septic shock, low cardiac output (hypoperfusion) states, congestive heart failure, cardiogenic shock

DOSAGE

Adult

• *Bronchospasm:* MDI 1-2 puffs 4-6 times/day; neb 0.25-0.5 ml of a 1% sol diluted in 2-3 ml normal saline or 0.25% and 0.5% undiluted, treatment may be repeated up to 5 times/day

• *Dysrhythmia/heart block:* IV 0.02-0.06 mg (1-3 ml of 1:50,000 dilution) bolus, followed by subsequent doses of 0.01-0.2 mg (0.5-10 ml of 1:50,000 dilution); IV INF 5 µg/min initially, titrate to desired response, usual range 2-20 µg/min; IM 0.2 mg (1 ml of 1:5,000 dilution) initially, subsequent doses of 0.02-1 mg (0.1-5 ml of 1:5,000 dilution); SC 0.2 mg (1 ml of 1:5,000 dilution) initially, subsequent doses of 0.15-0.2 mg (0.75-1 ml of 1:5,000 dilution); IC 0.02 mg (0.1 ml of 1:5,000 dilution)

• *Shock:* IV INF 0.5-5 µg/min (0.25-2.5 ml of 1:500,000 dilution), titrate to patient response

Child

• *Bronchospasm:* MDI 1-2 puffs up to 6 times/day; neb 0.01 ml/kg of 1% sol; min dose 0.1 ml, max dose 0.5 ml diluted in 2-3 ml normal saline

• *Shock:* IV INF 0.05-2 µg/kg/min, rate (ml/hr) = dose (µg/kg/min) × weight (kg) × 60 min/hr divided by concentration (µg/ml)

AVAILABLE FORMS/COST OF THERAPY

• Sol—INH: 0.25%, 15 ml: **$12.50**

• Inj, Sol—IV: 0.02 mg/ml, 10 ml: **$16.11;** 0.2 mg/ml, 5 ml: **$3.83-$21.78**

CONTRAINDICATIONS: Tachydysrhythmias, tachycardia or heart block caused by digitalis intoxication, ventricular dysrhythmias requiring inotropic therapy, angina pectoris

PRECAUTIONS: Hypovolemia, CAD, coronary insufficiency, diabetes, hyperthyroidism

PREGNANCY AND LACTATION: Pregnancy category C; no reports linking isoproterenol with congenital defects have been located; excretion into breast milk unknown; use caution in nursing mothers

SIDE EFFECTS/ADVERSE REACTIONS

CNS: Anxiety, dizziness, headache, *mild tremors,* nervousness, weakness

CV: Angina, hypertension, hypotension, palpitations, tachycardia, ***tachydysrhythmias, ventricular dysrhythmias***

GI: Nausea, vomiting

RESP: ***Pulmonary edema***

SKIN: Flushing of skin, sweating

INTERACTIONS

Drugs

▨ *Amitriptyline:* Combined use may result in predisposition to cardiac arrhythmias

▨ *Beta-blockers:* Reduced effec-

---

italic = common side effects   ***bold italic*** = life-threatening reactions

tiveness of isoproterenol in the treatment of asthma
Labs
• *False increase:* Serum AST, serum bilirubin, serum glucose

---

isosorbide
(eye-soe-sor'bide)
Rx: Ismotic
Chemical Class: Hexatol ester
Therapeutic Class: Antiglaucoma agent; osmotic diuretic

CLINICAL PHARMACOLOGY
Mechanism of Action: Induces diuresis by elevating the osmolarity of glomerular filtrate, thereby hindering the tubular reabsorption of water
Pharmacokinetics
PO: Onset 10-30 min, peak 1-1½ hr, duration 5-6 hr, excreted unchanged in urine; $t_{1/2}$ 5-9½ hr
INDICATIONS AND USES: Short-term reduction of intraocular pressure prior to and after intraocular surgery; acute attack of glaucoma
DOSAGE
Adult
• PO 1.5 g/kg initially, then 1-3 g/kg bid-qid prn
$ AVAILABLE FORMS/COST OF THERAPY
• Sol—Oral: 45%, 220 ml: **$306.75**
CONTRAINDICATIONS: Well-established anuria, severe dehydration, pulmonary edema, severe cardiac decompensation, hypersensitivity
PRECAUTIONS: Diseases associated with salt retention
PREGNANCY AND LACTATION: Pregnancy category B; excretion into breast milk unknown; use caution in nursing mothers

SIDE EFFECTS/ADVERSE REACTIONS
CNS: Confusion, disorientation, dizziness, headache, lethargy, lightheadedness
CV: Syncope
EENT: Vertigo
GI: Gastric discomfort, nausea, thirst, vomiting
METAB: Hypernatremia, hyperosmolarity
SKIN: Rash
MISC: Hiccups, irritability
SPECIAL CONSIDERATIONS
PATIENT/FAMILY EDUCATION
• Palatability may be improved if the medication is poured over cracked ice and sipped
MONITORING PARAMETERS
• Fluid and electrolyte balance; urine output

---

isosorbide dinitrate/mononitrate
(eye-soe-sor'bide dye-nye'-trate/mon-oh-nye'trate)
Rx: *Dinitrate (sublingual chewable):* Isordil, Sorbitrate, Dilatrate-SR
Monnitrate (oral): Monoket, ISMO, Imdur, Isotrate ER
Chemical Class: Organic nitrate
Therapeutic Class: Antianginal

CLINICAL PHARMACOLOGY
Mechanism of Action: Stimulation of c-GMP production yields vascular smooth muscle relaxation; venous dilation predominates but dose-dependent dilation of arterial beds occurs; dilation of postcapillary vessels promotes venous pooling, decreases venous return to the heart, reducing left ventricular end-diastolic pressure (preload); arteri-

---

* = non-FDA-approved use

olar relaxation reduces systemic vascular resistance and arterial pressure (afterload); myocardial oxygen consumption/demand is decreased; blood pressure decreases with reflex

Pharmacokinetics

Dinitrate

PO: Onset 20-40 min, duration 4-6 hr
PO SUS REL: Onset up to 4 hr, duration 6-8 hr
SL: Onset 2-5 min, duration 1-3 hr
Metabolized by liver in urine as metabolites

Mononitrate

PO: Onset 30-60 min
Not subject to 1st-pass metabolism; <4% bound to plasma proteins; metabolized to inactive metabolites; $t_{1/2}$ 5 hr

INDICATIONS AND USES: Prevention of angina pectoris; relief of acute anginal episodes and prophylaxis prior to events likely to provoke an attack (SL dinitrate formulation only); CHF,* hypertension (acute)*

DOSAGE

• Asymmetric dosing regimens provide a daily nitrate-free interval to minimize the development of tolerance

Adult

• *Dinitrate:* SL 2.5-5 mg initially, titrate upward until angina is relieved or side effects limit the dose; chewable tabs 5 mg initially, titrate upward until angina is relieved or side effects limit the dose; PO 5-20 mg bid-tid initially (last dose no later than 7 PM), maintenance 10-40 mg bid-tid (last dose no later than 7 PM); PO SUS REL 40 mg qd-bid initially (last dose no later than 2 PM), maintenance 40-80 mg qd-bid (last dose no later than 2 PM)
• *Mononitrate:* PO 5-20 mg bid (with the 2 doses 7 hr apart); PO

SUS REL 30-60 mg qd initially, titrate to 120-240 mg qd if necessary

🔳 AVAILABLE FORMS/COST OF THERAPY

Dinitrate:

• Tab, SL—Oral: 2.5 mg, 100's: **$2.00-$28.93;** 5 mg, 100's: **$2.50-$31.08;** 10 mg, 100's: **$32.38**
• Tab, Uncoated—Oral: 5 mg, 100's: **$2.10-$27.84;** 10 mg, 100's: **$2.75-$36.14;** 20 mg, 100's: **$3.16-$56.08;** 30 mg, 100's: **$7.09-$63.06;** 40 mg, 100's: **$42.96-$68.40**
• Tab, Chewable—Oral: 5 mg, 100's: **$19.99;** 10 mg: **$24.79**
• Cap, Gel, SUS Action—Oral: 40 mg, 100's: **$63.40**
• Tab, Coated, SUS Action—Oral: 40 mg, 100's: **$4.95-$63.40**

Mononitrate:

• Tab, Uncoated—Oral: 10 mg, 100's: **$65.45-$80.18;** 20 mg, 100's: **$71.56-$84.74**
• Tab, Coated, SUS Action—Oral: 30 mg, 100's: **$111.55-$136.54;** 60 mg, 100's: **$116.11-$143.70;** 120 mg, 100's: **$201.18**

CONTRAINDICATIONS: Hypersensitivity to nitrates, severe anemia, closed-angle glaucoma, postural hypotension, head trauma or cerebral hemorrhage (may increase intracranial pressure), acute MI or CHF (mononitrate)

PRECAUTIONS: Acute MI, hypertrophic cardiomyopathy, glaucoma, volume depletion, hypotension, abrupt withdrawal, continuous delivery without nitrate-free interval (tolerance will develop)

PREGNANCY AND LACTATION: Pregnancy category C; excretion into breast milk unknown; use caution in nursing mothers

SIDE EFFECTS/ADVERSE REACTIONS

CNS: Agitation, anxiety, apprehension, confusion, *dizziness,* dyscoordination, *headache,* hypoesthesia, hypokinesia, insomnia, nervousness, nightmares, restlessness, vertigo, weakness

CV: **Atrial fibrillation, cardiovascular collapse, crescendo angina, dysrhythmias,** edema, hypotension (sometimes with paradoxical bradycardia and increased angina), palpitations, *postural hypotension,* premature ventricular contractions, rebound hypertension, retrosternal discomfort, syncope, tachycardia

EENT: Blurred vision, diplopia

GI: Abdominal pain, diarrhea, dyspepsia, involuntary passing of feces, nausea, tenesmus, vomiting

GU: Dysuria, impotence, involuntary passing of urine, urinary frequency

HEME: **Hemolytic anemia, methemoglobinemia**

MS: Arthralgia, muscle twitching

SKIN: Cold sweat, crusty skin lesions, exfoliative dermatitis, *flushing,* pallor, perspiration, pruritis, rash

INTERACTIONS

Drugs

3 *Alcohol:* Exaggerated hypotension and cardiac collapse

3 *Calcium channel blockers:* Exaggerated symptomatic orthostatic hypotension

3 *Dihydroertotamine:* Increases the bioavailability of dihydroertotamine with resultant increase in mean standing systolic blood pressure; functional antagonism, decreasing effects

3 *Sildenafil:* Excessive hypotensive effects

SPECIAL CONSIDERATIONS PATIENT/FAMILY EDUCATION

• Headache may be a marker for drug activity; do not try to avoid by altering treatment schedule; contact clinician if severe or persistent; aspirin or acetaminophen may be used for relief

• Dissolve SL tablets under tongue; do not crush, chew, or swallow

• Do not crush chewable tablets before administering

• Avoid alcohol

• Make changes in position slowly to prevent fainting

---

isotretinoin
(eye-soe-tret'i-noyn)
Rx: Accutane
Chemical Class: Vitamin A derivative
Therapeutic Class: Antiacne agent

CLINICAL PHARMACOLOGY

Mechanism of Action: Exact mechanism unknown; reduces sebaceous gland size and inhibits gland activity thereby decreasing sebum secretion; indirectly decreases the number of *Propionibacterium acnes* organisms within the follicle; exhibits antikeratinizing and anti-inflammatory actions

Pharmacokinetics

PO: Peak 3 hr; 99.9% bound to plasma proteins (almost exclusively to albumin); metabolized in liver and possibly in gut wall to 4-oxo-isotretinoin (active), eliminated via the bile and urine; $t_{1/2}$ 10-20 hr

INDICATIONS AND USES: Severe recalcitrant cystic acne; keratinization disorders (keratosis follicularis, pityriasis rubra pilaris, lamellar ichthyosis, keratosis palmaris et plantaris, congenital ichthyosiform erythroderma, rosacea, lichen planus, psoriasis)*; cutaneous T-cell lymphoma (mycosis fungoides) and leukoplakia*; prevention of skin cancer in patients with xeroderma pigmentosum*; prevention of 2nd primary tumors in patients treated for squamous cell carcinoma of the head and neck*

---

* = non-FDA-approved use

DOSAGE
Adult
• PO 0.5-2 mg/kg/day divided bid for 15-20 wk or until total cyst count decreases by 70%; a 2nd course may be initiated after ≥2 mo off therapy if warranted by persistent or recurring severe cystic acne

💲 AVAILABLE FORMS/COST OF THERAPY
• Cap, Elastic—Oral: 10 mg, 100's: **$481.62;** 20 mg, 100's: **$571.14;** 40 mg, 100's: **$663.54**

CONTRAINDICATIONS: Pregnancy, hypersensitivity to parabens (preservative in gelatin capsule)

PRECAUTIONS: Diabetes, obesity, family history of hypertriglyceridemia, contact lens use, inflammatory bowel disease

PREGNANCY AND LACTATION: Pregnancy category X; isotretinoin is a potent human teratogen; excretion into breast milk unknown, but based on the close relationship to vitamin A, the presence of isotretinoin in breast milk should be expected; avoid use in nursing mothers

SIDE EFFECTS/ADVERSE REACTIONS
CNS: Depression, fatigue, headache, **pseudotumor cerebri** (headache, visual disturbances, papilledema)
CV: Edema, palpitations, tachycardia, transient chest pain, vasculitis
EENT: Cataracts, contact lens intolerance, *conjunctivitis,* corneal opacities, decreased night vision, *dry eyes, dry nose, epistaxis,* eyelid inflammation, optic neuritis, photophobia, visual disturbances
GI: Abdominal pain, anorexia, *dry mouth,* gingival bleeding and inflammation, **hepatotoxicity,** increased liver function tests, inflammatory bowel disease, *nausea, vomiting,* weight loss

GU: Abnormal menses, *hematuria, proteinuria,* pyuria
HEME: **Anemia, thrombocytopenia,** *thrombocytosis*
METAB: Glucose intolerance, *hypertriglyceridemia*
MS: Bone, joint, and muscle pain and stiffness
SKIN: Bruising, *cheilitis, drying of mucous membranes, dry skin,* erythema nodosum, exaggerated healing response, *facial skin desquamation,* hyperpigmentation, hypopigmentation, *nail brittleness,* paronychia, peeling of palms and soles, *petechiae,* photosensitivity, *pruritis,* pyogenic granuloma, *rash, skin fragility,* skin infections, thinning of hair, urticaria

INTERACTIONS
Drugs
ℝ *Carbamazepine:* Decreased concentrations of carbamazepine in one patient

SPECIAL CONSIDERATIONS
• Have patient complete consent form included with package insert prior to initiating therapy

PATIENT/FAMILY EDUCATION
• Administer with meals
• Avoid alcohol
• Do not take vitamin supplements containing vitamin A
• **Women of childbearing potential should practice contraception during therapy and for 1 mo before and after therapy,** a pregnancy test within 2 wk of starting therapy is advised, begin on day 2 or 3 of the next menstrual period
• Notify clinician immediately if pregnancy is suspected
• A transient exacerbation of acne may occur during the initiation of therapy
• Avoid prolonged exposure to sunlight or sunlamps
• Do not donate blood during and for 30 days after stopping therapy

---

italic = common side effects   ***bold italic*** = life-threatening reactions

- Use caution driving or operating any vehicle at night
- Discontinue drug if visual difficulties occur and have an ophthalmologic exam

MONITORING PARAMETERS
- CBC with differential, platelet count, baseline sedimentation rate, serum triglycerides (baseline and biweekly for 4 wk), liver enzymes

---

isoxsuprine
(eye-sox′syoo-preen)
Rx: Vasodilan, Voxsuprine
Chemical Class: Phenoxyiso-propdylnorsuprifen
Therapeutic Class: Peripheral vasodilator

CLINICAL PHARMACOLOGY
Mechanism of Action: Vasodilation by direct effect on vascular smooth muscle, primarily within skeletal muscle; little effect on cutaneous blood flow; α-adrenoreceptor antagonism and β-adrenoreceptor stimulation produce cardiac stimulation and uterine relaxation
Pharmacokinetics
PO: Onset 1 hr; partially conjugated in blood; eliminated primarily in urine; $t_{1/2}$ 1¼ hr

INDICATIONS AND USES: "Possibly effective" for cerebral vascular insufficiency, peripheral vascular disease or arteriosclerosis obliterans, thromboangiitis obliterans, and Raynaud's disease; dysmenorrhea*; threatened premature labor*

DOSAGE
Adult
- PO 10-20 mg tid-qid

💲 AVAILABLE FORMS/COST OF THERAPY
- Tab, Uncoated—Oral: 10 mg, 100's: **$5.79-$38.80;** 20 mg, 100's: **$7.95-$62.15**

CONTRAINDICATIONS: Immediately postpartum, arterial bleeding
PREGNANCY AND LACTATION: Pregnancy category C; has been used to prevent premature labor; excretion into breast milk unknown; use caution in nursing mothers
SIDE EFFECTS/ADVERSE REACTIONS
CNS: Dizziness, weakness
CV: Chest pain, *hypotension,* tachycardia
GI: Abdominal distress, nausea, vomiting
SKIN: Flushing, *severe rash*
INTERACTIONS
Labs
- *False positive:* Urine amphetamine
SPECIAL CONSIDERATIONS
PATIENT/FAMILY EDUCATION
- Avoid sudden changes in posture to avoid dizziness (orthostatic hypotension)

---

isradipine
(is-rad′i-peen)
Rx: DynaCirc
Chemical Class: Dihydropyridine
Therapeutic Class: Calcium channel blocker: antihypertensive; antianginal

CLINICAL PHARMACOLOGY
Mechanism of Action: Inhibits calcium ion influx across cell membrane in vascular smooth muscle and cardiac muscle; produces relaxation of coronary and peripheral vascular smooth muscle; hemodynamics: decreases myocardial contractility; increases cardiac output; significantly decreases peripheral vascular resistance
Pharmacokinetics
PO: Peak serum concentration 1½ hr, onset 2 hr; significant first pass

---

* = non-FDA-approved use

metabolism; oral bioavailability 17%, 95% bound to plasma proteins; metabolized in liver, excreted in urine and feces (metabolites); $t_{1/2}$ 5-11 hr

INDICATIONS AND USES: Hypertension, chronic stable angina*

DOSAGE

Adult

• PO 2.5 mg bid initially, increase in 2-4 wk intervals prn to max of 10 mg bid; SUS REL PO 5 mg qd, may increase by 5 mg increments at 2-4 wk intervals, max 20 mg/day

§ AVAILABLE FORMS/COST OF THERAPY

• Cap, Gel—Oral: 2.5 mg, 100's: **$73.61;** 5 mg, 100's: **$108.04**
• Tab, SUS REL—Oral: 5 mg, 100's: **$121.64;** 10 mg, 100's: **$193.82**

PRECAUTIONS: CHF, hypotension, hepatic insufficiency, aortic stenosis, elderly, children

PREGNANCY AND LACTATION: Pregnancy category C; excretion into breast milk unknown; use caution in nursing mothers

SIDE EFFECTS/ADVERSE REACTIONS

CNS: Anxiety, asthenia, depression, dizziness, fatigue, headache, insomnia, malaise, nervousness, paresthesia, somnolence, tremor

CV: Bradycardia, *dysrhythmia,* hypotension, palpitations, *peripheral edema,* syncope, tachycardia

EENT: Epistaxis, nasal congestion, tinnitus

GI: Abdominal cramps, constipation, diarrhea, dry mouth, flatulence, gastric upset, nausea, vomiting

GU: Nocturia, polyuria, sexual dysfunction

SKIN: Hair loss, pruritus, rash, urticaria

MISC: Cough, flushing, muscle cramps, shortness of breath, sweating, weight gain

INTERACTIONS

Drugs

3 *Digitalis glycosides:* Increased digitalis levels; increased risk of toxicity

3 *Fentanyl:* Severe hypotension or increased fluid volume requirements

3 *Histamine H_2 antagonists:* Increased blood levels of nifedipine with cimetidine

3 *Lovastatin:* Decreased lovastatin concentrations

---

itraconazole

(it-ra-con'a-zol)
Rx: Sporanox
Chemical Class: Triazole derivative
Therapeutic Class: Antifungal

CLINICAL PHARMACOLOGY

Mechanism of Action: Inhibits the cytochrome P-450-dependent synthesis of ergosterol, which is a vital component of fungal cell membranes

Pharmacokinetics

PO: Peak 3-5 hr, requires acid pH for absorption, distributed poorly to CSF; 98% bound to plasma proteins; metabolized in liver to hydroxyitraconazole (active) and other metabolites; excreted in urine, bile, and feces; $t_{1/2}$ 60 hr

INDICATIONS AND USES: Blastomycosis, histoplasmosis, aspergillosis, oropharyngeal candidiasis (sol), esophageal candidiasis (sol), superficial mycoses (dermatophytoses, pityriasis versicolor, sebopsoriasis, candidiasis*), onychomycosis, systemic mycoses (candidiasis,* cryptococcal infections, paracoccidioidomycosis, coccidioidomycosis),* subcutaneous mycoses (sporotrichosis, chromomycosis),* cutaneous leishmaniasis,* fungal keratitis,* alternariosis,* zygomycosis*

DOSAGE

Adult

• *Oropharyngeal candidiasis:* PO 200 mg sol (20 ml) qd for 1-2 wk
• *Oropharyngeal candidiasis refractory to fluconazole:* PO 100 mg sol (10 ml) bid
• *Esophageal candidiasis:* PO 100 mg sol (10 ml) qd for 3 wk, treat for at least 2 wk past resolution of symptoms
• *Blastomycosis/histoplasmosis:* PO 200 mg qd; may increase if evidence of progressive disease to 300-400 mg/day in 2 divided doses
• *Aspergillosis:* PO 200-400 mg/day; doses >200 mg/day should be given in 2 divided doses
• *Life-threatening situations:* PO loading dose of 200 mg tid should be given for 1st 3 days
• *Onychomycosis:* PO 200 mg qd for at least 3 mo or 200 mg qd × 1 wk/mo

💲 AVAILABLE FORMS/COST OF THERAPY

• Cap, Gel—Oral: 100 mg, 30's: **$190.38**
• Susp—Oral: 10 mg/ml, 150 ml: **$98.04**

PRECAUTIONS: Hypersensitivity to other azole antifungals; preexisting hepatic function abnormalities, children, hypochlorhydria (reduces drug absorption)

PREGNANCY AND LACTATION: Pregnancy category C; excreted into breast milk; do not administer to nursing mothers

SIDE EFFECTS/ADVERSE REACTIONS

CNS: Decreased libido, depression, dizziness, fatigue, fever, headache, insomnia, malaise, somnolence
CV: Edema, hypertension
GI: Abdominal pain, anorexia, diarrhea, hepatitis, liver function test abnormality, *nausea,* vomiting
GU: Albuminuria, impotence
METAB: Hypokalemia
SKIN: Pruritis, rash (more common in patients receiving immunosupressants)

INTERACTIONS

Drugs

3 *Alprazolam:* Increased plasma alprazolam concentration
3 *Aluminum:* Reduced itraconazole absorption
3 *Amprenavir:* Increased plasma amprenavir concentration
3 *Antacids:* Reduced itraconazole absorption
⚠ *Astemizole:* QT prolongation and life-threatening dysrhythmia
3 *Atevirdine:* Increased plasma atevirdine concentration
3 *Atorvastatin:* Increased plasma atorvastatin concentration with risk of rhabdomyolysis
3 *Buspirone:* Increased plasma buspirone concentration
3 *Calcium:* Reduced itraconazole absorption
3 *Cerivastatin:* Increased plasma cerivastatin concentration with risk of rhabdomyolysis
3 *Chlordiazepoxide:* Increased plasma chlordiazepoxide concentration
3 *Cimetidine:* Reduced itraconazole absorption
⚠ *Cisapride:* QT prolongation and life-threatening dysrhythmia
3 *Clarithromycin:* Increased plasma itraconazole concentration
3 *Cyclosporine:* Increased plasma cyclosporine concentration
3 *Diazepam:* Increased plasma diazepam concentration
3 *Digoxin:* Increased plasma digoxin concentration
3 *Didanosine:* Reduced itraconazole absorption

* = non-FDA-approved use

3 *Erythromycin:* Increased plasma itraconazole concentration

3 *Ethanol:* Disulfiram-like reaction possible

3 *Famotidine:* Reduced itraconazole absorption

3 *Felodipine:* Increased plasma felodipine concentration

3 *Fluvastatin:* Increased plasma fluvastatin concentration with risk of rhabdomyolysis

3 *Food:* Increased intraconazole absorption

3 *Indinavir:* Increased plasma indinavir concentration

3 *Lansoprazole:* Reduced itraconazole absorption

2 *Lovastatin:* Increased plasma lovastatin concentration with risk of rhabdomyolysis

3 *Magnesium:* Reduced itraconazole absorption

3 *Methadone:* Increased plasma methadone concentration

3 *Methylprednisolone:* Increased plasma methylprednisolone concentration

3 *Midazolam:* Increased plasma midazolam concentration

3 *Nelfinavir:* Increased plasma nelfinavir concentration

3 *Nizatidine:* Reduced itraconazole absorption

3 *Omeprazole:* Reduced itraconazole absorption

3 *Oral anticoagulants:* Increased hypoprothrombinemic response

2 *Phenytoin:* Markedly reduced plasma itraconazole concentration

⚠ *Pimozide:* Increased plasma pimozide concentration, QT prolongation and life-threatening dysrhythmia

3 *Pravastatin:* Increased plasma pravastatin concentration with risk of rhabdomyolysis

⚠ *Quinidine:* Increased plasma quinidine concentration, QT prolongation and life-threatening dysrhythmia

3 *Rifampin:* Decreased plasma itraconazole concentration; decreased plasma rifampin concentration

3 *Ritonavir:* Increased plasma ritonavir concentration

3 *Saquinavir:* Increased plasma saquinavir concentration

2 *Simvastatin:* Increased plasma simvastatin concentration with risk of rhabdomyolysis

3 *Sodium bicarbonate:* Reduced itraconazole absorption

3 *Sucralfate:* Reduced intraconazole absorption

3 *Tacrolimus:* Increased plasma tacrolimus concentration

⚠ *Terfenadine:* QT prolongation and life-threatening dysrhythmia

3 *Tolbutamide:* Increased plasma tolbutamide concentration

2 *Triazolam:* Increased plasma triazolam concentration

3 *Warfarin:* Increased hypoprothrombinemic response

SPECIAL CONSIDERATIONS
PATIENT/FAMILY EDUCATION
• Take with food to ensure maximal absorption
• Avoid antacids within 2 hr of itraconazole administration

MONITORING PARAMETERS
• Liver function tests in patients with pre-existing abnormalities

---

ivermectin
(eye-vir-mek'tin)
Rx: Mectizan, Stromectol
Chemical Class: Avermectin derivative
Therapeutic Class: Anthelmintic

CLINICAL PHARMACOLOGY
Mechanism of Action: Acts as a glutamate and gamma amino bu-

---

italic = common side effects   **bold italic** = life-threatening reactions

tyric acid agonist causing hyperpolarization of invertebrate nerve and muscle cells and death of susceptible organisms

Pharmacokinetics

PO: Peak plasma level 4 hr; does not cross blood-brain barrier; metabolized by liver; excreted in feces; $t_{1/2}$ 18-38 hr

INDICATIONS AND USES: Oncocerciasis, intestinal strongyloidiasis, ascariasis,* bancroftian filariasis,* enterobiasis,* trichuriasis,* scabies,* pediculosis*

DOSAGE

Adult and Child >15 kg

• *Strongyloidiasis:* PO 3 mg (15-24 kg), 6 mg (25-35 kg), 9 mg (36-50 kg), 12 mg (51-65 kg), 15 mg (66-79 kg), 200 µg/kg (>80 kg)

• *Oncocerciasis:* PO 3 mg (15-24 kg), 6 mg (25-35 kg), 9 mg (36-50 kg), 12 mg (51-65 kg), 15 mg (66-79 kg), 150 µg/kg (>80 kg)

• *Ascariasis:* PO 50-200 µg/kg

• *Enterobiasis:* PO 50-200 µg/kg

• *Trichuriasis:* PO 200 µg/kg qd × 2 days

• *Scabies:* TOP 0.8% solution applied to entire body; PO 12 mg

$ AVAILABLE FORMS/COST OF THERAPY

• Tab, Uncoated—Oral: 6 mg, 10's: **$9.38**

PRECAUTIONS: Rapid killing of microfilariae may induce systemic or ocular inflammatory response (Mazzotti reaction)

PREGNANCY AND LACTATION: Pregnancy category C; excreted in breast milk in low concentrations

SIDE EFFECTS/ADVERSE REACTIONS

CNS: Dizziness, somnolence, tremor, vertigo

GI: Anorexia, constipation, diarrhea, increased transaminase levels, nausea

HEME: **Leukopenia**

SKIN: Pruritus, rash, urticaria

MISC: Fatigue

PATIENT/FAMILY EDUCATION

• Rapid killing of microfilariae may induce systemic or ocular inflammatory response (Mazzotti reaction, manifest by pruritus, rash, lymphadenopathy, and fever)

MONITORING PARAMETERS

• Stool for parasites; blood for microfilaria and eosinophils

---

kanamycin

(kan-a-mye'sin)
Rx: Kantrex
Chemical Class: Aminoglycoside
Therapeutic Class: Antibiotic

CLINICAL PHARMACOLOGY

Mechanism of Action: Interferes with protein synthesis in bacterial cell by binding to 30S ribosomal subunit, which causes misreading of genetic code; inaccurate peptide sequence forms in protein chain, causing bacterial death

Pharmacokinetics

IM: Onset rapid, peak 1-2 hr

IV: Onset immediate

Plasma $t_{1/2}$ 2-3 hr; not metabolized, excreted unchanged in urine

INDICATIONS AND USES: Severe systemic infections of CNS, respiratory, GI, urinary tract, bone, skin, soft tissues caused by susceptible organisms; *Mycobacterium avium* complex infections (as part of a multiple-drug regimen),* cystic fibrosis (inhaled),* suppression of intestinal bacteria (PO), hepatic coma (PO)

Antibacterial spectrum usually includes

• Gram-positive organisms: penicillinase- and non-penicillinase-producing *Staphylococcus* spp. (in general, has a low order of activity against other Gram-positive organisms)

• Gram-negative organisms: *Escherichia coli, Proteus* spp. (indole-positive and indole-negative), *Providencia* spp., *Klebsiella-Enterobacter-Serratia* spp., *Acinetobacter* spp., *Citrobacter* spp., *Shigella* spp., *Yersinia pestis, Hemophilus influenzae, Neisseria* spp., *Salmonella* spp.

DOSAGE
Adult
• *Severe systemic infections:* IM/IV 15 mg/kg/day divided q8-12h; do not exceed 1.5 g/day
• *Suppression of intestinal bacteria:* PO 1g q1h for 4 hr, followed by 1 g q6h for 36-72 hr
• *Hepatic coma:* PO 8-12 g/day in divided doses
• *Aerosol treatment:* 250 mg bid-qid; withdraw 250 mg (1 ml) from 500 mg vial, dilute with 3 ml normal saline, and nebulize
• *Intraperitoneal:* 500 mg diluted in 20 ml sterile distilled water instilled through a polyethylene catheter into wound (absorption similar to IM use)
Child
• *Severe systemic infections:* IM/IV 15 mg/kg/day divided q8-12h; do not exceed 1.5 g/day

🔳 AVAILABLE FORMS/COST OF THERAPY
• Inj, Sol—IM, IV: 1 g/3 ml, 3 ml: **$2.50-$10.00;** 75 mg/2 ml, 2 ml: **$3.04-$3.50;** 500 mg/2 ml, 2 ml: **$3.36-$5.00**
• Cap, Gel—Oral: 0.5 g, 100's: **$198.25**

CONTRAINDICATIONS: Hypersensitivity to aminoglycosides
PRECAUTIONS: Neonates, renal disease, myasthenia gravis, hearing deficits, Parkinson's disease, elderly, dehydration

PREGNANCY AND LACTATION: Pregnancy category D; 8th cranial nerve toxicity in the fetus has been reported; excreted into breast milk in low concentrations; poor oral availability reduces potential for ototoxicity for the infant; compatible with breast feeding

SIDE EFFECTS/ADVERSE REACTIONS
CNS: Headache, ***neuromuscular blockade,*** paresthesia
EENT: Deafness, hearing loss, loss of balance, ototoxicity
GI: Diarrhea, nausea, vomiting
GU: Azotemia, hematuria, ***nephrotoxicity, oliguria, renal failure***
MS: ***Acute muscular paralysis***
RESP: Apnea
SKIN: Rash

INTERACTIONS
Drugs
🔳 *Amphotericin B:* Synergistic nephrotoxicity
❷ *Atracurium:* Kanamycin potentiates respiratory depression by atracurium
🔳 *Carbenicillin:* Potential for inactivation of kanamycin in patients with renal failure
🔳 *Carboplatin:* Additive nephrotoxicity or ototoxicity
🔳 *Cephalosporins:* Increased potential for nephrotoxicity in patients with preexisting renal disease
🔳 *Cisplatin:* Additive nephrotoxicity or ototoxicity
🔳 *Cyclosporine:* Additive nephrotoxicity
❷ *Ethacrynic acid:* Additive ototoxicity
🔳 *Indomethacin:* Reduced renal clearance of kanamycin in premature infants
🔳 *Methoxyflurane:* Additive nephrotoxicity

K

---

italic = common side effects   ***bold italic*** = life-threatening reactions

❷ *Neuromuscular blocking agents:* Kanamycin potentiates respiratory depression by neuromuscular blocking agents

▪ *NSAIDs:* May reduce renal clearance of kanamycin

▪ *Penicillins (extended spectrum):* Potential for inactivation of kanamycin in patients with renal failure

▪ *Piperacillin:* Potential for inactivation of kanamycin in patients with renal failure

❷ *Succinylcholine:* Kanamycin potentiates respiratory depression by succinylcholine

▪ *Ticarcillin:* Potential for inactivation of kanamycin in patients with renal failure

▪ *Vancomycin:* Additive nephrotoxicity or ototoxicity

❷ *Vecuronium:* Kanamycin potentiates respiratory depression by vecuronium

Labs
• *False increase:* Urine amino acids

SPECIAL CONSIDERATIONS
PATIENT/FAMILY EDUCATION
• Report headache, dizziness, loss of hearing, ringing, roaring in ears, or feeling of fullness in head
MONITORING PARAMETERS
• Urinalysis
• Urine output
• Serum peak drawn at 30-60 min after IV INF or 60 min after IM inj, trough level drawn just before next dose; adjust dosage per levels, especially in renal function impairment (usual therapeutic plasma levels; peak 15-30 mg/L, trough ≤10 mg/L)
• Serum creatinine for CrCl calculation
• Serum calcium, magnesium, sodium
• Audiometric testing; assess hearing before, during, after treatment

kaolin-pectin
(kay′o-lynn)
OTC: Kao-Spen, Kapectolin, Kaolinpec
Combinations
  OTC: with bismuth subcarbonate (K-C); with bismuth subsalicylate (Kaodene non-narcotic)
Chemical Class: Kaolin: hydrous magnesium aluminum silicate; pectin: purified carbohydrate product
Therapeutic Class: Antidiarrheal

CLINICAL PHARMACOLOGY
Mechanism of Action: May act as adsorbents and protectants; effects in the treatment of diarrhea remain to be clearly established
INDICATIONS AND USES: Diarrhea
DOSAGE
Adult
• PO 60-120 ml after each loose bowel movement
Child 6-12 yr
• PO 30-60 ml after each loose bowel movement
Child 3-6 yr
• PO 15-30 ml after each loose bowel movement
💲 **AVAILABLE FORMS/COST OF THERAPY**
• Susp—Oral: 5.2 g (kaolin)/260 mg (pectin)/30 ml, 480 ml: **$3.75-$4.61**
• Liq—Oral: 5.8 g (kaolin)/130 mg (pectin)/30 ml, 480 ml: **$4.00**
PRECAUTIONS: Infants, debilitated elderly patients
PREGNANCY AND LACTATION: Pregnancy category C; neither agent is systemically absorbed; should have no effect on lactation or nursing infant

---

* = non-FDA-approved use

SIDE EFFECTS/ADVERSE REACTIONS

GI: Constipation

INTERACTIONS

Drugs

❷ *Clindamycin, lincomycin:* Reduced antibacterial efficacy of these drugs

❸ *Digoxin:* Reduced bioavailability of digoxin tablets, capsules not affected

❸ *Lovastatin:* Pectin inhibits cholesterol lowering effects of lovastatin

❸ *Quinidine:* Reduced plasma quinidine concentrations

SPECIAL CONSIDERATIONS
PATIENT/FAMILY EDUCATION

• Do not self-medicate diarrhea for >48 hr without consulting a provider

---

ketoconazole

(kee-toe-koe′na-zole)

Rx: Nizoral

Chemical Class: Imidazole derivative

Therapeutic Class: Antifungal

CLINICAL PHARMACOLOGY

Mechanism of Action: Inhibits biosynthesis of ergosterol or other sterols, damaging the fungal cell membrane and altering its permeability with resultant loss of essential intracellular elements; inhibits several fungal enzymes resulting in build-up of toxic concentrations of hydrogen peroxide; inhibits biosynthesis of triglycerides and phospholipids by fungi

Pharmacokinetics

PO: Bioavailability decreases as gastric pH increases, peak 1-4 hr; partially metabolized by liver to inactive metabolites, excreted mainly in feces (57%) and urine (13%); $t_{1/2}$ 8 hr; CSF penetration poor

INDICATIONS AND USES: TAB:
candidiasis, chronic mucocutaneous candidiasis, oral thrush, candiduria, blastomycosis, coccidioidomycosis, histoplasmosis, chromomycosis, paracoccidioidomycosis; severe recalcitrant dermatophyte infections, onychomycosis,* pityriasis versicolor*; tinea corporis, pedis, capitus, cruris*; vaginal candidiasis,* advanced prostate cancer (high doses)*; Cushing's syndrome (high doses)*; CRE: tinea corporis, cruris, pedis; pityriasis versicolor, cutaneous candidiasis, seborrheic dermatitis, SHAMPOO: seborrhea

DOSAGE

Adult

• PO 200 mg qd initially, increase to 400 mg qd for serious infections or if clinical response insufficient; duration 1-2 wk (candidiasis), 6 mo (other indicated systemic mycoses)

• CRE: apply qd to affected area for 2 wk (bid for 4 wk for seborrheic dermatitis)

• Shampoo twice weekly for 4 wk with at least 3 days between each shampooing, then intermittently prn

Child >2 yr

• PO 3.3-6.6 mg/kg/day as a single dose

🔳 AVAILABLE FORMS/COST OF THERAPY

• Cre—Top: 2%, 15, 30, 60 g: **$25.63**/30 g

• Shampoo—Top: 2%, 120 ml: **$18.84**

• Tab, Uncoated—Oral: 200 mg, 100's: **$306.80**

CONTRAINDICATIONS: Fungal meningitis (poor CSF penetration)

PRECAUTIONS: Renal disease, hepatic disease, achlorhydria (drug-induced), children <2 yr, other hepatotoxic agents, sulfite sensitivity (CRE)

---

italic = common side effects   ***bold italic*** = life-threatening reactions

K

PREGNANCY AND LACTATION: Pregnancy category C; has been used, apparently without harm, for the treatment of vaginal candidiasis during pregnancy; not detected in plasma with chronic shampoo use; unknown if cre absorbed; oral ketoconazole probably excreted in breast milk; use in breast feeding not recommended

SIDE EFFECTS/ADVERSE REACTIONS

CNS: Dizziness, headache, somnolence

GI: Abdominal pain, anorexia, diarrhea, ***hepatotoxicity,*** nausea, vomiting

GU: Gynecomastia, impotence, oligospermia (high doses)

HEME: **Hemolytic anemia, leukopenia, thrombocytopenia**

SKIN: Dermatitis, pruritus, purpura, rash, urticaria

MISC: Chills, fever, photophobia

INTERACTIONS

Drugs

🔳 *Alprazolam:* Increased plasma alprazolam concentration

🔳 *Aluminum:* Reduced ketoconazole absorption

🔳 *Amprenavir:* Increased plasma amprenavir concentration

🔳 *Antacids:* Reduced ketoconazole absorption

🅰 *Astemizole:* QT prolongation and life-threatening dysrhythmia

🔳 *Atevirdine:* Increased plasma atevirdine concentration

🔳 *Atorvastatin:* Increased plasma atorvastatin concentration with risk of rhabdomyolysis

🔳 *Buspirone:* Increased plasma buspirone concentration

🔳 *Calcium:* Reduced ketoconazole absorption

🔳 *Chlordiazepoxide:* Increased plasma chlordiazepoxide concentration

🔳 *Cimetidine:* Reduced ketoconazole absorption

➋ *Cisapride:* QT prolongation and dysrhythmia

🔳 *Cyclosporine:* Increased plasma cyclosporine concentration

🔳 *Diazepam:* Increased plasma diazepam concentration

🔳 *Didanosine:* Reduced ketoconazole absorption

🔳 *Ethanol:* Disulfiram-like reaction possible

🔳 *Famotidine:* Reduced ketoconazole absorption

🔳 *Felodipine:* Increased plasma felodipine concentration

🔳 *Fluvastatin:* Increased plasma fluvastatin concentration with risk of rhabdomyolysis

🔳 *Indinavir:* Increased plasma indinavir concentration

🔳 *Lansoprazole:* Reduced ketoconazole absorption

➋ *Lovastatin:* Increased plasma lovastatin concentration with risk of rhabdomyolysis

🔳 *Magnesium:* Reduced ketoconazole absorption

🔳 *Methadone:* Increased plasma methadone concentration

🔳 *Methylprednisolone:* Increased plasma methylprednisolone concentration

🔳 *Midazolam:* Increased plasma midazolam concentration

🔳 *Nelfinavir:* Increased plasma nelfinavir concentration

🔳 *Nizatidine:* Reduced ketoconazole absorption

🔳 *Omeprazole:* Reduced ketoconazole absorption

🔳 *Oral anticoagulants:* Increased hypoprothrombinemic response

🔳 *Pravastatin:* Increased plasma pravastatin concentration with risk of rhabdomyolysis

🔳 *Quinidine:* Increased plasma quinidine concentration

3 *Rifampin:* Decreased plasma ketoconazole concentration; decreased plasma rifampin concentration

3 *Ritonavir:* Increased plasma ritonavir concentration

3 *Saquinavir:* Increased plasma saquinavir concentration

2 *Simvastatin:* Increased plasma simvastatin concentration with risk of rhabdomyolysis

3 *Sodium bicarbonate:* Reduced ketoconazole absorption

3 *Sucralfate:* Reduced ketoconazole absorption

3 *Tacrolimus:* Increased plasma tacrolimus concentration

⚠ *Terfenadine:* QT prolongation and life-threatening dysrhythmia

3 *Tolbutamide:* Increased plasma tolbutamide concentration

3 *Triazolam:* Increased plasma triazolam concentration

3 *Warfarin:* Increased hypoprothrombinemic response

SPECIAL CONSIDERATIONS
PATIENT/FAMILY EDUCATION

• For shampoo, moisten hair and scalp, apply shampoo, and gently massage over entire scalp for 1 min; rinse with warm water; repeat, leaving shampoo on scalp for additional 3 min

• Do not take tab with antacids or H_2-receptor antagonists; separate doses by at least 2 hr

• Take tablets with food

MONITORING PARAMETERS

• Liver function tests at baseline and periodically during treatment

---

ketoprofen
(kee-toe-proe'fen)
Rx: Orudis, Oruvail
OTC: Actron, Orudis KT
Chemical Class: Propionic acid derivative
Therapeutic Class: NSAID with analgesic and antipyretic activity

CLINICAL PHARMACOLOGY
Mechanism of Action: Reversible cyclooxygenase (i.e., prostaglandin synthetase) inhibitor; non-selectively decreases the formation of both prostaglandins and thromboxane A2; variable effects on lipoxygenase synthesis and subsequent leukotriene production; antiinflammatory, antipyretic, and analgesic activity; inhibits platelet aggregation

Pharmacokinetics
PO: Peak 0.5-2 hr, highly bound to plasma proteins; metabolized primarily in liver, excreted in urine (60%-75%) and feces; $t_{1/2}$ 1-4 hr

INDICATIONS AND USES: Biliary colic,* dysmenorrhea, fever, osteoarthritis, rheumatoid arthritis, renal colic,* soft tissue injuries,* ankylosing spondylitis,* prevention of cognitive decline,* pain—mild to moderate

DOSAGE
Adult

• PO 150-300 mg in divided doses tid-qid, not to exceed 300 mg/day; PO SUS 100-200 mg qd (not recommended for acute pain); PO (OTC) 12.5 mg q4-6h, if pain or fever persist for more than 1 hr, follow with additional 12.5 mg dose

💲 AVAILABLE FORMS/COST OF THERAPY

• Cap, Gel—Oral: 25 mg, 100's: **$65.68-$95.78;** 50 mg, 100's: **$89.25-$117.58;** 75 mg, 100's: **$98.40-$130.78**

• Cap, Gel, SUS Action—Oral: 100 mg, 100's: **$181.48-$219.78**; 150 mg, 100's: **$220.58-$267.13**; 200 mg, 100's: **$249.00-$301.61**

• Tab—Oral: 12.5 mg, 100's: **$7.90-$8.57** (OTC)

CONTRAINDICATIONS: Bronchospasm, nasal polyps, angioedema precipitated by aspirin or other NSAIDs

PRECAUTIONS: History of GI ulceration, bleeding, or perforation; renal dysfunction, hypertension or cardiac conditions aggravated by fluid retention and edema, history of liver dysfunction, history of coagulation

PREGNANCY AND LACTATION: Pregnancy category B (category D if used in 3rd trimester); could cause constriction of the ductus arteriosus *in utero;* persistent pulmonary hypertension of the newborn or prolonged labor; unknown if excreted into human breast milk

SIDE EFFECTS/ADVERSE REACTIONS

CNS: Dizziness, headache, lightheadedness

CV: Chest pain, ***CHF, dysrhythmias,*** edema, hypertension, hypotension, palpitation, tachycardia

EENT: Dry eyes, hearing disturbances, photophobia, tinnitus, visual disturbances

GI: Abdominal cramps, constipation, diarrhea, *dyspepsia,* flatulence, **gastric or duodenal ulcer with bleeding or perforation,** hepatitis, *nausea,* occult blood in stool, ***pancreatitis,*** vomiting

GU: **Acute renal failure**

HEME: **Agranulocytosis,** eosinophilia, **leukopenia, neutropenia, pancytopenia, thrombocytopenia**

METAB: Hyperglycemia, hyperkalemia, hypoglycemia, hyponatremia

RESP: Bronchospasm, dyspnea

SKIN: Photosensitivity, rash, urticaria

INTERACTIONS

Drugs

3 *Aminoglycosides:* Reduced clearance with elevated aminoglycoside levels and potential for toxicity (especially indomethacin in premature infants; other NSAIDs probably)

3 *Anticoagulants:* Excessive hypoprothrombinemia, decreased platelet aggregation with increased risk of GI bleeding

3 *Antihypertensives (α-blockers, angiotensin-converting enzyme inhibitors, angiotensin II receptor blockers, β-blockers, diuretics):* Inhibition of antihypertensive and other favorable hemodynamic effects

3 *Corticosteroids:* Increased risk of GI ulceration

3 *Cyclosporine:* Increased nephrotoxicity risk

3 *Lithium:* Decreased clearance of lithium (mediated via prostaglandins) resulting in elevated serum lithium levels and risk of toxicity

3 *Methotrexate:* Decreased renal secretion of methotrexate resulting in elevated methotrexate levels and risk of toxicity

3 *Phenylpropanolamine:* Possible acute hypertensive reaction

3 *Potassium-sparing diuretics:* Additive hyperkalemia potential

3 *Triamterene:* Acute renal failure reported with addition of indomethacin; caution with other NSAIDs

Labs

• *False decrease:* Serum ALT, AST; serum lactate dehydrogenase

SPECIAL CONSIDERATIONS

• No significant advantage over other NSAIDs; cost should govern use

---

* = non-FDA-approved use

PATIENT/FAMILY EDUCATION
• Avoid aspirin and alcoholic beverages
• Take with food, milk, or antacids to decrease GI upset

MONITORING PARAMETERS
• Initial hemogram and fecal occult blood test within 3 mo of starting regular chronic therapy; repeat every 6-12 mo (more frequently in high-risk patients (>65 years, peptic ulcer disease, concurrent steroids or anticoagulants); electrolytes, creatinine, and BUN within 3 mo of starting regular chronic therapy; repeat every 6-12 mo

---

ketorolac
(kee-toe'role-ak)
Rx: Systemic: Toradol
Ophthalmic: Acular, Acular PF
Chemical Class: Acetic acid derivative
Therapeutic Class: NSAID with analgesic and antipyretic activity

CLINICAL PHARMACOLOGY
Mechanism of Action: Reversible cyclooxygenase (i.e., prostaglandin synthetase) inhibitor; non-selectively decreases the formation of both prostaglandins and thromboxane A2; variable effects on lipoxygenase synthesis and subsequent leukotriene production; antiinflammatory, antipyretic, and analgesic activity; inhibits platelet aggregation

Pharmacokinetics
PO: Peak 0.5-1 hr
IM: Onset 10 min, duration up to 6 hr
99% bound to plasma proteins; metabolized in liver, excreted in urine (metabolites); $t_{1/2}$ 2.4-8.6 hr (increased in elderly, renal impairment)

INDICATIONS AND USES: Cancer pain,* cataract extraction—inflammation, cholecystectomy pain,* conjunctivitis—seasonal allergic, corneal abrasion,* cystoid macular edema,* fracture reduction—pain,* gouty arthritis,* headache,* narcotic sparing effect,* ocular pain, pain control with regional anesthesia,* pain—moderately severe

DOSAGE
Adult
• IM (single-dose treatment) one 60 mg dose; (multiple-dose treatment) 30 mg q6h for no more than 5 days, max 120 mg/day; IV (single-dose treatment) one 30 mg dose; (multiple-dose treatment) 30 mg q6h for no more than 5 days, max 120 mg/day; PO (indicated only as continuation therapy for parenteral ketorolac) 20 mg as a 1st dose then 10 mg q4-6h for no longer than 5 days (including parenteral therapy), max 40 mg/day

• *Elderly (>65 yr), renal impairment, weight <50 kg:* IM (single-dose treatment) one 30 mg dose; (multiple-dose treatment) 15 mg q6h for no more than 5 days, max 60 mg/day; IV (single-dose treatment) one 15 mg dose; (multiple-dose treatment) 15 mg q6h for no more than 5 days, max 60 mg/day; PO 10 mg q4-6h for no more than 5 days (including parenteral therapy), max 40 mg/day

• OPHTH 1 gtt qid

$ **AVAILABLE FORMS/COST OF THERAPY**
• Inj, Sol—IV/IM: 15 mg/ml, 1 ml: **$6.05-$80.00;** 30 mg/ml, 1 ml: **$6.35-$84.00**
• Sol—Ophth: 0.5%, 5 ml: **$40.90**
• Tab, Uncoated—Oral: 10 mg, 100's: **$92.97-$119.10**

CONTRAINDICATIONS: Bronchospasm, nasal polyps, angioedema

---

italic = common side effects   ***bold italic*** = life-threatening reactions

precipitated by aspirin or other NSAIDs; active peptic ulcer disease, recent GI bleeding or perforation; advanced renal impairment, volume depletion; before any major surgery; suspected or confirmed cerebrovascular bleeding, hemorrhagic diathesis, incomplete hemostasis, and those at high risk of bleeding; concurrent ASA or NSAIDs; neuraxial (epidural or intrathecal) administration due to its alcohol content; concomitant use of probenecid; while wearing soft contact lenses (ophth)

PRECAUTIONS: History of GI ulceration, bleeding, or perforation; renal dysfunction, hypertension or cardiac conditions aggravated by fluid retention and edema, history of liver dysfunction, history of coagulation

PREGNANCY AND LACTATION: Pregnancy category C; excreted into breast milk; not recommended in lactation

SIDE EFFECTS/ADVERSE REACTIONS

CNS: Dizziness, headache, lightheadedness

CV: Chest pain, ***CHF, dysrhythmias,*** edema, hypertension, palpitation, tachycardia

EENT: Dry eyes, hearing disturbances, photophobia, tinnitus; visual disturbances; *burning, stinging upon instillation (ophth)*

GI: Abdominal cramps, constipation, diarrhea, *dyspepsia,* flatulence, ***gastric or duodenal ulcer with bleeding or perforation,*** hepatitis, *nausea,* occult blood in stool, ***pancreatitis,*** vomiting

GU: ***Acute renal failure***

HEME: ***Agranulocytosis,*** eosinophilia, ***leukopenia, neutropenia, pancytopenia, thrombocytopenia***

METAB: Hyperglycemia, hyperkalemia, hypoglycemia, hyponatremia

RESP: ***Bronchospasm,*** dyspnea

SKIN: Photosensitivity, rash, urticaria

INTERACTIONS

Drugs

▨ *Aminoglycosides:* Reduced clearance with elevated aminoglycoside levels and potential for toxicity (especially indomethacin in premature infants; other NSAIDs probably)

▨ *Anticoagulants:* Excessive hypoprothrombinemia, decreased platelet aggregation with increased risk of GI bleeding

▨ *Antihypertensives (α-blockers, angiotensin-converting enzyme inhibitors, angiotensin II receptor blockers, β-blockers, diuretics):* Inhibition of antihypertensive and other favorable hemodynamic effects

▨ *Corticosteroids:* Increased risk of GI ulceration

▨ *Cyclosporine:* Increased nephrotoxicity risk

▨ *Lithium:* Decreased clearance of lithium (mediated via prostaglandins) resulting in elevated serum lithium levels and risk of toxicity

▨ *Methotrexate:* Decreased renal secretion of methotrexate resulting in elevated methotrexate levels and risk of toxicity

▨ *Phenylpropanolamine:* Possible acute hypertensive reaction

▨ *Potassium-sparing diuretics:* Additive hyperkalemia potential

▨ *Triamterene:* Acute renal failure reported with addition of indomethacin; caution with other NSAIDs

SPECIAL CONSIDERATIONS

PATIENT/FAMILY EDUCATION

• Not for chronic use

• No significant advantage over other oral NSAIDs; cost and clinical situation should govern use; no reason to continue parenteral course

---

* = non-FDA-approved use

of therapy with oral ketorolac (more expensive, more toxic)

• Combined use of ketorolac parenteral and oral should not exceed 5 days

---

labetalol
(la-bet´a-lole)

Rx: Normodyne, Trandate
Combinations
   Rx: with hydrochlorothiazide
   (Normozide, Trandate
   HCT)
Chemical Class: Nonselective β-adrenergic blocker; peripheral α-adrenergic blocker
Therapeutic Class: Antihypertensive

CLINICAL PHARMACOLOGY
Mechanism of Action: Combines both selective, competitive postsynaptic α_1-adrenergic blocking and nonselective, competitive β-adrenergic blocking activity; produces reduction in systemic arterial pressure and total peripheral resistance, without significant effects on resting heart rate or cardiac output; produces negative inotropic and chronotropic responses; slows AV nodal conduction; decreases heart rate; decreases myocardial oxygen consumption; antiarrhythmic effects (class II); reduction in platelet aggregation and blood viscosity; suppression of renin release; inhibition of central sympathetic outflow; decreases presynaptic receptor neurotransmitter release; weak intrinsic sympathomimetic activity; no membrane stabilizing activity; moderate lipid solubility
Pharmacokinetics
PO: Onset 20 min-2 hr, peak 1-4 hr, duration 8-24 hr
IV: Onset 5 min, peak 5-15 min, duration 2-4 hr

50% bound to plasma proteins; metabolized in liver, excreted in urine and feces (metabolites); $t_{1/2}$ 5.5-8 hr
INDICATIONS AND USES: Hypertension, eclampsia, preeclampsia, postmyocardial infarction,* supraventricular arrhythmias (atrial fibrillation, atrial flutter, paroxysmal supraventricular tachycardia),* aggressive behavior,* angina pectoris,* anxiety,* congestive heart failure,* tremor,* aortic dissection,* drug withdrawal syndromes (clonidine, alcohol)* electroconvulsive therapy-induced adverse effects,* hypertensive urgencies and emergencies,* stimulant drug overdoses (cocaine, epinephrine, pseudoephedrine),* pheochromocytoma,* post- and intraoperative hypertension,* Raynaud's phenomenon, tetanus, tyramine-monoamine oxidase inhibitor interaction*
DOSAGE
Adult and Child >16 yr
• *Angina pectoris:* PO 100-400 mg bid-tid
• *Hypertension:* PO 100 mg bid; increase q2-3 days in 100 mg bid increments; usually maintenance dose, 200-400 mg bid; max 1200-2400 mg bid dosing; IV bolus—1-2 mg/kg (may overshoot); alternate 20, 40, 80, 160 q1h or until satisfactory control; IV INF 2 mg/min allows for safe titration
• Reduce dose by 50% in patients with chronic liver disease
Child
• *Hypertension:* PO 0.2 to 1 mg/kg/day divided bid
§ AVAILABLE FORMS/COST OF THERAPY
• Inj, Sol—IV: 5 mg/ml, 20 ml: **$35.34-$40.09**
• Tab, Coated—Oral: 100 mg, 100's: **$48.00-$55.21**; 200 mg, 100's: **$68.10-$78.32**; 300 mg, 100's: **$90.59-$104.18**

L

---

italic = common side effects   ***bold italic*** = life-threatening reactions

CONTRAINDICATIONS: Bronchial asthma, cardiogenic shock, overt cardiac failure, second and third degree AV block, severe sinus bradycardia

PRECAUTIONS: Anesthesia/surgery (myocardial depression), avoid abrupt withdrawal, bronchospastic airways, congestive heart failure, diabetes mellitus, hyperthyroidism/thyrotoxicosis (labetolol, unlike propranolol, does not decrease T_3 levels), concurrent clonidine (discontinue labetolol several days prior to withdrawal of clonidine); peripheral vascular disease, renal disease

PREGNANCY AND LACTATION: Pregnancy category C; similar drug, atenolol, frequently used in the third trimester for treatment of hypertension (many studies of efficacy and safety of atenolol in pregnancy-induced hypertension); long-term use has been associated with intrauterine growth retardation; only a small amount of drug appears in milk (0.004% of dose); unlikely to be therapeutically significant

SIDE EFFECTS/ADVERSE REACTIONS

CNS: Anxiety, catatonia, depression, dizziness, drowsiness, fatigue, headache, lethargy, mental changes, nightmares, paresthesias (scalp tingling)

*CV: **AV block,** bradycardia, chest pain, **CHF,** orthostatic hypotension, ventricular dysrhythmias*

EENT: Double vision, dry burning eyes, sore throat, tinnitus, visual changes

GI: Diarrhea, nausea, vomiting

GU: Dysuria, ejaculatory failure, impotence, Peyronie's disease

*HEME: **Agranulocytosis, thrombocytopenic purpura*** (reported with other β-blockers only) (rare)

MS: Asthenia, muscle cramps, toxic myopathy

*RESP: **Bronchospasm,** dyspnea, wheezing*

SKIN: Alopecia, fever, pruritus, rash, urticaria

INTERACTIONS

Drugs

🔳 *α-1 adrenergic blockers:* Potential enhanced first dose response (marked initial drop in blood pressure, particularly on standing)

🔳 *Amiodarone:* Symptomatic bradycardia and sinus arrest; AV node refractory period prolonged and sinus node automaticity decreased, especially patients with bradycardia, sick sinus syndrome, or partial AV

🔳 *Cimetidine:* Increased plasma labetolol concentrations

🔳 *Clonidine:* Withdrawal of clonidine abruptly may exaggerate the hypertension due to unopposed alpha stimulation; safer than other β-blockers, however

🔳 *Digoxin:* Additive prolongation of atrioventricular (AV) conduction time

🔳 *Dihydropyridine calcium channel blockers:* Severe hypotension or impaired cardiac performance; most prevalent with impaired left ventricular function, cardiac arrhythmias, or aortic stenosis

🔳 *Diltiazem:* Potentiates β-adrenergic effects; hypotension, left ventricular failure, and AV conduction disturbances problematic in elderly, patients with left ventricular dysfunction, aortic stenosis, or with large doses of either drug

🔳 *Epinephrine:* Increased diastolic pressure and bradycardia during epinephrine infusions

🔳 *Hypoglycemic agents:* Masked hypoglycemia, hyperglycemia

🔳 *NSAIDs:* Reduced hypotensive effects of β-blockers

❷ *Theophylline:* Antagonistic pharmacodynamic effects

❸ *Verapamil:* Potentiates β-adrenergic effects; hypotension, left ventricular failure, and AV conduction disturbances problematic in elderly, patients with ventricular dysfunction, aortic stenosis, or with large doses of either drug

Labs
• *False positive:* Urine amphetamine
• *False increase:* Urinary catecholamines, plasma epinephrine

SPECIAL CONSIDERATIONS
PATIENT/FAMILY EDUCATION
• Do not discontinue abruptly; may require taper; rapid withdrawal may produce rebound hypertension or angina
• Transient scalp tingling may occur, especially when treatment is initiated
• May mask the symptoms of hypoglycemia, except for sweating, in diabetic patients

MONITORING PARAMETERS
• Angina: Reduction in nitroglycerin usage; frequency, severity, onset, and duration of angina pain; heart rate
• Arrhythmias: Heart rate
• Congestive heart failure: Functional status, cough, dyspnea on exertion, paroxysmal nocturnal dyspnea, exercise tolerance, and ventricular function
• Hypertension: Blood pressure
• Postmyocardial infarction: Left ventricular function, lower resting heart rate
• Toxicity: Blood glucose, bronchospasm, hypotension, bradycardia, depression, confusion, hallucination, sexual dysfunction

---

lactulose
(lak'tyoo-lose)
Rx: Cephulac, Cholac, Chronulac, Constilac, Constulose, Duphalac, Enulose, Generlac, Kristalose
Chemical Class: Synthetic disaccharide analog of lactose
Therapeutic Class: Ammonia detoxicant; laxative

CLINICAL PHARMACOLOGY
Mechanism of Action: Hydrolyzed by colonic bacteria to low molecular weight acids, which convert ammonia (NH_3) to ammonium ion (NH_4+), trapping it and preventing its absorption; laxative action due to increased osmotic pressure of colonic contents and increased stool water content

Pharmacokinetics
PO: Poorly absorbed, does not produce effect until reaching colon, 24-48 hr may be required to produce normal bowel movement

INDICATIONS AND USES: Constipation; portal-systemic encephalopathy

DOSAGE
Adult
• *Constipation:* PO 15-30 ml qd; increase to 60 ml qd if necessary
• *Portal-systemic encephalopathy:* PO 30-45 ml tid-qid, adjust dose to produce 2-3 soft stools/day; PR mix 300 ml lactulose with 700 ml water, instill 180 ml via rectal balloon catheter and retain for 30-60 min, repeat q4-6h

Child
• *Constipation:* PO 7.5 ml qd after breakfast
• *Portal-systemic encephalopathy:* PO 40-90 ml/day divided tid-qid; adjust dose to produce 2-3 soft stools/day

---

italic = common side effects   ***bold italic*** = life-threatening reactions

Infant
• *Portal-systemic encephalopathy:*
PO 2.5-10 ml/day divided tid-qid;
adjust dose to produce 2-3 soft
stools/day

🔋 **AVAILABLE FORMS/COST
OF THERAPY**

• Sol—Oral: 10 g/15 ml, 480 ml:
$10.94-$22.85
• Syr—Oral: 10 g/15 ml, 480 ml:
$26.05-$44.22
• Powder, Packet—Oral: 10 gm/
packet, 30's: **$75.25;** 20 gm/packet
30's: **$91.95**

CONTRAINDICATIONS: Patients
requiring a low galactose diet

PRECAUTIONS: Electrocautery
procedures (may spark explosion),
diabetes

PREGNANCY AND LACTATION:
Pregnancy category B; breast feeding risk to fetus and the newborn
negligible

**SIDE EFFECTS/ADVERSE REAC-
TIONS**

*GI: Abdominal discomfort, belch-
ing,* diarrhea, *flatulence, gaseous distension, nausea,* vomiting

INTERACTIONS
Labs
• *False increase:* Serum creatinine

SPECIAL CONSIDERATIONS
PATIENT/FAMILY EDUCATION
• May be mixed with fruit juice,
water, or milk to increase palatability
• Do not take other laxatives while
on lactulose therapy

MONITORING PARAMETERS
• Serum electrolytes, carbon dioxide periodically during chronic treatment

---

lamivudine (3TC)
(la-miv'yoo-deen)
Rx: Epivir, Epivir-HBV
Combinations
  Rx: with zidovudine: (Com-
    bivir)
Chemical Class: Nucleoside
analog
Therapeutic Class: Antiretro-
viral

CLINICAL PHARMACOLOGY
Mechanism of Action: Phosphorylated to active 5′-triphosphate metabolite, which inhibits HIV reverse
transcription via viral DNA chain
termination; also inhibits the RNA-
and DNA-dependent DNA polymerase activities of reverse transcriptase

Pharmacokinetics
PO: Rapidly absorbed, bioavailability 86%; <36% bound to plasma
proteins, 54%-57% bound to erythrocytes; majority eliminated unchanged in urine; $t_{1/2}$ 5-7 hr (prolonged in renal failure)

INDICATIONS AND USES: HIV infection in combination with zidovudine, chronic hepatitis B*

DOSAGE
Adult and Child ≥12 yr
• *HIV:* PO 150 mg bid in combination with zidovudine; in renal failure adjust dose as follows: CrCl
30-49 ml/min 150 mg qd; CrCl
15-29 ml/min 150 mg × 1, then 100
mg qd; CrCl 5-14 ml/min 150
mg × 1, then 50 mg qd; CrCl <5
ml/min 50 mg × 1, then 25 mg qd
• For latest treatment guidelines, see
www.hivatis.org
• *Chronic hepatitis B:* PO 100 mg
qd
Child 3 mo-11 yr
• *HIV:* PO 4 mg/kg bid (up to maximum of 150 mg bid) in combina-

---

* = non-FDA-approved use

tion with zidovudine; adjust dose in renal failure (see adult dose)

• For latest treatment guidelines, see www.hivatis.org

💲 **AVAILABLE FORMS/COST OF THERAPY**

• Tab, Film Coated—Oral: 150 mg, 60's: **$245.39**

• Sol—Oral: 10 mg/ml, 240 ml: **$65.43**

PRECAUTIONS: Impaired renal function; patients at risk for pancreatitis (especially in children)

PREGNANCY AND LACTATION: Pregnancy category C; not recommended in nursing mothers

SIDE EFFECTS/ADVERSE REACTIONS

CNS: Depression, dizziness, fatigue, *headache,* insomnia, neuropathy

EENT: Nasal signs and symptoms

GI: Abdominal cramps, abdominal pain, anorexia, *diarrhea,* dyspepsia, increased ALT/AST, *nausea,* **pancreatitis (incidence ~15% in children),** vomiting

HEME: **Anemia, neutropenia, thrombocytopenia**

MS: Arthralgia, musculoskeletal pain, myalgia

RESP: Cough

SKIN: Rash

---

lamotrigine

(la-moe-trih'jeen)

Rx: Lamictal, Lamictal CD

Chemical Class: Phenyltriazine derivative

Therapeutic Class: Anticonvulsant

CLINICAL PHARMACOLOGY

Mechanism of Action: Inhibits voltage-sensitive sodium channels thereby stabilizing neuronal membranes and consequently modulating presynaptic transmitter release

of excitatory amino acids (e.g., glutamate and aspartate)

Pharmacokinetics

PO: Peak 1.4-4.8 hr; 55% bound to plasma proteins; metabolized by glucuronic acid conjugation, eliminated in urine as unchanged drug (10%) and inactive glucuronides (86%); induces its own metabolism; $t_{1/2}$ 25.4-32.8 hr

INDICATIONS AND USES: Adjunctive therapy of partial seizures; generalized tonic-clonic,* absence,* atypical absence,* myoclonic seizures*; Lennox-Gastaut syndrome*

DOSAGE

Adult

• *Patients receiving enzyme-inducing antiepileptic drugs (AEDs) and no valproic acid:* PO 50 mg qd for 2 wk, followed by 50 mg bid for 2 wk, then 300-500 mg/day divided bid (escalate dose by 100 mg/day qwk)

• *Patients receiving enzyme-inducing AEDs plus valproic acid:* PO 25 mg qod for 2 wk, followed by 25 mg qd for 2 wk, then 100-150 mg/day divided bid (escalate dose by 25-50 mg/day q1-2 wk)

💲 **AVAILABLE FORMS/COST OF THERAPY**

• Tab, Uncoated—Oral: 25 mg, 100's: **$187.94;** 100 mg, 100's: **$199.50;** 150 mg, 60's: **$125.78;** 200 mg, 60's: **$131.86**

• Tab, Chewable—Oral: 5 mg, 100's: **$177.60;** 25 mg, 100's: **$186.00**

CONTRAINDICATIONS: Children <16 yr (high incidence of severe, potentially life-threatening rashes)

PRECAUTIONS: Abrupt discontinuation (reduce by 50% qwk over at least 2 wk), renal/hepatic function impairment, children, cardiac function impairment

PREGNANCY AND LACTATION: Pregnancy category C; passes into

L

---

breast milk, effects on infants exposed by this route are unknown

SIDE EFFECTS/ADVERSE REACTIONS

CNS: Anxiety, *ataxia,* chills, confusion, decreased memory, depression, *dizziness,* emotional lability, fever, *headache,* insomnia, irritability, **seizure exacerbation,** sleep disorder, *somnolence,* speech disorder, tremor, vertigo

CV: Hot flushes, palpitations

EENT: Blurred vision, diplopia, ear pain, tinnitus

GI: Abdominal pain, *nausea, vomiting*

GU: Amenorrhea, dysmenorrhea, vaginitis

MS: Arthralgia, joint disorder, myasthenia, neck pain

RESP: Dyspnea, increased cough, pharyngitis, rhinitis

SKIN: Acne, alopecia, angioedema, photosensitivity, pruritus, *rash,* **Stevens-Johnson syndrome, toxic epidermal necrolysis**

INTERACTIONS

Drugs

3 *Carbamazepine:* Increased carbamazepine epoxide levels; decreased lamotrigine levels

3 *Phenobarbital, primidone, phenytoin:* Decreased lamotrigine concentrations

3 *Valproic acid:* Increased lamotrigine concentration; decreased valproic acid concentration

SPECIAL CONSIDERATIONS
PATIENT/FAMILY EDUCATION

• Notify clinician immediately if a skin rash develops

• Avoid prolonged exposure to direct sunlight

lansoprazole

(lan-soe'pray-zole)
Rx: Prevacid
Chemical Class: Substituted benzimidazole derivative
Therapeutic Class: Gastrointestinal antisecretory agent

CLINICAL PHARMACOLOGY

Mechanism of Action: Irreversibly inactivates proton pump in gastric parietal cells, which blocks the final step in secretion of hydrochloric acid; acid secretion is inhibited until additional enzyme is synthesized; inhibits basal and stimulated gastric acid secretion

Pharmacokinetics

PO: Peak 1.7 hr, duration >24 hr; 97% bound to plasma proteins; extensively metabolized in the liver, eliminated as metabolites in urine (33%) and feces (66%); $t_{1/2}$ <2 hr (does not reflect duration of acid suppression)

INDICATIONS AND USES: Short-term treatment of duodenal ulcer; maintenance of healed duodenal ulcers (for up to 1 yr); in combination with clarithromycin and/or amoxicillin for the eradication of *H. pylori* infection in patients with active or recurrent duodenal ulcers; short-term treatment of benign gastric ulcer; short-term treatment of erosive esophagitis; maintenance of healed erosive esophagitis (for up to 1 yr); pathologic hypersecretory conditions (Zollinger-Ellison syndrome, multiple endocrine adenomas, systemic mastocytosis)

DOSAGE

Adult

• *Duodenal ulcer:* PO 15 mg qd before eating for 4 wk; maintenance 15 mg qd

• *H. pylori:* PO 30 mg plus 500 mg clarithromycin and 1 g amoxicillin all given bid for 14 days; or 30 mg plus 1 g amoxicillin given tid for 14 days (intolerance to clarithromycin)
• *Erosive esophagitis:* PO 30 mg qd before eating for 8 wk; may treat an additional 8 wk if complete healing not present; maintenance 15 mg qd
• *Zollinger-Ellison syndrome:* PO 60 mg qd initially; increase as needed up to 180 mg/day; doses >120 mg/day should be divided bid

$ **AVAILABLE FORMS/COST OF THERAPY**
• Cap, Gel, SUS Action—Oral: 15 mg, 100's: **$352.73**, 30 mg, 100's: **$359.44**

PRECAUTIONS: Children, maintenance therapy in duodenal ulcer; symptomatic response does not preclude gastric cancer

PREGNANCY AND LACTATION: Pregnancy category B; excretion into breast milk unknown

SIDE EFFECTS/ADVERSE REACTIONS
CNS: Headache
GI: Abdominal pain, diarrhea, increased ALT and AST, nausea

INTERACTIONS
Drugs
3 *Cefpodoxime, cefuroxime, ketoconazole, enoxacin:* Reduced concentrations of these drugs
3 *Digoxin, nifedipine:* Increased serum concentrations of these drugs
3 *Food:* 50% decrease in absorption if given 30 min after food compared to the fasting condition
3 *Glipizide, glyburide, tolbutamide:* Increased concentrations of these drugs, potential for hypoglycemia

SPECIAL CONSIDERATIONS
• For patients with a nasogastric tube, capsules may be opened and the intact granules mixed with 40 ml of apple juice and injected through tube into stomach
• For patients unable to swallow capsules, capsule can be opened and the intact granules sprinkled on 1 tablespoon of applesauce and swallowed immediately; do not crush or chew granules

---

latanoprost
(lah-tan′o-prost)
Rx: Xalatan
Chemical Class: Prostaglandin $F_{2-\alpha}$ analog
Therapeutic Class: Antiglaucoma agent

CLINICAL PHARMACOLOGY
Mechanism of Action: Increases aqueous humor outflow, reducing intraocular pressure
Pharmacokinetics
OPHTH: Absorbed through cornea, hydrolyzed to active acid; peak 2 hrs; intraocular pressure reduction starts in 3-4 hr, maximum effect 8-12 hr; plasma $t_{1/2}$ 17 min; hepatic metabolite cleared by kidneys

INDICATIONS AND USES: Ocular hypertension and open-angle glaucoma in patients intolerant or nonresponsive to another agent

DOSAGE
Adult
• *TOP:* apply 1 gtt in affected eye(s) each evening

$ **AVAILABLE FORMS/COST OF THERAPY**
• Sol—Top: 0.005% (50 µg/ml), 2.5 ml: **$45.03**

PRECAUTIONS: Concurrent corneal disease or disruption of ocular epithelial surface (risk bacterial keratitis with contaminated multi-dose container)

PREGNANCY AND LACTATION: Pregnancy category C; unknown if excreted into breast milk

L

SIDE EFFECTS/ADVERSE REACTIONS

CV: Angina, chest pain

EENT: Blurred vision, burning, conjunctival hyperemia, conjunctivitis, discharge from eye, dry eye, eye pain, *foreign body sensation, increased pigmentation of iris, itching,* kiplopia, lid crusting, lid discomfort, lid edema, lid erythema, photophobia, *punctate epithelial keratopathy,* retinal artery embolus, retinal detachment, *stinging,* tearing, vitreous hemorrhage from diabetic retinopathy

MS: Arthralgia, myalgia

SKIN: Rash

DRUG INTERACTIONS

Drugs

3 *Thimerisol:* Precipitate forms

SPECIAL CONSIDERATIONS

• May cause darkening of iris; may not be noticeable for months to years; may be permanent

• Darkening of iris caused by increased pigment in melanocytes; long-term significance unknown; monitor and consider stopping if occurs

• Does not cause darkening of freckles, nevi

• Administer with at least 5 min interval if drops containing thimerosal used

• Do not administer while wearing contact lenses; may reinsert 15 min later

• If other top ophth drugs used, administer ≥5 min apart

• To decrease risk of infection, do not allow tip of container to contact eye

---

leflunomide
(le-flu′na-mide)
Rx: Arava
Chemical Class: Isoxazole derivative
Therapeutic Class: Immunomodulatory agent; disease-modifying antirheumatic drug (DMARD)*

CLINICAL PHARMACOLOGY

Mechanism of Action: T-cell pyrimidine biosynthesis inhibitor—antiproliferative and antiinflammatory effects; disease-modifying antirheumatic effects not completely evaluated

Pharmacokinetics

PO: 80% bioavailable; no food effect on absorption; metabolized to active metabolite (which is responsibe for immunomodulating activity); peak metabolite levels at 6 to 12 hr with low Vd and extensive albumin binding (>93%); renal elimination following further hepatic metabolism (renal elimination predominates over the first 96 hr, after which fecal elimination becomes more prominent); elimination half-life of major metabolite, approximately 14 days (4-28 days)—long half-life mandates loading dose to facilitate rapid attainmnet of steady-state blood levels and clinical effects

INDICATIONS AND USES: Rheumatoid arthritis, organ transplantation*

DOSAGE

Adult and Child <18 yr

• *Rheumatoid arthritis: Loading dose* 100 mg qd for 3 days; *Maintenance dose* 20 mg daily (10 mg qd if side effects intolerable); *Drug elimination procedure:* cholestyramine 8 g tid × 11 days (consecu-

---

* = non-FDA-approved use

tive days not necessary); without these extra measures, nondetectable plasma levels would take ≤2 years, after drug discontinuation

§ AVAILABLE FORMS/COST OF THERAPY

• Tab, coated—Oral: 10 mg, 30's: **$244.80**; 20 mg, 30's: 100 mg, **$244.80**; 3's: **$122.40**

CONTRAINDICATIONS: Preexisting liver impairment

PRECAUTIONS: Hepatotoxicity, renal insufficiency, immunodeficiency, bone-marrow dysplasia, severe infections (potential for immunosuppression)

PREGNANCY AND LACTATION: Pregnancy category X; amount of excretion into breast milk unknown; use of leflunomide by nursing mothers is not recommended since the potential risk to nursing infants is considered serious

SIDE EFFECTS/ADVERSE REACTIONS

CNS: Headache, dizziness, paresthesia
CV: Hypertension
GI: Diarrhea, nausea, abdominal pain, hepatitis, abnormal liver enzymes
GU: Polyuria, dysuria
METAB: Weight loss
RESP: Respiratory infection, bronchitis
SKIN: Alopecia, rash, pruritis

INTERACTIONS

Drugs

3 *Cholestyramine, charcoal:* Coadministration results in rapid and significant decrease in active metabolite

3 *Nonsteroidal antiinflammatory drugs:* Inhibition of CYP 2C9, decreases the metabolism of many NSAIDS

3 *Rifampin:* Leflunomide levels increased 40%

SPECIAL CONSIDERATIONS

• Discuss potential risks of pregnancy and recommend appropriate contraception

PATIENT/FAMILY EDUCATION

MONITORING PARAMETERS

• *Efficacy:* ESR, C-reactive protein, platelet count, hemoglobin, improvement of RA; *toxicity:* LFTs (baseline, then monthly until stable)

---

lepirudin
(leh-peer'u-din)
Rx: Refludan
Chemical Class: Polypeptide
Therapeutic Class: Anticoagulant

CLINICAL PHARMACOLOGY

Mechanism of Action: Binds to and directly inhibits the thrombogenic activity of thrombin; a recombinant hirudin (natural hirudin is produced in trace amounts by the leech *Hirudo medicinalis*)

Pharmacokinetics

IV: Likely metabolized by catabolic hydrolysis; approximately 48% excreted in urine (35% as unchanged drug); terminal $t_{1/2}$ 1.3 hr (prolonged in patients with marked renal insufficiency)

INDICATIONS AND USES: Anticoagulation in patients with heparin-induced thrombocytopenia (HIT) and associated thromboembolic disease in order to prevent further thromboembolic complications

DOSAGE

Adult

• *Initial dose:* IV 0.4 mg/kg (max 44 mg) injected over 15-20 sec, followed by 0.15 mg/kg/hr (max 16.5 mg/hr) as continuous INF for 2-10 days or longer if clinically needed

• *Dose modifications:* If aPTT ratio is above target range (1.5-2.5), stop INF for 2 hr; at restart, decrease INF

L

rate by 50% (no additional IV bolus should be administered); determine aPTT ratio again in 4 hr; if aPTT ratio is below target range, increase INF rate in steps of 20%, determine aPTT again in 4 hr

• *Renal function impairment:* IV 0.2 mg/kg injected over 15-20 sec, followed by continuous INF based on creatinine clearance, 0.075 mg/kg/hr (creatine clearance 45-60 ml/min), 0.045 mg/kg/hr (30-44 mg/min), 0.0225 mg/kg/hr (15-29 ml/min); avoid if creatinine clearance <15 ml/min; additional aPTT monitoring is highly recommended

• *Concomitant use with thrombolytic therapy:* IV 0.2 mg/kg bolus, followed by 0.1 mg/kg/hr as continuous INF

• *Patients scheduled to switch to oral anticoagulation:* Gradually reduce lepirudin dose in order to reach an aPTT ratio just above 1.5 before initiating oral anticoagulation; stop lepirudin as soon as international normalized ratio (INR) of 2.0 is reached

$ **AVAILABLE FORMS/COST OF THERAPY**

• Inj, powder—IV: 50 mg, 1 vial: **$126.00**

PRECAUTIONS: Recent puncture of large vessels or organ biopsy; anomaly of vessels or organs; recent cerebrovascular accident, stroke, intracerebral surgery or other neuraxial procedures; severe uncontrolled hypertension; bacterial endocarditis; advanced renal impairment; hemorrhagic diathesis; recent major surgery; recent major bleeding; children; severe liver dysfunction; prolonged therapy

PREGNANCY AND LACTATION: Pregnancy category B; use caution in nursing mothers

SIDE EFFECTS/ADVERSE REACTIONS

CV: **Heart failure**
GI: Abnormal liver function
GU: Abnormal kidney function
HEME: **Bleeding**
SKIN: Allergic skin reactions
MISC: Fever, **multiorgan failure,** allergic reactions

INTERACTIONS

Drugs

3 *Thrombolytics (tPA, streptokinase, urokinase, reteplase):* Increased risk of bleeding complications; enhanced effect of lepirudin on aPTT prolongation

3 *Antithrombotic agents (warfarin, aspirin, ticlopidine, clopidogrel, persantine):* Inceased risk of bleeding

SPECIAL CONSIDERATIONS

• Untreated, HIT can lead to thrombosis, venous thromboembolism, acute MI, peripheral artery occlusion, and stroke; mortality rate approaches 20% to 30%

• All sources of heparin must be discontinued as soon as HIT is detected

• In clinical trials the cumulative risk of death 35 days after starting treatment was 9% in the lepirudin-treated patients, compared with 18% in historical controls; cumulative risk of new thromboembolic complications was 6% with lepirudin and 22% in historical controls

MONITORING PARAMETERS

• aPTT ratio (patient aPTT over median of laboratory normal range for aPTT); target range 1.5-2.5; do not start in patients with baseline aPTT ratio ≥2.5; determine aPTT ratio 4 hr following start of INF and at least daily thereafter

• CBC with platelet count (to detect bleeding complications and monitor recovery of platelets)

leucovorin
(loo-koe-vor'in)
Rx: Leucovorin
Chemical Class: Folic acid derivative
Therapeutic Class: Dihydrofolate reductase inhibitor antidote; hematinic

CLINICAL PHARMACOLOGY
Mechanism of Action: Reduced form of folic acid that does not require reduction by dihydrofolate reductase and, therefore, is not affected by blockage of this enzyme by dihydrofolate reductase inhibitors (e.g., methotrexate)

Pharmacokinetics
PO: Peak 1.72 hr, onset 20-30 min, duration 3-6 hr
IM: Peak 0.71 hr, onset 10-20 min, duration 3-6 hr
IV: Onset <5 min, duration 3-6 hr
Metabolized by liver and intestinal mucosa to active metabolite, eliminated in the urine (80%-90%) and feces (5%-8%); $t_{1/2}$ 6.2 hr

INDICATIONS AND USES: Rescue therapy following high-dose methotrexate therapy in osteosarcoma and inadvertant overdoses of dihydrofolate reductase inhibitors (methotrexate, pyrimethamine, trimetrexate, trimethoprim); megaloblastic anemias due to folic acid deficiency (parenteral); palliative therapy of advanced colorectal cancer in combination with 5-fluorouracil (parenteral)

DOSAGE
Adult and Child
• Give parenterally when individual doses are >25 mg
• *Folate deficient megaloblastic anemia:* IM 1 mg/day
• *Megaloblastic anemia secondary*
to congenital deficiency of dihydrofolate reductase: IM 3-6 mg/day
• *Rescue dose:* PO/IV/IM 15 mg (approximately 10 mg/m^2) every 6 hr for 10 doses starting 24 h after the beginning of the methotrexate INF (administer parenterally in the presence of GI toxicity, nausea, or vomiting); if serum creatinine is elevated >50% 24 hr after methotrexate **or** the 24 hr serum methotrexate level is $>5 \times 10^{-6}$M, increase dose to 100 mg/m^2/dose q3h until serum methotrexate level is $<5 \times 10^{-8}$M
• *Advanced colorectal cancer:* Consult current protocols

💲 **AVAILABLE FORMS/COST OF THERAPY**
• Inj, Sol—IV/IM: 50 mg/vial: **$18.40-$56.25;** 100 mg/vial: **$35.00-$56.25;** 200 mg/vial: **$78.00;** 350 mg/vial: **$137.94**
• Tab, Uncoated—Oral: 5 mg, 100's: **$209.93-$235.20;** 15 mg, 24's: **$200.96;** 25 mg, 25's: **$397.28-$600.00**

CONTRAINDICATIONS: Pernicious anemia and other megaloblastic anemias secondary to vitamin B$_{12}$ deficiency
PRECAUTIONS: Third-space fluid accumulation (i.e., ascites, pleural effusion), renal insufficiency, or inadequate hydration (may increase leucovorin requirement to prevent methotrexate toxicity)
PREGNANCY AND LACTATION: Pregnancy category C; has been used in the treatment of megaloblastic anemia during pregnancy; compatible with breast feeding
SIDE EFFECTS/ADVERSE REACTIONS
*RESP: **Anaphylactoid reactions,*** wheezing
SKIN: Urticaria
SPECIAL CONSIDERATIONS
• Administer as soon as possible fol-

L

---

lowing overdoses of dihydrofolate reductase inhibitors

MONITORING PARAMETERS

• CBC with differential and platelets, electrolytes, and liver function tests prior to each treatment with leucovorin/5-fluorouracil combination

• Plasma methotrexate concentrations as a therapeutic guide to high-dose methotrexate therapy with leucovorin rescue; continue leucovorin until plasma methotrexate concentrations are $<5 \times 10^{-8}$M (see dosage)

• Serum creatinine

---

leuprolide

(loo'proe-lide)

Rx: Lupron, Oaklide, Lupron Depot, Lupron Depot-Ped

Chemical Class: Synthetic gonadotropin-releasing hormone (GnRH)

Therapeutic Class: Antineoplastic; antiendometriosis agent

CLINICAL PHARMACOLOGY

Mechanism of Action: GnRH agonist; inhibits gonadotropin secretion when given continuously in therapeutic doses; after initial stimulation, chronic leuprolide results in suppression of ovarian and testicular steroidogenesis, which is reversible upon discontinuation

Pharmacokinetics

SC: Peak 3 hr

IM (depot): Peak 4 hr, duration >4 wk 7%-15% bound to plasma proteins; $t_{1/2}$ 3 hr

INDICATIONS AND USES: Advanced prostate cancer, endometriosis, central precocious puberty; breast, ovarian, and endometrial cancer*; leiomyoma uteri,* infertility,* prostatic hypertrophy*

DOSAGE

Adult

• *Advanced prostate cancer:* SC 1 mg qd; IM (depot) 7.5 mg/dose given qmo, or 22.5 mg/dose given q3mo, or 30 mg/dose given q4mo

• *Endometriosis/uterine leiomyomata:* IM (depot) 3.75 mg/dose given once qmo or 11.25 mg/dose given q3mo for 6 consecutive mo (3-6 mo for fibroids); repeated courses not recommended

Child

• *Precocious puberty:* SC 50 μg/kg/day, titrate upward by 10 μg/kg qd if total suppression of ovarian or testicular steroidogenesis is not achieved; IM/SC (depot) 7.5 mg q4wk (children <25 kg), 11.25 mg q4wk (children 25-37.5 kg), 15 mg q4wk (children >37.5 kg); titrate upward in 3.75 mg/dose increments q4wk until clinical or laboratory tests indicate no progression of disease

💲 **AVAILABLE FORMS/COST OF THERAPY**

• Inj, Sol—SC: 5 mg/ml, 2.8 ml: **$337.50**

• Inj, Susp (Depot)—IM: 3.75 mg/vial, 1's: **$478.01-$518.64**

• Inj, Susp (Depot)—IM: 7.5 mg/vial, 1's: **$594.65-$623.79**

• Inj, Susp (Depot-3)—IM: 11.25 mg/vial, 1's: **$1455.48-$1555.92;** 22.5 mg/vial, 1's: **$1783.95-$1871.37**

• Inj, Susp (Depot-4)—IM: 30 mg/vial, 1's: **$2378.60**

• Kit (Depot-Ped)—IM: 7.5 mg/vial, 1's: **$594.65-$623.79;** 11.25 mg/vial, 1's: **$1132.73;** 15 mg/vial, 1's: **$1247.58**

CONTRAINDICATIONS: Undiagnosed vaginal bleeding

PRECAUTIONS: Edema, hepatic disease, CVA, MI, seizures, hypertension, diabetes mellitus, thromboembolic disease

---

* = non-FDA-approved use

PREGNANCY AND LACTATION:
Pregnancy category X; spontaneous abortions or intrauterine growth retardation are possible; not recommended during lactation

SIDE EFFECTS/ADVERSE REACTIONS

CNS: Dizziness, headache, insomnia, pain, *hot flashes* (50%-80%)
CV: Cardiac murmurs, **CHF,** ECG changes, *edema, hypertension, ischemia,* thrombosis
GI: Anorexia, constipation, nausea, vomiting
GU: Amenorrhea, anovulation, urinary frequency, vaginal bleeding, vaginal discharge, vaginitis, *gynecomastia/breast tenderness*
METAB: Androgen-like effects, *decreased libido, decreased testicular size, impotence*
MS: Bone pain (with initiation in prostate cancer), myalgia
RESP: Dyspnea, sinus congestion

SPECIAL CONSIDERATIONS
PATIENT/FAMILY EDUCATION
• May cause increase in bone pain and difficulty urinating during 1st few wk of treatment for prostate cancer, may also cause hot flashes
• Gonadotropin and sex steroids rise above baseline initially; side effects greatest in 1st weeks
• Continuous therapy vital for treatment of central precocious puberty
• Females may experience menses or spotting during 1st 2 mo of therapy for central precocious puberty; notify provider if continues into 2nd treatment mo; non-hormonal contraception should be used

MONITORING PARAMETERS
• Monitor response to therapy for prostate cancer by measuring prostate specific antigen (PSA) levels
• GnRH stimulation test and sex steroid levels 1-2 mo after starting therapy for central precocious puberty, measurement of bone age for advancement q6-12mo

levetiracetam
(leva-tir-ass'eh-tam)
Rx: Keppra
Chemical Class: Pyrrolidone derivative
Therapeutic Class: Antiepileptic agent

CLINICAL PHARMACOLOGY
Mechanism of Action: S-enantiomer binds to the synaptic plasma membrane in the central nervous system and stimulates several neurochemical systems, including dopaminergic, cholinergic, and glutamanergic neurotransmission

Pharmacokinetics
PO: Onset 1 hr; duration 6-30 hr; peak plasma concentration 20-120 min; 100% bioavailability, not affected by food; minimal metabolism (no CYP systems), metabolites inactive; renal excretion of unchanged drug; $t_{1/2}$ 7 hr

INDICATIONS AND USES:
DOSAGE
Adult and Child >16 yr
• *Adjunctive therapy of partial onset seizures:* PO 1 g-4 g qd, given in 2 equally divided doses; initiate with 500 mg bid with dosing increments increased by 1000 mg/day at 2 wk intervals
• *Patients with renal impairment:* For CrCl 50-80 ml/min: 500-1000 mg bid; for CrCl 30-50 ml/min: 250-750 mg bid; for CrCl <30 ml/min 250-500 mg bid

AVAILABLE FORMS/COST OF THERAPY
• Tabs—Oral: 250 mg, 120's: **$168.72;** 500 mg, 120's: **$205.48**

PRECAUTIONS: Neuropsychiatric conditions (somnolence and fatigue, coordination difficulties, behavioral abnormalities); withdrawal seizures (withdraw slowly to minimize potential); hematologic abnormalities; hepatic abnormalities

PREGNANCY AND LACTATION: Pregnancy category C; developmental toxicity in animals

SIDE EFFECTS/ADVERSE REACTIONS

CNS: Asthenia, amnesia, anxiety, ataxia, depression, *dizziness, emotional lability,* hostility, *nervousness,* paresthesia, *somnolence,* vertigo, confusion, insomnia, tremor

CV: Chest pain

EENT: Diplopia, ambylopia, otitis media

GI: Abdominal pain, constipation, diarrhea, dyspepsia, gastroenteritis, gingivitis, nausea, vomiting, weight gain

HEME: Ecchymosis

MS: Arthralgia, back pain

RESP: Cough, *pharyngitis,* rhinitis, sinusitis, bronchitis

SKIN: Rash

MISC: Infection, fever, flu syndrome

SPECIAL CONSIDERATIONS
• Reserve as an alternative treatment for patients with partial onset seizures not responding to first-line agents

PATIENT/FAMILY EDUCATION
• Notify clinician if female patients intend to or become pregnant
• Caution about common adverse effects, i.e., dizziness and somnolence

MONITORING PARAMETERS
• Therapeutic plasma concentrations not established; base dosing on therapeutic response (reduction in severity and frequency of seizures)

---

levodopa
(lee-voe-doe′pa)
Rx: Larodopa
Combinations
  Rx: with Carbidopa
    (Sinemet, Sinemet CR)
Chemical Class: Catecholamine precursor
Therapeutic Class: Anti-Parkinson's agent; antidyskinetic

CLINICAL PHARMACOLOGY
Mechanism of Action: Decarboxylated to dopamine, which stimulates dopaminergic receptors in the basal ganglia, improving the balance between cholinergic and dopaminergic activity; improves modulation of voluntary nerve impulses transmitted to the motor cortex; carbidopa in combination product inhibits peripheral decarboxylation of levodopa making more levodopa available for transport to brain and conversion to dopamine

Pharmacokinetics
PO: Peak 1-3 hr, 0.7 hr (Sinemet), 2.4 hr (Sinemet CR); onset 2-3 wk, duration up to 5 hr/dose; 95% converted to dopamine by L-aromatic amino acid decarboxylase enzyme in the lumen of the stomach and intestines and on 1st pass through the liver (reduced by carbidopa); <1% reaches CNS due to extensive metabolism in the periphery and liver (improved by carbidopa); excreted by the kidneys as metabolites; $t_{1/2}$ 1-3 hr

INDICATIONS AND USES: Idiopathic Parkinson's disease, postencephalitic parkinsonism, symptomatic parkinsonism following injury to the nervous system by carbon monoxide or manganese intoxication, parkinsonism associated with

---

cerebral arteriosclerosis; herpes zoster,* restless legs syndrome*

DOSAGE

Adult

• Parkinson's disease (L-dopa): PO 0.5-1 g qd divided bid-qid with meals; may increase gradually by up to 0.75 g/day q3-7 days as tolerated, do not exceed 8 g/day unless closely supervised; (Sinemet) PO 1 tab of 25 mg carbidopa/100 mg levodopa tid or 10 mg/100 mg tid-qid; increase by 1 tab qd-qod prn until dosage of 8 tabs/day is reached; provide at least 70-100 mg of carbidopa/ day; (Sinemet CR) PO 1 tab bid at intervals of not <6 hr; usual dose is 2-8 tabs/day in divided doses at intervals of 4-8 hr while awake; allow at least 3 days between dosage adjustments

• Restless legs: PO 1 tab 25 mg/100 mg qhs

💲 AVAILABLE FORMS/COST OF THERAPY

• Tab, Uncoated—Oral: 100 mg, 100's: **$23.40;** 250 mg, 100's: **$37.36;** 500 mg, 100's: **$64.18**

• (Sinemet) Tab, uncoated—Oral: 10 mg/100 mg, 100's: **$25.53-$68.81;** 25 mg/100 mg 100's: **$27.54-$77.69;** 25 mg/250 mg, 100's: **$32.55-$99.00**

• (Sinemet CR): Tab, Time-Rel—Oral: 25 mg/100 mg, 100's: **$82.87;** 50 mg/200 mg, 100's: **$166.31**

CONTRAINDICATIONS: Narrow-angle glaucoma, concurrent MAOI therapy, history of melanoma or suspicious undiagnosed skin lesions (can activate malignant melanoma)

PRECAUTIONS: Severe cardiovascular or pulmonary disease, bronchial asthma, occlusive cerebrovascular disease; renal, hepatic, endocrine disease; affective disorders, major psychoses, cardiac dysrhythmias, history of peptic ulcer, wide-angle glaucoma

PREGNANCY AND LACTATION: Pregnancy category C; do not use in nursing mothers

SIDE EFFECTS/ADVERSE REACTIONS

CNS: Anxiety, ataxia, *choreiform or dystonic movements,* confusion, delusions, depression, dizziness, euphoria, hallucinations, headache, increased hand tremor, insomnia, mental changes, nightmares, "on-off" phenomenon

CV: Edema, hypertension, orthostatic hypotension, palpitations, phlebitis

EENT: Blepharospasm, blurred vision, dilated pupils, diplopia, hoarseness, oculogyric crisis

GI: Abdominal pain, anorexia, burning sensation of tongue, constipation, diarrhea, *dry mouth, dysgeusia, dysphagia,* flatulence, *GI bleeding, nausea,* sialorrhea, *vomiting*

GU: Dark urine, priapism, urinary incontinence, urinary retention

*HEME: **Agranulocytosis, hemolytic anemia, leukopenia***

RESP: Bizarre breathing patterns, hiccups

SKIN: Dark sweat, flushing, hot flushes, increased sweating, loss of hair, rash

MISC: Weight gain

INTERACTIONS

Drugs

3 *Benzodiazepines:* Diazepam and chlordiazepoxide have exacerbated parkinsonism in a few patients receiving levodopa, effect of other benzodiazepines not clinically established

3 *Food:* High-protein diets may inhibit the efficacy of levodopa

3 *Iron:* Reduced levodopa bioavailability possible

3 *Methionine, phenytoin, pyridoxine, spiramycin, tacrine:* Inhibited clinical response to levodopa

---

italic = common side effects   ***bold italic*** = life-threatening reactions

3 *Moclobemide:* Increased risk of adverse effects from levodopa

3 *MAOIs:* Hypertensive response

2 *Neuroleptics:* Inhibited clinical response to levodopa

Labs

• *False positive:* Urine ferric chloride test, urine ketones, urine glucose, Coombs test

• *False negative:* Urine glucose (glucose oxidase), urine guaiacols spot test

• *False increase:* Serum acid phosphatase, urine amino acids, serum AST, serum bilirubin, plasma catecholamines, serum cholinesterase, serum creatinine, urine creatinine, creatinine clearance, serum glucose, urine hydroxy-methoxymandelic acid, urine ketones, serum lithium, urine protein, urine sugar, serum uric acid, urine uric acid

• *False decrease:* Serum bilirubin (conjugated and unconjugated), serum glucose, urine glucose, serum triglycerides, serum urea nitrogen, serum uric acid, VMA

SPECIAL CONSIDERATIONS

• Combination with carbidopa is preferred preparation

PATIENT/FAMILY EDUCATION

• Full benefit may require up to 6 mo

• Take with food to minimize GI upset

• Avoid sudden changes in posture

• May cause darkening of the urine or sweat

MONITORING PARAMETERS

• CBC, renal function, liver function, ECG, intraocular pressure

levofloxacin
(levo-flox'a-sin)
Rx: Levaquin
Chemical Class: Fluoroquinolone derivative
Therapeutic Class: Antibiotic

CLINICAL PHARMACOLOGY

Mechanism of Action: Interferes with the enzyme DNA gyrase needed for the synthesis of bacterial DNA; bactericidal

Pharmacokinetics

PO: Rapidly and completely absorbed, peak 1-2 hr; can be administered without regard to food

IV: Interchangeable with PO route; Widespread distribution into body tissues; 24%-38% bound to plasma proteins; primarily excreted unchanged in the urine; $t_{1/2}$ 6-8 hr (prolonged in renal failure)

INDICATIONS AND USES: Acute maxillary sinusitis, acute bacterial exacerbation of chronic bronchitis, community acquired pneumonia, uncomplicated skin and skin structure infections, uncomplicated and complicated urinary tract infection, acute pyelonephritis

Antibacterial spectrum usually includes:

• Gram-positive organisms: *Enterococcus faecalis, Staphylococcus aureus, Streptococcus pneumoniae, S. pyogenes*

• Gram-negative organisms: *Enterobacter cloacae, Escherichia coli, Haemophilus influenzae, H. parainfluenzae, Klebsiella pneumoniae, Legionella pneumophila, Moraxella catarrhalis, Proteus mirabilis, Pseudomonas aeruginosa*

• Other organisms: *Chlamydia pneumoniae, Mycoplasma pneumoniae*

DOSAGE

Adult

• *Bronchitis, pneumonia, sinusitis,*

skin and skin structure infections: PO/IV 500 mg q24h

• *Complicated UTI, pyelonephritis:* PO/IV 250 mg q24h

• *Dosage in renal failure:* PO/IV CrCl 20-49 ml/min, 500 mg × 1, then 250 mg q24h; CrCl 10-19 ml/min, 500 mg × 1, then 250 mg q48h

$ AVAILABLE FORMS/COST OF THERAPY

• Tab, Film Coated—Oral: 250 mg, 50's: **$314.70**; 500 mg, 50's: **$367.57**
• Sol—IV: 500 mg/20 ml 1's: **$39.60**

PRECAUTIONS: Children (potential for arthropathy and osteochondrosis), renal disease, seizure disorders, diabetes mellitus

PREGNANCY AND LACTATION: Pregnancy category C; excretion into breast milk unknown; due to the potential for arthropathy and osteochondrosis, use extreme caution in nursing mothers

SIDE EFFECTS/ADVERSE REACTIONS

CNS: Anxiety, depression, dizziness, fatigue, headache, insomnia, *seizures,* somnolence

EENT: Dizziness, visual disturbances

GI: Abdominal pain, anorexia, diarrhea, dry mouth, flatulence, heartburn, increased AST, ALT; nausea, *pseudomembranous colitis,* vomiting

SKIN: Photosensitivity, pruritus, rash

INTERACTIONS

Drugs

3 *Aluminum:* Reduced absorption of levofloxacin; do not take within 4 hr of dose

3 *Antacids:* Reduced absorption of levofloxacin; do not take within 4 hr of dose

3 *Calcium:* Reduced absorption of levofloxacin; do not take within 4 hr of dose

3 *Cimetidine:* Reduced absorption of levofloxacin

3 *Didanosine:* Markedly reduced absorption of levofloxacin; take levofloxacin 2 hr before didanosine

3 *Famotidine:* Reduced absorption of levofloxacin

3 *Iron:* Reduced absorption of levofloxacin; do not take within 4 hr of dose

3 *Lansoprazole:* Reduced absorption of levofloxacin

3 *Magnesium:* Reduced absorption of levofloxacin; do not take within 4 hr of dose

3 *Nizatidine:* Reduced absorption of levofloxacin

3 *Omeprazole:* Reduced absorption of levofloxacin

3 *Ranitidine:* Reduced absorption of levofloxacin

3 *Sodium bicarbonate:* Reduced absorption of levofloxacin; do not take within 4 hr of dose

3 *Sucralfate:* Reduced absorption of levofloxacin; do not take within 4 hr of dose

3 *Warfarin:* May increase hypoprothrombinemic response to warfarin

3 *Zinc:* Reduced absorption of levofloxacin; do not take within 4 hr of dose

SPECIAL CONSIDERATIONS

• L-isomer of the racemate, ofloxacin (a commercially available quinolone antibiotic)

PATIENT/FAMILY EDUCATION

• Avoid direct exposure to sunlight (even when using sunscreen)
• Drink fluids liberally

L

levonorgestrel

(lee-voe-nor-jess'trel)
Rx: Norplant System, Plan B
Combinations
   Rx: See oral contraceptives
   monograph for combined
   oral contraceptives containing levonorgestrel
Chemical Class: 19-Nortestos-
terone derivative; progestin
Therapeutic Class: Contraceptive; progestin

CLINICAL PHARMACOLOGY

Mechanism of Action: Exerts a progestational effect on the endometrium, alters cervical mucus, suppresses ovulation in some patients,
renders the endometrium hostile to
implantation

Pharmacokinetics

IMPLANT: Max concentrations within
24 hr; duration 5 yr; concentrations
show considerable interindividual
variation depending on individual
clearance rates, body weight, and
possibly other factors; metabolized
by reduction followed by conjugation
PO: Peak 0.5-2 hr, $t_{1/2}$ 11-45 hr,
highly bound to albumin and sex
hormone binding globulin
INDICATIONS AND USES: Prevention of pregnancy (Norplant), emergency contraception (Plan B)

DOSAGE

Adult
• IMPLANT 216 mg (6×36 mg
caps) subdermally in the upper arm
during 1st 7 days after onset of menses; implantation should be fanlike,
15 degrees apart, 8 cm (3 in) above
the crease of the elbow
• *Emergency contraception:* PO
0.75 mg within 72 hr of unprotected
intercourse, followed by 0.75 mg
12 h later

💲 AVAILABLE FORMS/COST OF THERAPY

• Kit: 216 mg, 1 kit: **$491.25**
• Tab—Oral: 0.75 mg package of 2:
Price N/A
CONTRAINDICATIONS: Active
thrombophlebitis or thromboembolic
disorders, undiagnosed abnormal
genital bleeding, pregnancy, acute
liver disease, liver tumors, breast
cancer, hypersensitivity
PRECAUTIONS: Diabetes mellitus,
impaired liver function, conditions
aggravated by fluid retention, history of depression, contact lens wear-
ers
PREGNANCY AND LACTATION:
Pregnancy category X; compatible
with breast feeding

SIDE EFFECTS/ADVERSE REACTIONS

CNS: Dizziness, headache, nervousness
CV: Edema
EENT: Contact lens intolerance
GI: Weight gain, change of appetite,
nausea
GU: Ovarian cysts, amenorrhea, cervicitis, *irregular bleeding, many
bleeding days, prolonged bleeding,
spotting,* vaginitis, galactorrhea,
mastalgia
METAB: Altered glucose tolerance
MS: Musculoskeletal pain
SKIN: Acne, dermatitis, hirsutism,
hypertrichosis, infection at inj site;
pain, itching at inj site, scalp hair
loss

INTERACTIONS

Drugs
🛇 *Carbamazepine, phenobarbital,
phenytoin:* Decreased efficacy of
levonorgestrel, pregnancy has occurred

SPECIAL CONSIDERATIONS
PATIENT/FAMILY EDUCATION

• Most women can expect some variation in menstrual bleeding; these

---

* = non-FDA-approved use

irregularities should diminish with continued use

• Capsules can be removed at any time for any reason or at the end of 5 yr. Removal is more difficult than insertion.

• Failure rate 0.2-1.0%, increases to 5% in patients ≥70 kg (Norplant)

• Efficacy of emergency contraception is better as soon as possible after unprotected intercourse. Causes less nausea and vomiting than other products for emergency contraception. Decreases risk of pregnancy from 8% to 19%

---

levorphanol

(lee-vor'fa-nole)
Rx: Levo-Dromoran
Chemical Class: Synthetic opium alkaloid; phenanthrene derivative
Therapeutic Class: Narcotic analgesic
DEA Class: Schedule II

CLINICAL PHARMACOLOGY
Mechanism of Action: Narcotic agonist with activity at Mu receptors (supraspinal analgesia, euphoria, respiratory and physical depression, miosis, and reduced GI motility), Kappa receptors (pentazocine-like spinal analgesia, sedation, and miosis), and Delta receptors (dysphoria, psychotomimetic effects [e.g., hallucinations], and respiratory and vasomotor stimulation caused by drugs with antagonist activity); compared to morphine, equal analgesia, constipation, respiratory depression, and sedation; less emesis
Pharmacokinetics
PO/SC: Peak analgesia 1-1½ hr, duration 6-8 hr
IV: Peak analgesia 20 min, duration 6-8 hr

Metabolized by liver, excreted in urine as glucuronide conjugate; $t_{1/2}$ 11 hr
INDICATIONS AND USES: Moderate to severe pain, preoperative sedation (parenteral)
DOSAGE
Adult
• PO/SC/IV 2-3 mg q6-8h prn
🔢 **AVAILABLE FORMS/COST OF THERAPY**
• Inj, Sol—SC: 2 mg/ml: 1 ml, **$3.96**
• Tab, Uncoated—Oral: 2 mg, 100's: **$56.23-$75.44**
CONTRAINDICATIONS: Acute bronchial asthma, upper airway obstruction
PRECAUTIONS: Head injury, increased intracranial pressure, acute abdominal conditions, elderly, severe impairment of hepatic or renal function, hypothyroidism, Addison's disease, prostatic hypertrophy, urethral stricture, history of drug abuse
PREGNANCY AND LACTATION: Pregnancy category B (category D if used for prolonged periods or in high doses at term); use during labor produces neonatal depression
SIDE EFFECTS/ADVERSE REACTIONS
CNS: Agitation, dependency, dizziness, *drowsiness,* lethargy, restlessness, *sedation*
CV: Bradycardia, orthostatic hypotension, palpitations, tachycardia
GI: Anorexia, constipation, nausea, vomiting
GU: Urinary retention
RESP: **Respiratory depression, respiratory paralysis**
SKIN: Flushing, rash, urticaria
INTERACTIONS
Drugs
🔢 *Antihistamines, chloral hydrate, glutethimide, methocarbamol:* Enhanced depressant effects
🔢 *Barbiturates:* Additive respiratory and CNS depressant effects

---

italic = common side effects   ***bold italic*** = life-threatening reactions

3 Cimetidine: Increased respiratory and CNS depression

3 Ethanol: Additive CNS effects

Labs

• *False increase:* Amylase and lipase

SPECIAL CONSIDERATIONS

• Do not administer agonist/antagonist analgesics (i.e., pentazocine, nalbuphine, butorphanol, dezocine, buprenorphine) to patient who has received a prolonged course of levorphanol (a pure agonist). In opioid-dependent patients, mixed agonist/antagonist analgesics may precipitate withdrawal symptoms

PATIENT/FAMILY EDUCATION

• Physical dependency may result when used for extended periods

• Change position slowly; orthostatic hypotension may occur

• Minimize nausea by administering with food and remain lying down following dose

---

levothyroxine
(lee-voe-thye-rox′een)

Rx: Levo-T, Levothroid, Levoxine, Synthroid, Levoxyl

Combinations

Rx: with liothyronine (Euthroid, Thyrolar)

Chemical Class: Synthetic *levo* isomer of thyroxine (T_4)

Therapeutic Class: Thyroid hormone

CLINICAL PHARMACOLOGY

Mechanism of Action: Increases metabolic rate, increases cardiac output, O_2 consumption, body temperature, blood volume, growth, development at cellular level, metabolism of carbohydrates, lipids, and proteins; exerts profound effects on every organ system, especially CNS

Pharmacokinetics

IV: Onset 6-8 hr

PO: Extent of absorption increased by the fasting state, peak 12-48 hr; >99% bound to plasma proteins; 35% of T_4 is converted in the periphery to T_3; $t_{1/2}$ 6-7 days (3-4 days in hyperthyroidism, 9-10 days in myxedema)

INDICATIONS AND USES: Hypothyroidism (including cretinism, myxedema, non-toxic goiter), pituitary TSH suppression (thyroid nodules, Hashimoto's disease, multinodular goiter, thyroid cancer), thyrotoxicosis (with antithyroid drugs)

DOSAGE

Adult

• *Hypothyroidism:* PO 50 µg qd to start, increase by 25-50 µg/day at intervals of 2-4 wk, usual dose 100-200 µg/day; use ≤25 µg/day in patients with long-standing hypothyroidism if cardiovascular impairment present; IM/IV 50% of oral dose

• *Myxedema:* IV 200-500 µg 1 time, then 100-300 µg the next day prn; resume oral therapy as soon as clinical situation stabilized

• *TSH suppression:* PO larger amounts than needed for replacement are required; optimal dose determined by laboratory findings and clinical response

Child

• PO 8-10 µg/kg or 25-50 µg qd (0-6 mo); 6-8 µg/kg or 50-75 µg qd (6-12 mo); 5-6 µg/kg or 75-100 µg qd (1-5 yr); 4-5 µg/kg or 100-150 µg qd (6-12 yr); 2-3 µg/kg or ≥150 µg qd (>12 yr); IM/IV 50%-75% of oral dose

§ **AVAILABLE FORMS/COST OF THERAPY**

• Inj, Lyphl-Sol—IM, IV: 0.2 mg/vial: **$9.75-$47.90;** 0.5 mg/vial: **$11.25-$46.80**

• Tab, Uncoated—Oral: .025 mg, 100's: **$3.15-$25.44;** .05 mg, 100's: **$3.17-$25.44;** .075 mg, 100's: **$2.85-$30.90;** .088 mg, 100's: **$15.19-**

$32.28; 0.1 mg, 100's: **$2.52-$33.35;** 0.112 mg, 100's: **$16.32-$34.14;** 0.125 mg, 100's: **$3.28-$38.00;** 0.137 mg, 100's: **$18.11-$20.38;** 0.15 mg, 100's: **$3.52-$38.22;** 0.175 mg, 100's: **$21.84-$61.00;** 0.2 mg, 100's: **$3.00-$47.06;** 0.3 mg, 100's: **$4.10-$57.66**

CONTRAINDICATIONS: Adrenal insufficiency, MI, thyrotoxicosis

PRECAUTIONS: Cardiovascular disease, diabetes mellitus or insipidus, elderly

PREGNANCY AND LACTATION: Pregnancy category A; little or no transplacental passage at physiologic serum concentrations; excreted into breast milk in low concentrations (inadequate to protect a hypothyroid infant; too low to interfere with neonatal thyroid screening programs)

SIDE EFFECTS/ADVERSE REACTIONS

CNS: Headache, *insomnia,* nervousness, *tremors*

CV: Angina pectoris, **cardiac arrest, cardiac dysrhythmias,** *palpitations, tachycardia*

GI: Diarrhea, gastric intolerance, nausea

GU: Menstrual irregularities

METAB: Bone demineralization (osteoporosis)

MISC: Fever, heat intolerance, sweating, weight loss

INTERACTIONS

Drugs

🄳 *Bile acid sequestrants:* Reduced serum thyroid hormone concentrations

🄳 *Carbamazepine, phenytoin, rifampin:* Increased elimination of thyroid hormones; possible increased requirement for thyroid hormones in hypothyroid patients

🄳 *Oral anticoagulants:* Thyroid hormones increase catabolism of vitamin K-dependent clotting factors; an increase or decrease in clinical thyroid status will increase or decrease the hypoprothrombinemic response to oral anticoagulants

🄳 *Theophylline:* Reduced serum theophylline concentrations with initiation of thyroid therapy

Labs

• *False increase:* Serum triiodothyronine

SPECIAL CONSIDERATIONS

• Bioequivalence problems have been documented in the past for products marketed by different manufacturers; however, studies in patients have shown comparable clinical efficacy between brands based on the results of thyroid function tests; brand interchange should be limited to products with demonstrated therapeutic equivalence

PATIENT/FAMILY EDUCATION

• Transient, partial hair loss may be experienced by children in the 1st few mo of therapy

• Take as a single daily dose, preferably before breakfast

MONITORING PARAMETERS

• TSH

L

---

italic = common side effects   **bold italic** = life-threatening reactions

lidocaine (local, topical)

(lye'doe-kane)

Rx: *Local:* Dilocaine, Duo-Trach Kit, Lidoject, Nervocaine, Octocaine, Xylocaine
Topical: Anestacon, Xylocaine

OTC: *Topical:* DermaFlex, Solarcaine, Zilactin-L
Combinations

  Rx: with epinephrine (Xylocaine with Epinephrine); Prilocaine (EMLA)

Chemical Class: Aminoacyl amide

Therapeutic Class: Local anesthetic

CLINICAL PHARMACOLOGY

Mechanism of Action: Prevents the generation and conduction of nerve impulses by reducing sodium permeability, increasing electrical excitation threshold, slowing nerve impulse propagation, and reducing rate of rise of the action potential

Pharmacokinetics

TOP: Peak 2-5 min, duration 30-60 min

LOCAL: Onset 0.5-1 min (5-15 min for epidural), duration 0.5-1 hr (1-3 hr for epidural)

55%-65% bound to plasma proteins; metabolized primarily in the liver, excreted in urine and bile as metabolites

INDICATIONS AND USES: LOCAL: infiltration anesthesia, nerve block techniques (peripheral, sympathetic, epidural [including caudal], spinal), intraperitoneal anesthesia*; TOP (spray, oint, sol): anesthesia of skin and accessible mucous membranes

TOP (jelly): anesthesia of urethra, anesthetic lubricant for endotracheal intubation

DOSAGE

Adult and Child

• LOCAL varies with procedure, degree of anesthesia desired, vascularity of tissue, duration of anesthesia required, and physical condition of patient; max 4.5 mg/kg/dose, do not repeat within 2 hr

• TOP apply to affected area prn, max 3 mg/kg/dose, do not repeat within 2 hr

💲 AVAILABLE FORMS/COST OF THERAPY

Top

• Gel—Top; Oral: 2%, 30 g: **$14.90-$17.25**

• Oint—Top: 5%, 0.5, 3.5, 35, 50 g: **$2.50-$15.43**/37.5 g

• Sol—Top: 2%, 100 ml: **$2.70**

• Sol, Viscous—Top, Oral: 2%, 15, 20, 100, 240, 450 ml: **$2.63-$18.21**/100 ml

• Aer, Spray—Oral; Top: 10%, 30 ml: **$51.36**

Local

• Inj, Sol: 0.5%, 50 ml: **$3.73-$4.30;** 1%, 50 ml: **$3.49-$4.19;** 1.5%, 20 ml: **$9.76;** 2%, 50 ml: **$3.72-$5.25;** 4%, 25 ml: **$1.16;** 10%, 10 ml: **$9.07;** 20%, 10 ml: **$12.53**

• Kit—Intracavity, Intrathecal, misc: 1%, 2%, 4%, per kit: **$16.42-$19.45**

CONTRAINDICATIONS: Hypersensitivity to amide anesthetics, heart block (large doses), septicemia (spinal anesthesia), ophth use (top preparations), spinal anesthesia (preparations containing preservatives)

PRECAUTIONS: Inflammation, sepsis, shock, elderly, children, severe liver disease

PREGNANCY AND LACTATION: Pregnancy category C; has been used as a local anesthetic during labor and delivery; may produce CNS depression and bradycardia in the newborn with high serum levels; compatible with breast feeding

SIDE EFFECTS/ADVERSE REACTIONS

CNS: Anxiety, disorientation, drowsiness, loss of consciousness, restlessness, *seizures,* shivering, tremors

CV: Bradycardia, *cardiac arrest, dysrhythmias,* hypertension, hypotension, *myocardial depression*

EENT: Blurred vision, pupil constriction, tinnitus

GI: Nausea, vomiting

RESP: Respiratory arrest, status asthmaticus

SKIN: Allergic reactions, burning, edema, irritation, rash, sensitization (top), skin discoloration at inj site, tissue necrosis, urticaria

INTERACTIONS

Drugs

3 *Disopyramide:* Induction of dysrhythmia or heart failure in predisposed patients

3 *Metoprolol, nadolol, propranolol, cimetidine:* Increased serum lidocaine concentrations

Labs

• *False increase:* Serum creatinine, CSF protein

SPECIAL CONSIDERATIONS

PATIENT/FAMILY EDUCATION

• Do not ingest food for 60 min following oral use (impairs swallowing)

---

lidocaine (systemic)

(lye'doe-kane)

Rx: Xylocaine

Chemical Class: Aminoacyl amide

Therapeutic Class: Antidysrhythmic (Class IB)

CLINICAL PHARMACOLOGY

Mechanism of Action: Decreases depolarization, automaticity, and excitability in the ventricles during the diastolic phase by a direct action on the tissues, especially the Purkinje network, without involvement of the autonomic system; contractility, systolic arterial blood pressure, atrioventricular (AV) conduction velocity, absolute refractory period are not altered by usual therapeutic doses

Pharmacokinetics

IV: Onset immediate, duration 10-20 min

IM: Onset 5-15 min, duration 60-90 min

60%-80% bound to plasma proteins; metabolized by liver to active metabolites, eliminated in urine (10% as unchanged drug); $t_{1/2}$ 1-2 hr

INDICATIONS AND USES: Acute ventricular dysrhythmias

DOSAGE

Adult

• IV bolus 50-100 mg over 2-3 min, repeat q3-5 min, not to exceed 300 mg in 1 hr, begin IV INF; IV INF 20-50 µg/kg/min (1-4 mg/min); decrease the dose in patients with CHF, acute MI, shock, or hepatic disease; IM 200-300 mg in deltoid muscle, additional doses may be given after 60-90 min if necessary; ET 2-2.5 times the IV dose

Child

• IV/ET/IO 1 mg/kg loading dose, repeat if needed in 10-15 min × 2 doses, begin IV INF; IV INF 20-50 µg/kg/min

§ AVAILABLE FORMS/COST OF THERAPY

For direct IV administration:

• Inj, Sol—IV: 0.5%, 50 ml: **$3.92-$10.62;** 1%, 5 ml: **$0.65-$30.00;** 1.5%, 20 ml: **$7.24-$11.64** 2%, 5 ml: **$0.68-$30.00**

For IV admixture:

• Inj, Sol: 4%, 5 ml: **$3.63-$8.93;** 10%, 10 ml: **$10.50;** 20%, 10 ml: **$14.50-$19.17**

CONTRAINDICATIONS: Hypersensitivity to amide anesthetics, Stokes-Adams syndrome, Wolff-Parkinson-White syndrome, severe heart block (in absence of a pacemaker)

PRECAUTIONS: Children, renal disease, liver disease, CHF, reduced cardiac output, digitalis toxicity accompanied by AV block, respiratory depression, genetic predisposition to malignant hyperthermia, atrial fibrillation or flutter

PREGNANCY AND LACTATION: Pregnancy category C; compatible with breast feeding

SIDE EFFECTS/ADVERSE REACTIONS

CNS: Apprehension, confusion, *dizziness,* drowsiness, euphoria, hallucinations, lightheadedness, mood changes, nervousness, **seizures,** tremors, twitching, unconsciousness

CV: Bradycardia, **cardiovascular collapse,** edema, **heart block,** *hypotension*

EENT: Blurred or double vision, tinnitus

GI: Vomiting

*RESP: **Respiratory depression and arrest***

SKIN: Rash, swelling, urticaria

MISC: Febrile response, ***malignant hyperthermia,*** phlebitis at inj site

INTERACTIONS

Drugs

🔟 *Disopyramide:* Induction of dysrhythmia or heart failure in predisposed patients

🔟 *Metoprolol, nadolol, propranolol, cimetidine:* Increased serum lidocaine concentrations

Labs

• *False increase:* Serum creatinine, CSF protein

SPECIAL CONSIDERATIONS

MONITORING PARAMETERS

• Constant ECG monitoring, blood pressure

• Therapeutic serum concentrations

are 1.5-6 µg/ml (concentrations >6-10 µg/ml are usually associated with toxicity)

lindane (gamma benzene hexachloride)

(lin'dane)

Rx: Lindane

Chemical Class: Cyclic chlorinated hydrocarbon

Therapeutic Class: Scabicide/pediculicide

CLINICAL PHARMACOLOGY

Mechanism of Action: Absorbed through the exoskeleton of arthropods, stimulates the nervous system resulting in seizures and death

Pharmacokinetics

TOP: Slowly and incompletely absorbed through intact skin; stored in body fat; metabolized by the liver, excreted in urine and feces

INDICATIONS AND USES: *Pediculus capitis* (head lice), *Pediculus pubis* (crab lice) and their ova; *Sarcoptes scabiei* (scabies)

DOSAGE

Adult and Child

• *Lotion:* (Crab lice) apply sufficient quantity only to cover the hair and skin of the pubic area and adjacent infested areas, leave in place for 12 hr then wash thoroughly, may repeat in 7 days if necessary, treat sexual contacts concurrently; (head lice) apply a sufficient quantity to cover only the affected area, rub into scalp, and leave in place for 12 hr then wash thoroughly, may repeat in 7 days if necessary; (scabies) make total body application from neck down, leave on 8-12 hr (adults), 6-8 hr (children), 6 hr (infants), remove by thorough washing, 60 ml usually sufficient for adults

• *Shampoo:* (Head lice and crab lice) apply a sufficient quantity to dry hair, work thoroughly into hair and allow to remain in place for 4 min, add small quantities of water until a good lather forms, rinse hair thoroughly and towel briskly; comb with a fine-toothed comb or use tweezers to remove any remaining nits or nit shells, retreatment not usually necessary; short hair requires approximately 30 ml, long hair 60 ml

💲 **AVAILABLE FORMS/COST OF THERAPY**

• Lotion—Top: 1%, 60 ml: **$3.90-$7.98**
• Shampoo—Top: 1%, 60 ml: **$4.12-$8.55**

CONTRAINDICATIONS: Premature neonates, seizure disorder

PRECAUTIONS: Children, infants, avoid contact with eyes; inflammation of skin, abrasions, or breaks in skin

PREGNANCY AND LACTATION: Pregnancy category B; use no more than twice during a pregnancy; amounts excreted in breast milk probably clinically insignificant

SIDE EFFECTS/ADVERSE REACTIONS

CNS: Dizziness, *seizures,* stimulation

SKIN: Eczematous eruptions due to irritation

SPECIAL CONSIDERATIONS
PATIENT/FAMILY EDUCATION

• Do not exceed prescribed dosage
• Do not apply to face
• Avoid getting in eyes
• Wear rubber gloves for application
• Do not use oil-based hair products (e.g., conditioners) after using product
• Treat sexual and household contacts concurrently

---

liothyronine (T3)
(lye-oh-thye′roe-neen)
Rx: Cytomel, Triostat
Combinations
  Rx: with levothyroxine (Euthroid, Thyrolar)
Chemical Class: Synthetic triiodothyronine (T_3)
Therapeutic Class: Thyroid hormone

CLINICAL PHARMACOLOGY
Mechanism of Action: Increases metabolic rate, increases cardiac output, O_2 consumption, body temperature, blood volume, growth, development at cellular level, metabolism of carbohydrates, lipids and proteins; exerts profound effects on every organ system, especially CNS

Pharmacokinetics
PO: Peak 48-72 hr, duration following withdrawal of chronic therapy up to 72 hr; >99% bound to plasma proteins; $t_{1/2}$ 0.6-1.4 hr

INDICATIONS AND USES: Hypothyroidism (including cretinism, myxedema, non-toxic goiter), pituitary TSH suppression (thyroid nodules, Hashimoto's disease, multinodular goiter, thyroid cancer), T_3 suppression test

DOSAGE
Adult
• *Hypothyroidism:* PO 25 µg/day; increase by 12.5-25 µg q1-2 wk to max of 100 µg/day
• *T_3 suppression test:* PO 75-100 µg/day for 7 days
• *Myxedema coma:* IV 25-50 µg; repeat prn at 4-12 hr intervals
Elderly
• *Hypothyroidism:* PO 5 µg/day; increase by 5 µg/day q1-2wk; usual maintenance dose 25-75 µg/day
Child
• *Congenital hypothyroidism:* PO 5

---

italic = common side effects   ***bold italic*** = life-threatening reactions

µg/day, increase by 5 µg q3d to 20 µg/day (infants), 50 µg/day (child 1-3 yr), adult dose (child >3 yr)

$ AVAILABLE FORMS/COST OF THERAPY

• Tab, Uncoated—Oral: 5 µg, 100's: **$31.63;** 25 µg, 100's: **$38.10;** 50 µg, 100's: **$50.33**

• Inj, Sol—IV: 10 µg/ml, 1 ml 1's: **$359.88**

CONTRAINDICATIONS: Adrenal insufficiency, MI, thyrotoxicosis

PRECAUTIONS: Cardiovascular disease, diabetes mellitus or insipidus, elderly

PREGNANCY AND LACTATION: Pregnancy category A; little or no transplacental passage at physiologic serum concentrations; excreted into breast milk in low concentrations; (inadequate to protect a hypothyroid infant; too low to interfere with neonatal screening programs)

SIDE EFFECTS/ADVERSE REACTIONS

CNS: Headache, *insomnia,* nervousness, *tremors*

CV: Angina pectoris, **cardiac arrest, cardiac arrhythmias,** palpitations, *tachycardia*

GI: Diarrhea, gastric intolerance, vomiting

GU: Menstrual irregularities

METAB: Bone demineralization (osteoporosis)

MISC: Fever, heat intolerance, sweating, weight loss

INTERACTIONS

Drugs

3 *Bile acid sequestrants:* Reduced serum thyroid hormone concentrations

3 *Carbamazepine, phenytoin, rifampin:* Increased elimination of thyroid hormones; possible increased requirement for thyroid hormones in hypothyroid patients

3 *Oral anticoagulants:* Thyroid hormones increase catabolism of vitamin K-dependent clotting factors; an increase or decrease in clinical thyroid status will increase or decrease the hypoprothrombinemic response to oral anticoagulants

3 *Theophylline:* Reduced serum theophylline concentrations with initiation of thyroid therapy

SPECIAL CONSIDERATIONS

PATIENT/FAMILY EDUCATION

• Transient, partial hair loss may be experienced by children in the 1st few mo of therapy

• Other thyroid products have longer half-lives. Take this into consideration when switching from them to liothyronine.

• Take as single daily dose, preferably before breakfast

MONITORING PARAMETERS

• TSH

---

lisinopril
(ly-sin'oh-pril)
Rx: Prinivil, Zestril
Combinations
  Rx: with hydrochlorothiazide
    (Prinzide, Zestoretic)
Chemical Class: Nonsulfhydryl angiotensin-converting enzyme (ACE) inhibitor
Therapeutic Class: Antihypertensive

CLINICAL PHARMACOLOGY

Mechanism of Action: Antihypertensive, hypoproliferative, and cardioprotective effects attributable to competitive inhibition of angiotensin-converting enzyme (ACE) yielding decreased plasma concentrations of angiotensin II, plasma aldosterone concentrations, systemic vascular resistance, blood pressure, preload and afterload; not accompanied by changes in heart rate, pressor sensitivity to exogenous norepinephrine, or baroreceptor sensitivity

Pharmacokinetics

PO: Peak 7 hr, onset 1 hr, duration 24 hr; excreted unchanged in urine; $t_{1/2}$ 12 hr (prolonged in renal dysfunction)

INDICATIONS AND USES: Hypertension, CHF, MI, erythrocytosis,* nephropathy,* retinopathy*

DOSAGE

Adult and Child >16 yr

• *Hypertension:* PO 10 mg qd; usual dosage range 20-40 mg/day

• *CHF:* PO 5 mg qd; usual dosage range 5-20 mg/day

• *Acute MI:* PO in hemodynamically stable patients within 24 hr of acute MI, 5 mg followed by 5 mg after 24 hr, 10 mg after 48 hr, then 10 mg qd; continue for 6 wk (or longer if concurrent hypertension or CHF)

• *Nephropathy (proteinuria):* PO 5 to 20 mg qd; (dose titration maximal response is required)

• *Renal impairment:* PO initial dose 5 mg qd (serum creatinine ≥3 mg/dl); initial dose 2.5 mg qd (dialysis patients)

💲 AVAILABLE FORMS/COST OF THERAPY

• Tab, Uncoated—Oral: 2.5 mg, 100's: **$58.08-$58.94;** 5 mg, 100's: **$87.01-$88.27;** 10 mg, 100's: **$89.92-$91.26;** 20 mg, 100's: **$96.24-$97.68;** 30 mg, **$138.18;** 40 mg, 100's: **$140.66-$142.68**

PRECAUTIONS: Renal insufficiency (<30 ml/min), hypotension (CHF, elderly, volume depletion—diuretics, dialysis, cirrhosis), aortic stenosis, hyperkalemia (potassium supplements, potassium-sparing diuretics, renal disease, diabetes), neutropenia (autoimmune diseases, collagen vascular, febrile illness, immunosuppressant drug therapy), proteinuria, renal artery stenosis, surgery/anesthesia (excessive hypotension, correctable with fluids)

PREGNANCY AND LACTATION: Pregnancy category C (1st trimester), category D (2nd and 3rd trimesters); ACE inhibitors can cause fetal and neonatal morbidity and death when administered to pregnant women; when pregnancy is detected, discontinue ACE inhibitors as soon as possible; detectable in breast milk in trace amounts; a newborn would receive <0.1% of the mg/kg maternal dose; effect on nursing infant has not been determined

SIDE EFFECTS/ADVERSE REACTIONS

CNS: Anxiety, *dizziness, fatigue, headache,* insomnia, paresthesia

CV: Angina, hypotension, palpitations, postural hypotension, syncope (especially with 1st dose)

GI: Abdominal pain, constipation, melena, nausea, vomiting

GU: **Acute renal failure,** decreased libido, impotence, increased BUN, creatinine

HEME: **Agranulocytosis, neutropenia**

METAB: Hyperkalemia, hyponatremia

MS: Arthralgia, arthritis, myalgia

RESP: Asthma, bronchitis, *cough,* dyspnea, sinusitis

SKIN: **Angioedema,** flushing, rash, sweating

INTERACTIONS

Drugs

❷ *Allopurinol:* Predisposition to hypersensitivity reactions to ACE inhibitors

❸ *Aspirin, NSAIDs:* Inhibition of the antihypertensive response to ACE inhibitors

❸ *Azathioprine:* Increased myelosuppression

---

italic = common side effects   ***bold italic*** = life-threatening reactions

3 *Insulin:* Enhanced insulin sensitivity

3 *Lithium:* Increased risk of serious lithium toxicity

3 *Loop diuretics:* Initiation of ACE inhibitor therapy in the presence of intensive diuretic therapy results in a precipitous fall in blood pressure in some patients; ACE inhibitors may induce renal insufficiency in the presence of diuretic-induced sodium depletion

3 *Potassium-sparing diuretics:* Increased risk for hyperkalemia

3 *Prazosin, terazosin, doxazosin:* Exaggerated first-dose hypotensive response to α-blockers

3 *Trimethoprim:* Additive risk of hyperkalemia, especially in patient predisposed to renal insufficiency
Labs
ACE inhibition can account for approximately 0.5mEq/L rise in serum potassium

SPECIAL CONSIDERATIONS
PATIENT/FAMILY EDUCATION
• Caution with salt substitutes containing potassium chloride
• Rise slowly to sitting/standing position to minimize orthostatic hypotension
• Dizziness, fainting, lightheadedness may occur during 1st few days of therapy
• May cause altered taste perception or cough; persistent dry cough usually does not subside unless medication is stopped; notify clinician if these symptoms persist
MONITORING PARAMETERS
• BUN, creatinine, potassium within 2 wk after initiation of therapy (increased levels may indicate acute renal failure)

lithium
(li'thee-um)
Rx: *Tablets:* Eskalith, Lithane, Lithotabs, Lithobid
Capsules: Eskalith, Lithonate
Syrup: Cibalith-S
Chemical Class: Monovalent cation
Therapeutic Class: Antimanic; psychotherapeutic agent

CLINICAL PHARMACOLOGY
Mechanism of Action: Alters sodium transport in nerve and muscle cells; effects a shift toward intraneuronal metabolism of catecholamines; affects the synthesis, storage, release and reuptake of central monoamine neurotransmitters (norepinephrine, serotonin, dopamine, acetylcholine, and GABA); antimanic effects as a result of increases in norepinephrine uptake and increased serotonin receptor sensitivity
Pharmacokinetics
PO: Peak ½ hr (syr), 1-3 hr (cap or tabs), 3-4 hr (EXT REL formulations); onset 1-3 wk; not bound to plasma proteins; excreted unchanged in urine (95%); $t_{1/2}$ 18-36 hr
INDICATIONS AND USES: Manic episodes of bipolar affective disorder; prophylaxis of cluster headache,* premenstrual syndrome,* bulimia,* alcoholism,* SIADH,* tardive dyskinesia,* hyperthyroidism,* postpartum affective psychosis*
DOSAGE
Adult
• *Acute mania:* PO 600 mg tid or 900 mg bid (EXT REL formulations); determine serum lithium concentrations twice weekly until stabilized
• *Maintenance:* PO 300 mg tid-qid;

adjust to maintain therapeutic serum lithium concentration

Child

• PO 15-60 mg/kg/day in 3-4 divided doses; adjust to maintain therapeutic serum lithium concentration; do not exceed usual adult dose

$ AVAILABLE FORMS/COST OF THERAPY

• Lithium carbonate: Cap, Gel—Oral: 150 mg, 100's: **$13.97;** 300 mg, 100's: **$6.27-$19.40;** 600 mg, 100's: **$34.92**

• Tab, Uncoated—Oral: 300 mg, 100's: **$19.21**

• Tab, Coated, SUS Action—Oral: 300 mg, 100's: **$33.03;** 450 mg, 100's: **$43.10**

• Lithium citrate: Syr—Oral: 300 mg/5 ml, 480 ml: **$14.95-$19.82**

CONTRAINDICATIONS: Severe cardiovascular or renal disease

PRECAUTIONS: Toxicity closely related to serum levels (facilities for serum lithium determinations required to monitor therapy); dehydration, sodium depletion, elderly, children <12 yr, concomitant infection, thyroid disease, tartrazine sensitivity, diabetes mellitus

PREGNANCY AND LACTATION: Pregnancy category D; avoid use in pregnancy if possible, especially during the 1st trimester; contraindicated in nursing mothers

SIDE EFFECTS/ADVERSE REACTIONS

CNS: Ataxia, clonic movements, confusion, *dizziness, drowsiness, fine hand tremor, headache,* memory loss, ***pseudotumor cerebri,*** restlessness, ***seizures,*** slurred speech, stupor, twitching

CV: Bradycardia, ***circulatory collapse, dysrhythmias,*** ECG changes, edema, *hypotension*

EENT: Blurred vision, tinnitus

GI: Abdominal pain, *anorexia, diarrhea, dry mouth,* excessive salivation, flatulence, gastritis, metallic taste, *nausea, vomiting*

GU: Albuminuria, decreased creatinine clearance, glycosuria, polydipsia, *polyuria,* proteinuria, sexual dysfunction, symptoms of nephrogenic diabetes, urinary incontinence

METAB: Euthyroid goiter, hyperthyroidism (rare), hyponatremia, hypothyroidism, transient hyperglycemia

MS: Arthralgia

SKIN: Acne, anesthesia of skin, ***angioedema,*** chronic folliculitis, drying and thinning of hair, exacerbation of psoriasis, generalized pruritis

MISC: Excessive weight gain, thirst

INTERACTIONS

Drugs

🔳 *ACE inhibitors, methyldopa:* Increased risk of lithium toxicity

🔳 *Diltiazem, verapamil, amitriptyline, carbamazepine, fluoxetine, fluvoxamine:* Neurotoxicity, including seizures

❷ *MAOIs:* Malignant hyperpyrexia

🔳 *Neuroleptics:* Reduced neuroleptic response; severe neurotoxicity possible in acute manic patients receiving lithium and neuroleptics

🔳 *NSAIDs:* Increased lithium concentrations

🔳 *Phenytoin:* Development of lithium toxicity has been reported

🔳 *Potassium iodide:* Increased risk for hypothyroidism

🔳 *Sodium bicarbonate:* Decreased plasma lithium concentrations

🔳 *Sodium chloride:* High sodium intake may reduce serum lithium concentrations; sodium restriction may increase serum lithium

🔳 *Theophylline:* Increased lithium renal clearance, decreased lithium efficacy

---

italic = common side effects   ***bold italic*** = life-threatening reactions

3 *Thiazide diuretics:* Increased lithium concentrations
Labs
• *False increase:* Serum creatinine
SPECIAL CONSIDERATIONS
PATIENT/FAMILY EDUCATION
• Take with meals to avoid stomach upset
• Discontinue medication and contact clinician for diarrhea, vomiting, unsteady walking, coarse hand tremor, severe drowsiness, muscle weakness
• Drink 8-12 glasses of water or other liquid every day
• Do not restrict sodium in diet
MONITORING PARAMETERS
• Serum lithium concentrations drawn immediately prior to next dose (8-12 hr after previous dose), monitor biweekly until stable then q2-3mo; therapeutic range 0.8-1.2 mEq/L (acute), 0.5-1.0 mEq/L (maintenance)
• Serum creatinine, CBC, urinalysis, serum electrolytes, fasting glucose, ECG, TSH

---

lomefloxacin
(lome-flock'sa-sin)
Rx: Maxaquin
Chemical Class: Fluoroquinolone
Therapeutic Class: Antibiotic

CLINICAL PHARMACOLOGY
Mechanism of Action: Interferes with the enzyme DNA gyrase needed for synthesis of bacterial DNA; bactericidal
Pharmacokinetics
PO: Peak 1-2 hr, absorption decreased by coadministration with food; excreted in urine as active drug, metabolites; $t_{1/2}$ 6-8 hr
INDICATIONS AND USES: Infections of the lower respiratory tract, urinary tract; prevention of UTI in patients undergoing transurethral procedures; gonorrhea*
Antibacterial spectrum usually includes:
• Gram-positive organisms: *Staphylococcus saprophyticus*
• Gram-negative organisms: *Citrobacter diversus, Enterobacter cloacae, Escherichia coli, Haemophilus influenzae, Klebsiella pneumoniae, Moraxella catarrhalis, Proteus mirabilis, Pseudomonas aeruginosa* (urinary tract only)
DOSAGE
Adult
• *Lower respiratory tract:* PO 400 mg qd for 10 days
• *Urinary tract:* PO 400 mg qd for 3-14 days
• *Prophylaxis:* PO 400 mg as a single dose 2-6 hr prior to surgery
• *Gonorrhea:* PO 400 mg as a single dose
• *Renal function impairment:* PO 400 mg loading dose, then 200 mg qd for duration of treatment (CrCl <40 ml/min/1.73 m^2)
$ AVAILABLE FORMS/COST OF THERAPY
• Tab, Uncoated—Oral: 400 mg, 20's: **$132.08**
CONTRAINDICATIONS: Hypersensitivity to quinolones
PRECAUTIONS: Children (potential for arthropathy and osteochondrosis), elderly, renal disease, seizure disorders
PREGNANCY AND LACTATION: Pregnancy category C; excretion into breast milk unknown; due to the potential for arthropathy and osteochondrosis, use extreme caution in nursing mothers
SIDE EFFECTS/ADVERSE REACTIONS
CNS: Anxiety, depression, dizziness, fatigue, headache, insomnia, seizures, somnolence
EENT: Dizziness, visual disturbances

---

* = non-FDA-approved use

GI: Abdominal pain, anorexia, diarrhea, dry mouth, flatulence, heartburn, increased AST, ALT; *nausea,* ***pseudomembranous colitis,*** vomiting

SKIN: Photosensitivity, pruritus, rash

INTERACTIONS
Drugs
3 *Aluminum:* Reduced absorption of lomefloxacin; do not take within 4 hr of dose

3 *Antacids:* Reduced absorption of lomefloxacin; do not take within 4 hr of dose

3 *Calcium:* Reduced absorption of lomefloxacin; do not take within 4 hr of dose

3 *Cimetidine:* Reduced absorption of lomefloxacin

3 *Didanosine:* Markedly reduced absorption of lomefloxacin; take lomefloxacin 2 hr before didanosine

3 *Famotidine:* Reduced absorption of lomefloxacin

3 *Iron:* Reduced absorption of lomefloxacin; do not take within 4 hr of dose

3 *Lansoprazole:* Reduced absorption of lomefloxacin

3 *Magnesium:* Reduced absorption of lomefloxacin; do not take within 4 hr of dose

3 *Nizatidine:* Reduced absorption of lomefloxacin

3 *Omeprazole:* Reduced absorption of lomefloxacin

3 *Ranitidine:* Reduced absorption of lomefloxacin

3 *Sodium bicarbonate:* Reduced absorption of lomefloxacin; do not take within 4 hr of dose

3 *Sucralfate:* Reduced absorption of lomefloxacin; do not take within 4 hr of dose

3 *Warfarin:* May increase hypoprothrombinemic response to warfarin

3 *Zinc:* Reduced absorption of

lomefloxacin; do not take within 4 hr of dose

SPECIAL CONSIDERATIONS
PATIENT/FAMILY EDUCATION
• Avoid direct exposure to sunlight (even when using sunscreen)
• Drink fluids liberally
• Do not take antacids containing magnesium or aluminum or products containing iron or zinc within 4 hr before or 2 hr after dosing

---

loperamide
(loe-per'a-mide)
Rx: Imodium
OTC: Imodium A-D, Maalox Anti-Diarrheal
Combinations
  OTC: with simethicone (Imodium Advanced)
Chemical Class: Piperidine derivative
Therapeutic Class: Antidiarrheal

CLINICAL PHARMACOLOGY
Mechanism of Action: Direct action on intestinal muscles to decrease GI peristalsis
Pharmacokinetics
PO: 40% absorbed, onset 30-60 min, peak 5 hr (capsule) and 2½ hr (liquid); metabolized in liver; excreted in feces as unchanged drug, small amount in urine; $t_{1/2}$ 7-14 hr

INDICATIONS AND USES: Diarrhea (acute non-specific); chronic diarrhea (inflammatory bowel disease); reduction of volume from ileostomy; traveler's diarrhea

DOSAGE
Adult
• PO 4 mg, then 2 mg after each loose stool, max 16 mg/day; maintenance for chronic diarrhea usually 4-8 mg/day
Child
• <2 yr, use not recommended

• 13-20 kg PO 1 mg tid on day 1, then 0.1 mg/kg after each loose stool
• 20-30 kg PO 2 mg bid on day 1, then 0.1 mg/kg after each loose stool
• >30 kg PO 2 mg tid on day 1, then 0.1 mg/kg after each loose stool

💲 **AVAILABLE FORMS/COST OF THERAPY**
• Cap, Gel—Oral: 2 mg, 100's: **$14.55-$83.99**
• Tab (OTC)—Oral: 2 mg, 12's: **$4.87-$5.21**
• Liq (OTC)—Oral: 1 mg/5 ml, 120 ml: **$5.60-$6.47**

CONTRAINDICATIONS: Acute diarrhea due to invasive organisms (enteroinvasive *E. coli, Salmonella, Shigella*) or pseudomembranous colitis

PRECAUTIONS: Liver disease, dehydration, severe ulcerative colitis (toxic megacolon), children (greater variability in response)

PREGNANCY AND LACTATION: Pregnancy category B; unknown if excreted in breast milk; compatible with breast feeding

SIDE EFFECTS/ADVERSE REACTIONS
CNS: Fatigue, fever, dizziness, drowsiness
GI: Abdominal pain, anorexia, *constipation, dry mouth, nausea,* **toxic megacolon,** vomiting
RESP: Respiratory depression
SKIN: Rash

SPECIAL CONSIDERATIONS
PATIENT/FAMILY EDUCATION
• Do not self-medicate diarrhea for >48 hr without consulting provider

loracarbef
(lor-a-kar´bef)
Rx: Lorabid
Chemical Class: Carbacephem derivative (structurally related to cephalosporins, 2nd generation)
Therapeutic Class: Antibiotic

CLINICAL PHARMACOLOGY
Mechanism of Action: Inhibits bacterial cell wall synthesis
Pharmacokinetics
PO: Well absorbed from GI tract, slower with food; peak 1 hr (cap), ½ hr (susp); 25% bound to plasma proteins; excreted in urine as unchanged drug; $t_{1/2}$ 1 hr

INDICATIONS AND USES: Infections of the upper and lower respiratory tract (including pharyngitis and tonsillitis); urinary tract (cystitis, pyelonephritis), skin infections; otitis media, sinusitis

Antibacterial spectrum usually includes:
• Gram-positive organisms: *Streptococcus pneumoniae, Str. pyogenes, Staphylococcus aureus, S. saprophyticus*
• Gram-negative organisms: *Haemophilus influenzae, E. coli, Proteus mirabilis, Klebsiella* spp., *Moraxella catarrhalis*

DOSAGE
Adult
• *UTI:* PO 200 mg q24h for 7 days
• *Pyelonephritis:* PO 400 mg q12h for 14 days
• *Upper and lower respiratory tract:* PO 200-400 mg q12h
• *Skin:* PO 200 mg q12h
Child 6 mo-12 yr
• *Acute otitis media, sinusitis:* PO 15 mg/kg/day divided q12h for 10 days

---

• *Pharyngitis, skin infections:* PO 7.5 mg/kg q12h

• *Renal function impairment:* CrCl ≥50 ml/min, use regular dose; CrCl 10-49 ml/min, use half regular dose at regular interval; CrCl <10 ml/min, use regular dose q3-5d; repeat after hemodialysis

$ AVAILABLE FORMS/COST OF THERAPY

• Cap, Gel—Oral: 200 mg, 100's: **$314.45-$411.40;** 400 mg, 100's: **$480.73**

• Susp—Oral: 100 mg/5 ml, 100 ml: **$26.84-$56.58;** 200 mg/5 ml, 100 ml: **$40.28-$54.11**

CONTRAINDICATIONS: Hypersensitivity to cephalosporins

PRECAUTIONS: Children <6 mo, renal disease, hypersensitivity to penicillins (10% cross reactivity)

PREGNANCY AND LACTATION: Pregnancy category B; unknown if excreted into breast milk

SIDE EFFECTS/ADVERSE REACTIONS

CNS: Chills, confusion, dizziness, fatigue, fever, headache, paresthesia

GI: Abdominal pain, anorexia, ***bleeding,*** colitis, diarrhea, dysgeusia, flatulence, glossitis, heartburn, increased LFTs, jaundice, nausea, stomach cramps, vomiting, diarrhea

GU: Candidiasis, ***nephrotoxicity,*** pruritus, pyuria, reversible interstitial nephritis, vaginitis

HEME: ***Bone marrow suppression,*** eosinophilia, ***hemolytic anemia,*** leukocytosis, lymphocytosis

RESP: Dyspnea

SKIN: Dermatitis, rash, urticaria

SPECIAL CONSIDERATIONS

• Essentially same spectrum and utility as cefaclor

• Take 1h before eating or 2h after eating

---

loratadine
(loer-at'ah-deen)
Rx: Claritin, Claritin Reditabs
Combinations
  Rx: with pseudoephedrine (Claritin-D)
Chemical Class: Piperidine derivative
Therapeutic Class: Antihistamine

CLINICAL PHARMACOLOGY

Mechanism of Action: Decreases allergic response by blocking histamine at H_1-receptors; provides antihistamine action without sedation

Pharmacokinetics

PO: Absorption limited by food, peak 1-2 hr metabolized in liver to active metabolite (descarboethoxyloratadine), excreted in urine and feces; elimination $t_{1/2}$ 8.4 hr

INDICATIONS AND USES: Seasonal allergic rhinitis; idiopathic chronic urticaria

DOSAGE

Adult

• PO 10 mg qd; give qod in hepatic impairment or renal insufficiency (CrCl <30 ml/min)

$ AVAILABLE FORMS/COST OF THERAPY

• Syr—Oral: 5 mg/5 ml, 480 ml: **$122.40**

• Tab, Uncoated—Oral: 10 mg, 100's: **$218.87**

• Tab, Rapidly Disintegrating—Oral: 10 mg, 30's: **$75.71**

PRECAUTIONS: Increased intraocular pressure, hepatic disease, renal insufficiency

PREGNANCY AND LACTATION: Pregnancy category B; excreted into breast milk at levels equivalent to serum levels

---

italic = common side effects   ***bold italic*** = life-threatening reactions

SIDE EFFECTS/ADVERSE REACTIONS

CNS: Insomnia, sedation (more common with increased doses)
GI: Dry mouth

INTERACTIONS
Drugs

3 *Itraconazole, ketoconazole, miconazole:* Increased loratadine levels but no increase in toxicity reported

SPECIAL CONSIDERATIONS
• Effective, but expensive nonsedating antihistamine; reserve for patients unable to tolerate sedating antihistamines like chlorpheniramine

---

lorazepam
(lor-a'ze-pam)
Rx: Ativan
Chemical Class: Benzodiazepine
Therapeutic Class: Anxiolytic; sedative/hypnotic; anticonvulsant
DEA Class: Schedule IV

CLINICAL PHARMACOLOGY
Mechanism of Action: CNS depressants via facilitation of inhibitory GABA at benzodiazepine receptor sites (BZ_1—associated with sleep; BZ_2— associated with memory, motor, sensory, and cognitive function); effects include muscle relaxation (spinal cord), anticonvulsant activity (brain stem), ataxia (cerebellum), emotional behavior (limbic and cortical areas), and anxiolytic effects (separate from general CNS depression); other effects include sedative, appetite-stimulating and weak analgesic actions

Pharmacokinetics
PO: Peak 1-6 hr, duration 3-6 hr
IM: Peak 60-90 min
Metabolized by liver to inactive metabolites; excreted by kidneys; crosses placenta, breast milk; $t_{1/2}$ 10-20 hr

INDICATIONS AND USES: Anxiety disorders, preoperative sedation (inj); insomnia,* acute alcohol withdrawal symptoms,* initial treatment of status epilepticus (inj), adjunct in endoscopic procedures,* chemotherapy-induced nausea and vomiting*

DOSAGE
Adult
• *Anxiety:* PO 2-6 mg/day in divided doses bid-tid; largest dose at hs; not to exceed 10 mg/day
• *Insomnia:* PO 2-4 mg hs; only minimally effective after 2 wk continuous therapy
• *Elderly:* 1-2 mg/day in divided doses
• *Preoperatively:* IM 0.05 mg/kg to max 4 mg given ≥2 hr before procedure; IV 0.044-0.05 mg/kg, max 4 mg, 15-20 min before procedure
Child
• Not recommended IM/IV <18 yr, PO <12 yr

$ **AVAILABLE FORMS/COST OF THERAPY**
• Inj, Sol—IM, IV: 2 mg/ml, 1 ml: **$8.31-$13.51;** 4 mg/ml, 1 ml: **$10.18-$15.72**
• Tab, Uncoated—Oral: 0.5 mg, 100's: **$63.02-$77.90;** 1 mg, 100's: **$78.70-$101.45;** 2 mg, 100's: **$114.78-$147.89**
• Sol—Oral: 2 mg/ml, 30 ml: **$36.50**

CONTRAINDICATIONS: Acute narrow-angle glaucoma, psychosis
PRECAUTIONS: Elderly, debilitated, hepatic disease, renal disease, suicidal patients, COPD, history of drug abuse
PREGNANCY AND LACTATION: Pregnancy category D (other benzodiazepines associated with cleft lip, cleft palate, microcephaly, pyloric stenosis); neonatal withdrawal, hypotonia; excreted into breast milk

---

* = non-FDA-approved use

in low quantities; effect on infant unknown

SIDE EFFECTS/ADVERSE REACTIONS

CNS: Anxiety, confusion, depression, *dizziness, drowsiness,* fatigue, hallucinations, headache, insomnia, stimulation, tremors, unsteadiness

CV: ECG changes, *orthostatic hypotension,* tachycardia

EENT: Blurred vision, mydriasis, tinnitus

GI: Anorexia, constipation, diarrhea, dry mouth, nausea, vomiting

SKIN: Dermatitis, itching, rash

INTERACTIONS

Drugs

3 *Ethanol:* Increased adverse psychomotor effects of lorazepam

2 *Fluconazole:* Potential for increased lorazepam concentrations

3 *Itraconazole:* Potential for increased lorazepam concentrations

SPECIAL CONSIDERATIONS

• A good choice for elderly or patients with liver dysfunction who need benzodiazepines due to phase II metabolism to inactive metabolites (less likely to accumulate)

PATIENT/FAMILY EDUCATION

• Do not discontinue abruptly after long-term use, withdrawal syndrome (seizures, anxiety, insomnia, nausea, vomiting, flu-like illness, confusion, hallucinations, memory impairment) can occur

---

losartan

(lo-sar'tan)

Rx: Cozaar

Combinations

  Rx: with hydrochlorothiazide (Hyzaar)

Chemical Class: Angiotensin II receptor antagonist

Therapeutic Class: Antihypertensive

CLINICAL PHARMACOLOGY

Mechanism of Action: Antihypertensive (inhibition of vasoconstriction and aldosterone secretion), smooth muscle hypoproliferative, and cardioprotective effects are attributable to selective blockade of angiotensin II (AT1) receptors found throughout the cardiovascular and renal systems; effects independent of angiotensin II synthesis

Pharmacokinetics

PO: Peak, 1-1.5 hrs; peak response, 6 hrs

PO bioavailability, 25-35%, <10% food effect; 98+% protein bound (parent and active metabolite), extensively metabolized by liver (CYP2C9, 3A4) to active metabolite, minimal excretion via urine (13%); elimination $t_{1/2}$, 1.5-2 hrs (metabolite, 4-9 hrs)

INDICATIONS AND USES: Hypertension, CHF (left ventricular dysfunction),* myocardial infarction,* diabetic nephropathy*

DOSAGE

Adult >18 yr

• PO 25-50 mg qd; range 25-100 mg qd; divide bid if effect at trough inadequate

$ AVAILABLE FORMS/COST OF THERAPY

• Tab, Uncoated—Oral: 25, 50 mg; 100's: **$125.10**; 100 mg, 100's: **$187.50**; Hyzaar: 12.5-50 mg, 100's: **$125.10**; 25-100 mg, 100's: **$187.50**

---

italic = common side effects   ***bold italic*** = life-threatening reactions

PRECAUTIONS: Angioedema (associated with aspirin and/or penicillin allergy), aortic or mitral valve stenosis, biliary cirrhosis or biliary obstruction, breast feeding period, coronary artery disease, elderly patients, hepatic dysfunction (adjust dose), hypertrophic cardiomyopathy, hypotension (sodium or volume depleted patients), pregnancy, renal artery stenosis, solitary kidney, or congestive heart failure

PREGNANCY AND LACTATION: Pregnancy category C, first trimester—Category D, second and third trimesters; drugs acting directly on the renin-angiotensin-aldosterone system are documented to cause fetal harm (hypotension, oligohydramnios, neonatal anemia, hyperkalemia, neonatal skull hypoplasia, anuria, and renal failure; neonatal limb contractures, craniofacial deformities, and hypoplastic lung development)

SIDE EFFECTS/ADVERSE REACTIONS

CNS: Dizziness, insomnia
CV: Orthostatic effects, syncope
EENT: Nasal congestion, sinus disorder
GI: Diarrhea, dyspepsia, elevated liver enzymes
GU: Increased BUN, creatinine
HEME: Decreased hct, purpura
METAB: Hyperkalemia
MS: Back pain, leg pain, muscle cramps, myalgia
RESP: Cough
MISC: Angioedema

INTERACTIONS
Drugs
3 *Fluconazole:* Decreased conversion to active metabolite (CYP2C9 inhibition), loss of antihypertensive effects
2 *Lithium:* Increased renal lithium reabsorption at the proximal tubular site due to the natriuresis associated with the inhibition of aldosterone secretion; increased risk of lithium toxicity
3 *Rifampin:* Induced metabolism of losartan and metabolite, resulting in a decrease in the area under the concentration-time curve (AUC) and half-life of both compounds and reduced losartan efficacy

SPECIAL CONSIDERATIONS
• Potentially as or more effective than angiotensin-converting enzyme inhibitors, without cough; no evidence for reduction in morbidity and mortality as first line agents in hypertension, yet; whether they provide the same cardiac and renal protection also still tentative; Like ACE inhibitors, less effective in black patients

PATIENT/FAMILY EDUCATION
• Call your clinician immediately if note following side effects: wheezing; lip, throat or face swelling; hives or rash

MONITORING PARAMETERS
• Baseline electrolytes, urinalysis, blood urea nitrogen and creatinine with recheck at 2-4 weeks after initiation (sooner in volume depleted patients); monitor sitting blood pressure; watch for symptomatic hypotension, particularly in volume-depleted patients

---

loteprednol
(loh-teh-pred'nol)
Rx: Alrex (0.2%); Lotemax (0.5%)
Chemical Class: Glucocorticoid
Therapeutic Class: Ophthalmic corticosteroid

CLINICAL PHARMACOLOGY
Mechanism of Action: Suppresses

the inflammatory response to a variety of inciting agents of a mechanical, chemical, or immunological nature; inhibits edema, cellular infiltration, capillary dilation, fibroblastic proliferation, deposition of collagen, and scar formation associated with inflammation

Pharmacokinetics

OPHTHAL: Highly lipid soluble; limited systemic absorption; extensively metabolized to inactive carboxylic acid metabolites

INDICATIONS AND USES: Temporary relief of signs and symptoms of seasonal allergic conjunctivitis (0.2% susp); treatment of steroid-responsive inflammatory conditions of the palpebral and bulbar conjunctiva, cornea, and anterior segment of the globe (allergic conjunctivitis, acne rosacea, superficial punctate keratitis, herpes zoster keratitis, iritis, cyclitis, selected infective conjunctivitis), when the inherent hazard of corticosteroid use is accepted to obtain an advisable diminution in edema and inflammation (0.5% susp); treatment of postoperative inflammation following ocular surgery (0.5% susp)

DOSAGE

Adult

• 0.2% susp: 1 gtt into affected eye(s) qid

• 0.5% susp: (steroid-responsive disease) 1-2 gtt into affected eye(s) qid; may increase to 1 gtt q1h during initial week of treatment; (postoperative inflammation) 1-2 gtt into affected eye(s) qid beginning 24 hr after surgery and continuing throughout the first 2 wk of postoperative period

$ AVAILABLE FORMS/COST OF THERAPY

• Susp—Ophthal: 0.2%, 5, 10 ml: **$35.00**/10 ml; 0.5%, 5, 10, 15 ml: **$32.50**/10 ml

CONTRAINDICATIONS: Most viral diseases of the cornea and conjunctiva; mycobacterial infections of the eye; fungal infections of the eye

PRECAUTIONS: Glaucoma; prolonged use (may result in ocular hypertension/glaucoma, damage to optic nerve, defects in visual acuity and visual fields, and posterior subcapsular cataract formation)

PREGNANCY AND LACTATION: Pregnancy category C; use caution in nursing mothers

SIDE EFFECTS/ADVERSE REACTIONS

CNS: Headache

EENT: Blurred vision, burning, chemosis, discharge, dry eyes, epiphora, foreign body sensation itching, injection photophobia, conjunctivitis, corneal abnormalities, eyelid erythema, keratoconjunctivitis, ocular pain/irritation/discomfort, papillae, uveitis, rhinitis, pharyngitis, elevated intraocular pressure

SPECIAL CONSIDERATIONS

• Less effective than prednisolone acetate 1% in two 28-day controlled clinical studies in acute anterior uveitis

PATIENT/FAMILY EDUCATION

• Do not wear contact lenses if eyes are red; wait at least 10 min after instilling before inserting soft contact lenses

---

lovastatin

(lo′va-sta-tin)
Rx: Mevacor
Chemical Class: Substituted hexahydronaphthlene
Therapeutic Class: Antilipemic (HMG-CoA reductase inhibitor); "statin"

CLINICAL PHARMACOLOGY
Mechanism of Action: Competitively inhibits 3-hydroxy-3-methyl-

glutaryl-coenzyme A (HMG-CoA) reductase, an early rate-limiting step in cholesterol biosynthesis; increases HDL cholesterol mildly [2%-10%], significantly decreases total and LDL cholesterol [16%-29%, 21%-40% respectively], minimal lowering effect on triglycerides [6%-10%]

Pharmacokinetics

PO: Peak 2-4 hr; metabolized in liver (metabolites); highly protein bound (>95%); excreted in urine (10%), feces (83%); crosses placenta; excreted in breast milk; max effect on lipid levels in 4-6 wk

INDICATIONS AND USES: Primary hypercholesterolemia (heterozygous familial and nonfamilial hypercholesterolemia), mixed dyslipidemia (Fredrickson types IIa and IIb), and secondary prevention of cardiovascular events

DOSAGE

Adult

• PO 10-20 mg qd with evening meal; may increase to 20-80 mg/day in single or divided doses, not to exceed 80 mg/d; dosage adjustments should be made qmo; for cholesterol levels >300 mg/dl initiate at 40 mg/day

§ AVAILABLE FORMS/COST OF THERAPY

• Tab, Uncoated—Oral: 10 mg, 60's: **$82.23;** 20 mg, 60's: **$145.00;** 40 mg, 60's: **$261.03**

CONTRAINDICATIONS: Active liver disease

PRECAUTIONS: Past liver disease, alcoholics, severe acute infections, trauma, hypotension, uncontrolled seizure disorders, severe metabolic disorders, electrolyte imbalances

PREGNANCY AND LACTATION: Pregnancy category X (may produce skeletal malformations); not recommended in nursing mothers

SIDE EFFECTS/ADVERSE REACTIONS

CNS: Dizziness, headache, insomnia

EENT: Blurred vision, dysgeusia, lens opacities

GI: Abdominal pain, constipation, diarrhea, dyspepsia, flatus, heartburn, hepatotoxicity, increased transaminases, nausea

MS: Muscle cramps, myalgia, myositis, *rhabdomyolysis*

SKIN: Pruritus, rash

INTERACTIONS

Drugs

§ *Cholestyramine, colestipol:* Decreased bioavailability of lovastatin possible, effect likely overcome by additive lipid-lowering effects of concurrent therapy

§ *Clarithromycin, cyclosporine, danazol, erythromycin, niacin:* Severe myopathy or rhabdomyolysis

❷ *Clofibrate, gemfibrozil, nefazodone:* Severe myopathy or rhabdomyolysis with combination, especially at high doses

§ *Cyclosporine:* Concomitant administration increases risk of severe myopathy or rhabdomyolysis

❷ *Fluconazole, itraconazole:* Large increases in lovastatin concentration, myopathy or rhabdomyolysis possible

§ *Isradipine:* Reduction in lovastatin concentration

§ *Niacin:* Concomitant administration increases risk of severe myopathy or rhabdomyolysis

§ *Pectin:* Reduced cholesterol-lowering effect of lovastatin

§ *Warfarin:* Increased prothrombin times and bleeding reported with concomitant use

SPECIAL CONSIDERATIONS

• Less effective in homozygous familial hypercholesterolemia (lack of functional LDL receptors); these patients also more likely to have ad-

---

* = non-FDA-approved use

verse reaction of elevated transaminases

• Statin selection based on lipid-lowering prowess, cost, and availability

PATIENT/FAMILY EDUCATION

• Report symptoms of myalgia, muscle tenderness, or weakness

• Take daily doses in the evening for increased effect

MONITORING PARAMETERS

• Cholesterol (max therapeutic response 4-6 wk)

• LFTs (AST, ALT) at baseline and at 12 wk of therapy; if no change, no further monitoring necessary (discontinue if elevations persist $>3 \times$ upper limit of normal)

• CPK in patients complaining of diffuse myalgia, muscle tenderness, or weakness

---

loxapine
(lox′a-peen)
Rx: Loxitane
Chemical Class: Dibenzoxazepine derivative
Therapeutic Class: Antipsychotic

CLINICAL PHARMACOLOGY
Mechanism of Action: Dopamine receptor antagonist, with higher affinity for D_2- over D_1-receptors, and variable selectivity among the cortical dopamine tracts; also activity on nondopaminergic sites, i.e., cholinergic, alpha$_1$-adrenergic and histaminic receptors (explaining side effects); moderate risk extrapyramidal reactions; minimal sedation, orthostatic hypotension and anticholinergic effects
Pharmacokinetics
PO: Onset 20-30 min, peak 1-2 hr, duration 12 hr

IM: Onset 15-30 min, peak 5 hr, duration 12 hr

Metabolized by liver to active and inactive metabolites, excreted in urine (30%-40%) and feces (50%); crosses placenta; enters breast milk; terminal $t_{1/2}$ 19 hr

INDICATIONS AND USES: Psychotic disorders

DOSAGE
NOTE: 15 mg equivalent to chlorpromazine 100 mg
Adult and child>16yr

• PO 10 mg bid-qid initially, may be rapidly increased depending on severity of condition, range 60-100 mg/day divided bid-qid, reduce to maintenance 20-60 mg/day in divided doses; IM 12.5-50 mg q4-6 hr until desired response, then start PO form

💲 AVAILABLE FORMS/COST OF THERAPY

• Cap, Gel—Oral: 5 mg, 100's: **$53.81-$85.59**; 10 mg, 100's: **$94.80-$110.60**; 25 mg, 100's: **$143.24-$167.12**; 50 mg, 100's: **$191.12-$222.97**

• Liq—Oral: 25 mg/ml, 120 ml: **$246.24**

• Inj, Sol—IM: 50 mg/ml, 10 ml: **$105.98**

CONTRAINDICATIONS: Coma, severe drug-induced depressed states
PRECAUTIONS: Seizure disorders, hepatic disease, cardiac disease, prostatic hypertrophy, child <16 yr, glaucoma, COPD
PREGNANCY AND LACTATION: Pregnancy category C; no data in lactating women
SIDE EFFECTS/ADVERSE REACTIONS

CNS: Akathisia, confusion, *drowsiness,* dystonia, headache, pseudoparkinsonism, *seizures,* tardive dyskinesia

---

italic = common side effects   ***bold italic*** = life-threatening reactions

CV: **Cardiac arrest,** ECG changes, hypertension, *orthostatic hypotension,* tachycardia
EENT: Blurred vision, glaucoma
GI: Anorexia, *constipation,* diarrhea, *dry mouth,* jaundice, nausea, vomiting, weight gain
GU: Amenorrhea, enuresis, gynecomastia, impotence, urinary frequency, urinary retention
HEME: **Agranulocytosis, anemia, leukocytosis, leukopenia, thrombocytopenia**
RESP: Dyspnea, laryngospasm, **respiratory depression**
SKIN: Dermatitis, photosensitivity, rash

INTERACTIONS
Drugs

🔳 *Anticholinergics:* Decreased neuroleptic effect

🔳 *Bromocriptine:* Decreased lowering of prolactin by bromocriptine in patients with pituitary adenoma

🔳 *Lithium:* Increased neurotoxicity

🔳 *Lorazepam:* Isolated cases of respiratory depression, stupor and hypotension have been observed

---

lypressin
(lye-press′in)
Rx: Diapid
Chemical Class: Lysine vasopressin
Therapeutic Class: Antidiuretic

CLINICAL PHARMACOLOGY
Mechanism of Action: Promotes reabsorption of water by action on renal tubular epithelium, acts as antidiuretic hormone; little vasopressor or oxytocic effect
Pharmacokinetics
NASAL: Prompt onset, peak 30-120 min, duration 3-8 hr, $t_{1/2}$ 15 min;

metabolized in liver, kidneys; excreted in urine
INDICATION AND USES: Neurogenic diabetes insipidus
DOSAGE
Adult
• INTRANASAL 1-2 sprays in one or both nostrils qid prn excessive urination or thirst, extra dose hs if needed; reduce time between doses if >2 sprays q4-6h needed

💲 **AVAILABLE FORMS/COST OF THERAPY**
• Spray—Intranasal: 0.185 mg/ml, 8 ml: **$41.76**
PRECAUTIONS: CAD, upper respiratory tract infection (decreased effectiveness)
PREGNANCY AND LACTATION: Pregnancy category B; compatible with breast feeding
SIDE EFFECTS/ADVERSE REACTIONS
CNS: Headache
CV: **MI**
EENT: Congestion, conjunctivitis, nasal irritation, rhinitis, rhinorrhea
GI: Cramps, heartburn, nausea
RESP: Chest tightness, cough, dyspnea (when inhaled)
SPECIAL CONSIDERATIONS
• Useful in patients who have become unresponsive to other therapy or who have adverse reactions to products of animal origin

---

mafenide
(ma′fe-nide)
Rx: Sulfamylon
Chemical Class: Sulfonamide derivative
Therapeutic Class: Topical antibiotic

CLINICAL PHARMACOLOGY
Mechanism of Action: Reduces bacterial population present in avascular tissue of 2nd and 3rd degree

---

* = non-FDA-approved use

burns; permits spontaneous healing of deep partial-thickness burns; inhibits carbonic anhydrase

Pharmacokinetics

TOP: Absorbed through devascularized areas, peak concentration 24 hr after initial dose; rapidly metabolized to inactive metabolite, excreted in urine

INDICATIONS AND USES: Adjunctive treatment in burns (2nd, 3rd degree); bacteriostatic against many Gram-positive and Gram-negative organisms, including *Pseudomonas* and some anaerobes

DOSAGE

Adult and Child >2 mo

• TOP apply thin layer (1/16 in) to clean and debrided affected area qd-bid, reapply if washed off

[$] AVAILABLE FORMS/COST OF THERAPY

• Cre—Top: 85 mg/g, 60, 120, 454 g: **$18.50**/60 g

• Pow—Top: 50 g/packet: **$157.50**

PRECAUTIONS: Impaired pulmonary function, impaired renal function, G-6-PD deficiency, blood dyscrasias, inhalation injury

PREGNANCY AND LACTATION: Pregnancy category C; compatible with breast feeding except in G-6-PD deficiency and ill, jaundiced, or premature infants

SIDE EFFECTS/ADVERSE REACTIONS

HEME: **Bone marrow suppression,** eosinophilia, **fatal hemolytic anemia**

METAB: Metabolic acidosis

RESP: Tachypnea

SKIN: Bleeding, blisters, *burning,* erythema, excoriation of new skin, facial edema, hives, pruritus, rash, *stinging,* superinfections, urticaria

DRUG INTERACTIONS

Labs

• *False increase:* Urine amino acids

---

magaldrate

(mag'al-drate)

OTC: Riopan

Combinations

  OTC: with simethicone

  (Riopan Plus)

Chemical Class: Mixture of aluminum and magnesium hydroxide and sulfate

Therapeutic Class: Antacid

CLINICAL PHARMACOLOGY

Mechanism of Action: Neutralizes gastric acidity

Pharmacokinetics

PO: Duration 20-60 min (fasting), 1-3 hr (if given 1 hr after meals)

INDICATIONS AND USES: Hyperacidity; peptic ulcer disease,* GERD,* prevention of stress ulcer bleeding*

DOSAGE

Adult and Child

• *Peptic ulcer disease:* 5-10 ml 1 and 3 hr after meals and at hs for 4-6 wk

• *Gastroesophageal reflux:* 5-10 ml q30-60 min for severe symptoms, or as for peptic ulcer disease

• *GI bleeding:* Administer q hr to keep nasogastric aspirate pH >3.5

• *Before anesthesia:* 5-10 ml 30 min before anesthesia

[$] AVAILABLE FORMS/COST OF THERAPY

• Liq/Susp—Oral: 540 mg/5ml, 12 oz: **$2.98-$4.49**

PRECAUTIONS: Elderly, fluid restriction, decreased GI motility, GI obstruction, dehydration, renal disease, Na-restricted diets, CHF, edema, cirrhosis

PREGNANCY AND LACTATION: Pregnancy category C

SIDE EFFECTS/ADVERSE REACTIONS

GI: Constipation, diarrhea

METAB: Hypermagnesemia

M

---

italic = common side effects   ***bold italic*** = life-threatening reactions

INTERACTIONS

🄱 *Allopurinol, cefpodoxime, cipro-floxacin, isoniazid, ketoconazole, quinolones, tetracyclines, digoxin, iron salts, indomethacin:* Decreased GI absorption of these drugs

🄱 *Pseudoephedrine, enteric coated aspirin, diazepam:* Increased GI absorption of these drugs

🄱 *Quinidine:* Increased quinidine levels

🄱 *Salicylates:* Increased urinary excretion of salicylates

---

magnesium

Magnesium oxide:
OTC: Mag-Ox 400, Maox, Uro-Mag
Magnesium hydroxide:
OTC: Milk of Magnesia, Phillips' Chewable
Magnesium citrate:
OTC: Evac-Q-Mag, Citro-Nesia, Citroma
Magnesium sulfate:
OTC: Epsom Salts
Magnesium gluconate:
OTC: Almora, Magonate, Magtrate
Magnesium chloride:
OTC: Slow-Mag
Chemical Class: Divalent cation
Therapeutic Class: Antacid; laxative; antiarrhythmic, uterine relaxant, electrolyte supplement

---

CLINICAL PHARMACOLOGY

Mechanism of Action: Antacid products: neutralize gastric acidity magnesium citrate: causes osmotic retention of fluid in GI tract, increases peristalsis

Magnesium sulfate: decreases acetylcholine release at neuromuscular junction; slows rate of SA node impulse formation, prolongs conduction time

Pharmacokinetics

Magnesium citrate: renal excretion

Magnesium hydroxide/oxide: onset of laxative action 4-8 hr; renal excretion (30%), unabsorbed drug excreted in feces

Magnesium sulfate: PO onset of laxative action 1-2 hr; IM onset 1 hr, duration 3-4 hr; IV onset immediate, duration 30 min; excreted by kidneys and in stool

Magnesium gluconate: PO 15%-30% absorbed; renal excretion

INDICATIONS AND USES:

Magnesium citrate: bowel evacuation prior to procedures

Magnesium oxide/hydroxide/sulfate (PO): laxative

Magnesium hydroxide/oxide: antacid; hypomagnesemia (oxide)

Magnesium gluconate: hypomagnesemia

Magnesium sulfate (parenteral): hypomagnesemia, eclampsia prophylaxis, preterm labor,* cardiac dysrhythmias,* acute MI,* acute exacerbations of asthma*

DOSAGE

Adult

• Magnesium citrate: PO ½-1 full bottle

• Magnesium hydroxide: PO 30-60 ml qd (laxative); 5-15 ml or 622-1244 mg (tabs) up to qid (antacid)

• Magnesium oxide: PO 2-4 g hs with water (laxative); 140 mg (caps) tid-qid or 400-840 mg/day (tabs) (antacid)

• Magnesium gluconate: PO 1-2 tabs bid-tid

• Magnesium sulfate: IM 4-5 g of 50% Sol q4h prn; IV 4 g of a 10%-20% Sol initially then 4-5 g in 250 ml of D_5W or NS at a rate not exceeding 3 ml/min by infusion (preeclampsia); IM/IV 1 g q6h for 4 doses; for severe deficiency, 8-12

---

* = non-FDA-approved use

g/day in divided doses (hypomagnesemia); PO 10-15 g in a glass of water (laxative)

Child

• Magnesium citrate: PO (<6 yr) 0.5 ml/kg to max 200 ml repeated q 4-6 hr until clear; (6-12 yr) ⅓-½ bottle

• Magnesium hydroxide: Laxative PO (<2 yr) 0.5 ml/kg/dose, (2-5 yr) 5-15 ml/day or divided, (6-12 yr) 15-30 ml/day or divided; antacid PO 2.5-5 ml qd-qid as needed

• Magnesium gluconate: PO 3-6 mg/kg/d divided tid-qid, max 400 mg/day

• Magnesium sulfate: Neonate IV 25-50 mg/kg/dose q 8-12 hr for 2-3 doses; child IM/IV 25-50 mg/kg/dose q 4-6 hr for 3-4 doses, max single dose 2000 mg (hypomagnesemia); PO 5-10 g in a glass of water (laxative)

§ AVAILABLE FORMS/COST OF THERAPY

• Liq (citrate)—Oral: 10 oz: **$0.70-$1.17**

• Liq (hydroxide)—Oral: 16 oz: **$1.44-$3.60**

• Cap, Gel (hydroxide)—Oral: 30's: **$3.54**

• Tab (hydroxide)—Oral: 100's: **$4.09**

• Tab (gluconate)—Oral: 30 mg, 100's: **$3.56;** 500 mg, 100's: **$1.85-$2.39**

• Inj, Conc-Sol (sulfate)—IV; IM: 500 mg/ml, 10 ml: **$1.91-$18.44**

• Inj, Sol (sulfate)—IV; IM: 100 mg/ml, 20 ml: **$1.20-$5.75**

• Inj, Sol (sulfate)—IV: 2 meq/ml, 150 ml: **$1.15**

• Sol (sulfate)—IV: 1%, 100 ml: **$7.15;** 2%, 500 ml: **$7.51;** 4%, 100 ml: **$7.08;** 8%, 50 ml: **$7.08**

CONTRAINDICATIONS: Renal failure (Mg toxicity), hypermagnesemia; do not use cathartics in patients with appendicitis, impaction, intestinal obstruction, or perfora-

tion; do not use parenterally in patients with heart block, myocardial damage

PRECAUTIONS: Diarrhea, digitalized patients, impaired renal function (monitor Mg levels)

PREGNANCY AND LACTATION: Pregnancy category B; compatible with breast feeding

SIDE EFFECTS/ADVERSE REACTIONS

CNS: **Coma,** *depressed deep tendon reflexes, depression, lethargy, weakness*

CV: Decreased BP, **heart block,** *increased pulse*

GI: Belching, cramps, (PO) diarrhea, flatulence, impaction, nausea, obstruction, pain, vomiting

METAB: Hypermagnesemia

RESP: **Respiratory depression**

INTERACTIONS

Drugs

3 *Allopurinol, cefpodoxime, ciprofloxacin, atenolol, tetracyclines, iron salts, isoniazid, ketoconazole, lomefloxacin, norfloxacin, ofloxacin, pefloxacin, penicillamine, trovafloxacin:* Decreased PO effectiveness of these drugs with PO magnesium products

3 *Aspirin:* Decreased salicylate concentrations due to alkinization of urine with oral magnesium hydroxide

3 *Glipizide, glyburide:* Increased absorption of these drugs with oral magnesium hydroxide

3 *Nifedipine:* Decreased effect of nifedipine with parenteral magnesium sulfate

3 *Quinidine:* Increased quinidine concentrations with oral magnesium products

3 *Sodium polystyrene sulfonate:* Systemic alkalosis with oral magnesium products

3 *Succinylcholine:* Increased tox-

M

icity of these drugs with parenteral magnesium sulfate

Labs

• *False increase:* Serum alkaline phosphatase

SPECIAL CONSIDERATIONS
MONITORING PARAMETERS

• Parenteral magnesium: knee jerk reflexes prior to each dose (do not administer if absent), respiration rate (do not administer if <16/min), urine output (do not administer if <100 ml during 4 hr preceding each dose), serum magnesium concentrations (normal 1.5-3 mEq/L; therapeutic concentrations for preeclampsia, eclampsia, convulsions 4-7 mEq/L)

---

magnesium salicylate
Rx: Mobidin
OTC: Doan's pills
Chemical Class: Salicylic acid derivative
Therapeutic Class: Nonnarcotic analgesic; NSAID

CLINICAL PHARMACOLOGY
Mechanism of Action: Inhibits prostaglandin synthesis; analgesic, antiinflammatory, antipyretic actions

Pharmacokinetics

PO: Onset 15-30 min, peak 1-2 hr, duration 4-6 hr; 50%-90% bound to plasma proteins; metabolized in liver, eliminated in urine; $t_{1/2}$ 2 hr

INDICATIONS AND USES: Mild to moderate pain, rheumatoid arthritis, osteoarthritis, related rheumatic disorders

DOSAGE
Adult

• PO 650 mg q4h or 1090 mg tid, may increase to 3.6-4.8 g/day in 3-4 divided doses

💲 AVAILABLE FORMS/COST OF THERAPY

• Tab, Uncoated—Oral: (OTC) 325 mg, 24's: **$3.84;** 500 mg, 24's: **$4.61**

• Tab, Uncoated—Oral: 600 mg, 100's: **$23.22**

CONTRAINDICATIONS: Hypersensitivity to NSAIDs, hemophilia, bleeding ulcers, hemorrhagic states, advanced chronic renal insufficiency

PRECAUTIONS: Children; teenagers with chickenpox or influenza (association with Reye's syndrome); impaired hepatic function, history of peptic ulcer disease, diabetes mellitus, gout

PREGNANCY AND LACTATION: Pregnancy category C; excreted into breast milk; use caution in nursing mothers due to potential adverse effects in nursing infant

SIDE EFFECTS/ADVERSE REACTIONS

CNS: Confusion, dizziness, drowsiness, headache

EENT: Dimness of vision, reversible hearing loss, tinnitus

GI: Anorexia, diarrhea, *dyspepsia,* epigastric discomfort, **GI bleeding,** heartburn, hepatotoxicity, *nausea*

HEME: Decreased plasma iron concentration, **leukopenia,** prolonged bleeding time, shortened erythrocyte survival time, **thrombocytopenia**

METAB: Hypermagnesemia, hypoglycemia, hypokalemia, hyponatremia

RESP: Hyperpnea, wheezing

SKIN: Angioedema, bruising, hives, rash, urticaria

MISC: Fever, thirst

INTERACTIONS
Labs

• *False increase:* Serum bicarbonate, CSF protein, serum theophylline

• *False decrease:* Urine cocaine, urine estrogen, serum glucose, urine 17-hydroxycorticosteroids, urine opiates

---

* = non-FDA-approved use

- *False positive:* Urine ferric chloride test

SPECIAL CONSIDERATIONS
- Consider for patients with GI intolerance to aspirin or patients in whom interference with normal platelet function by aspirin or other NSAIDs is undesirable

MONITORING PARAMETERS
- AST, ALT, bilirubin, creatinine, CBC, hct if patient is on long-term therapy

mannitol
(man´i-tall)
Rx: Osmitrol, Resectisol
Chemical Class: Hexahydric alcohol
Therapeutic Class: Osmotic diuretic; genitourinary irrigant; antiglaucoma agent

CLINICAL PHARMACOLOGY
Mechanism of Action: Induces diuresis by elevating the osmolarity of the glomerular filtrate, thereby hindering the tubular reabsorption of water; excretion of sodium and chloride is increased

Pharmacokinetics
IV: Onset 30-60 min, peak 1 hr, duration 6-8 hr; mainly excreted unchanged in the urine; $t_{1/2}$ 15-100 min

INDICATIONS AND USES: Reduction of intracranial pressure associated with cerebral edema; reduction of intraocular pressure; improvement of renal function in oliguric phase of acute renal failure; irrigation in transurethral prostatic resection or other transurethral surgical procedures (2.5% only); promotion of urinary excretion of toxic substances

DOSAGE
Adult
- *Oliguria (prevention):* IV 50-100 g of 5%-25% sol

- *Oliguria (treatment):* IV 50-100 g of 15%-20% sol
- *Intraocular pressure, intracranial pressure:* IV 1.5-2 g/kg of 15%-25% sol over 30-60 min
- *Diuresis in drug intoxication:* IV 5%-10% sol continuously up to 200 g while maintaining urine output of 100-500 ml/hr
- *Urologic irrigation:* Add contents of two 50 ml vials of 25% mannitol to 900 ml sterile water for inj and use as irrigation

Child
- IV 0.5-1 g/kg initially, then 0.25-0.5 g/kg q4-6hr for maintenance

AVAILABLE FORMS/COST OF THERAPY
- Inj, Sol—IV: 5%, 1000 ml: **$38.59-$62.62**; 10%, 1000 ml: **$55.87-$89.11**; 15%, 500 ml: **$60.09-$76.69**; 20%, 500 ml: **$60.15-$89.70**; 25%, 50 ml: **$1.20-$6.13**

CONTRAINDICATIONS: Active intracranial bleeding, anuria, severe pulmonary congestion or edema, severe dehydration

PRECAUTIONS: Fluid and electrolyte imbalances, renal function impairment (consider use of 0.2 g/kg test dose followed by monitoring for increased urine flow), hepatic function impairment

PREGNANCY AND LACTATION: Pregnancy category C

SIDE EFFECTS/ADVERSE REACTIONS
CNS: Confusion, dizziness, headache, rebound increased intracranial pressure, *seizures*
CV: Angina-like chest pains, *CHF,* edema, hypertension, hypotension, tachycardia, thrombophlebitis
EENT: Blurred vision, loss of hearing, nasal congestion
GI: Diarrhea, dry mouth, *nausea, vomiting*

GU: Osmotic nephrosis, urinary retention

METAB: Acidosis, dehydration, electrolyte loss, fluid and electrolyte imbalances

SKIN: Skin necrosis, urticaria

MISC: Chills, fever

INTERACTIONS

Labs

• *False increase:* Serum osmolality, serum phosphate, CSF protein

• *False decrease:* Serum phosphate

SPECIAL CONSIDERATIONS

MONITORING PARAMETERS

• Serum electrolytes, urine output

---

maprotiline
(ma-proe'ti-leen)

Rx: Ludiomil

Chemical Class: Dibenzo-bicyclo-octadiene derivative

Therapeutic Class: Tetracyclic antidepressant

CLINICAL PHARMACOLOGY

Mechanism of Action: Blocks reuptake of norepinephrine presynaptically, prolonging neuronal activity; moderate-anticholinergic and sedative; slight orthostatic hypotensive activity

Pharmacokinetics

PO: Peak 9-16 hr, onset of therapeutic effect 2-3 wk; 88% bound to plasma proteins; metabolized in the liver, excreted in bile (30%) and urine (65%); $t_{1/2}$ 27-58 hr (active metabolite 60-90 hr)

INDICATIONS AND USES: Major depression, dysthymic disorder, anxiety associated with depression, depressive phase of bipolar disorder

DOSAGE

Adult

• PO 75 mg/day initially, increase by 25 mg q2 wk up to 150-225 mg/day divided qd-tid; elderly may require smaller doses

---

§ AVAILABLE FORMS/COST OF THERAPY

• Tab, Coated—Oral: 25 mg, 100's: **$27.95-$56.61**; 50 mg, 100's: **$40.95-$83.81**; 75 mg, 100's: **$71.48-$115.02**

CONTRAINDICATIONS: Acute recovery phase of MI, concurrent use of MAOIs, seizure disorder

PRECAUTIONS: Suicidal patients, prostatic hypertrophy, psychiatric disease, severe depression, increased intraocular pressure, narrow-angle glaucoma, urinary retention, cardiac disease; hepatic/renal disease; hyperthyroidism, electroshock therapy, elective surgery, elderly, abrupt discontinuation

PREGNANCY AND LACTATION: Pregnancy category B; excreted into breast milk, milk; plasma ratios of 1.5 and 1.3 have been reported, significance to the nursing infant unknown

SIDE EFFECTS/ADVERSE REACTIONS

CNS: Anxiety, confusion (especially in elderly), *dizziness, drowsiness,* EPS (elderly), fatigue, headache, increased psychiatric symptoms, insomnia, memory impairment, nervousness, nightmares, panic, *seizures* (dose related), stimulation, tremors, weakness

CV: **Dysrhythmias,** hypertension, *orthostatic hypotension,* palpitations, syncope, tachycardia

EENT: Blurred vision, increased intraocular pressure, mydriasis, nasal congestion, ophthalmoplegia, tinnitus

GI: Constipation, cramps, diarrhea, *dry mouth,* epigastric distress, hepatitis, increased appetite, jaundice, nausea, *paralytic ileus,* stomatitis, vomiting

GU: Urinary retention

HEME: **Agranulocytosis,** eosino-

---

philia, *leukopenia, thrombocytopenia*

SKIN: Photosensitivity, pruritus, rash, sweating, urticaria

INTERACTIONS

Drugs

3 *Barbiturates:* Reduced serum concentrations of cyclic antidepressants

2 *Bethanidine:* Reduced antihypertensive effect of bethanidine

3 *Carbamazepine:* Reduced cyclic antidepressant serum concentrations

3 *Cimetidine:* Increased maprotiline concentrations

2 *Clonidine:* Reduced antihypertensive response to clonidine; enhanced hypertensive response with abrupt clonidine withdrawal

3 *Debrisoquin:* Inhibited antihypertensive response of debrisoquin

2 *Epinephrine:* Markedly enhanced pressor response to IV epinephrine

3 *Ethanol:* Additive impairment of motor skills; abstinent alcoholics may eliminate cyclic antidepressants more rapidly than nonalcoholics

3 *Fluoxetine, fluvoxamine, grapefruit juice:* Marked increases in cyclic antidepressant plasma concentrations

3 *Guanethidine:* Inhibited antihypertensive response to guanethidine

2 *Moclobemide:* Potential association with fatal or non-fatal serotonin syndrome

A *MAOIs:* Excessive sympathetic response, mania, or hyperpyrexia possible

3 *Neuroleptics:* Increased therapeutic and toxic effects of both drugs

2 *Norepinephrine:* Markedly enhanced pressor response to norepinephrine

2 *Phenylephrine:* Enhanced pressor response to IV phenylephrine

3 *Propantheline:* Excessive anticholinergic effects

3 *Propoxyphene:* Enhanced effect of cyclic antidepressants

3 *Quinidine:* Increased cyclic antidepressant serum concentrations

3 *Tolazemide:* Enhanced hypoglycemic effects of tolazemide

Labs

• *False negative:* Serum tricyclic antidepressants screen

SPECIAL CONSIDERATIONS

• Not first-line agent due to risk of seizures

PATIENT/FAMILY EDUCATION

• Use caution in driving or other activities requiring alertness

• Do not discontinue abruptly after long-term use

MONITORING PARAMETERS

• CBC

• Weight

• Mental status: mood, sensorium, affect, suicidal tendencies

• Determination of maprotiline plasma concentrations is not routinely recommended, but may be useful in identifying toxicity, drug interactions, or noncompliance (adjustments in dosage should be made according to clinical response not plasma concentrations); therapeutic plasma levels 200-300 ng/ml (including active metabolite)

---

mazindol

(may´zin-dole)

Rx: Mazanor, Sanorex

Chemical Class: Imadazoline derivative

Therapeutic Class: Anorexiant

DEA Class: Schedule IV

CLINICAL PHARMACOLOGY

Mechanism of Action: Acts on adrenergic and dopaminergic pathways, directly stimulating the satiety center in the hypothalamic and

italic = common side effects   ***bold italic* = life-threatening reactions

limbic regions; produces CNS stimulation and blood pressure elevation; tolerance phenomenon demonstrated

Pharmacokinetics

PO: Onset 30-60 min, duration 8-15 hr; excreted primarily in urine as unchanged drug and conjugated metabolites

INDICATIONS AND USES: Exogenous obesity (as a short-term adjunct to caloric restriction)

DOSAGE

Adult

- PO 1 mg tid 1 hr ac, or 2 mg qd 1 hr before lunch

$ AVAILABLE FORMS/COST OF THERAPY

- Tab, Uncoated—Oral: 1 mg, 100's: **$154.25**; 2 mg, 100's: **$244.75**

CONTRAINDICATIONS: Hypersensitivity to sympathomimetic amines, glaucoma, history of drug abuse, cardiovascular disease, moderate to severe hypertension, advanced arteriosclerosis, agitated states, hyperthyroidism, within 14 days of MAOI administration

PRECAUTIONS: Diabetes mellitus, seizure disorders, mild hypertension, children

PREGNANCY AND LACTATION: Pregnancy category C

SIDE EFFECTS/ADVERSE REACTIONS

CNS: Dizziness, dysphoria, exacerbation of schizophrenia, headache, *insomnia,* mental depression, *nervousness, overstimulation, restlessness,* shivering, tremor

CV: Chest pain, palpitation, *tachycardia*

GI: Constipation, diarrhea, *dry mouth,* nausea, unpleasant taste

GU: Dysuria, impotence, pollakiuria

SKIN: Clamminess, excessive sweating, pallor, rash

INTERACTIONS
Drugs

3 *Furazolidone:* Hypertensive crisis

3 *Guanethidine:* Decreased antihypertensive effects

2 *MAOIs:* Hypertensive crisis

3 *Tricyclic antidepressants:* Decreased anorexiant effects

Labs

- *False positive:* Chlordiazepoxide, flurazepam, methadone, methapyrilene, methylphenidate, phendimetrazine

SPECIAL CONSIDERATIONS
PATIENT/FAMILY EDUCATION

- May cause insomnia; avoid taking late in the day
- Use caution while driving or performing other tasks requiring alertness; may cause dizziness or blurred vision
- Take with food if stomach upset occurs
- Do not discontinue abruptly

---

mebendazole

(me-ben′da-zole)

Rx: Vermox

Chemical Class: Benzimidazole derivative

Therapeutic Class: Anthelmintic

CLINICAL PHARMACOLOGY

Mechanism of Action: Causes degeneration of parasite's cytoplasmic microtubules and thereby selectively and irreversibly blocks glucose uptake in susceptible adult intestine-dwelling helminths and their tissue-dwelling larvae

Pharmacokinetics

PO: Poorly absorbed (5%-10%), peak 2-5 hr; 90%-95% bound to plasma proteins; metabolized by liver to inactive metabolites, eliminated primarily in feces (95%); $t_{1/2}$

2.5-5.5 hr (35 hr in liver dysfunction)

INDICATIONS AND USES: Single or mixed infections due to *Trichuris trichiura* (whipworm), *Enterobius vermicularis* (pinworm), *Ascaris lumbricoides* (roundworm), *Ancylostoma duodenale* (common hookworm), *Necator americanus* (American hookworm)

DOSAGE
Adult and Child
• *Pinworms:* PO 100 mg as a single dose; may need to repeat after 3 wk
• *Whipworms, roundworms, hookworms:* PO 100 mg bid for 3 consecutive days; repeat course in 3-4 wk if necessary

$ AVAILABLE FORMS/COST OF THERAPY
• Tab, Chewable—Oral: 100 mg, 12's: **$56.34-$62.60**

PRECAUTIONS: Child <2 yr

PREGNANCY AND LACTATION: Pregnancy category C; consider treatment if the parasite is causing clinical disease or may cause public health problems; it is doubtful that enough mebendazole is absorbed to be excreted into breast milk in significant quantities

SIDE EFFECTS/ADVERSE REACTIONS
CNS: Dizziness, fever
GI: Diarrhea, transient abdominal pain

INTERACTIONS
Drugs
3 *Carbamazepine:* Decreased mebendazole concentrations and effect via induction of metabolism
2 *Phenytoin:* Decreased mebendazole concentrations; possible impairment of therapeutic effect

SPECIAL CONSIDERATIONS
PATIENT/FAMILY EDUCATION
• Chew or crush tablets and administer with food
• Parasite death and removal from digestive tract may take up to 3 days after treatment
• Consult clinician if not cured in 3 wk
• For pinworms, all household contacts of patient should be treated
• Strict hygiene essential to prevent reinfection; disinfect toilet facilities, change and launder undergarments, bed linens, towels, and nightclothes

---

mecamylamine

(mek-a-mill'a-meen)
Rx: Inversine
Chemical Class: Ganglionic blocker
Therapeutic Class: Ganglionic blocker: antihypertensive

CLINICAL PHARMACOLOGY
Mechanism of Action: Blocks transmission of impulses at both sympathetic and parasympathetic ganglia; hypotensive effect is due to reduction in sympathetic tone, vasodilation, reduced cardiac output; predominantly orthostatic
Pharmacokinetics
PO: Onset 0.5-2 hr, duration 6-12 hr; mostly excreted unchanged in urine

INDICATIONS AND USES: Moderate to severe hypertension (not 1st line)

DOSAGE
Adult
• PO 2.5 mg bid initially, may increase in increments of 2.5 mg q2 days until desired response, usual maintenance dose 25 mg/day divided bid-qid

$ AVAILABLE FORMS/COST OF THERAPY
• Tab, Uncoated—Oral: 2.5 mg, 100's: **$13.03**

CONTRAINDICATIONS: Mild, labile hypertension; coronary insuf-

---

italic = common side effects   ***bold italic*** = life-threatening reactions

ficiency, recent MI; uremia; glaucoma; organic pyloric stenosis; patients receiving sulfonamides or antibiotics

PRECAUTIONS: Cerebral arteriosclerosis, recent CVA, renal insufficiency, abrupt discontinuation, prostatic hypertrophy, bladder neck obstruction, urethral stricture

PREGNANCY AND LACTATION: Pregnancy category C; not recommended in nursing mothers

SIDE EFFECTS/ADVERSE REACTIONS

CNS: Choreiform movements, *fatigue,* mental aberrations, paresthesia, *sedation,* **seizures,** tremor, weakness

CV: Orthostatic dizziness, syncope

EENT: Blurred vision, dilated pupils

GI: Anorexia, constipation, dry mouth, glossitis, nausea, *paralytic ileus,* vomiting

GU: Decreased libido, impotence, urinary retention

SPECIAL CONSIDERATIONS

PATIENT/FAMILY EDUCATION

• Take after meals

• Arise slowly from reclining position

• Orthostatic changes are exacerbated by alcohol, exercise, hot weather

MONITORING PARAMETERS

• Maintenance doses should be limited to dose that causes slight faintness or dizziness in the standing position

meclizine
(mek'li-zeen)
Rx: Antivert, Medivert, Meclicot, **OTC:** Bonine
Chemical Class: Piperazine derivative
Therapeutic Class: Antihistamine; antivertigo agent

CLINICAL PHARMACOLOGY

Mechanism of Action: Central anticholinergic actions; diminishes vestibular stimulation, depresses labyrinthine function; an action on medullary chemoreceptive trigger zone may also be involved in antiemetic effect; also has antihistaminic, CNS depressant, and local anesthetic effects

Pharmacokinetics

PO: Onset 1 hr, duration 8-24 hr, $t_{1/2}$ 6 hr

INDICATIONS AND USES: Motion sickness; "possibly effective" in vertigo associated with diseases affecting vestibular system

DOSAGE

Adult and Child >12 yr

• *Motion sickness:* PO 25-50 mg 1 hr prior to travel; may repeat qd for duration of journey

• *Vertigo:* PO 25-100 mg/day in divided doses, usually tid

§ AVAILABLE FORMS/COST OF THERAPY

• Tab, Uncoated—Oral: 12.5 mg, 100's: **$2.85-$40.04;** 25 mg, 100's: **$2.55-$69.56;** 30 mg, 100's: **$24.65;** 50 mg, 100's: **$120.31**

• Tab, Chewable—Oral: 25 mg, 100's: **$2.77**

PRECAUTIONS: Children <12 yr, glaucoma; obstructive GI, GU disease; prostatic hypertrophy

PREGNANCY AND LACTATION: Pregnancy category B; used for treatment of nausea and vomiting during pregnancy; excretion into breast milk unknown

SIDE EFFECTS/ADVERSE REACTIONS

CNS: Drowsiness, excitation (paradoxical reaction in children), restlessness

CV: Hypotension, palpitations, tachycardia

EENT: Blurred vision, diplopia, dry nose, dry throat

GI: Anorexia, constipation, diarrhea, *dry mouth,* nausea, vomiting

GU: Difficult urination, urinary frequency, urinary retention

SKIN: Rash, urticaria

---

meclofenamate
(me′kloe-fen′a-mate)

Rx: Meclomen, Meclodium

Chemical Class: Anthranilic acid derivative

Therapeutic Class: NSAID with analgesic and antipyretic activity

---

CLINICAL PHARMACOLOGY

Mechanism of Action: Reversible cyclooxygenase (i.e., prostaglandin synthetase) inhibitor; nonselectively decreases the formation of both prostaglandins and thromboxane A2; variable effects on lipoxygenase synthesis and subsequent leukotriene production; antiinflammatory, antipyretic, and analgesic activity; inhibits platelet aggregation

Pharmacokinetics

PO: Peak 0.5-2 hr (completely bioavailable); >90% bound to plasma proteins; metabolized by liver, excreted in urine (metabolites); $t_{1/2}$ 2-3.3 hr

INDICATIONS AND USES: Acute gouty arthritis,* menorrhagia, nephrotic syndrome,* dysmenorrhea, osteoarthritis, rheumatoid arthritis, ankylosing spondylitis,* pain—mild to moderate, psoriatic arthritis*

DOSAGE

Adult

• *Mild to moderate pain:* PO 50 mg q4-6h; max 400 mg/day

• *Primary dysmenorrhea:* PO 100 mg tid for up to 6 days; start at onset of menstrual flow

• *Arthritis:* PO 200-400 mg/day in 3-4 divided doses

💲 **AVAILABLE FORMS/COST OF THERAPY**

• Cap, Gel—Oral: 50 mg, 100's: **$39.80-$174.24;** 100 mg, 100's: **$60.36-$339.72**

CONTRAINDICATIONS: Bronchospasm, nasal polyps, angioedema precipitated by aspirin or other NSAIDs

PRECAUTIONS: History of GI ulceration, bleeding, or perforation; renal dysfunction, hypertension or cardiac conditions aggravated by fluid retention and edema, history of liver dysfunction, history of coagulation

PREGNANCY AND LACTATION: Pregnancy category B (category D if used in 3rd trimester); may implant labor and prolong pregnancy, cause constriction of the ductus arteriosus *in utero,* or cause persistent pulmonary hypertension of the newborn

SIDE EFFECTS/ADVERSE REACTIONS

CNS: Dizziness, headache, lightheadedness

CV: Chest pain, *CHF, dysrhythmias,* edema, hypertension, hypotension, palpitation, tachycardia

EENT: Dry eyes, hearing disturbances, photophobia, tinnitus, visual disturbances

GI: Abdominal cramps, constipation, *diarrhea, dyspepsia,* flatulence, *gastric or duodenal ulcer with bleeding or perforation,* hepatitis,

---

italic = common side effects   ***bold italic*** = life-threatening reactions

nausea, occult blood in stool, ***pancreatitis,*** vomiting

*GU: **Acute renal failure***

*HEME: **Agranulocytosis,*** eosinophilia, ***leukopenia, neutropenia, pancytopenia, thrombocytopenia***

METAB: Hyperglycemia, hyperkalemia, hypoglycemia, hyponatremia

RESP: Bronchospasm, dyspnea

SKIN: Photosensitivity, rash, urticaria

INTERACTIONS

Drugs

3 *Aminoglycosides:* Reduced clearance with elevated aminoglycoside levels and potential for toxicity (especially indomethacin in premature infants; other NSAIDs probably)

3 *Anticoagulants:* Excessive hypoprothrombinemia, decreased platelet aggregation with increased risk of GI bleeding

3 *Antihypertensives (α-blockers, angiotensin-converting enzyme inhibitors, angiotensin II receptor blockers, β-blockers, diuretics):* Inhibition of antihypertensive and other favorable hemodynamic effects

3 *Corticosteroids:* Increased risk of GI ulceration

3 *Cyclosporine:* Increased nephrotoxicity risk

3 *Lithium:* Decreased clearance of lithium (mediated via prostaglandins) resulting in elevated serum lithium levels and risk of toxicity

3 *Methotrexate:* Decreased renal secretion of methotrexate resulting in elevated methotrexate levels and risk of toxicity

3 *Phenylpropanolamine:* Possible acute hypertensive reaction

3 *Potassium-sparing diuretics:* Additive hyperkalemia potential

3 *Triamterene:* Acute renal failure reported with addition of indomethacin; caution with other NSAIDs

SPECIAL CONSIDERATIONS

• No significant advantage over other NSAIDs; cost should govern use

PATIENT/FAMILY EDUCATION
MONITORING PARAMETERS

• Initial hemogram and fecal occult blood test within 3 mo of starting regular chronic therapy; repeat every 6-12 mo (more frequently in high-risk patients (>65 years, peptic ulcer disease, concurrent steroids or anticoagulants); electrolytes, creatinine, and BUN within 3 mo of starting regular chronic therapy; repeat every 6-12 mo

---

medroxyprogesterone

(me-drox'ee-proe-jess'te-rone)
Rx: Amen, Curretab, Cycrin, Depo-Provera, Provera
Chemical Class: 17 α-hydroxyprogesterone derivative
Therapeutic Class: Progestin; contraceptive; antineoplastic

CLINICAL PHARMACOLOGY

Mechanism of Action: Exerts a progestational effect on the endometrium, alters cervical mucus, suppresses ovulation in some patients, renders the endometrium hostile to implantation

Pharmacokinetics

Metabolized in the liver

IM: Peak levels 3 wk, $t_{1/2}$-50 days

INDICATIONS AND USES: Dysfunctional uterine bleeding, secondary amenorrhea, endometrial cancer, renal cancer, contraception, menopause,* obesity-hypoventilation syndrome (Pickwickian syndrome),* obstructive sleep apnea,* hirsutism,* homozygous sickle-cell disease*

---

* = non-FDA-approved use

DOSAGE
Adult
• *Secondary amenorrhea:* PO 5-10 mg qd for 5-10 days; withdrawal bleeding usually occurs 3-7 days after therapy ends
• *Endometrial/renal cancer:* IM 400-1000 mg/wk; maintenance of improvement may require as little as 400 mg/mo
• *Uterine bleeding:* PO 5-10 mg qd for 5-10 days; withdrawal bleeding usually occurs 3-7 days after therapy ends
• *Contraceptive:* IM 150 mg q3 mo
• *Menopause:* PO 10 mg qd days 16-25 of month; or 2.5-5 mg qd (in combination with estrogen)

AVAILABLE FORMS/COST OF THERAPY
• Tab, Uncoated—Oral: 2.5 mg, 100's: **$29.34-$54.20;** 5 mg, 100's: **$22.50-$91.51;** 10 mg, 100's: **$16.31-$66.30**
• Inj, Susp—IM: 150 mg/ml, 1 ml: **$48.10;** 400 mg/ml, 2.5 ml: **$110.39-$156.44**

CONTRAINDICATIONS: Impaired liver function or disease, breast cancer, undiagnosed vaginal bleeding, missed abortion, use as a diagnostic test for pregnancy

PRECAUTIONS: Epilepsy, migraine, asthma, cardiac or renal dysfunction, depression, diabetes

PREGNANCY AND LACTATION: Pregnancy category X; compatible with breast feeding

SIDE EFFECTS/ADVERSE REACTIONS
CNS: Depression, *dizziness, headache, insomnia, fatigue*
CV: Edema
GI: **Cholestatic jaundice;** *increased weight (approx 4 lbs/yr), nausea, appetite changes*
GU: Amenorrhea, breakthrough bleeding, breast changes, decreased libido, delayed return to fertilty, hot flashes, leukorrhea
METAB: Decreased bone density
SKIN: Acne, alopecia, hirsutism, melasma, oily skin, photosensitivity, rash, melasma

INTERACTIONS
Drugs
3 *Aminoglutethimide:* Reduced plasma medroxyprogesterone concentrations
Labs
• *Feces:* Green color

SPECIAL CONSIDERATIONS
PATIENT/FAMILY EDUCATION
• Take protective measures against exposure to ultraviolet light
• Diabetic patients must monitor blood glucose carefully during therapy
• Take with food if GI upset occurs
• When used as contraceptive, menstrual cycle may be disrupted and irregular and unpredictable bleeding or spotting results; usually decreases to the point of amenorrhea as treatment continues (55% at 1 yr)
• After stopping injections, 50% of women who become pregnant will do so in about 10 mo after the last injection, 93% within 18 mo; not related to length of time drug used; women with lower body weights conceive sooner
• Failure rate 0.3% in first year of constant use

M

---

medrysone
(me'dri-sone)
Rx: HMS
Chemical Class: Glucocorticoid
Therapeutic Class: Ophthalmic corticosteroid

CLINICAL PHARMACOLOGY
Mechanism of Action: Suppresses aspects of the inflammatory process

---

italic = common side effects   **bold italic** = life-threatening reactions

such as hyperemia, cellular infiltration, vascularization, and fibroblastic proliferation

Pharmacokinetics

OPHTHAL: Absorbed through aqueous humor; metabolized in liver, excreted in urine and feces

INDICATIONS AND USES: Steroid-responsive inflammatory conditions of the palpebral and bulbar conjunctiva, lid, cornea, and anterior segment of the globe; corneal injury graft rejection following keratoplasty

DOSAGE

Adult and Child

• INSTILL 1 gtt q1h during the day and q2h during the night; reduce dosage to 1 gtt q4h when a favorable response is obtained

💲 **AVAILABLE FORMS/COST OF THERAPY**

• Susp—Ophth: 1%, 5, 10 ml: **$24.90**/10 ml

CONTRAINDICATIONS: Acute superficial herpes simplex keratitis; fungal diseases of ocular structures; vaccinia, varicella, and most other viral diseases of the cornea and conjunctiva; ocular TB; following uncomplicated removal of a superficial corneal foreign body

PRECAUTIONS: Prolonged use, infections of the eye, glaucoma

PREGNANCY AND LACTATION: Pregnancy category C

SIDE EFFECTS/ADVERSE REACTIONS

EENT: Cataracts, decreased acuity, glaucoma exacerbation, increased intraocular pressure, increased possibility of corneal infection, optic nerve damage, poor corneal wound healing, transient burning, stinging

SPECIAL CONSIDERATIONS PATIENT/FAMILY EDUCATION

• Do not discontinue use without consulting clinician

• Notify clinician if no improvement after 1 wk, if condition worsens, or if pain, itching, or swelling of the eye occurs

MONITORING PARAMETERS

• Check intraocular pressure and lens frequently during prolonged use

---

mefenamic acid

(me-fe-nam′ik)

Rx: Ponstel

Chemical Class: Anthranilic acid derivative

Therapeutic Class: NSAID with analgesic and antipyretic activity

CLINICAL PHARMACOLOGY

Mechanism of Action: Reversible cyclooxygenase (i.e., prostaglandin synthetase) inhibitor; nonselectively decreases the formation of both prostaglandins and thromboxane A2; variable effects on lipoxygenase synthesis and subsequent leukotriene production; antiinflammatory, antipyretic, and analgesic activity; inhibits platelet aggregation

Pharmacokinetics

PO: Peak 2-4 hr; >90% bound to plasma proteins; metabolized by liver, excreted in urine (metabolites); $t_{1/2}$ 2-4 hr

INDICATIONS AND USES: Dysmenorrhea, fever,* menorrhagia,* osteoarthritis,* pain, low back pain, premenstrual syndrome,* rheumatoid arthritis*

DOSAGE

Adult and Child >14 yr

• *Acute pain:* PO 500 mg, then 250 mg q6h prn; not to exceed 1 wk of therapy

• *Primary dysmenorrhea:* PO 500 mg, then 250 mg q6h; start with onset of bleeding and associated symptoms

---

* = non-FDA-approved use

§ AVAILABLE FORMS/COST OF THERAPY

• Cap, Gel—Oral: 250 mg, 100's: **$112.40**

CONTRAINDICATIONS: Bronchospasm, nasal polyps, angioedema precipitated by aspirin or other NSAIDs

PRECAUTIONS: History of GI ulceration, bleeding, or perforation; renal dysfunction, hypertension or cardiac conditions aggravated by fluid retention and edema, history of liver dysfunction, history of coagulation

PREGNANCY AND LACTATION: Pregnancy category C (category D if used in 3rd trimester)

SIDE EFFECTS/ADVERSE REACTIONS

CNS: Dizziness, headache, lightheadedness

CV: Chest pain, CHF, **dysrhythmias,** edema, hypertension, hypotension, palpitation, tachycardia

EENT: Dry eyes, hearing disturbances, photophobia, tinnitus, visual disturbances

GI: Abdominal cramps, constipation, *diarrhea, dyspepsia,* flatulence, **gastric or duodenal ulcer with bleeding or perforation, hepatitis,** *nausea,* occult blood in stool, pancreatitis, vomiting

GU: **Acute renal failure**

HEME: **Agranulocytosis,** eosinophilia, **leukopenia, neutropenia, pancytopenia, thrombocytopenia**

METAB: Hyperglycemia, hyperkalemia, hypoglycemia, hyponatremia

RESP: Bronchospasm, dyspnea

SKIN: Photosensitivity, rash, urticaria

INTERACTIONS

Drugs

§ *Aminoglycosides:* Reduced clearance with elevated aminoglycoside levels and potential for toxicity (especially indomethacin in premature infants; other NSAIDs probably)

§ *Anticoagulants:* Excessive hypoprothrombinemia, decreased platelet aggregation with increased risk of GI bleeding

§ *Antihypertensives (α-blockers, angiotensin-converting enzyme inhibitors, angiotensin II receptor blockers, β-blockers, diuretics):* Inhibition of antihypertensive and other favorable hemodynamic effects

§ *Corticosteroids:* Increased risk of GI ulceration

§ *Cyclosporine:* Increased nephrotoxicity risk

§ *Lithium:* Decreased clearance of lithium (mediated via prostaglandins) resulting in elevated serum lithium levels and risk of toxicity

② *Methotrexate:* Decreased renal secretion of methotrexate resulting in elevated methotrexate levels and risk of toxicity

§ *Phenylpropanolamine:* Possible acute hypertensive reaction

§ *Potassium-sparing diuretics:* Additive hyperkalemia potential

§ *Triamterene:* Acute renal failure reported with addition of indomethacin; caution with other NSAIDs

SPECIAL CONSIDERATIONS

• No significant advantage over other NSAIDs; cost should govern use

• Use of beyond 1 wk is not recommended

MONITORING PARAMETERS

• Initial hemogram and fecal occult blood test within 3 mo of starting regular chronic therapy; repeat 6-12 mo (more frequently in high-risk patients (>65 years, peptic ulcer disease, concurrent steroids or anticoagulants); electrolytes, creatinine, and BUN within 3 mo of starting

M

---

italic = common side effects   ***bold italic*** = life-threatening reactions

regular chronic therapy; repeat every 6-12 mo

mefloquine
(me'flow-quine)
Rx: Lariam
Chemical Class: Quinolinemethanol derivative
Therapeutic Class: Antimalarial

CLINICAL PHARMACOLOGY
Mechanism of Action: Blood schizonticide
Pharmacokinetics
PO: 98% bound to plasma proteins, concentrated in blood erythrocytes; metabolized in liver; $t_{1/2}$ 15-33 days
INDICATIONS AND USES: Treatment and prevention of *Plasmodium falciparum* and *P. vivax* malaria infections
DOSAGE
Adult
• *Treatment:* PO 1250 mg (5 tabs) as a single dose
• *Prevention:* PO 250 mg qwk for 4 wk, then 250 mg q2wk; CDC recommends 250 mg qwk starting 1 wk prior to travel, continued weekly during travel and for 4 wk after leaving endemic area
Child
• PO: CDC recommends following doses to be taken weekly starting 1 wk prior to travel, continued weekly during travel, and for 4 wk after leaving endemic area: 15-19 kg, ¼ tab; 20-30 kg, ½ tab; 31-45 kg, ¾ tab; >45 kg, 1 tab
$ AVAILABLE FORMS/COST OF THERAPY
• Tab, Uncoated—Oral: 250 mg, 25's: **$185.96**
PRECAUTIONS: Children, cardiac dysrhythmias, neurologic disease
PREGNANCY AND LACTATION: Pregnancy category C; use caution

during the 1st 12-14 wk of pregnancy; excreted in breast milk in amounts not thought to be harmful to the nursing infant and insufficient to provide adequate protection against malaria
SIDE EFFECTS/ADVERSE REACTIONS
CNS: Anxiety, *coma,* confusion, disorientation, dizziness, hallucinations, headache, *seizures,* syncope
CV: Bradycardia, extrasystole
EENT: Retinal, lens, corneal abnormalities (rats only), tinnitus
GI: Abdominal pain, diarrhea, loss of appetite, nausea, transiently increased transaminases, vomiting
HEME: **Leukopenia, thrombocytopenia**
MS: Myalgia
SKIN: Itching, rash
SPECIAL CONSIDERATIONS
PATIENT/FAMILY EDUCATION
• Do not take on an empty stomach
• Take medication with at least 8 oz water
• Caution, initially, when driving, operating machinery, where concentration necessary
MONITORING PARAMETERS
• Liver function tests and ophthalmic examinations during prolonged therapy

megestrol
(me-jess'trole)
Rx: Megace
Chemical Class: Progesterone derivative (methylpregnadienedione)
Therapeutic Class: Antineoplastic; appetite stimulant

CLINICAL PHARMACOLOGY
Mechanism of Action: Antineoplastic effect may result from suppression of luteinizing hormone by inhibition of pituitary function or a

local effect on cancerous cells; effects on weight gain may be related to appetite-stimulation or metabolic effects

Pharmacokinetics

PO: Peak 1-5 hr; metabolized in liver, eliminated in urine and feces; $t_{1/2}$ 60 min

INDICATIONS AND USES: Anorexia, cachexia, or unexplained weight loss in patients with AIDS (suspension); advanced breast or endometrial cancer

DOSAGE

Adult

• *Breast cancer:* PO 40 mg qid for at least 2 mo

• *Endometrial cancer:* PO 40-320 mg/day in divided doses for at least 2 mo

• *Anorexia, cachexia:* PO 800 mg/day (20 ml susp/day) initially; daily doses of 400-800 mg have been shown to be effective

💲 **AVAILABLE FORMS/COST OF THERAPY**

• Tab, Uncoated—Oral: 20 mg, 100's: **$52.50-$72.03;** 40 mg, 100's: **$75.52-$128.48**

• Susp—Oral: 40 mg/ml, 235.6 ml: **$137.24**

CONTRAINDICATIONS: As a diagnostic test for pregnancy, known or suspected pregnancy, prophylactic use to avoid weight loss

PRECAUTIONS: Children, HIV-infected women

PREGNANCY AND LACTATION: Pregnancy category X; not recommended during the 1st 4 mo of pregnancy

SIDE EFFECTS/ADVERSE REACTIONS

CNS: Headache, confusion, depression, hypesthesia, neuropathy, paresthesia

CV: Edema, palpitation

GI: Abdominal pain, nausea, vomiting, weight gain, flatulence

GU: Gynecomastia, breast tenderness, impotence, breakthrough bleeding

HEME: Thrombophlebitis, ***pulmonary embolism***

RESP: Dyspnea

SPECIAL CONSIDERATIONS

• Average weight gain in AIDS patients 11 lbs in 12 wk. Begin therapy only after treatable causes of weight loss are sought and addressed

---

menotropins

(men-oh-troe′pins)

Rx: Humegon, Pergonal, Repronex

Chemical Class: Purified preparation of human pituitary gonadotropins, (FSH and LH)

Therapeutic Class: Ovarian stimulant; fertility agent

CLINICAL PHARMACOLOGY

Mechanism of Action: Women: produces ovarian follicular growth in the absence of primary ovarian failure; does not induce ovulation; men: with human chorionic gonadotropin (HCG), induces spermatogenesis in the presence of primary or secondary pituitary hypofunction

Pharmacokinetics

IM: $t_{1/2}$ of FSH and LH 70 hr and 4 hr, respectively; 8% of dose excreted unchanged in urine

INDICATIONS AND USES: Stimulation of ovarian follicular growth prior to induction of ovulation by HCG; induction of multiple follicles in ovulatory patients participating in an *in vitro* fertilization program; stimulation of spermatogenesis in men with primary or secondary hypogonadotropic hypogonadism (in conjunction with HCG)

DOSAGE

Adult

• Women: IM 75 IU FSH/LH qd for

M

---

italic = common side effects   **bold italic** = life-threatening reactions

7-12 days, followed by 10,000 IU HCG 1 day after last dose of menotropins; repeat for at least 2 more cycles if evidence of ovulation, but no pregnancy, then increase to 150 IU FSH/LH qd for 7-12 days, followed by 10,000 IU HCG 1 day after last dose of menotropins, repeat as above
• Men: IM 75 IU FSH/LH 3 times/wk with HCG 2000 IU 2 times/wk for 4 mo (following pretreatment with HCG alone 5000 IU 3 times/wk for 4-6 mo)

$ **AVAILABLE FORMS/COST OF THERAPY**
• Inj, Sol—IM: 75 U, 1's: **$56.40-$71.60**

CONTRAINDICATIONS: Women: Primary ovarian failure, abnormal bleeding; thyroid, adrenal dysfunction; organic intracranial lesion, ovarian cysts, pregnancy; men: primary testicular failure, normal pituitary function, infertility disorder other than hyopgonadotropic hypogonadism

PREGNANCY AND LACTATION: Pregancy category X

SIDE EFFECTS/ADVERSE REACTIONS
CNS: Chills, dizziness, febrile reactions, headache, malaise, *stroke*
CV: Tachycardia, *venous, arterial thromboembolism*
GI: Abdominal pain, bloating, cramps, diarrhea, *nausea,* vomiting
GU: Adnexal torsion, *ectopic pregnancy, hemoperitoneum, hyperstimulation syndrome* (sudden ovarian enlargement and ascites, with or without pain or pleural effusion), ovarian cysts, *ovarian enlargement* (20%)
MS: Joint pains, musculoskeletal aches
RESP: Acute respiratory distress syndrome, atelectasis, dyspnea, tachypnea

SKIN: Body rashes, pain, rash, irritation at inj site
MISC: Gynecomastia (men)

SPECIAL CONSIDERATIONS
PATIENT/FAMILY EDUCATION
• Multiple births occur in approximately 20% of women treated with menotropins and HCG
• Couple should engage in intercourse daily, beginning on the day prior to HCG administration, until ovulation occurs
• Ovarian enlargement regresses without treatment in 2-3 wk

MONITORING PARAMETERS
• Urinary estrogen; do not administer HCG if >150 µg/24 hr (increased risk of hyperstimulation of ovaries syndrome)
• Sonographic visualization of ovaries; estradiol levels

---

mepenzolate
(me-pen'zoe-late)
Rx: Cantil
Chemical Class: Quaternary ammonium compound
Therapeutic Class: Gastrointestinal antispasmodic agent; gastrointestinal antiulcer agent (adjunct)

CLINICAL PHARMACOLOGY
Mechanism of Action: Inhibits GI motility and diminishes gastric acid secretion
Pharmacokinetics
PO: Onset 1 hr, duration 3-4 hr, poor lipid solubility; 3%-22% of dose excreted in urine, remainder excreted in feces (probably as unabsorbed drug)

INDICATIONS AND USES: Peptic ulcer disease (in combination with other drugs); functional GI disorders (diarrhea, pylorospasm, hypermotility, neurogenic colon)*; irritable bowel syndrome (spastic colon,

---

* = non-FDA-approved use

mucous colitis)*; acute enterocolitis,* ulcerative colitis,* diverticulitis,* mild dysenteries,* pancreatitis,* splenic flexure syndrome*

DOSAGE

Adult

• PO 25-50 mg qid with meals, hs

$ AVAILABLE FORMS/COST OF THERAPY

• Tab, Uncoated—Oral: 25 mg, 100's: **$94.08**

CONTRAINDICATIONS: Hypersensitivity to anticholinergic drugs, narrow-angle glaucoma, obstructive uropathy, obstructive disease of the GI tract, paralytic ileus, intestinal atony, unstable cardiovascular status in acute hemorrhage, severe ulcerative colitis, toxic megacolon complicating ulcerative colitis, myasthenia gravis

PRECAUTIONS: Hyperthyroidism, CAD, dysrhythmias, CHF, ulcerative colitis, hypertension, hiatal hernia, hepatic disease, renal disease, urinary retention, prostatic hypertrophy, elderly, children, glaucoma

PREGNANCY AND LACTATION: Pregnancy category C; excretion into breast milk unknown, although would be expected to be minimal due to quaternary structure

SIDE EFFECTS/ADVERSE REACTIONS

CNS: Anxiety, confusion, dizziness, drowsiness, hallucination, headache, insomnia, stimulation (especially in elderly), weakness

CV: Palpitations, tachycardia

EENT: Blurred vision, cycloplegia, increased ocular tension, mydriasis, photophobia

GI: Absence of taste, *constipation, dry mouth,* dysphagia, heartburn, nausea, ***paralytic ileus,*** vomiting

GU: Hesitancy, impotence, *retention*

SKIN: Allergic reactions, anhidrosis, fever, pruritis, rash, urticaria

SPECIAL CONSIDERATIONS
PATIENT/FAMILY EDUCATION

• Take drug 30-60 min before a meal

• Drug may cause drowsiness, dizziness, or blurred vision; use caution while driving or performing other tasks requiring alertness

• Notify clinician if eye pain occurs

---

meperidine
(me-per′i-deen)
Rx: Demerol
Combinations
  Rx: with promethazine
    (Mepergan)
Chemical Class: Synthetic opium alkaloid; phenylpiperidine derivative
Therapeutic Class: Narcotic analgesic
DEA Class: Schedule II

M

CLINICAL PHARMACOLOGY
Mechanism of Action: Narcotic agonist with activity at Mu receptors (supraspinal analgesia, euphoria, respiratory and physical depression, miosis, and reduced GI motility), Kappa receptors (pentazocine-like spinal analgesia, sedation, and miosis), and Delta receptors (dysphoria, psychtomimetic effects [e.g., hallucinations], and respiratory and vasomotor stimulation caused by drugs with antagonist activity); compared to morphine, equal analgesia, respiratory depression, and physical dependence; less antitussive, constipation, sedation

Pharmacokinetics
PO: Peak analgesia within 1 hr, duration 2-4 hr
IM: Peak analgesia 30-50 min, duration 2-4 hr
SC: Peak analgesia 40-60 min, duration 2-4 hr

---

italic = common side effects   ***bold italic*** = life-threatening reactions

IV: Peak analgesia 5-30 min, duration 2-4 hr

60%-80% bound to plasma proteins; metabolized by liver (normeperidine is an active metabolite with half the analgesic potency but twice the CNS stimulant potency of the parent drug), eliminated in urine; $t_{1/2}$ 3-5 hr (normeperidine $t_{1/2}$ 8-21 hr; may be prolonged in renal impairment)

INDICATIONS AND USES: Moderate to severe pain, preoperative sedation (parenteral)

DOSAGE

• Oral doses are about half as effective as parenteral doses

Adult

• *Analgesia:* PO/IM/IV/SC 50-150 mg q3-4h prn

• *Preoperative sedation:* IM/SC 50-100 mg 30-90 min before beginning anesthesia

Child

• *Analgesia:* PO/IM/IV/SC 1-1.5 mg/kg/dose q3-4h prn; max 100 mg/dose

• *Preoperative sedation:* IM/SC 1-2 mg/kg 30-90 min before beginning anesthesia

$ AVAILABLE FORMS/COST OF THERAPY

• Inj, Sol—IM, IV, SC: 10 mg per ml, 30 ml: **$17.00-$19.00;** 25 mg/ml, 1 ml: **$0.52-$1.14;** 50 mg/ml, 1 ml: **$0.50-$1.20;** 75 mg/ml, 1 ml: **$0.41-$1.22;** 100 mg/ml, 1 ml: **$0.63-$1.28**

• Syr—Oral: 50 mg/5ml, 480 ml: **$95.16**

• Tab, Uncoated—Oral: 50 mg, 100's: **$68.12-$84.79;** 100 mg, 100's: **$129.57-$161.25**

CONTRAINDICATIONS: Concurrent use and within 14 days of MAOI therapy

PRECAUTIONS: Head injury, increased intracranial pressure, acute abdominal conditions, asthma and respiratory conditions, elderly, renal function impairment (normeperidine may accumulate, resulting in increased CNS adverse reactions), hepatic impairment, hypothyroidism, Addison's disease, prostatic hypertrophy, urethral stricture, history of drug abuse

PREGNANCY AND LACTATION: Pregnancy category B (category D if used for prolonged periods or in high doses at term); use during labor may produce neonatal respiratory depression; compatible with breast feeding

SIDE EFFECTS/ADVERSE REACTIONS

CNS: Agitation, dependency, dizziness, *drowsiness,* lethargy, myoclonus, restlessness, *sedation,* **seizures,** tremors, twitches

CV: Bradycardia, orthostatic hypotension, palpitations, tachycardia

GI: Anorexia, constipation, increased amylase, lipase; *nausea, vomiting*

GU: Urinary retention

RESP: **Respiratory depression, respiratory paralysis**

SKIN: Flushing, rash, urticaria

INTERACTIONS

Drugs

3 *Antihistamines, chloral hydrate, glutethimide, methocarbamol:* Enhanced depressant effects

3 *Barbiturates:* Additive respiratory and CNS depressant effects

3 *Cimetidine:* Increased respiratory and CNS depression

3 *Ethanol:* Additive CNS effects

⚠ *MAOIs:* Accumulation of CNS serotonin leading to agitation, blood pressure changes, hyperpyrexia, seizures

3 *Neuroleptics:* Hypotension, excessive CNS depression

3 *Phenytoin:* Enhanced metabolism; reduced meperidine concentrations

2 *Selegiline:* Though primarily

---

* = non-FDA-approved use

MAO-B inhibitor, residual MAO-A activity; see MAOI description
Labs
• *False increase:* Amylase and lipase

SPECIAL CONSIDERATIONS
PATIENT/FAMILY EDUCATION
• Physical dependency may result when used for extended periods
• Do not administer agonist/antagonist analgesics (i.e., pentazocine, nalbuphine, butorphanol, dezocine, buprenorphine) to patient who has received a prolonged course of meperidine (a pure agonist). In opioid-dependent patients, mixed agonist/antagonist analgesics may precipitate withdrawal symptoms.
• Change position slowly; orthostatic hypotension may occur
• Avoid hazardous activities if drowsiness or dizziness occurs
• Avoid alcohol, other CNS depressants unless directed by clinician
• Minimize nausea by administering with food and remain lying down following dose

---

mephentermine
(me-fen'ter-meen)
Rx: Wyamine
Chemical Class: Amphetamine derivative
Therapeutic Class: Antihypotensive

CLINICAL PHARMACOLOGY
Mechanism of Action: Primarily an indirect sympathomimetic that releases norepinephrine from its storage sites; increases blood pressure by increasing cardiac output (positive inotropic effect) and, to a lesser degree, by increasing peripheral resistance due to vasoconstriction
Pharmacokinetics
IM: Onset 5-15 min, duration 1-4 hr

IV: Onset almost immediate, duration 15-30 min
Metabolized by liver, eliminated in urine
INDICATIONS AND USES: Hypotension during spinal anesthesia
DOSAGE
Adult
• *Prevention of hypotension during spinal anesthesia:* IM 30-45 mg 10-20 min prior to anesthesia
• *Hypotension following spinal anesthesia:* IV 30-45 mg, repeat doses of 30 mg prn to maintain blood pressure; IV INF use 0.1% sol in D_5W (1 mg/ml), titrate to patient response
[$] AVAILABLE FORMS/COST OF THERAPY
• Inj, Sol—IM, IV: 15 mg/ml, 2 ml: **$6.33**
CONTRAINDICATIONS: Hypotension induced by chlorpromazine, concurrent use with any MAOI
PRECAUTIONS: Cardiovascular disease, chronically ill patients, hemorrhagic shock, hyperthyroidism, hypertension
PREGNANCY AND LACTATION: Pregnancy category C
SIDE EFFECTS/ADVERSE REACTIONS
CNS: Anxiety, confusion, drowsiness, incoherence, tremors
CV: Hypertension, palpitations, tachycardia
INTERACTIONS
Drugs
3 *Halogenated hydrocarbon anesthetics:* Sensitization of myocardium to effects of catecholamines; serious dysrhythmia may result
3 *MAOIs:* Hypertensive crisis
Labs
• *Amphetamines:* False positive for amphetamine, methamphetamine in urine

M

---

italic = common side effects   ***bold italic*** = life-threatening reactions

mephenytoin
(me-fen'i-toyn)
Rx: Mesantoin
Chemical Class: Hydantoin derivative
Therapeutic Class: Anticonvulsive

CLINICAL PHARMACOLOGY
Mechanism of Action: Stabilizes neuronal membranes decreasing seizure activity by increasing efflux or decreasing influx of sodium ions across cell membranes in the motor cortex during generation of nerve impulses

Pharmacokinetics
PO: Onset 30 min, duration 24-48 hr; metabolized by liver to active metabolite, excreted in urine; $t_{1/2}$ 144 hr

INDICATIONS AND USES: Tonic-clonic, partial, Jacksonian, and psychomotor seizures in patients refractory to less toxic anticonvulsants

DOSAGE
Adult
• PO 50-100 mg/day initially, increase by 50-100 mg at weekly intervals; usual maintenance dose 200-600 mg/day divided tid; max 800 mg/day

Child
• PO 3-15 mg/kg/day divided tid; usual maintenance dose 100-400 mg/day divided tid

$ AVAILABLE FORMS/COST OF THERAPY
• Tab, Uncoated—Oral: 100 mg, 100's: **$34.69**

PRECAUTIONS: Abrupt withdrawal, elderly, impaired liver function, hyperglycemia, acute intermittent porphyria

PREGNANCY AND LACTATION: Pregnancy category C

SIDE EFFECTS/ADVERSE REACTIONS
CNS: Ataxia, choreiform movements, depression, dizziness, *drowsiness,* dysarthria, fatigue, insomnia, irritability, mental confusion, nervousness, psychotic disturbances, tremor
CV: Edema
EENT: Diplopia, nystagmus, photophobia
GI: Hepatitis, jaundice, nausea, vomiting
GU: Nephrosis
HEME: **Agranulocytosis, anemia, aplastic anemia, hemolytic anemia, leukopenia,** lymphadenopathy, **megaloblastic anemia, neutropenia, pancytopenia, thrombocytopenia**
METAB: Hyperglycemia
MS: Osteomalacia, polyarthropathy
RESP: **Pulmonary fibrosis**
SKIN: Alopecia, erythema multiforme, **exfoliative dermatitis,** maculopapular, morbilliform, scarlantiniform, urticarial, purpuric, and nonspecific skin rashes; **toxic epidermal necrolysis**
MISC: Lupus erythematosus syndrome, weight gain

INTERACTIONS
Drugs
3 *Acetaminophen:* Enhanced hepatotoxic potential of overdose
3 *Acetazolamide:* Increased risk of osteomalacia
3 *Antidepressants:* Increased mephenytoin concentrations; reduced cyclic antidepressant concentrations
3 *Antineoplastics (cisplatin), diazoxide, folic acid, rifampin:* Reduced plasma mephenytoin concentrations
3 *Carbamazepine:* Combined use may decrease serum concentrations of both drugs; mephenytoin may either increase or decrease when carbamazepine is added
3 *Chloramphenicol, cimetidine,*

disulfiram, felbamate, fluconazole, flouroquinolones, fluoxetine, isoniazid, omeprazole, sulfonamides, sulthiame: Increased serum mephenytoin concentrations

3 *Cyclosporine:* Reduced cyclosporine concentrations

3 *Loop diuretics:* Reduced diuretic response

3 *Mebendazole:* Reduced plasma mebendazole concentrations

3 *Methadone:* Reduced serum methadone concentrations

3 *Metyrapone:* Invalidated metyrapone test

3 *Mexiletine:* Reduced mexiletine concentrations

2 *Oral anticoagulants:* Transient increase followed by inhibition of hypoprothrombinemic response to oral anticoagulants

3 *Oral contraceptives:* Inhibited effect of oral contraceptives

3 *Primidone:* Enhanced conversion of primidone to phenobarbital

3 *Quinidine:* Decreased serum quinidine concentrations

3 *Theophylline:* Reduced serum theophylline concentrations

3 *Thyroid hormones:* Increased thyroid replacement dose requirements

3 *Valproic acid:* Increased, decreased, or unaltered plasma mephenytoin concentrations

Labs
• *Phenytoin:* Decreased serum level of phenytoin

SPECIAL CONSIDERATIONS
PATIENT/FAMILY EDUCATION
• Take with food
• Drug may cause drowsiness, dizziness, or blurred vision
• Avoid alcohol
• Notify clinician of skin rash, severe nausea or vomiting, swollen glands, bleeding, swollen or tender gums, yellowish discoloration of skin or eyes, joint pain, unexplained fever, sore throat, persistent headache, pregnancy

MONITORING PARAMETERS
• CBC with differential and platelet count at baseline, 2 wk after dosage changes, q1 mo for 1 yr, then q3 mo thereafter
• Therapeutic serum concentrations 25-40 µg/ml (mephenytoin plus active metabolite)

---

mephobarbital
(me'foe-bar'bi-tal)
Rx: Mebaral
Chemical Class: Barbituric acid derivative
Therapeutic Class: Sedative/hypnotic; anticonvulsant
DEA Class: Schedule IV

CLINICAL PHARMACOLOGY
Mechanism of Action: CNS depressant: depresses the sensory cortex, decreases motor activity, alters cerebellar function, produce drowsiness, sedation, and hypnosis; little analgesic action at subanesthetic doses (may increase reaction to painful stimuli); anticonvulsant activity in subhypnotic doses; dose-dependent respiratory depression (hypnotic doses produce respiratory depression similar to physiologic sleep)

Pharmacokinetics
PO: Onset 20-60 min, duration 10-16 hr; metabolized by the liver to phenobarbital, excreted in urine; $t_{1/2}$ 11-67 hr

INDICATIONS AND USES: Sedative (relief of anxiety, tension), partial and generalized tonic-clonic and cortical focal seizures

DOSAGE
Adult
• *Sedative:* PO 32-100 mg tid-qid
• *Epilepsy:* PO 400-600 mg/day in 2-4 divided doses

---

italic = common side effects   **bold italic** = life-threatening reactions

M

Child
- *Sedative:* PO 16-32 mg tid-qid
- *Epilepsy:* PO 4-10 mg/kg/day in 2-4 divided doses

$ AVAILABLE FORMS/COST OF THERAPY

- Tab, Uncoated—Oral: 32 mg, 250's: **$43.15-$51.10;** 50 mg, 250's: **$62.01-$73.14;** 100 mg, 250's: **$84.47-$98.03**

CONTRAINDICATIONS: Respiratory depression, severe liver impairment, porphyria

PRECAUTIONS: Myasthenia gravis, myxedema, anemia, hepatic disease, renal disease, elderly, mental depression, history of drug abuse, abrupt discontinuation, children, hyperthyroidism, fever, diabetes

PREGNANCY AND LACTATION: Pregnancy category D; has caused major adverse effects in some nursing infants; should be given with caution to nursing women

SIDE EFFECTS/ADVERSE REACTIONS

CNS: CNS depression, dizziness, *drowsiness, hangover,* headache, *lethargy,* lightheadedness, mental depression, physical dependence, slurred speech, stimulation in the elderly and children, vertigo

CV: Bradycardia, hypotension

GI: Constipation, diarrhea, nausea, vomiting

HEME: **Agranulocytosis,** megaloblastic anemia (long-term treatment), **thrombocytopenia**

RESP: **Apnea, bronchospasm, depression, laryngospasm**

SKIN: Abscesses at injection site, **angioedema,** erythema multiforme, pain, *rash,* **Stevens-Johnson syndrome,** thrombophlebitis, urticaria

MISC: Rickets, osteomalacia (prolonged use)

INTERACTIONS

Drugs

3 *Acetaminophen:* Enhanced hepatotoxic potential of acetaminophen overdoses

3 *Antidepressants:* Reduced serum concentration of cyclic antidepressants

3 *Beta-adrenergic blockers:* Reduced serum concentrations of beta-blockers which are extensively metabolized

3 *Calcium channel blockers:* Reduced serum concentrations of verapamil and dihydropyridines

3 *Chloramphenicol:* Increased barbiturate concentrations; reduced serum chloramphenicol concentrations

3 *Corticosteroids:* Reduced serum concentrations of corticosteroids; may impair therapeutic effect

3 *Cyclosporine:* Reduced serum concentration of cyclosporine

3 *Digitoxin:* Reduced serum concentration of digitoxin

3 *Disopyramide:* Reduced serum concentration of disopyramide

3 *Doxycycline:* Reduced serum doxycycline concentrations

3 *Estrogen:* Reduced serum concentration of estrogen

3 *Ethanol:* Excessive CNS depression

3 *Griseofulvin:* Reduced griseofulvin absorption

3 *Methoxyflurane:* Enhanced nephrotoxic effect

3 *MAOIs:* Prolonged effect of barbiturates

3 *Narcotic analgesics:* Increased toxicity of meperidine; reduced effect of methadone; additive CNS depression

3 *Neuroleptics:* Reduced effect of either drug

2 *Oral anticoagulants:* Decrease hypoprothrombinemic response to oral anticoagulants

3 *Oral contraceptives:* Reduced efficacy of oral contraceptives

3 *Phenytoin:* Unpredictable effect on serum phenytoin levels

3 *Propafenone:* Reduced serum concentration of propafenone

3 *Quinidine:* Reduced quinidine plasma concentrations

3 *Tacrolimus:* Reduced serum concentration of tacrolimus

3 *Theophylline:* Reduced serum theophylline concentrations

3 *Valproic acid:* Increased serum concentrations of amobarbital

2 *Warfarin:* See oral anticoagulants

Labs

• *Phenobarbital:* Falsely increased result

SPECIAL CONSIDERATIONS
PATIENT/FAMILY EDUCATION

• Avoid driving or other activities requiring alertness

• Avoid alcohol ingestion or CNS depressants

• Do not discontinue medication abruptly after long-term use

• Notify clinician of fever, sore throat, mouth sores, easy bruising or bleeding, broken blood vessels under skin

MONITORING PARAMETERS

• Periodic CBC, liver and renal function tests, serum folate, vitamin D during prolonged therapy

---

mepivacaine

(me-piv´a-kane)
Rx: Carbocaine, Polocaine, Polocaine-MPF
Chemical Class: Amide derivative
Therapeutic Class: Local anesthetic

CLINICAL PHARMACOLOGY
Mechanism of Action: Blocks the generation and conduction of nerve impulses; the order of loss of nerve function is: (1) pain, (2) temperature, (3) touch, (4) proprioception, and (5) skeletal muscle tone

Pharmacokinetics

Infiltrative anesthesia: Onset 3-5 min, duration 0.75-1.5 hr

Epidural: Onset 5-15 min, duration 1-3 hr

Spinal: Duration 0.5-1.5 hr

60%-85% bound to plasma proteins; metabolized by liver, excreted in urine (metabolites)

INDICATIONS AND USES: Nerve block, caudal anesthesia, epidural anesthesia, pain relief, paracervical block in obstetrics, transvaginal block, soft tissue infiltration anesthesia, anesthesia for dental procedures

DOSAGE
Adult

• Dose varies with procedure, depth of anesthesia, vascularity of tissues, duration of anesthesia, and condition of patient

• Max amount given per procedure should not exceed 400 mg; total dose/24 hr should not exceed 1 g

• *Nerve block:* 1% or 2% sol

• *Paracervical block:* 1% sol

• *Transvaginal block:* 1% sol

• *Caudal and epidural block:* 1%, 1.5%, or 2% sol

• *Infiltration:* 1% sol

• *Dental procedures:* 3% sol

$ **AVAILABLE FORMS/COST OF THERAPY**

• Inj, Sol: 1%, 30 ml: **$7.10-$11.54;** 1.5%, 30 ml: **$9.53-$15.75;** 2%, 20 ml: **$7.89-$12.96**

CONTRAINDICATIONS: Heart block (large doses), septicemia (spinal anesthesia)

PRECAUTIONS: Hepatic disease, use in head and neck area, children, inflammation, sepsis, elderly, neurologic disease, spinal deformities, septicemia, severe hypertension (epidural and caudal anesthesia); impaired cardiovascular function, renal disease

PREGNANCY AND LACTATION:
Pregnancy category C; epidural, caudal, or pudendal anesthesia during labor and delivery may alter the forces of parturition through changes in uterine contractility or maternal expulsive efforts; use caution in nursing mothers

SIDE EFFECTS/ADVERSE REACTIONS

CNS: Anxiety, disorientation, drowsiness, *loss of consciousness,* restlessness, *seizures,* shivering, tremors

CV: Bradycardia, *cardiac arrest, dysrhythmias, fetal bradycardia,* hypertension, hypotension, *myocardial depression*

EENT: Blurred vision, pupil constriction, tinnitus

GI: Nausea, vomiting

RESP: Anaphylaxis, respiratory arrest

SKIN: Allergic reactions, burning, edema, rash, skin discoloration at inj site, tissue necrosis, urticaria

INTERACTIONS

Drugs

3 *Beta-blockers:* Acute discontinuation of β-blockers before local anesthesia may increase the risk of side effects due to anesthetic

SPECIAL CONSIDERATIONS

• Amide-type local anesthetic

MONITORING PARAMETERS

• Blood pressure, pulse, respiration during treatment, ECG

• Fetal heart tones if used during labor

---

meprobamate
(me-proe′ba-mate)
Rx: Equanil, Miltown, Neuramate
Chemical Class: Carbamate derivative
Therapeutic Class: Anxiolytic; sedative/hypnotic
DEA Class: Schedule IV

CLINICAL PHARMACOLOGY
Mechanism of Action: CNS depressant activity at multiple sites in CNS including hypothalamus, thalamus, limbic system, and spinal cord; mildly tranquilizing; some anticonvulsant and muscle relaxant properties

Pharmacokinetics
PO: Onset 1 hr, peak concentration 1-3 hr; metabolized in liver, excreted in urine (metabolites); $t_{1/2}$ 6-17 hr

INDICATIONS AND USES: Anxiety disorders

DOSAGE

Adult

• PO 1.2-1.6 g/day divided tid-qid, do not exceed 2.4 g/day; sustained release 400-800 mg bid

Child 6-12 yr

• PO 100-200 mg bid-tid; SR 200 mg bid

$ **AVAILABLE FORMS/COST OF THERAPY**

• Tab, Uncoated—Oral: 200 mg, 100′s: **$4.71-$158.41;** 400 mg, 100′s: **$9.25-$194.24**

CONTRAINDICATIONS: Acute intermittent porphyria

PRECAUTIONS: History of drug abuse, renal and hepatic function impairment, elderly, children <6 yr, epilepsy

PREGNANCY AND LACTATION:
Pregnancy category D; excreted into breast milk in concentrations

---

2-4 times that of maternal plasma; effect on nursing infant unknown

SIDE EFFECTS/ADVERSE REACTIONS

CNS: Ataxia, *dizziness, drowsiness,* euphoria, fast EEG activity, headache, overstimulation, paradoxical excitement, *seizures,* slurred speech, vertigo, weakness

CV: Hypotensive crises, palpitations, peripheral edema, syncope, tachycardia, transient ECG changes, *various dysrhythmias*

EENT: Impairment of visual accommodation

GI: Diarrhea, nausea, proctitis, stomatitis, vomiting

GU: **Anuria, oliguria**

HEME: **Agranulocytosis, aplastic anemia, eosinophilia, leukopenia,** thrombocytopenic purpura

RESP: **Bronchospasm**

SKIN: Ecchymoses, **erythema multiforme, exfoliative dermatitis,** fixed drug eruption, petechiae, rash, **Stevens-Johnson syndrome**

MISC: Angioneurotic edema, exacerbation of porphyric symptoms

INTERACTIONS

Drugs

3 *Ethanol:* Enhanced CNS depression

Labs

• *17-Hydroxycorticosteroids:* Urine, increased

• *17-Ketogenic Steroids:* Urine, increased

SPECIAL CONSIDERATIONS

PATIENT/FAMILY EDUCATION

• Avoid alcohol

• Do not discontinue abruptly following long-term use

MONITORING PARAMETERS

• Periodic CBC with differential and platelets during prolonged therapy

mesalamine

(mez-al'a-meen)

Rx: Asacol, Pentasa, Rowasa

Chemical Class: 5-amino derivative of salicylic acid

Therapeutic Class: GI anti-inflammatory

CLINICAL PHARMACOLOGY

Mechanism of Action: May act by blocking cyclooxygenase and inhibiting prostaglandin production in the colon; appears to produce a local inhibitory effect on the mucosal production of arachidonic acid metabolites, which are increased in patients with chronic inflammatory bowel disease

Pharmacokinetics

PR: Poorly absorbed; excreted principally in feces

PO (TABS): Designed to release drug in terminal ileum and beyond; 28% absorbed; peak 4-12 hr

PO (CAPS): Designed to release drug throughout the GI tract; 20%-30% absorbed; peak 3 hr

Unabsorbed drug eliminated in feces; absorbed drug metabolized and eliminated in urine (metabolite); $t_{1/2}$ 42 min (following IV administration)

INDICATIONS AND USES: Remission and treatment of ulcerative colitis (oral); treatment of distal ulcerative colitis, proctosigmoiditis or proctitis (rectal)

DOSAGE

Adult

• PO (tabs) 800 mg tid for 6 wk; PO (caps) 1 g qid for up to 8 wk; PR (supp) 1 supp (500 mg) bid for 3-6 wk, retain supp in rectum for 1-3 hr if possible; PR (enema) 60 ml (4 g) instilled qd, preferably hs, and retained for 8 hr, treat for 3-6 wk

M

💲 AVAILABLE FORMS/COST OF THERAPY

• Tab, Enteric Coated—Oral: 400 mg, 100's: **$ 68.18**
• Cap, Gel, SUS Action—Oral: 250 mg, 240's: **$97.36**
• Enema—Rect: 4 g/60 ml, 60 ml; 7's: **$78.14**
• Supp—Rect: 500 mg/supp, 12's: **$44.20**

PRECAUTIONS: Hypersensitivity to sulfasalazine, renal function impairment, sulfite sensitivity (enema), children

PREGNANCY AND LACTATION: Pregnancy category B; has produced adverse effects in a nursing infant and should be used with caution during breast feeding; observe nursing infant closely for changes in stool consistency

SIDE EFFECTS/ADVERSE REACTIONS

CNS: Asthenia, fatigue, *headache,* insomnia, malaise, mental depression, weakness
*CV: **Pericarditis,*** peripheral edema
GI: Abdominal pain, colitis, constipation, *cramps,* difficulty retaining enema, *discomfort;* extension of inflammation to entire colon (rectal), flatulence, hemorrhoids, nausea, pain on enema insertion, ***pancreatitis,*** rectal pain, worsening diarrhea
GU: Urinary burning
MS: Back pain, leg or joint pain
SKIN: Acne, alopecia, pruritis, rash, ***Stevens-Johnson syndrome***
MISC: Acute intolerance syndrome (cramping, abdominal pain, bloody diarrhea, fever, headache, rash)

SPECIAL CONSIDERATIONS
PATIENT/FAMILY EDUCATION

• Swallow tabs whole, do not break the outer coating
• Intact or partially intact tabs may be found in stool; notify clinician if this occurs repeatedly
• Avoid excess handling of suppositories
• Lie on left side during enema administration (to facilitate migration into the sigmoid colon)

---

mesna
(mess'na)
Rx: Mesnex, Mesnex VHA Plus
Chemical Class: Thiol derivative
Therapeutic Class: Ifosfamide antidote

CLINICAL PHARMACOLOGY
Mechanism of Action: Binds with and detoxifies acrolein and other urotoxic metabolites of ifosfamide and cyclophosphamide
Pharmacokinetics
IV: Rapidly oxidized to mesna disulfide (dimesna); dimesna rapidly eliminated by kidneys; dimesna reduced to free thiol compound (mesna) in the kidney; $t_{1/2}$ 0.36 hr (dimesna 1.17 hr)

INDICATIONS AND USES: Prevention of ifosfamide-induced and (cyclophosphamide-induced)* hemorrhagic cystitis

DOSAGE
Adult and Child
• IV give 20% of ifosfamide dosage (by weight) at the time of ifosfamide administration and 4 and 8 hr after each dose of ifosfamide

💲 AVAILABLE FORMS/COST OF THERAPY

• Inj, Sol—IV: 100 mg/ml, 10 ml: **$174.30**

PRECAUTIONS: Children
PREGNANCY AND LACTATION: Pregnancy category B; use caution in nursing mothers

SIDE EFFECTS/ADVERSE REACTIONS
CNS: Fatigue, *headache*

---

* = non-FDA-approved use

CV: Hypotension
GI: Bad taste in mouth, diarrhea, nausea, soft stools, vomiting
MS: Limb pain

INTERACTIONS
Labs
• *False positive:* Urinary ketones, β-hydroxybutyrate

SPECIAL CONSIDERATIONS
MONITORING PARAMETERS
• Urinalysis each day prior to ifosfamide administration
• Reduction or discontinuation of ifosfamide may be initiated in patients developing hematuria (>50 RBC/hpf)

---

mesoridazine
(mez-oh-rid'a-zeen)
Rx: Serentil
Chemical Class: Piperidine phenothiazine derivative
Therapeutic Class: Antipsychotic

CLINICAL PHARMACOLOGY
Mechanism of Action: Dopamine receptor antagonist, with higher affinity for D_2- over D_1-receptors, and variable selectivity among the cortical dopamine tracts; also activity on nondopaminergic sites, i.e., cholinergic, α_1-adrenergic and histaminic receptors (explaining side effects); high rates of sedation and anticholinergic effects; moderate orthostatic hypotension; minimal risk of extrapyramidal reaction
Pharmacokinetics
PO: Peak 2-4 hr, onset 0.5-1 hr, duration 4-6 hr; 91%-99% bound to plasma proteins; metabolized in liver, eliminated mostly in urine; $t_{1/2}$ 24-48 hr

INDICATIONS AND USES: Schizophrenia; behavioral problems associated with mental deficiency and chronic brain syndrome; adjunctive treatment of alcoholism; personality disorders; anxiety and tension associated with neuroses

DOSAGE
NOTE: 50 mg equivalent to chlorpromazine 100 mg
Adult and Child>16yr
• *Schizophrenia:* PO 50 mg tid initially; usual range 100-400 mg/day
• *Mental deficiency, chronic brain syndrome:* PO 25 mg tid initially; usual range 75-300 mg/day
• *Alcoholism:* PO 25 mg bid initially; usual range 50-200 mg/day
• *Neuroses:* PO 10 mg tid initially; usual range 30-150 mg/day
• IM 25 mg as a single dose, may repeat in 30-60 min prn; do not exceed 200 mg/day

AVAILABLE FORMS/COST OF THERAPY
• Inj, Sol—IM: 25 mg/ml, 1 ml: **$5.31**
• Liq—Oral: 25 mg/ml, 120 ml: **$57.72**
• Tab, Plain Coated—Oral: 10 mg, 100's: **$66.73;** 25 mg, 100's: **$89.45;** 50 mg, 100's: **$100.88;** 100 mg, 100's: **$123.56**

CONTRAINDICATIONS: Severe CNS depression, coma
PRECAUTIONS: Children <12 yr, elderly, prolonged use, severe cardiovascular disorders, epilepsy, hepatic or renal disease, glaucoma, prostatic hypertrophy, hypocalcemia (increased susceptibility to dystonic reactions), COPD

PREGNANCY AND LACTATION: Pregnancy category C; bulk of evidence indicates that phenothiazines are safe for mother and fetus; effect on nursing infant is unknown, but may be of concern

SIDE EFFECTS/ADVERSE REACTIONS
CNS: Agitation, anxiety, confusion, depression, *drowsiness;* EPS (akathisia, dystonia, pseudoparkin-

---

italic = common side effects   ***bold italic*** = life-threatening reactions

sonism, tardive dyskinesia); euphoria, exacerbation of psychotic symptoms including catatonic-like behavioral states, hallucinations; heat or cold intolerance, *headache,* insomnia, lethargy, *neuroleptic malignant syndrome,* restlessness, *seizures*

CV: ECG changes, hypertension, hypotension, tachycardia

EENT: Blurred vision, cataracts, dry eyes, glaucoma, pigmentation of retina or cornea, retinopathy, vertigo

GI: Anorexia, constipation, diarrhea, *dry mouth,* dyspepsia, hypersalivation, increased LFTs, *nausea,* vomiting

GU: Priapism, sexual dysfunction, urinary retention

HEME: Agranulocytosis, anemia, *aplastic anemia, hemolytic anemia,* minimal decreases in red blood cell counts; transient leukopenia, leukocytosis

METAB: Breast engorgement, gynecomastia, hypercholestreolemia, hyperglycemia, hypoglycemia, hyponatremia, impotence, increased libido, lactation, mastalgia, menstrual irregularities

RESP: Bronchospasm, increased depth of respiration, laryngospasm

SKIN: Diaphoresis, loss of hair, maculopapular and acneiform skin reactions, photosensitivity

INTERACTIONS
Drugs

3️⃣ *Anticholinergics:* Inhibited therapeutic response to antipsychotic; enhanced anticholinergic side effects

3️⃣ *Antidepressants:* Increased serum concentrations of some cyclic antidepressants

3️⃣ *Antimalarials:* Mesoridazine serum levels increased

3️⃣ *Attapulgite:* Reduced mesoridazine via decreased absorption

3️⃣ *Barbiturates:* Reduced effect of antipsychotic

3️⃣ *Beta-blockers:* Enhanced effects of both drugs

3️⃣ *Bromocriptine, lithium:* Reduced effects of both drugs

3️⃣ *Clonidine:* Hypotension

3️⃣ *Epinephrine:* Reversed pressor response to epinephrine

3️⃣ *Guanadrel:* Mesoridazine inhibits antihypertensive response

3️⃣ *Guanethidine:* Inhibited antihypertensive response to guanethidine

2️⃣ *Levodopa:* Inhibited effect of levodopa on Parkinson's disease

3️⃣ *Narcotic analgesics:* Excessive CNS depression, hypotension, respiratory depression

3️⃣ *Orphenadrine:* Reduced serum neuroleptic concentrations; excessive anticholinergic effects

3️⃣ *Phenylpropanolamine:* Case report of patient death on combination of these two drugs

SPECIAL CONSIDERATIONS
PATIENT/FAMILY EDUCATION
• Do not discontinue abruptly
• Concentrate may be diluted just prior to administration with distilled water, acidified tap water, orange or grape juice

MONITORING PARAMETERS
• Observe closely for signs of tardive dyskinesia
• Periodic CBC with platelets during prolonged therapy

---

metaproterenol
(met-a-proe-ter′e-nole)
Rx: Alupent
Chemical Class: Sympathomimetic amine; β_2-adrenergic agonist
Therapeutic Class: Antiasthmatic, bronchodilator

CLINICAL PHARMACOLOGY
Mechanism of Action: Causes

bronchodilation by β_2-stimulation, resulting in relaxation of bronchial smooth muscle; inhibits mast cell degranulation; stimulates cilia to remove secretions

Pharmacokinetics

PO: Onset 15 min, peak 1 hr, duration 4 hr

INH: Onset 1 min (MDI), 5-30 min (neb), peak 1 hr, duration 4 hr

Metabolized in the liver, eliminated in urine (40% as unchanged drug)

INDICATIONS AND USES: Bronchial asthma, reversible bronchospasm associated with bronchitis and emphysema

DOSAGE

Adult

• PO 20 mg tid-qid; MDI 2-3 puffs q3-4h prn; NEB 5-15 inhalations of undiluted 5% sol or 0.2-0.3 ml of 5% sol diluted in 2.5-3 ml normal saline q4-6h (can be given more frequently according to need)

Child

• PO (<2 yr) 0.4 mg/kg/dose tid-qid, in infants the dose can be given q8-12h; (2-6 yr) 1-2.6 mg/kg/day divided q6-8h; (6-9 yr) 10 mg tid-qid; NEB 0.01-0.12 ml/kg of 5% sol (min dose 0.1 ml, max dose 0.3 ml) diluted in 2-3 ml normal saline q4-6h (may be given more frequently according to need)

$ **AVAILABLE FORMS/COST OF THERAPY**

• Sol—INH: 0.4%, 2.5 ml: **$1.38-$1.97;** 0.6%, 2.5 ml: **$1.38-$1.97;** 5%, 30 ml: **$37.70-$48.40**

• Syr—Oral: 10 mg/5 ml, 480 ml: **$6.43-$39.83**

• Tab, Uncoated—Oral: 10 mg, 100's: **$15.78-$36.47;** 20 mg, 100's: **$20.99-$51.80**

• MDI—INH: 0.65 mg/puff, 200 puffs: **$24.24**

CONTRAINDICATIONS: Pre-existing cardiac dysrhythmias associated with tachycardia

PRECAUTIONS: Ischemic heart disease, cardiac dysrhythmias, hypertension, hyperthyroidism, diabetes mellitus

PREGNANCY AND LACTATION: Pregnancy category C; has been used to prevent premature labor; long-term evaluation of infants exposed *in utero* to β-agonists has been reported, but not specifically for metaproterenol, no harmful effects were observed

SIDE EFFECTS/ADVERSE REACTIONS

CNS: Anxiety, dizziness, headache, insomnia, nervousness, stimulation, tremors

*CV: **Cardiac arrest, dysrhythmias,** hypertension, palpitations, tachycardia*

EENT: Throat irritation

GI: Bad taste, GI distress, nausea, vomiting

METAB: Hypokalemia

MS: Muscle cramps in extremities

RESP: Cough, dyspnea

INTERACTIONS

Drugs

3 *Furosemide:* Potential for additive hypokalemia

❷ β-*blockers:* Decreased action of metaproterenol, cardio selective beta-blockers preferable if concurrent use necessary

Labs

• *Glucose:* Urine, increase via Benedict's reagent

SPECIAL CONSIDERATIONS

PATIENT/FAMILY EDUCATION

• Proper inhalation technique is vital for MDIs

• Excessive use may lead to adverse effects

• Notify clinician if no response to usual doses

M

---

italic = common side effects   ***bold italic*** = life-threatening reactions

metaraminol

(met-ar-am´e-nol)
Rx: Aramine
Chemical Class: Synthetic catecholamine
Therapeutic Class: α-Adrenergic sympathomimetic amine; vasopressor

CLINICAL PHARMACOLOGY

Mechanism of Action: Increases both systolic and diastolic blood pressure, primarily by vasoconstriction, which is usually accompanied by marked reflex bradycardia; acts predominantly by a direct effect on α-adrenergic receptors; also has an indirect effect by releasing norepinephrine from its storage sites

Pharmacokinetics

IV: Onset 1-2 min, duration 20-60 min

IM: Onset 10 min, duration 20-60 min

SC: Onset 5-20 min, duration 20-60 min

Pharmacologic effect terminated principally by uptake into tissues and urinary excretion

INDICATIONS AND USES: Acute hypotensive states associated with spinal anesthesia, hemorrhage, reactions to medications, surgical complications; shock associated with brain damage resulting from trauma or tumor; "probably effective" in hypotension due to cardiogenic shock or septicemia

DOSAGE

Adult

• SC/IM 2-10 mg; IV INF dilute 15-500 mg in 500 ml of D_5W or normal saline, administer at a rate adjusted to maintain desired blood pressure; IV 0.5-5 mg as a single dose in severe shock, follow with IV INF

Child

• SC/IM 0.1 mg/kg or 3 mg/m²; IV INF 0.4 mg/kg or 12 mg/m², diluted and administered at a rate adjusted to maintain desired blood pressure; IV 0.01 mg/kg or 0.3 mg/m² as a single dose in severe shock, follow with IV INF

§ AVAILABLE FORMS/COST OF THERAPY

• Inj, Sol—IM, IV, SC: 10 mg/ml, 10 ml: **$12.26**

CONTRAINDICATIONS: Use with cyclopropane or halothane anesthesia

PRECAUTIONS: Prolonged administration, heart disease, thyroid disease, hypertension, diabetes, cirrhosis, extravasation (phentolamine is antidote), history of malaria (may provoke relapse), sulfite sensitivity

PREGNANCY AND LACTATION: Pregnancy category D; use could cause reduced uterine blood flow and fetal hypoxia

SIDE EFFECTS/ADVERSE REACTIONS

CNS: Apprehension, dizziness, headache, tremors

CV: **Cardiac arrest;** flushing, hypertension, hypotension (following cessation); palpitation; sinus tachycardia, **ventricular tachycardia, other dysrhythmias**

GI: Nausea

SKIN: Extravasation (abscess, tissue necrosis, sloughing at inj site), sweating

INTERACTIONS

Drugs

3 *Guanethidine:* Reversed antihypertensive effects

2 *Halogenated hydrocarbon anesthetics:* Sensitized myocardium to the effects of catecholamines, arrhythmias possible

⚠ *MAOIs:* Severe hypertensive response

3 *Oxytocic drugs:* Concomitant

use may cause severe persistent hypertension

3 *Tricyclic antidepressant:* Vasopressor response decreased; higher sympathomimetic may be necessary

SPECIAL CONSIDERATIONS
MONITORING PARAMETERS

• Maximum effect is not immediately apparent; allow at least 10 min to elapse before increasing the dose

• BP and pulse

---

metaxalone
(me-tax′a-lone)
Rx: Skelaxin
Chemical Class: Oxazolidinone derivative
Therapeutic Class: Skeletal muscle relaxant

CLINICAL PHARMACOLOGY
Mechanism of Action: General CNS depressant; has no direct action on contractile mechanism of striated muscle, the motor endplate, or nerve fiber

Pharmacokinetics
PO: Peak 2 hr, onset 1 hr, duration 4-6 hr; metabolites excreted in urine; $t_{1/2}$ 2-3 hr

INDICATIONS AND USES: Adjunctive therapy to rest and physical therapy for acute, painful musculoskeletal conditions

DOSAGE
Adult and Child >12 yr

• PO 800 mg tid-qid

[$] **AVAILABLE FORMS/COST OF THERAPY**

• Tab, Uncoated—Oral: 400 mg, 100's: **$52.54-$59.40**

CONTRAINDICATIONS: Tendency to drug-induced hemolytic or other anemia; significantly impaired renal or hepatic function

PRECAUTIONS: Liver function impairment, children

SIDE EFFECTS/ADVERSE REACTIONS

CNS: Dizziness, *drowsiness,* headache, irritability, nervousness

GI: GI upset, jaundice, nausea, vomiting

HEME: **Hemolytic anemia, leukopenia**

SKIN: Hypersensitivity reaction (light rash with or without pruritus)

DRUG INTERACTIONS
Labs

• *False positive:* Glucose, urine via Benedict's reagent

---

metformin
(met-for′min)
Rx: Glucophage
Chemical Class: Biguanide
Therapeutic Class: Antidiabetic

CLINICAL PHARMACOLOGY
Mechanism of Action: Potentiates the effect of insulin; decreases hepatic glucose production, decreases intestinal glucose absorption, and improves insulin sensitivity by increasing peripheral glucose uptake and utilization; does not stimulate pancreatic β-cells to increase secretion of insulin; does not produce hypoglycemia by itself

Pharmacokinetics
PO: Peak 1-3 hr; 50%-60% bioavailable; food decreases the extent and delays the time to achieve maximum absorption; peak serum concentrations may be 40% lower; 90% excreted unchanged in urine; $t_{1/2}$ 6.2 hr; crosses placenta

INDICATIONS AND USES: Diabetes mellitus, type 2; polycystic ovary syndrome[*]

DOSAGE
Adult

• PO 250-500 mg qd-bid with meals;

---

increase by 250-500 mg at 3-5 day-weekly intervals to 1000 mg bid
• Combination therapy: If after 4 wk and a 2 gm daily dose of metformin, there is an inadequate response, sulfonylurea should be added; if at maximum doses of a sulfonylurea and metformin the patient still has an inadequate response, both agents should be stopped, and insulin should be started
• Adding metformin to insulin therapy: Continue current insulin dose; initial recommended dosage of metformin is 250-500 mg daily; increased by 250-500 mg/day at intervals of 1 wk or more; max dose is 2,000 mg/day; fasting plasma glucose concentration below 120 mg/dL call for decreasing insulin dose by 10%-25% and closer monitoring
• Transferring metformin to sulfonylurea: (except chlorpropamide to metformin), no transition period is necessary; if transferring from chlorpropamide, careful monitoring for 2 wk due to an increased risk of hypoglycemia
• Geriatric dosing: Conservative initial and maintenance doses due to decreased renal function; dosage adjustments made carefully and conservatively; maximal doses should not be used

NOTE: Lower initiation doses (i.e., 250 mg qd) with gradual titration (i.e., 250 mg q3-5 days) may attenuate GI adverse effect

$ AVAILABLE FORMS/COST OF THERAPY
• Tab, Uncoated—Oral: 500 mg, 100's: **$60.39;** 850 mg, 100's: **$102.67;** 1000 mg, 100's: **$124.40**

CONTRAINDICATIONS: Congestive heart failure requiring drug therapy, acute or chronic metabolic acidosis, including ketoacidosis, renal impairment (e.g., serum creatinine > 1.5 mg/dL in males; 1.4 mg/dL in females); during (temporarily) radiology studies using iodinated contrast media

PRECAUTIONS: Hypoxemia, dehydration, hepatic disease, severe congestive failure, fever, trauma, infection, megaloblastic anemia, thyroid disease, excessive alcohol intake; during and after surgical procedures

PREGNANCY AND LACTATION: Pregnancy category B; breast milk excretion unknown

SIDE EFFECTS/ADVERSE REACTIONS
CNS: Headache
GI: Abdominal bloating, anorexia, diarrhea, flatulence, metallic taste, *nausea, vomiting*
HEME: Megaloblastic anemia (impaired vitamin B_{12} absorption)
METAB: Hypoglycemia (rare); *lactic acidosis (diarrhea; severe muscle pain, cramping; shallow and fast breathing, unusual tiredness and weakness, unusual sleepiness)*
SKIN: Dermatitis, rash

INTERACTIONS
Drugs
3 *Cimetidine:* Increased metformin AUC 50%, peak concentrations 81%, and decreased renal clearance 27%, increasing the risk of lactic acidosis
3 *Monoamine oxidase (MAO) inhibitors:* Stimulate insulin secretion via β-adrenergic stimulation; excessive and prolonged hypoglycemia may occur in some individuals

SPECIAL CONSIDERATIONS
• May also lower triglycerides
• May decrease insulin requirement in insulin-requiring diabetics

PATIENT/FAMILY EDUCATION
• Administer with food
• Avoid excessive alcohol
• Notify clinician of diarrhea, severe muscle pain or cramping, shallow and fast breathing, unusual tired-

ness and weakness, unusual sleepiness (signs of lactic acidosis)

MONITORING PARAMETERS

• Glycosylated hemoglobin q 3-6 mo (sub 7.0%); self-monitored preprandial blood sugars <150 mg/dL; absence of hyperglycemia (e.g., polyuria, polyphagia, polydipsia, blurred vision)

• Renal and hepatic function tests before and annually during therapy

• Serum vitamin B_{12} annually during chronic therapy

---

methacholine

(meth-a-ko'leen)

Rx: Provocholine

Chemical Class: Acetylcholine derivative

Therapeutic Class: Diagnostic agent

CLINICAL PHARMACOLOGY

Mechanism of Action: Causes bronchoconstriction; when inhaled in a sodium chloride solution, patients with asthma are significantly more sensitive to methacholine-induced bronchoconstriction than are healthy individuals

INDICATIONS AND USES: Diagnosis of bronchial airway hyperactivity in subjects who do not have clinically apparent asthma (methacholine challenge test)

DOSAGE

Adult and Child >5 yr

• INH 5 inhalations at each of 5 concentrations in ascending order as follows: 0.025 mg/ml, 0.25 mg/ml, 2.5 mg/ml, 10 mg/ml, and 25 mg/ml (see monitoring parameters); administer via nebulizer that permits intermittent delivery time of 0.6 sec by either a Y-tube or a breath-actuated timing device; following the procedure, a β-agonist inhalation may be administered to help

return FEV_1 to baseline and relieve patient discomfort

$ **AVAILABLE FORMS/COST OF THERAPY**

• Powder—INH: 100 mg, 1's: **$39.95**

CONTRAINDICATIONS: Repeated challenge tests on the same day; use in patients receiving any β-adrenergic blocking agent

PRECAUTIONS: Epilepsy; cardiovascular disease accompanied by bradycardia; vagotonia; peptic ulcer disease; thyroid disease; urinary tract obstruction; child <5 yr; **for diagnostic purposes only**

PREGNANCY AND LACTATION: Pregnancy category C

SIDE EFFECTS/ADVERSE REACTIONS

CNS: Headache, lightheadedness

EENT: Throat irritation

SKIN: Itching

INTERACTIONS

Drugs

3 *Beta-blockers:* Exaggerated response to methacholine challenge, prolonged recovery, poor response to treatment

SPECIAL CONSIDERATIONS

MONITORING PARAMETERS

• FEV_1 3-5 min after administration of each serial concentration; procedure is complete when there is a ≥20% reduction in FEV_1 compared to baseline (positive response) or when 5 inhalations have been administered at each concentration and FEV_1 has been reduced by ≤14% (negative response)

M

---

italic = common side effects **bold italic** = life-threatening reactions

methadone

(meth'a-done)
Rx: Dolophine
Chemical Class: Synthetic opium alkaloid; diphenylheptane derivative
Therapeutic Class: Narcotic analgesic
DEA Class: Schedule II

CLINICAL PHARMACOLOGY
Mechanism of Action: Narcotic agonist with activity at Mu receptors (supraspinal analgesia, euphoria, respiratory and physical depression, miosis, and reduced GI motility), Kappa receptors (pentazocine-like spinal analgesia, sedation, and miosis), and Delta receptors (dysphoria, psychotomimetic effects [e.g., hallucinations], and respiratory and vasomotor stimulation caused by drugs with antagonist activity); compared to morphine, equal analgesia, antitussive, constipation, respiratory depression; less sedation, emesis, and physical dependence
Pharmacokinetics
PO: Onset 30-60 min, prolonged duration compared to parenteral therapy
IM: Onset 10-20 min, peak 30-60 min, duration 4-6 hr (22-48 hr after repeated administration)
SC: Onset 10-20 min, peak 50-90 min, duration 4-6 hr (22-48 hr after repeated administration)
Highly bound to tissue protein; metabolized by liver, eliminated in urine and feces; $t_{1/2}$ 13-47 hr
INDICATIONS AND USES: Severe pain; detoxification and maintenance of opiate dependence
DOSAGE
Adult
• *Pain:* SC/IM 2.5-10 mg q3-4h prn; PO 2.5-10 mg q6h prn; adjust dose according to severity of pain and response, tolerance of patient
• *Detoxification:* PO 15-40 mg/day should suppress withdrawal symptoms; reductions of 10%-20% qod usually tolerated; treatment should not exceed 21 days and may not be repeated earlier than 4 wk after completion of preceding course
• *Maintenance of opiate dependence:* PO 20-120 mg/day
Child
• *Pain:* PO/SC/IM 0.7 mg/kg/day divided q4-6h prn or 0.1-0.2 mg/kg q4-12h prn; max 10 mg/dose

💲 AVAILABLE FORMS/COST OF THERAPY
• Conc—Oral: 10 mg/ml, 946 ml: **$79.88-$84.70**
• Sol—Oral: Sol—1 mg/ml, 500 ml: **$30.85;** 10 mg/5 ml, 500 ml: **$53.43**
• Tab, Uncoated—Oral: 5 mg, 100's: **$8.68-$34.16;** 10 mg, 100's: **$14.10-$38.86;** 40 mg, 100's: **$33.00-$37.26**
• Inj, Sol—IM, SC: 10 mg/ml, 20 ml: **$12.26-$15.89**

PRECAUTIONS: Head injury, increased intracranial pressure, acute abdominal conditions, elderly, severe impairment of hepatic or renal function, hypothyroidism, Addison's disease, prostatic hypertrophy, urethral stricture, history of drug abuse, acute asthma, upper airway obstruction

PREGNANCY AND LACTATION: Pregnancy category B (category D if used for prolonged periods or in high doses at term); compatible with breast feeding if mother consumes ≤20 mg/24 hr

SIDE EFFECTS/ADVERSE REACTIONS
CNS: Agitation, dependency, dizziness, *drowsiness,* lethargy, restlessness, *sedation*
CV: Bradycardia, orthostatic hypotension, palpitations, tachycardia

* = non-FDA-approved use

GI: *Anorexia, constipation,* increased amylase, *nausea, vomiting*
GU: Urinary retention
RESP: **Respiratory depression, respiratory paralysis**
SKIN: *Excessive sweating,* flushing, rash, urticaria
INTERACTIONS
Drugs
3 *Anticoagulants:* Potentiation of warfarin's anticoagulant effect
3 *Antihistamines, chloral hydrate, glutethimide, methocarbamol:* Enhanced depressant effects
3 *Barbiturates:* Additive respiratory and CNS depressant effects
3 *Carbamazepine, phenobarbital, primidone, rifampin:* Reduced serum methadone concentrations; increased symptoms associated with narcotic withdrawal
3 *Cimetidine:* Increased effect of narcotic analgesics
3 *Ethanol:* Additive CNS effects
3 *Neuroleptics:* Hypotension and excessive CNS depression
2 *Phenytoin:* As with carbamazepine above
3 *Protease inhibitors:* Increased respiratory and CNS depression
Labs
• *Morphine:* Urine, increased
• *Pregnancy tests:* Urine, false positive (Gravindex)
• *False increase:* Amylase and lipase
SPECIAL CONSIDERATIONS
When used for the treatment of narcotic addiction in detoxification or maintenance programs, can only be dispensed by approved hospital pharmacies, approved community pharmacies, and maintenance programs approved by the Food and Drug Administration and the designated state authority

• Do not administer agonist/antagonist analgesics (i.e., pentazocine, nalbuphine, butorphanol, dezocine, buprenorphine) to patient who has received a prolonged course of methadone (a pure agonist). In opioid-dependent patients, mixed agonist/antagonist analgesics may precipitate withdrawal symptoms.
PATIENT/FAMILY EDUCATION
• Change position slowly; orthostatic hypotension may occur
• Minimize nausea by administering with food and remain lying down following dose

methamphetamine
(meth-am-fet′a-meen)
Rx: Desoxyn
Chemical Class: Amphetamine derivative
Therapeutic Class: Anorexiant; CNS stimulant
DEA Class: Schedule II

CLINICAL PHARMACOLOGY
Mechanism of Action: Sympathomimetic amines with CNS stimulant activity increases release of norepinephrine from central noradrenergic neurons; at higher doses, dopamine may be released in the mesolimbic system; peripheral α- and β-activity includes elevation of systolic and diastolic blood pressures and weak bronchodilator and respiratory stimulation action; heart rate reflexly slowed at standard doses, arrhythmias with overdose
Pharmacokinetics
PO: Duration 8-24 hr; metabolized in liver to amphetamine (4%-7%) and other metabolites; eliminated in urine; biologic $t_{1/2}$ 4-5 hr (increased by alkaline urine)
INDICATIONS AND USES: Short-term adjunct to caloric restriction in exogenous obesity (**high potential**

for abuse, use only when alternative therapies have failed); attention deficit disorder with hyperactivity

DOSAGE

Adult

• *Obesity:* PO 5 mg 30 min before each meal; sustained release PO 10-15 mg qAM; treatment duration should not exceed a few weeks

Child

• *Attention deficit disorder with hyperactivity:* PO 5 mg qd-bid initially; increase in increments of 5 mg/day at weekly intervals until an optimum response is achieved; usual effective dose 20-25 mg/day (divided bid with conventional tablets or qd with sustained release formulations)

💲 **AVAILABLE FORMS/COST OF THERAPY**

• Tab, Uncoated—Oral: 5 mg, 100's: **$71.74**
• Tab, Uncoated, SUS Action—Oral: 5 mg, 100's: **$192.56;** 10 mg, 100's: **$258.76;** 15 mg, 100's: **$330.09**

CONTRAINDICATIONS: Hyperthyroidism, moderate to severe hypertension, glaucoma, severe arteriosclerosis, history of drug abuse, symptomatic cardiovascular disease, agitated states, within 14 days of MAOI administration

PRECAUTIONS: Mild hypertension, child <3 yr, Tourette's disorder, motor and phonic tics, tartrazine sensitivity (15 mg sustained release preparation)

PREGNANCY AND LACTATION: Pregnancy category C; use of amphetamine for medical indications does not pose a significant risk to the fetus for congenital anomalies; mild withdrawal symptoms may be observed in the newborn; illicit maternal use presents significant risks to the fetus and newborn including intrauterine growth retardation, premature delivery, and the potential for increased maternal, fetal, and neonatal morbidity; concentrated in breast milk; contraindicated during breast feeding

SIDE EFFECTS/ADVERSE REACTIONS

CNS: Addiction, aggressiveness, changes in libido, chills, dependence, dizziness, dyskinesia, dysphoria, euphoria, headache, *hyperactivity, insomnia,* irritability, overstimulation, psychotic episodes, *restlessness,* talkativeness, tremor

CV: **Arrhythmias** (at larger doses), dysrhythmias, hypertension, *palpitations,* reflex decrease in heart rate, *tachycardia*

GI: Anorexia, constipation, cramps, diarrhea, dry mouth, metallic taste, nausea, vomiting, weight loss

GU: Impotence

METAB: Reversible elevations in serum thyroxine (T_4) with heavy use

SKIN: Urticaria

DRUG INTERACTIONS

Drugs

🔳 *Acetazolamide:* Increased serum amphetamine concentrations and prolonged amphetamine effects

🔳 *Antidepressants:* Increased effect of amphetamines, clinical evidence lacking

🔳 *Furazolidone:* Hypertensive reactions

🔳 *Guanadrel, guanethidine:* Inhibition of the antihypertensive response

⚠ *MAOIs:* Severe hypertensive reactions possible

🔳 *Selegiline:* Potential for enhanced pressor effect if used in combination

🔳 *Sodium bicarbonate:* Large doses of sodium bicarbonate inhibit the elimination and increase the effect of amphetamines

---

* = non-FDA-approved use

Labs
- *Amino acids:* Urine, increased
- *Amphetamine:* Urine, positive at 1.0 µg/ml

SPECIAL CONSIDERATIONS
PATIENT/FAMILY EDUCATION
- Take early in the day
- Do not discontinue abruptly
- Avoid hazardous activities until stabilized on medication
- Avoid OTC preparations unless approved by clinician

---

methantheline
(meth-an'tha-leen)
Rx: Banthine
Chemical Class: Quaternary ammonium derivative
Therapeutic Class: Genitourinary antispasmodic; gastrointestinal antiulcer agent (adjunctive)

CLINICAL PHARMACOLOGY
Mechanism of Action: Inhibits GI propulsive motility and diminishes gastric acid secretion
Pharmacokinetics
PO: Incompletely absorbed from GI tract; excreted mainly in urine as unchanged drug and metabolites, remainder excreted in feces (probably as unabsorbed drug)
INDICATIONS AND USES: Adjunctive treatment of peptic ulcer; uninhibited hypertonic neurogenic bladder
DOSAGE
Adult
- *Peptic ulcer:* PO 50-100 mg q6h initially; decrease dose by half for maintenance therapy
- *Neurogenic bladder:* PO 50-100 mg qid; adjust dose according to patient response and tolerance
Child
- PO (<1 mo) 12.5 mg bid, increased to tid prn; (1-12 mo) 12.5 mg qid

increased to 25 mg qid prn; (>12 mo) 12.5-50 mg qid
🔋 AVAILABLE FORMS/COST OF THERAPY
- Tab, Uncoated—Oral: 50 mg, 100's: **$28.93**
CONTRAINDICATIONS: Narrow-angle glaucoma, obstructive uropathy, obstructive disease of the GI tract, intestinal atony, unstable cardiovascular status in acute hemorrhage, severe ulcerative colitis, toxic megacolon complicating ulcerative colitis, myasthenia gravis
PRECAUTIONS: Hyperthyroidism, CAD, dysrhythmias, CHF, ulcerative colitis, hypertension, hiatal hernia, hepatic disease, renal disease, urinary retention, prostatic hypertrophy, elderly, children, glaucoma, autonomic neuropathy
PREGNANCY AND LACTATION: Pregnancy category C; excretion into breast milk unknown, although would be expected to be minimal due to quaternary structure (see also atropine)
SIDE EFFECTS/ADVERSE REACTIONS
CNS: Anxiety, confusion, dizziness, drowsiness, hallucination, headache, insomnia, stimulation (especially in elderly), weakness
CV: Palpitations, tachycardia
EENT: Blurred vision, cyclopegia, increased ocular tension, mydriasis, photophobia
GI: Absence of taste, *constipation, dry mouth,* dysphagia, heartburn, nausea, **paralytic ileus,** vomiting
GU: Hesitancy, impotence, *retention*
SKIN: Allergic reactions, anhidrosis, fever, pruritus, rash, urticaria
DRUG INTERACTIONS
Drugs
3 *Amantadine, rimantadine:* Methantheline potentiates the CNS side effects of antivirals; antivirals po-

---

italic = common side effects   ***bold italic*** = life-threatening reactions

tentiate the anticholinergic side effects of other anticholinergics

3 *Antidepressants (amitriptylline, doxepin, imipramine, maprotiline, nortriptyline, protriptyline, trimipramine):* Excessive anticholinergic effects

3 *Neuroleptics (chlorpromazine, haloperidol):* Methantheline may inhibit the therapeutic response to neuroleptics; excessive anticholinergic effects with combination

3 *Tacrine:* Tacrine may inhibit the therapeutic effects of anticholinergic agents; centrally acting anticholinergics may inhibit the therapeutic effects of tacrine

Labs
• *Glucose:* Urine, false positive with Ames 2-drop clinitest method

SPECIAL CONSIDERATIONS
• Use in peptic ulcer disease largely replaced by more effective H_2-antagonists

PATIENT/FAMILY EDUCATION
• Drug is usually taken 30-60 min before a meal
• Notify clinician if eye pain occurs

---

methazolamide
(meth-ah-zole'ah-mide)
Rx: Neptazane
Chemical Class: Carbonic anhydrase inhibitor; sulfonamide derivative
Therapeutic Class: Antiglaucoma agent

CLINICAL PHARMACOLOGY
Mechanism of Action: Kidney: Increased excretion of sodium, potassium, bicarbonate, and water—alkaline diuresis; *CNS:* reduction in rate of aqueous humor formation—decreased intraocular pressure (IOP)
Pharmacokinetics
PO: Onset 2-4 hr, peak 6-8 hr, duration 10-18 hr; 55% bound to plasma proteins; partially metabolized in liver, excreted in urine; $t_{1/2}$ 14 hr

INDICATIONS AND USES: Adjunctive treatment of open-angle glaucoma; preoperatively in acute angle-closure glaucoma when delay of surgery is desired to lower intraocular pressure; acute mountain sickness

DOSAGE
Adult
• PO 50-100 mg bid-tid

$ **AVAILABLE FORMS/COST OF THERAPY**
• Tab, Uncoated—Oral: 25 mg, 100's: **$43.40-$66.39;** 50 mg, 100's: **$65.44-$74.23**

CONTRAINDICATIONS: Renal disease, severe hepatic disease, electrolyte imbalance (hyponatremia, hypokalemia, hyperchloremic acidosis), adrenalcortical insufficiency, cirrhosis, long-term use in angle-closure glaucoma

PRECAUTIONS: Children, severe loss of respiratory capacity, diabetes mellitus, hypercalciuria, gout

PREGNANCY AND LACTATION: Pregnancy category C

SIDE EFFECTS/ADVERSE REACTIONS
CNS: Ataxia, confusion, depression, dizziness, drowsiness, excitement, fatigue, flaccid paralysis, headache, irritability, lassitude, malaise, nervousness, *paresthesia*, sedation, *seizures,* tremor, vertigo
EENT: Altered smell, myopia, tinnitus
GI: Abdominal distention, altered taste, *anorexia,* constipation, diarrhea, dry mouth, excessive thirst, *nausea, vomiting,* weight loss
GU: Crystalluria, dysuria, glycosuria, hematuria, phosphaturia, polyuria, renal calculi, renal colic, sulfonamide-like renal lesions, *urinary frequency*

HEME: **Agranulocytosis, aplastic anemia, hemolytic anemia, leukopenia, thrombocytopenia**
METAB: Hyperglycemia, hypokalemia, increased serum uric acid
MS: Muscular weakness
SKIN: **Exfoliative dermatitis,** photosensitivity, pruritus, rash, skin eruptions, urticaria
INTERACTIONS
Drugs
3 *Amphetamines:* Increased amphetamine serum concentrations and prolonged effects
3 *Antiarrhythmics (flecainide, mexiletine):* Alkalinization of urine increases concentrations of these drugs
3 *Cyclosporine:* Increased trough cyclosporine levels with potential for neurotoxicity and nephropathy
3 *Ephedrine:* Increased ephedrine concentrations
3 *Methenamine compounds:* Interference with antibacterial activity
3 *Phenytoin:* Increased risk of osteomalacia with prolonged use of both agents
3 *Quinidine:* Alkalinization of urine increases quinidine concentrations
2 *Salicylates:* Increased concentrations of methazolamide leading to CNS toxicity; also see furosemide for other general diuretic interactions
Labs
• *Increase:* Blood glucose levels, bilirubin, blood ammonia, calcium, chloride
• *Decrease:* Urine citrate, serum potassium
• *False positive:* Urinary protein
SPECIAL CONSIDERATIONS
PATIENT/FAMILY EDUCATION
• Take with food if GI upset occurs
MONITORING PARAMETERS
• Intraocular pressure, reduction in AMS symptoms, serum electrolytes, creatinine, CO_2

---

methenamine
(meth-en'a-meen)
Rx: *Hippurate:* Hiprex, Urex
Mandelate: Mandelamine
Chemical Class: Formaldehyde precursors
Therapeutic Class: Urinary anti-infectives

CLINICAL PHARMACOLOGY
Mechanism of Action: Hydrolyzed by acids to form formaldehyde and ammonia; formaldehyde is a nonspecific antibacterial agent that is bactericidal in action; acid portions of methenamine salts (hippuric acid, mandelic acid) have some nonspecific bacteriostatic activity and may enhance liberation of formaldehyde by maintaining urinary acidity
Pharmacokinetics
PO: Peak formaldehyde concentrations in acid urine in 2-8 hr; some hepatic metabolism (10%-25%), 70%-90% excreted unchanged in urine; $t_{1/2}$ 3-6 hr
INDICATIONS AND USES: Prophylaxis or suppression of recurrent UTI **(should not be used alone for acute infections)**
DOSAGE
Adult
• *Hippurate:* PO 1 g bid
• *Mandelate:* PO 1 g qid ac and hs
Child 6-12 yr
• *Hippurate:* PO 25-50 mg/kg/day divided q12h
• *Mandelate:* PO 50-75 mg/kg/day divided q6h
$ **AVAILABLE FORMS/COST OF THERAPY**
• Tab, Uncoated (hippurate)—Oral: 1 g, 100's: **$113.16-$121.20**

- Susp (mandelate)—Oral: 250 mg/5 ml, 480 ml: **$53.88**; 500 mg/5 ml: **$37.50-$76.20**
- Tab, Enteric Coated (mandelate)—Oral: 500 mg, 100's: **$5.25-$32.92**; 1 g 100's: **$6.95-$52.63**

CONTRAINDICATIONS: Renal insufficiency, severe hepatic impairment (hippurate), severe dehydration (hippurate)

PRECAUTIONS: Tartrazine sensitivity (Hiprex tablets), patients susceptible to lipoid pneumonitis (mandelate susp)

PREGNANCY AND LACTATION: Pregnancy category C; excreted into breast milk; no adverse effects on nursing infants have been reported

SIDE EFFECTS/ADVERSE REACTIONS

CNS: Headache
CV: Edema
EENT: Tinnitus
GI: Abdominal cramps, anorexia, diarrhea, nausea, stomatitis; transient elevations in serum AST and ALT (hippurate), *vomiting*
GU: Dysuria, hematuria
MS: Muscle cramps
SKIN: Pruritus, rash, urticaria

INTERACTIONS
Drugs
🔳 *Acetazolamide:* Acetazolamide interferes with the urinary antibacterial activity of methenamine
🔳 *Antacids (magnesium, aluminum, sodium bicarbonate):* Interfere with urinary antibacterial activity of methenamine
🔳 *Sulfadiazine (sulfamethizole, sulfathiazole):* Combination may yield crystalluria
Labs
- *Catecholamines:* Plasma, increased
- *Estriol:* Urine, decreased
- *Estrogens:* Urine, decreased
- *PSP Excretion:* Urine, increased
- *Sugar:* Urine, increased via Benedict's reagent
- *Urobilinogen:* Urine, increased

SPECIAL CONSIDERATIONS
PATIENT/FAMILY EDUCATION
- Keep urine acidic (pH <5.5) by eating food that acidifies urine (meats, eggs, fish, gelatin products, prunes, plums, cranberries); may need to add ascorbic acid
- Fluids must be increased to 3 L/day to avoid crystallization in kidneys
- Take at evenly spaced intervals around clock for best results

MONITORING PARAMETERS
- Periodic liver function tests (hippurate); urine pH

---

methicillin
(meth-i-sill'in)
Rx: Staphcillin
Chemical Class: Semisynthetic penicillinase-resistant penicillin
Therapeutic Class: Antibiotic

CLINICAL PHARMACOLOGY
Mechanism of Action: Inhibits biosynthesis of cell wall mucopeptide in susceptible organisms; the cell wall, rendered osmotically unstable, swells and bursts from osmotic pressure; bactericidal when adequate concentrations are reached; resistant to inactivation by most staphylococcal penicillinases
Pharmacokinetics
IM: Peak 30-60 min, duration 4 hr
IV: Peak 15 min, duration 2 hr
30%-50% bound to plasma proteins; not metabolized to any appreciable extent, excreted in urine; $t_{1/2}$ 0.4-0.5 hr (normal renal function)

INDICATIONS AND USES: Infections of the upper and lower respiratory tract, skin and skin structures, bones and joints, urinary tract; meningitis, septicemia and endocarditis caused by penicillinase-producing staphylococci; perioperative prophylaxis*

Antibacterial spectrum usually includes:

Gram positive organisms: Penicillinase-producing and non-penicillinase-producing strains of *Staphylococcus aureus, S. epidermis, S. saprophyticus;* groups A, B, C, and G streptococci, *Streptococcus pneumoniae,* some viridans streptococci, *Bacillus anthracis*

DOSAGE
Adult
• IM 1 g q4-6h; IV 1 g q6h
• *Endocarditis, acute or chronic osteomyelitis:* IV 1.5-2 g q4h
• *Dose adjustment in renal impairment:* Administer q8-12h for CrCl <10 ml/min
Child
• IM/IV 150-200 mg/kg/day divided q6h, 200-400 mg/kg/day divided q4-6h has been used for severe infections, max 12 g/day

🚱 **AVAILABLE FORMS/COST OF THERAPY**
• Inj, Dry-Sol—IM, IV: 4 g/vial, 1's: **$20.15;** 1 g/vial, 1's: **$5.53**

PRECAUTIONS: Hypersensitivity to cephalosporins, renal insufficiency, prolonged or repeated therapy, neonates

PREGNANCY AND LACTATION: Pregnancy category B; potential exists for modification of bowel flora in nursing infant; allergy/sensitization and interference with interpretation of culture results if fever workup required

SIDE EFFECTS/ADVERSE REACTIONS
CNS: Chills, fever, headache

CV: Phlebitis, thrombophlebitis
GI: Increased AST, ALT
GU: Hemorrhagic cystitis, interstitial nephritis, nephropathy
HEME: ***Eosinophilia, granulocytopenia, hemolytic anemia, leukopenia, neutropenia,*** positive Coombs test, ***thrombocytopenia***
MS: Myalgia
SKIN: Pain at inj site, pruritis, rash, sterile abscess at inj site
MISC: Serum sickness-like reactions

INTERACTIONS
Drugs
🚱 *Chloramphenicol:* Inhibited antibacterial activity of methicillin; ensure adequate amounts of both agents are given and administer methicillin a few hours before chloramphenicol
🚱 *Macrolides (clarithromycin, erythromycin, azithromycin, dirithromycin):* Inhibit bacterial activity of methicillin
🚱 *Methotrexate:* Increased serum methotrexate concentrations
🚱 *Oral contraceptives:* Occasional impairment of oral contraceptive efficacy; consider use of supplementary contraception during cycles in which methicillin is used
🚱 *Probenecid:* Increased methicillin concentrations
🚱 *Tetracyclines:* Inhibited antibacterial activity of methicillin; ensure adequate amounts of both agents are given and administer methicillin a few hours before tetracycline
🚱 *Warfarin:* Inhibition of hypoprothrombinemic response via metabolism enhancement
Labs
• *Phosphate:* Serum, increased
• *Protein:* CSF, increased
• *Triglycerides:* Serum, increased

SPECIAL CONSIDERATIONS
• Because acute interstitial nephritis has been reported more frequently

italic = common side effects   **bold italic** = life-threatening reactions

with methicillin, nafcillin or oxacillin may be preferable
• Should not be used for organisms susceptible to penicillin G
MONITORING PARAMETERS
• Urinalysis, BUN, serum creatinine, CBC with differential, periodic liver function tests

---

methimazole
(meth-im'a-zole)
Rx: Tapazole
Chemical Class: Thioimidazole derivative
Therapeutic Class: Antithyroid agent

CLINICAL PHARMACOLOGY
Mechanism of Action: Inhibits synthesis of thyroid hormones by interfering with the incorporation of iodine into tyrosyl residues of thyroglobulin; does not inhibit action of already-formed or exogenously administered thyroid hormones; partially inhibits peripheral conversion of T_4 to T_3
Pharmacokinetics
PO: Peak 1 hr; onset 30-40 min; excreted in urine; $t_{1/2}$ 6-13 hr
INDICATIONS AND USES: Hyperthyroidism; preparation for thyroidectomy or radioactive iodine therapy
DOSAGE
Adult
• PO 15-60 mg/day divided q8h initially, 5-15 mg/day maintenance × 18-24 months; single daily doses (30-40 mg) are as effective as divided doses
Child
• PO 0.4 mg/kg/day in 3 divided doses initially, 0.2 mg/kg/day in 3 divided doses maintenance × 18-24 months; single daily doses (30-40 mg) are as effective as divided doses

§ AVAILABLE FORMS/COST OF THERAPY
• Tab, Uncoated—Oral: 5 mg, 100's: **$18.38-$37.83;** 10 mg, 100's: **$65.36**
PRECAUTIONS: Thyroid storm, infection, bone marrow depression, hepatic disease
PREGNANCY AND LACTATION: Pregnancy category D; use smallest possible dose to control maternal disease (propylthiouracil preferable, less likely to cross the placenta); excreted into breast milk
SIDE EFFECTS/ADVERSE REACTIONS
CNS: CNS stimulation, depression, drowsiness, headache, neuritis, neuropathies, paresthesias, vertigo
CV: Edema
GI: Epigastric distress, hepatitis, jaundice, loss of taste, *nausea,* sialadenopathy, *vomiting*
GU: Nephritis
*HEME: **Agranulocytosis, aplastic anemia, granulocytopenia, hypoprothrombinemia, leukopenia, thrombocytopenia,** lymphadenopathy*
METAB: Insulin autoimmune syndrome (may result in **hypoglycemic coma**)
MS: Arthralgia, myalgia
RESP: Interstitial pneumonitis
SKIN: Abnormal hair loss, erythema nodosum, **exfoliative dermatitis,** lupus-like syndrome, pruritis, skin pigmentation, rash, urticaria
INTERACTIONS
Drugs
3 *Oral anticoagulants:* Reduced hypoprothrombinemic response to oral anticoagulants
3 *Theophylline:* Physiologic response to antithyroid drug will increase theophylline concentrations via decreased clearance
Labs
• *False increase:* Glucose

SPECIAL CONSIDERATIONS
• Methimazole is the thioamide of choice based on improved patient adherence and outcomes
• Block-replace regimen-increase remission: iodine is added to fixed dose methimazole

PATIENT/FAMILY EDUCATION
• Notify clinician of fever, sore throat, unusual bleeding or bruising, rash, yellowing of skin, vomiting

MONITORING PARAMETERS
• CBC periodically during therapy (especially during initial 3 mo), TSH

---

methocarbamol
(meth-oh-kar´ba-mole)
Rx: Robaxin, Robaxin-750
Combinations
　Rx: with aspirin (Robaxisal)
Chemical Class: Carbamate derivative
Therapeutic Class: Skeletal muscle relaxant

CLINICAL PHARMACOLOGY
Mechanism of Action: General CNS depressant; no direct action on contractile mechanism of striated muscle, motor endplate, or nerve fiber
Pharmacokinetics
PO: Peak 2 hr, onset 30 min; extensively metabolized by liver, excreted in urine and small amounts in feces; $t_{1/2}$ 1-2 hr

INDICATIONS AND USES: Adjunctive therapy to rest and physical therapy for acute painful musculoskeletal conditions; tetanus

DOSAGE
Adult
• *Musculoskeletal conditions:* PO 1.5 g qid for 2-3 days, then decrease to 4-4.5 g/day in 3-6 divided doses; IM/IV 1 g q8h, max 3 g/day for 3 consecutive days (unless treating tet-

anus), may be reinstituted after 2 drug-free days
• *Tetanus:* IV 1-2 g, followed by additional 1-2 g (max 3 g total); repeat with 1-2 g q6h until nasogastric tube or PO therapy possible; total daily dose of up to 24 g may be needed
Child
• *Tetanus:* IV 15 mg/kg/dose or 500 mg/m^2/dose; may repeat q6h prn; max 1.8 g/m^2/day for 3 days only

$ **AVAILABLE FORMS/COST OF THERAPY**
• Inj, Sol—IM, IV: 100 mg/ml, 10 ml: **$4.49-$9.40**
• Tab, Plain Coated—Oral: 500 mg, 100's: **$7.75-$61.08;** 750 mg, 100's: **$10.40-$87.30**

CONTRAINDICATIONS: Known or suspected renal pathology (parenteral)
PRECAUTIONS: Child <12 yr, extravasation, seizure disorder (inj)
PREGNANCY AND LACTATION: Pregnancy category C; compatible with breast feeding

SIDE EFFECTS/ADVERSE REACTIONS
CNS: Dizziness, drowsiness, fever, headache, *lightheadedness,* **seizures** (IV administration), vertigo
CV: Bradycardia, flushing, hypotension, syncope
EENT: Blurred vision, conjunctivitis, diplopia, nasal congestion, nystagmus
GI: Anorexia, GI upset, metallic taste, nausea
HEME: **Leukopenia** (rare), small amount of hemolysis (IV administration)
SKIN: Extravasation (thrombophlebitis, sloughing, pain at injection site), pruritus, rash, skin eruptions, urticaria
MISC: Muscular incoordination

---

italic = common side effects　　　　　**bold italic** = life-threatening reactions

M

INTERACTIONS
Labs
• *Color:* Urine brown, green, blue or black on standing
• *5-hydroxyindole acetic acid:* Urine, increased
• *Vanillyl-mandelic acid:* Urine, increased

---

methotrexate
(meth-oh-trex'ate)
Rx: Folex, Rheumatrex, Mexate
Chemical Class: Dihydrofolate reductase inhibitor
Therapeutic Class: Antineoplastic; antipsoriatic; disease-modifying antirheumatic drug (DMARD)

CLINICAL PHARMACOLOGY
Mechanism of Action: Reversibly inhibits dihydrofolate reductase, the enzyme that reduces folic acid to tetrahydrofolic acid; limits the availability of one-carbon fragments necessary for synthesis of purines and the conversion of deoxyuridylate to thymidylate in the synthesis of DNA and cell reproduction; also has immunosuppressive activity
Pharmacokinetics
IM/IV: Peak 0.5-2 hr
PO: Peak 1-4 hr
Widely distributed into body tissues; 50% bound to plasma proteins; does not appear to be appreciably metabolized; excreted primarily by kidneys and small amounts in feces; $t_{1/2}$ 3-10 hr
INDICATIONS AND USES: Abortion—therapeutic,* arthritis-rheumatoid, asthma,* bladder carcinoma,* brain cancer,* breast cancer, bullous phemphigoid,* Burkitt's lymphoma, cardinomatous meningitis,* cerebral vasculitis,* cervical carcinoma,* choriocarcinoma,* cochleovestibu-

lar disorders,* Crohn's disease,* cutaneous lupus erythematosus,* dermatomyositis,* diffuse large cell lymphoma, ectopic pregnancy,* esophageal cancer,* Felty's syndrome,* gestational trophoblastic neoplasms, graft vs. host disease,* head and neck cancer, hepatitis—idiopathic granulomatous,* inflammatory bowel disease,* leukemia - acute lymphocytic,* acute myelogenous,* chronic myelogenous,* meningeal*; lymphona—Hodgkin's,* mantle cell,* meningeal,* non-Hodgkin's, intraocular*; lymphomatoid papulosis,* mesothelioma,* multiple sclerosis,* osteogenic sarcoma, polymyalgia rheumatica,* primary biliary cirrhosis,* primary sclerosing cholangitis,* psoriasis,* pyoderma gangrenosum,* rejection-cardiac transplant,* Reiter's syndrome,* reticulohistiocytosis—multicentric,* retinoblastoma,* sarcoidosis,* Sézary syndrome,* Still's disease,* Takayasu's disease,* toxoplasmosis chorioretinitis,* vasculitis,* Wegener's granuloma*
DOSAGE
NOTE: Administration and dosage vary significantly depending on the diagnosis and indication for drug use; check carefully
Adult
• *Abortion—therapeutic:* IM/PO 50 mg/m², followed by PV misoprostol 800 mg 7 days later; misoprostol may not be necessary
• *Trophoblastic neoplasms:* PO/IM 15-30 mg qd for 5 days; repeat 3-5 times as required, with rest periods of 1 or more wk interposed between courses
• *Acute lymphoblastic leukemias:* PO 3.3 mg/m² in combination with 60 mg/m² of prednisone qd for 4-6 wk to induce remission (not drug of choice for induction); IM/PO 20-30 mg/m²/wk divided twice weekly or

---

* = non-FDA-approved use

IV 2.5 mg/kg q14 days for maintenance therapy

• *Meningeal leukemia:* Intrathecal 12 mg/m^2; max 15 mg at 2-5 day intervals until the cell count of the CSF returns to normal, then 1 additional dose (use preservative-free preparation only)

• *Burkitt's lymphoma:* PO 10-25 mg/day for 4-8 days; usually given as several courses interposed with 7-10 day rest periods

• *Mycosis fungoides:* PO 2.5-10 mg/day for weeks to months; IM 50 mg qwk or 25 mg twice weekly

• *Psoriasis:* PO/IM/IV 10-25 mg qwk or PO 2.5 mg q12h for 3 doses each wk; adjust gradually to achieve optimal clinical response; max 30 mg/wk; once response achieved reduce to lowest possible effective dose

• *Rheumatoid arthritis:* PO 7.5 mg qwk or 2.5 mg q12h for 3 doses each wk; adjust gradually to achieve an optimal response; max 20 mg/wk; once response achieved reduce to lowest possible effective dose

Child

• *Acute lymphoblastic leukemias:* Same as adult

• *Meningeal leukemia:* Intrathecal (≤3 mo) 3 mg, (4-11 mo) 6 mg, (1 yr) 8 mg, (2 yr) 10 mg at 2-5 day intervals until the cell count of the CSF returns to normal, then 1 additional dose (use preservative-free preparation only)

• *Rheumatoid arthritis:* PO/IM 5-15 mg/m^2/wk as a single dose or in 3 divided doses given 12 hr apart

$ AVAILABLE FORMS/COST OF THERAPY

• Inj, Sol—Intra-articular: 2.5 mg/ml, 2 ml: **$78.75**

• Inj, Sol—IM, IV: 25 mg/ml, 2 ml, **$4.75-$6.88;** 4 ml: **$8.50-$8.75;** 8 ml: **$17.50;** 10 ml: **$20.48**

• Inj, Lyphl-Sol—Intrathecal: 25 mg/vial, 2 ml: **$4.75**

• Tab, Uncoated—Oral: 2.5 mg, 100's: **$269.45-$525.41**

CONTRAINDICATIONS: Severe renal or hepatic impairment, preexisting profound bone marrow depression

PRECAUTIONS: Infection, peptic ulcer, ulcerative colitis, elderly, preexisting bone marrow suppression, renal or hepatic impairment, ascites, pleural effusion, dehydration

PREGNANCY AND LACTATION: Pregnancy category D; contraindicated in breast feeding

SIDE EFFECTS/ADVERSE REACTIONS

CNS: Dizziness, drowsiness, headache, malaise, *seizures*

EENT: Blurred vision, eye discomfort, tinnitus

GI: Abdominal distress, *anorexia,* diarrhea, enteritis, gingivitis, glossitis, hematemesis, *hepatotoxicity,* melena, *nausea,* pharyngitis, *stomatitis,* ulcerations and bleeding of the mucous membranes of the mouth or other portion of the GI tract, *vomiting*

GU: Azotemia, defective spermatogenesis, hematuria, menstrual irregularities, *renal failure,* uric acid nephropathy, urinary retention

*HEME: **Anemia, hemorrhage, leukopenia, pancytopenia, thrombocytopenia***

METAB: Increased serum uric acid

MS: Arthralgia, myalgia, osteoporosis

RESP: Pneumonitis, *pulmonary fibrosis*

SKIN: Acne, *alopecia,* depigmentation, dermatitis, ecchymoses, *erythematous rashes,* folliculitis, furunculosis, hyperpigmentation, petechiae, photosensitivity, pruritus, telangiectasia, urticaria, vasculitis

M

MISC: Effects following intrathecal administration (headache, back pain, nuchal rigidity, fever, paresis, leukoencephalopathy)

INTERACTIONS

Drugs

3 *Aminoglycosides, oral (neomycin, vancomycin):* Reduction of 30-50% in methotrexate absorption in patient receiving concurrent oral aminoglycosides

3 *Antimalarials (chloroquine, hydroxychloroquine):* Methotrexate concentrations reduced by concurrent antimalarial administration

3 *Binding resins:* Reduced methotrexate concentrations

3 *Co-trimoxazole, omeprazole, penicillins:* Increased methotrexate concentrations, possible toxicity

3 *Cyclosporine:* Increased toxicity of both agents

3 *Ethanol:* Increased risk of methotrexate-induced liver injury

3 *Etretinate:* Increased risk of hepatotoxicity

2 *NSAIDs, probenecid, salicylates, sulfinpyrazone, trimethoprim/sulfamethoxazole:* Increased methotrexate concentrations, possible toxicity

⚠ *Vaccines:* Increased risk of infection following use of live vaccines; reduced seroconversion rate to vaccine

Labs

• *Alanine aminotransferase:* Serum, decreased
• *Alkaline phosphatase:* Serum, increased
• *Bilirubin:* Serum, increased
• *Cholesterol:* Serum, increased
• *Color:* Feces, black
• *Ethanol:* Serum, increased
• *Lactate dehydrogenase:* Serum, decreased
• *Phosphate:* Serum, increased
• *Protein:* CSF, increased
• *Triglycerides:* Serum, decreased
• *Uric acid:* Serum, decreased

SPECIAL CONSIDERATIONS

PATIENT/FAMILY EDUCATION

• Notify clinician of black, tarry stools, chills, fever, sore throat, bleeding, bruising, cough, shortness of breath, dark or bloody urine
• Hair may be lost during treatment
• Drink 10-12 glasses of fluid/day
• Avoid alcohol, salicylates

MONITORING PARAMETERS

• Tumor response: Objective remissions are usually associated with a 50% decrease in the size of solid tumor as measured by physical measurement or test parameter (e.g., chest X-ray). After intrathecal administration, clearing of malignant cells in the cerebrospinal fluid indicates a positive response
• Rheumatoid arthritis: Tender, swollen joints, visual analogue scale for pain; acute phase reactants (ESR, C-reactive protein), duration of early morning stiffness, preservation of function
• CBC and platelets at 7, 10, and 14 days postdrug administration/injection; due to the possibility of early-onset pancytopenia, a lower initial dose for rheumatoid arthritis treatment along with intensified monitoring during early therapy is recommended—CBC's at 1, 2, and 4 wk of treatment; if stable dose may be increased and subsequent CBC's should be performed at monthly intervals
• BUN, serum uric acid, urine ClCr, electrolytes before, during therapy
• Liver function tests before and during therapy

methotrimeprazine
(meth-oh-trye-mep'ra-zeen)
Rx: Levoprome
Chemical Class: Phenothiazine derivative
Therapeutic Class: Nonnarcotic analgesic; anxiolytic; sedative

CLINICAL PHARMACOLOGY
Mechanism of Action: Depresses subcortical area of the brain at the levels of the thalamus, hypothalamus, and reticular and limbic systems; suppresses sensory impulses, reduces motor activity, alters temperature regulation, causes sedation and tranquilization; appears to have some analgesic effects possibly by raising pain threshold

Pharmacokinetics
IM: Maximum analgesia 20-40 min, duration 4 hr; metabolized in liver, excreted primarily in urine (metabolites); $t_{1/2}$ 15-30 hr

INDICATIONS AND USES: Moderate to severe pain in nonambulatory patients; preoperative sedation; analgesia and sedation during labor

DOSAGE
Adult
• *Analgesia:* IM 10-20 mg q4-6h; max 40 mg/dose
• *Preoperative sedation:* IM 2-20 mg 0.75-3 hr prior to surgery
• *Labor:* IM 15-20 mg

$ AVAILABLE FORMS/COST OF THERAPY
• Inj, Sol—IM: 20 mg/ml, 10 ml: **$226.89**

CONTRAINDICATIONS: Severe renal, cardiac, or hepatic disease; seizure disorders; coma; during overdoses of CNS depressants; child <12 yr; clinically significant hypotension

PRECAUTIONS: Ambulatory patients (can cause substantial orthostatic hypotension), elderly, use for >30 days, sulfite sensitivity

PREGNANCY AND LACTATION: Pregnancy category C; does not affect force, duration, and frequency of uterine contractions during labor

SIDE EFFECTS/ADVERSE REACTIONS
CNS: Amnesia, disorientation, drowsiness, euphoria, excessive sedation, extrapyramidal reactions, headache, *seizures,* slurred speech, weakness
CV: Bradycardia, *orthostatic hypotension* (fainting, weakness, dizziness), palpitation, tachycardia
EENT: Blurred vision, nasal congestion
GI: Abdominal discomfort, anorexia, dry mouth, *hepatotoxicity,* jaundice, nausea, vomiting
GU: Dysuria, hematuria, hesitancy, retention, uterine inertia (rare)
HEME: Agranulocytosis, hemolytic anemia (long-term, high dose), *leukopenia, neutropenia, thrombocytopenia*
RESP: Respiratory depression
SKIN: Pain at inj site

INTERACTIONS
Drugs
⚠ *MAOIs:* Coadministration with pargyline associated with fatality in 1 reported case
Labs
• *Ferric chloride test:* Urine, positive
• *Phenylketones:* Urine, positive

SPECIAL CONSIDERATIONS
MONITORING PARAMETERS
• CBC with differential and platelets; liver function tests during prolonged therapy

M

methoxamine

(meth-ox'a-meen)
Rx: Vasoxyl
Chemical Class: Synthetic catecholamine
Therapeutic Class: Sympathomimetic amine, vasopressor

CLINICAL PHARMACOLOGY
Mechanism of Action: α-adrenergic receptor stimulant that produces prompt and prolonged rise in blood pressure; no β-adrenergic effects; minimal arrhythmogenic potential
Pharmacokinetics
IV: Onset immediate, peak 0.5-2 min, duration 5-15 min
IM: Peak 15-20 min, duration 60-90 min
Metabolic fate and route of excretion unknown
INDICATIONS AND USES: Hypotension during anesthesia; supraventricular paroxysmal tachycardia; hypotension and shock*; diagnosis of heart murmurs*
DOSAGE
Adult
• *During spinal anesthesia:* IM 10-20 mg shortly before or with spinal anesthesia; repeat prn
• *Emergencies:* IV 3-5 mg injected slowly
• *Supraventricular tachycardia:* IV 10 mg injected slowly
$ AVAILABLE FORMS/COST OF THERAPY
• Inj, Sol—IM, IV: 20 mg/ml, 1 ml ampul: **$24.42**
CONTRAINDICATIONS: Severe hypertension
PRECAUTIONS: Children, hypovolemia, extravasation (phentolamine can be used as antidote), hyperthyroidism, bradycardia, partial heart block, myocardial disease, se-

vere arteriosclerosis, sulfite sensitivity
PREGNANCY AND LACTATION: Pregnancy category C; could reduce uterine blood flow, thereby producing fetal hypoxia and bradycardia; may also interact with oxytocics or ergot derivatives to produce severe persistent maternal hypertension; ephedrine may be a more suitable pressor agent
SIDE EFFECTS/ADVERSE REACTIONS
CNS: Anxiety, headache (often severe)
CV: Excessive blood pressure elevation, ventricular ectopic beats
GI: Nausea, vomiting (often projectile)
GU: Fetal bradycardia, urinary urgency, uterine hypertonus
SKIN: Pilomotor response, sweating
DRUG INTERACTIONS
Drugs
3 β-*blockers (nadolol, pindolol, practolol, propranolol, timolol):* Non-cardioselective β-blockers enhance the pressor response to alpha stimulation, resulting in hypertension and bradycardia
⚠ *Bromocriptine:* Case report of hypertension and ventricular tachycardia with combination of a related sympathomimetic
3 *Furazolidone:* Enhanced hypertensive response when sympathomimetics used concurrently
3 *Guanadrel, guanethidine:* Reversal of antihypertensive effects
3 *Indomethacin:* Hypertensive reactions
2 *Moclobemide:* Enhanced pressor response to methoxamine (headache, palpitations, and lightheadedness)
⚠ *Monamine oxidase inhibitors (MAOI) (isocarboxazid, phenelzine, procarbazine, tranylcypromine):* Hypertensive reactions

* = non-FDA-approved use

3 *Oxytocic drugs:* May cause severe persistent hypertension

2 *Tricyclic antidepressants (imipramine, protriptyline):* Predisposition to cardiac arrhythmias; enhanced pressor response

SPECIAL CONSIDERATIONS
MONITORING PARAMETERS
• Blood pressure and pulse

methoxsalen
(meth-ox'a-len)
Rx: 8-Mop, Oxsoralen, Oxsoralen-Ultra
Chemical Class: Psoralen or Furocoumarin compound
Therapeutic Class: Pigmenting agent; antipsoriatic

CLINICAL PHARMACOLOGY
Mechanism of Action: Increases tyrosinase activity in melanin-producing cells, as well as inhibits DNA synthesis, cell division, and epidermal turnover; successful pigmentation requires the presence of functioning melanocytes
Pharmacokinetics
PO: Peak serum concentration 1.5-6 hr (hard gelatin capsule), 0.5-4 hr (soft gelatin capsule); peak photosensitivity 3.9-4.25 hr (hard capsule), 1.5-2.1 hr (soft capsule); duration approximately 8 hr; highly protein bound; activated by long-wavelength ultraviolet light (UVA), further metabolized by liver; eliminated mainly in urine as metabolites; $t_{1/2}$ 1.1 hr (hard capsule), 2 hr (soft capsule)
INDICATIONS AND USES: Severe, refractory, disabling psoriasis, in conjunction with UVA—treatment known as PUVA (psoralen plus ultraviolet light A); repigmentation in the treatment of vitiligo (PUVA); cutaneous T-cell lymphoma (in conjunction with photopheresis)

DOSAGE
Adult
• *Psoriasis:* PO (hard caps) administer with food or milk 2 hr before UVA exposure, separate doses by at least 48 hr, (<30 kg) 10 mg, (30-50 kg) 20 mg, (51-65 kg) 30 mg, (66-80 kg) 40 mg, (81-90 kg) 50 mg, (91-115 kg) 60 mg, (>115 kg) 70 mg; (soft caps) administer with low-fat food or milk 1.5-2 hr before UVA exposure, separate doses by at least 48 hr, (<30 kg) 10 mg, (30-50) kg) 10-20 mg, (51-65 kg) 20-30 mg, (66-80 kg) 20-40 mg, (81-90 kg) 30-50 mg, (91-115 kg) 30-60 mg, (>115 kg) 40-70 mg
• *Vitiligo:* PO 20 mg 2-4 hr before measured periods of UVA exposure, 2-3 times/wk (at least 48 hr apart); TOP apply to small, well-defined lesion, then expose to UVA light once/wk or less depending on results
• *Cutaneous T-cell lymphoma:* PO (hard capsules) 0.6 mg/kg administered 2 hr before obtaining blood for extracorporeal exposure of extracted leukocytes to high-intensity UVA light
$ **AVAILABLE FORMS/COST OF THERAPY**
• Cap, Gel—Oral: 10 mg, 50's: **$244.20** (soft caps); **$244.20** (hard caps)
• Lotion—Top: 1%, 30 ml: **$98.64 (do not dispense to patient)**
CONTRAINDICATIONS: Hypersensitivity to psoralens, diseases associated with photosensitivity, melanoma, invasive squamous cell carcinoma, aphakia (oral)
PRECAUTIONS: Cardiac disease, hepatic disease, children <12 yr, contains tartrazine (hard caps), photosensitizing agents
PREGNANCY AND LACTATION: Pregnancy category C; excretion into breast milk unknown

SIDE EFFECTS/ADVERSE REACTIONS

CNS: Dizziness, headache, insomnia, malaise, nervousness, psychological depression

CV: Edema, hypotension

EENT: Cataract formation

GI: Nausea

MS: Leg cramps

SKIN: Basal cell epitheliomas, cutaneous tenderness, *erythema,* extension of psoriasis, folliculitis, herpes simplex, hypopigmentation, nonspecific rash, *pruritus,* severe burns, urticaria, vesiculation and bullae formation

SPECIAL CONSIDERATIONS

• Hard and soft caps are not equivalent

PATIENT/FAMILY EDUCATION

• Do not sunbathe during 24 hr prior to methoxsalen ingestion and UVA exposure

• Wear UVA-absorbing sunglasses for 24 hr following treatment to prevent cataract

• Avoid sun exposure for at least 8 hr after methoxsalen ingestion

• Avoid concurrent photosensitizing drugs

• Avoid furocoumarin-containing foods (e.g., limes, figs, parsley, parsnips, mustard, carrots, celery)

• Repigmentation of vitiligo may require 6-9 mo

---

methscopolamine
(meth-skoe-pol′a-meen)

Rx: Pamine

Chemical Class: Quaternary ammonium derivative

Therapeutic Class: Gastrointestinal antiulcer agent (adjunctive)

CLINICAL PHARMACOLOGY

Mechanism of Action: Inhibits GI motility and diminishes gastric acid secretion

Pharmacokinetics

PO: Onset 1 hr, duration 4-6 hr; incompletely absorbed from GI tract, excreted mainly in urine as unchanged drug and metabolites, remainder excreted in feces (probably as unabsorbed drug)

INDICATIONS AND USES: Adjunctive treatment of peptic ulcer

DOSAGE

Adult

• PO 2.5-5 mg qid (½ hr ac, hs)

Child

• PO 0.2 mg/kg or 6 mg/m² daily, given in 4 equally divided doses

💲 AVAILABLE FORMS/COST OF THERAPY

• Tab, Uncoated—Oral: 2.5 mg, 100's: **$42.40**

CONTRAINDICATIONS: Narrow-angle glaucoma, obstructive uropathy, obstructive disease of the GI tract, paralytic ileus, intestinal atony, unstable cardiovascular status in acute hemorrhage, severe ulcerative colitis, toxic megacolon complicating ulcerative colitis, myasthenia gravis

PRECAUTIONS: Hyperthyroidism, CAD, dysrhythmias, CHF, ulcerative colitis, hypertension, hiatal hernia, hepatic disease, renal disease, urinary retention, prostatic hypertrophy, elderly, children, glaucoma

PREGNANCY AND LACTATION: Pregnancy category C; excretion into breast milk unknown, although would be expected to be minimal due to quaternary structure (see also atropine)

SIDE EFFECTS/ADVERSE REACTIONS

CNS: Anxiety, confusion, dizziness, drowsiness, hallucination, headache, insomnia, stimulation (especially in elderly), weakness

CV: Palpitations, tachycardia

---

* = non-FDA-approved use

EENT: Blurred vision, cycloplegia, increased ocular tension, mydriasis, photophobia

GI: Absence of taste, *constipation, dry mouth,* dysphagia, heartburn, nausea, ***paralytic ileus,*** vomiting

GU: Hesitancy, impotence, *retention*

SKIN: Allergic reactions, anhidrosis, fever, pruritus, rash, urticaria

INTERACTIONS

Drugs

3 *Amantadine, rimantadine:* Methscopolamine potentiates the CNS side effects of antivirals; antivirals potentiate the anticholinergic side effects of other anticholinergics

3 *Antidepressants (amitriptylline, doxepin, imipramine, maprotiline, nortriptyline, protriptyline, trimipramine):* Excessive anticholinergic effects

3 *Neuroleptics (chlorpromazine, haloperidol):* Methscopolamine may inhibit the therapeutic response to neuroleptics; excessive anticholinergic effects with combination

3 *Tacrine:* Tacrine may inhibit the therapeutic effects of anticholinergic agents; centrally acting anticholinergics may inhibit the therapeutic effects of tacrine

SPECIAL CONSIDERATIONS
• Has not been shown to be effective in contributing to the healing of peptic ulcer, decreasing the rate of recurrence, or preventing complications

methsuximide
(meth-sux'i-mide)
Rx: Celontin
Chemical Class: Succinimide derivative
Therapeutic Class: Anticonvulsant

CLINICAL PHARMACOLOGY
Mechanism of Action: Increases the seizure threshold and suppresses paroxysmal spike-and-wave pattern in absence seizures; depresses nerve transmission in the motor cortex

Pharmacokinetics
PO: Peak 1-3 hr; rapidly demethylated in liver to *N*-desmethyl-methsuximide (active), excreted in urine (metabolites); $t_{1/2}$ 2-4 hr (*N*-desmethylmethsuximide 26-80 hr)

INDICATIONS AND USES: Refractory absence (petit mal) seizures

DOSAGE
Adult
• PO 300 mg/day for 1st wk; may increase by 300 mg/day at weekly intervals up to 1.2 g/day divided bid-qid

Child
• PO 10-15 mg/kg/day divided tid-qid initially; increase weekly up to max of 30 mg/kg/day

☒ AVAILABLE FORMS/COST OF THERAPY
• Cap, Gel—Oral: 150 mg, 100's: **$52.75**; 300 mg, 100's: **$86.47**

PRECAUTIONS: Hepatic, renal function impairment; abrupt withdrawal; monotherapy with mixed types of epilepsy (may increase frequency of grand-mal seizures)

PREGNANCY AND LACTATION: Pregnancy category C

SIDE EFFECTS/ADVERSE REACTIONS
CNS: Aggressiveness, *ataxia,* confusion, depression, *dizziness,* dream-

M

like state, *drowsiness*, euphoria, fatigue, headache, hyperactivity, hypochondriacal behavior, inability to concentrate, insomnia, instability, irritability, lethargy, mental slowness, nervousness, night terrors

EENT: Blurred vision, myopia, periorbital edema, photophobia

GI: Anorexia, constipation, cramps, diarrhea, epigastric and abdominal pain, *nausea,* swelling of tongue, *vague gastric upset, vomiting,* weight loss

GU: Microscopic hematuria, renal damage, urinary frequency, vaginal bleeding

*HEME: **Agranulocytosis, eosinophilia, granulocytopenia, leukopenia, monocytosis, pancytopenia***

MS: Muscle weakness

SKIN: Alopecia, ***erythema multiforme,*** hirsutism, pruritic erythematous rashes, pruritus, skin eruptions, ***Stevens-Johnson syndrome,*** urticaria

MISC: Systemic lupus erythematosus

INTERACTIONS
Labs
• *Ethosuximide:* False positive metabolite cross-reacts

SPECIAL CONSIDERATIONS
PATIENT/FAMILY EDUCATION
• Take with food or milk
• Do not discontinue abruptly
MONITORING PARAMETERS
• CBC with differential; liver enzymes
• Serum *N*-desmethylmethsuximide concentrations at trough for efficacy (range 10-40 µg/ml) and 3 hr postdose for toxicity (>40 µg/ml)

---

methyclothiazide
(meth-ee-cloh-thye′a-zide)
Rx: Aquatensen, Enduron
Combinations
  Rx: with reserpine
    (Diutensen-R)
Chemical Class: Sulfonamide derivative
Therapeutic Class: Thiazide diuretic; antihypertensive

CLINICAL PHARMACOLOGY
Mechanism of Action: Inhibits reabsorption of sodium and chloride in cortical thick ascencing limb of the loop of Henle and the early distal tubules—increasing the urinary excretion of sodium and chloride; sulfonamide moiety provides some carbonic anhydrase inhibition activity; other actions—increased potassium and bicarbonate excretion; decreased calcium excretion; uric acid retention; antihypertensive action dependent on sodium depletion, drop in peripheral vascular resistance, and reduction in extracellular volume.

Pharmacokinetics
PO: Onset 2 hr, peak effect 6 hr, duration 24 hr; excreted in urine (inactive metabolite and unchanged drug)

INDICATIONS AND USES: Edema (CHF, hepatic cirrhosis, corticosteroid and estrogen therapy, nephrotic syndrome, acute glomerulonephritis); hypertension; calcium nephrolithiasis,* prevention of osteoporosis*; diabetes insipidus*

DOSAGE
NOTE: Equivalent hydrochlorothiazide dose: 5 mg = 50 mg
Adult
• *Edema:* PO 2.5-10 mg qd
• *Hypertension:* PO 2.5-5 mg qd

---

* = non-FDA-approved use

🔰 AVAILABLE FORMS/COST OF THERAPY

• Tab, Uncoated—Oral: 2.5 mg, 100's: **$8.25-$52.58;** 5 mg, 100's: **$9.98-$160.93**

CONTRAINDICATIONS: Anuria, renal decompensation

PRECAUTIONS: Fluid and electrolyte imbalance (including sodium, potassium, magnesium, calcium), renal disease, hepatic disease, gout, COPD, lupus erythematosus, diabetes mellitus, hyperparathyroidism, vomiting, diarrhea, elevated cholesterol/triglycerides, tartrazine sensitivity

PREGNANCY AND LACTATION: Pregnancy category B; therapy for preexisting hypertension can be continued throughout pregnancy with minimal risk; initiating for simple edema not recommended; few unequivocal indications for diuretic therapy in pregnancy except for pulmonary edema or congestive heart failure; excreted into breast milk in small amounts; considered compatible with breast feeding

SIDE EFFECTS/ADVERSE REACTIONS

CNS: Anxiety, depression, *dizziness,* drowsiness, *fatigue,* headache, paresthesia, *weakness*

CV: Arrhythmias, irregular pulse, orthostatic hypotension, palpitations, volume depletion, angina

EENT: Blurred vision, nasal congestion

GI: Anorexia, constipation, cramps, diarrhea, GI irritation, hepatitis, *nausea,* pancreatitis, *vomiting*

GU: Frequency, glucosuria, polyuria, uremia, increased creatinine, BUN

*HEME: **Agranulocytosis, aplastic anemia, hemolytic anemia, leukopenia, neutropenia, thrombocytopenia***

METAB: Hypercalcemia, *hyperglycemia, hyperuricemia;* hypochloremia, *hypokalemia,* hypomagnesemia, hyponatremia lipid abnormalities (increased total LDL-cholesterol, triglycerides

SKIN: Fever, photosensitivity, purpura, *rash,* urticaria

INTERACTIONS

Drugs

❷ *Angiotensin converting enzyme inhibitors:* Risk of postural hypotension when added to ongoing diuretic therapy; more common with loop diuretics; first dose hypotension possible in patients with sodium depletion or hypovolemia due to diuretics or sodium restriction; hypotensive response is usually transient; hold diuretic day of first dose

❸ *Calcium:* Large doses can lead to milk-alkali syndrome

❸ *Carbenoxolone:* Severe hypokalemia

❸ *Binding resins (cholestyramine, colestipol):* Reduces thiazide serum levels and lessened diuretic effects

❸ *Corticosteroids:* Concomitant therapy may result in excessive potassium loss

❸ *Diazoxide:* Hyperglycemia

❸ *Digitalis glycosides:* Diuretic-induced hypokalemia may potentiate the risk of digitalis toxicity

❸ *Hypoglycemic agents:* Thiazide diuretics tend to increase blood glucose; may increase dosage requirements of hypoglycemic agents.

❸ *Insulin:* Increased blood glucose, increased dosage requirement of antidiabetic drugs

❸ *Lithium:* Increased lithium concentrations

❸ *Methotrexate:* Increased methotrexate effects; potentiates bone marrow toxicity

❸ *Nonsteroidal antiinflammatory drugs:* Concurrent use may reduce diuretic and antihypertensive effects.

---

italic = common side effects   ***bold italic*** = life-threatening reactions

SPECIAL CONSIDERATIONS

- Doses above 2.5 mg provide no further blood pressure reduction, but are more likely to induce metabolic disturbance (i.e., hypokalemia, hyperuricemia, etc.)
- May protect against osteoporotic hip fractures
- Loop diuretics or metolazone more effective if CrCl <40-50 ml/min

PATIENT/FAMILY EDUCATION

- Will increase urination temporarily (approx. 3 weeks); take early in the day to prevent sleep disturbance
- May cause sensitivity to sunlight; avoid prolonged exposure to the sun and other ultraviolet light
- May cause gout attacks; notify clinician if sudden joint pain occurs

MONITORING PARAMETERS

- Weight, urine output, serum electrolytes, BUN, creatinine, CBC, uric acid, glucose, lipids

---

methylcellulose

(meth-ill-sell′yoo-lose)
OTC: Citrucel
Chemical Class: Hydrophilic semisynthetic cellulose derivative
Therapeutic Class: Bulk laxative

CLINICAL PHARMACOLOGY

Mechanism of Action: Attracts water, expands in intestine to increase peristalsis; also absorbs excess water in stool; decreases diarrhea

Pharmacokinetics
PO: Not absorbed, onset 12-24 hr, full effect may not be apparent for 2-3 days

INDICATIONS AND USES: Constipation

DOSAGE

Adult and Child >12 yr
- PO 1 heaping tablespoon in 8 oz cold water, 1-3 times daily

Child
- PO 1 level tablespoon in 4 oz cold water, 1-3 times daily

$ AVAILABLE FORMS/COST OF THERAPY
- Powder—Oral: 2 g/heaping tablespoon, 480 g: **$12.90**; packet, 120's: **$8.36**

CONTRAINDICATIONS: Nausea, vomiting, or other symptom of appendicitis; acute surgical abdomen; fecal impaction; intestinal obstruction; undiagnosed abdominal pain

PRECAUTIONS: Rectal bleeding; esophageal stricture; intestinal ulcerations, stenosis, or disabling adhesions

PREGNANCY AND LACTATION: Bulk forming laxatives are the laxative of choice during pregnancy; compatible with breast feeding

SIDE EFFECTS/ADVERSE REACTIONS
GI: Abdominal distension, obstruction

SPECIAL CONSIDERATIONS
PATIENT/FAMILY EDUCATION

- Notify clinician of unrelieved constipation, rectal bleeding
- Ensure adequate fluids, proper dietary fiber intake and regular exercise

---

methyldopa

(meth-ill-doe′pa)
Rx: Aldomet
Combinations
  Rx: with HCTZ (Aldoril); with chlorothiazide (Aldoclor)
Chemical Class: Catecholamine derivative
Therapeutic Class: Antihypertensive, centrally acting sympathoplegic

---

CLINICAL PHARMACOLOGY
Mechanism of Action: Stimulates

inhibitory central α_2-adrenergic receptors by false transmitter, α-methylnorepinephrine, resulting in reduced sympathetic outflow from the CNS to the heart, kidneys, and peripheral vasculature; reduced peripheral resistance and plasma renin activity levels may also contribute to its effect

Pharmacokinetics

PO: Peak effect 3-6 hr

IV (methyldopate): Onset 4-6 hr, duration 10-16 hr

50% of PO dose absorbed; weakly bound to plasma proteins; extensively metabolized in GI tract and liver, eliminated in urine; $t_{1/2}$ 7-16 hr (24% unchanged) and feces (50%)

INDICATIONS AND USES: Moderate to severe hypertension

DOSAGE

Adult

• PO 250 mg bid-tid, increase q2d prn, usual dose 1-1.5 g/day in 2-4 divided doses, max 3 g/day; IV (methyldopate) 250-1000 mg q6-8h, max 4 g/day

• *Dosing interval in renal impairment:* CrCl >50 ml/min q8h; CrCl 10-50 ml/min q8-12h; CrCl <10 ml/min q12-24h

Child

• PO 10 mg/kg/day in 2-4 divided doses, increase q2d prn to max dose of 65 mg/kg/day, do not exceed 3 g/day; IV 2-4 mg/kg/dose; if response not seen within 4-6 hr, may increase to 5-10 mg/kg/dose; administer doses q6-8h; max daily dose 65 mg/kg or 3 g, whichever is less

• *Dosing interval in renal impairment:* CrCl >50 ml/min q8h; CrCl 10-50 ml/min q8-12h; CrCl <10 ml/min q12-24h

$ AVAILABLE FORMS/COST OF THERAPY

• Inj, Sol—IV: 50 mg/ml, 5 ml: **$6.24-$10.17** (methyldopate)

• Susp—Oral: 250 mg/5 ml, 480 ml: **$60.53**

• Tab, Plain Coated—Oral: 125 mg, 100's: **$9.75-$30.83;** 250 mg, 100's: **$12.50-$39.25;** 500 mg, 100's: **$22.50-$71.73**

CONTRAINDICATIONS: Active hepatic disease

PRECAUTIONS: History of liver disease, pheochromocytoma, sulfite sensitivity, renal failure, autonomic dysfunction

PREGNANCY AND LACTATION: Pregnancy category B (oral); C (IV); no adverse reactions have been reported despite rather wide use during pregnancy; compatible with breast feeding

SIDE EFFECTS/ADVERSE REACTIONS

CNS: Asthenia, Bell's palsy, decreased mental acuity, depression, *dizziness, headache,* involuntary choreoathetotic movements, lightheadedness, paresthesias, parkinsonism, psychic disturbances, *sedation,* symptoms of cerebrovascular insufficiency

CV: Aggravation of angina pectoris, bradycardia, edema, myocarditis, orthostatic hypotension, paradoxical pressor response, pericarditis, prolonged carotid sinus hypersensitivity

EENT: Dry mouth, nasal stuffiness

GI: Abnormal liver function tests, colitis, constipation, diarrhea, distension, flatus, hepatitis, jaundice, nausea, ***pancreatitis,*** sialadenitis, vomiting

GU: Decreased libido, failure to ejaculate, impotence

HEME: ***Bone marrow depression,*** eosinophilia, ***granulocytopenia, hemolytic anemia,*** positive Coombs test (10-20%), positive tests for antinuclear antibody, LE cells, and rheumatoid factor

METAB: Amenorrhea, breast enlarge-

---

italic = common side effects   ***bold italic*** = life-threatening reactions

ment, galactorrhea, hyperprolactinemia

MS: Arthralgia, myalgia

SKIN: Rash, ***toxic epidermal necrolysis***

MISC: Fever, lupus-like syndrome

INTERACTIONS

Drugs

▨ β-*blockers:* Rebound hypertension from methyldopa withdrawal exacerbated by noncardioselective β-blockers

▨ *Iron:* Inhibited antihypertensive response to methyldopa

▨ *Lithium:* Lithium toxicity not necessarily associated with excessive lithium concentrations

▨ *Tricyclic antidepressants:* Inhibit the antihypertensive response

Labs

• *Interference:* Plasma and urine catecholamines, serum creatinine, glucose, serum, urine uric acid, and acetaminophen, AST

• *False increase:* Urine amino acids, serum bilirubin, urine ferric chloride test, urine ketones, metanephrines, VMA

• *False decrease:* Serum cholesterol, triglycerides

• *False positive:* Guaiacols spot test, urine melanogen, urine Thormahlen test

SPECIAL CONSIDERATIONS

• Perform both direct and indirect Coombs test if blood transfusion needed. If indirect Coombs test positive, interference may occur with cross match. Positive direct Coombs test will not interfere

PATIENT/FAMILY EDUCATION

• Urine exposed to air after voiding may darken

• Do not discontinue abruptly

• Initial sedation usually improves

MONITORING PARAMETERS

• CBC, liver function tests periodically during therapy

• Direct Coombs test before therapy and after 6-12 mo. If positive rule out hemolytic anemia

---

methylene blue

(meth'i-leen)

Rx: Urolene Blue

Chemical Class: Thiazine dye

Therapeutic Class: Antidote, cyanide; antidote, drug-induced methemoglobinemia; diagnostic agent

CLINICAL PHARMACOLOGY

Mechanism of Action: Combines with cyanide to form cyanmethemoglobin, preventing interference of cyanide with the cytochrome system (high concentrations only); directly inhibits calcium binding by oxalate; possesses weak antiseptic and tissue-staining properties

Pharmacokinetics

PO/IV: Rapidly reduced in tissues to leukomethylene blue, excreted in urine and bile

INDICATIONS AND USES: Methemoglobinemia; cyanide poisoning; urolithiasis (ineffective in dissolving previously formed stones); genitourinary antiseptic (use is obsolete); cutaneous viral infections (in conjunction with polychromatic light)*; diagnosis of gastroesophageal reflux in infants and children*; delineation of body structures and fistulas through dye effect*; diagnosis of premature rupture of membrane*

DOSAGE

Adult

• IV 1-2 mg/kg (0.1-0.2 ml/kg) or 25-50 mg/m² over several min, may be repeated after 1 hr if necessary; PO 65-130 mg tid with a full glass of water

Child

• IV 1-2 mg/kg (0.1-0.2 ml/kg) or

---

* = non-FDA-approved use

25-50 mg/m^2 over several min, may be repeated after 1 hr if necessary

$ AVAILABLE FORMS/COST OF THERAPY

• Inj, Sol—IV: 1%, 1 ml: **$4.50-$17.00**

• Tab, Uncoated—Oral: 65 mg, 100's: **$41.44**

CONTRAINDICATIONS: Renal insufficiency, instraspinal inj

PRECAUTIONS: G6PD deficiency, prolonged administration, analine-induced methemoglobinemia (may precipitate Heinz body formation and hemolytic anemia)

PREGNANCY AND LACTATION: Pregnancy category C (category D if inj intra-amniotically); deep blue staining of the newborn, hemolytic anemia, hyperbilirubinemia, and methemoglobinemia in the newborn may occur after inj into the amniotic fluid

SIDE EFFECTS/ADVERSE REACTIONS

CNS: Dizziness, fever, *headache,* mental confusion

GI: Abdominal pain, blue-green stool, diarrhea, *nausea, vomiting*

GU: Bladder irritation, blue-green urine

HEME: Hemolytic anemia, methemoglobinemia (large doses)

SKIN: Profuse sweating, stains skin blue (may be removed by hypochlorite solution)

SPECIAL CONSIDERATIONS
PATIENT/FAMILY EDUCATION

• Photosensitivity may occur

MONITORING PARAMETERS

• Hct

---

methylergonovine

(meth-ill-er-goe-noe'veen)

Rx: Methergine

Chemical Class: Ergot alkaloid

Therapeutic Class: Oxytocic

CLINICAL PHARMACOLOGY

Mechanism of Action: Partial agonist or antagonist at α-adrenergic, dopaminergic, and tryptaminergic receptors; increases the strength, duration, and frequency of uterine contractions and decreases uterine bleeding when used after placental delivery

Pharmacokinetics

IV: Onset immediate, duration 3 hr

IM: Onset 2-5 min, duration 3 hr

PO: Onset 5-10 min, duration 3 hr

Excretion partially renal and partially hepatic; t$_{1/2}$ 20-30 min

INDICATIONS AND USES: Postpartum, postabortal hemorrhage due to uterine atony; subinvolution; routine management after delivery of the placenta

DOSAGE

Adult

• IM/IV 0.2 mg after delivery of the placenta, after delivery of the anterior shoulder, or during the puerperium; repeat q2-4h prn; PO 0.2 mg tid-qid in the puerperium for a max of 1 wk

$ AVAILABLE FORMS/COST OF THERAPY

• Inj, Sol—IM, IV: 0.2 mg/ml, 1's: **$3.40**

• Tab, Coated—Oral: 0.2 mg, 100's: **$42.96-$120.08**

CONTRAINDICATIONS: Hypertension, toxemia, hypersensitivity to ergots

PRECAUTIONS: Rapid IV INF (may induce sudden hypertension and CVAs), sepsis, obliterative vas-

M

cular disease; hepatic/renal impairment

PREGNANCY AND LACTATION:
Pregnancy category C; small quantity appears in breast milk; adverse effects have not been described

SIDE EFFECTS/ADVERSE REACTIONS

CNS: Dizziness, hallucinations, *headache,* paresthesias, *seizure*
CV: Hypertension, palpitations, temporary chest pain, thrombophlebitis
EENT: Tinnitus
GI: Diarrhea, foul taste, nausea, vomiting
MS: Leg cramps
RESP: Dyspnea
SKIN: Diaphoresis

SPECIAL CONSIDERATIONS
PATIENT/FAMILY EDUCATION
• Report increased blood loss, severe abdominal cramps, increased temperature, or foul-smelling lochia.
• Symptoms of ergotism occur with overdosage (nausea, vomiting, diarrhea, seizure, hallucinations, delirium, numb/gangrenous extremities)

MONITORING PARAMETERS
• Blood pressure, pulse, and uterine response

---

methylphenidate

(meth-ill-fen'i-date)
Rx: Ritalin, Ritalin-SR
Chemical Class: Piperidine derivative of amphetamine
Therapeutic Class: Cerebral stimulant
DEA Class: Schedule II

CLINICAL PHARMACOLOGY
Mechanism of Action: Sympathomimetic amine with CNS stimulant activity; like amphetamines, increases release of norepinephrine from central noradrenergic neurons;

at higher doses, dopamine released in mesolimbic system; peripheral α- and β-activity includes elevation of systolic and diastolic blood pressures and weak bronchodilator and respiratory stimulation action; heart rate reflexly slowed at standard doses, arrhythmias with overdose

Pharmacokinetics
PO: Peak 1-3 hr (sustained release 4-7 hr), duration 3-6 hr (sustained release 8 hr); 80% metabolized to ritalinic acid, excreted in urine

INDICATIONS AND USES: Attention deficit disorders; narcolepsy; depression in elderly, cancer, and poststroke patients*

DOSAGE
Adult
• *Narcolepsy:* PO 10 mg bid-tid; 30-45 min ac; may increase up to 40-60 mg/day

Child ≥6 yr
• *Attention deficit disorder:* PO 0.3 mg/kg/dose or 2.5-5 mg/dose given before breakfast and lunch; increase by 0.1 mg/kg/dose or 5-10 mg/day at weekly intervals; usual dose 0.5-1 mg/kg/day; max 2 mg/kg/day or 60 mg/day; sustained release may be used when the 8 hr dosage of sustained release corresponds to the titrated 8 hr dose of immediate-release tabs

💲 **AVAILABLE FORMS/COST OF THERAPY**
• Tab, Plain Coated, SUS Action—Oral: 20 mg, 100's: **$105.65-$123.41**
• Tab, Uncoated—Oral: 5 mg, 100's: **$28.77-$38.76;** 10 mg, 100's: **$40.23-$55.26;** 20 mg, 100's: **$58.86-$79.46**

CONTRAINDICATIONS: Marked anxiety, tension, and agitation; glaucoma; history of Tourette's syndrome or motor tics, prevention of normal fatigue

PRECAUTIONS: Severe depres-

---

* = non-FDA-approved use

sion, seizure disorders, hypertension, history of drug abuse, children <6 yr, symptoms associated with acute stress reactions

PREGNANCY AND LACTATION: Pregnancy category C

SIDE EFFECTS/ADVERSE REACTIONS

CNS: Akathisia, dizziness, dyskinesia, fever, headache, *hyperactivity, insomnia, restlessness,* talkativeness, Tourette's syndrome (rare)

CV: Angina, blood pressure changes, *dysrhythmias, palpitations, tachycardia*

GI: Abdominal pain, anorexia, dry mouth, nausea, weight loss

GU: Uremia

HEME: **Anemia, leukopenia**

METAB: Growth retardation

MS: Arthralgia

SKIN: **Erythema-multiforme, exfoliative dermatitis,** rash, scalp hair loss, urticaria

INTERACTIONS

Drugs

3 *Guanethidine:* Inhibition of guanethidine antihypertensive effect

2 *MAOIs:* Hypertensive reactions

3 *Phenytoin:* Increased phenytoin levels with risk of toxicity

3 *Tricyclic antidepressants:* Increased serum concentrations of tricyclic antidepressants

Labs

• *False positive:* Urine amphetamine

SPECIAL CONSIDERATIONS

• Overdosage may cause vomiting, agitation, tremor, muscle twitching, seizures, confusion, tachycardia, hypertension, arrhythmias

PATIENT/FAMILY EDUCATION

• Take last daily dose prior to 6 PM to avoid insomnia

• Do not discontinue abruptly

• Avoid OTC preparations unless approved by clinician

• Do not crush or chew sustained release formulation

MONITORING PARAMETERS

• Periodic CBC with differential and platelet count

---

methylprednisolone

(meth-il-pred-niss'oh-lone)

Rx: *Methylprednisolone:* Medrol

Acetate: Depo-Medrol, depMedalone, Depoject, Depopred, D-Med, Duralone, Medralone, M-Prednisol, Rep-Pred

Sodium Succinate: A-Metha-Pred, Solu-Medrol

Chemical Class: Synthetic glucocorticoid

Therapeutic Class: Systemic corticosteroid

CLINICAL PHARMACOLOGY

Mechanism of Action: Decreases inflammation by depressing migration of polymorphonuclear leukocytes and activity of endogenous mediators of inflammation. Has many profound metabolic effects, does not possess mineralocorticoid activity

Pharmacokinetics

PO: Peak effect 1-2 hr, duration 30-36 hr

IM (acetate): Peak effect 4-8 days, duration 1-4 wk

Intra-articular: Peak effect 1 wk, duration 1-5 wk

Metabolized in liver, excreted in urine and bile; biologic $t_{1/2}$ 18-36 hr

INDICATIONS AND USES: *Systemic:* Antiinflammatory or immunosuppressant agent in the treatment of a variety of diseases of hematologic, allergic, inflammatory, neoplastic, and autoimmune origin

Intra-articular: Synovitis, osteoarthritis

M

---

italic = common side effects　　　　**bold italic** = life-threatening reactions

Intradermal: Keloids, alopecia areata, inflammatory skin lesions

DOSAGE

Adult

• PO 4-48 mg/day initially, adjust until satisfactory response is noted, taper gradually if used continuously for >10 days

• *Sodium succinate:* IM/IV 10-40 mg initially, may repeat q6h prn; for acute spinal cord injury, give 30 mg/kg IV over 15 min followed in 45 min by a continuous INF of 5.4 mg/kg/hr for 23 hr

• *Acetate:* IM 40-120 mg q1-2 wk; intra-articular/intralesional 4-40 mg, up to 80 mg for large joints q1-5 wk

Child

• PO/IM/IV 0.12-1.7 mg/kg/day or 5-25 mg/m^2/day in divided doses q6-12h

• *Status asthmaticus:* IV 2 mg/kg loading dose, then 0.5-1 mg/kg/dose q6h

AVAILABLE FORMS/COST OF THERAPY

• Tab, Uncoated—Oral: 4 mg, 21's: **$10.56-$20.03** (dose-pack)

• Tab, Uncoated—Oral: 2 mg, 100's: **$44.11;** 4 mg, 100's: **$36.60-$59.51;** 8 mg, 100's: **$117.16;** 16 mg, 100's: **$181.02;** 24 mg, 100's: **$221.44;** 32 mg, 100's: **$269.60**

• Inj, Sol (acetate)—IM, intraarticular, intralesional: 20 mg/ml, 10 ml: **$7.50;** 40 mg/ml, 10 ml: **$10.08-$40.36;** 80 mg/ml, 5 ml: **$9.75-$40.36**

• Inj, Lyphl-Sol (sodium succinate)—IM,IV: 40 mg/vial, 1's: **$2.13-$4.00;** 125 mg/vial, 1's: **$3.73-$12.50;** 500 mg/vial, 1's: **$8.37-$37.50;** 1 g/vial, 1's: **$31.80-$65.00**

• Inj, Sol (sodium succinate)—IM, IV: 2 g/vial, 1's: **$57.98**

CONTRAINDICATIONS: Systemic fungal infections, idiopathic thrombocytopenic purpura (IM), prema-

ture infants (sodium succinate, acetate, secondary gasping syndrome from benzyl alcohol), intrathecal administration

PRECAUTIONS: Psychosis, diabetes mellitus, glaucoma, osteoporosis, seizure disorders, ulcerative colitis (intestinal perforation), CHF, hypertension, myesthenia gravis (if used with anticholinesterase agents), renal disease, esophagitis, peptic ulcer, latent tuberculosis or amebiasis (reactivation of disease). Topical: use on face, groin, or axilla, ocular herpes simplex

PREGNANCY AND LACTATION: Pregnancy category C; excreted in breast milk, could suppress infant's growth and interfere with endogenous corticosteroid production

SIDE EFFECTS/ADVERSE REACTIONS

CNS: Depression, headache, *mood changes,* **seizures,** vertigo

CV: **CHF,** hypertension, tachycardia, thromboembolism, thrombophlebitis

EENT: Blurred vision, cataract, increased intraocular pressure

GI: Abdominal distension, diarrhea, **GI hemorrhage,** increased appetite, *nausea,* **pancreatitis**

METAB: Cushingoid state, decreased glucose tolerance, growth suppression in children, HPA suppression

MS: Aseptic necrosis of femoral and humeral heads, fractures, muscle mass loss, osteoporosis, weakness

SKIN: Acne, bruising, ecchymosis, petechiae, poor wound healing, striae, thin fragile skin

INTERACTIONS

Drugs

3 *Aminoglutethamide:* Enhanced elimination of corticosteroids; marked reduction in corticosteroid response; increased clearance of methylprednisolone; doubling of dose may be necessary

❸ *Antidiabetics:* Increased blood glucose

❸ *Barbiturates, carbamazepine:* Reduced serum concentrations of corticosteroids; increased clearance of methylprednisolone

❸ *Cholestyramine colestipol:* Possible reduced absorption of corticosteroids

❸ *Cyclosporine:* Possible increased concentration of both drugs, seizures

❸ *Erythromycin, troleandomycin, clarithromycin, ketoconazole:* Possible enhanced steroid effect

❸ *Estrogens, oral contraceptives:* Enhanced effects of corticosteroids

❸ *Isoniazid:* Reduced plasma concentrations of isoniazid

❸ *IUDs:* Inhibition of inflammation may decrease contraceptive effect

❸ *NSAIDs:* Increased risk GI ulceration

❸ *Rifampin:* Reduced therapeutic effect of corticosteroids; may reduce hepatic clearance of methylprednisolone

❸ *Salicylates:* Subtherapeutic salicylate concentrations possible

Labs

• *False increase:* Cortisol, digoxin, theophylline level

• *False decrease:* Urine glucose (Clinistix, Diastix only, Testape no effect)

• *False negative:* Skin allergy tests

SPECIAL CONSIDERATIONS
PATIENT/FAMILY EDUCATION

• Take single daily doses in AM

• May mask infections

• Increased dose of rapidly acting corticosteroids may be necessary in patients subjected to unusual stresses

• Signs of adrenal insufficiency include fatigue, anorexia, nausea, vomiting, diarrhea, weight loss, weakness, dizziness, and low blood sugar

• Avoid abrupt withdrawal of therapy following high dose or long-term therapy. Relative insufficiency may exist for up to 1 yr after discontinuation

• Patients on chronic steroid therapy should wear Medic Alert bracelet

• Do not give live virus vaccines to patients on prolonged therapy

MONITORING PARAMETERS

• Serum K and glucose

• Growth of children on prolonged therapy

---

methyltestosterone

(meth-ill-tess-toss'teh-rone)
Rx: Android, Methitest, Testred, Virilon
Chemical Class: Testosterone derivative
Therapeutic Class: Androgen; antineoplastic
DEA Class: Schedule III

M

CLINICAL PHARMACOLOGY

Mechanism of Action: Promotes weight gain via retention of nitrogen, potassium, and phosphorus, increased protein anabolism and decreased catabolism; endogenous androgens essential for normal growth and development of male sex organs and maintenance of secondary sex characteristics

Pharmacokinetics

PO: Half as potent as buccally administered tablets; metabolized in liver, excreted in urine

INDICATIONS AND USES: Males: primary hypogonadism (congenital or acquired), hypogonadotropic hypogonadism (congenital or acquired), delayed puberty; females: palliative therapy of metastatic breast cancer, postpartum breast pain, engorgement,* moderate to severe vasomotor symptoms of menopause (in conjunction with estrogens)

---

italic = common side effects   ***bold italic*** = life-threatening reactions

DOSAGE
Adult
• *Male hypogonadism:* PO 10-50 mg qd; buccal 5-25 mg qd
• *Delayed puberty:* PO 10 mg qd for 4-6 mo; buccal 5 mg qd for 4-6 mo
• *Breast cancer:* PO 50-200 mg qd; buccal 25-100 mg qd
• *Postpartum breast pain and engorgement:* PO 80 mg qd for 3-5 days after parturition; buccal 40 mg qd for 3-5 days after parturition
• *Menopause:* PO 1.25-10 mg qd (with estrogen)

$ AVAILABLE FORMS/COST OF THERAPY
• Cap, Gel—Oral: 10 mg, 100's: **$36.00-$170.38**
• Tab—Uncoated—Oral: 10 mg, 100's: **$171.17** 25 mg, 100's: **$223.13**

CONTRAINDICATIONS: Severe cardiac, hepatic, or renal disease; carcinoma of breast or prostate (males); pregnancy; enhancement of athletic performance

PRECAUTIONS: Epilepsy, migraine headaches, children, benign prostatic hypertrophy, acute intermittent porphyria, risk factors for atherosclerosis, coronary artery disease

PREGNANCY AND LACTATION: Pregnancy category X; causes virilization of female fetuses; excretion into breast milk unknown; use extreme caution in nursing mothers

SIDE EFFECTS/ADVERSE REACTIONS
CNS: Anxiety, decreased or increased libido, dizziness, emotional lability, fatigue, flushing, headache, insomnia, paresthesias, sweating, tremors
CV: Increased blood pressure, *CHF,* edema
EENT: Conjunctival edema, deepening of voice (women), nasal congestion

GI: Cholestatic jaundice, constipation, nausea, *peliosis hepatis,* stomatitis (buccal), vomiting, weight gain
GU: Amenorrhea, *clitoral hypertrophy,* excessive frequency and duration of erection, hematuria, libido changes, oligospermia, testicular atrophy, vaginitis, menstrual changes
HEME: Polycythemia, suppression of clotting factors II, V, VII, and X
METAB: Abnormal GTT; decreased TBG (causes decreased total T_4, increased T_3 resin uptake, but normal free T_4), hypercalcemia; increased serum cholesterol, retention of sodium, chloride, water, potassium, and inorganic phosphate
MS: Cramps, spasms
SKIN: Acneiform lesions, acne vulgaris, hirsutism, male pattern baldness, oily hair, skin, rash, sweating
MISC: Decreased breast size, gynecomastia, *virilization (females)*

INTERACTIONS
Drugs
3 *Cyclosporine:* Increased cyclosporine concentrations
2 *Warfarin:* Enhanced hypoprothrombinemic response to oral anticoagulants

SPECIAL CONSIDERATIONS
PATIENT/FAMILY EDUCATION
• Do not swallow buccal tablets, allow to dissolve between cheek and gum
• Avoid eating, drinking, or smoking while buccal tablet in place
MONITORING PARAMETERS
• LFTs, lipids, Hct
• Growth rate in children (Xrays for bone age q6 mo)

methysergide
(meth-i-ser′jide)
Rx: Sansert
Chemical Class: Semisynthetic ergot alkaloid
Therapeutic Class: Antimigraine agent

CLINICAL PHARMACOLOGY
Mechanism of Action: Exact mechanism of action in preventing migraine unknown; may be related to antiserotonin effect

Pharmacokinetics
PO: Onset of action 1-2 days, duration 1-2 days; metabolized in liver, excreted in urine (unchanged drug and metabolites); $t_{1/2}$ 10 hr

INDICATIONS AND USES: Prevention of vascular headache (not 1st-line); diarrhea in patients with carcinoid disease*

DOSAGE
Adult
• PO 4-8 mg/day in divided doses with meals; **a drug-free interval of 3-4 wk must follow each 6 mo course. Reduce dose gradually during last 2-3 wk to avoid "headache rebound"**

🚺 AVAILABLE FORMS/COST OF THERAPY
• Tab, Coated—Oral: 2 mg, 100's: **$210.79**

CONTRAINDICATIONS: Peripheral vascular disease; severe arteriosclerosis; severe hypertension; CAD; phlebitis or cellulitis of lower limbs; pulmonary disease; collagen diseases or fibrotic processes; impaired liver or renal function; valvular heart disease; peptic ulcer; debilitated states; serious infections
PRECAUTIONS: Tartrazine sensitivity, uninterrupted administration (increases risk of fibrotic complications)

PREGNANCY AND LACTATION: Contraindicated in pregnancy due to oxytocic properties; ergot derivatives in the milk of nursing mothers have caused symptoms of ergotism (e.g., vomiting, diarrhea) in the infant
SIDE EFFECTS/ADVERSE REACTIONS
CNS: Ataxia, dizziness, drowsiness, hyperesthesia, insomnia, lightheadedness, mild euphoria, unworldly feelings, weakness
CV: **Cardiac fibrosis,** edema, vasoconstriction of small and large arteries (chest pain, abdominal pain, cold, numb, painful extremities, diminished or absent pulses)
GI: Abdominal pain, constipation, diarrhea, heartburn, nausea, vomiting
GU: **Retroperitoneal fibrosis**
HEME: Eosinophilia, **neutropenia**
MS: Arthralgia, myalgia
RESP: **Pleuropulmonary fibrosis**
SKIN: Facial flush, increased hair loss, non-specific rashes, telangiectasia
MISC: Weight gain

SPECIAL CONSIDERATIONS
• Reserve for patients who have failed to respond to safer agents (e.g., β-blockers, TCAs, and calcium channel blockers)
PATIENT/FAMILY EDUCATION
• Continuous administration should not exceed 6 mo
• Notify clinician of cold, numb, or painful extremities; leg cramps when walking; girdle, flank, or chest pain; painful urination; or shortness of breath (i.e. fibrotic symptoms)
MONITORING PARAMETERS
• Consider baseline urography, repeated q6-12 mo during therapy
• Monitor for new cardiac murmurs

M

---

italic = common side effects   ***bold italic*** = life-threatening reactions

metipranolol

(met-ee-pran'oh-lol)

Rx: Optipranolol

Chemical Class: Nonselective β-adrenergic blocker

Therapeutic Class: Antiglaucoma agent

CLINICAL PHARMACOLOGY

Mechanism of Action: Reduces aqueous humor production; slight increase in outflow may be an additional mechanism; little or no effect on pupil size or accommodation

Pharmacokinetics

OPHTH: Onset ≤30 min, max effect by 2 hr, duration 12-24 hr, may be absorbed systemically

INDICATIONS AND USES: Chronic open-angle glaucoma; ocular hypertension; ocular conditions where lowering intraocular pressure would be of benefit

DOSAGE

Adult

• INSTILL 1 gtt in affected eye(s) bid

$ AVAILABLE FORMS/COST OF THERAPY

• Sol—Ophth: 0.3%, 5, 10 ml: **$15.68/5 ml**

CONTRAINDICATIONS: Asthma, severe COPD, sinus bradycardia, 2nd or 3rd degree AV block, overt cardiac failure, cardiogenic shock

PRECAUTIONS: Systemic absorption, major surgery, diabetes mellitus, hyperthyroidism, cerebrovascular insufficiency, children, angle-closure glaucoma

PREGNANCY AND LACTATION: Pregnancy category C

SIDE EFFECTS/ADVERSE REACTIONS

CNS: Anxiety, asthenia, depression, dizziness, headache

CV: Angina, *arrhythmia,* bradycardia, *cerebral ischemia, cerebral vascular accident, congestive heart failure,* heart block, hypertension, *MI,* palpitation, syncope

EENT: Blepharitis, blepharoptosis, browache, conjunctivitis, diplopia, epistaxis, eyelid dermatitis, keratitis, photophobia, ptosis, rhinitis, tearing, transient local discomfort, visual disturbances

GI: Nausea

METAB: Masked symptoms of hypoglycemia in diabetics (sweating excepted)

MS: Arthritis, myalgia

RESP: **Bronchospasm,** dyspnea, *respiratory failure*

SKIN: Hypersensitivity, localized and generalized rash

SPECIAL CONSIDERATIONS

PATIENT/FAMILY EDUCATION

• Apply pressure to lacrimal sac for 1 min following instillation to minimize systemic absorption

• Do not touch dropper to eye

metoclopramide

(met'oh-kloe-pra'mide)

Rx: Reglan

Chemical Class: Paraminobenzoic acid derivative

Therapeutic Class: Gastrointestinal prokinetic agent; antiemetic

CLINICAL PHARMACOLOGY

Mechanism of Action: Inhibits gastric smooth muscle relaxation produced by dopamine, thus enhancing cholinergic responses of GI smooth muscle; increases resting pressure of the lower esophageal sphincter, increases amplitude of esophageal peristaltic contractions; dopamine antagonist action raises the threshold of activity in the chemoreceptor trigger zone and decreases input from afferent visceral nerves; stimulates prolactin secretion

Pharmacokinetics

PO: Onset 30-60 min, duration 1-2 hr
IM: Onset 10-15 min, duration 1-2 hr
IV: Onset 1-3 min, duration 1-2 hr
13%-22% bound to plasma proteins; partially metabolized in liver, eliminated in urine; $t_{1/2}$ 4-6 hr

INDICATIONS AND USES: Gastroesophageal reflux disease (GERD); diabetic gastroparesis; chemotherapy-induced nausea and vomiting (parenteral); facilitation of small bowel intubation; postoperative nausea and vomiting; prevention of aspiration pneumonitis presurgery*; slow gastric emptying*; gastic stasis in preterm infants*; vascular headache*; lactation deficiency*; diabetic cystoparesis*; esophageal variceal bleeding*

DOSAGE

Adult

• *GERD/gastroparesis:* PO/IM/IV 10-15 mg 30 min ac and hs; PR 25 mg (5 oral tabs compounded in polyethylene glycol) 30 min ac and hs
• *Intubation of small bowel:* IV 10 mg.
• *Postoperative nausea and vomiting:* IM 10-20 mg near the end of surgery
• *Chemotherapy-induced nausea and vomiting:* IV 1-2 mg/kg/dose q2-4 hr; dilute in 50 ml of parenteral sol and infuse over at least 15 min
• *Dosing adjustment in renal failure:* CrCl 10-50 ml/min administer 75% of recommended dose; CrC1 <10 ml/min, administer 25%-50% of recommended dose

Child

• *GERD:* PO/IM/IV 0.4-0.8 mg/kg/day divided qid
• *Intubation of small bowel:* IV (<6 yr) 0.1 mg/kg; (6-14 yr) 2.5-5 mg
• *Chemotherapy-induced nausea and vomiting:* IV 1-2 mg/kg/dose q2-4 hr

💲 **AVAILABLE FORMS/COST OF THERAPY**

• Inj, Sol—IM, IV: 5 mg/ml, 2 ml: **$0.89-$2.10**
• Syr—Oral: 5 mg/5ml, 480 ml: **$12.00-$57.49**
• Conc—Oral: 10 mg/ml, 30 ml: **$19.49**
• Tab, Uncoated—Oral: 5 mg, 100's: **$9.87-$48.76;** 10 mg, 100's: **$1.88-$76.88**

CONTRAINDICATIONS: GI hemorrhage, mechanical obstruction or perforation of the GI tract, pheochromocytoma, seizure disorder

PRECAUTIONS: History of depression, Parkinson's disease, hypertension, anastomosis or closure of the gut

PREGNANCY AND LACTATION: Pregnancy category B; has been used during pregnancy as an antiemetic and to decrease gastric emptying time; excreted into milk; use during lactation a concern because of the potent CNS effects the drug is capable of producing

SIDE EFFECTS/ADVERSE REACTIONS

CNS: Dizziness, *drowsiness, EPS* (dystonia, parkinson-like symptoms, akathisia, tardive dyskinesia 1-9%), *fatigue,* hallucinations, *headache, restlessness, sedation,* **seizures,** *sleeplessness*

CV: Bradycardia, hypertension, hypotension, supraventricular tachycardia

EENT: Visual disturbances

GI: Bowel disturbances, *diarrhea,* nausea

GU: Incontinence, urinary frequency

HEME: **Agranulocytosis, leukopenia, methemoglobinemia** (especially overdoses in neonates), **neutropenia,** porphyria

METAB: Amenorrhea, elevated al-

dosterone, galactorrhea, gynecomastia, impotence (hyperprolactinemia)
SKIN: Rash, urticaria
MISC: **Neuroleptic malignant syndrome**

INTERACTIONS
Drugs
3 *Cyclosporine:* Increased bioavailability and serum concentrations of cyclosporine
3 *Digitalis glycosides:* Reduced serum digoxin concentration when coadministered with generic formulations
3 *Ethanol:* Increased sedative effects of ethanol

SPECIAL CONSIDERATIONS
• Dystonic reactions can be managed with 50 mg diphenhydramine or 1-2 mg benztropine IM

---

metolazone

(met-tole'a-zone)
Rx: Mykrox (rapid acting),
Zaroxolyn (slow acting)
Chemical Class: Quinazoline derivative
Therapeutic Class: Thiazide-like diuretic; antihypertensive

CLINICAL PHARMACOLOGY
Mechanism of Action: Structural and pharmacological similarities to thiazide diuretics; inhibits reabsorption of sodium and chloride in cortical thick ascending limb of the loop of Henle and the early distal tubules—increasing the urinary excretion of sodium and chloride; retains some proximal tubule activity via carbonic anhydrase inhibition activity; other actions—increased potassium and bicarbonate excretion; decreased calcium excretion; uric acid retention; antihypertensive action dependent on sodium depletion, drop in peripheral vascular resistance, and reduction in extracellular volume; more effective than thiazides in patients with impaired renal function (may produce diuresis with CrCl <20 ml/min)
Pharmacokinetics
PO: (Rapid acting) peak 2-4 hr, steady state within 4-5 days; (Slow acting) peak 8 hr; 50%-70% bound to erythrocytes, up to 33% bound to plasma proteins; 70%-95% excreted unchanged in urine by glomerular filtration and active tubular secretion; $t_{1/2}$ 8 hr

INDICATIONS AND USES: Slow acting: edema (CHF, nephrotic syndrome, hepatic cirrhosis, corticosteroid and estrogen therapy); potentiation of loop diuretics: concomitant with loop diuretic to induce diuresis in patients who did not respond to either diuretic alone; hypertension. Rapid acting: hypertension (not indicated for diuresis as dosage not established)

DOSAGE
NOTE: Equivalent hydrochlorothiazide dose: 5 mg-50 mg
Adult
• *Edema:* PO (Slow acting) 5-10 mg qAM; up to 20 mg qd may be required for edema associated with renal disease
• *Hypertension:* PO (Slow acting) 1.25-5 mg qAM; (Rapid acting) 0.5-1 mg qAM
Child
• PO (Slow acting) 0.2-0.4 mg/kg/day divided q12-24h

$ AVAILABLE FORMS/COST OF THERAPY
• Tab, Uncoated—Oral: 0.5 mg, 100's: **$89.50** (Mykrox)
• Tab, Uncoated—Oral: 2.5 mg, 100's: **$60.87;** 5 mg, 100's: **$69.19;** 10 mg, 100's: **$82.82** (Zaroxolyn)

CONTRAINDICATIONS: Anuria, hepatic coma or pre-coma
PRECAUTIONS: Fluid and electrolyte imbalance (including sodium,

potassium, chloride, magnesium, calcium), renal disease, hepatic disease, gout, COPD, lupus erythematosus, diabetes mellitus, hyperparathyroidism, vomiting, diarrhea, elevated cholesterol/triglycerides

PREGNANCY AND LACTATION: Pregnancy category B; therapy for preexisting hypertension can be continued throughout pregnancy with minimal risk; initiating for simple edema not recommended; few unequivocal indications for diuretic therapy in pregnancy except for pulmonary edema or congestive heart failure; excreted into breast milk in small amounts; considered compatible with breast feeding

SIDE EFFECTS/ADVERSE REACTIONS

CNS: Anxiety, depression, *dizziness, drowsiness, fatigue, headache,* paresthesia, *weakness,* neuropathy

CV: Chest pain, irregular pulse, ***arrhythmias,*** orthostatic hypotension, palpitations, volume depletion

EENT: Blurred vision, dry mouth

GI: Abdominal bloating, *anorexia,* jaundice, cholecystitis, constipation, cramps, diarrhea, GI irritation, hepatitis, *nausea,* **pancreatitis,** *vomiting*

GU: Frequency, glucosuria, impotence, polyuria

HEME: **Agranulocytosis, aplastic anemia, leukopenia**

METAB: Hypercalcemia, hyperglycemia, hyperuricemia, hypochloremia, *hypokalemia,* hypomagnesemia, hyponatremia, increased creatinine, BUN

MS: Muscle cramps, joint pain

SKIN: Fever, photosensitivity, pruritis, purpura, *rash,* urticaria

INTERACTIONS

Drugs

❷ *Angiotensin-converting enzyme inhibitors:* Risk of postural hypotension when added to ongoing diuretic therapy; more common with loop diuretics; first dose hypotension possible in patients with sodium depletion or hypovolemia due to diuretics or sodium restriction; hypotensive response is usually transient; hold diuretic day of first dose

❸ *Calcium:* Milk-alkali syndrome

❸ *Carbenoxolone:* Enhanced hypokalemia

❸ *Cholestyramine, colestipol:* Reduced serum concentrations of metolazone

❸ *Corticosteroids:* Concomitant therapy may result in excessive potassium loss

❸ *Diazoxide:* Hyperglycemia

❸ *Digitalis glycosides:* Diuretic-induced hypokalemia may increase the risk of digitalis toxicity

❸ *Hypoglycemic agents:* Metolazone increases blood glucose

❸ *Lithium:* Increased serum lithium concentrations, toxicity may occur

❸ *Methotrexate:* Enhanced bone marrow suppression

❸ *Nonsteroidal antiinflammatory drugs:* Concurrent use may reduce diuretic and antihypertensive effects

SPECIAL CONSIDERATIONS

• More effective than other thiazide-type diuretics in patients with impaired renal function

• Metolazone formulations are not bioequivalent or therapeutically equivalent at the same doses. Mykrox is more rapidly and completely bioavailable; Don't interchange brands.

PATIENT/FAMILY EDUCATION

• Will increase urination; take early in the day to prevent sleep disturbance

• May cause sensitivity to sunlight; avoid prolonged exposure to the sun and other ultraviolet light

• May cause gout attacks; notify clinician if sudden joint pain occurs

M

MONITORING PARAMETERS

• Weight, urine output, serum electrolytes, BUN, creatinine, CBC, uric acid, glucose, lipids

---

metoprolol

(me-toe'pro-lole)
Rx: Lopressor, Toprol XL
Combination
  Rx: with hydrochlorothiazide (Lopressor Hct)
Chemical Class: β_1-selective (cardioselective) adrenoreceptor blocker
Therapeutic Class: Antihypertensive; antianginal; postmyocardial infarction

---

CLINICAL PHARMACOLOGY

Mechanism of Action: PO competitive β-adrenergic antagonist; produces negative inotropic and chronotropic responses; slows AV nodal conduction; decreases heart rate; decreases myocardial oxygen consumption; antiarrhythmic effects (class II); reduction in platelet aggregation and blood viscosity; suppression of renin release; inhibition of central sympathetic outflow; decreases presynaptic receptor neurotransmitter release; no intrinsic sympathomimetic, weak membrane stabilizing activity; moderate lipid solubility

Pharmacokinetics

PO: Peak effect 1.5-4 hr, duration 10-20 hr (peak delayed with extended release)
IV: Peak effect 20 min, duration 5-8 hr
8%-12% bound to plasma proteins; extensively metabolized in liver, excreted in urine (3%-10% unchanged); $t_{1/2}$ 3-4 hr

INDICATIONS AND USES: Glaucoma,* migraine headache,* hypertension, postmyocardial infarction, supraventricular arrhythmias (atrial fibrillation, atrial flutter, paroxysmal supraventricular tachycardia),* aggressive behavior,* angina pectoris, anxiety,* cataract extraction prophylaxis,* congestive heart failure,* neuroleptic-induced akathisia,* retinal detachment,* tremor,* malignant vasovagal syncope or neurocardiogenic syncope*

DOSAGE

Adult

• *Hypertension:* PO 100 mg/day in single or divided doses, max 450 mg/day; SUS REL 50-100 mg qd, max 400 mg/day

• *Angina pectoris:* PO 50 mg bid, max 400 mg/day; SUS REL 100 mg qd, max 400 mg/day

• *MI:* (early treatment) IV 5 mg q2 min times 3 doses, then PO 25-50 mg q6h 15 min after last IV dose, continue for 48 hr; maintenance 100 mg bid; (late treatment) 100 mg bid as soon as clinical condition allows; continue for at least 3 mo

💲 AVAILABLE FORMS/COST OF THERAPY

• Inj, Sol—IV: 5 mg/5 ml, 1's: **$4.58-$7.43**
• Tab, Coated—Oral: 50 mg, 100's: **$12.75-$69.76**; 100 mg, 100's: **$62.75-$104.74**
• Tab, Coated, SUS Action—Oral: 50 mg, 100's: **$55.78**; 100 mg, 100's: **$83.81**; 200 mg, 100's: **$167.60**

CONTRAINDICATIONS: Bronchial asthma, cardiogenic shock, overt cardiac failure, 2nd and 3rd degree AV block, severe sinus bradycardia

PRECAUTIONS: Anesthesia/surgery (myocardial depression), avoid abrupt withdrawal, bronchospastic airways, congestive heart failure, diabetes mellitus, hyperthyroidism/thyrotoxicosis, concurrent clonidine (discontinue atenolol several days

---

* = non-FDA-approved use

prior to withdrawal of clonidine), peripheral vascular disease, renal disease

PREGNANCY AND LACTATION: Pregnancy category C; similar drug, atenolol, frequently used in the third trimester for treatment of hypertension (many studies of efficacy and safety of atenolol in pregnancy-induced hypertension; long-term use has been associated with intrauterine growth retardation; excreted into breast milk in insignificant concentrations; prudent to monitor infant for signs of β-blockade

SIDE EFFECTS/ADVERSE REACTIONS
CNS: Confusion, depression, *dizziness, fatigue,* headache, insomnia, memory loss, strange dreams
CV: Bradycardia, **CHF,** cold extremities, **heart block,** hypotension
EENT: Tinnitus, visual disturbances
GI: Constipation, *diarrhea,* dry mouth, heartburn, nausea
GU: Impotence, sexual dysfunction
HEME: **Agranulocytosis** (rare)
METAB: Hyperlipidemia (increased TG, total cholesterol, LDL; decreased HDL; masked hypoglycemic response to insulin (sweating excepted)
RESP: **Bronchospasm (1%),** dyspnea
SKIN: Alopecia, pruritis, rash
INTERACTIONS
Drugs
3 *α-adrenergic blockers:* Potential enhanced first dose response (marked initial drop in blood pressure) particularly on standing (especially prazocin)
3 *Amiodarone:* Bradycardia, cardiac arrest, or ventricular dysrhythmia
3 *Antidiabetics:* Altered response to hypoglycemia, prolonged recovery of normoglycemia, hypertension, blockade of tachycardia; may increase blood glucose and impair peripheral circulation
3 *Antipyrine:* Increased antipyrine concentrations
3 *Barbiturates:* Reduced β-blocker concentrations
2 *Beta agonists:* Antagonism of bronchodilating effect
3 *Bromazepam, diazepam, oxazepam:* Increased benzodiazepine effect (lorazepam and alprazolam unaffected)
3 *Cimetidine, etintidine, propafenone, propoxyphene, quinidine:* Increased plasma metoprolol concentration
3 *Clonidine:* Abrupt withdrawal of clonidine while on a β-blocker may exaggerate the rebound hypertension due to unopposed α stimulation
3 *Digoxin:* Additive prolongation of atrioventricular (AV) conduction time
3 *Dihydropyridines (nicardipine, nifedipine, felodipine, isradipine, nisoldipine):* Increased beta blocker effects
3 *Diltiazem:* Potentiates β-adrenergic effects; hypotension, left ventricular failure, and AV conduction disturbances problematic in elderly, patients with left ventricular dysfunction, aortic stenosis, or with large doses of either drug
3 *Dipyridamole, Tacrine:* Bradycardia
3 *Fluoxetine:* Enhanced effect of β-blocker
3 *Hypoglycemic agents:* Masked hypoglycemia, hyperglycemia
3 *Isoproterenol:* Potential reduction in effectiveness of isoproterenol in the treatment of asthma; less likely with cardioselective agents like metoprolol
3 *Local anesthetics:* Use of local

anesthetics containing epinephrine may result in hypertensive reactions in patients taking β-blockers

🔳 *NSAIDs:* Reduced hypotensive effects of β-blockers

🔳 *Phenylephrine:* Enhanced pressor response to phenylephrine, particularly when it is administered IV

🔳 *Prazosin:* First-dose response to prazosin may be enhanced by β-blockade

🔳 *Quinolones:* Inhibition of β-blocker metabolism, increased β-blocker effects

🔳 *Rifampin:* Reduced plasma metoprolol concentration

🔳 *Theophylline:* Antagonistic pharmacodynamic effects

🔳 *Verapamil:* Potentiates β-adrenergic effects; hypotension, left ventricular failure, and AV conduction disturbances problematic in elderly, patients with left ventricular dysfunction, aortic stenosis, or with large doses of either drug

MONITORING PARAMETERS

• Angina: Reduction in nitroglycerin usage; frequency, severity, onset, and duration of angina pain; heart rate

• Arrhythmias: heart rate

• Congestive heart failure: Functional status, cough, dyspnea on exertion, paroxysmal nocturnal dyspnea, exercise tolerance, and ventricular function

• Hypertension: Blood pressure

• Migraine headache: Reduction in the frequency, severity, and duration of attacks

• Postmyocardial infarction: Left ventricular function, lower resting heart rate

• Toxicity: Blood glucose, bronchospasm, hypotension, bradycardia, depression, confusion, hallucination, sexual dysfunction

PATIENT/FAMILY EDUCATION

• Do not discontinue abruptly; may

* = non-FDA-approved use

require taper; rapid withdrawal may produce rebound hypertension or angina

---

metronidazole
(me-troe-ni'da-zole)
Rx: Flagyl, Flagyl ER, Metro IV, MetroCream, MetroGel, Metrolotion, Noritate, Protostat
Kit: Helidac (metronidazole, bismuth subsalicylate, tetracycline)
Chemical Class: Nitroimidazole derivative
Therapeutic Class: Antibiotic; antiprotozoal; anthelmintic

CLINICAL PHARMACOLOGY
Mechanism of Action: Reduced metronidazole, which is cytotoxic but short-lived, interacts with DNA to cause a loss of helical structure, strand breakage, and resultant inhibition of nucleic acid synthesis and cell death
Pharmacokinetics
PO: Peak 1-3 hr
IV: Onset immediate
VAG: 20%-25% systemic bioavailability
<20% bound to plasma proteins; metabolized in liver; eliminated via urine (60%-80%) and feces (6%-15%); $t_{1/2}$ 6-8 hr
INDICATIONS AND USES: Trichomoniasis, amebiasis, giardiasis,* anaerobic bacterial infections, perioperative prophylaxis during colorectal surgery, bacterial vaginosis (VAG and PO*), acne rosacea, *Helicobacter pylori* infection associated with peptic ulcer disease (as part of a multidrug regimen), pseudomembranous colitis,* hepatic encephalopathy,* Crohn's disease*
Antibacterial spectrum usually includes:

• Anaerobic Gram-negative bacilli: *Bacteroides* spp. including the *B. fragilis* group (*B. fragilis, B. distasonis, B. ovatus, B. thetaiotaomicron, B. vulgatus), Fusobacterium* spp.

• Anaerobic Gram-positive bacilli: *Clostridium* spp., susceptible strains of *Eubacterium*

• Anaerobic Gram-positive cocci: *Peptococcus* spp., *Peptostreptococcus* spp.

Protozoa: *Entamoeba histolytica, Trichomonas vaginalis, Giardia lamblia, Balantidium coli*

DOSAGE

Adult

• *Amebiasis:* PO 500-750 mg q8h

• *Trichomoniasis:* PO 250 mg q8h for 7 days or 2 g as a single dose

• *Anaerobic infections:* PO/IV 7.5 mg/kg q6h; do not exceed 4 g/day

• *Pseudomembranous colitis:* PO 250-500 mg tid-qid for 10-14 days; IV 500 mg q8h for 10-14 days

• *Rosacea:* TOP apply to affected areas bid

• *Bacterial vaginosis:* Vag 5 g (1 applicatorful) bid for 5 days; PO 500 mg bid for 7-10 days

• *H. pylori:* PO 250 mg qid or 500 mg bid in combination with omeprazole and clarithromycin, omeprazole and amoxicillin or bismuth subsalicylate and clarithromycin

Child

• *Amebiasis:* PO 35-50 mg/kg/day divided q8h; do not exceed 4 g/day

• *Other parasitic infections:* PO 15-30 mg/kg/day divided q8h

• *Anaerobic infections:* PO/IV 30 mg/kg/day divided q6h; do not exceed 4 g/day

• *Pseudomembranous colitis:* PO 20 mg/kg/day divided q6h

$ AVAILABLE FORMS/COST OF THERAPY

• Inj, Sol—IV: 500 mg/100 ml, 100 ml: **$3.79-$9.65**

• Tab, Plain Coated—Oral: 250 mg, 100's: **$2.99-$148.29;** 500 mg, 100's: **$5.93-$270.14**

• Tab, Ext Rel—Oral: 750 mg, 30's: **$171.00**

• Cap, Gel—Oral: 375 mg, 100's: **$223.92**

• Kit, Blister card—Oral: **$77.70**

• Gel—Top: 0.75%, 28, 45 g: **$38.25**/45 g

• Cream—Top: 0.75%, 45 g: **$38.25**

• Gel—Vag: 0.75%, 70 g: **$30.48**

PRECAUTIONS: History of blood dyscrasias, severe hepatic impairment, CNS disease, severe renal failure

PREGNANCY AND LACTATION: Pregnancy category B; use in pregnancy controversial; use in 1st trimester and single-dose therapy often avoided; use with caution during breast feeding; if single-dose therapy is used, discontinue breast feeding for 12-24 hr to allow excretion of the drug

SIDE EFFECTS/ADVERSE REACTIONS

CNS: Ataxia, confusion, depression, dizziness, headache, incoordination, insomnia, irritability, peripheral neuropathy, *seizures,* vertigo, weakness

CV: T-wave flattening

EENT: Furry tongue, glossitis, stomatitis

GI: Abdominal discomfort, *anorexia,* constipation, diarrhea, *dry mouth,* epigastric distress, *metallic taste, nausea, **pancreatitis*** (rare), pseudomembranous colitis, vomiting

GU: Cystitis, decreased libido, discoloration of urine (IV), dyspareunia, dysuria, incontinence, polyuria, sense of pelvic pressure, urethral burning, vaginal dryness

HEME: Transient thrombocytopenia, leukopenia

MS: Fleeting joint pains

M

---

italic = common side effects   ***bold italic*** = life-threatening reactions

SKIN: Erythematous rash, flushing, pruritus, urticaria

INTERACTIONS

Drugs

3 *Carbamazepine:* Increased carbamazepine levels

3 *Cholestyramine, colestipol:* Reduced metronidazole absorption

3 *Disulfiram:* CNS toxicity

3 *Ethanol:* Disulfiram-like reaction

2 *Fluorouracil:* Enhanced toxicity of fluorouracil

3 *IV phenytoin, phenobarbital, diazepam, nitroglycerine, trimethoprim-sulfamethoxazole:* Disulfiram-like reaction due to ethanol in IV preparations

2 *Oral anticoagulants:* Increased hypoprothrombinemic response to warfarin

3 *Phenytoin:* Increased phenytoin levels

Labs

• *Interference:* Glucose

• *False decrease:* AST, zidovudine level

• *False positive increase:* Clindamycin, erythromycin, polymyxin, tetracycline, and trimethoprim assays

SPECIAL CONSIDERATIONS

• Treat sexual partner(s) for trichomoniasis

PATIENT/FAMILY EDUCATION

• Drug may cause GI upset; take with food

• Avoid alcoholic beverages during therapy and for at least 24 hr following last dose (disulfiram-like reaction possible)

• Drug may cause darkening of urine

• May cause an unpleasant metallic taste

• H_2 blocker must be prescribed with Helidac kit

MONITORING PARAMETERS

• CBC

metyrosine

(me-tye'roe-seen)

Rx: Demser

Chemical Class: α-methyl-L-tyrosine

Therapeutic Class: Agent for pheochromocytoma

CLINICAL PHARMACOLOGY

Mechanism of Action: Inhibitor of tyrosine hydroxylase, the rate-limiting step in catecholamine biosynthesis; decreases endogenous catecholamine concentrations by 35%-80%

Pharmacokinetics

PO: Peak 1-3 hr, onset within 1st 2 days of therapy; excreted unchanged in urine; $t_{1/2}$ 3.4-7.2 hr

INDICATIONS AND USES: Pheochromocytoma (preoperative preparation for surgery; patients in whom surgery is contraindicated; chronic treatment in malignant neoplasm), adjunct to neuroleptics in chronic schizophrenia*

DOSAGE

Adult and Child >12 yr

• PO 250 mg qid, may increase by 250-500 mg qd up to max of 4 g/day in divided doses

AVAILABLE FORMS/COST OF THERAPY

• Cap, Gel—Oral: 250 mg, 100's: **$163.46**

PRECAUTIONS: Impaired hepatic or renal function, children <12 yr

PREGNANCY AND LACTATION: Pregnancy category C

SIDE EFFECTS/ADVERSE REACTIONS

CNS: Anxiety, confusion, depression, disorientation, drooling, hallucinations, headache, insomnia and psychic stimulation upon drug withdrawal, parkinsonism, *sedation, speech difficulty,* tremor, trismus

CV: Peripheral edema

EENT: Nasal stuffiness

GI: Abdominal pain, *diarrhea (10%)*, dry mouth, increased AST, nausea, vomiting

GU: Crystalluria, urolithiasis, failure to ejaculate, hematuria, impotence, transient dysuria

HEME: Anemia, eosinophilia, ***thrombocytopenia***, thrombocytosis

METAB: Breast swelling, galactorrhea

MISC: Hypersensitivity reactions (urticaria, pharyngeal edema)

INTERACTIONS

Drugs

3 *Phenothiazines, haloperidol:* Potentiation of EPS

Labs

• *False increase:* Urinary catecholamines (due to presence of metyrosine metabolites)

SPECIAL CONSIDERATIONS
PATIENT/FAMILY EDUCATION

• Maintain a daily liberal fluid intake

• Avoid alcohol or CNS depressants

MONITORING PARAMETERS

• Blood pressure, ECG

---

mexiletine

(mex-il'e-teen)
Rx: Mexitil
Chemical Class: Lidocaine derivative
Therapeutic Class: Antidysrhythmic (Class IB)

CLINICAL PHARMACOLOGY
Mechanism of Action: Blocks the fast sodium channel in cardiac tissues; reducing rate of rise and amplitude of the action potential, and decreasing the effective refractory period in Purkinje fibers; does not significantly alter sinus node automaticity, left ventricular function,

systolic arterial blood pressure, AV conduction velocity, QRS or QT intervals

Pharmacokinetics

PO: Onset 0.5-2 hr, peak 2-3 hr; 60%-75% bound to plasma proteins; metabolized in liver, eliminated via bile and urine; $t_{1/2}$ 10-12 hr (prolonged in hepatic or renal failure, reduced cardiac output, acute MI)

INDICATIONS AND USES: Documented, life-threatening ventricular dysrhythmia; diabetic neuropathy*

DOSAGE

Adult

• PO 200 mg q8h initially, adjust in 50-100 mg increments q2-3 days, do not exceed 1200 mg/day

Child

• PO 1.4-5 mg/kg/dose q8h

• *Dosing adjustment in renal impairment:* Administer 50%-75% of normal dose if CrCl <10 ml/min

• *Dosing adjustment in hepatic disease:* Administer 25%-30% of normal dose

5 **AVAILABLE FORMS/COST OF THERAPY**

• Cap, Gel—Oral: 150 mg, 100's: **$69.06-$97.63;** 200 mg, 100's: **$82.22-$116.21;** 250 mg, 100's: **$95.25-$133.87**

CONTRAINDICATIONS: Cardiogenic shock, pre-existing 2nd or 3rd degree AV block (if pacemaker not present)

PRECAUTIONS: Structural heart disease, hepatic disease, renal function impairment, children, 1st degree AV block, pre-existing sinus node dysfunction, intraventricular conduction abnormalities, hypotension, severe CHF, seizure disorder

PREGNANCY AND LACTATION: Pregnancy category C; limited data do not suggest significant risk to the

M

---

italic = common side effects   ***bold italic*** = life-threatening reactions

fetus; compatible with breast feeding

SIDE EFFECTS/ADVERSE REACTIONS

CNS: Changes in sleep habits, confusion, *coordination difficulties,* depression, *dizziness,* fatigue, fever, hallucinations, headache, *lightheadedness,* nervousness, paresthesias, psychosis, **seizures,** short-term memory loss, speech difficulties, *tremor,* weakness

CV: Angina, atrial dysrhythmias, AV block, bradycardia, **cardiogenic shock,** chest pain, **CHF,** conduction disturbances, edema, hot flashes, hypertension, hypotension, **increased ventricular dysrhythmias,** palpitations, PVCs, syncope

EENT: Blurred vision, tinnitus

GI: Abdominal pain, altered taste, changes in appetite, constipation, diarrhea, dry mouth, dysphagia, esophageal ulceration, hepatitis, oral mucous membrane changes, peptic ulcer, pharyngitis, salivary changes, **upper GI bleeding,** *upper GI distress* (nausea, vomiting, heartburn, 40%)

GU: Decreased libido, impotence, urinary hesitancy

HEME: **Agranulocytosis, leukopenia,** positive ANA, **thrombocytopenia** (rare)

MS: Arthralgia

RESP: Dyspnea, hiccups

SKIN: Diaphoresis, dry skin, **exfoliative dermatitis,** hair loss, rash

INTERACTIONS

Drugs

3 *Acetazolamide, sodium bicarbonate:* Alkalinization of urine retards mexiletine elimination

3 *Phenytoin, rifampin:* Reduced mexiletine concentrations

3 *Quinidine:* Elevated mexiletine concentrations

2 *Theophylline:* Elevated theophylline serum concentrations and toxicity

SPECIAL CONSIDERATIONS
- Because of proarrhythmic effects, not recommended for non-life threatening arrhythmias
- Antiarrhythmic drugs have not been shown to increase survival of patients with ventricular arrhythmias
- Initiate therapy in facilities capable of providing continuous ECG monitoring and managing life-threatening dysrhythmias

PATIENT/FAMILY EDUCATION
- Take with food or antacid

MONITORING PARAMETERS
- Therapeutic mexiletine concentrations 0.5-2 μg/ml

---

mezlocillin
(mez'-loe-sill-in)
Rx: Mezlin
Chemical Class: Semisynthetic acylaminopenicillin
Therapeutic Class: Antibiotic

CLINICAL PHARMACOLOGY

Mechanism of Action: Inhibits bacterial wall synthesis; bactericidal

Pharmacokinetics

IM: Peak 45-90 min; 16%-42% bound to plasma proteins; 15% metabolized to inactive metabolites; excreted principally in urine by tubular secretion and glomerular filtration, partly excreted via bile; $t_{1/2}$ 0.7-1.3 hr (prolonged in severe renal impairment)

INDICATIONS AND USES: Treatment of infections caused by susceptible gram-negative aerobic bacilli and mixed aerobic-anaerobic bacterial infections including serious intra-abdominal infections, UTIs, gynecologic infections, respiratory tract infections, skin and skin stucture infections, bone and joint infections, and septicemia; uncomplicated gonorrhea; perioperative prophylaxis

Antibacterial spectrum usually includes:

• Gram-positive organisms: *Staphylococcus aureus* (non-penicillinase-producing strains), β-hemolytic streptococci (Groups A and B), *Streptococcus pneumoniae, S. faecalis* (enterococcus)

• Gram-negative organisms: *Escherichia coli, Klebsiella* spp. (including *K. pneumoniae), Proteus mirabilis, P. vulgaris, Enterobacter* spp., *Shigella* spp., *Morganella morganii, Pseudomonas aeruginosa, Providencia rettgeri, H. influenzae, H. parainfluenzae, Providencia stuartii, Citrobacter* spp., *Neisseria* spp., many strains of *Serratia, Salmonella,* and *Acinetobacter* are also susceptible

• Anaerobes: *Peptococcus* spp., *Peptostreptococcus* spp., *Clostridium* spp., *Bacteroides* sp. (including *B. fragilis* group), *Fusobacterium* spp., *Veillonella* spp., *Eubacterium* spp.

DOSAGE

Adult

• IM/IV 3 g q4h or 4 g q6h, do not exceed 24 g/day; IM doses should not exceed 2 g/injection

• *Uncomplicated UTI:* IM/IV 1.5-2 g q6h

• *Complicated UTI:* IM/IV 3 g q6h

• *Uncomplicated gonococcal urethritis:* IM/IV 1-2 g in conjunction with 1 g of probenecid

• *Perioperative prophylaxis:* IV 4 g 0.5-1.5 hr prior to surgery

Child 1 mo-12 yr

• IM/IV 50 mg/kg q4h

§ AVAILABLE FORMS/COST OF THERAPY

• Inj, Dry-Sol—IM, IV: 1 g/vial:

$4.94; 2 g/vial: $8.94; 3 g/vial: $14.80

• Inj, Dry-Sol—IV: 4 g/vial: **$17.94-$18.84**

PRECAUTIONS: Hypersensitivity to cephalosporins, renal insufficiency, prolonged or repeated therapy, sodium restricted patients

PREGNANCY AND LACTATION: Pregnancy category B; excreted into breast milk in low concentrations; no adverse effects have been observed

SIDE EFFECTS/ADVERSE REACTIONS

CNS: Fever, headache, neuromuscular hyperirritability, *seizures*

GI: Abdominal pain, colitis, *diarrhea;* glossitis; increased AST, ALT; *nausea, pseudomembranous colitis,* vomiting

GU: Acute interstitial nephritis, transient increases in serum creatinine and BUN

HEME: Bleeding abnormalities, bone marrow depression, eosinophilia

METAB: Hypernatremia, hypokalemia

RESP: Respiratory distress

SKIN: Erythema multiforme, pain at inj site, rash, urticaria

INTERACTIONS

Drugs

3 *Aminoglycosides:* Potential for inactivation of aminoglycosides in patients with severe renal impairment

3 *Chloramphenicol:* Possible inhibition of penicillin antibacterial activity

3 *Methotrexate:* Increased methotrexate concentrations, possible toxicity

Labs

• *False increase:* Urine glucose (with Clinitest; Diastix and TesTape do not interfere), urine protein

---

italic = common side effects   **bold italic** = life-threatening reactions

SPECIAL CONSIDERATIONS
MONITORING PARAMETERS

- Renal, hepatic, and hematologic systems during prolonged therapy
- Serum electrolytes

---

mibefradil
(me-biff'ra-dill)
Rx: Posicor
Chemical Class: Benz-dimidazolyl-substituted tetra-line derivative; calcium channel blocker
Therapeutic Class: Antihypertensive; antianginal

CLINICAL PHARMACOLOGY
Mechanism of Action: Inhibits calcium ion influx across cell membranes (i.e., calcium channel antagonist); higher affinity for T-type (transient, low-voltage activated) vs. the L-type (long-lasting, high-voltage activated) calcium channels at therapeutic doses; T-type channel function may be involved in regulation of pacemaker function and ventricular hypertrophy; high vascular affinity, vascular smooth muscle and cardiac muscle; less negative inotropic effect; reduces total peripheral resistance (afterload) without reflex tachycardia; decreases myocardial oxygen demand

Pharmacokinetics
PO: Peak plasma level 1-2 hr; peak blood pressure lowering effect 3-4 hr; duration >24 hr; well-absorbed (PO); bioavailability 70%; metabolized in liver, metabolites excreted in urine; highly protein bound (99%); inhibits cytochrome P450-2D6, 3A4; $t_{1/2}$ 17-25 hr; crosses placenta

INDICATIONS AND USES: Hypertension; chronic stable angina pectoris, vasospastic angina,* CHF,* dysrhythmias

DOSAGE
Adult

- *Hypertension and angina:* 50-100 mg qd (dosage adjustments not necessary with renal dysfunction or in elderly patients)

$ AVAILABLE FORMS/COST OF THERAPY

- Tab—Oral: 50 mg, 100's: **$120;** 100 mg, 100's: **$199**

CONTRAINDICATIONS: Sick sinus syndrome, 2nd or 3rd degree heart block

PRECAUTIONS: Causes dose-related ECG changes, T and U waves, interferes with measurement of QT_c interval

PREGNANCY AND LACTATION: Pregnancy category C; animal data suggest nursing infant would develop serum levels slightly lower than mother, but no human data available

SIDE EFFECTS/ADVERSE REACTIONS
CNS: Lightheaded feeling
CV: Dizziness (7%), *ECG changes* (8%), 1st degree heart block, flushing, headache, lengthened QT_c intervals, palpitations, sinus bradycardia (5%)
EENT: Rhinitis
GI: Abdominal pain, gastralgia, heartburn
HEME: Intravascular hemolysis after IV administration

DRUG INTERACTIONS
Drugs

3 *Antidepressants, tricyclics:* Increased levels of imipramine and desipramine reported via inhibition of CYP2D6; dosage adjustments of tricyclic antidepressants necessary

A *Astemizole:* Increased astemizole concentrations via inhibition of CYP3A4; prolonged QT_c intervals expected

A *Cisapride:* Increased cisapride concentrations via inhibition of

---

* = non-FDA-approved use

CYP3A4; prolonged QT_c intervals expected

3 *Cyclosporine or tacrolimus (FK-506):* Increased immunosuppressant levels via inhibition of CYP3A4; monitor cyclosporine A levels and adjust accordingly

3 *HMG-CoA reductase inhibitors:* Increased risk of rhabdomyolysis

⚠ *Terfenadine:* Increased terfenadine concentrations via CYP3A4 inhibition; prolonged QT_c intervals reported

SPECIAL CONSIDERATIONS
• Promoted as inducing less reflex tachycardia, edema, negative inotropism than previous calcium channel blockers; clinical advantages and safety compared to other calcium channel antagonists may be more clearly determined by the results of the Mortality Assessment in Congestive Heart Failure Trial (MACH 1), which is currently underway

---

miconazole
(mi-kon′a-zole)
Rx: *IV:* Monistat
Top: Micatin, Monistat-Derm, Fungoid Tincture Nail Kit
Vag: Monistat 3, Monistat 5, Monistat 7, Monistat Dual-Pak, Femizol-7
Chemical Class: Imidazole derivative
Therapeutic Class: Antifungal

CLINICAL PHARMACOLOGY
Mechanism of Action: Alters permeability of fungal cell membrane
Pharmacokinetics
TOP: Small amounts absorbed systemically
IV: Onset immediate; distributed into inflamed joints, vitreous humor, peritoneal cavity; limited crossing of blood-brain barrier, terminal $t_{1/2}$ 24 hr; metabolized in liver, excreted in feces, urine (inactive metabolites); >90% protein binding

INDICATIONS AND USES: *IV:* Second line drug in treatment of severe systemic fungal infections such as coccidioidomycosis, candidiasis, cryptococcoses, paracoccidioidomycosis, fungal meningitis, fungal UTI; *TOP:* Tinea pedis, tinea cruris, tinea corporis, tinea versicolor; *Vag:* vulvovaginal candidiasis

DOSAGE
Adult
• IV INF initial test dose of 200 mg, then 200-3600 mg/day; may be divided in 3 INF 200-1200 mg/INF for 1-20 wk
• *Fungal meningitis:* Supplement IV INF with intrathecal miconazole 20 mg q3-7 days
• *Bladder mycoses:* Supplement IV INF with bladder irrigation of miconazole 200 mg bid-qid or as continuous INF
• *Vulvovaginal candidiasis:* Vag (cr) 1 applicatorful qhs for 7 days; (supp) 200 mg (1 supp) qhs for 3 days
• *Tinea:* Top apply to affected area bid for 2-4 wk
Child >1 yr
• IV 20-40 mg/kg/day, not to exceed 15 mg/kg/dose
• *Tinea:* Top same as adult

💲 AVAILABLE FORMS/COST OF THERAPY
• Inj, Sol—Intrathecal, IV: 10 mg/ml, 20 ml: **$38.47**
• Cre—Top: 2%, 15, 30, 60, 85 g: **$2.36-$16.61**/15 g
• Vag Supp—Top: 100 mg, 7's: **$8.49-$22.81;** 200 mg, 3's: **$20.89-$29.70**
• Vag, Cre—Top: 2%, 45 g: **$6.60**
• Kit—Top Cre, Vag Supp: 100 mg: **$15.97;** 200 mg: **$26.52**
• Lot—Top: 2%, 56 g: **$10.00**
• Oint—Top: 2%, 30, 60 g: **$2.77**/30g

M

---

italic = common side effects   ***bold italic*** = life-threatening reactions

- Powder/Top: 2%, 90 gm: **$4.55-$5.36**
- Aer, Spray—Top: 2%, 90, 109, 120 ml; **$2.50-$4.25**/90 ml
- Tampon—Vag: 100 mg: 5's: **$15.96**
- Tincture—Top: 2%, 30 ml: **$11.50**

PRECAUTIONS: Renal disease, hepatic disease

PREGNANCY AND LACTATION: Pregnancy category C (Top category B); unknown if excreted into breast milk

SIDE EFFECTS/ADVERSE REACTIONS

CNS: Drowsiness, headache

CV: **Dysrhythmias** (rapid IV), tachycardia

GI: Anorexia, cramps, diarrhea, nausea, vomiting (IV)

GU: Hyponatremia, itching, pelvic cramps (topical forms), vulvovaginal burning

HEME: **Thrombocytopenia**

METAB: Hyperlipidemia (due to vehicle in IV prep)

SKIN: Fever, flushing, hives, *phlebitis* (IV), pruritus, rash

INTERACTIONS

- The base in suppository products may interfere with latex; do not use these with contraceptive diaphragms, condoms

Drugs

3 *Aminoglycosides:* Decreased antibiotic peak levels

A *Astemizole:* QT prolongation and arrhythmia

2 *Cisapride:* Increased cisapride concentrations, toxicity and arrhythmias

3 *Coumarin drugs:* Enhanced anticoagulant effect

3 *Cyclosporine:* Possible increased cyclosporine levels

3 *Felodipine:* Enhanced vasodilation, hypotension

2 *HMG-CoA reductase inhibitors* (*e.g. lovastatin*): Increased toxicity, rhabdomyolysis

3 *Loratadine:* Increased loratadine concentrations

3 *Midazolam:* Reduced midazolam metabolism

3 *Quinidine:* Increased quinidine concentrations

3 *Tacrolimus:* Possible increased tacrolimus levels

3 *Tolbutamide:* Inhibition of tolbutamide metabolism

3 *Triazolam:* Reduced triazolam metabolism

3 *Warfarin:* Enhanced anticoagulant effect

---

midazolam

(mid-az'zoe-lam)
Rx: Versed
Chemical Class: Benzodiazepine
Therapeutic Class: Sedative
DEA Class: Schedule IV

CLINICAL PHARMACOLOGY

Mechanism of Action: CNS depressants via facilitation of inhibitory GABA at benzodiazepine receptor sites (BZ_1—associated with sleep; BZ_2—associated with memory, motor, sensory, and cognitive function); effects include muscle relaxation (spinal cord), anticonvulsant activity (brain stem), ataxia (cerebellum), emotional behavior (limbic and cortical areas), and anxiolytic effects (separate from general CNS depression)

Pharmacokinetics

IM: Onset 15 min, peak serum concentration $\frac{1}{2}$-1 hr

IV: Onset 3-5 min, onset of anesthesia $1\frac{1}{2}$-5 min

Protein binding 97%; $t_{\frac{1}{2}}$ 1.2-12.3 hr; metabolized in liver, metabolites excreted in urine; crosses placenta, blood-brain barrier

---

* = non-FDA-approved use

INDICATIONS AND USES: Preoperative sedation (IM); general anesthesia induction, sedation for diagnostic endoscopic procedures, intubation (IV)

DOSAGE

Adult

• *Preoperative sedation:* IM 70-80 µg/kg 30-60 min before general anesthesia

• *Conscious sedation:* IV using 1 mg/ml dilution, titrate slowly to desired effect (e.g., slurred speech); give no more than 2.5 mg over at least 2 min; wait at least 2 min to fully evaluate effect; administer small doses to appropriate level of sedation prn

• *Induction of general anesthesia:* IV 150-350 µg/kg over 30 sec, wait 2 min, follow with 25% of initial dose if needed; use lower doses for patients who are >55 yrs age, premedicated, debilitated, or severe systemic disease

Child

• *Preoperative sedation:* IM 80-200 µg/kg

• *General anesthesia:* IV 50-200 µg/kg

$ AVAILABLE FORMS/COST OF THERAPY

• Inj, Sol—IM, IV: 1 mg/ml, 2 ml: **$5.55;** 5 mg/ml, 2 ml: **$21.81-$27.40**

• Syrup: 2 mg/ml, 118 ml: **$522.50**

CONTRAINDICATIONS: Shock, coma, alcohol intoxication, acute narrow-angle glaucoma

PRECAUTIONS: COPD, CHF, chronic renal failure, hepatic disease, elderly, debilitated, myasthenia gravis, other muscular dystrophies and myotonias

NOTE: Associated with respiratory depression and respiratory arrest, especially when used IV for conscious sedation; death and hypoxic encephalopathy have resulted; reserve use for settings that provide for continuous monitoring of respiratory and cardiac function and immediate availability of resuscitative drugs, equipment, and personnel

PREGNANCY AND LACTATION: Pregnancy category D; excreted in breast milk, use with caution in nursing mothers

SIDE EFFECTS/ADVERSE REACTIONS

CNS: Anxiety, confusion, euphoria, headache, insomnia, paresthesia, retrograde amnesia, slurred speech, tremors, weakness

CV: Bigeminy, hypotension, nodal rhythm, PVCs, tachycardia

EENT: Blocked ears, blurred vision, diplopia, loss of balance, nystagmus

GI: Hiccups, increased salivation, nausea, vomiting

RESP: Apnea, ***bronchospasm,*** coughing, dyspnea, ***laryngospasm, respiratory depression***

SKIN: Pain, pruritus, rash, swelling at inj site, urticaria

INTERACTIONS

Drugs

3 *Calcium channel blockers, erythromycin, ketoconazole, itraconazole:* Increased midazolam levels; increased sedation; respiratory depression

3 Additive effects with other CNS depressants

---

midodrine

(mid′o-dreen)

Rx: ProAmatine

Chemical Class: Synthetic catecholamine

Therapeutic Class: α-adrenergic sympathomimetic; vasopressor

CLINICAL PHARMACOLOGY

Mechanism of Action: Long-acting, selective α-adrenergic agonist;

---

italic = common side effects   ***bold italic*** = life-threatening reactions

M

activity in both venous and arterial systems

Pharmacokinetics

PO: Peak 30 min, onset 45-90 min, duration 4-6 hr

Rapid oral absorption; essentially a "pro-drug," i.e., hydrolyzed enzymatically to active metabolite (desglymidodrine: peak 1 hr); renal excretion; $t_{1/2}$'s, 0.5 hr and 3 hr (parent and metabolite, respectively)

INDICATIONS AND USES: Orthostatic hypotension, secondary hypotension,* ejaculation disorders,* female stress incontinence,* urinary incontinence

DOSAGE

Adult

• *Orthostatic hypotension:* 2.5 mg PO bid-tid, increasing gradually to a maximum recommended dose of 40 mg daily

• Give upon arising then q3-4 hr during daytime

• *Psychotropic drug-induced hypotension:* 6.7-15 mg/day

• *Ejaculatory incompetence:* 5 mg tid

⑤ AVAILABLE FORMS/COST OF THERAPY

• Tab—Oral: 2.5 mg, 100's: **$98.75**; 5 mg, 100's: **$171.09**

CONTRAINDICATIONS: Hypertension, severe organic heart disease or congestive heart failure, acute renal disease, acute nephritis, or urinary retention, pheochromocytoma, thyrotoxicosis

PREGNANCY AND LACTATION: Pregnancy category C; unknown if excreted in breast milk

SIDE EFFECTS/ADVERSE REACTIONS

CNS: Dizziness, drowsiness, excitability, headache, irritability, *paresthesia (18%)*, restlessness

CV: Supine hypertension (25%)

GI: Nausea, vomiting

GU: Dysuria, urinary frequency, urinary retention

METAB: Changes in blood glucose, increase in body weight

SKIN: Chills, diaphoresis, *paresthesia* (18%), *piloerection* (13%)

INTERACTIONS

Drugs

❷ *Alpha adrenergic agonists:* Enhanced pressor response

❸ *Alpha adrenergic antagonists:* Antagonism of midodrines effects

❸ *Cardiac glycosides, Beta blockers:* Increased risk of bradycardia, AV block, arrhythmia

SPECIAL CONSIDERATIONS

• Advantages include rapid and nearly complete absorption, a long elimination $t_{1/2}$, lack of central nervous system (CNS) penetration, and minimal to no cardiac effects

• Supine hypertension has been a therapy-limiting complication

PATIENT/FAMILY EDUCATION

• To minimize supine hypertension, avoid taking drug after the evening meal

---

milrinone

(mill're-none)

Rx: Primacor

Chemical Class: Bipyridine derivative

Therapeutic Class: Cardiac inotropic agent

CLINICAL PHARMACOLOGY

Mechanism of Action: Positive inotropic agent with vasodilator properties; selective inhibitor of peak III cAMP phosphodiesterase isozyme in cardiac and vascular muscle; reduces preload and afterload by direct relaxation of vascular smooth muscle

Pharmacokinetics

IV: Onset 2-5 min, peak 10 min, duration variable, $t_{1/2}$ 2-4 hr; metab-

---

* = non-FDA-approved use

olized in liver, excreted in urine as drug (83%) and metabolites

INDICATIONS AND USES: Short-term management of CHF not responsive to other medication (can be used with digitalis)

DOSAGE

Adult

• IV bolus 50 µg/kg given over 10 min; start INF of 0.375-0.75 µg/kg/min

• Reduced dose in renal impairment:

CREATININE CLEARANCE (ml/min/1.73 m 2)	INFUSION RATE (µg/kg/min)
5	0.20
10	0.23
20	0.28
30	0.33
40	0.38
50	0.43

§ AVAILABLE FORMS/COST OF THERAPY

• Inj, Sol—IV: 1 mg/ml, 5 ml: **$42.95-$43.28**

CONTRAINDICATIONS: Severe aortic stenosis, severe pulmonic stenosis, acute MI

PRECAUTIONS: Children, renal disease, hepatic disease; atrial flutter, fibrillation; outflow tract obstruction in hypertrophic subaortic stenosis, elderly

PREGNANCY AND LACTATION: Pregnancy category C; caution with breastfeeding until more known about excretion in breast milk

SIDE EFFECTS/ADVERSE REACTIONS

CNS: Headache, tremor

CV: Chest pain, ***dysrhythmias*** (12%), hypotension

GI: Abdominal pain, anorexia, hepatotoxicity, jaundice, nausea, vomiting

HEME: ***Thrombocytopenia***

METAB: Hypokalemia

SPECIAL CONSIDERATIONS

MONITORING PARAMETERS

• Fluid and electrolyte changes, renal function

• Improvement in cardiac output may increase diuresis, and K$^+$ loss

---

minocycline

(mi-noe-sye'kleen)

Rx: Dynacin, Minocin

Chemical Class: Semisynthetic tetracycline

Therapeutic Class: Antibiotic

CLINICAL PHARMACOLOGY

Mechanism of Action: Inhibits protein synthesis, phosphorylation in microorganisms by binding to 30S and possibly the 50S ribosomal subunits; bacteriostatic

Pharmacokinetics

PO: Peak 2-3 hr; t$_{1/2}$ 11-17 hr; biliary and urinary excretion; crosses placenta; excreted in breast milk; 76% protein bound

INDICATIONS AND USES: Syphilis; non-gonococcal urethritis; endocervical and rectal infections caused by *C. trachomatis, U. urealyticum;* gonorrhea; lymphogranuloma venereum; rickettsial infections (Rocky Mountain spotted fever, typhus fever, Q fever, rickettsialpox, tick fevers); inflammatory acne; skin granulomas caused by *Mycobacterium marinum;* respiratory tract infections caused by susceptible organisms; skin and skin structure infections; UTI; treatment of asymptomatic meningococcal carriers when rifampin contraindicated; tularemia; cholera; plague; chancroid; psittacosis; brucellosis (with streptomycin); yaws; anthrax; actinomycosis; trachoma, relasping fever, granuloma inguinale, listeriosis; sclerosing agent in malignant pleural effusions

M

---

italic = common side effects   ***bold italic*** = life-threatening reactions

Antibacterial specturm usually includes:

• Gram-positive organisms: *Streptococcus pneumoniae, Str. pyogenes,* alpha hemolytic streptococci; many strains strep resistant, demonstrate susceptibility

• Gram-negative organisms: *Bartonella bacilliformis, Brucella, Campylobacter fetus, Francisella tularensis, Haemophilus influenzae, H. ducreyi, Listeria monocytogenes, Neisseria gonorrhea, Vibrio cholera; some strains of E. coli, Klebsiella, Shigella, Bacteroides, Enterobacter aerogenes, Acinetobacter*

• Other organisms: *Bacillus anthracis, Balantidium coli, Borrelia recurrentis, Chlamydia psittoci, C. trachomatis, Clostridium, Fusobacterium fusiforme, Mycoplasma pneumoniae, Propionibacterium acnes, Rickettsiae, Treponema pallidum, Ureaplasma urealyticum*

DOSAGE
Adult

• PO/IV 200 mg, then 100 mg q12h or 50 mg q6h, not to exceed 400 mg/24h IV

• *Gonorrhea* (not drug of choice): PO 200 mg, then 100 mg q12h for 4 days

• *Chlamydia trachomatis, Ureaplasma urealyticum:* PO 100 mg bid for 7 days

• *Syphilis* (PCN allergic patients): PO 200 mg, then 100 mg q12h for 10-15 days

• *Acne:* 50 mg 1-3 times/day

• *Skin granulomas from M. marinum:* 100 mg bid for 6-8 wk

• *Sclerosing agent:* 300 mg diluted with 50 ml 0.9% NaCl inj instilled via thoracostomy tube

Child >8 yr

• PO/IV 4 mg/kg then 2 mg/kg q12h

💲 AVAILABLE FORMS/COST OF THERAPY

• Inj, Lyphl-Sol—IV: 100 mg/vial: **$38.86**

• Susp—Oral: 50 mg/5 ml, 60 ml: **$36.49**

• Cap, Gel—Oral: 50 mg, 100's: **$40.43-$195.49;** 100 mg, 100's: **$80.84-$325.66**

CONTRAINDICATIONS: Children <8 yr

PRECAUTIONS: Hepatic disease

PREGNANCY AND LACTATION: Pregnancy category D; not recommended in last half of pregnancy secondary to adverse effects on fetal teeth; not recommended in breast feeding

SIDE EFFECTS/ADVERSE REACTIONS

CNS: Dizziness, fever, lightheadedness, pseudotumor cerebri, vertigo,
CV: Pericarditis
EENT: Decreased calcification of deciduous teeth, dysphagia, oral candidiasis
GI: Abdominal cramps, abdominal pain, anorexia, *diarrhea,* enterocolitis, epigastric burning, flatulence, glossitis, hepatotoxicity, *nausea,* stomatitis, *vomiting*
GU: Increased BUN
HEME: Eosinophilia, ***hemolytic anemia, neutropenia, thrombocytopenia***
SKIN: Angioedema, blue-gray color of skin and mucous membranes, ***exfoliative dermatitis,*** *increased pigmentation, photosensitivity,* pruritus, *rash, urticaria*

INTERACTIONS
Drugs

3 *Antacids:* Decreased effect of minocycline

3 *Barbiturates:* Decreased effect of minocycline

2 *Bismuth:* Inhibited antibiotic absorption

---

* = non-FDA-approved use

3 *Carbamazepine:* Decreased effect of minocycline

3 *Colestipol, cholestyramine:* Inhibited antibiotic absorption

3 *Digoxin:* Increased digoxin levels in 10% of patients

3 *Iron:* Decreased minocycline absorption

2 *Methoxyflurane:* Renal toxicity

3 *Oral contraceptives:* Decreased contraceptive efficacy

3 *Penicillins:* Antagonizes antibacterial effect of penicillins

3 *Warfarin:* Possible increase in hypoprothrombinemic response

SPECIAL CONSIDERATIONS
PATIENT/FAMILY EDUCATION
• May take with food
• Avoid sun exposure

---

minoxidil
(min-nox′i-dill)
Rx: *Oral:* Loniten
OTC: Rogaine
Chemical Class: Piperidinopyrimidine derivative
Therapeutic Class: Direct vasodilator: antihypertensive (oral use); hair growth stimulant (topical use)

CLINICAL PHARMACOLOGY
Mechanism of Action: Relaxes arteriolar smooth muscle, causes vasodilation with reflex increase in heart rate, cardiac output; increases cutaneous blood flow, stimulate hair follicles

Pharmocokinetics
PO: Onset 30 min, peak 2-3 hr, duration 24-48 hr, t₁/₂ 4.2 hr; metabolized in liver, 97% renal excretion (metabolites); excreted in breast milk
TOP: Small amounts absorbed (0.3%-4.5%), absorption increased through inflamed skin; onset of action min 4 mo; growth peaks at 1 yr

INDICATIONS AND USES: Severe hypertension not responsive to other therapy, in conjunction with diuretic; topically to treat alopecia androgenetica (less effective in frontal hair loss), alopecia areata*

DOSAGE
Adult and Adolescents
• PO 2.5-5 mg/day as single dose or divided bid not to exceed 100 mg/day, usual range 10-40 mg/day; double dose q3 days to appropriate response; for rapid control adjust q6h, monitor closely
• TOP 1 ml (2% sol) bid regardless of size of area, max 2 ml qd
Child <12 yr
• Initial dose PO 0.2 mg/kg/day (max 5 mg), effective range 0.25-1 mg/kg/day in 1 or 2 doses, max 50 mg/day

💲 AVAILABLE FORMS/COST OF THERAPY
• Tab, Uncoated—Oral: 2.5 mg, 100's: **$22.01-$66.04;** 10 mg, 100's: **$40.00-$129.14**
• Sol—Top: 2%, 60 ml: **$6.10-$22.56;** 5%, 60 ml: **$24.00-$28.32**

CONTRAINDICATIONS: Acute MI, dissecting aortic aneurysm, pheochromocytoma (PO)

PRECAUTIONS: Children, renal disease, CAD, CHF (PO)

PREGNANCY AND LACTATION: Pregnancy category C; compatible with breast feeding

SIDE EFFECTS/ADVERSE REACTIONS
CV: Angina, *CHF,* edema, ***pericardial effusion, pericarditis, pulmonary edema,*** severe rebound hypertension, sodium and water retention, tachycardia, *T wave changes* (direction and magnitude, 60%)
GI: Nausea, vomiting
GU: Breast tenderness, gynecomastia

---

italic = common side effects   ***bold italic*** = life-threatening reactions

HEME: Decreased Hct (hemodilution), *leukopenia, thrombocytopenia*

SKIN: Hypertrichosis (80% of patients, resolves 1-6 months after discontinuation of drug), pruritus, rash, *Stevens-Johnson syndrome*

SKIN: Contact dermatitis, hypertrichosis; irritant

INTERACTIONS
Drugs
❷ *Guanethidine:* Orthostatic hypotension, may be severe

• No known interactions with top sol

SPECIAL CONSIDERATIONS
• Must be used in conjunction with diuretic (except dialysis patients) and β-blocker or other sympathetic nervous system depressant (to prevent reflex tachycardia)

PATIENT/FAMILY EDUCATION
• At least 4 mo of bid application necessary before evidence of hair growth with topical solution
• Continued treatment necessary to maintain or increase hair growth with topical solution

---

mirtazapine
(mir-taz′a-peen)
Rx: Remeron
Chemical Class: Tetracyclic piperazino-azepine derivative
Therapeutic Class: Antidepressant

CLINICAL PHARMACOLOGY
Mechanism of Action: Enhances central noradrenergic and serotonergic activity by blocking central presynaptic alpha-2 inhibitory receptors and postsynaptic serotonin receptors; has anxiolytic properties; moderate anticholinergic and orthostatic hypotensive effects; high sedative activity

Pharmacokinetics
PO: Peak 2 hr, completely absorbed; elimination $t_{1/2}$ 20-40 hr (longer in females than males); 85% protein bound; extensive hepatic metabolism; excretion 75% by kidney, 15% in feces

INDICATIONS AND USES: Depression, preoperative insomnia/anxiety*

DOSAGE
Adult
• *Depression:* PO 15 mg qhs to start, increase q1-2 wk; effective dosage range 15-45 mg qd
• *Preoperative insomnia:* PO 15 mg

💲 AVAILABLE FORMS/COST OF THERAPY
• Tab—Oral: 15 mg, 30's: **$69.72;** 30 mg, 30's: **$71.83;** 45 mg, 30's: **$76.50**

CONTRAINDICATIONS: Concurrent MAO inhibitor therapy

PRECAUTIONS: Elderly, hepatic insufficiency, renal insufficiency, mania or hypomania, seizure disorder

PREGNANCY AND LACTATION: Unknown if excreted in breast milk

SIDE EFFECTS/ADVERSE REACTIONS
CNS: Abnormal dreams, anxiety, cerebral ischemia, confusion, *dizziness* (7%), *drowsiness* (54%), EPS, hallucinations, migraine, *seizures* (<0.01%), tremor, vertigo
CV: Angina, bradycardia, CHF, hypertension, hypotension, MI, syncope, ventricular extrasystoles
EENT: Dry mouth
GI: Constipation (13%), increased appetite, weight gain
HEME: Agranulocytosis and neutropenia (0.1%), anemia, lymphadenopathy, lymphocytosis, *pancytopenia,* thrombocytopenia
METAB: Elevated cholesterol

INTERACTIONS
Drugs
⚠ *MAOIs:* Possible serotonin syn-

---

* = non-FDA-approved use

drome (hyperthermia, autonomic instability, seizures, death)

SPECIAL CONSIDERATIONS
• Chemical structure unrelated to TCAs, SSRIs, MAOIs
• Shown to be an effective antidepressant in several trials but place in therapy not yet determined
• Manufacturer recommends stopping MAOI 14 days before initiating therapy secondary to interactions between MAOIs and other antidepressants

---

misoprostol
(me-soe-prost'ole)
Rx: Cytotec
Combinations
  Rx: with diclofenac
    (Arthrotec)
Chemical Class: Prostaglandin E_1 analog
Therapeutic Class: Gastrointestinal protectant; abortifacient

CLINICAL PHARMACOLOGY
Mechanism of Action: Inhibits gastric acid secretion; may protect gastric mucosa; can increase bicarbonate and mucus production; stimulates uterine contractions
Pharmacokinetics
PO: Rapidly metabolized to active metabolite; peak 12 min; plasma steady state achieved within 2 days; excreted in urine; $t_{1/2}$ 20-40 min; unknown if metabolite excreted in breast milk

INDICATIONS AND USES: Prevention of nonsteroidal anti-inflammatory drug (NSAID)-induced gastric ulcers; treatment of duodenal ulcer*; abortifacient in early pregnancies (with methotrexate or mifepristone)*; morning after contraception*

DOSAGE
Adult
• *Gastric ulcer prophylaxis:* PO 200 μg qid with food for duration of NSAID therapy; if drug not tolerated, decrease to 100 μg qid or 200 μg bid

🔋 **AVAILABLE FORMS/COST OF THERAPY**
• Tab, Uncoated—Oral: 100 μg, 60's: **$37.04;** 200 μg, 60's: **$53.93**
CONTRAINDICATIONS: Pregnancy (unless used as abortifacient)
PRECAUTIONS: Women of childbearing age, children
PREGNANCY AND LACTATION: Pregnancy category X; do not use in breast feeding (possible diarrhea in infant)
SIDE EFFECTS/ADVERSE REACTIONS
CNS: Headache
GI: Abdominal pain, constipation, *diarrhea,* dyspepsia, flatulence, nausea, vomiting
GU: Cramps, spotting, vaginal bleeding
INTERACTIONS
Drugs
🔳 *Phenylbutazone:* Increase in adverse effects (headache, flushes, dizziness, nausea)
SPECIAL CONSIDERATIONS
• Reserve use for those patients at high risk for NSAID-induced ulcer (e.g., elderly, history of previous ulcer)
• Does not prevent NSAID-associated GI pain or discomfort

M

---

italic = common side effects   ***bold italic*** = life-threatening reactions

modanfinil

(moe-daf'ih-nil)

Rx: Provigil

Chemical Class:
Benzhydrylsulfinylacetamide
compound; (bears a distant
similarity to
dextroamphetamine)

Therapeutic Class: Central
nervous system stimulant

CLINICAL PHARMACOLOGY

Mechanism of Action: Mechanism
of CNS stimulation unknown; does
not bind to potentially relevant receptors (norepinephrine, serotonin,
dopamine, GABA, adenosine, his-
tamine-3, melatonin, or benzodiazepines); not a direct or indirect dopamine receptor or α-1 adrenergic
agonist; no peripheral sympathomimetic effects as observed with amphetamines; however, does require
an intact sympathomimetic nervous
system for activity

Pharmacokinetics

PO: Peak conc 2-4 hr; absorption is
rapid, not affected by food; metabolized by liver (metabolites inactive), protein binding 60%; Vd 0.9 L/
kg; metabolites renally excreted
(10% unchanged in urine); $t_{1/2}$ 7.5-
12 hr

INDICATIONS AND USES: Narcolepsy, idiopathic hypersomnia,* obstructive sleep apnea (hypopnea syndrome),* organic brain syndrome,*
sleep deprevation

DOSAGE

Adult and Child >16 yr

• *Narcolepsy:* 200 mg qam (400 mg
daily doses fail to provide further
benefits); *Idiopathic hypersomnia:*
200-300 mg qam (up to 500 mg)/
day divided bid—qam and noon);
reduce 50% for severe hepatic insufficiency

$ **AVAILABLE FORMS/COST OF THERAPY**

• Tab—Oral: 200 mg, 100's: **$290;**
300 mg, 100's: **$388.00**

PRECAUTIONS: Cardiovascular
disease (left ventricular hypertrophy, ischemic ECG changes, chest
pain, arrhythmia, mitral valve prolapse, recent myocardial infarction,
unstable angina); elderly patients
(possible dose reductions); history
of emotional instability, drug abuse
or psychosis, hypertension (periodic
monitoring is advised); severe hepatic disease (50% dose reduction);
severe renal impairment; risk of
pregnancy with concurrent oral contraceptives use

PREGNANCY AND LACTATION:
Pregnancy category C; no mutagenic or clastogenic potential in several in vitro assays; in vivo mouse
bone marrow micronucleus assays
were also negative for mutagenic-
ity; not fully evaluated; breast milk
excretion unknown

**SIDE EFFECTS/ADVERSE REAC-
TIONS**

CNS: Headache (50%) nervousness
(8%), dizziness (5%), depression
(4%), anxiety (4%), and insomnia
(3%), delayed sleep; euphoria, motor excitation reported with 500 mg
daily doses

CV: Minimal effects on blood pressure and pulse

GI: Hypersalivation, nausea (13%),
diarrhea (8%), dry mouth (5%)

SPECIAL CONSIDERATIONS

• Comparisons of modanfinil with
agents that have proven effective in
narcolepsy, including methylphenidate, pemoline, and dextroamphetamine, are needed to clarify its relative safety and efficacy, and place
in therapy

MONITORING PARAMETERS

• *Efficacy:* Daytime sleepiness, day-

---

* = non-FDA-approved use

time sleep episodes, and overall daily performance
• *Toxicity:* Blood pressure

moexipril
(moe-ex′a-prile)
Rx: Univasc
Combinations
  Rx: with hydrochlorothiazide (Uniretic)
Chemical Class: Nonsulfhydryl angiotensin-converting enzyme (ACE) inhibitor
Therapeutic Class: Antihypertensive

CLINICAL PHARMACOLOGY
Mechanism of Action: Antihypertensive, hypoproliferative, and cardioprotective effects attributable to competitive inhibition of angiotensin-converting enzyme (ACE) yielding decreased plasma concentrations of angiotensin II, plasma aldosterone concentrations, systemic vascular resistance, blood pressure, preload, and afterload, not accompanied by changes in heart rate, pressor sensitivity to exogenous norepinephrine, or baroreceptor sensitivity

Pharmacokinetics
PO: Prodrug, requiring hepatic conversion to active metabolite (moexiprilat); bioavailability 13%; onset 1 hr, duration 24 hr; fecal excretion 50% (13% renal excretion); $t_{1/2}$ 2-10 hr

INDICATIONS AND USES: Hypertension, CHF (left ventricular dysfunction),* MI (left ventricular salvage),* erythrocytosis,* nephropathy,* retinopathy*

DOSAGE
Adult
PO 7.5 mg (3.75 mg with concomitant diuretic) qd; maintenance 7.5-30 mg qd or divided bid

• *Dosage in renal failure:* PO 3.75 mg qd; max maintenance 15 mg/day

💲 AVAILABLE FORMS/COST OF THERAPY
• Tab, Uncoated—Oral: 7.5, 15 mg, 100's: **$59.18**

PRECAUTIONS: History of anaphylaxis, renal insufficiency (<30 ml/min), hypotension (CHF, elderly, volume depletion—diuretics, dialysis, cirrhosis), aortic stenosis, hyperkalemia (potassium supplements, potassium-sparing diuretics, renal disease, diabetes), neutropenia (autoimmune diseases, collagen vascular, febrile illness, immunosuppressant drug therapy), proteinuria, renal artery stenosis, surgery/anesthesia (excessive hypotension, correctable with fluids)

PREGNANCY AND LACTATION: Pregnancy category D; ACE inhibitors can cause fetal and neonatal morbidity and death when administered to pregnant women; when pregnancy is detected, discontinue ACE inhibitors as soon as possible

SIDE EFFECTS/ADVERSE REACTIONS
CNS: Dizziness, fatigue, headache, insomnia, peripheral neuropathy
CV: ***CHF, dysrhythmia,*** *hypotension,* Raynaud's syndrome
GI: Abdominal pain, aphthous ulcers, diarrhea, dysgeusia, gastric irritation, nausea, vomiting, weight loss
GU: Nephrotic syndrome, polyuria, proteinuria, renal insufficiency
HEME: ***Agranulocytosis,*** decreased hemoglobin, ***neutropenia, pancytopenia, thrombocytopenia***
METAB: Electrolyte disturbance (hyperkalemia, hyponatremia)
RESP: ***Cough***
SKIN: Alopecia, pemphigus, pruritus, rash, scalded-mouth sensation

---

italic = common side effects   ***bold italic*** = life-threatening reactions

INTERACTIONS
Drugs
❷ *Allopurinol:* Combination may predispose to hypersensitivity reactions

▪ *Alpha adrenergic blockers:* Exaggerated first dose hypotensive reactions when added to moexipril

▪ *Aspirin:* May reduce hemodynamic effects of moexipril; less likely at doses under 236 mg; less likely with nonacetylated salicylates

▪ *Azathioprine:* Increased myelosuppression

▪ *Cyclosporine:* Combination may cause renal insufficiency

▪ *Insulin:* Moexipril may enhance insulin sensitivity

▪ *Iron:* Moexipril may increase chance of systemic reaction to IV iron

▪ *Lithium:* Reduced lithium clearance

▪ *Loop diuretics:* Initiation of moexipril may cause hypotension and renal insufficiency in patients taking loop diuretics

▪ *NSAIDs:* May reduce hemodynamic effects of moexipril

▪ *Potassium-sparing diuretics:* Increased risk of hyperkalemia

▪ *Trimethoprim:* Additive risk of hyperkalemia, especially in patient predisposed to renal insufficiency

Labs
• ACE inhibition can account for approximately 0.5mEq/L rise in serum potassium

SPECIAL CONSIDERATIONS
PATIENT/FAMILY EDUCATION
• Caution with salt substitutes containing potassium chloride

• Rise slowly to sitting/standing position to minimize orthostatic hypotension

• Dizziness, fainting, lightheadedness may occur during 1st few days of therapy

• May cause altered taste perception or cough; persistent dry cough usually does not subside unless medication is stopped; notify clinician if these symptoms persist

MONITORING PARAMETERS
• BUN, creatinine, potassium within 2 wk after initiation of therapy (increased levels may indicate acute renal failure)

---

molindone
(moe-lin'done)
Rx: Moban
Chemical Class: Dihydroindolone derivative
Therapeutic Class: Antipsychotic

CLINICAL PHARMACOLOGY
Mechanism of Action: Dopamine receptor antagonist, with higher affinity for D_2 over D_1 receptors, and variable selectivity among the cotical dopamine tracts; also activity on nondopaminergic sites, i.e., cholinergic, α_1-adrenergic and histamine receptors (explaining side effects); moderate risk extrapyramidal reactions and sedation; minimal orthostatic hypotension and anticholinergic effects

Pharmacokinetics
PO: Onset erratic, peak 1½ hr, duration 24-36 hr
Metabolized by liver (36 recognized metabolites); excreted in urine and feces; $t_{1/2}$ 1½ hr

INDICATIONS AND USES: Psychotic disorders

DOSAGE
Note: 10 mg equivalent to chlorpromazine 100 mg
Adult
• PO initial dose 50-75 mg/day increasing to 225 mg/day if needed; maintenance dose, mild, 5-15 mg tid-qid; moderate, 10-25 mg tid-

---

* = non-FDA-approved use

qid; severe 225 mg/day may be required

$ AVAILABLE FORMS/COST OF THERAPY

• Conc—Oral: 20 mg/ml, 120 ml: **$190.88**

• Tab, Uncoated—Oral: 5 mg, 100's: **$89.94;** 10 mg, 100's: **$129.25;** 25 mg, 100's: **$192.75;** 50 mg, 100's: **$257.44;** 100 mg, 100's: **$343.88**

CONTRAINDICATIONS: Coma, children

PRECAUTIONS: Hypertension, hepatic disease, cardiac disease, Parkinson's disease, brain tumor, glaucoma, urinary retention, diabetes mellitus, respiratory disease, prostatic hypertrophy, geriatric patients

PREGNANCY AND LACTATION: Pregnancy category C

SIDE EFFECTS/ADVERSE REACTIONS

CNS: Akathisia, drowsiness, dystonia, extrapyramidal symptoms including pseudoparkinsonism, headache, *seizures,* tardive dyskinesia

CV: Cardiac arrest, ECG changes, hypertension, *orthostatic hypotension,* tachycardia

EENT: Blurred vision, glaucoma

GI: Anorexia, constipation, diarrhea, *dry mouth,* jaundice, *nausea, vomiting,* weight gain

GU: Amenorrhea, enuresis, gynecomastia, impotence, urinary frequency, urinary retention

HEME: Agranulocytosis, anemia, leukocytosis, leukopenia

RESP: Dyspnea, *laryngospasm, respiratory depression*

SKIN: Dermatitis, photosensitivity, rash

MISC: Decreased sweating

DRUG INTERACTIONS

Drugs

🔳 *Barbiturates:* Reduce serum levels of molindone

🔳 *Benztropine:* May inhibit therapeutic response to molindone

🔳 *Bromocriptine:* May inhibit therapeutic response to molindone; molindone may inhibit therapeutic effect of bromocriptine on hyperprolactinemia

🔳 *Carbamazepine:* Reduces serum levels of molindone

🔳 *Fluoxetine:* Increases serum levels of molindone

🔳 *Guanethidine:* Reduced antihypertensive effect of guanethidine

🔳 *Indomethacin:* May increase risk of CNS side effects of molindone

② *Levodopa:* Molindone reduces antiparkinsonian effects of levodopa

🔳 *Lithium:*May reduce serum levels of lithium

🔳 *Orphenadrine:* Reduces serum levels of molindone

🔳 *Paroxetine:* Increases serum levels of molindone

🔳 *Quinidine:* Increases serum levels of molindone

🔳 *Trihexyphenidyl:* May inhibit therapeutic response to molindone

SPECIAL CONSIDERATIONS

• Neuroleptic structurally different from the phenothiazines, thioxanthenes, and butyrophenones

• High potency with high incidence of EPS, but a low incidence of sedation, anticholinergic effects, and cardiovascular effects

---

mometasone

(mo-met'a-sone)

Rx: Elocon, Nasonex

Chemical Class: Synthetic glucocorticoid

Therapeutic Class: Topical corticosteroid, intermediate potency; nasal corticosteroid

---

CLINICAL PHARMACOLOGY

Mechanism of Action: Depresses formation, release, and activity of endogenous mediators of inflam-

M

italic = common side effects   ***bold italic*** = life-threatening reactions

mation such as prostaglandins, kinins, histamine, liposomal enzymes, and the complement system resulting in decreased edema, erythema, and pruritus

Pharmacokinetics

TOP: Absorbed systemically across stratum corneum, extent dependent on dosage form and condition of the skin; hepatic metabolism (resistant to skin metabolism)

INDICATIONS AND USES: Topical: symptomatic relief of inflammation and/or pruritus associated with acute and chronic corticosteroid-responsive skin disorders Nasal spray: prophylaxis and treatment of the nasal symptoms of allergic rhinitis

DOSAGE

Adult

• TOP apply qd-bid, rub completely into skin

• Nasal spray: 1 spray in each nostril qd-bid

$ **AVAILABLE FORMS/COST OF THERAPY**

• Cre—Top: 0.1%, 15, 45 g: **$19.26**/15 g

• Lotion—Top: 0.1%, 30, 60 ml: **$20.88**/30 ml

• Oint—Top: 0.1%, 15, 45 g: **$19.26**/15 g

• Spray—Nasal: 0.05 mg/inh, 17 g: **$49.92**

PRECAUTIONS: Skin lesions covering large surface areas or involving thin-skinned areas; children, adolescents, geriatrics

PREGNANCY AND LACTATION: Pregnancy category C; systemic corticosteroids are excreted into breast milk in quantities not likely to have deleterious effects in breast-feeding infants; no information on topical steroids

SIDE EFFECTS/ADVERSE REACTIONS

CV: Hypertension

EENT: Glaucoma, subcapsular cataracts

METAB: Cushing's syndrome, glucose intolerance, hypokalemic syndrome

SKIN: Acneiform eruptions, allergic contact dermatitis; folliculitis, furunculosis, *hair loss,* hyperesthesia, *hypopigmentation,* pustules, pyoderma, secondary skin infection, skin atrophy, *striae,* vesiculation

DRUG INTERACTIONS

Labs

• *Interference:* With adrenal function as assessed by corticotropin stimulation, 24-hr urine-free cortisol measurements; plasma cortisol

---

monobenzone

(mono-ben′zone)

Rx: Benoquin

Chemical Class: Hydroquinone derivative

Therapeutic Class: Depigmenting agent

CLINICAL PHARMACOLOGY

Mechanism of Action: Decreases the number of functional melanocytes and inhibits the process of pigmentation (inhibition of tyrosinase, which catalyzes the oxidation of tyrosine to dihydroxyphenylalanine, a precursor of melanin)

Pharmacokinetics

TOP: Depigmentation is usually observed after 1-4 mo of therapy (discontinue if satisfactory results are not observed in 4 mo); complete depigmentation may require 9-12 mo

INDICATIONS AND USES: Final depigmentation in extensive vitiligo

DOSAGE

Adult

• TOP apply and rub into pigmented areas 2-3 times daily

---

* = non-FDA-approved use

Child
- Safety in children <12 not established

§ **AVAILABLE FORMS/COST OF THERAPY**
- Cre—Top: 20%, 37.5 g: **$41.34**

CONTRAINDICATIONS: Freckling; hyperpigmentation due to photosensitization; melasma (cholasma) of pregnancy; cafe-au-lait spots; pigmented nevi; malignant melanoma; pigment resulting from pigments other than melanin (i.e., bile, silver)

PREGNANCY AND LACTATION: Pregnancy category C; excretion into breast milk unknown

SIDE EFFECTS/ADVERSE REACTIONS
SKIN: Burning, *dermatitis,* irritation

SPECIAL CONSIDERATIONS
PATIENT/FAMILY EDUCATION
- Drug is not a mild cosmetic bleach; treated areas should not be exposed to sunlight (protect with a topical sunscreen)

---

moricizine

(mor-iss´i-zeen)
Rx: Ethmozine
Chemical Class: Phenothiazine derivative
Therapeutic Class: Antidysrhythmic (Class I)

CLINICAL PHARMACOLOGY
Mechanism of Action: Decreases rate of rise of action potential, prolongs refractory period, and shortens the action potential duration; depression of inward influx of sodium mediates these effects; slows atrial and AV nodal conduction; increase in resting blood pressure and heart rate; inhibits platelet aggregation; anticholinergic effects

Pharmacokinetics
PO: Peak 0.5-2.2 hr
Well absorbed; metabolized by the liver, metabolites are excreted in feces and urine; protein binding >90%; $t_{1/2}$ 1.5-3.5 hr

INDICATIONS AND USES: Symptomatic, life-threatening ventricular dysrhythmias

DOSAGE
Adult
- PO 600-900 mg/day in 2-3 divided doses; increase dosage in 150 mg increments at 3-day intervals up to 900 mg/day; decrease dose in patients with significant liver and renal dysfunction

§ **AVAILABLE FORMS/COST OF THERAPY**
- Tab, Coated—Oral: 200 mg, 100's: **$114.86;** 250 mg, 100's: **$137.14;** 300 mg, 100's: **$156.13**

CONTRAINDICATIONS: 2nd-3rd degree AV block; right bundle branch block when associated with left hemiblock (bifascicular block) unless a pacemaker is present; cardiogenic shock

PRECAUTIONS: CHF, hypokalemia, hyperkalemia, sick sinus syndrome, children, impaired hepatic and renal function, cardiac dysfunction

PREGNANCY AND LACTATION: Pregnancy category B; secreted into breast milk (1 patient); potential for serious adverse effects exists

SIDE EFFECTS/ADVERSE REACTIONS
CNS: Depression, *dizziness,* euphoria, fatigue, headache, nervousness, perioral numbness, sleep disorders, tinnitus
CV: Bradycardia, chest pain, ***CHF, dysrhythmias,*** hypertension, ***MI, palpitations,*** syncope, thrombophlebitis
GI: Abdominal pain, diarrhea, *nausea,* vomiting
GU: Difficult urination, dysuria, incontinence, sexual dysfunction

M

---

italic = common side effects   **bold italic** = life-threatening reactions

RESP: **Apnea,** asthma, cough, *dyspnea,* hyperventilation, pharyngitis
MISC: Musculoskeletal pain, sweating

DRUG INTERACTIONS
3 *Cimetidine:* Increases serum moricizine concentrations
3 *Theophylline:* Reduces serum theophylline levels by increasing clearance

SPECIAL CONSIDERATIONS
• Antidysrhythmic therapy has not been proven to be beneficial in terms of improving survival among patients with asymptomatic or mildly symptomatic ventricular dysrhythmias
• Studied in the CAST (Cardiac Arrhythmia Suppression Trial, I and II) with findings of excessive cardiac mortality and no benefit on long-term survival compared to placebo
• Initiate therapy in facilities capable of providing continuous ECG monitoring and managing life threatening dysrhythmias

---

morphine
(mor´feen)
Rx: Astramorph, Duramorph, Infumorph, Kadian, MS Contin, MSIR, Oramorph SR, RMS, Roxanol
Chemical Class: Natural opium alkaloid; phenanthrene derivative
Therapeutic Class: Narcotic analgesic
DEA Class: Schedule II

CLINICAL PHARMACOLOGY
Mechanism of Action: Narcotic agonist with activity at μ-receptors (supraspinal analgesia, euphoria, respiratory and physical depression, miosis, and reduced GI motility), κ-receptors (pentazocine-like spinal analgesia, sedation, and miosis), and Δ-receptors (dysphoria, psychotomimetic effects [e.g., hallucinations], and respiratory and vasomotor stimulation caused by drugs with antagonist activity); Standard pharmacologic comparator for analgesic, antitussive, constipation, respiratory depression, sedation, emesis, and physical dependence effects.

Pharmacokinetics
PO: 60 mg = 10 IM morphine; duration of action: 8-12 hr (EXT REL preps); 4-5 hr (other oral dosage forms)
SC: Onset 10-30 min, peak analgesia 50-90 min, duration 4-5 hr
IM: Onset 10-30 min, peak analgesia 30-60, duration 4.5 hr
IV: Peak analgesia 20 min
Metabolized by liver; 85% excreted by kidneys, 7%-10% biliary; $t_{1/2}$ 2½-3 hr

INDICATIONS AND USES: Severe pain; anesthesia (adjunct); diarrhea*; cough*; acute pulmonary edema*

DOSAGE
Adult
• *Chronic pain:* SC/IM 4-15 mg q4h prn; PO 5-30 mg q4h prn; EXT REL 15-60 mg q8-12h (base dose on 24-hr requirement of immediate-release morphine); Rec 10-20 mg q4h prn
• IV 4-15 mg diluted in 4-5 ml H_2O for inj, over 5 min
Child
• *Analgesia:* SC 0.1-0.2 mg/kg, not to exceed 15 mg

AVAILABLE FORMS/COST OF THERAPY
• Inj, Sol—Epidural, Intrathecal, IV: 0.5 mg/ml, 10 ml: **$14.38;** 1 mg/ml, 10 ml (preservative free): **$15.34**
• Inj, Sol—IM; IV; SC: 2 mg/ml, 1 ml: **$0.70-$0.77;** 4 mg/ml, 1 ml: **$0.73-$0.80;** 5 mg/ml, 30 ml: **$25.16-$25.29;** 8 mg/ml, 1 ml: **$0.61-$1.24;** 10 mg/ml, 1 ml: **$0.58-$1.28;** 15 mg/ml, 1 ml: **$0.70-$1.42**

- Inj, Sol—IV: 25 mg/ml, 4 ml: **$13.88-$85.80;** 50 mg/ml, 10 ml: **$28.68-$112.50**
- Cap, Gel—Oral: 15 mg, 50's: **$37.19;** 20 mg, 60's: **$82.99;** 30 mg, 100's: **$69.40;** 50 mg, 60's: **$200.39;** 100 mg, 60's: **$348.12**
- Conc—Oral: 100 mg/5 ml, 120 ml: **$51.85-$81.90**
- Sol—Oral: 10 mg/5 ml, 500 ml: **$23.40-$32.00;** 20 mg/5 ml, 500 ml: **$52.61-$53.00;** 20 mg/ml, 120 ml: **$40.00-$75.69**
- Supp—Rect: 5 mg, 12's: **$14.66-$14.82;** 10 mg, 12's: **$17.33-$17.47;** 20 mg, 12's: **$20.93-$21.06;** 30 mg, 12's: **$29.02-$29.44**
- Tab, Coated, SUS Action—Oral: 15 mg, 100's: **$84.45-$99.63;** 30 mg, 100's: **$160.50-$189.34;** 60 mg, 100's: **$313.15-$369.44;** 100 mg, 100's: **$479.58-$546.99;** 200 mg, 100's: **$1001.71**
- Tab, Soluable—IM, SC: 10 mg, 100's: **$22.03;** 15 mg, 100's: **$27.95**
- Tab, Uncoated—Oral: 15 mg, 100's: **$18.32-$34.45;** 30 mg, 100's: **$31.22-$57.80**

CONTRAINDICATIONS: Respiratory depression, hemorrhage, acute asthma attack, paralytic ileus, convulsive states (injection)

PRECAUTIONS: Addictive personality, elderly, hepatic disease, renal disease, child <18 yr, head injury, acute abdominal conditions, hypothyroidism, prostatic hypertrophy, Addison's disease

PREGNANCY AND LACTATION: Pregnancy category B; trace amounts enter breast milk; compatible with breast feeding

SIDE EFFECTS/ADVERSE REACTIONS

CNS: Addiction, confusion, *dizziness, drowsiness,* euphoria, headache, *sedation*

CV: Bradycardia, *hypotension,* palpitations

EENT: Blurred vision, diplopia, *miosis,* tinnitus

GI: Anorexia, biliary tract pressure, *constipation,* cramps, *nausea,* vomiting

GU: Urinary retention

RESP: **Respiratory depression**

SKIN: Bruising, diaphoresis, flushing, pruritus, rash, urticaria

MISC: Histamine release (decreased blood pressure, fast heartbeat, increased sweating, redness or flushing of face, wheezing or troubled breathing)

INTERACTIONS

Drugs

3 *Amitryptylline:* Additive respiratory and CNS-depressant effects

3 *Antihistamines, chloroal hydrate, gluethimide, methocarbamol:* Enhanced depressant effects

3 *Barbiturates:* Additive respiratory and CNS-depressant effects

3 *Cimetidine:* Increased respiratory and CNS depression

3 *Cloimipramine:* Additive respiratory and CNS-depressant effects

3 *Ethanol:* Additive CNS effects

3 *MAOI's:* Markedly potentiate the actions of morphine

3 *Nortriptylline:* Additive respiratory and CNS-depressant effects

Labs

- *Increase:* Urine glucose, urine 17-ketosteroids
- False elevations of amylase and lipase

SPECIAL CONSIDERATIONS

- Treatment of overdose: Naloxone (Narcan) 0.2-0.8 mg IV
- Remains the strong analgesic of choice for acute, severe pain, acute MI pain, and the agent of choice for chronic cancer pain
- 200 mg EXT REL tablet for use only in opioid-tolerant patients
- Do not administer agonist/antagonist analgesics (i.e., pentazocine, nalbuphine, butorphanol, de-

M

---

italic = common side effects   ***bold italic*** = life-threatening reactions

zocine, buprenorphine) to patient who has received a prolonged course of morphine (a pure agonist). In opioid-dependent patients, mixed agonist/anagonist analgesics may precipitate withdrawal symptoms

PATIENT/FAMILY EDUCATION

• Change position slowly to avoid orthostasis

• Avoid alcohol and other CNS depressants

• Physical dependency may result

• Do not chew or crush EXT REL preparations

---

mupirocin
(mew-per′o-sen)
Rx: Bactroban
Chemical Class: Pseudomonic acid derivative
Therapeutic Class: Topical antibiotic

CLINICAL PHARMACOLOGY
Mechanism of Action: Inhibits bacterial protein synthesis; shows no cross-resistance with chloramphenicol, erythromycin, fusidic acid, gentamicin, lincomycin, methicillin, neomycin, novobiocin, penicillin, streptomycin, and tetracycline
Pharmacokinetics
No measurable systemic absorption
INDICATIONS AND USES: Impetigo caused by *Staphylococcus aureus* (including methicillin-resistant and β-lactamase producing strains), *S. epidermidis, S. saprophyticus,* β-hemolytic *Streptococcus, Str. pyogenes;* eradication of nasal colonization with methicillin-resistant *S. aureus;* secondarily infected traumatic skin lesions
DOSAGE
Impetigo: TOP—Apply small amount to affected area tid

Nasal: Divide ½ the ointment from single-use tube between the nostrils and apply bid for 5 days

$ AVAILABLE FORMS/COST OF THERAPY
• Cre—Top: 2%, 15, 30 g: **$26.05/ 15 g**
• Oint—Top: 2%, 15, 30 g: **$19.05/15 g**
• Oint—Nasal: 2%, 1 g: 10's, **$49.40**
PREGNANCY AND LACTATION:
Pregnancy category B; excretion into breast milk unknown
SIDE EFFECTS/ADVERSE REACTIONS
SKIN: Burning, contact dermatitis, dry skin, erythema, increased exudate, *itching,* rash, *stinging,* swelling, tenderness
SPECIAL CONSIDERATIONS
• Comparable efficacy to systemic semisynthetic penicillins and erythromycin in impetigo and infected wounds

---

muromonab-CD3
(mur-oo-mon′ab)
Rx: Orthoclone OKT3
Chemical Class: Murine monoclonal antibody
Therapeutic Class: Immunosuppressant

CLINICAL PHARMACOLOGY
Mechanism of Action: Blocks graft rejection by blocking T-cell function
Pharmacokinetics
IV: Trough levels after 5 mg/day rose over the 1st 3 days and then averaged 900 ng/ml on days 3 to 14; therapeutic levels >800 ng/ml block the function of cytotoxic T cells *in vitro* and *in vivo*
INDICATIONS AND USES: Acute allograft rejection in renal, cardiac and hepatic transplant patients

---

* = non-FDA-approved use

DOSAGE

Adult

• IV bolus 5 mg/day × 10-14 days

$ **AVAILABLE FORMS/COST OF THERAPY**

• Inj, Sol—IV: 1 mg/ml ampule: **$750.24**

CONTRAINDICATIONS: Hypersensitivity to murine products; antimouse antibody titers ≥1 : 1000, uncompensated heart failure, seizure disorder; fluid overload

PRECAUTIONS: Child <2 yr, fever, unstable angina, recent MI, compensated heart failure, COPD, intravascular volume overload, increased risk of infection when used with immunosuppressant agents

PREGNANCY AND LACTATION: Pregnancy category C

SIDE EFFECTS/ADVERSE REACTIONS

CNS: Chills, headache, pyrexia, tremor

CV: Chest pain (angina, MI)

GI: Abdominal pain, diarrhea, nausea, vomiting

GU: Increased creatinine

MS: Generalized weakness, muscle, joint aches and pains

*RESP: Dyspnea, **pulmonary edema**, wheezing*

MISC: Cytokine release syndrome (CRS) (ranges from "flu-like" illness to life-threatening shock-like syndrome), infection

DRUG INTERACTIONS

Drugs

3 *Vaccines, live virus:* Increased side effects; decreased antibody response

SPECIAL CONSIDERATIONS

• Effective for reversal of resistant renal, hepatic, cardiac, and kidney or pancreas transplant rejection and is an important alternative to retransplantation

• No advantage over other immunosuppressive agents for prevention of rejection

• Manifestations of CRS may be prevented or minimized by pretreatment with methylprednisolone (8 mg/kg) 1-4 hr prior to administration of the 1st dose

MONITORING PARAMETERS

• BUN, serum creatinine, transaminases, WBCs and differential with platelet counts

• Chest x-ray within 24 hr (CHF)

M

mycophenolate

(my-co-fen'o-late)

Rx: CellCept

Chemical Class: Mycophenolic acid derivative

Therapeutic Class: Immunosuppressant

CLINICAL PHARMACOLOGY

Mechanism of Action: Mycophenolic acid (MPA), the active metabolite, inhibits T- and B-lymphocytes by interfering with purine synthesis; prolongs the survival of allogeneic transplants and reverses ongoing acute rejection

Pharmacokinetics

PO: Peak 6 hr; rapid absorption (94% bioavailable); presystemic metabolism to MPA (active metabolite); immediately posttransplant (<40 days), mean AUC, C_{max} approximately 50% lower than healthy volunteers or stable renal transplant patients; MPA 97% bound to plasma albumin; excreted as inactive metabolite in urine; not removed by hemodialysis; $t_{1/2}$ 17 hr

INDICATIONS AND USES: Primary maintenance immunosuppression and/or rescue or rejection therapy following renal, heart, and liver transplantation; rheumatoid arthritis*; psoriasis*

---

italic = common side effects   ***bold italic*** = life-threatening reactions

DOSAGE
Adult
• PO 1.0 g bid (on empty stomach) starting 72 hr after renal transplant; usually given with corticosteroids and cyclosporine
• With severe chronic renal impairment (glomerular filtration rate <25 ml/min/1.73m^2) outside of the immediate posttransplant period, doses >1 g should be avoided
Child
• PO 15 mg/kg bid (on empty stomach)

🛈 AVAILABLE FORMS/COST OF THERAPY
• Cap, Gel—Oral: 250 mg, 100's: **$225.00**
• Tab—Oral: 500 mg, 100's: **$449.96**
• Susp—Oral: 200 mg/ml 175 ml: **$314.98**

PRECAUTIONS: Peptic ulcer disease, history of GI bleeding, decreased renal function

PREGNANCY AND LACTATION: Pregnancy category C; mycophenolic acid excreted in milk; not recommended during breast feeding

SIDE EFFECTS/ADVERSE REACTIONS
CNS: Headache, pain
CV: Hypertension
GI: Constipation, *diarrhea,* dyspepsia, nausea, oral moniliasis, *vomiting*
GU: Hematuria, UTI
HEME: **Anemia,** leukocytosis, **leukopenia, thrombocytopenia**
METAB: Fever, hypercholesteremia, hyperkalemia, hypokalemia, hypophosphatemia, peripheral edema
MS: Back pain
MISC: **Malignancy, infection (opportunistic), sepsis**

DRUG INTERACTIONS
Drugs
🔢 *Acyclovir:* Increased serum acyclovir concentrations

🔢 *Aluminum-containing antacids:* Decreased mycophenolate bioavailability
🔢 *Cholestyramine:* Decreased mycophenolate bioavailability
🔢 *Ganciclovir:* Increased serum ganciclovir concentrations
🔢 *Magnesium containing antacids:* Decreased mycophenolate bioavailability
🔢 *Probenecid:* Increased serum mycophenolate concentrations

SPECIAL CONSIDERATIONS
• Drug can be given concurrently with cyclosporine, which may enable reduced cyclosporine doses and lower toxicity, or potential cyclosporine substitute in patients developing cyclosporine toxicity
• Drug is less likely than azathioprine to induce severe bone marrow depression, and may replace azathioprine in conventional maintenance immunosuppression regimens

MONITORING PARAMETERS
• CBC qwk × 1 mo, then q2wk × 2 mo, then monthly

---

nabumetone
(na-byu-me-tone)
Rx: Relafen
Chemical Class: Acetic acid derivative
Therapeutic Class: NSAID with analgesic and antipyretic activity

CLINICAL PHARMACOLOGY
Mechanism of Action: Reversible cyclooxygenase (i.e., prostaglandin synthetase) inhibitor; nonselectively decreases the formation of both prostaglandins and thromboxane A2; variable effects on lipoxygenase synthesis and subsequent leukotriene production; antiinflammatory, antipyretic, and analgesic activity; inhibit platelet aggregation

---

* = non-FDA-approved use

Pharmacokinetics

PO: Peak 2½-4 hr; plasma protein binding >99%; $t_{1/2}$ 22-30 hr; parent drug is a prodrug, which is metabolized in liver to active metabolite 6-methoxy-2-naphthylacetic acid (6 MNA); excreted in urine (metabolites)

INDICATIONS AND USES: Prevention of cognitive decline,* osteoarthritis, pain—mild to moderate, rheumatoid arthritis, soft tissue injuries*

DOSAGE

Adult

• PO 1 g as a single dose; may increase to 1.5-2 g/day if needed; may give qd or bid

$ AVAILABLE FORMS/COST OF THERAPY

• Tab, Uncoated—Oral: 500 mg, 100's: **$102.20-111.10;** 750 mg, 100's: **$131.25**

CONTRAINDICATIONS: Bronchospasm, nasal polyps, angioedema precipitated by aspirin or other NSAIDs

PRECAUTIONS: History of GI ulceration, bleeding, or perforation; renal dysfunction, hypertension or cardiac conditions aggravated by fluid retention and edema, history of liver dysfunction, history of coagulation

PREGNANCY AND LACTATION: Pregnancy category C

SIDE EFFECTS/ADVERSE REACTIONS

CNS: Anxiety, confusion, depression, dizziness, drowsiness, fatigue, headache, insomnia, nervousness, tremors

CV: **CHF, dysrhythmias,** edema, palpitations, peripheral, tachycardia

EENT: Blurred vision, hearing loss, tinnitus

GI: Anorexia, cholestatic hepatitis, constipation, cramps, diarrhea, dry mouth, flatulence, gastritis, jaundice, nausea, peptic ulcer, ***perforation, ulceration,*** vomiting

GU: Azotemia, cystitis, dysuria, hematuria, ***nephrotoxicity,*** oliguria

HEME: **Blood dyscrasias**

RESP: **Bronchospasm,** dyspnea, pharyngitis

SKIN: Photosensitivity, pruritus, purpura, rash, sweating

INTERACTIONS

Drugs

■ *Aminoglycosides:* Reduced clearance with elevated aminoglycoside levels and potential for toxicity (especially indomethacin in premature infants; other NSAIDs probably)

■ *Antihypertensives:* (alpha blockers, angiotensin converting enzyme inhibitors, angiotensin II receptor blockers, beta blockers, diuretics) inhibition of antihypertensive and other favorable hemodynamic effects

■ *Corticosteroids:* Increased risk of GI ulceration

■ *Anticoagulants:* Excessive hypoprothrombinemia, decreased platelet aggregation with increased risk of GI bleeding

■ *Cyclosporine:* Increased nephrotoxicity risk

■ *Lithium:* Decreased clearance of lithium (mediated via prostaglandins) resulting in elevated serum lithium levels and risk of toxicity

■ *Methotrexate:* Decreased renal secretion of methotrexate resulting in elevated methotrexate levels and risk of toxicity

■ *Phenylpropanolamine:* Possible acute hypertensive reaction

■ *Potassium-Sparing Diuretics:* Additive hyperkalemia potential

■ *Triamterene:* Acute renal failure reported with addition of indomethacin; caution with other NSAIDs

N

---

italic = common side effects   **bold italic** = life-threatening reactions

SPECIAL CONSIDERATIONS
• No significant advantage over other NSAIDs; cost should govern use

MONITORING PARAMETERS
• Initial hemogram and fecal occult blood test within 3 months of starting regular chronic therapy; repeat every 6-12 months (more frequently in high risk patients (>65 years, peptic ulcer disease, concurrent steroids or anticoagulants); electrolytes, creatinine, and BUN within 3 months of starting regular chronic therapy; repeat every 6-12 months

---

nadolol
(nay-doe'lole)
Rx: Corgard
Combinations
  Rx: With Bendroflumenthiazide (Corzide)
Chemical Class: Nonselective, β-adrenergic blocker
Therapeutic Class: Antihypertensive; antianginal; antiglaucoma agent

CLINICAL PHARMACOLOGY
Mechanism of Action: PO: Competitive beta-adrenergic antagonist; produces negative inotropic and chronotropic responses; slows AV nodal conduction; decreases heart rate; decreases myocardial oxygen consumption; antiarrhythmic effects (class II); reduction in platelet aggregation and blood viscosity; suppression of renin release; inhibition of central sympathetic outflow; decreases presynaptic receptor neurotransmitter release; no intrinsic sympathomimetic or membrane stabilizing activity; low to moderate lipid solubility

Pharmacokinetics
PO: Onset variable, peak 3-4 hr, duration 17-24 hr, t₁/₂ 16-20 hr; not metabolized, excreted in urine (unchanged)

INDICATIONS AND USES: Glaucoma,* migraine headache, hypertension, post-myocardial infarction, supraventricular arrhythmias (atrial fibrillation, atrial flutter, paroxysmal supraventricular tachycardia),* aggressive behavior,* angina pectoris, anxiety,* cataract extraction prophylaxis,* congestive heart failure,* hyperthyroidism,* neuroleptic-induced akathisia,* retinal detachment,* tremor,* gastrointestinal tract bleeding*

DOSAGE
Adult and Child >16 yr
• *Angina Pectoris:* PO 40 mg qd; increase by 40-80 mg q3-7 days; maintenance 40-240 mg/day
• *Arrhythmias:* PO 60-160 mg qd for supraventricular arrhythmias
• *Hypertension:* PO 40 mg qd; increase by 40-80 mg q3-7 days; maintenance 40-320 mg qd
• *Hyperthyroidisms:* PO 80-160 mg qd
• *Migraine headache prophylaxis:* PO 80-24 mg qd
• *Tremor:* PO 80-240 mg qd

💲 **AVAILABLE FORMS/COST OF THERAPY**
• Tab, Uncoated—Oral: 20 mg, 100's: **$74.42-$130.72;** 40 mg, 100's: **$84.67-$153.25;** 80 mg, 100's: **$116.09-$210.13;** 120 mg, 100's: **$174.99-$273.86;** 160 mg, 100's: **$189.99-$304.60**

CONTRAINDICATIONS: Bronchial asthma, cardiogenic shock, overt cardiac failure, second and third degree AV block, severe sinus bradycardia

PRECAUTIONS: Anesthesia-surgery (myocardial depression), avoid abrupt withdrawal, Bronchospastic airways, congestive heart failure, diabetes mellitus, hyperthyroidism/thyrotoxicosis, concurrent clonidine

---

(discontinue nadolol several days prior to withdrawal of clonidine, peripheral vascular disease, renal disease

PREGNANCY AND LACTATION: Pregnancy category C; similar drug, atenolol, frequently used in the third trimester for treatment of hypertension (many studies of efficacy and safety of atenolol in pregnancy-induced hypertension); long-term use has been associated with intrauterine growth retardation; mean milk: plasma ratio, 0.80 in one study; quantity of drug ingested by breast feeding infant unlikely to be therapeutically significant

SIDE EFFECTS/ADVERSE REACTIONS

CNS: Depression, dizziness, fatigue, hallucinations, headache, lethargy, paresthesias

CV: AV block, *bradycardia,* chest pain, ***CHF,*** conduction disturbances, edema, flushing, *hypotension,* palpitations, peripheral ischemia, vasodilation

EENT: Sore throat

GI: Colitis, constipation, cramps, diarrhea, dry mouth, flatulence, hepatomegaly, increased transaminases, serum alkaline phosphatase; nausea, pancreatitis, taste distortion, vomiting

HEME: ***Agranulocytosis, thrombocytopenia***

METAB: Hyperkalemia, hyperuricemia

RESP: ***Bronchospasm,*** cough, dyspnea, ***laryngospasm,*** nasal stuffiness, pharyngitis, respiratory dysfunction, wheezing

SKIN: Fever, pruritus, rash

INTERACTIONS

Drugs

3 *Adenosine:* Bradycardia aggravated

3 *α-1 adrenergic blockers:* Potential enhanced first dose response (marked initial drop in blood pressure, particularly on standing (especially prazocin).

3 *Amiodarone:* Symptomatic bradycardia and sinus arrest; caution in patients with bradycardia, sick sinus syndrome, or partial AV block when either amiodarone or β-blocking drug is used

3 *Ampicillin:* Reduced nadolol bioavailability

3 *Antacids:* Reduced nadolol absorption

3 *Calcium channel blockers:* See dihydropyridine and verapamil

3 *Clonidine:* Exacerbation of rebound hypertension upon discontinuation of clonidine

3 *Digoxin:* Additive prolongation of atrioventricular (AV) conduction time

3 *Dihydropyridine calcium channel blockers:* Severe hypotension or impaired cardiac performance; most prevalent with impaired left ventricular function, cardiac arrhythmias, or aortic stenosis

3 *Diltiazem:* Potentiates beta-adrenergic effects; hypotension, left ventricular failure, and AV conduction disturbances problemmatic in elderly, patients with left ventricular dysfunction, aortic stenosis, or with large doses of either drug

3 *Dipyridamole:* Bradycardia aggravated

3 *Hypoglycemic agents:* Masked hypoglycemia, hyperglycemia

3 *Lidocaine:* Increased serum lidocaine concentrations possible

3 *Neostigmine:* Bradycardia aggravated

3 *NSAIDs:* Reduced antihypertensive effect of nadolol

3 *Physostigmine:* Bradycardia aggravated

3 *Prazosin:* First-dose response to

N

prazosin may be enhanced by β-blockade

3 *Tacrine:* Bradycardia aggravated

2 *Theophylline:* Antagonistic pharmacodynamic effects

3 *Verapamil:* Potentiates beta-adrenergic effects; hypotension, left ventricular failure, and AV conduction disturbances problemmatic in elderly, patients with left ventricular dysfunction, aortic stenosis, or with large doses of either drug

SPECIAL CONSIDERATIONS
• No unique advantage over less expensive β-blockers

PATIENT/FAMILY EDUCATION
• Do **not** discontinue abruptly; may require taper; rapid withdrawal may produce rebound hypertension or angina

MONITORING PARAMETERS
• Angina: reduction in nitroglycerin usage; frequency, severity, onset, and duration of angina pain; heart rate
• Arrhythmias: heart rate
• Congestive heart failure: functional status, cough, dyspnea on exertion, paroxysmal nocturnal dyspnea, exercise tolerance, and ventricular function
• Hypertension: Blood pressure
• Migraine headache: reduction in the frequency, severity, and duration of attacks
• Post myocardial infarction: left ventricular function, lower resting heart rate
• Toxicity: blood glucose, bronchospasm, hypotension, bradycardia, depression, confusion, hallucination, sexual dysfunction

---

nafarelin
(na-far'eh-lin)
Rx: Synarel
Chemical Class: Synthetic gonadotropin-releasing hormone analog
Therapeutic Class: Gonadotropin

CLINICAL PHARMACOLOGY
Mechanism of Action: Stimulates release of LH and FSH resulting in a temporary increase of ovarian steroidogenesis; repeated dosing abolishes stimulatory effects on the pituitary gland with decreased secretion of gonadal steroids and consequent pseudomenopause

Pharmacokinetics
Nasal: Peak 10-40 min, $t_{1/2}$ 3 hr; rapidly absorbed intranasally, 2.8% bioavailability; 80% bound to plasma proteins; metabolized and excreted in urine and feces

INDICATIONS AND USES: Endometriosis; central precocious puberty in both sexes

DOSAGE
Adult
• *Endometriosis:* 400 µg/day; 200 µg (1 spray) in 1 nostril qAM, 200 µg in other nostril qPM; start treatment between days 2 and 4 of menstrual cycle; may increase to 800 µg/day; recommended duration of treatment is 6 mo

Child
• *Central precocious puberty:* 1600 µg/day (2 sprays in each nostril bid); may increase to 1800 µg/day if adequate suppression is not achieved

$ AVAILABLE FORMS/COST OF THERAPY
• Sol—Nasal: 200 µg/inh, 10 ml: **$453.36** (30 day supply for endometriosis)

---

* = non-FDA-approved use

CONTRAINDICATIONS: Undiagnosed abnormal vaginal bleeding
PRECAUTIONS: Ovarian cysts, persistent menstruation (menstruation should cease during therapy for endometriosis), osteoporosis risk factors (chronic alcohol and/or tobacco use, strong family history of osteoporosis, or chronic use of drugs that can reduce bone mass such as anticonvulsants or corticosteroids)
PREGNANCY AND LACTATION: Pregnancy category X; not recommended in nursing mothers
SIDE EFFECTS/ADVERSE REACTIONS
CNS: Depression, emotional lability, flushing, headache, insomnia
EENT: Rhinitis
GU: Breast tenderness, decreased libido; increased pubic hair, transient breast enlargement, vaginal dryness, bleeding
METAB: Bone density changes (8.7% decrease in trabecular bone density after 6 mo), *hot flashes*
SKIN: Acne, increased body hair
MISC: Body odor, seborrhea
DRUG INTERACTIONS
Drugs
3 *Decongestants, nasal/topical:* Potential interference with absorption; allow 30 min after use of nafarelin before applying a topical decongestant
Labs
• *Interference:* Gonadal and gonadotropic function tests conducted during treatment and for 4-8 wk after treatment may be misleading
SPECIAL CONSIDERATIONS
• Alternative to danazol and oophorectomy in the treatment of endometriosis; more tolerable adverse effect profile compared to danazol for some patients
• Agent of choice in patients concerned about future fertility
• Benefits are temporary

nafcillin
(naf'sill'in)
Rx: Nallpen
Chemical Class: Semisynthetic penicillinase-resistant penicillin
Therapeutic Class: Antibiotic

CLINICAL PHARMACOLOGY
Mechanism of Action: Inhibits bacterial wall synthesis; bactericidal
Pharmacokinetics
IV: Peak 5 min
IM/PO: Peak 30-60 min, duration 4-6 hr
Poor/erratic oral absorption; 90% bound to plasma proteins; metabolized by the liver, elimination 30% as unchanged drug in urine, primarily eliminated by nonrenal routes (namely hepatic inactivation and excretion in bile); $t_{1/2}$ 1 hr
INDICATIONS AND USES: Infections caused by penicillinase-producing staphylococci, which have demonstrated sensitivity to the drug Antibacterial spectrum usually includes:
• Gram-positive organisms: *Staphylococcus aureus, Streptococcus pyogenes, S. viridans, S. bovis, S. pneumoniae,* including penicillinase producing strains
DOSAGE
Adult
• PO/IM/IV 2-6 g/day in divided doses q4-6h (IV doses should be administered over 60 min to minimize vein irritation)
Child
• IM 25 mg/kg q12h; PO 25-50 mg/kg/day in divided doses q6h
Neonates
• IM 10 mg/kg bid
$ AVAILABLE FORMS/COST OF THERAPY
• Inj, Dry-Sol—IM, IV: 1 g: **$2.27-**

$3.16; 2 g: **$4.40-$6.60;** 500 mg: **$1.20**

• Cap, Gel—Oral: 250 mg, 100's: **$110.10**

PRECAUTIONS: Hypersensitivity to cephalosporins (5%-16% cross-allergenicity), neonates, hepatic and renal insufficiency

PREGNANCY AND LACTATION: Pregnancy category B; excreted into breast milk

SIDE EFFECTS/ADVERSE REACTIONS

CNS: Anxiety, coma, depression, hallucinations, lethargy, *seizures,* twitching

CV: Phlebitis or thrombophlebitis

GI: Abdominal pain, colitis, *diarrhea;* glossitis (black or hairy tongue), increased LFTs, *vomiting*

GU: Glomerulonephritis, hematuria, interstitial nephritis, *moniliasis,* oliguria, proteinuria, *vaginitis*

HEME: **Bone marrow depression,** increased bleeding time

DRUG INTERACTIONS

Drugs

🔳 *Chloramphenicol:* Inhibited antibacterial activity of nafcillin; administer nafcillin 3 hr before chloramphenicol

🔳 *Cyclosporine:* Reduced serum cyclosporine concentrations

🔳 *Macrolide antibiotics:* Inhibited antibacterial activity of nafcillin; administer nafcillin 3 hr before macrolides

🔳 *Methotrexate:* Increased serum methotrexate concentrations

🔳 *Oral contraceptives:* Occasional impairment of oral contraceptive efficacy; consider use of supplemental contraception during cycles in which nafcillin is used

🔳 *Tacrolimus:* Reduced serum tacrolimus concentrations

🔳 *Tetracyclines:* Inhibited antibacterial activity of nafcillin; administer nafcillin 3 hr before tetracyclines

🔳 *Warfarin:* May inhibit hypoprothrombinemic response to warfarin

Labs

• *Increase:* Serum protein

SPECIAL CONSIDERATIONS
MONITORING PARAMETERS

• Oral nafcillin absorption is erratic (consider alternate oral penicillinase-resistant penicillins)

• CBC, creatinine and UA for eosinophils during therapy to monitor for adverse effects

---

naftifine
(naf'te-feen)
Rx: Naftin
Chemical Class: Synthetic allylamine derivative
Therapeutic Class: Antifungal

CLINICAL PHARMACOLOGY
Mechanism of Action: Fungicidal, fungistatic; interferes with sterol biosynthesis by inhibiting the enzyme squalene 2,3-epoxidase

Pharmacokinetics

TOP: Systemic absorption 6% (cream), 4.2% (gel); excreted via urine and feces; $t_{1/2}$ 2-3 days

INDICATIONS AND USES: Topical fungal infections (i.e., tinea cruris, tinea corporis, tinea pedis) caused by the following susceptible organisms: *Trichophyton rubrum, T. mentagrophytes, T. tonsurans, Epidermophyton floccosum, Microsporum canis, M. audouini, M. gypseum;* fungistatic against *Candida* spp.

DOSAGE

Adult

• TOP apply qd (cream) or bid (gel) to affected area; reevaluate if no improvement after 4 wk of therapy

---

* = non-FDA-approved use

💲 AVAILABLE FORMS/COST OF THERAPY

• Cre—Top: 1%, 15, 30, 60 g: **$35.35**/30 g
• Gel—Top: 1%, 20, 40, 60 g: **$47.59**/40 g

PREGNANCY AND LACTATION: Pregnancy category B; excretion into breast milk unknown

SIDE EFFECTS/ADVERSE REACTIONS

SKIN: Burning, dryness, *itching,* local irritation, redness, *stinging*

SPECIAL CONSIDERATIONS

• First of a new class of antifungals (allylamine derivatives) unrelated to imidazoles
• Because of fungicidal activity at low concentrations may provide quicker onset of healing, enhance patient compliance with qd therapy

---

nalbuphine
(nal'byoo-feen)
Rx: Nubain
Chemical Class: Synthetic opiate derivative-Phenanthrene derivative
Therapeutic Class: Narcotic agonist-antagonist analgesic

CLINICAL PHARMACOLOGY

Mechanism of Action: Analgesia via μ-subclass opiate receptor binding in CNS; μ-receptors mediate morphine-like supraspinal analgesia, euphoria, and respiratory and physical depression; narcotic antagonist activity is approx. $10 \times$ pentazocine

Pharmacokinetics

IV: Onset 2-3 min, duration 3-6 hr
SC/IM: Onset <15 min, duration, 3-6 hr
Metabolized by liver, excreted by kidneys; $t_{1/2}$, 5 hr

INDICATIONS AND USES: Moderate to severe pain; can be used for supplement to balanced anesthesia, for preoperative and postoperative analgesia, and for obstetrical analgesia during labor and delivery

DOSAGE

Note: 3-6 mg IM is equivalent to 10 mg IM morphine

Adult

• *Pain:*SC/IM/IV 10-20 mg q3-6h prn, not to exceed 160 mg/day
• *Supplement to balanced anesthesia:* Induction 0.3-3 mg/kg IV administered over 10-15 min period; maintenance 0.25-0.50 mg/kg as required

💲 AVAILABLE FORMS/COST OF THERAPY

• Inj, Sol—IM, IV, SC:10 mg/ml, 1 ml: **$1.52-$6.09;** 20 mg/ml, 1 ml: **$2.28-$7.48**

CONTRAINDICATIONS: Narcotic addiction

PRECAUTIONS: Addictive personality, increased intracranial pressure, MI (acute), severe heart disease, respiratory depression, hepatic disease, renal disease, sulfite sensitivity

PREGNANCY AND LACTATION: Pregnancy category B

SIDE EFFECTS/ADVERSE REACTIONS

CNS: Confusion, crying, *dizziness,* dreams, dysphoria (high doses), euphoria, *headache, sedation; vertigo*
CV: Bradycardia, change in blood pressure, palpitations
EENT: Blurred vision, diplopia, miosis, tinnitus
GI: Anorexia, constipation, cramps, dry mouth, nausea, vomiting
GU: Dysuria, increased urinary output, urinary retention, urinary urgency
*RESP: **Respiratory depression***
SKIN: Bruising, diaphoresis, flushing, pruritus, *rash,* urticaria
MISC: Flushing, speech difficulty, warmth

---

italic = common side effects   ***bold italic*** = life-threatening reactions

N

INTERACTIONS
Drugs
3 *Barbiturates:* Additive respiratory and CNS depression

3 *Cimetidine:* Inhibition of narcotic hepatic metabolism; additive CNS effects

3 *Rifampin:* May reduce narcotic concentrations and precipitate withdrawal

Labs
• *Increase:* Amylase

SPECIAL CONSIDERATIONS
• Proposed, but not significant, advantages include low abuse potential, low respiratory depressant effects, low incidence of psychomimetic toxicity, and a lower incidence of hemodynamic toxicity

---

nalidixic acid
(nal-i-dix'ik)
Rx: NegGram
Chemical Class: Synthetic naphthyridine derivative
Therapeutic Class: Antibiotic

CLINICAL PHARMACOLOGY
Mechanism of Action: Inhibits DNA polymerization, primarily single-stranded DNA precursors in late stages of chromosomal replication; bactericidal

Pharmacokinetics
PO: Peak (serum) 1-2 hr, peak (urine) 3-4 hr; rapid absorption; 90% protein bound; metabolized in liver, excreted in urine (unchanged, hydroxynalidixic acid, similar antibacterial activity, and conjugates); serum $t_{1/2}$ 90 min, urine $t_{1/2}$ 6 hr; crosses placenta, enters breast milk

INDICATIONS AND USES: UTI caused by *E. coli, Klebsiella, Enterobacter, Proteus mirabilis, P. vulgaris, P. morganii*

DOSAGE
Adult
• PO 1 g qid × 1-2 wk, 2 g/day for long-term treatment
Child >3 mo
• PO 55 mg/kg/day in 4 divided doses for 1-2 wk; 33 mg/kg/day in 4 divided doses for long-term treatment

$ **AVAILABLE FORMS/COST OF THERAPY**
• Tab, Uncoated—Oral: 250 mg, 56's: **$46.74;** 500 mg, 100's: **$43.45-$81.68;** 1 g, 100's: **$65.45-$208.03**
• Susp-Oral: 250 mg/5 ml, 480 ml: **$120.22**

CONTRAINDICATIONS: Seizure disorder, infants <3 mo

PRECAUTIONS: Elderly, renal disease, hepatic disease, severe cerebral arteriosclerosis

PREGNANCY AND LACTATION: Pregnancy category B (safe last 2 trimesters); excreted into breast milk in low concentrations

SIDE EFFECTS/ADVERSE REACTIONS
CNS: Dizziness, drowsiness, *headache,* increased intracranial pressure, insomnia, *seizures;* toxic psychosis
EENT: Blurred vision, change in color perception, sensitivity to light
GI: Abdominal pain, diarrhea, increased transaminase levels, *nausea, vomiting*
SKIN: Photosensitivity, pruritus, rash, urticaria

INTERACTIONS
Drugs
3 *Warfarin:* Enhanced hypoprothrombinemic effects
Labs
• *False positive:* Urinary glucose
• *Increase:* Serum glucose, urine 17-ketogenic steroids, urine 17-ketosteroids, urine porphyrins, urine VMA

*= non-FDA-approved use

SPECIAL CONSIDERATIONS
• Resistance occurs in 2%-14% of patients during treatment

---

nalmefene
(nal'me-feen)
Rx: Revex
Chemical Class: Naltrexone derivative
Therapeutic Class: Opiate antidote

CLINICAL PHARMACOLOGY
Mechanism of Action: Prevents or reverses the effects of opioids, including respiratory depression; no opioid agonist activity
Pharmacokinetics
IV: Peak 5 min, duration is as long as most opioids; distribution to CNS rapid; 45% bound to plasma proteins; metabolized by the liver, excreted in urine; $t_{1/2}$ 10.8-9.4 hr

INDICATIONS AND USES: Complete or partial reversal of opioid drug effects, including respiratory depression; management of known or suspected opioid overdose
DOSAGE
Adult
• *Postoperative opioid depression:* Use 100 µg/ml dosage strength (blue label): IV initial dose 0.25 µg/kg, then 0.25 µg/kg incremental doses at 2-5 min intervals, stopping as soon as the desired degree of opioid reversal is obtained; cumulative total doses above 1 µg/kg do not provide additional therapeutic effects
• *Management of known or suspected opioid overdose:* Use 1 mg/ml dosage strength (green label): IV initial dose 0.5 mg/70 kg, then, if needed, a second dose of 1 mg/70 kg 2-5 min later (if a total dose of 1.5 mg/70 kg has been administered without clinical response,

additional drug is unlikely to have an effect)
• *Reasonable suspicion of opioid dependency:* Challenge dose of 0.1 mg/70 kg initially; if no evidence of withdrawal in 2 min, follow recommended dosing
💲 AVAILABLE FORMS/COST OF THERAPY
• Inj—Sol: 100 µg/ml, 1 ml (blue label): **$3.42;** 1 mg/ml, 2 ml (green label): **$47.93**
PRECAUTIONS: Pre-existing cardiac disease; known risk of precipitated withdrawal (like other opioid antagonists, is known to produce acute withdrawal symptoms and, therefore, should be used with extreme caution in patients with known physical dependence on opioids or following surgery involving high doses of opioids)
PREGNANCY AND LACTATION: Pregnancy category B; excretion into breast milk unknown, use caution in nursing mothers
SIDE EFFECTS/ADVERSE REACTIONS
CNS: Dizziness, headache, postoperative pain, withdrawal syndrome
CV: Hypertension, tachycardia
GI: Nausea, vomiting
METAB: Chills, fever
SPECIAL CONSIDERATIONS:
• Longer duration of action than naloxone at fully reversing doses; agent of choice in instances where prolonged opioid effects are predicted, including overdose with longer-acting opioids (e.g., methadone, propoxyphene), patients given large doses of opioids, and those with liver disease or renal failure (eliminating the need for continuous infusions of naloxone and prolonged observation periods after outpatient procedures)

---

italic = common side effects   ***bold italic*** = life-threatening reactions

naloxone
(nal-oks'one)
Rx: Narcan
Combinations
  Rx: with pentazocine (Talwin NX)
Chemical Class: Thebaine derivative
Therapeutic Class: Opiate antidote

CLINICAL PHARMACOLOGY
Mechanism of Action: Prevents or reverses the effects of opioids, including respiratory depression; no opioid agonist activity
Pharmacokinetics
IV: Onset 2 min
SC/IM: Onset slightly less rapid than IV
Metabolized in liver, excreted in urine; $t_{1/2}$ 64 min
INDICATIONS AND USES: Complete or partial reversal of narcotic depression, including respiratory depression; diagnosis of suspected acute opioid overdosage; reversal of alcoholic coma,* refractory shock,* Alzheimer's type dementia,* schizophrenia,* anaphylaxis*
DOSAGE
Adult
• *Narcotic overdose (known or suspected):* SC/IM/IV 0.4-2 mg initially, repeat at 2-3 min intervals up to 10 mg, if no response after 10 mg reevaluate diagnosis
• *Postoperative narcotic depression (partial reversal):* IV 0.1-0.2 mg at 2-3 min intervals to desired level of reversal (adequate ventilation and alertness without significant pain or discomfort); repeat doses may be required within 1-2 hr intervals
Child
• *Narcotic overdose (known or suspected):* SC/IM/IV 0.01 mg/kg initially, give subsequent doses of 0.01 mg/kg prn at 2-3 min intervals
• *Postoperative narcotic depression (partial reversal):* IV 0.005-0.01 mg q2-3 min to desired degree of reversal

💲 AVAILABLE FORMS/COST OF THERAPY
• Inj, Sol—IM, IV, SC: 0.02 mg/ml, 2 ml: **$1.95-$3.09;** 0.4 mg/ml, 1 ml: **$0.83-$5.49;** 1 mg/ml, 1 ml: **$3.41-$4.43**
PRECAUTIONS: Physical narcotic dependency, pre-existing cardiovascular disorders
PREGNANCY AND LACTATION: Pregnancy category B; excretion into breast milk unknown, use caution in nursing mothers
SIDE EFFECTS/ADVERSE REACTIONS
CNS: **Seizures,** tremulousness
CV: Hypertension, hypotension, tachycardia, ***ventricular dysrhythmia***
GI: Nausea, vomiting
RESP: **Pulmonary edema**
SKIN: Sweating
MISC: Reversal of analgesia
SPECIAL CONSIDERATIONS
• Duration of action of some narcotics may exceed that of naloxone; repeat doses prn
MONITORING PARAMETERS
• ECG, blood pressure, respiratory rate, mental status, pupil dilation

naltrexone
(nal-trex'one)
Rx: ReVia
Chemical Class: Thebaine derivative
Therapeutic Class: Opiate antidote; alcohol deterrent

CLINICAL PHARMACOLOGY
Mechanism of Action: Prevents or reverses the effects of opioids in-

* = non-FDA-approved use

cluding respiratory depression; no opioid agonist activity; mechanism of action in alcoholism not understood, may block the effects of endogenous opioids; does not cause disulfiram-like reaction

Pharmacokinetics

PO: Peak 1 hr; duration: 50 mg blocks 25 mg IV heroin × 24 hr, 100-150 mg blocks narcotic doses × 48-72 hr; significant 1st-pass metabolism; 21% bound to plasma proteins; metabolized to active metabolite (6-β-naltrexol), excreted primarily by kidney; t₁/₂ 10 hr (13 hr for 6-β-naltrexol)

INDICATIONS AND USES: Alcohol dependence, narcotic addiction, eating disorders,* postconcussional syndrome*

DOSAGE

Adult

• *Alcoholism:* PO 50 mg qd

• *Narcotic dependence:* PO 25 mg initially, observe for 1 hr, administer remaining 25 mg if no withdrawal signs occur (**do not attempt treatment until patient has remained opioid-free for 7-10 days; verify by analyzing urine for opioids and performing naloxone challenge test**); maintenance 50 mg qd or 100-150 mg q2-3 days

$ AVAILABLE FORMS/COST OF THERAPY

• Tab, Uncoated—Oral: 50 mg, 100's:**$427.51-$466.20**

CONTRAINDICATIONS: Current use of opioid analgesics, opioid dependency, acute opioid withdrawal, positive urine screen for opioids, failed naloxone test, acute hepatitis, liver failure

PRECAUTIONS: Active liver disease, children

PREGNANCY AND LACTATION: Pregnancy category C

SIDE EFFECTS/ADVERSE REACTIONS

CNS: Anxiety, attempted suicide, chills, confusion, *depression, difficulty sleeping,* disorientation, dizziness, fatigue, feeling down, hallucinations, *headache,* irritability, *nervousness,* nightmares, paranoia, restlessness

CV: Edema, increased blood pressure, non-specific ECG changes, palpitations, phlebitis, tachycardia

EENT: Blurred vision, clogged ears, excess mucus or phlegm, itching, nasal congestion, nose bleeds, photophobia, rhinorrhea, sinus trouble, sneezing, sore throat, tinnitus

GI: Abdominal pain, constipation, *cramps;* diarrhea, excessive gas, hemorrhoids, **hepatotoxicity,** increased thirst, loss of appetite, *nausea,* ulcer, *vomiting*

GU: Delayed ejaculation; decreased potency, discomfort during urination; increased, decreased sexual interest; increased urinary frequency

MS: Joint, muscle pain; painful shoulders, legs, or knees

RESP: Cough, heavy breathing, hoarseness, shortness of breath

SKIN: Acne, alopecia, athlete's foot, cold sores, oily skin, pruritus, skin rash

SPECIAL CONSIDERATIONS
PATIENT/FAMILY EDUCATION

• Wear ID tag indicating naltrexone use

• Do not try to overcome reversal of opiate effects by self-administration of large doses of narcotic

• Do not exceed recommended dose

MONITORING PARAMETERS

• Liver function tests

N

---

italic = common side effects   ***bold italic*** = life-threatening reactions

nandrolone
(nan'droe-lone)
Decanoate **Rx:** Deca-Durabolin, Hybolin Decanoate, Kabolin, Nandrolone Decanoate
Chemical Class: Halogenated testosterone derivative
Therapeutic Class: Androgen; antineoplastic
DEA Class: Schedule III

CLINICAL PHARMACOLOGY
Mechanism of Action: Promotes body tissue-building processes and reverses catabolic processes when administered with adequate calories and protein; inhibits endogenous testosterone release
Pharmacokinetics
IM: Metabolized in liver, excreted in urine
INDICATIONS AND USES: Anemia of renal insufficiency
DOSAGE
Adult
• *Anemia of renal disease:* IM 50-100 mg qwk (women); 100-200 mg qwk (men)
Child 2-13 yr
• *Anemia of renal disease:* IM 25-50 mg q3-4 wk

$ **AVAILABLE FORMS/COST OF THERAPY**
• Inj, Sol (decanoate)—IM: 50 mg/ml, 2 ml: **$10.95-$14.95;** 100 mg/ml, 2 ml: **$13.31-$29.02;** 200 mg/ml, 1 ml: **$24.46-$27.80**
CONTRAINDICATIONS: Male patients with prostate or breast cancer, hypercalcemia in females with breast cancer, nephrosis, nephrotic phase of nephritis, enhancement of physical appearance or athletic performance
PRECAUTIONS: Elderly, children, cardiac disease or risk factors for atherosclerosis, renal disease, hepatic disease, seizure disorder, migraine headache, diabetes
PREGNANCY AND LACTATION: Pregnancy category X, use extreme caution in nursing mothers
SIDE EFFECTS/ADVERSE REACTIONS
CNS: Choreiform movement, depression, excitation, habituation, insomnia
CV: Edema
EENT: Deepening of voice, hoarseness
GI: Cholestatic jaundice, diarrhea, *hepatic necrosis, hepatocellular neoplasms,* nausea, *peliosis hepatis,* vomiting
GU: Amenorrhea, clitoral hypertrophy, decreased breast size, decreased libido, testicular atrophy, vaginitis, virilization
METAB: Decreased glucose tolerance, decreased HDL cholesterol, increased LDL cholesterol, increased serum cholesterol, retention of sodium, chloride, water, potassium, phosphates, calcium
MS: Premature closure of epiphyses in children
SKIN: Acne, alopecia, flushing, hirsutism, rash, sweating
DRUG INTERACTIONS
Drugs
3 *Antidiabetic agents:* Enhanced hypoglycemic effects
2 *Cyclosporine:* Increased cyclosporine concentrations, potential for toxicity
3 *HMG-CoA reductase inhibitors (lovastatin, pravastatin):* Myositis risk increased
2 *Oral anticoagulants:* Enhanced hypoprothrombinemic response
3 *Tacrolimus:* Increased tacrolimus concentrations, potential for toxicity

SPECIAL CONSIDERATIONS
• Anabolic steroids have potential for abuse, especially in the athlete

MONITORING PARAMETERS
• Women should be observed for signs of virilization
• Liver function tests, lipids, Hct
• Growth rate in children (X-rays for bone age q 6 mo)

---

naphazoline
(naf-az'oh-leen)

Rx: (Ophthalmic); AK-Con, Albalon, Allersol, Naphcon-Forte, Nafazair, Ocu-Zoline, Vasocon

OTC: (Ophthalmic); Allerest, Clear Eyes, Naphcon, Vaso-Clear

Combinations

OTC: (Ophthalmic); with pheniramine (Naphcon-A)

Chemical Class: Imidazoline derivative

Therapeutic Class: Decongestant

CLINICAL PHARMACOLOGY
Mechanism of Action: Vasoconstriction through a local adrenergic mechanism on dilated conjunctival and nasal mucosal blood vessels

Pharmacokinetics

TOP: Onset 10 min, duration 2-6 hr, some systemic absorption

INDICATIONS AND USES: Nasal congestion, superficial corneal vascularity (congestion, itching, minor irritation, hyperemia)

DOSAGE
Adult
• NASAL 2 sprays of 0.05% sol instilled into each nostril q3-6h; do not exceed 3-5 days duration
• CONJUNCTIVAL 1 gtt q3-4h; do not exceed 3-4 days duration

💲 AVAILABLE FORMS/COST OF THERAPY
• Sol—Ophth: 0.012%, 15 ml: **$2.94-$13.50;** 0.02%, 15 ml: **$8.44;** 0.1%, 15 ml: **$4.73-$18.43**

• Spray—Nasal: 0.05%, 15 ml: **$3.55**

CONTRAINDICATIONS: Angle-closure glaucoma

PRECAUTIONS: Children <6 yr, hyperthyroidism, heart disease, hypertension, diabetes mellitus

PREGNANCY AND LACTATION: Pregnancy category C

SIDE EFFECTS/ADVERSE REACTIONS
CNS: Dizziness, headache, nervousness, weakness

CV: Cardiac irregularities, hypertension

EENT: Anosmia; blurred vision, dryness, hyperemia, increased, decreased intraocular pressure; irritation, mild transient stinging, mydriasis; rebound congestion, sneezing, stinging, transient burning, ulceration of nasal mucosa

GI: Nausea

SKIN: Sweating

SPECIAL CONSIDERATIONS
PATIENT/FAMILY EDUCATION
• Discontinue ophthalmic preparations if ocular pain or visual changes occur
• Drug may produce increased nasal congestion or redness of the eye if overused
• Do not use longer than 3-5 days unless under the direction of a clinician

N

---

italic = common side effects   **bold italic** = life-threatening reactions

naproxen

(na-prox'en)
Sodium salt: **Rx:** Anaprox, Anaprox DS, Naprelan
Rx: EC-Naprosyn
OTC: Aleve
Chemical Class: Propionic acid derivative
Therapeutic Class: NSAID with analgesic and antipyretic activity

CLINICAL PHARMACOLOGY
Mechanism of Action: Reversible cyclooxygenase (i.e., prostaglandin synthetase) inhibitor; non-selectively decreases the formation of both prostaglandins and thromboxane A2; variable effects on lipoxygenase synthesis and subsequent leukotriene production; antiinflammatory, antipyretic, and analgesic activity; inhibits platelet aggregation

Pharmacokinetics
PO: Onset 1 hr, peak 2-4 hr, duration up to 7 hr; >99% bound to plasma proteins; metabolized in liver, excreted by kidney; $t_{1/2}$ 12-15 hr

INDICATIONS AND USES: Bursitis, dysmenorrhea, ergotamine withdrawal,* erythema nodosum,* fever, gouty arthritis, headache, menorrhagia,* musculoskeletal disorders,* osteoarthritis, rheumatoid arthritis, soft tissue injuries,* ankylosing spondylitis, prevention of cognitive decline,* prevention of colon cancer,* pain—mild to moderate

DOSAGE
Adult
• *Arthritis:* PO 250-500 mg (275-550 mg naproxen sodium) bid, may increase to 1.5 g/day (1.65 g/day naproxen sodium) for limited periods; SUS REL PO 750-1000 mg qd; max 1000 mg/d

• *Acute gout:* PO 750 mg (825 mg naproxen sodium), followed by 250 mg (275 mg naproxen sodium) q8h until attack subsides; SUS REL PO 1000 mg qd, may increase to 1500 mg qd for brief period if needed

• *Mild to moderate pain, primary dysmenorrhea:* PO 500 mg (550 mg naproxen sodium) at earliest symptoms of menses, followed by 250 mg (275 mg naproxen sodium) q6-8h; do not exceed 1.25 g/day (1.375 g/day naproxen sodium)

• Minor aches and pains (OTC): PO 220 mg q12h prn

Child
• *Juvenile arthritis:* PO 10 mg/kg divided bid

$ **AVAILABLE FORMS/COST OF THERAPY**
• Tab, Uncoated—Oral: 220 mg, 100's: **$6.37-$11.87;** 250 mg, 100's: **$13.65-$85.04;** 275 mg, 100's: **$60.00-$83.94;** 375 mg, 100's: **$85.40-$109.31;** 500 mg, 100's: **$104.30-$149.67;** 550 mg, 100's: **$90.00-$138.01**

• Tab, Enteric Coated—Oral: 375 mg, 100's: **$93.37-$112.58;** 500 mg, 100's: **$114.04-$137.51**

• Tab, controlled release—oral: 375 mg, 100's: **$127.94;** 500 mg, 75's: **$117.02**

• Susp—Oral: 125 mg/5 ml, 500 ml: **$38.23**

CONTRAINDICATIONS: Bronchospasm, nasal polyps, angioedema precipitated by aspirin or other NSAIDs

PRECAUTIONS: History of GI ulceration, bleeding, or perforation; renal dysfunction, hypertension or cardiac conditions aggravated by fluid retention and edema, history of liver dysfunction, history of coagulation

PREGNANCY AND LACTATION: Pregnancy category B (category D if used in 3rd trimester); could cause

---

* = non-FDA-approved use

constriction of the ductus arteriosus *in utero,* persistent pulmonary hypertension of the newborn, or prolonged labor; passes into breast milk in small quantities; compatible with breast feeding

SIDE EFFECTS/ADVERSE REACTIONS

CNS: Dizziness, drowsiness, headache, lightheadedness

CV: Chest pain, **CHF, dysrhythmias, edema,** hypertension, palpitation, tachycardia

EENT: Hearing disturbances, *tinnitus,* visual disturbances

GI: Abdominal cramps, *constipation, diarrhea, dyspepsia,* flatulence, **gastric or duodenal ulcer with bleeding or perforation,** heartburn, hepatitis, *nausea,* occult blood in stool, **pancreatitis,** *stomatitis,* vomiting

GU: **Acute renal failure**

HEME: **Agranulocytosis,** eosinophilia, **leukopenia, neutropenia, pancytopenia, thrombocytopenia**

METAB: Hyperglycemia, hyperkalemia, hypoglycemia, hyponatremia

RESP: **Bronchospasm,** dyspnea, pulmonary infiltrates

SKIN: *Ecchymoses,* photosensitivity, *pruritus, rash,* urticaria

INTERACTIONS

Drugs

🔟 *Aminoglycosides:* Reduced clearance with elevated aminoglycoside levels and potential for toxicity (especially indomethacin in premature infants; other NSAIDs probably)

🔟 *Anticoagulants:* Excessive hypoprothrombinemia, decreased platelet aggregation with increased risk of GI bleeding

🔟 *Antihypertensives (α-blockers, angiotensin-converting enzyme inhibitors, angiotensin II receptor blockers, β-blockers, diuretics):* Inhibition of antihypertensive and other favorable hemodynamic effects

🔟 *Corticosteroids:* Increased risk of GI ulceration

🔟 *Cyclosporine:* Increased nephrotoxicity risk

🔟 *Lithium:* Decreased clearance of lithium (mediated via prostaglandins) resulting in elevated serum lithium levels and risk of toxicity

🔟 *Methotrexate:* Decreased renal secretion of methotrexate resulting in elevated methotrexate levels and risk of toxicity

🔟 *Phenylpropanolamine:* Possible acute hypertensive reaction

🔟 *Potassium-sparing diuretics:* Additive hyperkalemia potential

🔟 *Triamterene:* Acute renal failure reported with addition of indomethacin; caution with other NSAIDs

Labs

• *False increase:* Serum bicarbonate, urine 5-HIAA

SPECIAL CONSIDERATIONS

• No significant advantage over other NSAIDs; cost should govern use

PATIENT/FAMILY EDUCATION

• Avoid concurrent use of aspirin and alcoholic beverages

• Take with food, milk, or antacids to decrease GI upset

• Notify clinician if edema, black stools, or persistent headache occur

MONITORING PARAMETERS

• Initial hemogram and fecal occult blood test within 3 mo of starting regular chronic therapy; repeat every 6-12 mo (more frequently in high-risk patients (>65 years, peptic ulcer disease, concurrent steroids or anticoagulants); electrolytes, creatinine, and BUN within 3 mo of starting regular chronic therapy; repeat every 6-12 mo

N

---

italic = common side effects　　　　**bold italic** = life-threatening reactions

naratriptan
(nare-a-trip'tan)
Rx: Amerge
Chemical Class: Serotonin derivative
Therapeutic Class: Antimigraine agent

CLINICAL PHARMACOLOGY
Mechanism of Action: Selectively activates vascular 5-HT$_1$-receptors in cranial arteries causing vasoconstriction and inhibition of proinflammatory neuropeptide release, actions correlating with the relief of migraine in humans

Pharmacokinetics
PO: 70% bioavailability, peak 2-3 hr, onset 3 hr; 28%-31% bound to plasma proteins; metabolized by various cytochrome P-450 isozymes to inactive metabolites; 50% excreted unchanged in urine; t$_{1/2}$ 6 hr (11 hr in moderate renal impairment; 16 hr in severe hepatic impairment)

INDICATIONS AND USES: Acute migraine headache with or without aura.

DOSAGE
Adult
• PO 1-2.5 mg at first sign of headache; may repeat after 4 hr if partial response or headache returns (max 5 mg/24 hr)
• Mild to moderate renal or hepatic impairment: Do not exceed 2.5 mg/24 hr

💲 AVAILABLE FORMS/COST OF THERAPY
• Tab, film coated—PO: 1 mg, 9's: **$139.61**; 2.5 mg, 9's: **$139.61**

CONTRAINDICATIONS: Severe renal impairment (creatinine clearance <15 ml/min) or severe hepatic impairment; ischemic heart disease, hemiplegic or basilar migraine; Prinzmetal's angina; uncontrolled hypertension; within 24 hr of ergotamine-containing products; concurrent use of MAO inhibitor therapy (or within 2 wk of discontinuing an MAO inhibitor)

PRECAUTIONS: Atypical headache; mild to moderate renal or hepatic impairment; elderly; children

PREGNANCY AND LACTATION:
Pregnancy category C; use caution in nursing mothers

SIDE EFFECTS/ADVERSE REACTIONS
CNS: Paresthesia, dizziness, fatigue, drowsiness, vertigo, tremors, cognitive function disorders, sleep disorders, equilibrium disorders
CV: Palpitations, increased blood pressure, tachyarrhythmias, abnormal ECG, syncope
EENT: Photophobia, blurred vision, tinnitus
GI: Nausea, hyposalivation, vomiting, dyspeptic symptoms, diarrhea, constipation
GU: Bladder inflammation, polyuria, diuresis
HEME: Increased white cells
METAB: Thirst, polydipsia, dehydration, fluid retention
MS: Muscle pain, arthralgia, articular rheumatism, muscle cramps/spasms, joint/muscle stiffness, tightness, rigidity
RESP: Bronchitis, cough, pneumonia
SKIN: Sweating, rash, pruritus, urticaria
MISC: Pain/pressure sensations in neck/throat/jaw; chills, fever

INTERACTIONS
Drugs
⚠ *Ergotamine containing drugs:* Increased vasoconstriction
⚠ *MAO inhibitors:* Potential for decreased metabolism of naratriptan

---

* = non-FDA-approved use

❷ *Sibutramine:* Increased risk of serotonin syndrome

SPECIAL CONSIDERATIONS
• Longer acting than sumatriptan and zolmitriptan so recurrent headaches requiring a second dose less likely; slower onset than sumatriptan and zolmitriptan; should probably be reserved for patients who get recurrent headaches
• Safety of treating, on average, more than 4 headaches in a 30-day period has not been established

PATIENT/FAMILY EDUCATION
• Use only to treat migraine headache, not for prevention

---

natamycin
(na-ta-mye′sin)
Rx: Natacyn
Chemical Class: Tetraene polyene derivative
Therapeutic Class: Ophthalmic antifungal

CLINICAL PHARMACOLOGY
Mechanism of Action: Binds to fungal cell membrane, altering membrane permeability; depletes essential cellular constituents; fungicidal
Pharmacokinetics
OPHTHAL: Produces effective concentrations within corneal stroma; systemic absorption should not occur after topical administration

INDICATIONS AND USES: Fungal blepharitis, conjunctivitis, keratitis caused by susceptible organisms Antifungal spectrum usually includes: *Candida, Aspergillus, Cephalosporium, Fusarium, and Penicillium;* initial drug of choice in *Fusarium solani* keratitis

DOSAGE
ADULT
• *Fungal keratitis:* 1 gtt into conjunctival sac q1-2h, decrease to 1

gtt 6-8 times/day after 3-4 days; continue therapy for 14-21 days
• *Fungal blepharitis, conjunctivitis:* 1 gtt 4-6 times/day

💲 **AVAILABLE FORMS/COST OF THERAPY**
• Susp—Ophth: 5%, 15 ml: **$111.25**

PRECAUTIONS: Fungal endophthalmitis (effectiveness as single agent not established)

PREGNANCY AND LACTATION: Pregnancy category C

SIDE EFFECTS/ADVERSE REACTIONS
EENT: Conjunctival chemosis, conjunctival hyperemia

SPECIAL CONSIDERATIONS
PATIENT/FAMILY EDUCATION
• Shake well before using

MONITORING PARAMETERS
• Failure of keratitis to improve following 7-10 days of administration suggests infection not susceptible to natamycin

---

N

nedocromil
(ned-oh-crow′mil)
Rx: Tilade
Chemical Class: Pyranoquinoline dicarboxylic acid derivative
Therapeutic Class: Antiasthmatic, inhaled

CLINICAL PHARMACOLOGY
Mechanism of Action: Inhibits activation and release of inflammatory mediators from cells involved in asthmatic inflammation, including eosinophils, neutrophils, macrophages, mast cells, monocytes, and platelets; inhibits both early and late asthmatic responses to inhaled antigen and irritants
Pharmacokinetics
INH: Low systemic bioavailability; duration 4-6 hr; 89% bound to

---

italic = common side effects   ***bold italic*** = life-threatening reactions

plasma proteins; excreted unchanged in urine; $t_{1/2}$ 1.5-3.3 hr

INDICATIONS AND USES: Maintenance therapy in mild to moderate bronchial asthma, prevention of exercise-induced asthma,* prevention of acute bronchospasm induced by environmental pollutants*

DOSAGE

Adult and Child ≥6 yr

• INH 2 inhalations qid at regular intervals; may reduce to bid-tid in patients under good control

§ AVAILABLE FORMS/COST OF THERAPY

• Aer—INH: 1.75 mg/spray, 112 sprays: **$33.76**

PRECAUTIONS: Acute bronchospasm **(not a bronchodilator)**

PREGNANCY AND LACTATION: Pregnancy category B; excretion into breast milk unknown

SIDE EFFECTS/ADVERSE REACTIONS

CNS: Dizziness, *headache*
CV: Chest pain
EENT: Burning eyes, nasal congestion, *pharyngitis,* rhinitis, throat irritation, upper respiratory infection
GI: Abdominal pain, diarrhea, dry mouth, dyspepsia, nausea, *unpleasant taste,* vomiting
RESP: **Bronchospasm,** *coughing*

SPECIAL CONSIDERATIONS
PATIENT/FAMILY EDUCATION

• Must be used regularly to achieve benefit, even during symptom-free periods

• Therapeutic effect may take up to 4 wk

• Not to be used to treat acute asthmatic symptoms

---

nefazodone
(neh-faz'oh-doan)
Rx: Serzone
Chemical Class: Phenylpiperazine derivative
Therapeutic Class: Antidepressant

CLINICAL PHARMACOLOGY
Mechanism of Action: Inhibits neuronal uptake of serotonin (significant) and norepinephrine (slight); antagonizes α_1-adrenergic receptors, minimal anticholinergic, moderate sedative, and slight orthostatic hypotensive effects

Pharmacokinetics
PO: Absolute bioavailability low (about 20%); peak 1 hr; >99% bound to plasma proteins; extensively metabolized (active metabolite hydroxynefazodone), $t_{1/2}$ 2-4 hr

INDICATIONS AND USES: Depression

DOSAGE
Adult

• PO 200 mg/day in 2 divided doses, increase in increments of 100-200 mg/day in intervals of no less than 1 wk; max dose, 600 mg/day

• *Elderly:* PO 100 mg/day bid with gradual titration

§ AVAILABLE FORMS/COST OF THERAPY

• Tab, Uncoated—Oral: 50, 100, 150, 200, 250 mg, 60's: **$69.32**

CONTRAINDICATIONS: Coadministration with terfenadine or astemizole (see drug interactions)

PRECAUTIONS: Elderly, children, cardiovascular disease, cerebrovascular disease, dehydration, hypovolemia, history of mania, suicidal ideation, seizure disorder, cirrhosis

PREGNANCY AND LACTATION: Pregnancy category C

SIDE EFFECTS/ADVERSE REACTIONS

CNS: Abnormal dreams, agitation, *asthenia,* ataxia, *confusion, dizziness, headache,* insomnia, *lightheadedness,* memory impairment, paresthesia, *somnolence,* tremor

CV: Peripheral edema, postural hypotension, sinus bradycardia

EENT: Abnormal vision, blurred vision, pharyngitis, taste perversion, tinnitus, visual field defect

GI: Constipation, diarrhea, dry mouth, dyspepsia, increased appetite, nausea

GU: Impotence, urinary frequency, urinary retention, vaginitis

RESP: Cough

SKIN: Pruritus, rash

DRUG INTERACTIONS

Drugs

❷ *Astemizole, terfenadine:* Theoretical potential for QT prolongation and dysrhythmia

❸ *Atorvastatin, fluvastatin, lovastatin, pravastatin, simvastatin:* Potential for development of myositis with rhabdomyolysis

❷ *MAOIs:* Serious adverse reactions possible including hyperthermia, rigidity, myoclonus, autonomic instability, mental status changes, seizures; observe a 14-day washout period between discontinuing one drug and starting the other

SPECIAL CONSIDERATIONS

• Priapism reported with a similar drug; educate and monitor appropriately

PATIENT/FAMILY EDUCATION

• Therapeutic effect may not be apparent for several weeks

• Drug may cause drowsiness, use caution driving or performing other tasks where alertness is required

---

nelfinavir
(nel-fin'eh-veer)

Rx: Viracept

Chemical Class: HIV protease inhibitor

Therapeutic Class: HIV infection

CLINICAL PHARMACOLOGY

Mechanism of Action: By inhibiting the HIV protease, nelfinavir causes immature and noninfectious virus to be produced

Pharmacokinetics

PO: Onset 1 hr, peak 2-4 hr, bioavailability better with food; 98% protein bound; metabolized in liver by cytochrome P450 system including CYP3A, some metabolites active; $t_{1/2}$ 3.5-5 hr, 98% excreted in feces as unchanged drug and metabolites

INDICATIONS AND USES: Combination therapy for HIV-1

DOSAGE

Adult and Child >14 yr

• PO: 750 mg tid with food

Child 2-13 yr

• PO: 20-30 mg per dose, taken tid with food

• Adjust dose when used with indinavir, rifabutin, ritonavir

• For latest treatment guidelines see www.hivatis.org

🔟 **AVAILABLE FORMS/COST OF THERAPY**

• Powder—Oral: 50 mg nelfinavir base per g, 144 g: **$59.45**

• Tab, Uncoated—Oral: 250 mg, 270's: **$609.12-$619.79**

CONTRAINDICATIONS: Concurrent use of rifampin

PRECAUTIONS: Phenylketonuria, hepatic insufficiency, hemophilia; do not administer concurrently with terfenadine, astemizole, or cisapride;

N

---

avoid coadministration with rifampin, midazolam, or triazolam

PREGNANCY AND LACTATION: Pregnancy category B; excreted in breast milk; breast feeding not recommended for HIV-infected women

SIDE EFFECTS/ADVERSE REACTIONS

CNS: Dizziness, headache

EENT: Iritis, rhinitis

GI: Diarrhea (20%), dyspepsia, *nausea*

GU: Nephrolithiasis, sexual dysfunction

HEME: Anemia, leukopenia, thrombocytopenia

METAB: Hyperlipidemia, hyperuricemia, increased alkaline phosphatase, transaminases, CPK, LDH

MS: Arthralgia, myalgia, myopathy

RESP: Dyspnea

SKIN: Folliculitis, pruritus, rash

MISC: Weakness

INTERACTIONS

Drugs

⚠ *Astemizole:* Increased plasma levels of astemizole

3 *Barbiturates:* Increased clearance of nelfinavir; reduced clearance of barbiturates

2 *Carbamazepine:* Increased clearance of nelfinavir; reduced clearance of carbamazepine

⚠ *Cisapride:* Increased plasma levels of cisapride

⚠ *Ergot alkaloids:* Increased plasma levels of ergot alkaloids

3 *Erythromycin:* Reduced clearance of nelfinavir; nelfinavir reduces clearance of erythromycin

⚠ *Lovastatin:* Nelfinavir reduces clearance of lovastatin

⚠ *Midazolam:* Increased plasma levels of midazolam and prolonged effect

3 *Nevirapine:* Reduces plasma nelfinavir levels; increase nelfinavir dose to 1000 mg tid

3 *Oral contraceptives:* Nelfinavir may reduce efficacy

3 *Phenytoin:* Increased clearance of nelfinavir; reduced clearance of phenytoin

2 *Rifabutin:* Increased clearance of nelfinavir; reduced clearance of rifabutin—reduce rifabutin dose to 150 mg qd and increase nelfinavir dose to 1000 mg tid

⚠ *Rifampin:* Increased clearance of nelfinavir

3 *Ritonavir:* Decreased clearance of nelfinavir; decrease nelfinavir dose to 750 mg bid

3 *Saquinavir:* Decreased clearance of saquinavir; reduce dose of Fortovase (saquinavir soft gel capsule) to 800 mg tid

⚠ *Simvastatin:* Nelfinavir reduces clearance of simvastatin

⚠ *Terfenadine:* Increased plasma levels of terfenadine

⚠ *Triazolam:* Increased plasma levels of triazolam and prolonged effect

SPECIAL CONSIDERATIONS
• Positive results of treatment are based on surrogate markers only
• Take with meal or snack

PATIENT/FAMILY EDUCATION
• Contains phenylalanine, take with food

MONITORING PARAMETERS
• CBC, electrolytes, renal function, liver enzymes, CPK

neomycin

(nee-oh-mye'sin)
Rx (Oral): Mycifradin, Neo-
Fradin
OTC (Topical): Myciguent
Combinations
  Rx: with polymyxin B
   (Neosporin G.U. irrigant)
  OTC: with polymyxin B,
   bacitracin (Neosporin,
   Mycitracin)
Chemical Class: Aminoglyco-
side
Therapeutic Class: Antibiotic

CLINICAL PHARMACOLOGY
Mechanism of Action: Interferes
with protein synthesis in bacterial
cell by binding to 30S ribosomal
subunit, which causes misreading
of genetic code, inaccurate peptide
sequence forms in protein chain,
causing bacterial death
Pharmacokinetics
PO: Poorly absorbed, small absorbed
fraction rapidly excreted via kidney, unabsorbed fraction eliminated
unchanged in feces; intestinal bacteria suppressed for 48-72 hr after
oral administration
INDICATIONS AND USES: (Oral)
preoperative bowel preparation, adjunctive therapy of hepatic coma,
hypercholesterolemia*; (topical) minor skin infections
Antibacterial spectrum usually includes:
E. coli and the *Klebsiella-Entero-
bacter* group; no anaerobic coverage; minimal coverage of gram-
positive organisms
DOSAGE
Adult
• *Preoperative bowel preparation:*
PO 1 g q1h for 4 doses then 1 g q4h
for 5 doses; or 1 g at 1, 2, and 11 PM
on day preceding surgery as an ad-

junct to cathartics, enema, and oral
erythromycin; or 6 g/day divided
q4h for 2-3 days
• *Hepatic coma:* PO 4-12 g/day di-
vided q4-6h
• TOP apply to affected area qd-tid
Child
• *Preoperative bowel preparation:*
PO 90 mg/kg/day divided q4h for 2
days; or 25 mg/kg at 1, 2, and 11 PM
on the day preceding surgery as an
adjunct to cathartics, enema, and oral
erythromycin
• *Hepatic coma:* 2.5-7 g/m^2/day divided q4-6h for 5-6 days, not to
exceed 12 g/day
• TOP apply to affected area qd-tid
**⟡ AVAILABLE FORMS/COST
OF THERAPY**
• Tab, Uncoated—Oral: 500 mg,
100's: **$11.51-36.63**
• Sol—Oral: 125 mg/5 ml, 480 ml:
$25.05
• Cre—Top: 0.5%, 15 g: **$2.98**
• Oint—Top: 0.5%, 30 g: **$3.50**
CONTRAINDICATIONS: Intestinal obstruction, inflammatory or ulcerative gastrointestinal disease
PRECAUTIONS: Hepatic disease,
renal disease, prolonged treatment,
application to extensive burns or
large surface area, children <18 yr,
myasthenia gravis, parkinsonism
PREGNANCY AND LACTATION:
Pregnancy category D; ototoxicity
has not been reported as an effect of
in utero exposure; 8th cranial nerve
toxicity in the fetus is well known
following exposure to other aminoglycosides and could potentially
occur with neomycin
**SIDE EFFECTS/ADVERSE REAC-
TIONS**
EENT: Ototoxicity (prolonged and
high-dose therapy)
GI: Diarrhea, malabsorption syndrome has occurred during prolonged therapy; *nausea, **pseudomembranous colitis,** vomiting*

N

---

italic = common side effects   ***bold italic*** = life-threatening reactions

*GU: **Nephrotoxicity** (prolonged and high-dose therapy)*

SKIN: Sensitization (low-grade reddening with swelling, dry scaling, and itching or a failure to heal)

INTERACTIONS

Drugs

3 *Digitalis glycosides:* Reduced serum digoxin concentration

2 *Ethacrynic acid:* Increased risk of ototoxicity, especially in patients with renal impairment

3 *Oral anticoagulants:* Enhanced hypoprothrombinemic response; more common with large doses of neomycin, dietary vitamin K deficiency, impaired hepatic function

A *Methotrexate:* Oral absorption of methotrexate reduced 30%-50%

3 *Penicillin V:* Reduced concentrations of penicillin V, possible reduced efficacy

3 *Warfarin:* Enhanced hypoprothrombinemic response

SPECIAL CONSIDERATIONS
• Inform patient and family about possible toxic effects on the 8th cranial nerve; monitor for loss of hearing, ringing or roaring in ears, or a feeling of fullness in head

PATIENT/FAMILY EDUCATION
• Drink plenty of fluids

MONITORING PARAMETERS
• Renal function, audiometric testing during extended therapy or with application to extensive burns or large surface area

---

netilmicin

(ne-til-mye'sin)
Rx: Netromycin
Chemical Class: Aminoglycoside
Therapeutic Class: Antibiotic

CLINICAL PHARMACOLOGY
Mechanism of Action: Interferes with protein synthesis in bacterial cell by binding to 30S ribosomal subunit, which causes misreading of genetic code; inaccurate peptide sequence forms in protein chain, causing bacterial death

Pharmacokinetics

IM: Onset rapid, peak 30-60 min
IV: Onset immediate, peak 30 min after a 30 min inf
<30% bound to plasma proteins; duration 6-8 hr; not metabolized, eliminated unchanged in urine via glomerular filtration; plasma $t_{1/2}$ 2-3 hr; (antibacterial effect may persist after drug levels decline)

INDICATIONS AND USES: Serious or life-threatening bacterial infections of the urinary tract, skin and skin structures, lower respiratory tract, septicemia, intraabdominal infections

Antibacterial spectrum usually includes:
• Gram-positive organisms: *Staphylococcus* spp. (including penicillinase and non-penicillinase-producing strains), *Streptococcus faecalis* (in combination with cell wall synthesis inhibitor)
• Gram-negative organisms: *Acinetobacter* spp., *Escherichia coli*, *Proteus* spp. (indole-positive and indole-negative), *Pseudomonas aeruginosa*, *Klebsiella* spp., *Enterobacter* spp., *Serratia* spp., *Citrobacter* spp., *Providencia* spp., *Salmonella* spp., *Shigella* spp., *Yersinia pestis*

DOSAGE
Use ideal body weight for dosage calculations

Adult
• *Serious systemic infections:* IM/IV 1.3-2.2 mg/kg diluted in 50-100 ml NS or D_5W and infused over 30-60 min q8h or 2-3.25 mg/kg q12h; adjust dosage based on results of netilmicin serum peak and trough levels

---

* = non-FDA-approved use

• *Complicated UTI:* IM/IV 1.5-2 mg/kg q12h

Child 6 wk-12 yr

• IM/IV 1.8-2.7 mg/kg q8h or 2.7-4 mg/kg q12h

$ **AVAILABLE FORMS/COST OF THERAPY**

• Inj, Sol—IM, IV: 100 mg/ml, 1.5 ml: **$15.10**

PRECAUTIONS: Neonates, renal disease, myasthenia gravis, hearing deficits, Parkinson's disease, elderly, dehydration, hypokalemia

PREGNANCY AND LACTATION: Pregnancy category D; ototoxicity has not been reported as an effect of *in utero* exposure; 8th cranial nerve toxicity in the fetus is well known following exposure to other aminoglycosides and could potentially occur with netilmicin; potentiation of magnesium sulfate-induced neuromuscular weakness in neonates has been reported, use caution during the last 32 hr of pregnancy; excreted in breast milk in small amounts

SIDE EFFECTS/ADVERSE REACTIONS

CNS: Confusion, depression, dizziness, muscle twitching, myasthenia gravis-like syndrome, neurotoxicity, numbness, ***seizures,*** tremors, vertigo

CV: Hypertension, palpitations

EENT: Deafness, ototoxicity, tinnitus, visual disturbances

GI: Anorexia, hepatomegaly, increased ALT, AST, bilirubin; *nausea,* splenomegaly, *vomiting*

*GU: **Azotemia,** hematuria, **nephrotoxicity, oliguria, renal damage, renal failure***

*HEME: **Agranulocytosis,** anemia, eosinophilia, **leukopenia, thrombocytopenia***

METAB: Decreased serum calcium, sodium, potassium, magnesium

*RESP: **Respiratory depression***

SKIN: Alopecia, burning, dermatitis, *rash,* urticaria

INTERACTIONS

Drugs

3 *Amphotericin B:* Synergistic nephrotoxicity

2 *Atracurium:* Netilmicin potentiates respiratory depression by atracurium

3 *Carbenicillin:* Potential for inactivation of netilmicin in patients with renal failure

3 *Carboplatin:* Additive nephrotoxicity or ototoxicity

3 *Cephalosporins:* Increased potential for nephrotoxicity in patients with preexisting renal disease

3 *Cisplatin:* Additive nephrotoxicity or ototoxicity

3 *Cyclosporine:* Additive nephrotoxicity

2 *Ethacrynic acid:* Additive ototoxicity

3 *Indomethacin:* Reduced renal clearance of netilmicin in premature infants

3 *Methoxyflurane:* Additive nephrotoxicity

2 *Neuromuscular blocking agents:* Netilmicin potentiates respiratory depression by neuromuscular blocking agents

3 *NSAIDs:* May reduce renal clearance of netilmicin

3 *Penicillins (extended spectrum):* Potential for inactivation of netilmicin in patients with renal failure

3 *Piperacillin:* Potential for inactivation of netilmicin in patients with renal failure

2 *Succinylcholine:* Netilmicin potentiates respiratory depression by succinylcholine

3 *Ticarcillin:* Potential for inactivation of netilmicin in patients with renal failure

3 *Vancomycin:* Additive nephrotoxicity or ototoxicity

2 *Vecuronium:* Netilmicin poten-

N

---

italic = common side effects   ***bold italic*** = life-threatening reactions

tiates respiratory depression by ve-curonium

SPECIAL CONSIDERATIONS
PATIENT/FAMILY EDUCATION
• Inform patient and family about possible toxic effects on the 8th cranial nerve; monitor for dizziness, loss of hearing, ringing or roaring in ears, or feeling of fullness in head
MONITORING PARAMETERS
• Urinalysis for proteinuria, cells, casts; urine output
• Serum peak drawn at 30-60 min after IV inf or 60 min after IM inj, trough level drawn just before next dose; adjust dosage per levels usual therapeutic plasma levels; peak 4-12 µg/ml, trough ≤2 µg/ml
• Serum creatinine for CrCl calculation
• Serum calcium, magnesium, sodium
• Audiometric testing; assess hearing before, during, after treatment

---

nevirapine
(neh-veer´a-peen)
Rx: Viramune
Chemical Class: Dipyridodiaz-epinone derivative
Therapeutic Class: Antiviral

CLINICAL PHARMACOLOGY
Mechanism of Action: Directly reactive non-competitive inhibitor of HIV-1 reverse transcriptase; does not require intracellular phosphorylation; not active against HIV-2 reverse transcriptase
Pharmacokinetics
PO: Onset 15 min, peak 2 hr with 2nd peak at 3-14 hr due to enterohepatic circulation; elimination $t_{1/2}$ 20-40 hr; protein binding 50%-60%; distributed into CNS; metabolized in liver primarily by hydroxylation with enterohepatic recycling; self-induces cytochrome P450 isoenzymes over period of 2 wk; minimal excretion in urine

INDICATIONS AND USES: HIV-1 infection as part of a multidrug treatment regimen

DOSAGE
Adult
• PO 200 mg qd for 14 days, then 200 mg bid in combination with nucleoside analogue antiretroviral agents
• For latest treatment guidelines, see www.hivatis.org

Ⓢ AVAILABLE FORMS/COST OF THERAPY
• Cap—Oral: 200 mg, 100's: **$424.80**

PRECAUTIONS: Stevens-Johnson syndrome, liver disease, CNS disorders

PREGNANCY AND LACTATION: Pregnancy category C; excreted in breast milk, breastfeeding not recommended

SIDE EFFECTS/ADVERSE REACTIONS
CNS: Fatigue (63%), headache (33%), sedation
GI: Diarrhea (37%), increased GGTP levels (10%), nausea (20%)
SKIN: Rash (17%), **Stevens-Johnson syndrome**
MISC: Fever (40%)

INTERACTIONS
Drugs
③ *Clarithromycin:* 26% increase in plasma nevirapine level by clarithromycin; 30% decrease in plasma clarithromycin level by nevirapine; dose adjustment not recommended
③ *Erythromycin:* Mild increase in plasma nevirapine level by erythromycin; dose adjustment not recommended
③ *Indinavir:* 28% decrease in indinavir AUC by nevirapine; dose adjustment not recommended

---

* = non-FDA-approved use

❷ *Ketoconazole:* 63% reduction in plasma ketoconazole level by nevirapine; 15%-30% increase in plasma nevirapine level by ketoconazole; coadministration not recommended

❸ *Methadone:* Marked decrease in methadone level by nevirapine; dose adjustment recommended

❸ *Nelfinavir:* 10% increase in nelfinavir AUC by nevirapine; dose adjustment not recommended

❸ *Rifabutin:* 16% reduction in plasma nevirapine level by rifabutin

❷ *Rifampin:* 37% reduction in plasma nevirapine level by rifampin; coadministration not recommended

❸ *Ritonavir:* 11% decrease in ritonavir AUC by nevirapine; dose adjustment not recommended

❸ *Saquinavir:* 25% decrease in saquinavir AUC by nevirapine; dose adjustment not recommended

❸ *Troleandomycin:* Mild increase in plasma nevirapine level by troleandomycin; dose adjustment not recommended

SPECIAL CONSIDERATIONS
• 2-week lead in period with qd dosing decreases the potential for development of rash; stop therapy in any patient developing a severe rash or rash with constitutional symptoms

MONITORING PARAMETERS
• CBC, ALT, AST, renal function

niacin (vitamin B₃; nicotinic acid)
(nye'a-sin)

Rx: Niacor, Niaspan, Nicolor;
OTC: Nia-Bid, Nia-C, Niacels, Nico-400, Nicotinex, Slo-Niacin

Chemical Class: B complex vitamin
Therapeutic Class: Vitamin; antilipemic

CLINICAL PHARMACOLOGY
Mechanism of Action: Necessary for lipid metabolism, tissue respiration, and glycogenolysis; lowers total serum cholesterol, low-density lipoprotein (LDL) cholesterol and triglyceride concentrations by inhibiting the synthesis of very-low-density lipoproteins (VLDL), which are precursors to the formation of cholesterol; raises high-density lipoprotein (HDL) cholesterol

Pharmacokinetics
PO: Readily absorbed from GI tract; peak 45 min; metabolized in liver, eliminated in urine (almost entirely as metabolites); t₁/₂ 45 min

INDICATIONS AND USES: Vitamin deficiency (pellagra); types IIa, IIb, IV and V, hyperlipidemia as an adjunct to a low-cholesterol diet; to reduce risk of recurrent MI in patients with history of MI and hypercholesterolemia; reduction of atherosclerotic disease in patients with a history of CAD

DOSAGE
Adult
• *Recommended daily allowance PO:* Males 19-50 yr 19 mg/day; males >51 yr 15 mg/day; females 11-50 yr 15 mg/day; females >51 yr 13 mg/day
• *Pellagra:* PO 50-100 mg tid-qid; max 500 mg/day

N

---

italic = common side effects   ***bold italic*** = life-threatening reactions

• *Niacin deficiency:* PO 10-20 mg/day; max 100 mg/day
• *Hyperlipidemia:* PO 1.5-6 g/day divided bid-tid with or after meals (start at 100-250 mg/day and titrate gradually)
Child
• *Recommended daily allowance PO:* 0-0.5 yr 5 mg/day; 0.5-1 yr 6 mg/day; 1-3 yr 9 mg/day; 4-6 yr 12 mg/day; 7-10 yr 13 mg/day; males 11-14 yr 17 mg/day; males 15-18 yr 20 mg/day
• *Pellagra:* PO 50-100 mg tid

💲 **AVAILABLE FORMS/COST OF THERAPY**
• Tab, Uncoated—Oral: 50 mg, 100's: **$1.35-$3.78**; 100 mg, 100's: **$1.04-$3.75**; 500 mg, 100's: **$3.10-$28.17**
• Tab, ER—Oral: 250 mg, 100's: **$2.92-$6.29**; 500 mg, 100's: **$2.96-$53.47**; 750 mg, 100's: **$7.42-$68.92**; 1000 mg, 100's: **$8.25-$92.83**
• Cap, Gel, SUS Action—Oral: 100 mg, 100's: **$1.69**; 125 mg, 100's: **$3.23-$6.15**; 250 mg, 100's: **$2.70-$8.42**; 400 mg, 100's: **$4.03-$74.65**; 500 mg, 100's: **$4.29-$11.21**
• Elixir—Oral: 50 mg/5 ml, 480 ml: **$8.25**

CONTRAINDICATIONS: Hepatic dysfunction, active peptic ulcer, severe hypotension, hemorrhage
PRECAUTIONS: Unstable CAD, gallbladder disease, history of jaundice or liver disease, history of peptic ulcer, history of arterial bleeding, gout, diabetes mellitus, tartrazine sensitivity
PREGNANCY AND LACTATION: Pregnancy category A (category C if used in doses greater than recommended daily allowance); actively excreted in human breast milk; recommended daily allowance during lactation is 18-20 mg

SIDE EFFECTS/ADVERSE REACTIONS
CNS: Transient headache
CV: Atrial fibrillation, hypotension, orthostasis
EENT: Cystoidmacular edema, toxic amblyopia
GI: Abdominal pain, activation of peptic ulcer, diarrhea, *GI distress,* **hepatotoxicity** (more common with sustained-release formulations), *nausea,* vomiting
METAB: Decreased glucose tolerance, hyperuricemia
MS: Myopathy, myositis, ***rhabdomyolysis***
SKIN: Dry skin, keratosis nigricans, *pruritus, sensation of warmth, severe generalized flushing,* skin rash, tingling
INTERACTIONS
Drugs
🔟 *Lovastatin:* Isolated cases of myopathy and rhabdomyolysis have occurred, causality not established
Labs
• *Interference:* Plasma and urine catecholamines, urine glucose with Benedict's reagent
SPECIAL CONSIDERATIONS
• In 1 g doses: 10%-20% reduction of total plus LDL-cholesterol, 30%-70% reduction in triglycerides, and a 20%-35% increase in HDL-cholesterol
• Increased risk of hepatotoxicity with sustained release products
PATIENT/FAMILY EDUCATION
• Gradual dosage titration lessens flushing, adverse effects
• Avoid alcohol and hot beverages (increases flushing)
• Administer with meals and 2 glasses of water
• 125-350 mg of aspirin 20-30 min prior to dose may lessen flushing
• Do not miss any doses (flushing may return)

---

* = non-FDA-approved use

MONITORING PARAMETERS
• Liver function tests, blood glucose, uric acid regularly
• Fasting lipid profile q3-6 mo

---

nicardipine
(nye-card'i-peen)
Rx: Cardene, Cardene SR
Chemical Class: Dihydropyridine
Therapeutic Class: Calcium channel blocker: antihypertensive; antianginal

---

CLINICAL PHARMACOLOGY
Mechanism of Action: Inhibits calcium ion influx across cell membrane in vascular smooth muscle and cardiac muscle; produces relaxation of coronary and peripheral vascular smooth muscle; slight increase in AV conduction; hemodynamics: no effect on myocardial contractility; increases cardiac output; significantly decreases peripheral vascular resistance
Pharmacokinetics
PO: Onset 20 min, peak serum concentration 0.5-2 hr; >95% bound to plasma proteins, significant 1st-pass effect (35% systemic bioavailability); kinetics nonlinear; excreted in urine (60%) and feces (35%); $t_{1/2}$ 8.6 hr (steady state)

INDICATIONS AND USES: Chronic stable angina,* hypertension, Raynaud's disease*
DOSAGE
Adult
• *Angina:* PO 20 mg tid, may increase after 3 days to 40 mg tid
• *Hypertension:* PO 20 mg tid, may increase to 40 mg tid; SR 30 mg bid, may increase to 60 mg bid; IV INF 5 mg/hr initially, may be increased by 2.5 mg/hr q5-15 min up to maximum of 15 mg/hr; following achievement of goal blood pressure, decrease inf rate to 3 mg/hr, then adjust rate as needed to maintain desired response

$ **AVAILABLE FORMS/COST OF THERAPY**
• Cap—Oral: 20 mg, 100's: **$38.81-$44.20;** 30 mg, 100's: **$61.72-$71.09**
• Cap, Gel, SUS Action—Oral: 30 mg, 60's: **$41.92;** 45 mg, 60's: **$66.55;** 60 mg, 60's: **$79.68**
• Inj, Sol—IV: 25 mg/10 ml ampul, **$26.84**
CONTRAINDICATIONS: Advanced aortic stenosis
PRECAUTIONS: CHF,* hypotension, hepatic insufficiency, renal function impairment, aortic stenosis, elderly, children
PREGNANCY AND LACTATION: Pregnancy category C; significant excretion into rat maternal milk
SIDE EFFECTS/ADVERSE REACTIONS
CNS: Anxiety, *asthenia,* depression, *dizziness,* fatigue, *headache,* insomnia, malaise, nervousness, paresthesia, somnolence, tremor
CV: Angina, bradycardia, **dysrhythmia,** hypotension, palpitations, *peripheral edema,* syncope, tachycardia
GI: Abdominal cramps, constipation, diarrhea, dry mouth, flatulence, gastric upset, nausea, vomiting
GU: Nocturia, polyuria
SKIN: Hair loss, pruritus, rash, urticaria
MISC: Cough, epistaxis, flushing, muscle cramps, nasal congestion, sexual dysfunction, shortness of breath, sweating, tinnitus, weight gain
INTERACTIONS
Drugs
3 *Cyclosporine, tacrolimus:* Increased blood cyclosporine concentrations, increased risk of nephrotoxicity
3 *Histamine H$_2$-antagonists:* In-

N

---

italic = common side effects   ***bold italic*** = life-threatening reactions

creased blood levels of nicardipine with cimetidine and ranitidine

3 *Fentanyl:* Severe hypotension or increased fluid volume requirements

3 *Neuromuscular blocking agents:* Prolongation of neuromuscular blockade

---

nicotine

(nik'o-teen)

Rx: *Nasal Spray:* Nicotrol NS; Inhaler: Nicotrol Inhaler
OTC: *Chewing Gum:* Nicorette; *Transdermal:* Nicoderm CQ, Nicotrol, Habitrol
Chemical Class: Pyridine alkaloid
Therapeutic Class: Smoking deterrent

CLINICAL PHARMACOLOGY
Mechanism of Action: Agonist at the nicotinic receptors at the autonomic ganglia in the adrenal medulla, at neuromuscular junctions, and in the brain, producing reinforcing properties: stimulating effect (locus ceruleus)—increased alertness and cognitive performance; reward effect (limbic system); stimulant effects predominate at low doses; at high doses, reward effects predominate

Pharmocokinetics
BUCCAL: Peak 15-30 min, $t_{1/2}$ 30-60 min
TOP: Peak 4-9 hr, $t_{1/2}$ 3-4 hr
NASAL SPRAY: Peak 4-15 min, $t_{1/2}$ 2 hr
INH: 50% bioavailable (absorbed activity); peak 15 min, $t_{1/2}$ 2 hr
<5% bound to plasma proteins, metabolized by liver to cotinine and nicotine-*N*-oxide, eliminated in urine (10%-30% as unchanged drug)
INDICATIONS AND USES: Smoking cessation (temporary adjunct in conjunction with behavior modification), hemidystonia,* ulcerative colitis*

DOSAGE
Adult
• *Gum:* Chew 9-12 pieces of gum (2 mg for regular smokers, 4 mg for heavy smokers) at 1-2 hr intervals daily; do not exceed 80 mg/day; gradually reduce number of pieces/day; use longer than 3 mo is discouraged

• *Transdermal systems:* Apply qd, discard system in use and apply new system at different site; wear for 16 hr (Nicotrol) or 24 hr (Habitrol, Nicoderm CQ, ProStep); initiate therapy at highest available dosage of nicotine for all patients except those weighing <45 kg, those who smoke <10 cigarettes/day, and/or those who have cardiovascular disease (should receive lower initial doses); maintain initial dose for 4-12 wk; reduce doses for 1 or more periods of therapy in patients who have abstained from smoking over next 2-8 wk

• *Nasal spray:* One dose = 1 mg (1 spray in each nostril); individualize dose; 1-2 doses/hr to a max of 5 doses/hr or 40 doses/day; duration of treatment should not exceed 3 months

• *Inhaler:* 10 inhalations provide approx the same amount of nicotine as one puff on average cigarette; continuous puffing × 20 min—6-16 cartridges/day × 12 wk; then gradual tapering over 12 wk; individualize dose to control "urge to smoke"; recommended max cartridges/day:16

$ **AVAILABLE FORMS/COST OF THERAPY**
• Film, CONT REL—Percutaneous: 15 mg/16 hr, 7's: **$24.71-$25.76** (Nicotrol-OTC); 7, 14, 21/24 hr, 7's: **$28.50;** (Nicoderm CQ-OTC); 7, 14,

---

* = non-FDA-approved use

21 mg/24 hr, 30's: **$120.52, $127.22, $133.87,** respectively (Habitrol)
• Tab, Chewing Gum—Buccal: 2 mg, 48's: **$28.50** (Nicorette-OTC); 4 mg, 48's: **$32.07** (Nicorette-OTC)
• Sol—Nasal Spray: 0.5 mg/INH, 10 ml: **$40.80** (Nicotrol NS)
• Aerosol—INH: 10 mg/ml, 10 ml **$40.80**

CONTRAINDICATIONS: Temporomandibular joint disease (chewing gum)

PRECAUTIONS: Cardiovascular disease (history of MI, angina pectoris), serious cardiac dysrhythmias or vasospastic diseases, hypertension, hyperthyroidism, pheochromocytoma, insulin-dependent diabetes; hepatic, renal function impairment; elderly, children, oral or pharyngeal elimination (chewing gum), esophagitis, peptic ulcer disease, skin disease (transdermal), dental problems (chewing gum)

PREGNANCY AND LACTATION: Pregnancy category D; use of nicotine gum during last trimester has been associated with decreased fetal breathing movements; passes freely into breast milk; however, lower concentrations in milk can be expected with transdermal systems than cigarette smoking when used as directed

SIDE EFFECTS/ADVERSE REACTIONS

CNS: Abnormal dreams, confusion, depression, *dizziness,* euphoria, *headache,* impaired concentration, *insomnia,* lightheadedness, *nervousness,* numbness, paresthesia, ***seizures,*** syncope, weakness

CV: Edema, flushing, hypertension, palpitations, tachycardia, ***tachydysrhythmias***

EENT: Pharyngitis, *sinusitis,* tinnitus

GI: Abdominal pain, altered liver function tests, anorexia, aphthous ulcers (chewing gum); *constipation, diarrhea,* dry mouth, *dyspepsia,* eructation secondary to air swallowing, gingivitis, glossitis, jaw ache, *nausea,* stomatitis, *taste perversion,* traumatic injury to oral mucosa or teeth, vomiting

GU: Dysmenorrhea

MS: Arthralgia, *asthenia, back pain, myalgia*

RESP: Breathing difficulty, *cough, hiccups,* hoarseness, sneezing, wheezing

SKIN: Burning at application site, erythema, itching, *pruritus,* rash, sweating, urticaria

INTERACTIONS

Drugs

▣ *Adenosine:* Increased hemodynamic and AV blocking effects of adenosine

▣ *Cimetidine:* Increased blood nicotine concentration, may reduce the amount of gum or patches needed

▣ Coffee, cola: Reduced absorption of nicotine from chewing gum

SPECIAL CONSIDERATIONS
• Drugs that may require dosage reduction with smoking cessation: acetaminophen, caffeine, imipramine, oxazepam, pentazocine, propranolol, theophylline, insulin, prazocin, labetalol
• Drugs that may require an increase in dose with smoking cessation: isoproterenol, phenylephrine

PATIENT/FAMILY EDUCATION
• Chew gum slowly until burning or tingling sensation is felt, then park gum between cheek and gum until tingling sensation goes away
• Chew <30 min/piece
• Avoid coffee and cola drinks while chewing gum or using inhaler
• **Do not smoke while utilizing nicotine replacement therapy**
• Apply new transdermal system daily

N

---

italic = common side effects   ***bold italic*** = life-threatening reactions

• Rotate sites; apply to non-hairy area on upper torso

---

nifedipine
(nye-fed'i-peen)
Rx: Adalat, Adalat CC, Procardia; Procardia XL
Chemical Class: Dihydropyridine
Therapeutic Class: Calcium channel blocker: antihypertensive; antianginal

---

CLINICAL PHARMACOLOGY
Mechanism of Action: Inhibits calcium ion influx across cell membrane in vascular smooth muscle and cardiac muscle; produces relaxation of coronary and peripheral vascular smooth muscle; hemodynamics: decreases myocardial contractility; increases cardiac output; significantly decreases peripheral vascular resistance

Pharmacokinetics
PO: Peak serum concentration 30 min, onset within 20 min (1-5 min if capsule bitten and swallowed)
SUS REL: Peak 6 hr
50%-60% bioavailable, 92%-98% bound to plasma proteins; metabolized by liver to inactive V_d l4-2.2 L/kg metabolites, excreted by kidneys; $t_{1/2}$ 2-5 hr

INDICATIONS AND USES: Vasospastic (Prinzmetal's or variant) angina, chronic stable angina, hypertension, prevention of migraine headache,* preterm labor,* primary pulmonary hypertension,* esophageal disorders,* high altitude pulmonary edema*; Raynaud's disease,* CHF,* cardiomyopathy (diastolic dysfunction)

DOSAGE
Adult
• PO 10 mg tid initially, usual range 10-20 mg tid; doses >120 mg/day

are rarely necessary; PO XL 30-60 mg qd, titration to doses >120 mg/day is not recommended; PO CC 30 mg qd, titration to doses >90 mg/day not recommended

Child
• *Hypertensive urgencies:* PO 0.25-0.5 mg/kg/dose

$ AVAILABLE FORMS/COST OF THERAPY
• Cap, Gel—Oral: 10 mg, 100's: **$15.78-$68.05;** 20 mg, 100's: **$23.17-$122.45**
• Tab, Coated, SUS Action—Oral: 30 mg, 100's: **$112.30-$138.36;** 60 mg, 100's: **$192.43-$239.44;** 90 mg, 100's: **$233.46-$276.26**

CONTRAINDICATIONS: Use of immediate-release preparations in patients with severe obstructive CAD or recent MI, hypertensive emergencies

PRECAUTIONS: CHF, hypotension, hepatic insufficiency, renal function impairment, aortic stenosis, elderly, children, recent β-blocker withdrawal

PREGNANCY AND LACTATION: Pregnancy category C; has been used for tocolysis and as an antihypertensive agent in pregnant women; compatible with breast feeding

SIDE EFFECTS/ADVERSE REACTIONS
(NOTE: Usually less frequent with extended-release preparations)
CNS: Anxiety, asthenia, depression, *dizziness,* fatigue, *headache,* insomnia, malaise, nervousness, paresthesia, somnolence, tremor
CV: Bradycardia, *dysrhythmia, hypotension,* palpitations, *peripheral edema,* syncope, tachycardia
GI: Abdominal cramps, constipation, diarrhea, dry mouth, flatulence, gastric upset, *nausea,* vomiting
GU: Nocturia, polyuria
SKIN: Hair loss, pruritus, rash, urticaria

---

* = non-FDA-approved use

MISC: Cough, epistaxis, *flushing,* muscle cramps, nasal congestion, sexual dysfunction, shortness of breath, sweating, tinnitus, weight gain

INTERACTIONS

Drugs

3 *Barbiturates, rifampin, rifabutin:* Reduced plasma concentrations of nifedipine

3 *Beta-blockers:* Enhanced effects of β-blockers, hypotension; increased metoprolol and propanolol concentrations; additive negative effects on myocardial contractility

3 *Cimetidine, ranitidine, famotidine:* Increased nifedipine concentrations possible

3 *Digitalis glycosides:* Increased digitalis levels; increased risk of toxicity

3 *Diltiazem:* Increased serum concentrations of nifedipine

3 *Doxazosin:* Enhanced hypotensive effects

3 *Fentanyl:* Severe hypotension or increased fluid volume requirements

3 *Food:* Increased absorption of Adalat CC

3 *Grapefruit juice:* Increased serum nifedipine concentrations

3 *Histamine H_2-antagonists:* Increased blood levels of nifedipine with cimetidine

3 *Lansoprazole:* Increased nifedipine absorption

3 *Magnesium:* Potential for transient hypotensive effect

3 *Phenytoin:* Increased phenytoin concentration

3 *Quinidine:* Reduced blood concentrations of quinidine

3 *Vincristine:* Marked increase in vincristine half-life, clinical significance unknown

SPECIAL CONSIDERATIONS

• Given the seriousness of the reported adverse events and the lack of any clinical documentation attesting to a benefit, the use of nifedipine capsules for hypertensive urgencies or emergencies should be abandoned (*JAMA* 1996; 276:1328-1331)

PATIENT/FAMILY EDUCATION

• Administer Adalat CC on an empty stomach

• Do not crush or chew sustained release dosage forms

• Empty Procardia XL tablets may appear in stool, this is no cause for concern

nimodipine
(nye-mode′i-peen)
Rx: Nimotop
Chemical Class: Dihydropyridine
Therapeutic Class: Calcium channel blocker: cerebral vasodilator

CLINICAL PHARMACOLOGY

Mechanism of Action: Inhibits calcium ion influx across membranes of vascular smooth muscle; greater effect on cerebral arteries

Pharmacokinetics

PO: Peak 1 hr; >95% bound to plasma proteins; extensively metabolized in liver to inactive metabolites, excreted in urine (50%) and feces (32%); $t_{1/2}$ 1.7-9 hr

INDICATIONS AND USES: Subarachnoid hemorrhage, acute ischemic stroke,* prevention of migraine headache*

DOSAGE

Adult

• *Subarachnoid hemorrhage:* PO 60 mg q4h for 21 consecutive days beginning within 96 hr of occurrence of hemorrhage, reduce to 30 mg q4h in patients with hepatic failure; for patients unable to swallow oral capsules, the capsule may be punctured at both ends with an 18-gauge nee-

N

dle and the contents emptied directly into nasogastric tube, which is then flushed with 30 ml of normal saline

• *Prevention of migraine headache**
PO 120 mg/day in divided doses; response may not be apparent for 1-2 mo

$ **AVAILABLE FORMS/COST OF THERAPY**

• Cap, Elastic—Oral: 30 mg, 100's: **$647.17**

PRECAUTIONS: Impaired hepatic, renal function; children <18 yr

PREGNANCY AND LACTATION: Pregnancy category C

SIDE EFFECTS/ADVERSE REACTIONS

CNS: Dizziness, headache, lightheadedness, mental depression

CV: ECG abnormalities, edema, flushing, hypotension, palpitations

GI: Constipation, hepatitis, jaundice, lower abdominal discomfort

HEME: Anemia, ***thrombocytopenia***

MS: Muscle pain

RESP: Dyspnea

SKIN: Rash

INTERACTIONS

Drugs

3   *Cimetidine:* Increased serum nimodipine concentrations

3   *Omeprazole:* Increased serum nimodipine concentrations

3   *Valproic acid:* Increased oral bioavailability of nimodipine

SPECIAL CONSIDERATIONS
MONITORING PARAMETERS

• Blood pressure

---

nisoldipine
(nye-sold′i-peen)
Rx: Sular
Chemical Class: Dihydropyridine
Therapeutic Class: Calcium channel blocker: antihypertensive

CLINICAL PHARMACOLOGY
Mechanism of Action: Inhibits calcium ion influx across cell membrane in vascular smooth muscle and cardiac muscle; produces relaxation of coronary and peripheral vascular smooth muscle; hemodynamics: no effect on myocardial contractility and cardiac output; significantly decreases peripheral vascular resistance

Pharmacokinetics
PO: Systemic bioavailability 5% significant 1st pass metabolism; peak serum concentration, 1.5 hr; high-fat meal increases peak concentration by ~300%; highly metabolized in liver, excreted in urine; $t_{1/2}$ 2-14 hr

INDICATIONS AND USES: Hypertension

DOSAGE
Adult

• PO 20 mg qd; may increase by 10 mg/wk or longer intervals to maximum of 60 mg/day

$ **AVAILABLE FORMS/COST OF THERAPY**

• Tab, Coated—Oral: 10, 20, 30, 40 mg, 100's: **$96.38**

PRECAUTIONS: CHF, hypotension, following myocardial infarction, hepatic insufficiency, aortic stenosis, elderly, children

PREGNANCY AND LACTATION: Pregnancy category C

SIDE EFFECTS/ADVERSE REACTIONS

CNS: Anxiety, asthenia, depression, dizziness, fatigue, *headache,* insomnia, malaise, nervousness, paresthesia, somnolence, tremor

CV: Bradycardia, **dysrhythmia,** flushing, hypotension, palpitations, *peripheral edema,* syncope, tachycardia

EENT: Epistaxis, nasal congestion, sore throat, tinnitus

GI: Abdominal cramps, constipation, diarrhea, dry mouth, flatulence, gastric upset, nausea, vomiting

GU: Nocturia, polyuria, sexual dysfunction

MS: Muscle cramps

RESP: Cough, shortness of breath

SKIN: Hair loss, pruritus, sweating, urticaria

MISC: Weight gain

INTERACTIONS

Drugs

3 *Beta-adrenergic blockers:* Increased propranolol concentration

3 *Cimetidine, famotidine, nizatidine, omeprazole, ranitidine:* Increased nisoldipine concentrations possible

3 *Fentanyl:* Severe hypotension or increased fluid volume requirements

3 *Food:* Increased absorption with high-fat meal or grapefruit juice

SPECIAL CONSIDERATIONS

• No significant advantages over other dihydropyridine calcium channel blockers

PATIENT/FAMILY EDUCATION

• Do not take with high-fat meal or grapefruit juice

---

nitrofurantoin

(nye-troe-fyoor′an-toyn)
Rx: Furadantin, Macrodantin
Combinations
  Rx: nitrofurantoin macrocrystals with nitrofurantoin monohydrate (Macrobid)
Chemical Class: Synthetic nitrofuran derivative
Therapeutic Class: Antibiotic

CLINICAL PHARMACOLOGY

Mechanism of Action: May inhibit acetylcoenzyme A, interfering with bacterial carbohydrate metabolism; may also disrupt bacterial cell wall formation; bactericidal in urine at therapeutic doses

Pharmacokinetics

PO: Therapeutic concentrations achieved only in urine, macrocrystalline formulation slows absorption causing less GI irritation, food increases absorption, 60% bound to plasma proteins, partially inactivated in most body tissues, eliminated in urine (30%-50% unchanged), $t_{1/2}$ 20-60 min

INDICATIONS AND USES: UTIs Antibacterial spectrum usually includes:

• Gram-positive organisms: *Staphylococcus aureus, S. saprophyticus, Enterococcus faecalis, Streptococcus agalactiae,* group D streptococci, viridans streptococci, *Corynebacterium*

• Gram-negative organisms: *Citrobacter amalonaticus, C. diversus, C. freundii, Klebsiella oxytoca, K. ozaenae, Enterobacter, Escherichia coli, Neisseria, Salmonella, Shigella*

• NOTE: Not active against *Proteus* spp., *Serratia* spp., or *Pseudomonas* spp.

DOSAGE

Adult

• PO 50-100 mg qid; (Macrobid)

N

---

100 mg bid with food; for long-term suppressive therapy, 50-100 mg qhs

Child >1 mo

• PO 5-7 mg/kg/day divided qid × 1 week; for long-term suppressive therapy 1 mg/kg/day divided qd-bid

💲 AVAILABLE FORMS/COST OF THERAPY

• Cap, Gel—Oral: 25 mg, 100's: **$41.70-$61.08;** 50 mg, 100's: **$58.20-$82.84;** 100 mg, 100's: **$98.50-$142.49**

• CAP—PO: 50 mg, 100's: **$50.84;** 100 mg, 100's: **$127.91** (Macrobid)

• Susp—Oral: 25 mg/5ml, 60 ml: **$21.76** (Susp not macro crystals)

CONTRAINDICATIONS: CrCl <60 ml/min (inadequate antibacterial concentrations achieved in urine), children <1 mo, during labor and delivery (glutathione instability)

PRECAUTIONS: G-6-PD deficiency, renal impairment, anemia, diabetes, electrolyte imbalance, vitamin B deficiency, debilitating disease

PREGNANCY AND LACTATION: Pregnancy category B; compatible with breast feeding in infants >1 mo

SIDE EFFECTS/ADVERSE REACTIONS

CNS: Asthenia, chills, confusion, depression, dizziness, drowsiness, euphoria, headache, nystagmus, peripheral neuropathy (including optic neuritis), psychotic reactions (rare), vertigo

CV: ECG changes

GI: Abdominal pain, anorexia, cholestatic jaundice, chronic active hepatitis, diarrhea, **hepatic necrosis,** hepatitis, *nausea, **pancreatitis,*** parotitis, *vomiting*

GU: Superinfection of GU tract

*HEME: **Agranulocytosis, aplastic anemia,*** eosinophilia, ***granulocytopenia, hemolytic anemia,*** leukopenia, *megaloblastic anemia, **thrombocytopenia***

MS: Arthralgia, myalgia

*RESP: **Acute and chronic pulmonary hypersensitivity reactions*** (dyspnea, chest pain, cough, pulmonary infiltration)

SKIN: Angioedema, ***erythema multiforme, exfoliative dermatitis,*** pruritus, rash, transient alopecia, urticaria

INTERACTIONS

Labs

• *Interference:* Urine alkaline phosphatase, urine lactate dehydrogenase

• *False positive:* Urine glucose (not with glucose enzymatic tests)

• *False increase:* Serum bilirubin, serum creatinine

• *False decrease:* Serum unconjugated bilirubin

SPECIAL CONSIDERATIONS

PATIENT/FAMILY EDUCATION

• Food or milk may decrease GI upset

• May cause brown discoloration of urine

MONITORING PARAMETERS

• Periodic liver function tests during prolonged therapy

• CBC with differential and platelets during prolonged therapy

• Pulmonary review of systems

---

nitrofurazone

(nye-troe-fyoor′a-zone)

Rx: Furacin

Chemical Class: Synthetic nitrofuran derivative

Therapeutic Class: Topical antibiotic

CLINICAL PHARMACOLOGY

Mechanism of Action: Exact mechanism of action unknown; appears to inhibit bacterial enzymes involved in carbohydrate metabo-

---

lism; antibacterial action inhibited by organic matter (e.g., blood, pus, serum) and *p*-aminobenzoic acid

INDICATIONS AND USES: Topical adjunct in 2nd and 3rd degree burns when bacterial resistance is a potential problem; prevention of infection of skin grafts and/or donor sites prior to or following surgery Antibacterial spectrum usually includes:

• *S. aureus, Streptococcus, E. coli, Clostridium perfringens, Aerobacter aerogenes, Proteus* spp.

DOSAGE
Adult and Child
• TOP apply to affected area qd or every few days, depending on dressing technique; apply directly or place on gauze; flushing with sterile saline facilitates removal

💲 AVAILABLE FORMS/COST OF THERAPY
• Oint—Top: 0.2%, 30, 454 g: **$7.58-$91.69**/454 g
• Cre—Top: 0.2%, 28 g: **$19.15**
• Sol—Top: 0.2%, 480 ml: **$14.65-$73.30**

PRECAUTIONS: Renal function impairment (ointment contains polyethylene glycol); children; superinfection with non-susceptible organisms possible; no evidence of efficacy in minor burns, surface bacterial infection involving wounds, cutaneous ulcers, or the various pyodermas

PREGNANCY AND LACTATION: Pregnancy category C; excretion into breast milk unknown

SIDE EFFECTS/ADVERSE REACTIONS
SKIN: Contact dermatitis (rash, pruritus, local edema)

INTERACTIONS
Labs
• *False increase:* Urine creatinine, urine glucose via Benedict's reagent

nitroglycerin
(nye-troe-gli'ser-in)
Rx: *(Translingual): Buccal/ Sublingual/Translingual:* Nitrolingual, Nitroquick, Nitrostat
Oral: Nitro-Bid, Nitrocap TD, Nitrocine, Nitrogard, Nitroglyn, Nitrong, Nitro TD, Nitro-Time
Topical: Nitr-Bid, Nitrol
Transdermal: Deponit, Minitran, Nitrodisc, Nitro-Dur, Transderm-Nitro
IV: Nitro-Bid, Nitrostat IV, Tridil
Chemical Class: Organic nitrate
Therapeutic Class: Vasodilator: antianginal

CLINICAL PHARMACOLOGY
Mechanism of Action: Stimulation of c-GMP production yields vascular smooth muscle relaxation; venous dilation predominates but dose-dependent dilation of arterial beds occurs; dilation of postcapillary vessels promotes venous pooling, decreases venous return to the heart, reducing left ventricular end-diastolic pressure (preload); arteriolar relaxation reduces systemic vascular resistance and arterial pressure (afterload); myocardial oxygen consumption/demand is decreased; blood pressure decreases with reflex tachycardia; dilates coronary arteries and improves collateral flow to ischemic regions
Pharmacokinetics
SL: Onset 1-3 min, peak 4-8 min, duration 30-60 min
LINGUAL SPRAY: Onset 2 min, peak 4-10 min, duration 30-60 min
BUCCAL: Onset 2-5 min, peak 4-10 min, duration 2 hr
PO: Onset 20-45 min, peak 45-120 min, duration 4-8 hr

TOP: Onset 15-60 min, peak 30-120 min, duration 2-12 hr

TRANSDERMAL: Onset 40-60 min, peak 60-180 min, duration 8-24 hr

IV: Onset immediate, peak immediate, duration 3-5 min

60% bound to plasma proteins, metabolized by liver to inorganic nitrate (extensive 1st-pass effect), eliminated in urine; $t_{1/2}$ 1-4 min

INDICATIONS AND USES: Acute angina (SL, translingual spray, buccal), angina prophylaxis (top, transdermal, translingual spray, buccal, oral), perioperative hypertension (IV), congestive heart failure associated with MI (IV), unresponsive angina pectoris (IV), acute MI (SL, top),* Raynaud's disease (top),* hypertensive crisis (IV)*

DOSAGE

Adult

• BUCCAL 1 mg q3-5h while awake initially, titrate dosage upward if angina occurs with tab in place

• PO 2.5-9 mg bid-qid, up to 26 mg qid

• IV 5 µg/min via continuous inf, increase by 5 µg/min q3-5 min to 20 µg/min; if no response, increase by 10 µg/min q3-5 min up to 200 µg/min

• TOP 1-2 inches q8h, up to 4-5 inches q4h

• TRANSDERMAL 0.2-0.4 mg/hr initially, titrate to 0.4-0.8 mg/hr; apply new patch daily; tolerance is minimized by removing patch for 10-12 hr/day

• SL 0.2-0.6 mg q5 min for max of 3 doses in 15 min; may also use prophylactically 5-10 min prior to activities that provoke angina attack

• TRANSLINGUAL 1-2 sprays under tongue q3-5 min for max of 3 doses in 15 min; may also use prophylactically 5-10 min prior to activities that provoke angina attack

Child

• IV 0.25-0.5 µg/kg/min, titrate by 0.5-1 µg/kg/min q3-5 min prn; usual dose 1-3 µg/kg/min; max 20 µg/kg/min

§ AVAILABLE FORMS/COST OF THERAPY

• Aer Spray—Oral: 0.4 mg/spray, 14.49 g: **$31.23**

• Tab—SL: 0.3 mg, 100's: **$7.42-$8.34**; 0.4 mg, 100's: **$7.42-$18.18** 0.6 mg, 100's: **$7.42-$8.34**

• Tab, Uncoated, SUS Action—Buccal: 2 mg, 100's: **$42.10**; 3 mg, 100's: **$45.50**

• Cap, Gel, SUS Action—Oral: 2.5 mg, 100's: **$6.00-$11.45**; 6.5 mg, 100's: **$7.35-$17.38**; 9 mg, 100's: **$8.25-$18.69**

• Oint—Percutaneous: 2%; 1, 3, 30, 60 g: **$8.50-$16.33**/60 g

• Inj, Sol—IV: 5 mg/ml, 10 ml: **$12.72-$47.63**

• Transdermal: 0.1 mg/hr, 30's: **$45.10-$50.15**; 0.2 mg/hr, 30's: **$33.06-$61.84**; 0.4 mg/hr, 30's: **$39.33-$68.52**; 0.6 mg/hr, 30's: **$50.50-$64.66**; 0.8 mg/hr, 30's: **$60.32**

CONTRAINDICATIONS: Severe anemia, closed-angle glaucoma, postural hypotension, early MI (SL), head trauma, cerebral hemorrhage, hypotension or uncorrected hypovolemia, inadequate cerebral circulation, increased intracranial pressure, constrictive pericarditis, pericardial tamponade (IV)

PRECAUTIONS: Early days of MI, hypertrophic cardiomyopathy; severe hepatic, renal disease; children, glaucoma, abrupt withdrawal, continuous delivery (tolerance develops rapidly, IV excepted)

PREGNANCY AND LACTATION: Pregnancy category C; use of SL for angina during pregnancy without fetal harm has been reported

* = non-FDA-approved use

SIDE EFFECTS/ADVERSE REACTIONS

CNS: Agitation, anxiety, apprehension, confusion, *dizziness,* dyscoordination, *headache,* hypoesthesia, hypokinesia, insomnia, nervousness, nightmares, restlessness, vertigo, weakness

CV: Atrial fibrillation, ***collapse,*** crescendo angina, ***dysrhythmias,*** palpitations, *postural hypotension,* premature ventricular contractions, rebound hypertension, retrosternal discomfort, syncope, tachycardia

EENT: Blurred vision

GI: Abdominal pain, diarrhea, dyspepsia, fecal incontinence, nausea, tenesmus, tooth disorder, vomiting

GU: Dysuria, impotence, urinary frequency

HEME: ***Hemolytic anemia, methemoglobinemia***

MS: Arthralgia

SKIN: Allergic reactions (ointment), contact dermatitis (transdermal), crusty skin lesions, *cutaneous vasodilation with flushing,* ***exfoliative dermatitis,*** pallor, pruritus, rash, sweating

INTERACTIONS

Drugs

❷ *Ergot alkaloids:* Opposition to coronary vasodilatory effects of nitrates

❸ *Ethanol:* Additive vasodilation could cause hypotension

❸ *Metronidazole:* Ethanol contained in IV nitroglycerine preparations could cause disulfiram-like reaction in some patients

❸ *Sildenafil:* Excessive hypotensive effects

Labs

• *False increase:* Serum triglycerides

SPECIAL CONSIDERATIONS

• 10-12 hr drug-free intervals prevent development of tolerance

PATIENT/FAMILY EDUCATION

• Avoid alcohol
• Notify clinician if persistent headache occurs
• Take oral nitrates on empty stomach with full glass of water
• Keep tablets and capsules in original container, keep container closed tightly
• Dissolve SL tablets under tongue, lack of burning does not indicate loss of potency, use when seated, take at 1st sign of anginal attack, activate emergency response system if no relief after 3 tablets spaced 5 min apart
• Spray translingual spray onto or under tongue, do not inhale spray
• Place buccal tablets under upper lip or between cheek and gum, permit to dissolve slowly over 3-5 min, do not chew or swallow
• Spread thin layer of ointment on skin using applicator or dose-measuring papers, do not use fingers, do not rub or massage
• Apply transdermal systems to nonhairy area on upper torso, remove for 10-12 hr/day (usually hs)

MONITORING PARAMETERS

• Blood pressure, heart rate at peak effect times

N

---

nitroprusside
(nye-troe-pruss'ide)
Rx: Nitropress
Chemical Class: Cyanonitrosylferrate derivative
Therapeutic Class: Antihypertensive

CLINICAL PHARMACOLOGY

Mechanism of Action: Relaxes vascular smooth muscle and dilates peripheral arteries and veins; more active on veins than arteries; reduces left ventricular end-diastolic pressure and pulmonary capillary wedge

---

italic = common side effects   ***bold italic*** = life-threatening reactions

pressure (preload); reduces systemic vascular resistance, systolic arterial pressure, and mean arterial pressure (afterload); dilates coronary arteries

Pharmacokinetics

IV: Onset immediate; rapidly metabolized by interaction with sulfhydryl groups in erythrocytes and tissues (cyanogen is produced and converted to thiocyanate in liver), eliminated via urine (metabolites); circulating $t_{1/2}$ 2 min

INDICATIONS AND USES: Hypertensive crisis, controlled hypotension during surgery, severe refractory congestive heart failure (in combination with dopamine),* acute MI*

DOSAGE

Adult

• IV INF 2 µg/kg/min initially, increase in increments of 2-4 µg/kg/min (up to 20 µg/kg/min), then in increments of 10-20 µg/kg/min; cyanide toxicity more likely when >500 µg/kg is administered by prolonged infusion (>8 hr) of greater than 20 µg/kg/min

Child

• IV INF 1 µg/kg/min initially, increase in increments of 1 µg/kg/min at intervals of 20-60 min; do not exceed 10 µg/kg/min

🖫 AVAILABLE FORMS/COST OF THERAPY

• Inj, Lyphl-Sol—IV: 50 mg/2 ml: **$9.80-$10.38**

CONTRAINDICATIONS: Decreased cerebral perfusion, arteriovenous shunt or coarctation of the aorta (i.e., compensatory hypertension), congenital (Leber's) optic atrophy, tobacco amblyopia

PRECAUTIONS: Hepatic disease, decreased renal function, prolonged infusion, elevated intracranial pressure, anemia, hypovolemia, poor surgical risks, hypothyroidism, hyponatremia

PREGNANCY AND LACTATION: Pregnancy category C

SIDE EFFECTS/ADVERSE REACTIONS

CNS: Apprehension, *dizziness, headache,* increased intracranial pressure

CV: Bradycardia, ECG changes, hypotension, palpitations, retrosternal discomfort, tachycardia

GI: Abdominal pain, ileus, nausea, retching

HEME: Decreased platelet aggregation, *methemoglobinemia*

METAB: Hypothyroidism

MS: Muscle twitching

SKIN: Diaphoresis, flushing, irritation at INF site, rash

MISC: **Thiocyanate or cyanide toxicity**

INTERACTIONS

Drugs

3 *Clonidine:* Severe hypotensive reactions have been reported

3 *Diltiazem:* Reduction in the dose of nitroprusside required to produce hypotension

3 *Guanabenz, guanfacine:* Potential for severe hypotensive reactions

SPECIAL CONSIDERATIONS
MONITORING PARAMETERS

• Blood pressure, arterial blood gases, oxygen saturation, cyanide and thiocyanate concentrations, anion gap, lactate levels

---

nizatidine
(ni-za'ti-deen)
Rx: Axid
OTC: Axid AR
Chemical Class: Ethenediamine derivative
Therapeutic Class: Gastrointestinal antiulcer agent

CLINICAL PHARMACOLOGY
Mechanism of Action: Competitive, reversible inhibitor of hista-

mine at gastric H_2-receptors; reduces gastric acid secretion

Pharmacokinetics

PO: Onset 30-60 min, peak 0.5 to 3 hr, duration 4-8 hr, oral bioavailability 70%; protein binding 35%; metabolized in liver, 60% of drug excreted unchanged in urine, 6% eliminated in feces; $t_{1/2}$ 1-2 hr

INDICATIONS AND USES: Short-term treatment of duodenal and benign gastric ulcers; maintenance therapy for duodenal ulcer; gastroesophageal reflux disease (GERD); heartburn, acid indigestion, sour stomach due to overindulgence (OTC); gastritis*

DOSAGE

Adult

• *Heartburn, acid indigestion, sour stomach due to overindulgence:* PO 75 mg bid (OTC)

• *Active duodenal or benign gastric ulcer:* PO 300 mg hs or 150 mg bid × 4-8 wk

• *Maintenance of healed duodenal ulcer:* PO 150 mg hs

• *Gastroesophageal reflux disease:* PO 150 mg bid

• *Dosage adjustment for renal insufficiency (active ulcer disease),* CrCl 20-50 ml/min, 150 mg qd; CrCl <20 ml/min, 150 mg qod

$ **AVAILABLE FORMS/COST OF THERAPY**

• Cap, Gel—Oral: 75 mg, 30's: **$8.99 (OTC);** 150 mg, 100's: **$169.64;** 300 mg, 30's: **$95.75**

PRECAUTIONS: Renal insufficiency

PREGNANCY AND LACTATION: Pregnancy category B; excreted in breast milk (0.1% of dose)

SIDE EFFECTS/ADVERSE REACTIONS

CNS: Dizziness, drowsiness, headache

CV: Bradycardia, palpitation, tachycardia

EENT: Rhinitis

GI: Constipation, diarrhea, flatulence, hepatitis, nausea

HEME: Anemia, ***thrombocytopenia***

METAB: Gynecomastia, hyperuricemia

MS: Myalgia

SKIN: Acne, pruritus, sweating, urticaria

INTERACTIONS

Drugs

3 *Cefpodoxime, cefuroxime; enoxacin; ketoconazole:* Reduction in gastric acidity reduces absorption, decreases plasma levels, potential for therapeutic failure

3 *Glipizide, glyburide tolbutamide:* Increased absorption of these drugs, potential for hypoglycemia

3 *Nifedipine; Nitrendipine; nisoldipine:* Increased concentrations of these drugs

SPECIAL CONSIDERATIONS

• No advantage over other agents of this class, base selection on cost

PATIENT/FAMILY EDUCATION

• Stagger doses of nizatidine and antacids

---

norepinephrine

(nor-ep-i-nef′rin)

Rx: Levophed

Chemical Class: Synthetic catecholamine

Therapeutic Class: α- & β-Adrenergic sympathomimetic; vasopressor

CLINICAL PHARMACOLOGY

Mechanism of Action: Stimulates β_1- and α-adrenergic receptors causing increased myocardial contractility and heart rate as well as vasoconstriction; increases blood pressure and coronary artery blood flow; marked pressor effect primarily due to increased peripheral resistance

Pharmacokinetics

IV: Onset rapid, duration 1-2 min after INF discontinued; metabolized in liver and other tissues by monoamine oxidase (MAO) and catechol-*O*-methyltransferase (COMT) to inactive metabolites; pharmacologic action terminated mainly by uptake and metabolism in sympathetic nerve endings; excreted in urine (metabolites)

INDICATIONS AND USES: Acute hypotensive states, adjunct in treatment of cardiac arrest and profound hypotension

DOSAGE

Adult

• IV INF 8-12 µg/min; initiate at 4 µg/min and titrate to desired response

Child

• IV INF 0.05-0.1 µg/kg/min initially, titrate to desired effect

§ AVAILABLE FORMS/COST OF THERAPY

• Inj, Sol—IV: 0.1%, 4 ml: **$16.63-$23.63**

CONTRAINDICATIONS: Hypotension from blood volume deficits (except as an emergency measure until volume replacement can be completed), mesenteric or peripheral vascular thrombosis, cyclopropane and halothane anesthesia

PRECAUTIONS: Atherosclerosis, arteriosclerosis, diabetic endarteritis, Buerger's disease, elderly, extravasation (may cause necrosis and sloughing of surrounding tissue), sulfite sensitivity

PREGNANCY AND LACTATION: Pregnancy category D

SIDE EFFECTS/ADVERSE REACTIONS

CNS: Anxiety, *headache*

CV: Bradycardia, **cardiac dysrhythmias,** *chest pain,* hypertension, palpitations, tachycardia

EENT: Photophobia

GI: Nausea, vomiting

RESP: Respiratory distress

SKIN: Diaphoresis, gangrene, necrosis and sloughing following extravasation, pallor

MISC: Organ ischemia (due to vasocontriction of renal and mesenteric arteries)

INTERACTIONS

Drugs

❷ *Amitriptyline, desipramine, imipramine, protriptyline:* Marked enhancement of pressor response to norepinephrine

❸ *Guanadrel, guanethidine:* Exaggerated pressor response to norepinephrine

❸ *MAOIs:* Slight increase in the pressor response to norepinephrine

❸ *Methyldopa:* Prolongation of the pressor response to norepinephrine

SPECIAL CONSIDERATIONS

• Antidote for extravasation ischemia: infiltrate with 10-15 ml of saline containing 5-10 mg of phentolamine

MONITORING PARAMETERS

• Blood pressure, heart rate, ECG, urine output, peripheral perfusion

---

norethindrone

(nor-eth'in-drone)

Rx: Micronor, Nor-Q.D.

Acetate: **Rx:** Aygestin

Combinations

Rx: with ethinyl estradiol (see oral contraceptives)

Chemical Class: 19-nortestosterone derivative

Therapeutic Class: Progestin; contraceptive

CLINICAL PHARMACOLOGY

Mechanism of Action: Exerts a progestational effect on the endometrium, alters cervical mucus, suppresses ovulation in some patients, renders the endometrium hostile to implantation

Pharmacokinetics

PO: 80% bound to plasma proteins; metabolized in liver; $t_{1/2}$ 10 hr

INDICATIONS AND USES: Prevention of conception, secondary amenorrhea, abnormal uterine bleeding, endometriosis, prevention of endometrial hyperplasia during postmenopausal estrogen therapy

DOSAGE

Adult and Adolescents

• *Amenorrhea and abnormal uterine bleeding:* PO 2.5-10 mg acetate on days 5-25 of menstrual cycle **or** to induce optimum secretory transformation of estrogen-primed endometrium 2.5-10 mg of acetate for 5-10 days during the latter half of menstrual cycle

• *Endometriosis:* PO 5 mg acetate qd for 14 consecutive days; increase by 2.5 mg/day at 14 day intervals until max 15 mg/day is reached; daily therapy may then be continued consecutively (no drug-free intervals) for 6-9 mo

• *Contraception:* PO 0.35 mg qd beginning on first day of menses

• *Prevention of endometrial hyperplasia in conjunction with estrogen:* 5 mg × 10-13 days/mo

💲 AVAILABLE FORMS/COST OF THERAPY

• Tab, Uncoated—Oral: 0.35 mg, 28's: **$31.92-$33.48**

• Tab, Uncoated (acetate)—Oral: 5 mg, 100s: **$132.42**

CONTRAINDICATIONS: Active thrombophlebitis or thromboembolic disorders, cerebral hemorrhage, impaired liver function or disease, breast cancer, undiagnosed vaginal bleeding, missed abortion, use as a diagnostic test for pregnancy

PRECAUTIONS: Asthma, cardiac or renal dysfunction, depression, diabetes, epilepsy, migraine

PREGNANCY AND LACTATION: Pregnancy category X; compatible with breast feeding

SIDE EFFECTS/ADVERSE REACTIONS

CNS: Depression, dizziness, fatigue, headache

CV: Edema

GI: Anorexia, *cholestatic jaundice,* cramps, increased weight, *nausea,* vomiting

GU: Amenorrhea, breakthrough bleeding, spotting, breast changes, dysmenorrhea, endometriosis

METAB: Hyperglycemia

SKIN: Acne, alopecia, hirsutism, melasma, rash

SPECIAL CONSIDERATIONS

PATIENT/FAMILY EDUCATION

• Missed dose: one tablet—Take as soon as remembered, or take 2 tablets at next regular time

Missed 2 consecutive tablets— take 2 tablets at next 2 regular times

Three missed tablets—Discontinue, restart after menses appear or pregnancy is ruled out

Note: Use an additional method of contraception if 2 or more tablets are missed until menses appear or pregnancy ruled out

• Progestin only pills have slightly higher failure rate than combination oral contraceptives

• When used as contraceptive, menstrual cycle may be disrupted and irregular and unpredictable bleeding or spotting may result

N

---

italic = common side effects   ***bold italic*** = life-threatening reactions

norfloxacin

(nor-flox'a-sin)

Rx: Noroxin; (Ophthalmic): Chibroxin

Chemical Class: Fluoroquinolone derivative

Therapeutic Class: Antibiotic

CLINICAL PHARMACOLOGY

Mechanism of Action: Interferes with the enzyme DNA gyrase needed for the synthesis of bacterial DNA; bactericidal

Pharmacokinetics

PO: Peak 1-2 hr; 10%-15% bound to plasma proteins; partially metabolized, excreted in urine (60%) and feces (30%); $t_{1/2}$ 3-4 hr

INDICATIONS AND USES: Complicated and uncomplicated UTIs, uncomplicated gonorrhea (urethral, cervical), conjunctivitis (ophth), gastroenteritis,* travelers' diarrhea* Antibacterial spectrum usually includes:

• Gram-positive organisms: *Enterococcus faecalis, Staphylococcus aureus, S. epidermidis, S. saprophyticus, Streptococcus agalactiae*

• Gram-negative organisms: *Citrobacter freundii, Enterobacter aerogenes, E. cloacae, Escherichia coli, Klebsiella pneumoniae, Neisseria gonorrhoeae, Proteus mirabilis, P. vulgaris, Pseudomonas aeruginosa, Serratia marcescens*

Conjunctivitis due to *Acinetobacter calcoaceticus,* Aeromonas hydrophila,* Haemophilus influenzae, Proteus mirabilis,* Serratia marcescens,* Staphylococcus aureus, Staphylococcus epidermidis, Staphylococcus warnerii,* Streptococcus pneumoniae*

DOSAGE

Adult

• *Urinary tract infection:* PO 400 mg bid on an empty stomach for 3-10 days (uncomplicated) or 10-21 days (complicated)

• *Gonorrhea:* PO 800 mg as a single dose followed by doxycycline 100 mg bid for 7 days

• *Gastroenteritis:* PO 400 mg bid for 5 days

• *Travelers' diarrhea:* PO 400 mg bid for up to 3 days until symptoms resolve

• Dosage in renal impairment, administer 400 mg qd in patients with CrCl <30 ml/min/1.73 m^2

• *Conjunctivitis:* Ophth 1 drop qid

▧ AVAILABLE FORMS/COST OF THERAPY

• Sol—Ophth: 0.3%, 5 ml: **$20.01**

• Tab, Plain Coated—Oral: 400 mg, 20's: **$62.73**

PRECAUTIONS: Children (potential for arthropathy and osteochondrosis), elderly, renal disease, seizure disorders, dehydration (potential for crystalluria)

PREGNANCY AND LACTATION: Pregnancy category C; excretion into breast milk unknown; due to the potential for arthropathy and osteochondrosis use extreme caution in nursing mothers

SIDE EFFECTS/ADVERSE REACTIONS

CNS: Anxiety, depression, dizziness, fatigue, headache, insomnia, *seizures,* somnolence

EENT: Visual disturbances

GI: Abdominal pain, anorexia, diarrhea, dry mouth, flatulence, heartburn, increased AST, ALT; *nausea, pseudomembranous colitis,* vomiting

GU: Crystalluria

HEME: Eosinophilia, *leukopenia*

SKIN: Photosensitivity, pruritus, rash

INTERACTIONS

Drugs

▤ *Aluminum:* Reduced absorption

of norfloxacin; do not take within 4 hr of dose

3 *Antacids:* Reduced absorption of norfloxacin; do not take within 4 hr of dose

3 *Antipyrine:* Inhibits metabolism of antipyrine; increased plasma antipyrine level

3 *Caffeine:* Inhibits metabolism of caffeine; increased plasma caffeine level

3 *Calcium:* Reduced absorption of norfloxacin; do not take within 4 hr of dose

3 *Diazepam:* Inhibits metabolism of diazepam; increased plasma diazepam level

3 *Didanosine:* Markedly reduced absorption of norfloxacin; take norfloxacin 2 hr before didanosine

3 *Foscarnet:* Coadministration increase seizure risk

3 *Iron:* Reduced absorption of norfloxacin; do not take within 4 hr of dose

3 *Magnesium:* Reduced absorption of norfloxacin; do not take within 4 hr of dose

3 *Metoprolol:* Inhibits metabolism of metoprolol; increased plasma metoprolol level

3 *Pentoxifylline:* Inhibits metabolism of pentoxifylline; increased plasma pentoxifylline level

3 *Phenytoin:* Inhibits metabolism of phenytoin; increased plasma phenytoin level

3 *Propranolol:* Inhibits metabolism of propranolol; increased plasma propranolol level

3 *Ropinirole:* Inhibits metabolism of ropinirole; increased plasma ropinirole level

3 *Sodium bicarbonate:* Reduced absorption of norfloxacin; do not take within 4 hr of dose

3 *Sucralfate:* Reduced absorption of norfloxacin; do not take within 4 hr of dose

3 *Theobromine:* Inhibits metabolism of theobromine; increased plasma theobromine level

3 *Theophylline:* Inhibits metabolism of theophylline; cut maintenance theophylline dose in half during therapy with norfloxacin

3 *Warfarin:* Inhibits metabolism of warfarin; increases hypoprothrombinemic response to warfarin

3 *Zinc:* Reduced absorption of norfloxacin; do not take within 4 hr of dose

Labs

• *False increase:* Uroporphyrin

SPECIAL CONSIDERATIONS
PATIENT/FAMILY EDUCATION

• Administer on an empty stomach (1 hr before or 2 hr after meals)

• Drink fluids liberally

• Do not take antacids containing magnesium or aluminum or products containing iron or zinc within 4 hr before or 2 hr after dosing

• Avoid excessive exposure to sunlight

N

---

norgestrel
(nor-jess′trel)
Rx: Ovrette, Plan B
Combinations
   Rx: with ethinyl estradiol
   (see oral contraceptives)
Chemical Class: 19-nortestosterone derivative
Therapeutic Class: Progestin; contraceptive

CLINICAL PHARMACOLOGY
Mechanism of Action: Exerts a progestational effect on the endometrium, alters cervical mucus, suppresses ovulation in some patients, renders the endometrium hostile to implantation

Pharmacokinetics
PO: 93%-95% bound to plasma pro-

---

italic = common side effects   ***bold italic*** = life-threatening reactions

teins; metabolized in liver, excreted in urine and feces; $t_{1/2}$ 11-45 hr

INDICATIONS AND USES: Prevention of conception; emergency contraception* (morning-after pill)

DOSAGE

Adult

• *Contraception:* PO 0.075 mg qd beginning on 1st day of menses

• *Emergency contraception:* 2 doses, 1st dose within 72 hr of unprotected intercourse, 2nd dose 12 hr later:

FORMULATION	TABLETS/DOSE
Norgestrel 0.5 mg + ethinyl estradiol 50 mcg (Ovral)	2
Levonorgestrel 0.15 mg or norgestrel 0.3 mg + ethinyl estradiol 30 mcg (Nordette, Lo/Ovral, Levlen, Levora)	4
Norgestrel 0.075 mg (Ovrette)	20
Norgestrel 0.75 mg (Plan B)	1

$ AVAILABLE FORMS/COST OF THERAPY

• Tab, Uncoated—Oral: 0.075 mg, 28's: **$30.85**; 0.75 mg, 2's: **$21.95**

CONTRAINDICATIONS: Active thrombophlebitis or thromboembolic disorders, cerebral hemorrhage, impaired liver function or disease, breast cancer, undiagnosed vaginal bleeding, missed abortion, use as a diagnostic test for pregnancy

PRECAUTIONS: Epilepsy, migraine, asthma, cardiac or renal dysfunction, depression, diabetes

PREGNANCY AND LACTATION: Pregnancy category X; compatible with breast feeding

SIDE EFFECTS/ADVERSE REACTIONS

CNS: Depression, dizziness, fatigue, headache, migraines

CV: Edema

GI: Anorexia, *cholestatic jaundice,* cramps, increased weight, *nausea,* vomiting

GU: Amenorrhea, breakthrough bleeding, breast changes, dysmenorrhea, spotting

METAB: Hyperglycemia

SKIN: Acne, alopecia, hirsutism, melasma, rash

SPECIAL CONSIDERATIONS PATIENT/FAMILY EDUCATION

• Missed dose: One tablet—Take as soon as remembered, take next tablet at regular time; Two consecutive tablets—Take 1 of the missed tablets, discard the other

Three missed tablets—Discontinue Use an additional method of contraception if 2 or more tablets are missed until menses appear or pregnancy ruled out.

• Progestin only pills have slightly higher failure rate than combination oral contraceptives

• Take with food if GI upset occurs

• Menstrual cycle may be disrupted and irregular and unpredictable bleeding or spotting can result

• Based on WHO study, preferred emergency contraception; equal efficacy and 50% less nausea, vomiting compared to combined regimen

nortriptyline

(nor-trip'ti-leen)

Rx: Aventyl, Pamelor

Chemical Class: Dibenzocycloheptene derivative: secondary amine

Therapeutic Class: Tricyclic antidepressant

CLINICAL PHARMACOLOGY

Mechanism of Action: Inhibits reuptake of norepinephrine and serotonin (blocking activity moderate and high, respectively) at the presynaptic neuron prolonging neuronal activity; inhibits histamine and acetylcholine activity; mild peripheral vasodilator effects and possible "quinidine-like" actions on cardiac

* = non-FDA-approved use

conduction, moderate anticholinergic and sedative, slight orthostatic hypotensive side effects

Pharmacokinetics

PO: Peak 7-8.5 hr; 93%-95% bound to plasma proteins; metabolized in liver, excreted in urine, small amounts excreted in bile; $t_{1/2}$ 28-31 hr

INDICATIONS AND USES: Depression, panic disorder,* premenstrual depression,* dermatologic disorders (chronic urticaria and angioedema, nocturnal pruritis in atopic eczema),* nocturnal enuresis*

DOSAGE

Adult

• PO 25 mg qhs initially, increase at 3-5 day increments to 75-150 mg/day divided qd-qid

Elderly and Adolescents

• PO 30-50 mg/day in divided doses

Child

• *Nocturnal enuresis:* PO, 6-7 yr 10 mg/day; 8-11 yr 10-20 mg/day; >11 yr 25-35 mg/day

[$] AVAILABLE FORMS/COST OF THERAPY

• Cap, Gel—Oral: 10 mg, 100's: **$38.65-$58.55;** 25 mg, 100's: **$77.20-$116.83;** 50 mg, 100's: **$145.55-$220.15;** 75 mg, 100's: **$221.36-$335.57**

• Sol—Oral: 10 mg/5 ml, 480 ml: **$42.95-$67.17/480 ml**

CONTRAINDICATIONS: Acute recovery phase of MI, concurrent use of MAOIs

PRECAUTIONS: Suicidal patients, convulsive disorders, prostatic hypertrophy, psychiatric disease, severe depression, increased intraocular pressure, narrow-angle glaucoma, urinary retention, cardiac disease, hepatic disease, renal disease, hyperthyroidism, electroshock therapy, elective surgery, elderly, abrupt discontinuation

PREGNANCY AND LACTATION: Pregnancy category D; effect on nursing infant unknown but may be of concern, especially after prolonged exposure

SIDE EFFECTS/ADVERSE REACTIONS

CNS: Anxiety, confusion (especially in elderly), *dizziness,* extrapyramidal symptoms (elderly), fatigue, headache, increased psychiatric symptoms, insomnia, memory impairment, nervousness, nightmares, panic, *seizures,* stimulation, tremors, weakness

CV: **Dysrhythmias,** ECG changes, hypertension, *orthostatic hypotension,* palpitations, syncope, tachycardia

EENT: Blurred vision, mydriasis, nasal congestion, ophthalmoplegia, tinnitus

GI: Constipation, cramps, diarrhea, *dry mouth,* epigastric distress, hepatitis, increased appetite, jaundice, nausea, paralytic ileus, stomatitis, vomiting

GU: Urinary retention

HEME: **Agranulocytosis,** eosinophilia, **leukopenia, thrombocytopenia**

SKIN: Photosensitivity, pruritus, rash, sweating, urticaria

INTERACTIONS

Drugs

[3] *Anticholinergics:* Excessive anticholinergic effects

[3] *Barbiturates:* Reduced serum concentrations of cyclic antidepressants

[3] *Carbamazepine, rifampin:* Reduced cyclic antidepressant serum concentrations

[3] *Chlorpropamide:* Enhanced by hypoglycemic effects of chlorpropamide

[3] *Cimetidine:* Increased serum nortriptyline concentrations

[3] *Clonidine:* Reduced antihyper-

N

---

italic = common side effects   **bold italic** = life-threatening reactions

tensive response to clonidine; enhanced hypertensive response with abrupt clonidine withdrawal

❷ *Epinephrine:* Markedly enhanced pressor response to IV epinephrine

❸ *Ethanol:* Additive impairment of motor skills; abstinent alcoholics may eliminate cyclic antidepressants more rapidly than nonalcoholics

❸ *Fluoxetine:* Marked increases in cyclic antidepressant plasma concentrations

❷ *Guanethidine:* Inhibited antihypertensive response to guanethidine

❷ *Moclobemide:* Potential association with fatal or non-fatal serotonin syndrome

⚠ *MAOIs:* Excessive sympathetic response, mania or hyperpyrexia possible

❸ *Neuroleptics:* Increased therapeutic and toxic effects of both drugs

❷ *Norepinephrine:* Markedly enhanced pressor response to norepinephrine

❸ *Phenylephrine:* Enhanced pressor response to IV phenylephrine

❸ *Propoxyphene:* Enhanced effect of cyclic antidepressants

❸ *Quinidine:* Increased cyclic antidepressant serum concentrations

Labs

• *False increase:* Serum carbamazepine

SPECIAL CONSIDERATIONS
PATIENT/FAMILY EDUCATION

• Therapeutic effects may take 2-3 wk

• Avoid rising quickly from sitting to standing, especially elderly

• Avoid alcohol and other CNS depressants

• Do not discontinue abruptly after long-term use

• Wear sunscreen or large hat to prevent sunburn

MONITORING PARAMETERS

• CBC, weight, ECG, mental status (mood, sensorium, affect, suicidal tendencies)

• Determination of nortriptyline plasma concentrations is not routinely recommended but may be useful in identifying toxicity, drug interactions, or noncompliance (adjustments in dosage should be made according to clinical response not plasma concentrations), therapeutic range 50-150 ng/ml

nystatin

(nye-stat'in)
Rx: (Troche): Mycostatin; (Oral): Mycostatin, Nilstat, Nystex
(Topical): Mycostatin, Nystex, Nystop, Pedi-Dry
Combinations
Rx: (Topical) with triamcinolone (Mycolog-II, Mycomer, Mycasone, Myco Biotic II, Tri-Statin II, Mytrex, Myco-Triacet II, Mycogen II)

Chemical Class: Amphoteric polyene macrolide
Therapeutic Class: Antifungal

CLINICAL PHARMACOLOGY
Mechanism of Action: Binds to sterols in the fungal cell membrane, which results in loss of potassium and other cellular constituents; fungicidal/static

Pharmacokinetics

PO: Poorly absorbed; excreted almost entirely in feces as unchanged drug

TOP: Not absorbed from intact skin or mucous membranes

INDICATIONS AND USES: Cutaneous, mucocutaneous, and oral cavity candidal infections; candidal vulvovaginitis; intestinal candidiasis

DOSAGE

Adult

• *Oral candidiasis:* PO 400,000-600,000 U susp, swish and swallow qid; Troche 200,000-400,000 U 4-5 times/day

• *Cutaneous candidal infections:* Top apply ointment, cream, or powder to affected area tid-qid

• *Intestinal candidal infections:* PO 500,000-1,000,000 U q8h

• *Vaginal candidal infections:* Insert 1-2 vaginal tablets qhs for 2 wk

Child

• *Oral candidiasis:* PO 200,000 U qid or 100,000 U to each side of mouth qid

• *Cutaneous candidal infections:* Top apply ointment, cream, or powder to affected area tid-qid

Neonate

• *Oral candidiasis:* PO 100,000 U qid or 50,000 U to each side of mouth qid

💲 AVAILABLE FORMS/COST OF THERAPY

• Cre—Top: 100,000 U/g 15, 30 g: **$2.17-$24.74**/30 g

• Oint—Top: 100,000 U/g, 15, 30 g: **$3.00-$20.86**/30 g

• Powder—Top: 100,000 U/g, 15 g: **$25.41**

• Susp—Oral: 100,000 U/ml, 60, 480 ml: **$3.12-$24.00**/60 ml

• Tab, Plain Coated—Oral: 500,000 U, 100's: **$11.93-$62.00**

• Cap, Gel—Oral: 1,000,000 U 100's: **$43.75;** 300,000 U 100's: **$12.95;** 500,000 U 100's: **$30.00**

• Lozenge—Oral: 200,000 U 30's: **$31.40**

• Tab, Uncoated—Vag: 100,000 U, 15's: **$10.63-$32.31**

PREGNANCY AND LACTATION: Pregnancy category A/C; due to poor bioavailability, serum and breast milk levels do not occur

SIDE EFFECTS/ADVERSE REACTIONS

GI: Diarrhea, GI distress, nausea, vomiting

SKIN: Burning, rash, stinging, urticaria

SPECIAL CONSIDERATIONS

PATIENT/FAMILY EDUCATION

• Do not use troches in child <5 yr

---

octreotide

(ok-tree'oh-tide)

Rx: Sandostatin, Sandostatin Lar Depot

Chemical Class: Somatostatin analog

Therapeutic Class: Antidiarrheal; acromegaly agent

CLINICAL PHARMACOLOGY

Mechanism of Action: Actions similar to somatostatin; inhibits growth hormone, glucagon, and insulin more than somatostatin; suppresses LH response to gonadotropin releasing hormone; decreases splanchnic blood flow; inhibits release of serotonin, gastrin, vasoactive intestinal peptide (VIP), secretin, motilin, and pancreatic polypeptide

Pharmacokinetics

SC: Onset 0.4 hr, duration 12 hr; IV and SC doses bioequivalent; 65% protein bound; elimination $t_{1/2}$ 1.7 hr; metabolized by liver, 32% of dose excreted unchanged in urine; in dialysis patients, clearance is half of normals

INDICATIONS AND USES: Acromegaly, carcinoid syndrome (associated with metastatic carcinoid tumors), vasoactive intestinal peptide tumors (VIPomas), insulinoma,* HIV-associated secretory diarrhea,* cryptosporidiosis in HIV-infected persons,* control of bleeding esoph-

O

---

ageal varices,* irritable bowel syndrome,* dumping syndrome*
DOSAGE
Adult
• *Acromegaly:* SC or IV 0.05-0.1 mg tid
• *Carcinoid syndrome:* SC or IV 0.1-0.6 mg/day in 2-4 divided doses (mean daily dosage is 0.3 mg; max daily dose 1.5 mg)
• *VIPomas:* SC or IV 0.2-0.3 mg/day in 2-4 divided doses (range 0.15-0.75 mg)
• *HIV-associated diarrhea:* SC or IV 0.15-1.8 mg/day in 2-4 divided doses
• *Bleeding esophageal varices:* IV 0.05-0.1 mg bolus then 0.025-0.05 mg/hr continuous INF; 0.1 mg q8h as adjunct to sclerotherapy
Child
• SC 0.001-0.01 mg/kg/day in 2-4 divided doses
• For IV use, may be diluted in 50-200 ml of D_5NS and given IV over 15-30 min or given by IV push over 3 min

💲 **AVAILABLE FORMS/COST OF THERAPY**
• Inj, Sol—IV: 10 mg: **$1368.75;** 20 mg: **$1368.75;** 30 mg: **$2053.12**
• Inj, Sol—SC: 0.05 mg/ml, 1 ml: **$121.44;** 0.1 mg/ml, 1 ml: **$235.54;** 0.5 mg/ml, 1 ml: **$1136.08**

PRECAUTIONS: Gallbladder disease (stones or sludge in 48% of patients treated for 12 mo; in 2% of patients treated for 1 mo); may affect glycemic control in diabetics
PREGNANCY AND LACTATION: Pregnancy category B; breast milk excretion unknown
SIDE EFFECTS/ADVERSE REACTIONS
CNS: Dizziness, fatigue, headache, weakness
CV: Bradycardia (21% in acromegalies), conduction abnormalities, dysrhythmias

GI: Abdominal discomfort, *constipation,* diarrhea, distension, flatulence, nausea, *pancreatitis,* vomiting
HEME: Vitamin B_{12} deficiency
METAB: Goiter, hyperglycemia, hypoglycemia, *hypothyroidism*
MS: Bell's palsy, leg cramps
SKIN: Alopecia
MISC: Local pain on inj
SPECIAL CONSIDERATIONS:
MONITORING PARAMETERS
• Thyroid function, serum glucose (especially in drug-treated diabetics), vitamin B_{12} levels
• Heart rate (especially in persons taking β-blockers and calcium channel blockers)

---

ofloxacin

(o-flox'a-sin)
Rx: (Oral): Floxin;
(Ophthalmic): Ocuflox
Chemical Class: Fluoroquinolone derivative
Therapeutic Class: Antibiotic

CLINICAL PHARMACOLOGY
Mechanism of Action: Interferes with the enzyme DNA gyrase needed for the synthesis of bacterial DNA; bactericidal
Pharmacokinetics
PO: Peak 1-2 hr; 98% oral bioavailability; 32% bound to plasma proteins; excreted primarily unchanged in urine; $t_{1/2}$ 5-10 hr
INDICATIONS AND USES: Lower respiratory tract infections, uncomplicated urethral and cervical gonorrhea; non-gonococcal urethritis; cervicitis; skin and skin structure infections, UTIs, prostatitis; superficial ocular infections involving the conjunctiva or cornea (ophthalmic preparation)
Antibacterial spectrum usually includes:
• Gram-positive organisms: *Staph-*

---

* = non-FDA-approved use

ylocaccus aureus, S. epidermidis, S. saprophyticus, Enterococcus faecalis

• Gram-negative organisms: *Acinetobacter* spp., *Aeromonas* spp., *Campylobacter* spp., *Citrobacter* spp., *Enterobacter* spp., *Escherichia coli, Haemophilus influenzae, H. parainfluenzae, Klebsiella pneumoniae, Klebsiella* spp., *Legionella* spp., *Listeria monocytogenes, Moraxella catarrhalis, Morganella morganii, Neisseria gonorrhoeae, N. meningitidis, Plesiomonas shigelloides, Proteus mirabilis, P. vulgaris, Providencia rettgeri, P. stuartii, Pseudomonas aeruginosa, P. fluorescens, Salmonella* spp., *Serratia* spp., *Shigella* spp., *Vibrio* spp., *Xanthomonas maltophilia, Yersinia enterocolitica*

DOSAGE

Adult

• *Lower respiratory tract infections:* PO/IV 400 mg q12h for 10 days

• *Uncomplicated gonorrhea:* PO 400 mg as a single dose plus doxycycline 100 mg bid for 7 days

• *Nongonococcal urethritis, cervicitis:* PO/IV 300 mg q12h for 7 days

• *Skin and skin structure infections:* PO/IV 400 mg q12h for 10 days

• *UTI:* PO/IV 200 mg q12h for 3-10 days

• *Prostatitis:* PO/IV 300 mg q12h for 6 wk (do not continue IV therapy for >10 days, switch to PO)

• *Renal function impairment:* CrCl 10-50 ml/min use 24 hr dosage interval; CrCl <10 ml/min, 50% of recommended dose given q24h

• *Superficial ocular infections:* Ophth 1 gtt q2-4h for 1st 2 days, then qid for additional 5 days

Child >1 yr

• *Superficial ocular infections:* Ophth 1 gtt q2-4h for 1st 2 days, then qid for additional 5 days

💲 AVAILABLE FORMS/COST OF THERAPY

• Inj, Sol—IV: 40 mg/ml, 10 ml: **$26.40**

• Sol—Ophth: 0.3%, 5, 10 ml: **$25.58**/5 ml

• Tab, Plain Coated—Oral: 200 mg, 100's: **$346.20;** 300 mg, 100's: **$412.00;** 400 mg, 100's: **$434.52**

PRECAUTIONS: Children (potential for arthropathy and osteochondrosis), elderly, renal disease, seizure disorders

PREGNANCY AND LACTATION: Pregnancy category C; excreted into breast milk in quantities approximating maternal plasma concentrations; due to the potential for arthropathy and osteochondrosis, use extreme caution in nursing mothers

SIDE EFFECTS/ADVERSE REACTIONS

CNS: Anxiety, depression, dizziness, fatigue, headache, insomnia, *seizures,* somnolence

EENT: Dizziness, visual disturbances

GI: Abdominal pain, anorexia, diarrhea, dry mouth; flatulence, heartburn, increased AST, ALT; *nausea, pseudomembranous colitis,* vomiting

SKIN: Photosensitivity, pruritus, rash

INTERACTIONS

Drugs

3 *Aluminum:* Reduced absorption of ofloxacin; do not take within 4 hr of dose

3 *Antacids:* Reduced absorption of ofloxacin; do not take within 4 hr of dose

3 *Calcium:* Reduced absorption of ofloxacin; do not take within 4 hr of dose

3 *Iron:* Reduced absorption of ofloxacin; do not take within 4 hr of dose

3 *Magnesium:* Reduced absorption of ofloxacin; do not take within 4 hr of dose

---

italic = common side effects   ***bold italic*** = life-threatening reactions

3 *Procainamide:* Ofloxacin competitively inhibits renal tubular excretion of procainamide

3 *Sodium bicarbonate:* Reduced absorption of ofloxacin; do not take within 4 hr of dose

3 *Sucralfate:* Reduced absorption of ofloxacin; do not take within 4 hr of dose

3 *Warfarin:* Inhibits metabolism of warfarin; increases hypoprothrombinemic response to warfarin

3 *Zinc:* Reduced absorption of ofloxacin; do not take within 4 hr of dose

Labs

• *False increase:* Uroporphyrin

SPECIAL CONSIDERATIONS
PATIENT/FAMILY EDUCATION

• Administer on an empty stomach (1 hr before or 2 hr after meals)

• Drink fluids liberally

• Do not take antacids containing magnesium or aluminum or products containing iron or zinc within 4 hr before or 2 hr after dosing

• Avoid excessive exposure to sunlight

---

olanzapine
(oh-lan'za-peen)

Rx: Zyprexa

Chemical Class: Thienbenzodiazepine derivative

Therapeutic Class: Antipsychotic

CLINICAL PHARMACOLOGY

Mechanism of Action: Serotonin 5-HT$_2$ > dopamine-(D$_2$-) receptor antagonist; activity against several neurotransmitter systems: selective antagonist at limbic dopamine receptors (D$_1$, D$_2$, D$_4$, D$_5$) and serotonin receptors (5-HT$_2$, 5-HT$_6$, 5-HT$_7$); antagonism at α-$_1$-adrenergic receptors; and activity at muscarinic, histamine H$_1$, or nicotinic receptors; high sedation and anticholinergic effects; moderate orthostatic hypotension and weight gain risk; minimal risk of extrapyramidal symptoms

Pharmacokinetics

PO: Peak 6 hr, extensive first pass metabolism (40%), absorption unaffected by food; 93% bound to plasma proteins; highly metabolized by the liver; excreted in urine (57%) and feces (30%); t$_{1/2}$ 30 hr (21-54 hr)

INDICATIONS AND USES: Management of psychotic disorders

DOSAGE

Adult

• PO 5-10 mg qd; dosage may be increased in 5 mg/day increments if needed in intervals not <1 wk; maximum 20 mg/day; initiate with 5 mg qd in debilitated patients

$ **AVAILABLE FORMS/COST**
OF THERAPY

• Tab, Film-coated—Oral: 2.5 mg, 60's: **$280.70;** 5 mg, 7.5 mg, 60's: **$331.54;** 10 mg, 60's: **$504.02**

PRECAUTIONS: Hepatic function impairment; children <18 yr; history of myocardial infarction, heart failure, cardiac conduction abnormalities; cerebrovascular disease; seizure disorders; patients at risk for aspiration pneumonia; prostatic hypertrophy, narrow-angle glaucoma, history of paralytic ileus

PREGNANCY AND LACTATION: Pregnancy category C; excretion into human breast milk unknown; excreted in the milk of treated rats

SIDE EFFECTS/ADVERSE REACTIONS

CNS: Agitation, akathisia, amnesia, *anxiety,* articulation impairment, *dizziness,* euphoria, *headache, hostility,* hypertonia, *insomnia, nervousness, somnolence,* stuttering, tardive dyskinesia, tremor

CV: Chest pain, edema, hypotension, *postural hypotension,* tachycardia

---

* = non-FDA-approved use

EENT: Amblyopia, blepharitis, pharyngitis, *rhinitis*

GI: Abdominal pain, *constipation, dry mouth,* increased appetite, transaminase elevations

GU: Premenstrual syndrome

METAB: Weight gain

MS: Back pain, joint pain, twitching

SKIN: Rash

MISC: Fever, ***neuroleptic malignant syndrome***

INTERACTIONS

Drugs

3 *Carbamazepine:* Decreased olanzapine concentrations

3 *Levodopa:* Antagonism of the effects of levodopa due to dopamine receptor blockade

PATIENT/FAMILY EDUCATION

• Avoid exposure to extreme heat

MONITORING PARAMETERS

• Periodic assessment of liver transaminases in patients with significant hepatic disease

---

olopatadine
(oh-loe-pa-ta′deen)

Rx: Patanol

Chemical Class: Propilidinedibenzoxypin derivative

Therapeutic Class: Antihistamine

CLINICAL PHARMACOLOGY

Mechanism of Action: Selective histamine H_1-receptor antagonist; leukotriene B4 antagonist; inhibits histamine release from mast cells; also inhibits platelet-activating factor, IgE, and antigen-induced effects; devoid of alpha-adrenergic, dopaminergic, muscarinic type 1 and 2, and serotonergic effects

Pharmacokinetics

OPHTHAL: Low systemic exposure; excreted 60-70% in urine unchanged; $t_{1/2}$ 3 hr

INDICATIONS AND USES: Allergic conjunctivitis

DOSAGE

Adult and Child >3 yr

• INSTILL 1 gtt bid, in q6-8h intervals

§ AVAILABLE FORMS/COST OF THERAPY

• Sol—Ophth: 0.1%, 5 ml: **$50.00**

PRECAUTIONS: Should not be instilled while wearing contact lenses

PREGNANCY AND LACTATION: Pregnancy category C; excreted into milk after oral administration; doubtful ocular administration could result in sufficient quantities to produce detectable quantities

SIDE EFFECTS/ADVERSE REACTIONS

EENT: Blepharedema, burning, foreign body sensation, hyperemia, keratitis, pruritis, stinging, xerophthalmia

SPECIAL CONSIDERATIONS

• Combination effects: both inhibits mast cell degranulation (like cromolyn) and antagonizes histamine receptor (antihistamine); appears effective and well-tolerated for the topical treatment of allergic conjunctivitis from limited clinical data; compare with other topical ophthalmic and oral antihistamines

---

olsalazine
(ohl-sal′ah-zeen)

Rx: Dipentum

Chemical Class: Salicylate derivative

Therapeutic Class: GI anti-inflammatory agent

CLINICAL PHARMACOLOGY

Mechanism of Action: Bioconverted by colonic bacteria to 5-aminosalicylic acid (mesalamine), which may act by blocking cyclooxygenase and inhibiting pros-

---

italic = common side effects   ***bold italic*** = life-threatening reactions

taglandin production in the colon; local, mucosal anti-inflammatory effect in patients with chronic inflammatory bowel disease

Pharmacokinetics

PO: Limited systemic bioavailability (2.4% of 1 g dose absorbed); peak 1 hr; >99% bound to plasma proteins; <1% recovered in urine; serum $t_{1/2}$ 0.9 hr

INDICATIONS AND USES: Maintenance of remission of ulcerative colitis in patients intolerant of sulfasalazine

DOSAGE

Adult

• PO 1 g/day in 2 evenly divided doses

💲 **AVAILABLE FORMS/COST OF THERAPY**

• Cap, Gel—Oral: 250 mg, 100's: **$89.94**

PRECAUTIONS: Children, preexisting renal disease

PREGNANCY AND LACTATION: Pregnancy category C; mesalamine has produced adverse effects in a nursing infant and should be used with caution during breast feeding, observe nursing infant closely for changes in stool consistency

SIDE EFFECTS/ADVERSE REACTIONS

CNS: Depression, drowsiness, headache

GI: Anorexia, bloating, *cramping, diarrhea,* dyspepsia, nausea, stomatitis, vomiting

MS: Arthralgia

SKIN: Itching, rash

SPECIAL CONSIDERATIONS
PATIENT/FAMILY EDUCATION

• Take with food. Notify clinician if diarrhea occurs

MONITORING PARAMETERS

• BUN, urinalysis, serum creatinine in patients with pre-existing renal disease

---

omeprazole
(om-eh-pray′zole)

Rx: Prilosec

Chemical Class: Benzimidazole derivative

Therapeutic Class: Gastrointestinal antisecretory agent

CLINICAL PHARMACOLOGY

Mechanism of Action: Irreversibly inactivates proton pump in gastric parietal cells, which blocks the final step in secretion of hydrochloric acid; acid secretion is inhibited until additional enzyme is synthesized; inhibits basal and stimulated gastric acid secretion

Pharmacokinetics

PO: Peak 0.5-3½ hr; 95% bound to plasma proteins; metabolized in liver to inactivate metabolites, excreted in urine (77%) and feces (23%); $t_{1/2}$ ½-1 hr (does not reflect duration of acid suppression)

INDICATIONS AND USES: Active duodenal ulcer; short-term treatment of active benign gastric ulcers, in combination with clarithromycin for the treatment of *H. pylori;* gastroesophageal reflux disease (GERD) (including maintenance therapy); erosive esophagitis (including maintenance therapy); pathological hypersecretory conditions (e.g., Zollinger-Ellison syndrome, multiple endocrine adenomas, systemic mastocytosis); NSAID-induced ulcer*; posterior laryngitis*; treatment of steatorrhea in cystic fibrosis patients (enhances efficacy of pancreatic enzymes)

DOSAGE

Adult

• *Active duodenal ulcer:* PO 20 mg qd for 4-8 wk

• *H. Pylori:* PO 20 mg bid in combination with clarithromycin 500 mg

---

* = non-FDA-approved use

bid and amoxicillin 1 g bid for 7 days (other regimens have also been used)
• *Gastric ulcer:* PO 40 mg qd for 4-8 wk
• *GERD:* PO 20 mg qd for 4-8 wk
• *Maintenance of healing in erosive esophagitis:* 10-20 mg qd
• *Pathological hypersecretory conditions:* PO 60 mg qd initially, doses up to 120 mg tid have been administered (administer doses >80 mg/day in divided doses)

💲 **AVAILABLE FORMS/COST OF THERAPY**
• Cap, Gel, SUS Action—Oral: 10 mg, 100's: **$346.68;** 20 mg, 100's: **$386.99;** 40 mg, 100's: **$594.00**

PRECAUTIONS: Not for maintenance therapy of duodenal ulcer or GERD; elderly; children; symptomatic response does not preclude gastric malignancy

PREGNANCY AND LACTATION: Pregnancy category C; suppression of gastric acid secretion is potential effect in nursing infant, clinical significance unknown

SIDE EFFECTS/ADVERSE REACTIONS
CNS: Asthenia, dizziness, headache
GI: Abdominal pain, constipation, diarrhea, flatulence, nausea
MS: Back pain
RESP: Cough
SKIN: Rash

INTERACTIONS
Drugs
🔳 *Carbamazepine, diazepam, digoxin, glipizide, glyburide, nifedipine, nimodipine, nisoldipine, nitrendipine:* Increased concentrations of these drugs
🔳 *Cefpodoxime, cefuroxime, enoxacin, ketoconazole:* Decreased concentrations of these drugs
🔳 *Glipizide, glyburide, tolbutamide:* Increased absorption of these drugs, potential of hypoglycemia

🔳 *Methotrexate:* Case report of elevated methotrexate concentration
🔳 *Phenytoin:* Increased phenytoin concentration

SPECIAL CONSIDERATIONS
• Some patients on maintenance therapy may respond to 10 mg qd or 20 mg qod

PATIENT/FAMILY EDUCATION
• Take before eating
• Swallow capsule whole; do not open, chew, or crush

---

ondansetron
(on-dan-seh′tron)
Rx: Zofran, Zofran ODT
Chemical Class: Carbazole derivative
Therapeutic Class: Antiemetic

CLINICAL PHARMACOLOGY
Mechanism of Action: Selectively blocks the action of serotonin at 5-HT_3 receptors; cytotoxic chemotherapy appears to be associated with release of serotonin from enterochromaffin cells of the small intestine which may stimulate vagal afferents through 5-HT_3 receptors, initiating the vomiting reflex

Pharmacokinetics
IV: Peak immediate
PO: Peak 1.7-2 hr; bioavailability 56%
70%-76% bound to plasma proteins; extensively metabolized, excreted in urine and feces (metabolites); $t_{1/2}$ 4 hr (2-3 hr in children <15 yr; 5.5 hr in adults >75 yr)

INDICATIONS AND USES: Prevention of nausea and vomiting associated with emetogenic cancer chemotherapy, total body irradiation, and postoperative nausea and vomiting

---

italic = common side effects   **bold italic** = life-threatening reactions

DOSAGE

Adult

• *Emetogenic chemotherapy:* PO 8 mg 30 min before chemotherapy, repeat 8 hr after initial dose; then bid for 1-2 days after completion of chemotherapy; IV 0.15 mg/kg/dose infused 30 min before start of chemotherapy, repeat 4 and 8 hr after initial dose, or single 32 mg dose beginning 30 min before chemotherapy

• *Total body irradiation:* PO 8 mg 1-2 hr before each fraction of radiotherapy administered qd

• *Postoperative nausea or vomiting:* IV 4 mg over ≥30 sec immediately prior to induction of anesthesia or postoperatively; PO 16 mg as a single dose 1 hr prior to induction of anesthesia

Child

• PO 4 mg 30 min before chemotherapy, repeat 4 and 8 hr after initial dose then tid for 1-2 days after completion of chemotherapy; IV 0.15 mg/kg/dose infused 30 min before start of chemotherapy, repeat 4 and 8 hr after initial dose

💲 AVAILABLE FORMS/COST OF THERAPY

• Inj, Sol—IV: 2 mg/ml, 20 ml: **$244.43;** 32 mg/50 ml, 50 ml: **$206.41**

• Sol—Oral: 4 mg/5 ml, 50 ml: **$155.30**

• Tab Coated—Oral: 4 mg, 3's: **$45.72;** 8 mg, 3's: **$76.14**

• Tab ODT (dissolving)—Oral: 4 mg, 3's: **$45.72;** 8 mg, 3's: **$76.14**

PRECAUTIONS: Abdominal surgery (may mask ileus or gastric distension), children ≤3 yr

PREGNANCY AND LACTATION: Pregnancy category B; has been used in the treatment of hyperemesis gravidarum

SIDE EFFECTS/ADVERSE REACTIONS

CNS: Headache, lightheadedness, ***seizures***

CV: Angina, bradycardia, syncope, tachycardia

EENT: Blurred vision

GI: Constipation, diarrhea, transient elevation in liver enzymes

METAB: Hypokalemia

RESP: ***Bronchospasm***

SKIN: Rash

---

opium

(oh'pee-um)

Rx: Opium Tincture Combinations

   Rx: with belladonna alkaloids (B&O Suppositories)

Chemical Class: Natural alkaloid

Therapeutic Class: Narcotic analgesic; antidiarrheal

DEA Class: Schedule II

CLINICAL PHARMACOLOGY

Mechanism of Action: Narcotic agent with some activity at Mu receptors (supraspinal analgesia, euphoria, respiratory and physical depression, miosis, and reduced GI motility), Kappa receptors (pentazocine-like spinal analgesia, sedation, and miosis), and Delta receptors (dysphoria, psychotomimetic effects [e.g., hallucinations], and respiratory and vasomotor stimulation caused by drugs with antagonist activity); standard pharmacologic comparator for analgesic, antitussive, constipation, respiratory depression, sedation, emesis, and phyiscal dependence effects

GI: Decreases gastric motility; decreases biliary, pancreatic, and intestinal secretions and delays digestion of food in the small intestine;

resting tone increases and periodic spasms occur; decreases propulsive peristaltic waves in the large intestine; constricts sphincter of Oddi

Pharmacokinetics

PO: Variably absorbed from GI tract; metabolized in liver, excreted in urine

INDICATIONS AND USES: Symptomatic treatment of diarrhea; relief of severe pain in place of morphine; narcotic abstinence syndrome suppressant in neonates*

DOSAGE

Adult

• PO (tincture) 0.6 ml qid

Child

• PO (tincture) for diarrhea 0.005-0.01 ml/kg/dose q3-4h; for analgesia 0.01-0.02 ml/kg/dose q3-4h

$ AVAILABLE FORMS/COST OF THERAPY

• Tincture—Oral: 10%, 118 ml: **$53.00**

CONTRAINDICATIONS: Acute bronchial asthma, upper airway obstruction, glaucoma, respiratory depression, acute alcoholism, delerium tremens, premature labor

PRECAUTIONS: Head injury, increased intracranial pressure, acute abdominal conditions, elderly, severe impairment of hepatic or renal function, hypothyroidism, Addison's disease, prostatic hypertrophy, urethral stricture, history of drug abuse; seizure disorder

PREGNANCY AND LACTATION: Pregnancy category B (category D if used for prolonged periods or in high doses at term); compatible with breast feeding

SIDE EFFECTS/ADVERSE REACTIONS

CNS: Agitation, dependency, dizziness, *drowsiness,* lethargy, restlessness, *sedation*

CV: Bradycardia, orthostatic hypotension, palpitations, tachycardia

GI: Anorexia, constipation, dry mouth, *nausea, vomiting*

GU: Urinary retention

RESP: **Respiratory depression, respiratory paralysis**

SKIN: Flushing, rash, urticaria

INTERACTIONS

Drugs

▣ *Barbiturates:* Additive CNS depression

▣ *Cimetidine:* Increased effect of narcotic analgesics

▣ *Ethanol:* Additive CNS effects

▣ *Neuroleptics:* Hypotension and excessive CNS depression

Labs

• *False increase:* Amylase and lipase

SPECIAL CONSIDERATIONS

• Opium has been replaced by safer, more effective analgesics and sedative/hypnotics for diagnostic or operative medication; useful as an antidiarrheal

• Do not administer agonist/antagonist analgesics (i.e., pentazocine, nalbuphine, butorphanol, dezocine, buprenorphine) to patient who has received a prolonged course of opium (a pure agonist). In opioid-dependent patients, mixed agonist/antagonist analgesics may precipitate withdrawal symptoms

PATIENT/FAMILY EDUCATION

• Drug may be addictive if used for prolonged periods

O

---

italic = common side effects   ***bold italic*** = life-threatening reactions

oral contraceptives (combined)

Monophasic: **Rx:** Alesse, Brevicon, Demulen 1/35, Demulen 1/50, Desogen, Genora 0.5/35, Genora 1/35, Genora 1/50, Jenest-28, Levite, Levlen, Levora, Loestrin Fe 1/20, Loestrin Fe 1.5/30, Lo/Ovral, Low-Ogestrel, Modicon, Necon 1/50, Nelova 0.5/35, Nelova 1/35, Nelova 1/50, Nordette, Norethin 1/35, Norethin 1/50, Norinyl 1+35, Norinyl 1+50, Ortho-Cept, Ortho-Cyclen, Ortho-Novum 1/35, Ortho-Novum 1/50, Ovcon-35, Ovcon-50, Ovral, Zovia 1/35E, Zovia 1/50E

Biphasic: **Rx:** Necon 10/11, Ortho-Novum 10/11, Mircette

Triphasic: **Rx:** Ortho-Novum 7/7/7, Ortho Tri-Cyclen, Tri-Levlen, Tri-Norinyl, Triphasil

Chemical Class: Synthetic estrogen/progestin combinations

Therapeutic Class: Contraceptives

CLINICAL PHARMACOLOGY

Mechanism of Action: Inhibit ovulation by suppressing the gonadotropins, FSH and LH; alter cervical mucus (inhibiting sperm penetration) and endometrium (reducing likelihood of implantation)

Pharmacokinetics

• *Estrogens*

PO: Ethinyl estradiol (EE) peak 1.3 hr; mestranol demethylated to ethinyl estradiol (slight delay in subsequent peak, 1.9 hr); 98% bound to plasma proteins; metabolized in liver; excreted in urine and bile; undergoes some enterohepatic recirculation; $t_{1/2}$ 13-27 hr

• *Progestins*

PO: Bound both to albumin (79%-95%) and sex hormone-binding globulin; metabolized in liver, excreted in urine and bile; $t_{1/2}$ norethindrone 5-14 hr, levonorgestrel 11-45 hr; desogestrel metabolite 38±20 hr, norgestimate metabolite 12-30 hr

INDICATIONS AND USES: Prevention of pregnancy; emergency contraception (postcoital contraception or "morning after" pill)*; dysmenorrhea*; dysfunctional uterine bleeding,* endometriosis*

DOSAGE

Adult and Adolescent

• *21-day regimen:* PO 1 tab qd for 21 days beginning (a) 1st Sunday after menstruation begins or (b) day 5 of cycle, or (c) day 1 of cycle (consult instructions on dispensers or packs); no tabs are taken for next 7 days (withdrawal flow will normally occur about 3 days following last tab)

• *28-day regimen:* PO 1 tab qd for 28 days continuously beginning (a) 1st Sunday after menstruation begins, or (b) day 5 of cycle, or (c) day 1 of cycle (consult instructions on dispensers or packs); start new pack of tabs after completing 28-day course

• *Emergency contraception:* 2 doses, 1st dose within 72 hr of unprotected intercourse; 2nd dose 12 hr later:

FORMULATION	TABLETS/DOSE
Norgestrel 0.5 mg + ethinyl estradiol 50 µg (Ovral)	2
Levonorgestrel 0.15 mg or norgestrel 0.3 mg + ethinyl estradiol 30 µg (Nordette, Lo/Ovral, Levlen, Levora)	4

• Norgestrel-only regimens preferred because of less nausea and vomiting with equal efficacy (see Norgestrel)

---

* = non-FDA-approved use

💲 AVAILABLE FORMS/COST OF THERAPY

• Tab, Uncoated—Oral: 0.035 mg EE/1 mg ethynodiol diacetate, 28's: **$27.05** (Demulen 1/35, Zovia 1/35E); 0.05 mg/1 mg, 28's: **$30.07** (Demulen 1/50, Zovia 1/50E)

• Tab, Uncoated—Oral: 0.03 mg EE/0.15 mg levonorestrel, 28's: **$28.92** (Levora, Nordette, Levlen); 0.03 mg/0.05, 0.075, 0.125 mg, 28's: **$26.72** (Tri-Levlen, Triphasil); 0.02 mg/0.1 mg, 28's: **$28.68** (Alesse, Levite)

• Tab, Uncoated—Oral: 0.035 mg EE/0.5, 1 mg norethindrone, 28's: **$13.97-$25.36** (Necon 10/11, Ortho-Novum 10/11, Jenest-28); 0.035 mg/0.5 mg, 28's: **$22.38-$31.45** (Nelova 0.5/35E, Brevicon, Modicon, Genora 0.5/35); 0.035 mg/1mg, 28's: **$1.33-$28.83** (Norinyl 1+35, Genora 1/35, Nelova 1/35E, Ortho-Novum 1/35, N.E.E. 1/35, Norethin 1/35E); 0.035 mg/0.4 mg, 28's: **$31.00** (Ovcon-35); 0.05 mg/1 mg, 28's: **$39.30** (Ovcon-50); 0.035 mg/0.5, 1, 0.5 mg, 28's: **$25.72** (Tri-Norinyl); 0.035 mg/0.5, 0.75, 1 mg, 28's: **$28.83** (Ortho-Novum 7/7/7)

• Tab, Uncoated—Oral: 0.02 mg EE/1 mg norethindrone acetate, 28's: **$29.39** (Loestrin Fe 1/20); 0.03 mg/1.5 mg, 28's: **$29.39** (Loestrin Fe 1.5/30)

• Tab, Uncoated—Oral: 0.03 mg EE/0.3 mg norgestrel, 28's: **$28.74-$30.61** (Lo/Ovral, Low-Ogestrel); 0.05 mg/0.5 mg, 28's: **$46.86** (Ovral)

• Tab, Uncoated—Oral: 0.035 mg EE/0.25 mg norgestimate, 28's: **$28.06** (Ortho-Cyclen); 0.035 mg/0.18, 0.215, 0.25 mg, 28's: **$28.70** (Ortho Tri-Cyclen)

• Tab, Uncoated—Oral: 0.03 mg EE/0.15 mg desogestrel, 28's: **$24.88-$28.83** (Desogen, Ortho-Cept); .02 mg EE/.01 mg EE/ 0.15 mg desogestrel, 28's: **$28.60** (Mircette)

• Tab, Uncoated—Oral: 0.05 mg mestranol/1 mg norethindrone, 28's: **$16.40-$28.83** (Genora 1/50, Nelova 1/50M, Necon 1/50, Ortho-Novum 1/50, Norinyl 1/50)

CONTRAINDICATIONS: Thrombophlebitis, thromboembolic disorders, history of deep vein thrombophlebitis, cerebrovascular disease, MI, CAD, known or suspected breast carcinoma or estrogen-dependent neoplasia, carcinoma of endometrium; hepatic adenomas, carcinomas; past or present angina pectoris, undiagnosed abnormal vaginal bleeding, cholestatic jaundice

PRECAUTIONS: Hypertension, gallbladder disease, CHF, diabetes mellitus, depression, migraine headache, seizure disorders, hepatic disease, family history of breast or endometrial cancer, history of thromboembolic disorders, uterine fibroids, hypertriglyceridemia, hypercalcemia, cigarette smoking (especially >35 yr)

PREGNANCY AND LACTATION: Pregnancy category X; may decrease quantity and quality of breast milk

SIDE EFFECTS/ADVERSE REACTIONS

CNS: Depression, migraine headache, emotional lability

*CV: **Arterial thromboembolism, pulmonary embolism, CVA, MI,** hypertension, venous thrombosis edema

EENT: Contact lens intolerance, ***retinal thrombosis***

GI: Nausea and vomiting, gallbladder disease, bloating, benign hepatic tumors ***mesenteric thrombosis***

GU: Breakthrough bleeding (80% resolve in 3 mo), *spotting,* amenorrhea, change in cervical secretions,

---

italic = common side effects   ***bold italic*** = life-threatening reactions

breast enlargement, breast tenderness

METAB: Hyperglycemia, hypertriglyceridemia, hypercalcemia, vitamin B-6 deficiency

SKIN: Melasma

INTERACTIONS

Drugs

3 *Barbiturates, carbamazepine, griseofulvin, phenytoin, penicillins, rifampin; rifabutin, ritonavir, tetracyclines:* Reduced efficacy of oral contraceptives

3 *Corticosteroids:* Enhanced effect of corticosteroids

3 *Cyclosporine:* Elevated cyclosporine concentrations

3 *Grapefruit juice:* Increased ethinyl estradiol concentration

⚠ *Smoking:* Increased risk of oral contraceptive-induced adverse cardiovascular events

❷ *Warfarin:* Increased risk of thromboembolic disease with oral contraceptives

Labs

• *False positive:* Serum antinuclear antibodies

SPECIAL CONSIDERATIONS

PATIENT/FAMILY EDUCATION

• Take at same time each day with food

• Notify clinician if breakthrough bleeding/spotting lasts more than a few days or persists in the 3rd cycle

• Use additional methods of birth control until after the 1st week of administration in the initial cycle or for entire cycle if diarrhea or vomiting occurs

• Does not protect against sexually transmitted diseases (provide condoms additionally where appropriate)

• Notify clinician immediately of severe headache, chest pain, abdominal pain, eye pain or blurred vision, calf pain

• Take a missed pill as soon as remembered, use backup contraception for remainder of cycle

MONITORING PARAMETERS

• Blood pressure

---

orphenadrine

(or-fen'a-dreen)

Rx: Antiflex, Banflex, Mio-rel, Myotrol, Norflex, Orfro, Orphenate

Combinations

> **Rx:** with aspirin, caffeine (Norgesic, Norgesic Forte, Orphengesic, Orphengesic Forte)

Chemical Class: Tertiary amine

Therapeutic Class: Skeletal muscle relaxant

CLINICAL PHARMACOLOGY

Mechanism of Action: Probable central action at brain stem; does not directly relax tense skeletal muscle; possesses anticholinergic actions

Pharmacokinetics

PO: Peak 2 hr, duration 4-6 hr; metabolized to 8 known metabolites, excreted in urine and feces; $t_{1/2}$ 14 hr

INDICATIONS AND USES: Adjunctive therapy to rest and physical therapy for painful acute musculoskeletal conditions, quinine-resistant leg cramps*

DOSAGE

Adult

• PO 100 mg bid; IM/IV 60 mg, may repeat q12h prn

$ AVAILABLE FORMS/COST OF THERAPY

• Inj, Sol—IM, IV: 30 mg/ml, 10 ml: **$9.30-$19.75**

• Tab, Plain Coated, SUS Action—Oral: 100 mg, 100's: **$165.03-$210.00**

CONTRAINDICATIONS: Glaucoma, pyloric or duodenal obstruction, stenosing peptic ulcer, prostatic hypertrophy, obstruction of bladder neck, cardiospasm, myasthenia gravis

PRECAUTIONS: Children, cardiac decompensation, coronary insufficiency, cardiac dysrhythmia, tachycardia, sulfite sensitivity

PREGNANCY AND LACTATION: Pregnancy category C; excretion into breast milk unknown, use caution in nursing mothers

SIDE EFFECTS/ADVERSE REACTIONS

CNS: Agitation, confusion, *dizziness, drowsiness,* hallucinations, headache, *lightheadedness,* tremor, weakness

CV: Palpitation, tachycardia, transient syncope

EENT: Blurred vision, increased ocular tension, pupil dilation

GI: Constipation, dry mouth, gastric irritation, nausea, vomiting

GU: Urinary hesitancy, urinary retention

*HEME: **Aplastic anemia** (rare)*

SKIN: Urticaria and other dermatoses

INTERACTIONS

Drugs

3 *Neuroleptics:* Lower serum neuroleptic concentrations, excessive anticholinergic effects

---

oseltamivir

(ah-suhl-tahm'ah-veer)
Rx: Tamiflu
Chemical Class: Carboxylic acid ethyl ester
Therapeutic Class: Antiviral

CLINICAL PHARMACOLOGY
Mechanism of Action: Inhibits influenza virus neuraminidase; may alter virus particle aggregation and release

Pharmacokinetics
PO: Peak 1 hr; oral bioavailability 75%; converted by hepatic esterase hydrolysis to the active form, oseltamivir carboxylate with $t_{1/2}$ 1-3 hr; oseltamivir 42% protein bound, oseltamivir carboxylate 3% protein bound; oseltamivir carboxylate excreted in urine with $t_{1/2}$ 6-10 hr; crosses placenta, excreted in breast milk

INDICATIONS AND USES: Treatment of uncomplicated influenza infection in adults who have been symptomatic for no more than 2 days; reduces median time to improvement of symptoms by 1.3 days

DOSAGE
Adult and Child >16 yr
• PO 75 mg bid for 5 days; dose adjustment for renal insufficiency: if CrCl < 30 ml/min, give 75 mg q day for 5 days

💲 AVAILABLE FORMS/COST OF THERAPY
• Cap—Oral: 75 mg, 10's: **$53.00**

PRECAUTIONS: Children under age 18 yr, renal insufficiency

PREGNANCY AND LACTATION: Pregnancy category C; excreted in breast milk of animals

SIDE EFFECTS/ADVERSE REACTIONS

CNS: Insomnia, vertigo
GI: Nausea (10%)

SPECIAL CONSIDERATIONS
PATIENT/FAMILY EDUCATION
• May administer without regard for food
• When started within 40 hr of onset of symptoms, there was a 1.3 day reduction in the median time to improvement in influenza-infected subjects receiving osteltamivir compared to subjects receiving placebo

---

italic = common side effects   ***bold italic*** = life-threatening reactions

oxacillin

(ox-a-sill'in)
Rx: Bactrocill
Chemical Class: Semisynthetic penicillin, (penicillinase-resistant)
Therapeutic Class: Antibiotic

CLINICAL PHARMACOLOGY
Mechanism of Action: Inhibits bacterial wall synthesis; bactericidal
Pharmacokinetics
PO: Peak 0.5-2 hr, duration 4-6 hr
IM: Peak 30 min, duration 4-6 hr 89%-94% bound to plasma proteins; partially metabolized to active and inactive metabolites, rapidly excreted in urine; $t_{1/2}$ 0.3-0.8 hr
INDICATIONS AND USES: Infections of the upper and lower respiratory tract, skin and skin structures, bones and joints; meningitis, septicemia, and endocarditis caused by penicillinase-producing staphylococci; perioperative prophylaxis*
Antibacterial spectrum usually includes:

• Gram-positive organisms: penicillinase-producing and non-penicillinase-producing strains of *Staphylococus aureus, S. epidermidis, S. saprophyticus;* groups A, B, C, and G streptococci; *Streptococcus pneumoniae,* some viridans streptococci, *Bacillus anthracis*
DOSAGE
Adult
• PO 500-1000 mg q4-6h; IM/IV 250-1000 mg q4-6h; max 12 g/day
Child
• PO/IM/IV 50-100 mg/kg/day divided q4-6h; max 300 mg/kg/day
$ AVAILABLE FORMS/COST OF THERAPY
• Powder, Reconst—Oral: 250 mg/5 ml, 100 ml: **$3.75-$14.58**

• Cap, Gel—Oral: 250 mg, 100's: **$11.00-$28.40;** 500 mg, 100's: **$19.00**
• Inj, Dry-Sol—IM, IV: 500 mg/vial: **$1.37-$3.75;** 1 g/vial: **$2.68-$3.60;** 2 g/vial: **$5.14-$6.06**
PRECAUTIONS: Hypersensitivity to cephalosporins, renal insufficiency, prolonged or repeated therapy, neonates
PREGNANCY AND LACTATION: Pregnancy category B; potential exists for modification of bowel flora in nursing infant, allergy or sensitization, and interference with interpretation of culture results if fever workup required
SIDE EFFECTS/ADVERSE REACTIONS
CNS: Chills, fever, headache
CV: Phlebitis, thrombophlebitis
GI: Increased AST, ALT
GU: **Hemorrhagic cystitis, interstitial nephritis, nephropathy**
HEME: Eosinophilia, **bone marrow suppression,** positive Coombs test, **thrombocytopenia**
MS: Myalgia
SKIN: Pain at inj site, pruritus, rash, sterile abscess at inj site
MISC: Serum sickness-like reactions
INTERACTIONS
Drugs
3 *Chloramphenicol:* Inhibited antibacterial activity of oxacillin, ensure adequate amounts of both agents are given and administer oxacillin a few hours before chloramphenicol
3 *Methotrexate:* Increased serum methotrexate concentrations
3 *Tetracyclines:* Inhibited antibacterial activity of oxacillin, ensure adequate amounts of both agents are given and administer oxacillin a few hours before tetracycline
SPECIAL CONSIDERATIONS
• Sodium content of 1 g = 2.8-3.1 mEq

PATIENT/FAMILY EDUCATION
• Administer on an empty stomach (1 hr before or 2 hr after meals)

MONITORING PARAMETERS
• Urinalysis, BUN, serum creatinine, CBC with differential, periodic liver function tests

---

oxamniquine
(ox-am'ni-kwin)
Rx: Vansil
Chemical Class: Tetrahydroquinoline derivative
Therapeutic Class: Anthelmintic

CLINICAL PHARMACOLOGY
Mechanism of Action: Dislodges schistosomes from usual site of residence in mesenteric veins to liver where they are retained and subsequently killed by host tissue reactions; causes contraction and paralysis of musculature and subsequent immobilization of the worm's suckers; laying of eggs by females ceases within 24-48 hr substantially reducing egg load and eliminating principal cause of pathology associated with schistosomal infection

Pharmacokinetics
PO: Peak 1-1½ hr; extensively metabolized to inactive metabolites, excreted in urine; t₁/₂ 1-2½ hr

INDICATIONS AND USES: All stages of *Schistosoma mansoni* infection; single-dose treatment of neurocysticercosis (in combination with praziquantel)*

DOSAGE
Adult
• PO 12-15 mg/kg as a single dose (Western Hemisphere strains of *Schistosoma mansoni*); 30-60 mg/kg given in 2-4 equally divided doses of 15 mg/kg bid for 1-2 days (African and Middle Eastern strains of *Schistosoma mansoni*)
Child <30 kg
• PO 20 mg/kg given in 2 divided doses of 10 mg/kg with 2-8 hr between doses

💲 AVAILABLE FORMS/COST OF THERAPY
• Cap, Gel—Oral: 250 mg, 24's: **$106.79**
PRECAUTIONS: Seizure disorder
PREGNANCY AND LACTATION: Pregnancy category C
SIDE EFFECTS/ADVERSE REACTIONS
CNS: Dizziness, drowsiness, headache, **seizures (rare)**
GI: Abdominal pain, anorexia, mild to moderate liver enzyme elevations, nausea, vomiting
GU: Orange-red discoloration of urine
SKIN: Urticaria

SPECIAL CONSIDERATIONS
• Alternate to praziquantel for *Schistosoma mansoni;* little effect against other *Schistosoma*

PATIENT/FAMILY EDUCATION
• Take with food
• May cause orange-red discoloration of urine

---

oxandrolone
(ox-an'droe-lone)
Rx: Oxandrin
Chemical Class: Halogenated testosterone derivative
Therapeutic Class: Androgen
DEA Class: Schedule III

CLINICAL PHARMACOLOGY
Mechanism of Action: Promotes body tissue-building processes and reverses catabolic processes when administered with adequate calories and protein; inhibits endogenous testosterone release

---

italic = common side effects   ***bold italic*** = life-threatening reactions

Pharmacokinetics

PO: Metabolized in liver, excreted in urine

INDICATIONS AND USES: Promotion of weight gain following extensive surgery, chronic infection, or severe trauma; protein catabolism associated with prolonged administration of corticosteroids; bone pain associated with osteoporosis; alcololic hepatitis;* short stature associated with Turner's syndrome;* HIV wasting syndrome and HIV-associated muscle weakness;* constitutional delay of growth and puberty,* severe refractory hypertriglyceridemia*

DOSAGE

Adult

• PO 2.5 mg bid-qid for 2-4 wk; repeat intermittently prn; range of effective doses 2.5-20 mg/day

Child

• PO total daily dose is ≤0.1 mg/kg or ≤0.045 mg/lb; repeat intermittently prn

$ AVAILABLE FORMS/COST OF THERAPY

• Tab, Uncoated—Oral: 2.5 mg, 100's: **$375.00**

CONTRAINDICATIONS: Male patients with prostate or breast cancer, hypercalcemia in females with breast cancer, nephrosis, nephrotic phase of nephritis, hypercalcemia, enhancement of physical appearance or athletic performance

PRECAUTIONS: Elderly, children, cardiac disease, renal disease, hepatic disease, seizure disorder, migraine headache, diabetes

PREGNANCY AND LACTATION: Pregnancy category X; use extreme caution in nursing mothers

SIDE EFFECTS/ADVERSE REACTIONS

CNS: Choreiform movement, depression, excitation, habituation, insomnia

CV: Edema, *CHF*

EENT: Deepening of voice, hoarseness

GI: Cholestatic jaundice, diarrhea, *hepatic necrosis, hepatocellular neoplasms,* nausea, *peliosis hepatis,* vomiting

GU: Amenorrhea, clitoral hypertrophy, decreased breast size, decreased libido, menstrual irregularities, testicular atrophy, vaginitis, virilization

METAB: Decreased glucose tolerance, decreased HDL, increased LDL, increased serum cholesterol, retention of sodium, chloride, water, potassium, phosphates, calcium

MS: Premature closure of epiphyses in children

SKIN: Acne, alopecia, flushing, hirsutism, male pattern baldness, rash, sweating

DRUG INTERACTIONS

Drugs

3 *Antidiabetic agents:* Enhanced hypoglycemic effects

2 *Cyclosporine:* Increased cyclosporine concentrations, toxicity

3 *HMG-CoA reductase inhibitors (lovastatin, pravastatin):* Myositis risk increased

3 *Tacrolimus:* Increased tacrolimus concentrations, toxicity

2 *Oral anticoagulants:* Enhanced hypoprothrombinemic response

SPECIAL CONSIDERATIONS

• Anabolic steroids have potential for abuse, especially in the athlete

PATIENT/FAMILY EDUCATION

• Adequate dietary intake of calories and protein essential for successful treatment

MONITORING PARAMETERS

• LFTs, lipids

• Growth rate in children (X-rays for bone age q 6 mos)

• Serum calcium in breast cancer patients

* = non-FDA-approved use

oxaprozin
(ox-a-pro'zin)
Rx: Daypro
Chemical Class: Propionic acid derivative
Therapeutic Class: NSAID with analgesic and antipyretic activity

CLINICAL PHARMACOLOGY
Mechanism of Action: Reversible cyclooxygenase (i.e., prostaglandin synthetase) inhibitor; nonselectively decreases the formation of both prostaglandins and thromboxane A2; variable effects on lipoxygenase synthesis and subsequent leukotriene production; antiinflammatory, antipyretic, and analgesic activity; inhibits platelet aggregation
Pharmacokinetics
PO: Peak 3-5 hr; 99.9% bound to plasma proteins; metabolized in liver to inactive metabolites, excreted in urine (65%) and feces (35%); $t_{1/2}$ 42-50 hr

INDICATIONS AND USES: Osteoarthritis, rheumatoid arthritis, prevention of cognitive decline,* acute gout,* pain—mild to moderate, tendonitis/bursitis*

DOSAGE
Adult
• PO 600-1200 mg qd, individualize dosage to lowest effective dose; max 1800 mg/day or 26 mg/kg/day, whichever is lower

$ AVAILABLE FORMS/COST OF THERAPY
• Tab, Uncoated—Oral: 600 mg, 100's: **$153.15**

CONTRAINDICATIONS: Bronchospasm, nasal polyps, angioedema precipitated by aspirin or other NSAIDs

PRECAUTIONS: History of GI ulceration, bleeding, or perforation; renal dysfunction, hypertension or cardiac conditions aggravated by fluid retention and edema, history of liver dysfunction, history of coagulation

PREGNANCY AND LACTATION: Pregnancy category C (category D if used in 3rd trimester); could cause constriction of the ductus arteriosus *in utero,* persistent pulmonary hypertension of the newborn, or prolonged labor

SIDE EFFECTS/ADVERSE REACTIONS
CNS: Dizziness, headache, lightheadedness
CV: Chest pain, **CHF, dysrhythmias,** edema, hypertension, hypotension, palpitation, tachycardia
EENT: Dry eyes, hearing disturbances, photophobia, tinnitus, visual disturbances
GI: Abdominal cramps, constipation, diarrhea, *dyspepsia,* flatulence, **gastric or duodenal ulcer with bleeding or perforation,** hepatitis, *nausea,* occult blood in stool, **pancreatitis,** vomiting
GU: **Acute renal failure**
HEME: **Agranulocytosis,** eosinophilia, **leukopenia, neutropenia, pancytopenia, thrombocytopenia**
METAB: Hyperglycemia, hyperkalemia, hypoglycemia, hyponatremia
RESP: **Bronchospasm,** dyspnea, pulmonary infiltrates
SKIN: Photosensitivity, rash, urticaria

INTERACTIONS
Drugs
3 *Aminoglycosides:* Reduced clearance with elevated aminoglycoside levels and potential for toxicity (especially indomethacin in premature infants; other NSAIDs probably)
3 *Anticoagulants:* Excessive hypoprothrombinemia, decreased

---

italic = common side effects   ***bold italic*** = life-threatening reactions

platelet aggregation with increased risk of GI bleeding

3 *Antihypertensives (α-blockers, angiotensin-converting enzyme inhibitors, angiotensin II receptor blockers, β-blockers, diuretics):* Inhibition of antihypertensive and other favorable hemodynamic effects

3 *Corticosteroids:* Increased risk of GI ulceration

3 *Cyclosporine:* Increased nephrotoxicity risk

3 *Lithium:* Decreased clearance of lithium (mediated via prostaglandins) resulting in elevated serum lithium levels and risk of toxicity

3 *Methotrexate:* Decreased renal secretion of methotrexate resulting in elevated methotrexate levels and risk of toxicity

3 *Phenylpropanolamine:* Possible acute hypertensive reaction

3 *Potassium-sparing diuretics:* Additive hyperkalemia potential

3 *Triamterene:* Acute renal failure reported with addition of indomethacin; caution with other NSAIDs

SPECIAL CONSIDERATIONS
• No significant advantage over other NSAIDs; cost should govern use

PATIENT/FAMILY EDUCATION
• Avoid aspirin and alcoholic beverages
• Take with food, milk, or antacids to decrease GI upset

MONITORING PARAMETERS
• Initial hemogram and fecal occult blood test within 3 mo of starting regular chronic therapy; repeat every 6-12 mo (more frequently in high-risk patients (>65 years, peptic ulcer disease, concurrent steroids or anticoagulants); electrolytes, creatinine, and BUN within 3 mo of starting regular chronic therapy; repeat every 6-12 mo

---

oxazepam
(ox-a'ze-pam)
Rx: Serax
Chemical Class: Benzodiazepine
Therapeutic Class: Anxiolytic
DEA Class: Schedule IV

CLINICAL PHARMACOLOGY
Mechanism of Action: CNS depressant via facilitation of inhibitory GABA at benzodiazepine receptor sites (BZ_1—associated with sleep; BZ_2—associated with memory, motor, sensory, and cognitive function); effects include muscle relaxation (spinal cord), anticonvulsant activity (brain stem), ataxia (cerebellum), emotional behavior (limbic and cortical areas), and anxiolytic effects (separate from general CNS depression)

Pharmacokinetics

PO: Peak 2-4 hr, onset of action intermediate compared to other benzodiazepines; 86%-96% bound to plasma proteins; metabolized via conjugation to inactive metabolites, excreted in urine as unchanged drug (50%) and metabolites; $t_{1/2}$ 5-15 hr

INDICATIONS AND USES: Anxiety disorders; management of anxiety, tension, agitation, irritability in older patients; alcohol withdrawal; irritable bowel*

DOSAGE
Adult
• PO 10-30 mg tid-qid

AVAILABLE FORMS/COST OF THERAPY
• Cap, Gel—Oral: 10 mg, 100's: **$23.34-$87.40;** 15 mg, 100's: **$34.16-$109.88;** 30 mg, 100's: **$42.78-$158.93**
• Tab, Uncoated—Oral: 15 mg, 100's: **$109.88**

---

* = non-FDA-approved use

CONTRAINDICATIONS: Narrow-angle glaucoma, psychosis
PRECAUTIONS: Elderly, debilitated, hepatic disease, renal disease, history of drug abuse, abrupt withdrawal, respiratory depression
PREGNANCY AND LACTATION: Pregnancy category D; may cause fetal damage when administered during pregnancy; excreted into breast milk, may accumulate in breast-fed infants and is therefore not recommended
SIDE EFFECTS/ADVERSE REACTIONS
CNS: Abnormal thinking, agitation, amnesia, anxiety, apathy, *asthenia,* ataxia, decreased libido, decreased reflexes, emotional lability, hangover, hostility, *hypokinesia,* neuritis, seizure, sleep disorder, *somnolence,* stupor, twitch
CV: **Dysrhythmia,** syncope
EENT: Ear pain; epistaxis, eye irritation, pain, pharyngitis, photophobia, rhinitis, sinusitis, swelling
GI: Abdominal pain, decreased, increased appetite; dyspepsia; enterocolitis, flatulence, gastritis, melena, mouth ulceration
GU: Frequent urination, hematuria, itching; menstrual cramps; nocturia, oliguria, penile discharge, urinary hesitancy, urgency; urinary incontinence, vaginal discharge
HEME: **Agranulocytosis**
MS: Back pain, lower extremity pain
RESP: Asthma, cold symptoms, cough, dyspnea, hyperventilation
SKIN: Acne, dry skin, photosensitivity, urticaria
INTERACTIONS
Drugs
3 *Ethanol:* Enhanced adverse psychomotor effects of benzodiazepines
Labs
• *False increase:* Serum glucose
SPECIAL CONSIDERATIONS
• Niche compared to other benzo-

diazepines: treatment of anxiety in patients with hepatic disease; consider for alcohol withdrawal
PATIENT/FAMILY EDUCATION
• Avoid alcohol and other CNS depressants
• Do not discontinue abruptly after prolonged therapy
• Inform clinician if planning to become pregnant, pregnant, or become pregnant while taking this medicine
• May be habit forming
MONITORING PARAMETERS
• Periodic CBC, UA, blood chemistry analyses during prolonged therapy

---

oxiconazole
(ox-i-con′a-zole)
Rx: Oxistat
Chemical Class: Synthetic imidazole derivative
Therapeutic Class: Antifungal

CLINICAL PHARMACOLOGY
Mechanism of Action: Alteration of the fungal cell membrane, which allows leakage of essential intracellular components
Pharmacokinetics
TOP: Low systemic absorption
INDICATIONS AND USES: Tinea pedis (athlete's foot), tinea cruris (jock itch), and tinea corporis (ringworm) due to *Trichophyton rubrum, T. mentagrophytes,* and *Epidermophyton floccosum;* tinea (pityriasis) versicolor
DOSAGE
Adult and Child
• TOP apply to affected area(s) qd for 2 wk (jock itch, ringworm) or 4 wk (athlete's foot)

---

italic = common side effects   ***bold italic*** = life-threatening reactions

**$ AVAILABLE FORMS/COST
OF THERAPY**
- Cre—Top: 1%, 15, 30, 60 g:
$26.84/30 g
- Lotion—Top: 1% 30 ml: **$26.84**
PREGNANCY AND LACTATION:
Pregnancy category B; excreted in
breast milk
**SIDE EFFECTS/ADVERSE REAC-
TIONS**
SKIN: Burning, contact dermatitis,
dyshidrotic eczema, erythema, fis-
suring, folliculitis, irritation, mac-
eration, nodules, pain, papules, pru-
ritus, rash, scaling, stinging, tin-
gling
SPECIAL CONSIDERATIONS
- Niche: once daily imadazole; base
choice on cost and convenience
PATIENT/FAMILY EDUCATION
- For external use only, avoid con-
tact with eyes or vagina

---

oxtriphylline
(ox-trye'fi-lin)
Rx: Choledyl SA
Chemical Class: Xanthine
derivative (64% theophylline)
Therapeutic Class: Antiasthmatic, bronchodilator; COPD
agent

CLINICAL PHARMACOLOGY
Mechanism of Action: Directly relaxes bronchial and pulmonary blood
vessel smooth muscle; stimulates
CNS; induces diuresis; increases
gastric acid secretion, lowers lower
esophageal sphincter pressure; is a
central respiratory stimulant; exact
mechanism unproven but may involve antagonism of pulmonary
adenosine receptors
Pharmacokinetics
PO: Peak 4 hr; metabolized by liver,
excreted in urine; $t_{1/2}$ 3-12 hr; $t_{1/2}$
increased in geriatric patients, hepatic disease, cor pulmonale, and

CHF, decreased in children and
smokers
INDICATIONS AND USES: Asthma,
reversible bronchospasm associated
with chronic bronchitis and emphysema
DOSAGE
Adult
- PO 800-1200 mg/d divided q12h;
smokers may require more frequent
dosing; adjust dose based on measurement of serum theophylline concentrations
**$ AVAILABLE FORMS/COST
OF THERAPY**
- Tab, Coated, SUS Action—Oral:
400 mg, 100's: **$41.15;** 600 mg,
100's: **$49.37**
CONTRAINDICATIONS: Active
peptic ulcer, underlying seizure disorder (not on anticonvulsant therapy)
PRECAUTIONS: Elderly, CHF, cor
pulmonale, hepatic disease, pre-
existing dysrhythmias, hypertension,
hypoxemia, sustained high fever, history of peptic ulcer, alcoholism
PREGNANCY AND LACTATION:
Pregnancy category C; pharmacokinetics of theophylline may be altered during pregnancy, monitor serum concentrations carefully; excreted into breast milk, may cause
irritability in the nursing infant, otherwise compatible with breast feeding
**SIDE EFFECTS/ADVERSE REAC-
TIONS**
CNS: Anxiety, *dizziness,* headache,
insomnia, lightheadedness, muscle
twitching, reflex hyperexcitability,
restlessness, *seizures*
CV: Circulatory failure, extrasystoles, flushing, hypotension, *palpitations, sinus tachycardia, ventricular dysrhythmias*
GI: Anorexia, bitter taste, diarrhea,
dyspepsia, epigastric pain, esopha-

geal reflux, hematemesis, *nausea, vomiting*

GU: Proteinuria, urinary frequency

METAB: Hyperglycemia

RESP: Tachypnea

SKIN: Alopecia, urticaria

INTERACTIONS

Drugs

3 *Adenosine:* Inhibited hemodynamic effects of adenosine

3 *Allopurinol, amiodarone, cimetadine, ciprofloxacin, disulfiram, erythromycin, interferon alfa, isoniazid, methimazole, metoprolol, norfloxacin, pefloxacin, pentoxifylline, propafenone, propylthiouracil, radioactive iodine, tacrine, thiabendazole, ticlopidine, verapamil:* Increased theophylline concentrations

3 *Aminoglutethimide, barbiturates, carbamazepine, moricizine, phenytoin, rifampin, ritonavir, thyroid hormone:* Reduced theophylline concentrations; decreased serum phenytoin concentrations

2 *Enoxacin, fluvoxamine, mexiletine, propanolol, troleandomycin:* Increased theophylline concentrations

3 *Imipenem:* Some patients on oxtriphylline have developed seizures following the addition of imipenem

3 *Lithium:* Reduced lithium concentrations

3 *Smoking:* Increased oxtriphylline dosing requirements

Labs

• *False increase:* Serum barbiturate concentrations, urinary uric acid

• *False decrease:* Serum bilirubin

• *Interference:* Plasma somatostatin

SPECIAL CONSIDERATIONS

• Touted to produce less GI side effects; if dosed equipotently based on theophylline equivalents (oxtriphylline = 64% theophylline) no difference; compare costs as well as other characteristics

PATIENT/FAMILY EDUCATION

• Avoid large amounts of caffeine-containing products (tea, coffee, chocolate, colas)

MONITORING PARAMETERS

• Serum theophylline concentrations (therapeutic level is 8-20 µg/ml); toxicity may occur with small increase above 20 µg/ml, especially in the elderly

---

oxybutynin

(ox-i-byoo'ti-nin)

Rx: Ditropan, Ditropan XL

Chemical Class: Synthetic tertiary amine

Therapeutic Class: Genitourinary muscle relaxant; GI antispasmodic

CLINICAL PHARMACOLOGY

Mechanism of Action: Exerts direct antispasmodic effect on smooth muscle and inhibits action of acetylcholine at postganglionic cholinergic sites; increases bladder capacity and delays initial desire to void by reducing number of motor impulses reaching the detrusor muscle

Pharmacokinetics

PO: Peak 3-6 hr, onset ½-1 hr, duration 6-10 hr; metabolized in liver, eliminated via kidneys

INDICATIONS AND USES: Antispasmodic in uninhibited neurogenic or reflex neurogenic bladder, primary nocturnal enuresis,* antispasmodic in various GI disorders,* diabetic diarrhea,* postgustatory sweating*

DOSAGE

Adult

• PO 5 mg bid-tid; do not exceed 5 mg qid

Child

• PO 1-5 yr 0.2 mg/kg/dose divided bid-qid; >5 yr 5 mg bid, up to 5 mg tid

---

italic = common side effects   ***bold italic*** = life-threatening reactions

$ AVAILABLE FORMS/COST OF THERAPY

• Tab, Uncoated—Oral: 5 mg, 100's: **$15.90-$64.32**
• Syr—Oral: 5 mg/5 ml, 473 ml: **$39.99-$69.72**

CONTRAINDICATIONS: Angle-closure glaucoma, myasthenia gravis, partial or complete obstruction of the GI tract, adynamic ileus, megacolon, severe colitis, intestinal atony, obstructive uropathy, unstable cardiovascular status

PRECAUTIONS: Elderly, autonomic neuropathy, hepatic or renal disease, hyperthyroidism, CHD, prostatic hypertrophy, reflux esophagitis, ulcerative colitis

PREGNANCY AND LACTATION: Pregnancy category B; may suppress lactation

SIDE EFFECTS/ADVERSE REACTIONS

CNS: Asthenia, dizziness, *drowsiness,* hallucinations, insomnia, restlessness
CV: Palpitations, tachycardia, vasodilation
EENT: Amblyopia, blurred vision, cycloplegia, decreased lacrimation, mydriasis
GI: Constipation, decreased GI motility, *dry mouth,* nausea, vomiting
GU: Impotence, urinary hesitancy and retention
METAB: Suppression of lactation
SKIN: Decreased sweating, rash

SPECIAL CONSIDERATIONS

• Reported anticholinergic side effects not clinically or significantly different from other agents (i.e., propantheline); compare costs

PATIENT/FAMILY EDUCATION

• Avoid prolonged exposure to hot environments, heat prostration may result

---

oxycodone
(ox-ee-koe′done)
Rx: Oxycontin, Oxy IR, Percolone Oxyfast, Roxicodone
Combinations:
Rx: with aspirin (Percodan, Endodan, Roxiprin); with acetaminophen (Percocet, Endocet, Tylox, Roxicet, Roxilox)
Chemical Class: Semisynthetic opium alkaloid; phenanthrene derivative
Therapeutic Class: Narcotic analgesic
DEA Class: Schedule II

CLINICAL PHARMACOLOGY
Mechanism of Action: Narcotic agonist with activity at Mu receptors (supraspinal analgesia, euphoria, respiratory and physical depression, miosis, and reduced GI motility), Kappa receptors (pentazocine-like spinal analgesia, sedation, and miosis), and Delta receptors (dysphoria, psychotomimetic effects [e.g., hallucinations], and respiratory and vasomotor stimulation caused by drugs with antagonist activity); compared to morphine, equal analgesic, antitussive, constipation, respiratory depression, sedation, emesis, and physical dependence effects
Pharmacokinetics
PO: Onset 10-15 min, peak 30-60 min, duration 3-6 hr; metabolized in liver and kidneys, excreted primarily in urine

INDICATIONS AND USES: Moderate to moderately severe pain

DOSAGE
Adult
• PO 5 mg q6h prn
• SUS REL: PO (opioid-naive patients) 10 mg q12h, titrate to adequate pain relief; (patients on fixed

---

ratio opioid/APAP or ASA combinations) 10-20 mg q12h (if taking 1-5 tabs/caps daily of fixed ratio dmg), 20-30 mg q12h (6-9 tabs/caps each day), 30-40 mg q12h (10-12 tabs/caps each day), titrate to adequate pain relief; (patients currently on opioid therapy) calculate the total mg amount of current opioid and convert to oxycodone equivalent using conversion chart supplied by manufacturer; (patients on transdermal fentanyl therapy) 18 hours after stopping transdermal fentanyl, initiate 10 mg q12h for every 25 µg/hr fentanyl patch, titrate to adequate pain relief

Child
• PO 6-12 yr 1.25 mg q6h prn; >12 yr 2.5 mg q6h prn

$ AVAILABLE FORMS/COST OF THERAPY
• Sol—Oral: 5 mg/5 ml, 500 ml: **$41.65;** 20 mg/ml, 30 ml: **$33.75-$40.56**
• Tabs, SUS REL—Oral; 10 mg, 100's: **$117.10;** 20 mg, 100's: **$224.11;** 40 mg, 100's: **$397.66;** 80 mg, 100's: **$747.79**
• Tab, Uncoated—Oral: 5 mg, 100's: **$27.00-$68.75**
• Cap—Oral: 5 mg, 100's: **$24.44-$30.61**

CONTRAINDICATIONS: Acute bronchial asthma, upper airway obstruction

PRECAUTIONS: Head injury, increased intracranial pressure, acute abdominal conditions, elderly, severe impairment of hepatic or renal function, hypothyroidism, Addison's disease, prostatic hypertrophy, urethral stricture, history of drug abuse

PREGNANCY AND LACTATION: Pregnancy category B (category D if used for prolonged periods or in high doses at term); excreted into breast milk

SIDE EFFECTS/ADVERSE REACTIONS
CNS: Agitation, dependency, dizziness, *drowsiness,* lethargy, restlessness, *sedation*
CV: Bradycardia, orthostatic hypotension, palpitations, tachycardia
GI: Anorexia, constipation, nausea, vomiting
GU: Urinary retention
*RESP: **Respiratory depression, respiratory paralysis***
SKIN: Flushing, rash, urticaria

INTERACTIONS
Drugs
▣ *Amitriptylline:* Additive respiratory and CNS-depressant effects
▣ *Antihistamines, chloral hydrate, glutethimide, methocarbamol:* Enhanced depressant effects
▣ *Barbiturates:* Additive respiratory and CNS depressant effects
▣ *Cimetidine:* Increased respiratory and CNS depression
▣ *Clomipramine:* Additive respiratory and CNS depressant effects
▣ *Ethanol:* Additive CNS effects
▣ *MAOI's:* Markedly potentiate the actions of morphine
▣ *Nortriptyline:* Additive respiratory and CNS depressant effects
▣ *Protease inhibitors:* Increased CNS and respiratory depression
Labs
• *False increase:* Amylase and lipase

SPECIAL CONSIDERATIONS
PATIENT/FAMILY EDUCATION
• Physical dependency may result when used for extended periods
• Change position slowly, orthostatic hypotension may occur
• Do not administer agonist/antagonist analgesics (i.e., pentazocine, nalbuphine, butorphanol, dezocine, buprenorphine) to patient who has received a prolonged course of oxycodone (a pure agonist). In opioid-dependent patients, mixed agonist/

---

italic = common side effects　　**bold italic** = life-threatening reactions

antagonist analgesics may precipitate withdrawal symptoms

---

oxymetazoline
(ox-ee-met-az'oh-leen)
OTC: (Nasal): 4-way long lasting, Afrin 12-Hour, Benzedrex 12 hr, Cheracol, Dristan 12-hour, Duramist Plus, Duration, Genasal, Neo-Synephrine 12-Hour, Oxymata 12, Vicks Sinex 12-Hour Ultra Fine Mist (Ophthalmic): Ocu Clear, Visine L.R.
Chemical Class: Imidazoline derivative
Therapeutic Class: Decongestant

CLINICAL PHARMACOLOGY
Mechanism of Action: Local α-adrenergic-mediated vasoconstriction on dilated conjunctival and nasal mucosal blood vessels
Pharmacokinteics
TOP: Onset 5-10 min, duration 5-6 hr; some systemic absorption
INDICATIONS AND USES: Nasal congestion; eye redness due to minor eye irritations
DOSAGE
Adult and Child ≥6 yr
• NASAL 2-3 gtt or sprays of 0.05% sol instilled into each nostril bid; do not exceed 3-5 days duration
• CONJUNCTIVAL 1 gtt q6h; do not exceed 3-4 days duration
Child 2-5 yr
• NASAL 2-3 gtt of 0.025% sol instilled into each nostril bid; do not exceed 3-5 days duration
$ AVAILABLE FORMS/COST OF THERAPY
• Sol—Ophth: 0.025%, 15, 30 ml: **$3.07-$5.33**
• Sol—Nasal: 0.025%, 20 ml: **$3.35**; 0.05%, 15, 20, 30 ml: **$1.46-$7.24**

CONTRAINDICATIONS: Angle-closure glaucoma
PRECAUTIONS: Children <2 yr, hyperthyroidism, heart disease, hypertension, diabetes mellitus
PREGNANCY AND LACTATION: Pregnancy category C
SIDE EFFECTS/ADVERSE REACTIONS
CNS: Dizziness, headache, nervousness, weakness
CV: Cardiac irregularities, hypertension
EENT: Anosmia; blurred vision, dryness, increased or decreased intraocular pressure; irritation, mild transient stinging, mydriasis, rebound congestion/hyperemia ("rhinitis medicamentosa"), sneezing, stinging, transient burning, ulceration of nasal mucosa
GI: Nausea
SKIN: Sweating

SPECIAL CONSIDERATIONS
• Manage rebound congestion by stopping oxymetazoline: one nostril at a time, substitute systemic decongestant, substitute inhaled steroid
PATIENT/FAMILY EDUCATION
• Do not use for > 3-5 days or rebound congestion may occur

---

oxymetholone
(ox-ee-meth'oh-lone)
Rx: Anadrol-50
Chemical Class: Halogenated testosterone derivative
Therapeutic Class: Androgen; hematopoietic agent
DEA Class: Schedule III

CLINICAL PHARMACOLOGY
Mechanism of Action: Promotes body tissue-building processes and reverses catabolic processes when administered with adequate calories

---

* = non-FDA-approved use

and protein; inhibits endogenous testosterone release

Pharmacokinetics

PO: Metabolized in liver, excreted in urine

INDICATIONS AND USES: Anemias caused by deficient red cell production, acquired or congenital aplastic anemia, myelofibrosis and hypoplastic anemias due to administration of myelotoxic drugs

DOSAGE

Adult

• PO 1-5 mg/kg/day

💲 **AVAILABLE FORMS/COST OF THERAPY**

• Tab, Uncoated—Oral: 50 mg, 100's: **$1288.88**

CONTRAINDICATIONS: Hypersensitivity, male patients with prostate or breast cancer, hypercalcemia in females with breast cancer, nephrosis, nephrotic phase of nephritis, enhancement of physical appearance or athletic performance

PRECAUTIONS: Elderly, children, cardiac disease, renal disease, hepatic disease, seizure disorder, migraine headache, diabetes

PREGNANCY AND LACTATION: Pregnancy category X; use extreme caution in nursing mothers

SIDE EFFECTS/ADVERSE REACTIONS

CNS: Choreiform movement, depression, excitation, habituation, insomnia

CV: Edema, ***CHF***

EENT: Deepening of voice, hoarseness

GI: Cholestatic jaundice, diarrhea, ***hepatic necrosis, hepatocellular neoplasms,*** nausea, ***peliosis hepatis,*** vomiting

GU: Amenorrhea, clitoral hypertrophy, decreased breast size, decreased libido, testicular atrophy, vaginitis, virilization

HEME: ***Leukemia*** (observed in several patients with aplastic anemia, role of oxymetholone unclear)

METAB: Decreased glucose tolerance, decreased HDL cholesterol, increased LDL cholesterol, increased serum cholesterol; retention of sodium, chloride, water, potassium, phosphates, calcium

MS: Premature closure of epiphyses in children

SKIN: Acne, alopecia, flushing, hirsutism, rash, sweating

INTERACTIONS

Drugs

3 *Antidiabetic agents:* Enhanced hypoglycemic effects

2 *Cyclosporine:* Increased cyclosporine concentrations, toxicity

3 *HMG-CoA reductase inhibitors (lovastatin, prevastatin):* Myositis risk increased

3 *Tacrolimus:* Increased tacrolimus concentrations, potential for toxicity

2 *Oral anticoagulants:* Enhanced hypoprothrombinemic response

SPECIAL CONSIDERATIONS

• Anabolic steroids have potential for abuse, especially in the athlete

• Comparative advantages include less potential for virilization in women, convenience of oral administration; disadvantage includes increased risk of hepatotoxicity

PATIENT/FAMILY EDUCATION

• Hematologic response is often not immediate, needs minimum trial of 3-6 mo

MONITORING PARAMETERS

• LFTs, lipids, Hct

• Serum calcium in breast cancer patients

• Growth rate in children (X-rays for bone age q 6 mo)

---

italic = common side effects   ***bold italic*** = life-threatening reactions

oxymorphone

(ox-ee-mor´fone)
Rx: Numorphan
Chemical Class: Synthetic
opium alkaloid; phenanthrene
derivative
Therapeutic Class: Narcotic
analgesic
DEA Class: Schedule II

CLINICAL PHARMACOLOGY
Mechanism of Action: Narcotic agonist with activity at Mu receptors
(supraspinal analgesia, euphoria,
respiratory and physical depression,
miosis, and reduced GI motility),
Kappa receptors (pentazocine-like
spinal analgesia, sedation, and miosis), and Delta receptors (dysphoria, psychotomimetic effects [e.g.,
hallucinations], and respiratory and
vasomotor stimulation caused by
drugs with antagonist activity); compared to morphine, equal analgesia,
and constipation; less antitussive;
more emesis, respiratory depression, and physical dependence
Pharmacokinetics
PR: Onset 15-30 min, duration 3-6 hr
IV: Onset 5-10 min, duration 3-6 hr
SC/IM: Onset 10-15 min, duration
3-6 hr
Metabolized primarily in liver, excreted mainly in urine
INDICATIONS AND USES: Moderate to severe pain, preoperative sedation, analgesia during labor, pulmonary edema (not arising from
chemical respiratory irritant)
DOSAGE
Adult
• SC/IM 1-1.5 mg q4-6h prn; IV 0.5
mg; PR 5 mg q4-6h prn
• *Analgesia during labor:* IM
0.5-1 mg

🅢 **AVAILABLE FORMS/COST
OF THERAPY**
• Inj, Sol—IM, IV, SC: 1 mg/ml, 1

ml: **$2.86;** 1.5 mg/ml, 10 ml:
$33.50
• Supp—Rect: 5 mg, 6's: **$28.31**
CONTRAINDICATIONS: Acute
bronchial asthma, upper airway obstruction
PRECAUTIONS: Head injury, increased intracranial pressure, acute
abdominal conditions, elderly, severe impairment of hepatic or renal
function, hypothyroidism, Addison's
disease, prostatic hypertrophy, urethral stricture, history of drug abuse,
children
PREGNANCY AND LACTATION:
Pregnancy category B (category D
if used for prolonged periods or in
high doses at term); use during labor produces neonatal respiratory
depression
**SIDE EFFECTS/ADVERSE REAC-
TIONS**
CNS: Agitation, dependency, dizziness, *drowsiness,* lethargy, restlessness, *sedation*
CV: Bradycardia, orthostatic hypotension, palpitations, tachycardia
*GI: Anorexia, constipation, nausea,
vomiting*
GU: Urinary retention
*RESP: **Respiratory depression, respiratory paralysis***
SKIN: Flushing, rash, urticaria
INTERACTIONS
Drugs
❸ *Barbiturates:* Additive CNS depression
❸ *Cimetidine:* Increased effect of
narcotic analgesics
❷ *Ethanol:* Additive CNS effects
❸ *Neuroleptics:* Hypotension and
excessive CNS depression
Labs
• *False increase:* Amylase and lipase
SPECIAL CONSIDERATIONS
• Do not administer agonist/antag-
onist analgesics (i.e., pentazocine,

---

* = non-FDA-approved use

nalbuphine, butorphanol, dezocine, buprenorphine) to patient who has received a prolonged course of oxymorphone (a pure agonist). In opioid-dependent patients, mixed agonist/antagonist analgesics may precipitate withdrawal symptoms.

PATIENT/FAMILY EDUCATION
• Physical dependency may result when used for extended periods
• Change position slowly, orthostatic hypotension may occur

---

oxytetracycline
(ox'ee-tet-tra-sye'kleen)
Rx: Terramycin
Combinations
  Rx: with polymyxin (Terek); with phenazopyridine, sulfamethizole (Urobiotic-250, Tija)
Chemical Class: Tetracycline derivative
Therapeutic Class: Antibiotic

CLINICAL PHARMACOLOGY
Mechanism of Action: Inhibits protein synthesis in microorganisms by binding at the bacterial 30S ribosomal subunit; bacteriostatic
Pharmacokinetics
PO: Peak 2-4 hr; absorption 50%, decreased by food; 20%-40% protein bound; $t_{1/2}$ 6-10 hr; excreted in urine, bile, feces in active form
INDICATIONS AND USES: Treatment of infections caused by the following susceptible organisms:
• Gram-positive organisms: *Streptococcus* spp. (44%-74% resistant), *Diplococcus pneumoniae*
• Gram-negative organisms: *E. coli, Enterobacter aerogenes, Shigella* spp., *Actinobacter calcoaceticus, Haemophilus influenzae, H. ducreyi, Klebsiella* spp., *Yersinia pestis, Francisella tularensis, Bartonella bacilliformis, Bacteroides* spp.,

Campylobacter fetus, Brucella spp. (in conjunction with streptomycin)
• Miscellaneous organisms: *Treponema pallidum, T. pertenue* (syphilis and yaws), *Chlamydia trachomatis,* agents of lymphogranuloma venereum and granuloma inguinale, rickettsial infections, agents of psittacosis and ornithosis, *Mycoplasma pneumoniae, Borrelia recurrentis, Neisseria gonorrhoeae, N. meningitidis* (IV only), *Listeria monocytogenes, Clostridium* spp., *Bacillus anthracis, Fusobacterium fusiforme, Actinomyces* spp.

DOSAGE
Adult
• *Moderate to severe infections:* PO 250-500 mg q6h; IM 100 mg q8h or 150 mg q12h
• *Gonorrhea:* PO 1.5 g, then 500 mg qid for a total of 9 g
• *Chlamydia trachomatis:* PO 500 mg qid × 7 days
• *Syphilis:* PO 2-3 g in divided doses × 10-15 days up to 30-40 g total (not agent of first choice)
• *Acne:* PO 250 mg qid × 2 wk; then 250-500 mg qd
• Dosage adjustment necessary in renal impairment
Child >8 yr
• *Moderate to severe infections:* PO 25-50 mg/kg/day in divided doses q6h; IM 15-25 mg/kg/day in divided doses q8-12h

🔢 AVAILABLE FORMS/COST OF THERAPY
• Inj, Sol—IM: 50 mg/ml, 5's: **$47.18**
• Cap—Oral: 250 mg, 100's: **$85.50**
PRECAUTIONS: Renal disease, hepatic disease, last trimester of pregnancy, neonatal period and early childhood (may cause permanent tooth discoloration in children <8 yr), direct sunlight exposure, outdated products (have been associ-

---

ated with Fanconi's syndrome), sulfite sensitivity, hiatal hernia

PREGNANCY AND LACTATION:
Pregnancy category D; excreted into breast milk; milk:plasma ratio: 0.6-0.8; theoretically, may cause dental staining, but usually undetectable in infant serum (<0.05 µg/ml)

SIDE EFFECTS/ADVERSE REACTIONS

CNS: Fever, pseudotumor cerebri
CV: Pericarditis
EENT: Decreased calcification of deciduous teeth, dysphagia, glossitis, oral candidiasis
GI: Abdominal cramps, abdominal pain, anorexia, black, hairy tongue; *diarrhea,* dysphagia, enterocolitis, epigastric burning, fatty liver, flatulence, ***hepatotoxicity,*** *nausea,* proctitis, pruritus ani, sore throat; stomatitis, vomiting
GU: Increased BUN
HEME: Eosinophilia, ***hemolytic anemia, leukocytosis, neutropenia, thrombocytopenia***
SKIN: Angioedema, ***exfoliative dermatitis,*** *increased pigmentation,* onycholysis and discoloration of nails, pain at inj site, *photosensitivity,* pruritus, *rash, urticaria*
MISC: Tooth discoloration in children <8 yr

INTERACTIONS

Drugs

❷ *Antacids:* Reduced absorption of oxytetracycline
❸ *Bismuth salts:* Reduced absorption of oxytetracycline
❸ *Calcium:* See antacids
❸ *Food:* Reduced absorption of oxytetracycline
❸ *Iron:* Reduced absorption of oxytetracycline
❸ *Magnesium:* See antacids
❷ *Methoxyflurane:* Increased risk of nephrotoxicity
❸ *Oral contraceptives:* Interrup-

tion of enterohepatic circulation of estrogens, reduced oral contraceptive effectiveness
❸ *Zinc:* Reduced absorption of oxytetracycline

Labs

• *False negative:* Urine glucose with Clinistix or TesTape
• *Interference:* Uroporphyrin
• *False increase:* Urinary and plasma catecholamines, serum billirubin, CFS protein, urine glucose, serum uric acid, urine vanillylmandelic acid

SPECIAL CONSIDERATIONS:
• Offers no significant advantage over tetracycline; shares similar spectrum of activity (may be slightly less active than tetracycline and has longer dosage interval)

PATIENT/FAMILY EDUCATION
• Avoid milk products, take with a full glass of water

---

oxytocin
(ox-ee-toe'sin)
Rx: Pitocin, Syntocinon
Chemical Class: Synthetic polypeptide
Therapeutic Class: Oxytocic, galactokinetic

CLINICAL PHARMACOLOGY
Mechanism of Action: Produced by the posterior pituitary, augments the number of contracting myofibrils in the uterus, producing contraction; induces alveolar milk ejection (not production); has weak antidiuretic effects

Pharmacokinetics
IM: Onset 3-5 min, duration 3-5 hr
IV: Onset immediate, duration 30-60 min
Not absorbed orally; $t_{1/2}$<10 min; elimination via liver, kidneys, and oxytocinase

INDICATIONS AND USES: Induction and augmentation of labor; missed or incomplete abortion (adjunctive); postpartum bleeding; postpartum breast engorgement,* antepartum fetal heart rate testing (oxytocin challenge test)*

DOSAGE

Adult

• *Labor induction:* IV dilute 10 U/L of 0.9% NS or D₅NS, run at 1-2 mU/min at 15-30 min intervals to begin normal labor

• *Augmentation of labor:* IV INF in D₅W or 0.9% NaCl at 1-2 mU/min; may increase q15-30 min; not to exceed 20 mU/min

• *Incomplete abortion:* IV INF 10 U/500 ml D₅W or 0.9% NaCl given at 20-40 mU/min

• *Control of postpartum bleeding:* IV dilute 10-40 U/L, run at 10-20 mU/min, adjust rate as needed; IM 10 U following delivery of placenta

$ AVAILABLE FORMS/COST OF THERAPY

• Inj, Sol—IM, IV: 10 U/ml, 1 ml: **$1.22-$3.50**

CONTRAINDICATIONS: Cephalopelvic disproportion; fetal distress where delivery is not imminent; hypertonic uterus, contraindication to vaginal delivery (i.e., active herpes genitalis, placenta previa, cord presentation, or prolapse)

PRECAUTIONS: Cervical or uterine surgery, uterine sepsis, fetal distress, partial placenta previa, prematurity, cyclopropane anesthesia (maternal bradycardia), water intoxication

PREGNANCY AND LACTATION: Nasal oxytocin contraindicated during pregnancy; only minimal amounts pass into breast milk

SIDE EFFECTS/ADVERSE REACTIONS

CNS: Hypertension, *seizures,* tetanic contractions

CV: Bradycardia, *dysrhythmias,* hypotension, increased pulse, premature ventricular contractions, tachycardia

FETUS: **Dysrhythmias, hypoxia, intracranial hemorrhage,** jaundice

GI: Anorexia, constipation, nausea, vomiting

GU: **Abruptio placentae,** decreased uterine blood flow

METAB: Anuria, confusion, drowsiness, headache, water intoxication

RESP: Asphyxia

SKIN: Rash

SPECIAL CONSIDERATIONS

• Routinely used for the induction of labor at term and postpartum for the control of uterine bleeding; not the drug of choice for induction of labor for abortion

MONITORING PARAMETERS

• Continuous monitoring necessary for IV use (length, intensity, duration of contractions); fetal heart rate—acceleration, deceleration, fetal distress

---

pamidronate
(pam-id'drow-nate)
Rx: Aredia
Chemical Class: Synthetic analog of pyrophosphate
Therapeutic Class: Bisphosphonate

P

CLINICAL PHARMACOLOGY

Mechanism of Action: Binds to hydroxyapatite at sites of bone resorption, inhibiting normal and abnormal bone resorption ("crystal poison"); minimal secondary reduction in bone formation (resorption coupled to formation)

Pharmacokinetics

IV: Taken up by bones (49% of dose); 51% excreted unchanged in urine within 72 hr; $t_{1/2}$ 27.2 hr

INDICATIONS AND USES: Paget's disease; hypercalcemia of malig-

---

italic = common side effects   ***bold italic*** = life-threatening reactions

nancy; osteolytic bone lesions of multiple myeloma;* heterotropic ossification caused by spinal cord injury or complicating total hip replacement,* hyperparathyroidism,* bone pain in prostatic carcinoma and metastatic breast cancer,* prevention of glucocorticoid-induced osteoporosis*

DOSAGE

Adult

• *Severe hypercalcemia of malignancy* (corrected serum calcium >13.5 mg/dl): IV INF 90 mg over 24 hr

• *Moderate hypercalcemia of malignancy* (corrected serum calcium 12-13.5 mg/dl): IV INF 60 mg over at least 4 hr or 90 mg over 24 hr

• *Paget's disease:* IV INF 30 mg over 4 hr on 3 consecutive days (total 90 mg)

• *Osteolytic bone lesions of multiple myeloma:* IV 90 mg over 4 hr once monthly

$ AVAILABLE FORMS/COST OF THERAPY

• Inj, Sol—IV: 30 mg, 1's: **$244.75**; 90 mg, 1's: **$678.31**

PRECAUTIONS: Renal dysfunction

PREGNANCY AND LACTATION: Pregnancy category C; caution with administration to a nursing mother

SIDE EFFECTS/ADVERSE REACTIONS

CNS: Headache, *seizures*

CV: Hypertension

EENT: Iritis, uveitis

GI: Abdominal pain, anorexia, constipation, nausea, vomiting

GU: Fluid overload, UTI

HEME: Anemia

METAB: Hyperpyrexia, hypokalemia, hypomagnesemia, hypophosphatemia

MS: Bone pain

SKIN: Induration, pain on palpita-

tion at site of catheter insertion, redness, swelling

SPECIAL CONSIDERATIONS

• "Second-generation" bisphosphonate that offers potential advantages over etidronate (as does alendronate) in that it inhibits bone resorption at doses that do not impair bone mineralization, and is less likely than etidronate to produce osteomalacia

• Allow at least 7 days between initial treatment for patients requiring retreatment for hypercalcemia

---

pancrelipase
(pan-kre-li'pase)

Rx: Cotazym, Cotazym-S, Creon, Ilozyme, Ku-Zyme HP, Lipram, Pancrease, Pancrease MT, Protilase, Ultrase MT, Viokase, Zymase

Chemical Class: Pancreatic enzymes

Therapeutic Class: Digestant

CLINICAL PHARMACOLOGY

Mechanism of Action: Pancreatic enzymes: hydrolyze fats to glycerol and fatty acids; change protein to proteoses; convert starch into dextrins and sugars

INDICATIONS AND USES: Exocrine pancreatic secretion insufficiency due to cystic fibrosis (digestive aid), chronic pancreatitis, postpancreatectomy, ductal obstructions caused by cancer; steatorrhea due to malabsorption syndrome and postgastrectomy, or post-GI surgery

DOSAGE

Adjust dosage according to severity of symptoms (steatorrhea)

Adult

• 4000-48,000 U lipase with each meal/snack; may increase to 64,000-80,000 U with meals or increase to hourly intervals in severe deficiencies provided adverse GI effects do not occur; powder 0.7 g with meals and snacks

Child

• 6 mo-1 yr, 2000 U lipase per meal
• 1-6 yr, 4000-8000 U lipase with each meal; 4000 U with snacks
• 7-12 yr, 4000-12,000 U lipase with each meal and snacks

$ AVAILABLE FORMS/COST OF THERAPY

• Cap, Enteric Coated—Oral: 4000 U lipase/12,000 U protease/12,000 U amylase, 100's: **$31.76;** 4000/25,000/20,000, 100's: **$28.24-$32.80;** 5000/20,000/20,000, 100's: **$31.61;** 8000/30,000/30,000, 100's: **$23.37-$47.08;** 10,000/30,000/30,000, 100's: **$68.49;** 3,000/67,500/33,200, 100's: **$68.49;** 12,000/24,000/24,000, 100's: **$56.16;** 12,000/39,000/39,000, 100's: **$58.10;** 16,000/48,000/48,000, 100's: **$127.50;** 20,000/65,000/65,000, 100's: **$158.81;** 20,000/75,000/66,400, 100's: **$125.30**

• Tab, uncoated—Oral: 8000 U lipase/30,000 U protease/30,000 U amylase, 100's: **$33.60;** 11,000/30,000/30,000, 250's: **$132.60**

• Powder—Oral: 16,800 U lipase/70,000 U protease/70,000 U amylase, 8 oz: **$138.10**

CONTRAINDICATIONS: Hypersensitivity to pork, acute pancreatitis and exacerbations of chronic pancreatic disease

PREGNANCY AND LACTATION: Pregnancy category C

SIDE EFFECTS/ADVERSE REACTIONS

EENT: Buccal soreness

GI: Anal soreness, anorexia, diarrhea, glossitis, nausea, vomiting

METAB: Hyperuricemia, hyperuricuria

SKIN: Rash

SPECIAL CONSIDERATIONS

• Substitution at dispensing should be avoided

• Enteric-coated pancreatic enzymes are more effective than regular formulations; individual variations may require trials with several enzymatic preparations

• For patients who do not respond appropriately, adding antacid or H_2-antagonist may provide better results

• Preparations high in lipase concentration seem to be more effective for reducing steatorrhea

PATIENT/FAMILY EDUCATION

• Advise patient to take before or with meals

• Protect enteric coating; advise patient not to crush or chew microspheres in caps or tabs

MONITORING PARAMETERS

• Growth curves in children

---

pantoprazole

(pan-toe-pra′zole)

Rx: Prontonix

Chemical Class: Substituted benzimidazole

Therapeutic Class: Gastrointestinal antiulcer agent

CLINICAL PHARMACOLOGY

Mechanism of Action: Suppresses gastric acid secretion by inhibiting the parietal cell H^+/K^+ ATP pump

Pharmacokinetics

PO: Bioavailability 77%; 98% bound to plasma proteins; extensively metabolized by liver cytochrome P450 enzymes; metabolites primarily eliminated in the urine; $t_{1/2}$ 2 hr (does not reflect duration of acid suppression)

INDICATIONS AND USES: Short-term treatment of duodenal ulcers; short-term treatment of gastric ulcers; moderate to severe GERD; eradication of *H. pylori* infection (in combination with clarithromycin and metronidazole)

---

italic = common side effects   ***bold italic*** = life-threatening reactions

DOSAGE

Adult

• PO 40 mg qd taken before or with breakfast

💲 **AVAILABLE FORMS/COST OF THERAPY**

• *Not available*

PRECAUTIONS: Symptomatic response does not rule out gastric malignancy; hepatic insufficiency

PREGNANCY AND LACTATION: Pregnancy category C; excretion into breast milk unknown, use caution in nursing mothers

SIDE EFFECTS/ADVERSE REACTIONS

CNS: Headache, dizziness, depression

CV: Edema

EENT: Visual disturbances

GI: Diarrhea, nausea, abdominal pain, flatulence

SKIN: Rash, pruritis

MISC: Fever

INTERACTIONS

Drugs

❸ *Ketoconazole:* Decreased bioavailability of ketoconazole

MONITORING PARAMETERS

• Symptom relief, mucosal healing

---

papaverine

(pa-pav′er-een)

Rx: Papacon, Pavabid Plateau, Pava-Time S.R., Pavacot, Pavagen T.D.

Chemical Class: Benzylisoquinoline alkaloid

Therapeutic Class: Peripheral vasodilator

CLINICAL PHARMACOLOGY

Mechanism of Action: Relaxes all smooth muscle; inhibits cyclic nucleotide phosphodiesterase, which increases intracellular cAMP, causing vasodilation; increases cerebral blood flow and decreases cerebral vascular resistance in normal subjects

Pharmacokinetics

SUS REL: Poor and erratic absorption; oral bioavailability 54%; 90% bound to plasma proteins; metabolized in liver, excreted in urine (inactive metabolites) $t_{1/2}$ varies widely; peak plasma levels 1-2 hr

INDICATIONS AND USES: Arterial spasm resulting in cerebral and peripheral ischemia*; myocardial ischemia associated with vascular spasm or dysrhythmias*

DOSAGE

Adult

• PO SUS REL 150-300 mg q8-12h

💲 **AVAILABLE FORMS/COST OF THERAPY**

• Cap, Gel, SUS Action—Oral: 150 mg, 100's: **$6.75-$11.35**

• Inj, sol—30 mg/ml 2 ml: **$3.75-$10.00**

CONTRAINDICATIONS: Complete AV heart block

PRECAUTIONS: Cardiac dysrhythmias, glaucoma

PREGNANCY AND LACTATION: Pregnancy category C

SIDE EFFECTS/ADVERSE REACTIONS

CNS: Dizziness, drowsiness, headache, malaise, sedation, vertigo

CV: Increased blood pressure, tachycardia

GI: Abdominal pain, altered liver enzymes, anorexia, constipation, diarrhea, hepatotoxicity, jaundice, nausea

RESP: Increased depth of respirations

SKIN: Flushing, rash, *sweating*

INTERACTIONS

Drugs

❸ *Levodopa:* Loss of control of Parkinson's disease

---

* = non-FDA-approved use

SPECIAL CONSIDERATIONS
• No objective evidence of *any* therapeutic value

---

paregoric
(par-e-gor'ik)
Rx: Paregoric
Chemical Class: Opiate (most preparations also contain camphor and ethanol)
Therapeutic Class: Antidiarrheal
DEA Class: Schedule III

CLINICAL PHARMACOLOGY
Mechanism of Action: Direct effect on circular smooth muscle of the bowel that prolongs GI transit time; reduces GI secretions
Pharmacokinetics
PO: Onset 20-30 min, peak 60 min, duration 4 hr; metabolized in liver by glucuronidation; metabolites excreted in urine (90% within 24 hr), 10% excreted in bile
INDICATIONS AND USES: Diarrhea; neonatal opioid withdrawal syndrome*
DOSAGE
Adult
• PO 5-10 ml up to qid
Child
• *Antidiarrheal:* Age >2 yr, PO 0.25-0.5 ml/kg up to qid
• *Opioid withdrawal syndrome:* Neonate, PO 0.2 ml q3h, increase dose by 0.05 ml q3h until symptoms controlled (max dose of 0.7 ml)
• NOTE: 4 ml of paregoric equal to 2.5 mg diphenoxylate, 1.6 mg morphine sulfate
💲 AVAILABLE FORMS/COST OF THERAPY
• Liq—Oral: 0.4 mg/ml, 480 ml: **$7.30-$10.13**
CONTRAINDICATIONS: Diarrhea due to poisoning, infectious diarrhea

PRECAUTIONS: Respiratory disease, elderly patients
PREGNANCY AND LACTATION: Pregnancy category B; excreted in breast milk
SIDE EFFECTS/ADVERSE REACTIONS
CNS: Depression, *dizziness, drowsiness,* fatigue, restlessness, withdrawal syndrome (with prolonged use at high dose)
CV: Hypotension, orthostatic hypotension
EENT: Miosis
GI: Abdominal cramping, *constipation*
GU: Urinary retention
RESP: Respiratory depression
SKIN: Pruritus
INTERACTIONS
Drugs
3 *Barbiturates, rifampin:* Increased metabolism of paregoric
3 *Cimetidine:* Decreased metabolism of paregoric
SPECIAL CONSIDERATIONS
• Contains ethanol

---

paricalcitol
(pare-i-cal'sih-tal)
Rx: Zemplar
Chemical Class: Synthetic vitamin D analog
Therapeutic Class: Fat-soluble vitamin

CLINICAL PHARMACOLOGY
Mechanism of Action: Suppresses parathyroid hormone (PTH) levels in patients with chronic renal failure (CRF)
Pharmacokinetics
IV: Peak 5 min; approximately 50% metabolized; eliminated primarily by hepatobiliary excretion, 74% of dose recovered in feces, 16% recovered in urine; $t_{1/2}$ 15 hr
INDICATIONS AND USES: Preven-

---

italic = common side effects   ***bold italic*** = life-threatening reactions

tion and treatment of secondary hyperparathyroidism associated with CRF

DOSAGE
Adult
• IV bolus 0.04 to 0.2 mcg/kg no more frequently than qod at any time during dialysis; max 0.24 mcg/kg if satisfactory response not observed, dose may be increased by 2-4 mcg at 2-4 wk intervals

$ AVAILABLE FORMS/COST OF THERAPY
• Inj—IV 5 mcg/ml, 1 ml: **$26.48**
CONTRAINDICATIONS: Evidence of vitamin D toxicity, hypercalcemia
PRECAUTIONS: Children
PREGNANCY AND LACTATION: Pregnancy category C; use caution in nursing mothers
SIDE EFFECTS/ADVERSE REACTIONS
CNS: Lightheadedness
CV: Palpitation, edema
*GI: **GI bleeding**, nausea,* vomiting, dry mouth
RESP: Pneumonia
MISC: Chills, feeling unwell, fever, flu, sepsis
INTERACTIONS
Drugs
3 *Digoxin:* Hypercalcemia produced by paricalcitol may potentiate digoxin toxicity

SPECIAL CONSIDERATIONS
• Phosphate-binding compounds may be needed to control serum phosphorus levels
PATIENT/FAMILY EDUCATION
• Adhere to a dietary regimen of calcium supplementation and phosphorus restriction; avoid excessive use of aluminum-containing compounds
MONITORING PARAMETERS
• Serum calcium and phosphorus twice weekly during initial phase of therapy, then at least monthly once

dosage has been established; if an elevated calcium level or a Ca × P product > 75 is noted, immediately reduce or interrupt dosage until parameters are normalized, then reinitiate at lower dose; intact PTH assay every 3 mo (target range in CRF patients ≤ 1.5-3 × the nonuremic upper limit of normal)

---

paromomycin
(par-oh-moe-mye′sin)
Rx: Humatin
Chemical Class: Aminoglycoside
Therapeutic Class: Amebicide; antibiotic

CLINICAL PHARMACOLOGY
Mechanism of Action: Direct action in intestinal lumen
Pharmacokinetics
PO: Poor absorption; 100% excreted in feces
INDICATIONS AND USES: Intestinal amebiasis; adjunct in hepatic coma; other parasitic infections* *(Dientamoeba fragilis, Diphyllobothrium latum, Taenia saginata, T. solium, Dipylidium caninum, Hymenolepis nana)*
DOSAGE
Adult
• *Intestinal amebiasis:* PO 25-35 mg/kg/day in 3 divided doses pc for 5-10 days
• *Hepatic coma:* 4 g qd in divided doses for 5-6 days
Child
• *Intestinal amebiasis:* PO 25-35 mg/kg/day in 3 divided doses pc for 5-10 days
$ AVAILABLE FORMS/COST OF THERAPY
• Cap, Gel—Oral: 250 mg, 100's: **$190.08**
CONTRAINDICATIONS: GI obstruction

---

* = non-FDA-approved use

PRECAUTIONS: GI ulcerations, superinfection

PREGNANCY AND LACTATION: Pregnancy category C; poor oral bioavailability and lipid solubility limit passage into breast milk

SIDE EFFECTS/ADVERSE REACTIONS

EENT: Ototoxicity

GI: Anorexia, diarrhea, epigastric distress, nausea, pruritus ani, steatorrhea, *vomiting*

GU: Hematuria, ***nephrotoxicity***

---

paroxetine
(par-ox′e-teen)

Rx: Paxil, Paxil CR

Chemical Class: Phenylpiperidine

Therapeutic Class: Selective serotonin reuptake inhibitor (SSRI) antidepressant

---

CLINICAL PHARMACOLOGY

Mechanism of Action: Inhibits CNS neuronal uptake of serotonin (5HT); no significant activity for histaminergic, α- or β-adrenergic, muscarinic, or dopaminergic receptors

Pharmacokinetics

PO: Peak 5.2 hr; protein binding 93%-95%; metabolized in liver (CYP2D6), unchanged drugs and metabolites excreted in feces (36%) and urine (64%); $t_{1/2}$ 21 hr

INDICATIONS AND USES: Major depressive disorder; obsessive-compulsive disorder; panic disorder; social phobia

DOSAGE

Adult

• *Depression:* PO 20 mg qd in AM; after 4 wk if no clinical improvement is noted, dose may be increased by 10 mg/day qwk to desired response, not to exceed 50 mg/day

• *Obsessive-compulsive disorder:* PO 20 mg qd, increase in 1 wk increments by 10 mg/day; usual dose requirement 40 mg/day, maximum 60 mg/day

• *Panic disorder:* PO 10 mg qd, increase by 10 mg/day qwk prn; maximum 60 mg/day

§ AVAILABLE FORMS/COST OF THERAPY

• Tab, Uncoated—Oral: 10 mg, 30's: **$66.95;** 20 mg, 30's: **$69.85;** 30 mg, 30's: **$71.95;** 40 mg, 30's: **$76.00**

• Suspension: 10 mg/5 ml, 250 ml: **$111.40**

CONTRAINDICATIONS: Patients taking MAOIs (or within 14 days of discontinuing an MAOI)

PRECAUTIONS: History of mania; renal and hepatic disease

PREGNANCY AND LACTATION: Pregnancy category B; limited information; milk concentrations similar to plasma following a single oral dose; thus <1% of the daily dose would be transferred to a breast-feeding infant

SIDE EFFECTS/ADVERSE REACTIONS

CNS: Agitation, *anxiety,* asthenia, delusions, dizziness, euphoria, fatigue, hallucinations, headache, insomnia, myoclonus, nervousness, psychosis, sedation, tremor

CV: Palpitations, postural hypotension, vasodilation

EENT: Pharyngitis, visual changes

GI: Anorexia, constipation, cramps, *decreased appetite,* diarrhea, dry mouth, dyspepsia, flatulence, *nausea,* taste changes, vomiting

GU: Abnormal ejaculation, urinary frequency

MS: Arthritis, myalgia, myasthenia, myopathy, pain

RESP: Cough, dyspnea, infection, nasal congestion, pharyngitis, sinus headache, sinusitis

P

---

italic = common side effects   ***bold italic*** = life-threatening reactions

SKIN: Rash, sweating
MISC: Fever
INTERACTIONS
Drugs

3 *Beta-blockers (metroprolol, propranolol, sotalol):* Inhibition of metabolism (CYP2D6) leads to increased plasma concentrations of selective beta blockers and potential cardiac toxicity; atenolol may be safer choice

3 *Carbamazepine:* Inhibition of hepatic metabolism of carbamazepine, but the formation of carbamazepine epoxide is not inhibited, contributing to increased toxicity

3 *Cyproheptadine:* Serotonin antagonist may partially reverse antidepressant and other effects

2 *Dexfenfluramine:* Duplicate effects on inhibition of serotonin reuptake; inhibition of dexfenfluramine metabolism (CYP2D6) exaggerates effect; both mechanisms increase risk of serotonin syndrome

3 *Dextromethorphan:* Inhibition of dextromethorphan's metabolism (CYP2D6) by paroxetine and additive serotonergic effects

3 *Diuretics, loop (bumetanide, furosemide, torsemide):* Possible additive hyponatremia; two fatal case reports with furosemide and paroxetine

2 *Fenfluramine:* Duplicate effects on inhibition of serotonin reuptake; inhibition of dexfenfluramine metabolism (CYP2D6) exaggerates effect; both mechanisms increase risk of serotonin syndrome

3 *Haloperidol:* Inhibition of haloperidol's metabolism (CYP2D6) may increase risks of extrapyramidal symptoms

2 *HMG-Co A reductase inhibitors (atorvastatin, lovastatin, simvastatin):* Inhibition of statin metabolism (CYP3A4), by paroxetine, may lead to rhabdomyolysis

3 *Lithium:* Neurotoxicity (tremor, confusion, ataxia, dizziness, dysarthria, and absence seizures) reported in patients receiving this combination; mechanism unknown

⚠ *MAOI's (isocarboxazid, phenelzine, tranylcypromine):* Increased CNS serotonergic effects have been associated with severe or fatal reactions with this combination

3 *Selegiline:* Sporadic cases of mania and hypertension

3 *Tricyclic antidepressants (clomipramine, desipramine, doxepin, imipramine, nortriptyline, trazodone):* Marked increases in tricyclic antidepressant levels due to inhibition of metabolism (CYP2D6)

2 *Tryptophan:* Additive serotonergic effects

3 *Warfarin:* Increased risk of bleeding

SPECIAL CONSIDERATIONS
• Somewhat sedating compared to fluoxetine and sertraline

---

pemoline
(pem'oh-leen)
Rx: Cylert
Chemical Class: Oxazolidine derivative
Therapeutic Class: CNS stimulant; anorexiant
DEA Class: Schedule IV

CLINICAL PHARMACOLOGY
Mechanism of Action: Cerebral stimulation via dopaminergic mechanisms; minimal sympathomimetic effects

Pharmacokinetics
PO: Peak 2-4 hr, duration 8 hr, gradual onset of action (3-4 wk to effect); 50% protein bound; metabolized (50%) by liver, excreted (40%) by kidneys; $t_{1/2}$ 12 hr

INDICATIONS AND USES: Atten-

tion deficit disorder with hyperactivity; narcolepsy*
DOSAGE
Child >6 yr
• *Attention deficit disorder:* 37.5 mg in AM, increasing by 18.75 mg/wk, not to exceed 112.5 mg/day

[$] AVAILABLE FORMS/COST OF THERAPY
• Tab, Chewable—Oral: 37.5 mg, 100's: **$157.88**
• Tab, Uncoated—Oral: 18.75 mg, 100's: **$92.15**; 37.5 mg, 100's: **$144.84**; 75 mg, 100's: **$250.10**

CONTRAINDICATIONS: Hepatic insufficiency

PRECAUTIONS: Renal disease, drug abuse, child <6 yr

PREGNANCY AND LACTATION: Pregnancy category B

SIDE EFFECTS/ADVERSE REACTIONS

CNS: Aggressiveness, depression, dizziness, drowsiness, dyskinetic movements, Gilles de la Tourette's disorder, hallucinations, headache, *hyperactivity, insomnia,* irritability, *restlessness,* **seizures,** stimulation
GI: Abdominal pain, anorexia, diarrhea, hepatitis, increased liver enzymes, jaundice, nausea
MISC: Growth suppression in children, rashes

SPECIAL CONSIDERATIONS
MONITORING PARAMETERS
• LFTs periodically

---

penbutolol
(pen-bute'o-loll)
Rx: Levatol
Chemical Class: Nonselective β-adrenergic blocker
Therapeutic Class: Antihypertensive; antianginal

CLINICAL PHARMACOLOGY
Mechanism of Action: Competitive, nonselective, β-receptor antagonist; some intrinsic sympathomimetic activity; no membrane stabilizing activity; high lipid solubility

Pharmacokinetics

PO: Peak 1½-3 hr, duration >20 hr; absorption 100% bioavailability; metabolized by hepatic conjugation and oxidation; 80%-98% protein bound; metabolites excreted mainly in urine; $t_{½}$ 5 hr

INDICATIONS AND USES: Hypertension; angina pectoris*; MI*; migraine (prophylaxis)*; alcohol withdrawal syndrome*; aggressive behavior*; antipsychotic-induced akathisia*

DOSAGE
Adult
• *Hypertension:* 20 mg qd (flat dose-response curve)

[$] AVAILABLE FORMS/COST OF THERAPY
• Tab, Uncoated—Oral: 20 mg, 100's: **$136.81**

CONTRAINDICATIONS: Cardiogenic shock, sinus bradycardia, 2nd and 3rd degree atrioventricular conduction block, asthma

PRECAUTIONS: Anesthesia and major surgery; diabetes mellitus; abrupt withdrawal with concurrent CAD or thyrotoxicosis

PREGNANCY AND LACTATION: Pregnancy category C

SIDE EFFECTS/ADVERSE REACTIONS

CNS: Dizziness, fatigue, headache, insomnia
CV: Bradycardia, CHF
GI: Diarrhea, dyspepsia, nausea
GU: Impotence
RESP: Cough, dyspnea
SKIN: Excessive sweating

INTERACTIONS
Drugs
3 *Adenosine:* Bradycardia aggravated
3 *Amiodarone:* Bradycardia, car-

P

---

italic = common side effects   ***bold italic*** = life-threatening reactions

diac arrest, ventricular arrhythmia risk after initiation of penbutolol

3 *Antacids:* Reduced penbutolol absorption

3 *Calcium channel blockers:* See dihydropyridine calcium channel blockers and verapamil

3 *Clonidine, guanabenz, guanfacine:* Exacerbation of rebound hypertension upon discontinuation of clonidine

3 *Cocaine:* Cocaine-induced vasoconstriction potentiated; reduced coronary blood flow

3 *Contrast media:* Increased risk of anaphylaxis

3 *Digitalis:* Enhances bradycardia

3 *Dihydropyridine, calcium channel blockers:* Additive pharmacodynamic effects

3 *Dipyridamole:* Bradycardia aggravated

3 *Epinephrine, isoproterenol, phenylephrine:* Potentiates pressor response; resultant hypertension and bradycardia

3 *Flecainide:* Additive negative inotropic effects

3 *Fluoxetine:* Increased β-blockade activity

3 *Fluoroquinolones:* Reduced clearance of penbutolol

3 *Insulin:* Altered response to hypoglycemia; increased blood glucose concentrations; impaired peripheral circulation

3 *Lidocaine:* Increased serum lidocaine concentrations possible

3 *Neostigmine:* Bradycardia aggravated

3 *Neuroleptics:* Both drugs inhibit each other's metabolism; additive hypotension

3 *NSAIDs:* Reduced antihypertensive effect of penbutolol

3 *Physostigmine:* Bradycardia aggravated

3 *Prazosin:* First-dose response to prazosin may be enhanced by β-blockade

3 *Tacrine:* Bradycardia aggravated

2 *Terbutaline:* Antagonized bronchodilating effects of terbutaline

2 *Theophylline:* Antagonistic pharmacodynamic effects

3 *Verapamil:* Enhanced effects of both drugs; particularly AV nodal conduction slowing; reduced penbutolol clearance

SPECIAL CONSIDERATIONS
• Exacerbation of ischemic heart disease following abrupt withdrawal due to hypersensitivity to catecholamines possible
• Comparative trials indicate that penbutolol is as effective as propranolol and atenolol in the treatment of hypertension; may have fewer adverse CNS effects than propranolol

---

penciclovir
(pen-sye'kloe-veer)
Rx: Denavir
Chemical Class: Synthetic acyclic guanine derivative
Therapeutic Class: Antiviral

CLINICAL PHARMACOLOGY
Mechanism of Action: Inhibitory activity against herpes simplex virus types 1 (HSV-1) and 2 (HSV-2); phosphorylated to penciclovir triphosphate in HSV-infected cells, inhibiting viral DNA synthesis to penciclovir triphosphate
Pharmacokinetics
• *TOP:* Measurable concentrations not found in plasma or urine
INDICATIONS AND USES: Recurrent herpes labialis (cold sores)
DOSAGE
Adult
• TOP apply to affected area q2h during waking hours for 4 days; start treatment as early as possible (i.e.,

---

* = non-FDA-approved use

during prodrome or when lesions first appear)

$ AVAILABLE FORMS/COST OF THERAPY

• Cre—Top: 10 mg/g (1%), 2 g: **$22.90**

PRECAUTIONS: Immunocompromised patients

PREGNANCY AND LACTATION: Pregnancy category B; no data in nursing mothers, but milk concentrations should be low due to apparent lack of systemic absorption

SIDE EFFECTS/ADVERSE REACTIONS

SKIN: Application site reaction, pruritus, rash

SPECIAL CONSIDERATIONS

• In clinical trials, shortened the duration of lesions by approximately ½ day compared to placebo (4½ vs. 5 days); duration of pain was also shortened by approximately ½ day

---

penicillamine
(pen-i-sill'a-meen)
Rx: Cuprimine, Depen
Chemical Class: Thiol derivative
Therapeutic Class: Heavy metal antidote; disease-modifying antiarthritic drug (DMARD)

CLINICAL PHARMACOLOGY

Mechanism of Action: Binds with ions of lead, mercury, copper, iron, zinc to form a water-soluble complex excreted by kidneys; improves lymphocyte function, markedly reduces IgM rheumatoid factor and immune complexes, depresses T-cell but not B-cell activity; combines with cystine to form disulfide, which is more soluble, reduces excess cystine excretion in cystinuria

Pharmacokinetics

PO: Peak 1 hr, onset of action (Wilson's disease, 1-3 mo, rheumatoid arthritis, 2-3 mo); metabolized in liver; renal and fecal elimination

INDICATIONS AND USES: Wilson's disease; rheumatoid arthritis; cystinuria; lead poisoning,* primary biliary cirrhosis,* scleroderma*

DOSAGE

Adult

• *Wilson's disease:* 250 mg tid-qid, maximum 2 g/day

• *Rheumatoid arthritis:* 125-250 mg/day, increase 250 mg q2-3 mo prn, max 1 g/day; doses >500 mg/d should be administered in divided doses

• *Cystinuria:* PO 250 mg qid ac, not to exceed 5 g/day

Child

• *Chelating agent and cystinuria:* 20-30 mg/kg/day in divided doses qid ac

$ AVAILABLE FORMS/COST OF THERAPY

• Cap, Gel—Oral: 125 mg, 100's: **$72.05;** 250 mg, 100's: **$102.88**

• Tab, Coated—Oral: 250 mg, 100's: **$197.66**

CONTRAINDICATIONS: Penicillamine-related aplastic anemia or agranulocytosis; severe renal disease; pregnancy (except Wilson's disease or certain cases of cystinuria)

PRECAUTIONS: Renal insufficiency

PREGNANCY AND LACTATION: Pregnancy category D (continued therapy in Wilson's disease and cystinuria probably OK, not rheumatoid arthritis)

SIDE EFFECTS/ADVERSE REACTIONS

CV: Hypotension, tachycardia
EENT: Optic neuritis, tinnitus
GI: Abdominal cramping, anorexia, *diarrhea,* hepatotoxicity, *nausea,* pain, peptic ulcer, *vomiting*

---

italic = common side effects   **bold italic** = life-threatening reactions

P

GU: Glomerulonephritis, nephrotic syndrome, proteinuria
HEME: Aplastic anemia, eosinophilia, *granulocytopenia, hemolytic anemia,* increased sedimentation rate, *leukopenia,* lupus syndrome, *thrombocytopenia*
MS: Arthralgia
RESP: Asthma, pneumonitis, *pulmonary fibrosis*
SKIN: Alopecia, ecchymosis, *erythema,* fever, *pruritus, urticaria*

INTERACTIONS

Drugs

■ *Antacids:* Magnesium-aluminum hydroxides reduce bioavailability
■ *Digoxin:* Reduced digoxin concentrations
■ *Iron:* Oral iron substantially reduces plasma penicillamine concentration, with reduced therapeutic response

Labs

• *Cholesterol:* Decreased serum levels
• *Fructoseamine:* Decreased serum levels
• *Iron:* Decreased serum levels
• *Ketones:* Increased false-positive reactions with legal reaction

SPECIAL CONSIDERATIONS

• Because penicillamine can cause severe adverse reactions, restrict its use in rheumatoid arthritis to patients who have severe, active disease and who have failed to respond to an adequate trial of conventional therapy

PATIENT/FAMILY EDUCATION

• Should be administered on empty stomach, ½-1 hr before meals or at least 2 hr after meals
• Urine may become discolored (red)
• Patients with cystinuria should drink large amounts of water

• Therapeutic effect may take 1-3 mo

MONITORING PARAMETERS

• Hepatic, renal studies: CBC, urinalysis, skin for rash
• Urinary copper excretion

---

penicillin

(pen-i-sill'in)
Rx: *Penicillin G (Aqueous Pen G):* Pfizerpen
Rx: *Penicillin G: Pentids*
Rx: *Penicillin V:* (Phenoxymethyl Penicillin), Beepen VK, Pen-V, Pen-Vee K, Truxcillin VK, Veetids
Rx: *Penicillin G Benzathine:* Bicillin L-A, Permapen
Rx: *Penicillin G Procaine:* Crysticillin, Wycillin
Rx: *Penicillin G Benzathine and Procaine combined:* Bicillin C-R
Chemical Class: Natural penicillin
Therapeutic Class: Antibiotic

CLINICAL PHARMACOLOGY

Mechanism of Action: Inhibits bacterial wall synthesis; bactericidal
Pharmacokinetics
Excreted in urine and breast milk, crosses placenta
• *Penicillin G:* IV immediate peak; IM peak 15-30 min; PO duration 6 hr, peak 1 hr
• *Penicillin V:* PO peak 30-60 min, duration 6-8 hr, $t_{1/2}$ 30 min
• *Benzathine Penicillin:* IM very slow absorption, duration 21-28 days, $t_{1/2}$ 30-60 min
• *Procaine Penicillin:* IM peak 1-4 hr, duration 15 hr

INDICATIONS AND USES: For infections caused by susceptible organisms: *Penicillin G:* meningococcal meningitis, syphilis, anthrax, streptococcal infections, botulism, diphtheria, listeria, pasteurella infections, Lyme disease*; *Penicillin V:* scarlet fever; erysipelas; skin and soft-tissue infections; Vincent's gingivitis and pharyngitis; strep pharyngitis; rheumatic fever prophylaxis; endocarditis prophylaxis; *Benzathine penicillin:* Group A strep respiratory tract infection; syphilis; yaws; prophylaxis of rheumatic fever and/or chorea; *Procaine penicillin:* otitis media; skin and soft-tissue infections; scarlet fever; erysipelas; Vincent's gingivitis and pharyngitis; syphilis; gonorrhea; endocarditis prophylaxis; yaws; anthrax; erysipeloid; *Benzathine and procaine penicillin combined:* moderately severe streptococcal and pneumococcal infections. Do not use for severe infections, syphilis, gonorrhea, or yaws.

Antibacterial spectrum includes non–penicillinase-producing strains of:

• Gram-positive organisms: *Staphylococcus aureus, Streptococcus pyogenes, Str. viridans, Str. faecalis, Str. bovis, Str. pneumoniae, Bacillus anthracis, Listeria monocytogenes, Corynebacterium diphtheriae*

• Gram-negative organisms: *Neisseria gonorrhoeae, N. meningitidis, E. coli, Proteus mirabilis, Salmonella, Shigella, Enterobacter, S. moniliformis*

• Anaerobes: *Clostridium* sp., *Peptococcus* sp., *Peptostreptococcus* sp., *Bacteroides* sp. (except *B. fragilis*), *Fusobacterium* sp., *Eubacterium* sp.,

• Other organisms: *Treponema pallidum, Actinomyces bovis*

DOSAGE

Penicillin G (aqueous)

Adult

• *Moderate to severe infections:* IM/IV 12-30 million U/day in divided doses q4h

• *Endocarditis prophylaxis:* IM/IV 2 million U 30-60 min before dental procedure; 1 million U 6 hr after procedure

Child

• *Moderate to severe infections:* IM/IV 25,000-300,000 U/day in divided doses q4-12h

Penicillin G

Adult

• *Pneumococcal/streptococcal infections:* PO 400,000-500,000 U q6-8h for 10 days

• *Rheumatic fever prophylaxis:* PO 200,000-250,000 U bid continuously

• *Meningococcal meningitis:* IM 1-2 million U q2h; IV 20-30 million U/day continuous drip for 14 day or until afebrile for 7 day

• *Pneumococcal empyema:* IV 5-24 million U/day in divided doses q4-6h

• *Pneumococcal meningitis:* IV 20-24 million U/day in divided doses q4-6h for 14 day

• *Pasturella infections:* IV 4-6 million U/day in divided doses for 2 wk

• *Listeria infections:* IV 15-20 million U/day in divided doses for 2 wk (meningitis) or 4 wk (endocarditis)

• *Neurosyphilis:* IV 2-4 million U q4h for 10-14 days (many recommend following with Pen G Benzathine 2.4 million U IM qwk for 3 doses)

Child

• *Pneumococcal/streptococcal infections:* PO 25,000-90,000 U/kg/day in 3-6 divided doses

• *Rheumatic fever prophylaxis:* PO 25,000-90,000 U/kg/day in 3-6 divided doses; IV 100,000-250,000 U/kg/day in divided doses q4h

Infant (use larger doses for meningitis)

• >7 days and >2000 g, IV 100,000-200,000 U/kg/day in divided doses q6h

• >7 days and <2000 g, IV 75,000-

P

150,000 U/kg/day in divided doses q8h
• <7 days and >2000 g, IV 50,000-150,000 U/kg/day in divided doses q8h
• <7 days and <2000 g, IV 50,000-100,000 U/kg/day in divided doses q12h

Penicillin V

Adult

• *Pneumococcal infections:* PO 250-500 mg q6h
• *Streptococcal infections:* PO 125-250 mg q6-8h for 10 days
• *Strep pharyngitis:* PO 500 mg bid for 10 days
• *Rheumatic fever prophylaxis:* PO 125-250 mg bid continuously

Child

• PO 15-50 mg/kg/day in divided doses q6h

Benzathine penicillin

Adult

• *Early syphilis:* IM 2.4 million U in single dose
• *Syphilis >1 yr duration:* IM 2.4 million U in single dose
• *Neurosyphilis:* To follow up treatment with Pen G procaine or Pen G potassium as below
• *Group A strep URI:* IM 1.2 million U in single dose
• *Rheumatic fever:* IM 1.2 million U in single dose q mo or 600,000 U q2 wk

Child

• *Congenital syphilis (<2 yr):* IM 50,000 U/kg in single dose
• *Rheumatic fever/glomerulonephritis prophylaxis (<60 lb):* IM 600,000 U in single dose
• *Group A strep URI (>27 kg):* IM 900,000 U in single dose; (<27 kg) 50,000 U/kg in single dose

Procaine penicillin

Adult

• *Moderate to severe infections:* IM 600,000-1.2 million U/day in divided doses

• *Gonorrhea:* IM 4.8 million U in two inj given 30 min after probenecid 1 g
• *Syphilis (primary, secondary, latent with neg CSF):* IM 600,000 U/day for 8 days
• *Neurosyphilis:* IM 2-4 million U/day with probenecid 500 mg qid for 10-14 days (many recommend following with Pen G benzathine 2.4 million U q wk for 3 doses)

Child

• *Moderate to severe infections:* Same as adult; avoid in newborn (risk procaine toxicity, sterile abscess)
• *Congenital syphilis:* IM 50,000 U/kg qd for 10-14 days

Benzothaine and procaine penicillin combined

Adult

• *Moderate infections:* 2.4 million U IM once or q2-3 days until temperature normalizes

Child

• *Moderate infections:* (30-60 pounds) 900,000-1.2 million U; (<30 pounds) 600,000 units U once or q2-3 days until temperature normalizes

💲 **AVAILABLE FORMS/COST OF THERAPY**

Penicillin G (aqueous)
• Inj, Sol—IV: 1,000,000 U/vial, 10 ml: **$0.89;** 2,000,000 U, 50 ml, 1500 ml: **$324.48;** 3,000,000 U, 50 ml, 1500 ml: **$336.72;** 5,000,000 U/vial: **$2.51;** 10,000,000 U/vial: **$6.40;** 20,000,000 U/vial: **$10.09**

Penicillin G
• Inj, Dry-Sol—IM, IV: 5,000,000 U: **$6.34**

Penicillin V
• Tab, Uncoated—Oral: 250 mg, 100's: **$5.50-$8.12;** 500 mg, 100's: **$9.24-$15.30**
• Powder, Reconst—Oral: 125 mg/5 ml, 100 ml: **$1.67-$6.25;** 250 mg/5 ml, 100 ml: **$2.16-$5.98**

* = non-FDA-approved use

Benzathine penicillin G
• Inj, Susp—IM: 600,000 U/ml, 1 ml: **$9.72**
Procaine penicillin G
• Inj, Sol—IM: 600,000 U/ml, 1 ml: **$6.58**
Benzathine/procaine penicillin G combined
• Inj, Susp—IM: 150,000 U/150,000 U/ml, 10 ml: **$18.55-$19.36;** 300,000 U/300,000 U/ml, 2 ml: **$12.86-$13.43;** 900,000 U/300,000 U/2 ml, 2 ml: **$13.97**
PRECAUTIONS: Hypersensitivity to cephalosporins
PREGNANCY AND LACTATION: Pregnancy category B; may cause diarrhea, candidiasis, or allergic response in nursing infant
SIDE EFFECTS/ADVERSE REACTIONS
CNS: Anxiety, coma, depression, hallucinations, lethargy, *seizures,* twitching
GI: Abdominal pain, colitis, *diarrhea,* glossitis, *nausea, vomiting*
GU: Glomerulonephritis, hematuria, oliguria, proteinuria, vaginitis
HEME: **Bone marrow depression,** increased bleeding time
METAB: Alkalosis, hyperkalemia, hypernatremia, hypokalemia
SKIN: Rash
MISC: Jarisch-Herxheimer reaction (Benzathine penicillin E)
INTERACTIONS
Drugs
🛇 *Chloramphenicol:* Inhibited antibacterial activity of penicillin; administer penicillin 3 hr before chloramphenicol
🛇 *Macrolide antibiotics:* Inhibited antibacterial activity of penicillin; administer penicillin 3 hr before macrolides
🛇 *Methotrexate:* Penicillin in large doses may increase serum methotrexate concentrations
🛇 *Oral contraceptives:* Occasional impairment of oral contraceptive efficacy; consider use of supplemental contraception during cycles in which penicillin is used
🛇 *Tetracyclines:* Inhibited antibacterial activity of penicillin; administer penicillin 3 hr before tetracyclines
Labs
• *Albumin:* Decreased serum levels at very high penicillin levels
• *Aminoglycosides:* Decreased serum levels if specimen stored for a prolonged period of time
• *Folate:* Decreased serum levels
• *17-ketogenic steroids:* Increased urine concentrations
• *17-ketosteroids:* Increased urine concentrations
• *Protein:* Increased CSF concentrations
• *Protein electrophoresis:* False positives; causes bisalbuminemia
• *Sugar:* False positive with copper reduction procedures
• *Piperacillin:* False positive in the presence of penicillin V
• *Amdinocillin:* False positive in the presence of penicillin G
• *Methicillin:* False positive in the presence of penicillin G
SPECIAL CONSIDERATIONS
• Cross reactivity with cephalosporins is approx 10%

pentamidine
(pen-tam′i-deen)
Rx: NebuPent, Pentam
Chemical Class: Aromatic diamidine derivative
Therapeutic Class: Antiprotozoal

CLINICAL PHARMACOLOGY
Mechanism of Action: Interferes with protozoal nuclear metabolism; inhibits RNA/DNA, phospholipid, and protein synthesis

italic = common side effects   ***bold italic*** = life-threatening reactions

Pharmacokinetics

INH: Peak plasma levels minimally detected; bronchoalveolar lavage levels > than those obtained by injection (5-43 ng/ml vs. 1.5-4.0 ng/ml)

IV/IM: peak within 60 min

69% bound to plasma proteins; 33%-66% excreted in urine unchanged; $t_{1/2}$ 6.4-9.4 hr

INDICATIONS AND USES: Treatment of *Pneumocystis carinii* pneumonia (PCP) (IM/IV); prevention of PCP in high-risk, HIV-infected patients with a history of ≥1 episode of PCP and/or peripheral CD4+ lymphocyte count ≤200/mm³ (INH); trypanosomiasis*; visceral leishmaniasis*; amebic meningoencephalitis*; babesiosis*

DOSAGE

Adult

• *Treatment:* IM/IV 4 mg/kg qd for 14 days (reduce dosage, use a longer infusion time, or extend dosing interval in renal failure)

• *Prevention:* INH 300 mg q4 wk via Respirgard II nebulizer by Marquest

Child

• *Treatment:* IM/IV 4 mg/kg qd for 10-14 days

• *Prevention:* IM/IV 4 mg/kg q2-4 wk; INH (≥5 yr) 300 mg q3 wk via Respirgard II nebulizer

💲 AVAILABLE FORMS/COST OF THERAPY

• Aer—INH: 300 mg, 1's: **$98.75**
• Inj, Sol—IV: 300 mg, 1's: **$99.00**

PRECAUTIONS: Children (INH), hypertension, hypotension, hypoglycemia, hyperglycemia, hypocalcemia, leukopenia, thrombocytopenia, anemia, hepatic or renal dysfunction, ventricular tachycardia, pancreatitis, Stevens-Johnson syndrome

PREGNANCY AND LACTATION: Pregnancy category C; since aerosolized pentamidine results in very low systemic concentrations, fetal exposure to the drug is probably negligible; breast milk levels following aerosolized administration are likely nil

SIDE EFFECTS/ADVERSE REACTIONS

CNS: (Inj) Confusion/hallucination, dizziness, fever, neuralgia; (INH) anxiety, *chills,* confusion, depression, *dizziness,* drowsiness, emotional lability, *fatigue,* hallucination, headache, insomnia, memory loss, neuralgia, neuropathy, paranoia, paresthesia, *seizures,* tremors, unsteady gait, vertigo

CV: (Inj) hypotension, *ventricular tachycardia;* (INH) *chest pain/ congestion, CVA, edema,* hypertension, palpitations, syncope, tachycardia, vasculitis, vasodilation

EENT: (INH) Blepharitis, blurred vision, conjunctivitis, eye discomfort, loss of taste or smell, *pharyngitis*

GI: (Inj) Anorexia, bad taste in mouth, diarrhea, elevated liver function tests nausea; (INH) abdominal pain, colitis, diarrhea, dry mouth, dyspepsia, esophagitis, gastric ulcer, gastritis, gingivitis, hematochezia, hepatic dysfunction, hepatitis, hepatomegaly, hypersalivation, melena, *nausea,* oral ulcer, *pancreatitis,* splenomegaly

GU: (Inj) Flank pain, *increased serum creatinine;* nephritis, *renal failure*

HEME: (Inj and INH) *Anemia, leukopenia, thrombocytopenia*

METAB: (Inj) Hyperkalemia, hypocalcemia, hypoglycemia

MS: (INH) arthralgia, myalgia

RESP: (INH) *Bronchospasm,* cough, cyanosis, hemoptysis, hyperventilation, pleuritis, pneumonitis, pneumothorax, rales, *shortness of breath,* tachypnea

SKIN: (Inj) Rash, sterile abscess and

---

* = non-FDA-approved use

pain at IM inj site; ***Stevens-Johnson syndrome;*** (INH) desquamation, dry skin, erythema, pruritis, rash, urticaria

SPECIAL CONSIDERATIONS

• Considered 2nd line for *P. carinii* pneumonia, following cotrimoxazole (unresponsive to or intolerant of cotrimoxazole)

MONITORING PARAMETERS

• BUN, serum creatinine, blood glucose daily

• CBC and platelets; liver function tests, including bilirubin, alkaline phosphatase, AST, and ALT; and serum calcium before, during, and after therapy

• ECG at regular intervals

---

pentazocine

(pen-taz´oh-seen)

Rx: Talwin, Talwin NX (with Naloxone)

Combinations
  with ASA (Talwin Compound)
  with APAP (Talacen)

Chemical Class: Synthetic opiate of benzomorphan series
Therapeutic Class: Narcotic agonist-antagonist analgesic
DEA Class: Schedule IV

CLINICAL PHARMACOLOGY

Mechanism of Action: Has analgesic and very weak opiate antagonistic effects; binds to opiate receptors in the CNS causing inhibition of ascending pain pathways, altering the perception of and response to pain; believed to be a competitive antagonist at μ opiate receptors and an agonist at κ and σ opiate receptors

Pharmacokinetics

PO: Onset 15-30 min, duration 4-5 hr
IM/SC: Onset 15-30 min, duration 2-3 hr
IV: Onset 2-3 min, duration 2-3 hr

61% bound to plasma proteins, large 1st-pass effect, metabolized in liver, eliminated mainly in urine, small amounts eliminated in feces, $t_{1/2}$ 2-3 hr (prolonged in hepatic failure)

INDICATIONS AND USES: Moderate to severe pain

DOSAGE

Adult

• PO 50 mg q3-4h prn, may increase to 100 mg/dose prn, do not exceed 600 mg/day; IM/SC 30-60 mg q3-4h prn, do not exceed 360 mg/day; IV 30 mg q3-4h prn, do not exceed 360 mg/day

Child

• PO (>12 yr) same as adult; IM/SC (5-8 yr) 15 mg; (8-14 yr) 30 mg

AVAILABLE FORMS/COST OF THERAPY

• Syr: 6.25 mg/5 ml, 480 ml: **$180.00**

• Tab, Uncoated—Oral: 50 mg pentazocine/0.5 mg naloxone, 100's: **$104.17**

• Inj, Sol—IV, IM, SC: 30 mg/ml, 10 ml: **$38.77**; 50 mg/ml, 10 ml: **$2.60**

PRECAUTIONS: Head injury, increased intracranial pressure, acute abdominal conditions, elderly, severe impairment of hepatic or renal function, hypothyroidism, Addison's disease, prostatic hypertrophy, urethral stricture, history of drug abuse, impaired respiration, bronchial asthma, cyanosis, obstructive respiratory conditions, acute MI (see Special Considerations), chronic opiate use (may precipitate withdrawal symptoms), children

PREGNANCY AND LACTATION: Pregnancy category B (category D if used for prolonged periods or in high doses at term); use during labor may produce neonatal respiratory depression

---

italic = common side effects   ***bold italic*** = life-threatening reactions

SIDE EFFECTS/ADVERSE REACTIONS

CNS: Agitation, dependency, *dizziness, drowsiness, euphoria,* lethargy, restlessness, *sedation*

CV: Circulatory depression, increased blood pressure, *shock,* tachycardia

EENT: Blurred vision, diplopia, miosis, nystagmus

GI: Anorexia, constipation, nausea, vomiting

GU: Urinary retention

HEME: Eosinophilia, *granulocytopenia, leukopenia*

RESP: Respiratory depression, respiratory paralysis

SKIN: Flushing, rash, urticaria

INTERACTIONS

Drugs

🔢 *Aspirin:* Increased risk of papillary necrosis

🔢 *Barbiturates:* Additive CNS depression

🔢 *Phenothiazines:* Additive CNS depression

Labs

• *Increase:* Amylase

SPECIAL CONSIDERATIONS

• Naloxone 0.5 mg added to oral tablets to discourage misuse via parenteral inj

• Less effective compared to morphine, but less respiratory depression and opposite cardiovascular pharmacodynamics; increases pulmonary, arterial, and central venous pressure

PATIENT/FAMILY EDUCATION

• Report any symptoms of CNS changes, allergic reactions

• Physical dependency may result when used for extended periods

• Change position slowly, orthostatic hypotension may occur

• Avoid hazardous activities if drowsiness or dizziness occurs

• Avoid alcohol, other CNS depressants unless directed by clinician

---

pentobarbital

(pen-toe-bar'bi-tal)

Rx: Nembutal

Chemical Class: Barbituric acid derivative

Therapeutic Class: Sedative/hypnotic; anticonvulsant

DEA Class: Schedule II (oral, parenteral), schedule III (rectal)

CLINICAL PHARMACOLOGY

Mechanism of Action: CNS depressant: depresses the sensory cortex, decreases motor activity, alters cerebellar function, produces drowsiness, sedation, and hypnosis; little analgesic action at subanesthetic doses (may increase reaction to painful stimuli); anticonvulsant activity in anesthetic doses; dose-dependent respiratory depression (hypnotic doses produce respiratory depression similar to physiologic sleep)

Pharmacokinetics

PO: Onset 15-60 min, peak 30-60 min, duration 3-4 hr

PR: Onset 20-60 min, peak, duration 3-4 hr

IM: Onset 10-25 min

IV: Onset 1 min, duration 15 min 35%-45% bound to plasma proteins; metabolized in liver, excreted in urine (metabolites); $t_{1/2}$ 22-50 hr

INDICATIONS AND USES: Insomnia (short term), status epilepticus, facilitation of intubation and anesthesia, increased intracranial pressure,* cerebral ischemia,* drownings,* emesis,* psychiatric interviews*

DOSAGE

Adult

• *Hypnotic:* PO 100-200 mg hs or 20 mg tid-qid for daytime sedation;

---

* = non-FDA-approved use

IM 150-200 mg; IV 100 mg initially, may repeat q1-3 min up to 200-500 mg total; PR 120-200 mg hs

• *Preoperative sedation:* IM 150-200 mg

• *Pentobarbital coma for increased intracranial pressure:* IV 10-15 mg/kg over 1-2 hr loading dose, then 1 mg/kg/hr INF, increase to 2-3 mg/kg/hr if necessary; maintain burst suppression on EEG

Child

• *Sedative:* PO 2-6 mg/kg/day divided tid; max 100 mg/day

• *Hypnotic:* IM 2-6 mg/kg; max 100 mg/dose; PR <4 yr 3-6 mg/kg/dose, >4 yr 1.5-3 mg/kg/dose

• *Preoperative sedation:* PO/IM/PR 2-6 mg/kg; max 100 mg/dose; IV 1-3 mg/kg to a max of 100 mg until asleep

• *Pentobarbital coma for increased intracranial pressure:* Same as adult

$ AVAILABLE FORMS/COST OF THERAPY

• Cap, Gel—Oral: 50 mg, 100's: **$38.74;** 100 mg, 100's: **$60.68**

• Supp—Rect: 60 mg, 12's: **$56.58;** 200 mg, 12's: **$77.58**

• Inj, Sol—IM, IV: 50 mg/ml, 2 ml: **$4.00**

CONTRAINDICATIONS: Respiratory depression, severe liver impairment, porphyria

PRECAUTIONS: Myasthenia gravis, myxedema, anemia, hepatic disease, renal disease, hypertension, elderly, acute or chronic pain, mental depression, history of drug abuse, abrupt discontinuation, children, hyperthyroidism, fever, diabetes

PREGNANCY AND LACTATION: Pregnancy category D; excreted in breast milk; effect on nursing infant unknown

SIDE EFFECTS/ADVERSE REACTIONS

CNS: CNS depression, dizziness, *drowsiness, hangover,* headache, *lethargy,* lightheadedness, mental depression, physical dependence, slurred speech, stimulation in the elderly and children, vertigo

CV: Bradycardia, hypotension

GI: Constipation, diarrhea, nausea, vomiting

HEME: **Agranulocytosis, megaloblastic anemia** (long-term treatment), **thrombocytopenia**

RESP: **Apnea, bronchospasm, depression, laryngospasm**

SKIN: Abscesses at inj site, **angioedema,** erythema multiforme, pain, **rash, Stevens-Johnson syndrome,** thrombophlebitis, urticaria

MISC: Osteomalacia (prolonged use), rickets

INTERACTIONS

Drugs

3 *Acetaminophen:* Enhanced hepatotoxic potential of acetaminophen overdoses

3 *Antidepressants, cyclic:* Reduced serum concentrations of cyclic antidepressants

3 β-*adrenergic blockers:* Reduced serum concentrations of β-blockers which are extensively metabolized

3 *Calcium channel blockers:* Reduced serum concentrations of verapamil and dihydropyridines

3 *Chloramphenicol:* Increased barbiturate concentrations; reduced serum chloramphenicol concentrations

3 *Corticosteroids:* Reduced serum concentrations of corticosteroids; may impair therapeutic effect

3 *Cyclosporine:* Reduced serum concentration of cyclosporine

3 *Digitoxin:* Reduced serum concentration of digitoxin

P

italic = common side effects   ***bold italic*** = life-threatening reactions

🔳 *Disopyramide:* Reduced serum concentration of disopyramide

🔳 *Doxycycline:* Reduced serum doxycycline concentrations

🔳 *Estrogen:* Reduced serum concentration of estrogen

🔳 *Ethanol:* Excessive CNS depression

🔳 *Griseofulvin:* Reduced griseofulvin absorption

🔳 *Methoxyflurane:* Enhanced nephrotoxic effect

🔳 *MAOIs:* Prolonged effect of barbiturates

🔳 *Narcotic analgesics:* Increased toxicity of meperidine; reduced effect of methadone; additive CNS depression

🔳 *Neuroleptics:* Reduced effect of either drug

② *Oral anticoagulants:* Decreased hypoprothrombinemic response to oral anticoagulants

🔳 *Oral contraceptives:* Reduced efficacy of oral contraceptives

🔳 *Phenytoin:* Unpredictable effect on serum phenytoin levels

🔳 *Propafenone:* Reduced serum concentration of propafenone

🔳 *Quinidine:* Reduced quinidine plasma concentration

🔳 *Tacrolimus:* Reduced serum concentration of tacrolimus

🔳 *Theophylline:* Reduced serum theophylline concentrations

🔳 *Valproic acid:* Increased serum concentrations of amobarbital

🔳 *Warfarin:* See oral anticoagulants

SPECIAL CONSIDERATIONS
PATIENT/FAMILY EDUCATION
• Avoid driving or other activities requiring alertness
• Avoid alcohol ingestion or CNS depressants
• Do not discontinue medication abruptly after long-term use

MONITORING PARAMETERS
• Excessive usage; hypnotic hangover

---

pentosan polysulfate
(pen'toe-san)
Rx: Elmiron
Chemical Class: Sulfated glycosaminoglycan (heparin derivative)
Therapeutic Class: Anticoagulant, fibrinolytic

CLINICAL PHARMACOLOGY
Mechanism of Action: Anticoagulant, fibrinolytic and anti-inflammatory effects; biochemical properties of sulfated glycosaminoglycans may replace or augment natural surface glycosaminoglycans in interstitial cystitis patients
Pharmacokinetics
PO: Poorly/erratically absorbed (bioavailability 3%); metabolized in liver and excreted in urine; $t_{1/2}$ 1 hr after IV dose

INDICATIONS AND USES: Interstitial cystitis, urolithiasis,* nonbacterial prostatitis,* prophylaxis of DVT*

DOSAGE
Adult
• *Interstitial cystitis:* PO 100 mg tid with water on an empty stomach

💲 AVAILABLE FORMS/COST OF THERAPY
• Cap—Oral: 100 mg, 100's: **$154.50**

PRECAUTIONS: Bleeding complications, thrombocytopenia, hepatic insufficiency, transient elevations in liver transaminases

PREGNANCY AND LACTATION: Pregnancy category B; no data in nursing mothers

SIDE EFFECTS/ADVERSE REACTIONS
CNS: Dizziness, headache (3%)

---

* = non-FDA-approved use

EENT: Amblyopia, conjunctivitis, optic neuritis, tinnitus

GI: Abdominal pain, diarrhea (4%), dyspepsia, LFT abnormalities, nausea (4%)

HEME: Anemia, ecchymosis, ***leukopenia,*** prolonged PT and PTT, ***thrombocytopenia***

RESP: Dyspnea, epistaxis, pharyngitis, rhinitis

SKIN: Alopecia (4%), pruritus, rash, urticaria

MISC: Peripheral edema

---

pentoxifylline
(pen-tox-if'ih-lin)
Rx: Trental
Chemical Class: Dimethylxanthine derivative
Therapeutic Class: Hemorheologic agent

CLINICAL PHARMACOLOGY
Mechanism of Action: Thought to improve blood flow by decreasing blood viscosity and improving erythrocyte flexibility; increases blood flow to affected microcirculation, enhancing tissue oxygenation

Pharmacokinetics
PO: Peak 1 hr; undergoes 1st-pass metabolism in liver to active metabolites; excreted mainly in urine (95%) and feces (5%); $t_{1/2}$ 24-48 min (metabolites 60-96 min)

INDICATIONS AND USES: Intermittent claudication, cerebrovascular insufficiency,* diabetic angiopathies and neuropathies,* transient ischemic attack,* leg ulcers,* sickle cell thalassemias,* stroke,* high-altitude sickness,* asthenozoospermia,* acute and chronic hearing disorders,* eye circulation disorders,* Raynaud's phenomenon,* apththous ulcers*

DOSAGE
Adult
• PO 400 mg tid with meals; decrease to 400 mg bid if GI and CNS side effects occur

§ AVAILABLE FORMS/COST OF THERAPY
• Tab, Coated, SUS Action—Oral: 400 mg, 100's: **$55.45-$63.48**

PRECAUTIONS: Impaired renal function, children, chronic occlusive arterial disease of limbs

PREGNANCY AND LACTATION: Pregnancy category C; excreted in breast milk

SIDE EFFECTS/ADVERSE REACTIONS
CNS: Anxiety, confusion, dizziness, headache, tremor

CV: Angina or chest pain, dyspnea, edema, hypotension

EENT: Blurred vision, conjunctivitis, earache, epistaxis, laryngitis, nasal congestion, scotomata, sore throat, swollen neck glands

GI: Anorexia, bad taste, belching, bloating, cholecystitis, constipation, dry mouth, dyspepsia, excessive salivation, flatus, nausea, thirst, vomiting

HEME: ***Leukopenia***

SKIN: Brittle fingernails, pruritus, rash, urticaria

MISC: Malaise, weight change

INTERACTIONS
Drugs
3 *Fluoroquinolones (ciprofloxin, enoxacin, norfloxacin, pefloxacin, pipemidic acid):* Increased pentoxyphylline concentrations with subsequent side effects

3 *Theophylline:* Increased plasma theophylline concentrations

SPECIAL CONSIDERATIONS
• Statistically, but not always, clinically significant effects in intermittent claudication, however, other

---

italic = common side effects   ***bold italic*** = life-threatening reactions

drugs less impressive; will not replace surgical options

PATIENT/FAMILY EDUCATION
• Therapeutic effect may require 2-4 wk
• Stop smoking

---

pergolide

(per'go-lide)
Rx: Permax
Chemical Class: Ergoline derivative
Therapeutic Class: Antiparkinson's agent, dopaminergic

CLINICAL PHARMACOLOGY
Mechanism of Action: Potent dopamine receptor agonist at both D_1- and D_2-receptor sites; directly stimulates postsynaptic dopamine receptors in nigrostriatal system; inhibits prolactin
Pharmacokinetics
PO: 90% bound to plasma proteins; metabolized to at least 10 metabolites (some with dopamine agonist activity), excreted by kidney

INDICATIONS AND USES: Parkinson's disease (adjunct to levodopa/carbidopa)

DOSAGE
Adult
• PO 0.05 mg qd for 1st 2 days; increase gradually by 0.1 or 0.15 mg/day every 3rd day over next 12 days; subsequent increases by 0.25 mg/day every 3rd day until optimal therapeutic response obtained; divide total daily dose tid; doses >5 mg/day have not been systematically evaluated

$ AVAILABLE FORMS/COST OF THERAPY
• Tab, Uncoated—Oral: 0.05 mg, 30's: **$23.61;** 0.25 mg, 100's: **$120.32;** 1 mg, 100's: **$381.34**

PRECAUTIONS: Hypotension, children, cardiac dysrhythmia, pre-existing dyskinesia; coadministration with drugs affecting protein binding

PREGNANCY AND LACTATION: Pregnancy category B; may interfere with lactation

SIDE EFFECTS/ADVERSE REACTIONS
CNS: Akathisia, anxiety, confusion, *dizziness, dyskinesia,* dystonia, *hallucination, insomnia,* personality disorder, psychosis, somnolence, uncoordination
CV: Hypertension, hypotension, palpitation, peripheral edema, postural hypotension, syncope, vasodilation
EENT: Epistaxis, *rhinitis*
GI: Anorexia, *constipation,* diarrhea, dry mouth, *dyspepsia, nausea*
GU: Hematuria
RESP: Abnormal vision, dyspnea, hiccups
SKIN: Rash
MISC: Pain

INTERACTIONS
Drugs
3 *Lisinopril:* Additive hypotension
3 *Neuroleptics:* Potentially antagonistic pharmacodynamic effects

SPECIAL CONSIDERATIONS
• Adjunct to levodopa/carbidopa in Parkinson's disease; longer acting than bromocriptine

PATIENT/FAMILY EDUCATION
• Hypotensive cautions

---

permethrin

(per-meth'ren)
Rx: Acticin, Elimite; **OTC:** Nix
Chemical Class: Synthetic pyrethroid derivative
Therapeutic Class: Pediculicide; scabicide

CLINICAL PHARMACOLOGY
Mechanism of Action: Acts on parasite nerve cell membranes; dis-

---

rupts sodium channel current; delays repolarization and paralyzes pest; pediculicidal and ovicidal activity

Pharmacokinetics

TOP: Less than 2% of amount applied systemically absorbed; rapidly metabolized to inactive metabolites, excreted in urine; residual detectable on hair for at least 10 days following single application

INDICATIONS AND USES: Single application treatment of infestation with *Pediculus humanus capitis* (head louse) and its nits, or *Sarcoptes scabiei* (scabies)

DOSAGE

Adult and Child

• *Head lice (1%):* Top apply after hair has been shampooed, rinsed, and towel dried; apply sufficient volume of liquid to saturate hair and scalp; leave on hair for 10 min before rinsing with water; remove remaining nits; may repeat in 1 wk if necessary (1 application generally sufficient)

• *Scabies (5%):* Top apply cream from head to toe; leave on for 8-14 hr before washing off with water; may repeat in 1 wk if live mites reappear

💲 **AVAILABLE FORMS/COST OF THERAPY**

• Cre—Top: 5%, 60 g: **$23.62-$26.99**

• Liq—Top: 1%, 60 ml: **$8.93**

PRECAUTIONS: Children <2 mo

PREGNANCY AND LACTATION: Pregnancy category B; excretion into breast milk unknown

SIDE EFFECTS/ADVERSE REACTIONS

SKIN: Edema, numbness, *pruritus* (difficult to distinguish from infestation itself), rash, tingling, transient burning and stinging, transient erythema

SPECIAL CONSIDERATIONS

PATIENT/FAMILY EDUCATION

• For external use only; shake well

• Avoid contact with eyes, mucous membranes

• Itching may be temporarily aggravated following application

• Do not repeat administration sooner than 1 wk

• Itching from allergic reaction caused by mite may persist for several weeks even though infestation is cured

---

perphenazine

(per-fen′a-zeen)

Rx: Trilafon

Chemical Class: Piperazine phenothiazine derivative

Therapeutic Class: Antipsychotic; antiemetic

CLINICAL PHARMACOLOGY

Mechanism of Action: Dopamine receptor antagonist, with higher affinity for D_2- over D_1-receptors, and variable selectivity among the cortical dopamine tracts; also activity on nondopaminergic sites, i.e., cholinergic, α_1-adrenergic and histamine receptors (explaining side effects); moderate incidence of sedation and extrapyramidal reactions; minimal orthostatic hypotension and anticholinergic effects

Pharmacokinetics

PO: Onset ½-1 hr, peak 4-8 hr

IM: Onset 10 min, peak 1-2 hr, duration 6 hr

90% bound to plasma proteins; metabolized in liver, excreted in urine and bile; $t_{1/2}$ 9 hr

INDICATIONS AND USES: Psychotic disorders, severe nausea and vomiting,* intractable hiccups,* hemiballismus,* aggressive behavior,* tricyclic-induced tremor,* organic mental syndromes*

---

italic = common side effects **bold italic** = life-threatening reactions

DOSAGE
NOTE: 10 mg equivalent to chlorpromazine 100 mg

Adult
• *Psychosis:* PO 4-16 mg bid-qid; do not exceed 64 mg/day; IM 5 mg q6h up to 15 mg/day in ambulatory patients, 30 mg/day in hospitalized patients
• *Nausea/vomiting:* PO 8-16 mg/day in divided doses up to 24 mg/day; IM 5-10 mg q6h up to 15 mg/day in ambulatory patients, 30 mg/day in hospitalized patients; IV 1 mg at 1-2 min intervals up to 5 mg total

Child
• Not established <12 yr; use lowest adult dose >12 yr
• *Nausea/vomiting:* IM 5 mg q6h

🔋 AVAILABLE FORMS/COST OF THERAPY
• Tab, Coated—Oral: 2 mg, 100's: **$40.55-$78.34;** 4 mg, 100's: **$54.70-$107.17;** 8 mg, 100's: **$64.95-$130.03;** 16 mg, 100's: **$95.18-$174.92**
• Liq—Oral: 16 mg/5 ml, 120 ml: **$44.64**
• Inj, Sol—IM, IV: 5 mg/ml, 1 ml: **$6.64**

CONTRAINDICATIONS: Severe toxic CNS depression, coma, subcortical brain damage, bone marrow depression

PRECAUTIONS: Children <12 yr, elderly, prolonged use, severe cardiovascular disorders, epilepsy, hepatic or renal disease, glaucoma, prostatic hypertrophy, severe asthma, emphysema, hypocalcemia (increased susceptibility to dystonic reactions), COPD

PREGNANCY AND LACTATION: Pregnancy category C; has been used as an antiemetic during normal labor without producing any observable effect on newborn; excreted into human breast milk; effects on nursing infant unknown, but may be of concern

SIDE EFFECTS/ADVERSE REACTIONS
CNS: Agitation, anxiety, catatonic-like behavioral states, confusion, depression, *drowsiness, EPS (pseudoparkinsonism, akathisia, dystonia,* tardive dyskinesia), euphoria, exacerbation of psychotic symptoms including hallucinations, *headache,* heat or cold intolerance, insomnia, lethargy, *neuroleptic malignant syndrome,* restlessness, *seizures,* vertigo
CV: ECG changes, hypotension, *tachycardia*
EENT: Blurred vision, cataracts, dry eyes, glaucoma, pigmentation of retina or cornea, retinopathy
GI: Anorexia, constipation, diarrhea, *dry mouth,* dyspepsia, hypersalivation, increased LFTs, *nausea,* vomiting
GU: Priapism, urinary retention
HEME: **Agranulocytosis,** anemia, **aplastic anemia, hemolytic anemia,** leukocytosis, minimal decreases in red blood cell counts, transient leukopenia
METAB: Breast engorgement, gynecomastia, hyperglycemia, hypoglycemia, hyponatremia, impotence, increased libido, lactation, mastalgia, menstrual irregularities
RESP: Bronchospasm, increased depth of respiration, laryngospasm
SKIN: Diaphoresis, loss of hair, maculopapular and acneiform skin reactions, photosensitivity

INTERACTIONS
Drugs
3 *Amodiaquine, chloroquine, sulfadoxine-pyrimethamine:* Increased chlorpromazine concentrations
3 *Anticholinergics:* May inhibit neuroleptic response; excess anticholinergic effects

3 *Antidepressants:* Potential for increased therapeutic and toxic effects from increased levels of both drugs

3 *Barbiturates:* Decreased neuroleptic levels

3 *Clonidine, guanadrel, granethidine:* Severe hypotensive episodes possible

3 *Epinephrine:* Blunted pressor response to epinephrine

3 *Ethanol:* Additive CNS depression

2 *Levodopa:* Inhibited antiparkinsonian effect of levodopa

3 *Lithium:* Lowered levels of both drugs, rarely neurotoxicity in acute mania

3 *Narcotic analgesics:* Hypotension and increased CNS depression

3 *Orphenadrine:* Lowered neuroleptic concentrations, excessive anticholinergic effects

3 *Propranolol:* Increased plasma

Labs

• *Creatinine:* Decreased serum levels

SPECIAL CONSIDERATIONS

PATIENT/FAMILY EDUCATION

• Arise slowly from reclining position

• Do not discontinue abruptly

• Use a sunscreen during sun exposure to prevent burns, take special precautions to stay cool in hot weather

• Concentrate may be diluted just prior to administration with distilled water, acidified tap water, orange or grape juice

MONITORING PARAMETERS

• Observe closely for signs of tardive dyskinesia (abnormal involuntary movement scale)

• Periodic CBC with platelets during prolonged therapy

phenazopyridine
(fen-az'o-peer'i-deen)
Rx: Azo-Standard, Baridium, Eridium, Geridium, Phenazodine, Pyridiate, Pyridium, Urodine, Urogesic, Viridium
Combinations
  Rx: with sulfamethoxazole (Azo-Gantanol); with sulfisoxazole (Azo-Gantrisin)
Chemical Class: Azo dye
Therapeutic Class: Urinary tract analgesic

CLINICAL PHARMACOLOGY
Mechanism of Action: Exerts topical analgesic effect on urinary tract mucosa
Pharmacokinetics
PO: Rapidly excreted by kidneys, 65% excreted unchanged in urine
INDICATIONS AND USES: Symptomatic relief of urinary burning, itching, frequency, and urgency associated with UTI, or following urologic procedures
DOSAGE
Adult
• PO 100-200 mg tid after meals; do not exceed 2 days when used concomitantly with antibacterial agents for UTI
Child
• PO 12 mg/kg/day divided tid after meals
AVAILABLE FORMS/COST OF THERAPY
• Tab, Coated—Oral: 100 mg, 100's: **$1.49-$57.62;** 200 mg, 100's: **$2.09-$111.04**
CONTRAINDICATIONS: Renal insufficiency
PRECAUTIONS: Chronic use in undiagnosed urinary tract pain, children <12 yr
PREGNANCY AND LACTATION: Pregnancy category B

SIDE EFFECTS/ADVERSE REAC-TIONS

CNS: Headache

EENT: Staining of contact lenses, yellowish tinge of sclera

GI: GI disturbances, **hepatitis,** jaundice

GU: Orange-red discoloration of urine, renal stones, **transient acute renal failure**

HEME: **Hemolytic anemia, methemoglobinemia**

SKIN: Pruritus, rash, yellowish tinge of skin

MISC: **Anaphylactoid-like reaction**

INTERACTIONS

Labs

• *Albumin:* Increased serum concentrations

• *Bacteria:* False negatives on Microstix

• *Bile:* False positive with Ictotest, BiliLabstix

• *Bilirubin, conjugated:* False elevations in serum

• *Bilirubin, unconjugated:* False serum concentration elevations

• *BSP Retention:* False negatives

• *Cholinesterase:* Adds 34% negative bias to Ectachem method

• *Urine:* Yellow-orange color

• *Feces:* Orange-red color

• *Glucose:* Decreased serum levels

• *17-ketogenic steroids:* False positives in urine

• *Ketones:* Nitroprusside reactions masked by color; false negatives

• *17-ketosteroids:* Increase in urine

• *Porphyrins:* False positive

• *Pregnanediol:* Increased urine levels

• *Protein:* Increased serum levels

• *PSP excretion:* False positive in alkaline pH

• *Urobilinogen:* False positive urine test

• *Vanillylmandelic acid:* Increased urine concentrations

• *Xylose excretion:* Increased urine concentrations

SPECIAL CONSIDERATIONS

PATIENT/FAMILY EDUCATION

• May cause GI upset

• Take after meals

• May cause reddish-orange discoloration of urine; may stain fabric; may also stain contact lenses

---

phendimetrazine

(fen-dye-me′tra-zeen)

Rx: Adipost, Bontril, Dital Rexigen, Dyrexan-OD, Melfiat-105, Plegine, Prelu-2

Chemical Class: Morpholine
Therapeutic Class: Anorexiant
DEA Class: Schedule III

CLINICAL PHARMACOLOGY

Mechanism of Action: Acts on adrenergic and dopaminergic pathways, directly stimulating the satiety center in the hypothalamic and limbic regions

Pharmacokinetics

PO: Onset 30 min, peak 1-3 hr, duration 4-20 hr; metabolized by liver, excreted by kidneys; $t_{1/2}$ 2-10 hr

INDICATIONS AND USES: Exogenous obesity (as a short-term adjunct to caloric restriction)

DOSAGE

Adult

• PO 35 mg bid-tid, 1 hr ac, not to exceed 70 mg tid; PO SUS REL 105 mg qAM before breakfast

$ AVAILABLE FORMS/COST OF THERAPY

• Cap, Gel, SUS REL—Oral: 105 mg, 100's: **$14.01-$98.54**

• Tab, Uncoated—Oral: 35 mg, 100's: **$7.50-$12.99**

CONTRAINDICATIONS: Moderate to severe hypertension, children, glaucoma, history of drug abuse, cardiovascular disease, advanced arteriosclerosis, agitated states, hyperthyroidism, within 14 days of MAOI administration

PRECAUTIONS: Diabetes mellitus, convulsive disorders, mild hypertension

PREGNANCY AND LACTATION: Pregnancy category C

SIDE EFFECTS/ADVERSE REACTIONS

CNS: Dizziness, drowsiness, dysphoria, exacerbation of schizophrenia, headache, *insomnia,* mental depression, *nervousness, overstimulation, restlessness,* shivering, tremor, weakness

CV: Chest pain, palpitation, ***tachycardia***

GI: Constipation, diarrhea, dry mouth, nausea, unpleasant taste

GU: Impotence, testicular pain, urinary hesitancy

SKIN: Clamminess, excessive sweating, pallor, rash

SPECIAL CONSIDERATIONS
PATIENT/FAMILY EDUCATION
• May cause insomnia; avoid taking late in the day
• Weight reduction requires strict adherence to caloric restriction
• Do not discontinue abruptly

---

phenelzine

(fen'el-zeen)
Rx: Nardil
Chemical Class: Hydrazine derivative
Therapeutic Class: Monoamine oxidase (MAO) inhibitor antidepressant

CLINICAL PHARMACOLOGY
Mechanism of Action: MAOI resulting in increased endogenous concentrations of serotonin, norepinephrine, epinephrine, and dopamine in the CNS; chronic administration results in down regulation (desensitization) of α_2- or β-adrenergic and serotonin receptors, which may correlate with antidepressant activity

Pharmacokinetics
PO: Onset of action 4-8 wk, duration of MAO inhibition at least 10 days, peak serum concentration 2-4 hr, metabolized in liver, excreted in urine as metabolites and unchanged drug

INDICATIONS AND USES: Treatment-resistant depression, including patients characterized as atypical, nonendogenous, or neurotic

DOSAGE
Adult
• PO 15 mg tid initially, increase as tolerated to 60-90 mg/day; following achievement of maximal benefit, reduce dosage slowly over several weeks to lowest effective dose that maintains response

💲 AVAILABLE FORMS/COST OF THERAPY
• Tab, Sugar Coated—Oral: 15 mg, 100's: **$47.07**

CONTRAINDICATIONS: Pheochromocytoma, congestive heart failure, liver disease, severe renal function impairment, cerebrovascular defect, cardiovascular disease, hypertension, history of headache, age >60 yr

PRECAUTIONS: Children <16 yr, hypotension, bipolar affective disorder, agitation, schizophrenia, hyperactivity, diabetes mellitus, seizure disorder, angina, hyperthyroidism, suicidal ideation

PREGNANCY AND LACTATION: Pregnancy category C

SIDE EFFECTS/ADVERSE REACTIONS

CNS: Agitation, akathisia, ataxia, chills, coma, confusion, *dizziness, drowsiness,* euphoria, fatigue, headache, hyperreflexia, hypomania, jitteriness, mania, memory impairment, muscle twitching, myoclonic movements, neuritis, overactivity, overstimulation, restlessness, ***sei-***

---

zures, sleep disturbance, tremors, vertigo, weakness

*CV: **Dysrhythmias,** edema, **hypertension,** orthostatic hypotension,* palpitations, tachycardia

EENT: Blurred vision, glaucoma, nystagmus

GI: Abdominal pain, anorexia, black tongue, constipation, diarrhea, dry mouth, elevated transaminases, hepatitis, nausea

GU: Dysuria, incontinence, sexual disturbance, urinary retention

*HEME: **Agranulocytosis,** anemia, spider telangiectases, **thrombocytopenia***

METAB: Hypermetabolic syndrome, hypernatremia, SIADH-like syndrome

SKIN: Hyperhydrosis, photosensitivity, rash

MISC: Weight gain

INTERACTIONS

Drugs

⚠ *Amphetamines, alcoholic beverages containing tyramine, metaraminol, phenylephrine, phenylpropanolamine, pseudoephedrine, tyramine:* Severe hypertensive reaction

❷ *Antidepressants, cyclic:* Excessive sympathetic response, mania, hyperpyrexia

❸ *Barbiturates:* Prolonged effect of some barbiturates

⚠ *Clomipramine:* Death

⚠ *Dexfenfluramine, dextromethorphan, fenfluramine, meperidine:* Agitation, blood pressure changes, hyperpyrexia, convulsions

⚠ *Fluoxetine, Sertraline:* Hypomania, confusion, hypertension, tremor

⚠ *Food:* Foods containing large amounts of tyramine can result in hypertensive reactions

❸ *Guanadrel, guanethidine:* May inhibit antihypertensive effects

❸ *Levodopa:* Severe hypertensive reaction

❷ *Lithium:* Malignant hyperpyrexia

❸ *Neuromuscular blocking agents:* Prolonged muscle relaxation caused by succinylcholine

❸ *Reserpine:* Hypertensive reaction

❸ *Sumatriptan:* Increased sumatriptan plasma concentrations

Labs

• *Aspartate aminotransferase:* Increased serum levels

• *Bilirubin:* False-positive increases in serum

• *Uric acid:* False-positive increases in serum

SPECIAL CONSIDERATIONS
PATIENT/FAMILY EDUCATION

• Avoid tyramine-containing foods, beverages, and OTC products containing decongestants or dextromethorphan and products such as diet aids

• May cause drowsiness, dizziness, blurred vision

• Use caution driving or performing other tasks requiring alertness

• Arise slowly from reclining position

• Therapeutic effect may require 4-8 wk

phenobarbital

(fee-noe-bar´bi-tal)

Rx: Bellatal, Luminal, Solfoton

Combinations

Rx: with atropine, hyoscyamine, scopolamine (Donnatal); with belladonna, ergotamine (Bellergal Spacetabs)

Chemical Class: Barbituric acid derivative

Therapeutic Class: Sedative/hypnotic; anticonvulsant

DEA Class: Schedule IV

CLINICAL PHARMACOLOGY

Mechanism of Action: CNS depressant: depresses the sensory cortex, decreases motor activity, alters cerebellar function, produces drowsiness, sedation, and hypnosis; little analgesic action at subanesthetic doses (may increase reaction to painful stimuli); anticonvulsant activity in subhypnotic doses; dose-dependent respiratory depression (hypnotic doses produce respiratory depression similar to physiologic sleep)

Pharmacokinetics

PO: Onset 20-60 min, peak 1-6 hr, duration 10-16 hr

IV: Onset within 5 min, peak effect within 30 min, duration 4-10 hr 20%-50% bound to plasma proteins; metabolized in liver, excreted in urine (20%-50% unchanged); $t_{1/2}$ 53-140 hr (prolonged in overdose)

INDICATIONS AND USES: Routine and preoperative sedation, tonic-clonic (grand mal) seizures, partial seizures, prevention of febrile seizures (controversial), status epilepticus (not 1st line), neonatal hyperbilirubinemia,* congenital nonhemolytic unconjugated hyperbilirubinemia,* chronic intrahepatic cholestasis*

DOSAGE

Adult

• *Anticonvulsant:* PO/IV 1-3 mg/kg/day in divided doses or 50-100 mg bid-tid

• *Status epilepticus:* IV 300-800 mg initially followed by 120-240 mg at 20 min intervals until seizures are controlled or a total dose of 1-2 g

• *Sedation:* PO/IM 30-120 mg/day in 2-3 divided doses

• *Hypnotic:* PO/IM/IV/SC 100-320 mg/kg hs

• *Preoperative sedation:* IM 100-200 mg 1-1½ hr before procedure

Child

• *Anticonvulsant:* PO/IV neonates 2-4 mg/kg/day in 1-2 divided doses; infants 5-8 mg/kg/day in 1-2 divided doses; 1-5 yr 6-8 mg/kg/day in 1-2 divided doses; 5-12 yr 4-6 mg/kg/day in 1-2 divided doses

• *Status epilepticus:* IV neonates 15-20 mg/kg in a single or divided dose; infants and children 10-20 mg/kg in a single or divided dose, may give additional 5 mg/kg/dose q15-30 min until seizure is controlled or a total dose of 40 mg/kg is reached

• *Sedation:* PO 2 mg/kg tid

• *Hypnotic:* IM/IV/SC 3-5 mg/kg hs

• *Preoperative sedation:* PO/IM/IV 1-3 mg/kg 1-1½ hr before procedure

💲 AVAILABLE FORMS/COST OF THERAPY

• Inj, Sol—IM, IV: 30 mg/ml, 1 ml: **$3.28;** 60 mg/ml, 1 ml: **$3.05-$3.35;** 65 mg/ml, 1 ml: **$1.31;** 130 mg/ml, 1 ml: **$1.56-$7.70**

• Tab, Uncoated—Oral: 15 mg, 100's: **$1.59-$8.59;** 30 mg, 100's: **$1.80-$5.18;** 60 mg, 100's: **$3.25-$5.34;** 100 mg, 100's: **$3.75-$6.76**

• Tabs: 16.2 mg, 100's: **$3.57-$3.80;**

P

32.4 mg, 100's: **$3.90**; 64.8 mg, 100's: **$5.41**; 97.2 mg, 100's: **$6.92**
• Elixir—Oral: 20 mg/5 ml, 480 ml: **$3.65-$13.31**

CONTRAINDICATIONS: Respiratory depression, severe liver impairment, porphyria

PRECAUTIONS: Myasthenia gravis, myxedema, anemia, hepatic disease, renal disease, hypertension, elderly, acute or chronic pain, mental depression, history of drug abuse, abrupt discontinuation, children, hyperthyroidism, fever, diabetes

PREGNANCY AND LACTATION: Pregnancy category D; risks to fetus include minor congenital defects, hemorrhage at birth, addiction; risk to mother may be greater if seizure control is lost due to stopping drug; use at lowest possible level to control seizures; excreted into breast milk, has caused major adverse effects in some nursing infants, use caution in nursing women

SIDE EFFECTS/ADVERSE REACTIONS

CNS: CNS depression, dizziness, *drowsiness, hangover,* headache, *lethargy,* lightheadedness, mental depression, physical dependence, slurred speech, stimulation in the elderly and children, vertigo

CV: Bradycardia, hypotension

GI: Constipation, diarrhea, nausea, vomiting

HEME: Agranulocytosis, megaloblastic anemia (long-term treatment), *thrombocytopenia*

RESP: Apnea, bronchospasm, depression, laryngospasm

SKIN: Abscesses at injection site, *angioedema,* erythema multiforme, pain, *rash, Stevens-Johnson syndrome,* thrombophlebitis, urticaria

MISC: Osteomalacia (prolonged use), rickets

INTERACTIONS

Drugs

🔳 *Acetaminophen:* Enhanced hepatotoxic potential of acetaminophen overdoses

🔳 *Antidepressants:* Reduced serum concentrations of cyclic antidepressants

🔳 *Beta-blockers:* Reduced serum concentrations of β-blockers, which are extensively metabolized (metoprolol, propranolol, sotalol)

🔳 *Calcium channel blockers:* Reduced concentrations of verapamil and nifedipine

🔳 *Chloramphenicol:* Increased barbiturate concentrations; reduced serum chloramphenicol concentrations

🔳 *Corticosteroids:* Reduced serum concentrations of corticosteroids, may impair therapeutic effect

🔳 *Cyclosporine:* Reduced serum concentration of cyclosporine

🔳 *Digitoxin:* Reduced serum concentration of digitoxin

🔳 *Disopyramide:* Reduced serum concentration of disopyramide

🔳 *Doxycycline:* Reduced serum doxycycline concentrations

🔳 *Estrogen:* Reduced serum concentration of estrogen

🔳 *Ethanol:* Excessive CNS depression

🔳 *Felbamate:* Increased phenobarbital concentrations; increased risk of toxicity

🔳 *Furosemide:* Decreased diuretic effect

🔳 *Griseofulvin:* Reduced griseofulvin absorption

🔳 *Lamotrigine:* Lower lamotrigine plasma levels and decreased elimination $t_{1/2}$

🔳 *Methoxyflurane:* Enhanced nephrotoxic effect

🔳 *Narcotic analgesics:* Increased toxicity of meperidine; reduced effect of methadone; additive CNS depression

3 *Neuroleptics:* Reduced effect of either drug

2 *Oral anticoagulants:* Decreased hypoprothrombinemic response to oral anticoagulants

3 *Oral contraceptives:* Reduced efficacy of oral contraceptives

3 *Phenytoin:* Unpredictable effect on serum phenytoin levels

3 *Primidone:* Excessive phenobarbital concentrations

3 *Propafenone:* Reduced serum concentration of propafenone

3 *Quinidine:* Reduced quinidine plasma concentration

3 *Tacrolimus:* Reduced serum concentration of tacrolimus

3 *Theophylline:* Reduced serum theophylline concentrations

3 *Valproic acid:* Increased serum phenobarbital concentrations

Labs

• *Amino acids:* Increase in urine collection measurements

• *Calcium:* False increases with Technicon SRA-2000

• *Glucose:* False negatives with Clinistix, Diastix

• *5-Hydroxyindoleacetic acid:* False high colorimetric values

• *Lactate dehydrogenase:* Increased serum levels

• *Protein:* False elevations at high concentrations

SPECIAL CONSIDERATIONS
PATIENT/FAMILY EDUCATION

• Avoid driving or other activities requiring alertness

• Avoid alcohol ingestion or CNS depressants

• Do not discontinue medication abruptly after long-term use

MONITORING PARAMETERS

• Periodic CBC, liver and renal function tests, serum folate, vitamin D during prolonged therapy

• Serum phenobarbital concentra-

tion (therapeutic range for seizure disorders 20-40 µg/ml)

---

phenoxybenzamine
(fen-ox-ee-ben′za-meen)
Rx: Dibenzyline
Chemical Class: Haloalkylamine derivative
Therapeutic Class: Sympatholytic: Agent for pheochromocytoma

CLINICAL PHARMACOLOGY

Mechanism of Action: Irreversible α-adrenergic receptor (both pre- and postsynaptic) blocker; produces "chemical sympathectomy"; increases blood flow to skin, mucosa, abdominal viscera; lowers supine and standing blood pressure

Pharmacokinetics

PO: Incomplete oral absorption (20%-30%) onset gradual over several hours, duration 3-4 days; metabolized via dealkylation, excreted in urine and bile; $t_{1/2}$ 24 hr

INDICATIONS AND USES: Pheochromocytoma (control of episodes of hypertension and sweating), micturition disorders (neurogenic bladder, functional outlet obstruction, partial prostatic obstruction),* peripheral vasospastic disorders*

DOSAGE

Adult

• PO 10 mg bid initially, increase dosage qod until optimal response obtained as judged by blood pressure; usual dosage range 20-40 mg bid-tid

Child

• PO 1-2 mg/kg/day divided q6-8h

🔓 AVAILABLE FORMS/COST OF THERAPY

• Cap, Gel—Oral: 10 mg, 100's: **$85.05**

CONTRAINDICATIONS: Condi-

P

tions where a fall in blood pressure may be undesirable

PRECAUTIONS: Marked cerebral or coronary arteriosclerosis, renal damage, respiratory infection

PREGNANCY AND LACTATION: Pregnancy category C; indicated in hypertension secondary to pheochromocytoma during pregnancy, especially after 24 wk gestation when surgical intervention is associated with high rates of maternal and fetal mortality; no adverse fetal effects due to this treatment have been observed

SIDE EFFECTS/ADVERSE REACTIONS

CNS: Confusion, *dizziness,* drowsiness, sedation

CV: Palpitations, *postural hypotension, tachycardia*

EENT: Miosis, nasal congestion

GI: GI irritation, nausea, vomiting

GU: Inhibition of ejaculation

MISC: Fatigue

SPECIAL CONSIDERATIONS
PATIENT/FAMILY EDUCATION

• Avoid alcohol; avoid sudden changes in posture, dizziness may result

• Avoid cough, cold, or allergy medications containing sympathomimetics

---

phentermine

(fen′ter-meen)

Rx: Adipex-P, Fastin, Ionamin, Obe-Nix, Supramine, Tara-30, T-Diet, Teramin, Termene, Tora, Umi-Pex 30, Zantryl

Chemical Class: Phenethylamine analog (amphetamine-like

Therapeutic Class: Anorexiant

DEA Class: Schedule IV

CLINICAL PHARMACOLOGY
Mechanism of Action: Acts on ad-

renergic and dopaminergic pathways, directly stimulating the satiety center in the hypothalamic and limbic regions

Pharmacokinetics

PO, SUS REL: Duration 10-14 hr; metabolized by liver, excreted by kidney

INDICATIONS AND USES: Exogenous obesity

DOSAGE

Adult (>16 years)

• PO 8 mg tid ½ hr ac, or 15-37.5 mg as single daily dose before breakfast or 10-14 hr before retiring

§ AVAILABLE FORMS/COST OF THERAPY

• Cap, Gel—Oral: 15 mg, 100's: **$34.07;** 18.75 mg, 100's: **$28.95-$66.84;** 30 mg, 100's: **$11.96-$98.90;** 37.5 mg, 100's: **$34.95-$122.55**

• Tab, Uncoated—Oral: 8 mg, 100's: **$10.80-$54.07;** 37.5 mg, 100's: **$39.80-$120.39**

CONTRAINDICATIONS: Glaucoma, history of drug abuse, cardiovascular disease, moderate to severe hypertension, advanced arteriosclerosis, agitated states, hyperthyroidism, within 14 days of MAOI administration

PRECAUTIONS: Diabetes mellitus, convulsive disorders, hypertension, children

PREGNANCY AND LACTATION: Pregnancy category C

SIDE EFFECTS/ADVERSE REACTIONS

CNS: Dizziness, drowsiness, dysphoria, exacerbation of schizophrenia, headache, *insomnia,* mental depression, *nervousness, overstimulation, restlessness,* shivering, tremor, weakness

CV: Chest pain, palpitation, *tachycardia*

GI: Constipation, diarrhea, dry mouth, nausea, unpleasant taste

---

** = non-FDA-approved use

GU: Impotence, testicular pain, urinary hesitancy

SKIN: Clamminess, excessive sweating, pallor, rash

INTERACTIONS

Drugs

3 *Furazolidone:* Increased pressor response

3 *Guanethidine:* Decreased hypotensive effect

A *MAO Inhibitors:* Increased pressor response

3 *Tricyclic antidepressants:* Decreased anorexiant effect

Labs

• *Drugs of abuse:* Urine screen; false positive for amphetamines

• *Phenmetrazine:* False positive urine

• *Quinine:* False positive urine

SPECIAL CONSIDERATIONS
PATIENT/FAMILY EDUCATION

• May cause insomnia, avoid taking late in the day

• Weight reduction is facilitated by adherence to caloric restriction and exercise

---

phentolamine
(fen-tole′a-meen)
Rx: Regitine
Chemical Class: Imidazoline
Therapeutic Class: Sympatholytic: Agent for pheochromocytoma

CLINICAL PHARMACOLOGY
Mechanism of Action: α-adrenergic receptor (both pre- and postsynaptic) blocker; produces immediate onset and short duration "chemical sympathectomy"; acts at both the arterial and venous level; lowers supine and standing blood pressure; causes cardiac stimulation

Pharmacokinetics

IV: Onset of action immediate, duration 10-15 min

IM: Onset 15-20 min, duration 3-4 hr Metabolized in liver, excreted in urine (10% as unchanged drug)

INDICATIONS AND USES: Diagnosis of and treatment of hypertension associated with pheochromocytoma, treatment of dermal necrosis following extravasation of α-adrenergic drugs (norepinephrine, epinephrine, dobutamine, dopamine), hypertensive crises secondary to MAOI or sympathomimetic amine interactions and rebound hypertension on withdrawal of antihypertensives,* with papaverine as intracavernous injection for impotence*

DOSAGE
Adult

• *Diagnosis of pheochromocytoma:* IM/IV 5 mg

• *Hypertension, surgery for pheochromocytoma:* IM/IV 5 mg 1-2 hr before procedure, repeat q2-4h as needed

• *Drug extravasation:* Dilute 5-10 mg in 10 ml NS, infiltrate area with sol within 12 hr (blanching resolves within 1 hr if successful)

Child

• *Diagnosis of pheochromocytoma:* IM/IV 0.05-0.1 mg/kg/dose, max single dose 5 mg

• *Hypertension, surgery for pheochromocytoma:* IM/IV 0.05-0.1 mg/kg/dose 1-2 hr before procedure, repeat q2-4h as needed

• *Drug extravasation:* 0.1-0.2 mg/kg diluted in 10 ml NS infiltrated into area of extravasation within 12 hr

$ **AVAILABLE FORMS/COST OF THERAPY**

• Inj, Sol—IM, IV: 5 mg/ml; 1 ml vial: **$33.60**

CONTRAINDICATIONS: Angina, MI

PRECAUTIONS: Peptic ulcer disease (may exacerbate)

P

---

italic = common side effects   ***bold italic*** = life-threatening reactions

PREGNANCY AND LACTATION:
Pregnancy category C; unknown if
excreted in breast milk

**SIDE EFFECTS/ADVERSE REAC-
TIONS**

*CNS: **Cerebrovascular occlusion,***
dizziness, flushing, severe headache, weakness

*CV: Angina, **dysrhythmias,** hypotension, **MI,** reflex tachycardia*

EENT: Nasal congestion

*GI: Abdominal pain, diarrhea, dry
mouth, nausea, vomiting*

INTERACTIONS

Drugs

▣ *Epinepherine, ephedrine:* Vasoconstricting and hypertensive effects of these drugs are antagonized

Labs

• *5-hydroxyindoleacetic acid:* Urine,
falsely high colorimetric values

SPECIAL CONSIDERATIONS
• Urinary catecholamines preferred
over phentolamine for screening for
pheochromocytoma

**phenylephrine
(systemic)**
(fen-ill-ef'rin)

Rx: Neo-Synephrine,
AH-Chew D

Combinations

Rx: with chlorpheniramine
(Ed A-Hist, Prehist, Hista-
tab); with brompheni-
ramine (Dimetane); with
chlorpheniramine, phenyl-
propanolamine (Hista-
Vadrin); with chlorpheniramine, phenyltoloxamine
(Comhist); with bromphe-
niramine, phenylpropanol-
amine (Bromophen T.D.,
Tamine S.R.); with chlor-
pheniramine, phenyltolox-
amine, phenylpropanol-
amine (Decongestabs,
Naldecon, Nalgest, Tri-
phen, Uni-decon); with
chlorpheniramine, pyril-
amine, phenylpropanol-
amine (Vanex, Histalet);
with chlorpheniramine,
pyrilamine (R-tannate,
Rhinatate, R-tannamine,
Rynatan, Tanoral, Triotann,
Tritan, Tri-tannate)

Chemical Class: Substituted
phenylethylamine

Therapeutic Class: Vasopressor

CLINICAL PHARMACOLOGY

Mechanism of Action: Selective
postsynaptic α_1-receptor agonist;
causes vasoconstriction with increase in blood pressure and reflex
bradycardia

Pharmacokinetics

IV: Duration 20-30 min

IM/SC: Duration 45-60 min

PO: Biodegraded in gut wall (c-o-
methyltransferase); essentially, not
bioavailable

Excreted in urine; $t_{1/2}$ 2½ hr

INDICATIONS AND USES: Hypotension, shock, paroxysmal supraventricular tachycardia (PSVT), prolongation of spinal anesthesia, vasoconstriction in regional analgesia

DOSAGE

Adult

• *Decongestant:* PO 10 mg q4-6hr, PRN

• *Hypotension:* SC/IM 2-5 mg, may repeat q10-15 min if needed; IV 0.1-0.5 mg, may repeat q10-15 min if needed; IV INF 10 mg/500 ml D_5W given 100-180 gtt/min (based on 20 gtt/ml), then 40-60 gtt/min titrated to BP

• *PSVT:* IV bolus 0.5 mg given rapidly; subsequent doses should not exceed previous dose by >0.1-0.2 mg; max single dose 1 mg

• *Prolongation of spinal anesthesia:* Add 2-5 mg to anesthetic solution; increases duration of block by 50%

• *Prevention of hypotension in spinal anesthesia:* SC/IM 2-3 mg 3-4 min before anesthetic inj

• *Vasoconstriction in regional anesthesia:* Add 1 mg to 20 ml anesthetic sol

Child

• *Hypotension:* SC/IM 0.1 mg/kg/dose q1-2h (max 5 mg); IV bolus 5-20 μg/kg/dose q10-15 min; IV INF 0.1-0.5 μg/kg/min

• *PSVT:* IV 5-10 μg/kg/dose over 20-30 sec

• *Prevention of hypotension in spinal anesthesia:* SC/IM 0.05-0.1 mg/kg/dose

§ AVAILABLE FORMS/COST OF THERAPY

• Inj, Sol—IM, IV, SC: 10 mg/ml, 1 ml: **$0.72-$9.12**

• Tab-chewable 10 mg, 100's: **$26.10-$57.60**

• Liq-5 mg/5 mL, 120 mL: **$10.98**

• Suppository-0.25% 12's: **$2.95-$5.50**

CONTRAINDICATIONS: Ventricular fibrillation/tachycardia, pheochromocytoma, narrow-angle glaucoma, severe hypertension

PRECAUTIONS: Arterial embolism, peripheral vascular disease, elderly, hyperthyroidism, bradycardia, myocardial disease, severe arteriosclerosis

PREGNANCY AND LACTATION: Pregnancy category C; unknown if excreted in breast milk

SIDE EFFECTS/ADVERSE REACTIONS

CNS: Anxiety, dizziness, headache, insomnia, tremor

CV: Angina, ectopic beats, hypertension, palpitations, reflex bradycardia, tachycardia

GI: Nausea, vomiting

SKIN: **Gangrene,** necrosis, tissue sloughing with extravasation

INTERACTIONS

Drugs

3 *Beta-Blockers (non-selective):* Predisposed to hypertensive episodes

3 *Guanethidine:* Enhanced pupillary response to phenylephrine

3 *Imipramine:* Enhanced pressor response

1 *MAOIs:* Hypertensive episodes

Labs

• *Amino acids:* Increased in urine

• *Metanephrines, total:* Increased in urine

SPECIAL CONSIDERATIONS

• Antidote to extravasation: 5-10 ml phentolamine in 10-15 ml saline infiltrated throughout ischemic area

• Not indicated for hypotension secondary to hypovolemia

• As not bioavailable orally (see pharmacokinetics), combination products essentially lack decongestant. Only available by prescription, as lack effectiveness data required by FDA OTC panels

P

---

italic = common side effects   ***bold italic*** = life-threatening reactions

phenylephrine (topical)

(fen-ill-ef'rin)

Rx: *Ophthalmic:* Ak-Dilate, Ak-Nefrin, Mydfrin, Neo-Synephrine, Prefrin Liquifilm, Relief

OTC: *Nasal:* Alconefrin, Alconefrin, Neo-Synephrine, Nostril, Rhinall, Sinex, *Anorectal:* Medicone, Hem-Prep,

Combinations

  Rx (Nasal): with zinc (Zincfrin); with pheniramine (Dristan Nasal);

  Rx (Ophthalmic); with tropicamide (Diophenyl-t); with pyrilamine (Prefrin-A)

Chemical Class: Substituted phenylethylamine

Therapeutic Class: Decongestant; mydriatic

CLINICAL PHARMACOLOGY

Mechanism of Action: Postsynaptic α-receptor agonist; produces vasoconstriction (rapid, long-acting) of arterioles, decreasing fluid exudate, mucosal engorgement; stimulation of α-adrenergic receptors of the dilator muscle of the pupil, produce contraction, thus pupillary dilation

Pharmacokinetics

NASAL: May be systemically absorbed; duration of action 30 min-4 hr

OPHTH: Peak effect of mydriasis 15-60 min (2.5% sol), 10-90 min (10% sol); duration of action 3 hr (2.5% sol), 3-7 hr (10% sol)

INDICATIONS AND USES: Nasal congestion; mydriasis, uveitis with synechiae, and ocular decongestion

DOSAGE

Adult

• *Nasal:* Instill 2-3 gtt or sprays to nasal mucosa bid (0.25% sol, use 0.5%-1% sol in resistant only)

• *Ophth:* Mydriasis: 1 gtt to conjunctival sac (2.5% or 10% sol) after giving top anesthetic; ocular decongestant: 1 gtt to conjunctiva q3-4 hr as needed (0.12% sol)

• *Anorectal:* Apply PR after bowel movement, or bid

Child

• *Nasal:* 6-12 yr instill 1-2 gtt or sprays (0.25%) q3-4h prn; <6 yr instill 2-3 gtt or sprays (0.125%) q3-4h prn

• *Ophth:* 1 gtt of 2.5% sol to conjunctiva; ocular decongestant: 1 gtt to conjunctiva q3-4 hr as needed (0.08%-0.12% sol)

💲 AVAILABLE FORMS/COST OF THERAPY

• Sol—Nasal: 1% drops, 15 ml: **$3.90;** 1% spray, 15 ml: **$4.05;** 0.5% spray, 15 ml: **$3.72;** 0.25% drops, 15 ml, **$3.38;** 0.25% spray, 15 ml: **$3.45;** 0.125% drops, 15 ml: **$3.38**

• Sol—Ophth: 10%, 5 ml: **$3.00-$22.39;** 2.5%, 5 ml: **$2.63-$15.13**

• Ophth Sol—0.12%, 15 ml: **$3.56**

CONTRAINDICATIONS: Ten percent ophth sol not recommended in infants (hypertension)

PRECAUTIONS: Child <6 yr, elderly, diabetes, cardiovascular disease, hypertension, hyperthyroidism, increased intracranial pressure, prostatic hypertrophy, glaucoma

PREGNANCY AND LACTATION: Pregnancy category C; no breast feeding data, use caution

SIDE EFFECTS/ADVERSE REACTIONS

CNS: Anxiety, dizziness, fever, headache, insomnia, restlessness, tremors, weakness

EENT: Burning, dryness, irritation, rebound congestion, sneezing, stinging, visual blurring (ophth)

GI: Anorexia, nausea, vomiting

SKIN: Contact dermatitis
INTERACTIONS
Drugs, Lab
See interactions under systemic phenylephrine; interactions less likely than with systemic administration if given in proper dosage
SPECIAL CONSIDERATIONS
• Do not administer for more than 3-5 days (nasal product) or 2-3 days (ocular product used as decongestant) due to rebound congestion

phenylpropanolamine
(fen-ill-pro-pa-nole'a-mine)
OTC: Acutrim, Dexatrim, Propagest, Unitrol
Rx: Rhindecon
Combinations
(Phenylpropanolamine is available in many prescription and over-the-counter combinations; the following list is not all-inclusive.)
Rx: with antihistamines (Ornade) with antihistamines and other decongestants (Naldecon); with antihistamines and anticholinergics (Rhinolar); with antitussives (Tuss-Ornade, Drixoral Cough and Sore Throat, Hycomine); with antitussives and antihistamines (Dimetane DC); with expectorant (Entex)
OTC: with analgesics such as acetaminophen and aspirin (Rhino Capsules, St. Joseph's Cold); with antihistamines and analgesics (Coricidin, Tylenol Severe Allergy Capsules); with antihistamines (Contac Maximum Strength 12-Hour, Teldrin, Dimetapp, Tavist-D); with antitussive and antihistamine (Triaminicol Multi-Symptom, Comtrex)
Chemical Class: Sympathomimetic
Therapeutic Class: Anorexiant, decongestant

CLINICAL PHARMACOLOGY
Mechanism of Action: Suppresses appetite control center in hypothalamus, acts on α-adrenergic receptors to produce mucosal vasocon-

---

italic = common side effects   ***bold italic*** = life-threatening reactions

striction of respiratory tract, stimulates α-adrenergic receptors, causing contraction of bladder neck and urethral smooth muscle

Pharmacokinetics
PO: Onset 15-30 min; duration of action 3 hr (tab), 12-16 hr (extended-release); readily absorbed; hepatic metabolism, renal excretion

INDICATIONS AND USES: Exogenous obesity (short-term use, 6-12 wk, with diet, exercise, behavior modification); nasal congestion; urinary incontinence*

DOSAGE
Adult
• *Appetite suppressant:* PO 25 mg tid (tab, cap, gum); 75 mg qd (extended-release)
• *Decongestant:* PO 25 mg qid (tab, cap); 75 mg q12h (extended-release); max 150 mg/day
• *Urinary incontinence:* PO 50-150 mg/day in divided doses

Child
• *Decongestant:* PO 6.25 mg q4h, max 37.5 mg/day (2-6 yr); 12.5 mg q4h, max 75 mg/day (6-12 yr)

[$] AVAILABLE FORMS/COST OF THERAPY
• Cap, Gel, SUS Action—Oral: 75 mg, 60's: **$20.20**
• Tab—Oral: 25 mg, 100's: **$1.80-$7.65;** 37.5 mg, 100's: **$3.13;** 50 mg, 100's: **$2.71**
• Tab, SUS Action—Oral: 75 mg, 20's: **$2.29-$5.29**

CONTRAINDICATIONS: Severe CAD, severe hypertension, dysrhythmias, within 14 days of MAOI use, renal disease, glaucoma, depression

PRECAUTIONS: Postpartum women and children (increased psychiatric side effects), mild hypertension, hyperthyroidism, prostatic hypertrophy

PREGNANCY AND LACTATION: Pregnancy category C; possible increase in minor malformations with 1st trimester use; no data on breast feeding available

SIDE EFFECTS/ADVERSE REACTIONS
CNS: Confusion, dizziness, hallucinations, *headache,* insomnia, nervousness, *seizures*
CV: Chest tightness, *dysrhythmias,* hypertension
EENT: Dryness of nose and mouth
GI: Abdominal pain, nausea, vomiting
GU: Difficulty, pain with urination, *renal failure*

INTERACTIONS
Drugs
[3] *Antacids:* pH-dependent excretion; large antacid doses may inhibit the elimination of phenylpropanolamine
[A] *Bromocriptine:* Increased risk of hypertension and seizures
[3] *Furazolidone:* Increased risk of hypertensive response
[3] *Indomethacin:* Increased risk of hypertensive reactions
[A] *MAOIs:* Increased risk of hypertensive reactions
[3] *Thioridazine:* One patient on thioridazine died after single dose of phenylpropanolamine

SPECIAL CONSIDERATIONS
• Present in combination in many OTC products; some products may contain tartrazine, which may cause asthma in susceptible individuals (e.g., patients with aspirin sensitivity)

---

* = non-FDA-approved use

phenytoin
(fen'i-toy-in)
Rx: Dilantin
fosphenytoin
(foss-fen'i-toy-in)
Rx: Cerebyx
Chemical Class: Hydantoin
derivative
Therapeutic Class: Anticonvulsant

CLINICAL PHARMACOLOGY
Mechanism of Action: Inhibits spread of seizure activity in motor cortex by promoting sodium efflux, which stabilizes the threshold against hyperexcitability; fosphenytoin is pro-drug form of phenytoin; see Special Considerations
Pharmacokinetics
PO: Slow and variable absorption among products; peak 1½-3 hr (prompt cap), 4-12 hr (extended cap)
IV (As phenytoin): Immediate onset
IM (As phenytoin): Slow but complete (92%) absorption
IM/IV (As fosphenytoin): Completely bioavailable after IM Inj; 95-99% protein bound (decreases as plasma concentrations increase); conversion to phenytoin is complete; conversion $t_{1/2}$, 15 min

$t_{1/2}$ changes with dose and serum concentration secondary to saturation of hepatic metabolic enzyme systems; (mean, 12-28 hr) biotransformation increased in younger children, pregnant women, trauma; metabolites excreted in urine
INDICATIONS AND USES: Generalized tonic-clonic seizures; simple or complex partial seizures (psychomotor or temporal lobe); status epilepticus; nonepileptic seizures associated with Reye's syndrome or after head trauma; fosphenytoin—substitute for oral phenytoin when PO administration not feasible; migraines; trigeminal neuralgia*; Bell's palsy; ventricular dysrhythmias, especially related to digitalis toxicity*; epidermolysis bullosa*; diabetic neuropathy pain*
DOSAGE
NOTE: Fosphenytoin 75 mg equivalent to 50 mg phenytoin, after administration; the dose of IV fosphenytoin is expressed as phenytoin equivalents (PE) to avoid the need to perform molecular weight-based adjustments when converting between fosphenytoin and phenytoin doses
Adult
Phenytoin:
• *Seizures:* IV loading dose 15-20 mg/kg based on recent dosing history and serum levels, followed by 100 mg PO or IV q6-8h; PO loading dose 1 g divided 400 mg, 300 mg, 300 mg given q2h; if load not necessary, may give 100 mg tid, follow levels; maintenance dose: 300 mg/day or 5-6 mg/kg/day in divided doses; once dosage established may use extended caps and dose qd
• *Neuritic pain:* PO 200-400 mg/day
Fosphenytoin
• *Status epilepticus:* IV 15-20 mg PE/kg loading dose administered at 100-150 mg PE/min
• *Nonemergent and maintenance dosing:* IM/IV 10-20 mg PE/kg loading dose administered at a rate ≤150 mg PE/min: maintenance 4-6 mg PE/kg/day
Child
Phenytoin:
• *Seizures:* IV loading dose 15-20 mg/kg in divided doses of 5-10 mg/kg; PO 5 mg/kg/day in 2 or 3 divided doses to max 300 mg/day; daily maintenance dose 4-8 mg/kg

P

italic = common side effects   ***bold italic*** = life-threatening reactions

$ AVAILABLE FORMS/COST OF THERAPY

Phenytoin
- Inj, Sol—IM, IV: 50 mg/ml, 2 ml: **$0.62-$5.88**
- Susp—Oral: 125 mg/5 ml, 240 ml: **$29.98**
- Tab, Chewable—Oral: 50 mg, 100's: **$23.23**
- Cap, Gel—Oral: 100 mg, 100's: **$6.80**
- Cap, Sus Action: 30 mg, 100's: **$22.40;** 100 mg, 100's: **$23.36-$27.65**

Fosphenytoin
- Sol—IV, IM: 150 mg (100 mg phenytoin sodium)/2 ml, **$18.00**

CONTRAINDICATIONS: Bradycardia, 2nd and 3rd degree AV block, Stokes-Adams syndrome, sinoatrial block

PRECAUTIONS: Hepatic disease, renal disease, diabetes mellitus

PREGNANCY AND LACTATION: Pregnancy category D (risk of congenital defects increased 2-3 times; fetal hydantoin syndrome includes craniofacial abnormalities, hypoplasia, ossification of distal phalanges; may also be transplacental carcinogen); compatible with breast feeding

SIDE EFFECTS/ADVERSE REACTIONS

CNS: Ataxia, confusion, *dizziness,* drowsiness, fatigue, headache, insomnia, nystagmus, paresthesias, *psychiatric changes, slurred speech*
CV: **CV collapse** (when drug administered too rapidly IV), hypotension, *ventricular fibrillation*
EENT: Blurred vision, diplopia, *gingival hyperplasia,* nystagmus
GI: Anorexia, *constipation,* **hepatitis,** jaundice, *nausea, vomiting,* weight loss
GU: **Nephritis**
HEME: **Agranulocytosis, aplastic anemia, leukopenia,** lymphadenopathy, **megaloblastic anemia, thrombocytopenia**
METAB: Hyperglycemia
SKIN: Alopecia, hirsutism, **lupus erythematosus,** rash, **Stevens-Johnson syndrome**

INTERACTIONS
Drugs

3 *Acetaminophen:* Enhances the hepatotoxic potential of acetaminophen overdoses; may reduce the therapeutic response to acetaminophen

3 *Acetazolamide:* Osteomalacia

3 *Amiodarone:* Increased phenytoin levels; decreased amiodarone levels

3 *Azole-antifungals (fluconazole):* Phenytoin induces metabolism (CYP3A4) reducing antifungal effects

3 *Benzodiazepines (alprazolam, diazepam, midazolam, triazolam):* Enhanced metabolism (CYP3A4) phenytoin reduces benzodiazepine effects

3 *Carbamazepine:* Combined use usually decreases levels of both drugs

3 *Chloramphenicol, disulfiram, fluoxetine, isoniazid, omeprazole, sulfonamides:* Increased phenytoin levels

3 *Cimetidine, cisplatin, diazoxide, folate, rifampin:* Decreased phenytoin levels

3 *Clozapine:* Reduced levels via phenytoin induced enhanced metabolism

3 *Corticosteroids:* Decreased therapeutic effect of steroids

3 *Cyclic antidepressants:* Increased antidepressant levels

3 *Cyclosporine:* Reduced cyclosporine levels

3 *Dicumarol:* Increased anticoagulant effect, increased phenytoin levels

---

* = non-FDA-approved use

3 *Digitalis glycosides:* Lower digitalis levels

3 *Disopyramide:* Reduced efficacy, increased toxicity of disopyramide

3 *Dopamine:* More susceptible to hypotension after IV phenytoin

3 *Doxycycline:* Reduced doxycycline concentrations

3 *Felbamate:* Felbamate consistently increases phenytoin levels

3 *Furosemide:* Decreased diuretic effect

2 *Itraconazole:* Phenytoin induces metabolism (CYP3A4) reducing antifungal effects

3 *Lamotrigine:* Phenytoin stimulates metabolism-lower plasma levels; decreased $t_{1/2}$

3 *Levodopa:* Decreased antiparkinsonian effect

3 *Lithium:* Increased risk of lithium intoxication; causal explanation not known

2 *Mebendazole in high doses:* Decreased mebendazole levels

2 *Methadone:* Withdrawal

3 *Metyrapone:* Invalidates test

3 *Mexiletine:* Decreased mexiletine levels

3 *Oral contraceptives:* Decreased contraceptive effect

3 *Primidone:* Enhanced conversion to phenobarbital

3 *Pyridoxine:* Large doses may decrease phenytoin levels

3 *Quinidine:* Decreased quinidine levels

3 *Quinolone antibiotics (ciprofloxacin, enoxacin, norfloxacin, pefloxacin):* Elevates phenytoin concentrations

3 *Sucralfate:* Phenytoin reduces GI absorption

3 *Tacrolimus:* Reduced tacrolimus levels

3 *Theophylline:* Reduced theophylline levels

3 *Thyroid hormone:* Increased thyroid replacement dose requirements

3 *Tolbutamide:* Phenytoin inhibits insulin release, may result in hyperglycemia; tolbutamide displaces phenytoin from protein-binding sites; monitor for alterations in glucose control

3 *Trimethoprim:* Increased phenytoin concentrations

3 *Valproic acid:* Variable effects on phenytoin levels; decreased valproic acid levels

3 *Warfarin:* Transient increased hypoprothrombinemic response followed by inhibition of hypoprothrombinemic response

Labs

• *False positive:* Barbiturates, urine

• *Increased:* Cholesterol, serum; thyroxine, serum

SPECIAL CONSIDERATIONS

• Pro-drug, fosphenytoin rapidly converted to phenytoin *in vivo:* minimal activity before conversion; water soluble, thus more suitable for parenteral applications: doesn't require cardiac monitoring; can be administered at faster rate; no IV filter required; compatible with both saline and dextrose mixtures; requires refrigeration

MONITORING PARAMETERS

• Therapeutic range 10-20 µg/ml; nystagmus appears at 20 µg/ml, ataxia at 30 µg/ml, dysarthria and lethargy at levels above 40 µg/ml; lethal dose 2-5 g

P

---

italic = common side effects   ***bold italic*** = life-threatening reactions

physostigmine

(fi-zoe-stig'meen)

Rx: Antilirium

Chemical Class: Alkaloid; cholinesterase inhibitor

Therapeutic Class: Antiglaucoma agent; miotic; cholinergic

CLINICAL PHARMACOLOGY

Mechanism of Action: Inactivates acetylcholinesterase, potentiates acetylcholine at sites of cholinergic transmission; results in miosis, which increases outflow of aqueous humor, fall in intraocular pressure, and potentiation of accommodation; antagonizes anticholinergics

Pharmacokinetics

OPHTH: Onset 20-30 min, duration 12-36 hr (miosis); peak 2-6 hr, duration 12-36 hr (intraocular pressure)

IV/IM: Crosses blood-brain barrier; peak effect 20-30 min (IM), 5 min (IV); duration of action 30-60 min; destroyed in body by hydrolysis, very small amounts excreted in urine

INDICATIONS AND USES: Open-angle glaucoma (ophth), treatment of anticholinergic toxicity (systemic, including tricyclic antidepressants)

DOSAGE

Adult

• *Glaucoma:* Instill ¼ inch strip of 0.25% oint in conjunctival sac qd-tid; instill 1 gtt of a 0.25%-0.5% sol in conjunctival sac qd-qid

• *Anticholinergic toxicity:* IM/IV 0.5 mg-2 mg given at rate not greater than 1 mg/min; repeat q 20-30 min; max single dose 4 mg, as needed

Child

• *Glaucoma:* See adult

• *Anticholinergic toxicity:* IV 0.02 mg (20 µg)/kg over at least 1 min; may repeat q5-10min; max dose 2 mg

AVAILABLE FORMS/COST OF THERAPY

• Inj, Sol—IM, IV: 1 mg/ml, 2 ml: **$3.19-$11.12**

• Oint—Ophth: 0.25%, 3.5 g: **$1.62-$6.98**

CONTRAINDICATIONS: Inflammatory disease of iris or ciliary body, newborn (parenteral solution contains benzyl alcohol, toxic to neonate), organophosphate poisoning, intestinal or urogenital tract obstruction, asthma, diabetes mellitus, patients receiving choline esters or depolarizing neuromuscular blocking agents (decamethonium, succinylcholine)

PRECAUTIONS: Epilepsy, parkinsonism, bradycardia, bronchitis, CV disease

PREGNANCY AND LACTATION: Pregnancy category C; no data on breast feeding available

SIDE EFFECTS/ADVERSE REACTIONS

CNS: Anxiety, delirium, disorientation, hallucinations, headache, hyperactivity, *seizures*

CV: Bradycardia, hypertension, hypotension, irregular pulse

EENT: Blurred vision, conjunctivitis, decreased secretion in salivary and sweat glands; decreased secretions in pharynx, nasal passages, lacrimation, rhinorrhea, salivation, twitching of eyelids

GI: Abdominal cramps, diarrhea, nausea, vomiting

RESP: **Bronchospasm,** decreased bronchial secretions, dyspnea, *pulmonary edema*

MISC: Hyperpyrexia

INTERACTIONS

Drugs

β-*blockers:* Additive bradycardia

SPECIAL CONSIDERATIONS
• Atropine is antidote

---

phytonadione (vitamin K₁)
(fye-toe-na-dye'one)
Rx: AquaMEPHYTON, Mephyton
Chemical Class: Naphthoquinone fat-soluble vitamin
Therapeutic Class: Vitamin, antihemorrhagic

CLINICAL PHARMACOLOGY
Mechanism of Action: Normally synthesized by intestinal flora; promotes hepatic formation of clotting factors II, VII, IX, and X and anticoagulants protein C and protein S
Pharmacokinetics
PO, INJ: Readily absorbed from normal duodenum, bile salts required; rapid hepatic metabolism; onset of action 6-12 hr oral, 1-2 hr IV; prothrombin time normalizes in 12-14 hr following administration of adequate doses; excreted in urine, bile
INDICATIONS AND USES: Vitamin K malabsorption; hypoprothrombinemia; hemorrhagic disease of the newborn (prophylaxis); does not reverse hypoprothrombinemia due to hepatocellular damage
DOSAGE
Adult
• *Hypoprothrombinemia:* PO 2.5-10 mg (up to 25 mg) may repeat in 12 hr; IV/SC 1-10 mg (up to 25 mg), may repeat in 6-8 hr; NOTE: overzealous use during anticoagulant therapy may restore conditions which originally permitted thromboembolic phenomena, use doses >2.5 mg only if prothrombin time severely elevated, or if active bleeding present
• *Hypoprothrombinemia prevention during total parenteral nutrition:* IM 5-10 mg qwk
Child
• *Hypoprothrombinemia:* PO/IV/SC 1-10 mg; NOTE: overzealous use during anticoagulant therapy may restore conditions which originally permitted thromboembolic phenomena
• *Hypoprothrombinemia prevention during total parenteral nutrition:* IV 2-5 mg q wk
Infants
• *Hypoprothrombinemia:* PO/IV/SC 1-2 mg
• *Prevention of hemorrhagic disease of the newborn (HDN):* IM/SC 0.5-1 mg after birth, repeat in 6-8 hr if required (e.g., mother received anticonvulsants, rifampin, isoniazid during pregnancy)
💲 AVAILABLE FORMS/COST OF THERAPY
• Inj, Emulsion—IM, IV, SC: 1 mg/0.5 ml: **$2.22-$6.00**; 10 mg/ml, 1 ml: **$4.32-$5.49**
• Tab, Uncoated—Oral: 5 mg, 100's: **$56.29**
CONTRAINDICATIONS: Severe hepatic disease
PRECAUTIONS: G-6-PD deficiency; premature infants; correction of anticoagulant-induced hypoprothrombinemia in patients with continued needs for anticoagulation should be approached cautiously; consider mini-dosing (1-2.5 mg)
PREGNANCY AND LACTATION: Pregnancy category C; oral supplementation of women on anticonvulsants during last 2 weeks of pregnancy has been done to prevent HDN, but effectiveness unproven; compatible with breast feeding
SIDE EFFECTS/ADVERSE REACTIONS
CNS: Headache, **kernicterus** (premature infants, high doses)
HEME: **Hemoglobinuria, hemolytic**

---

anemia, hyperbilirubinemia (newborn)

SKIN: Flushing sensation, rash, urticaria

MISC: Anaphylaxis

INTERACTIONS

Drugs

3   *Oral anticoagulants:* Decreased anticoagulant effect

SPECIAL CONSIDERATIONS

• IV doses should be diluted and infused slowly over 20-30 min

---

pilocarpine
(pye-loe-kar´peen)

Rx: *Ophthalmic:* Akarpine, Isopto Carpine, Ocu-Carpine, Ocusert, Pilocar, Pilopine-HS, Piloptic

Oral: Salagen

Combinations

  Rx: with epinephrine
   (E-Pilo-6)

Chemical Class: Choline ester

Therapeutic Class: Miotic; ophthalmic cholinergic; antiglaucoma agent; salivation stimulant

---

CLINICAL PHARMACOLOGY

Mechanism of Action: Produces pupillary constriction by duplicating muscarinic effects of acetylcholine; increases aqueous humor outflow, intraocular pressure (IOP) decreases; orally increases exocrine gland secretion

Pharmacokinetics

OPHTH: Onset 10-30 min, duration 4-8 hr (sol, gel); Ocusert system onset 1½-2 hr, duration 7 days

PO: Onset 20 min, peak 1 hr, duration 3-5 hr; excreted in urine

INDICATIONS AND USES: Ophth: open-angle glaucoma, chronic angle-closure glaucoma, acute angle-closure glaucoma (in combination with other agents to decrease IOP before surgery), reversal of mydriasis, pre- and postoperative increased IOP; oral: xerostomia from salivary gland hypofunction secondary to radiotherapy for head and neck cancer

DOSAGE

Adult

• *Glaucoma:* Instill 1-2 gtt of 1% or 2% sol in eye q6-8h; instill 20-40 µg/hr (Ocusert) in cul-de-sac of eye, replace q7d; instill ½ inch ribbon of gel in conjunctival sac qhs

• *Xerostomia:* PO 5-10 mg tid

§   **AVAILABLE FORMS/COST OF THERAPY**

• Tab, Coated—Oral: 5 mg, 100's: **$119.28**

• Gel—Ophth: 4%, 3.5 g: **$28.75**

• Sol, Ophth: 0.5%, 15 ml: **$1.68-$11.63;** 1.0%, 15 ml: **$1.95-$16.50;** 2.0%, 15 ml: **$2.02-$16.75;** 3.0%, 15 ml: **$2.17-$12.75;** 4.0%, 15 ml: **$2.35-$17.75;** 5.0%, 15 ml: **$2.60;** 6.0%, 15 ml: **$2.95-$20.00;** 8.0%, 15 ml: **$22.25**

• Insert—Ophth: 20 µg/hr, 8's: **$45.13;** 40 µg/hr, 8's: **$45.13**

CONTRAINDICATIONS: Acute iritis, or other condition where acute miosis undesirable

PRECAUTIONS: Bronchial asthma, hypertension, bradycardia, hyperthyroidism, CV disease, biliary disease, renal colic (nephrolithiasis), epilepsy, parkinsonism, asthma

PREGNANCY AND LACTATION: Pregnancy category C

SIDE EFFECTS/ADVERSE REACTIONS

CNS: Headache

CV: AV block, bradycardia, *dysrhythmia,* hypertension, hypotension, *shock,* tachycardia

EENT: Blurred vision, conjunctival irritation (Ocusert), eye pain with change in focus, retinal detachment, stinging, tearing, twitching of eyelids

GI: Abdominal cramps, diarrhea, nausea, vomiting
GU: Bladder tightness, frequency, urgency
RESP: **Bronchospasm**
SPECIAL CONSIDERATIONS
• Antidote is atropine
PATIENT/FAMILY EDUCATION
• Miotics cause poor dark adaptation, use caution with night driving

---

pimozide
(pi'moe-zide)
Rx: Orap
Chemical Class: Diphenylbutylpiperidine derivative
Therapeutic Class: Antipsychotic

CLINICAL PHARMACOLOGY
Mechanism of Action: Dopamine receptor antagonist, with higher affinity for D_2- over D_1-receptors, and variable selectivity among the cortical dopamine tracts; also activity on nondopaminergic sites, i.e., cholinergic, α_1-adrenergic and histaminic receptors (explaining side effects); high risk extrapyramidal reactions; minimal orthostatic hypotension; moderate sedation and anticholinergic effects
Pharmacokinetics
PO: $t_{1/2}$ 19-39 hr, peak 4-12 hr 50% absorbed; hepatic metabolism, excreted in urine and stool
INDICATIONS AND USES: Gilles de la Tourette's syndrome (patients nonresponsive to haloperidol), chronic schizophrenia without excitement, agitation, or hyperactivity*
DOSAGE
NOTE: 0.3-0.5 mg equivalent to chlorpromazine 100 mg
Adult
• *Tourette's:* PO 1-2 mg qd in divided doses, increase qod as needed (usual dose 200 µg/kg/day or 10 mg

qd, whichever is less); max 300 µg/kg/day or 20 mg qd
• *Psychotic disorders:* PO 2-4 mg qd, increase qwk by 2-4 mg qd
$ **AVAILABLE FORMS/COST OF THERAPY**
• Tab, Uncoated—Oral: 2 mg, 100's: **$83.71**
CONTRAINDICATIONS: Simple tics other than Tourette's, history of cardiac dysrhythmias
PRECAUTIONS: Breast cancer (increased prolactin levels), liver disease, renal disease, hypokalemia (dysrhythmias), sensitivity to other neuroleptics
PREGNANCY AND LACTATION: Pregnancy category C
SIDE EFFECTS/ADVERSE REACTIONS
CNS: Akathisia, dizziness, *drowsiness, extra-pyramidal effects,* headache, mood or behavior changes, **neuroleptic malignant syndrome, parkinsonism, tardive dyskinesia**
CV: Hypotension, **prolonged QT interval,** tachycardia, **ventricular dysrhythmias**
EENT: Blurred vision, dryness of mouth
GI: Anorexia, *constipation,* diarrhea, nausea, obstructive jaundice, vomiting
GU: Loss of bladder control
HEME: **Blood dyscrasias**
SKIN: Itching, rash
MISC: Galactorrhea, mastalgia
INTERACTIONS
Drugs
3 *Anticholinergics (benztropine, trihexyphenidyl):* Antagonistic pharmacodynamic effects; excessive anticholinergic effects
3 *Bromocriptine:* Antagonistic pharmacodynamic effects
3 *Carbamazepine:* Decreased antipsychotic drug concentrations; decreased therapeutic response

---

italic = common side effects   **bold italic** = life-threatening reactions

3 *Clonidine:* Exaggerated hypotension

3 *Fluoxetine:* Increased risk of extrapyramidal symptoms

3 *Indomethacin:* Exaggerated side effects: drowsiness, tiredness, confusion

2 *Levodopa:* Antagonistic effects on the antiparkinsonian effects

3 *Lithium:* Reduced serum concentrations of both drugs; neurotoxic reactions reported in manic patients (delirium, seizures, encephalopathy, extrapyramidal symptoms)

3 *Meperidine:* Excessive hypotension and CNS depression

3 *Paroxetine:* Increased risk of extrapyramidal symptoms

3 *Phenobarbital:* Reduced pimozide concentrations; increased risk of hyperthermia associated with phenobarbital withdrawal

3 *Quinidine:* Increased pimozide concentrations and risk or subsequent toxicity

3 *Trazodone:* Additive hypotension

---

pindolol

(pin´doe-loll)
Rx: Visken

Chemical Class: Nonselective β-adrenergic blocker
Therapeutic Class: Antihypertensive; antianginal

CLINICAL PHARMACOLOGY
Mechanism of Action: Competitive, nonselective, β-adrenergic antagonist at β-receptors; produces negative inotropic and chronotropic responses; slows AV nodal conduction; decreases heart rate; decreases myocardial oxygen consumption; antiarrhythmic effects (class II); reduction in platelet aggregation and blood viscosity; suppression of renin release; inhibition of central sympathetic outflow; decreases presynaptic receptor neurotransmitter release; high intrinsic sympathomimetic activity; low membrane stabilizing activity; moderate lipid solubility

Pharmacokinetics
PO: Incomplete GI absorption (40%-60% bioavailable); peak serum concentrations, 2-4 hr; not metabolized by liver; excreted unchanged in urine and feces; $t_{1/2}$ 6-7 hr; crosses placenta in measurable, but not significant concentrations

INDICATIONS AND USES: Hypertension, angina pectoris,* migraine headache,* postmyocardial infarction,* alcohol withdrawal syndrome,* hyperthyroidism,* syncope, neuroleptic-induced akathesia*

DOSAGE
Adult and Child >16 yr
• *Hypertension:* PO 5-30 mg bid
• *Angina pectoris:* PO 2.5-5 mg/day initially; titrate gradually to 10-40 mg divided bid
• *Hyperthyroidism:* 15-30 mg/day
Child
• PO initial 1-1.2 mg/kg/dose qd; maximum 2 mg/kg/day qd

$ **AVAILABLE FORMS/COST OF THERAPY**
• Tab, Uncoated—Oral: 5 mg, 100's: **$59.98-$98.71;** 10 mg, 100's: **$79.51-$130.73**

CONTRAINDICATIONS: Cardiogenic shock; 2nd, 3rd degree heart block; severe bradycardia; overt cardiac failure; bronchial asthma

PRECAUTIONS: Anesthesia/surgery (myocardial depression), avoid abrupt withdrawal, bronchospastic airways, congestive heart failure, diabetes mellitus, concurrent clonidine (discontinue pindolol several days prior to withdrawal of clonidine), peripheral vascular disease, renal disease

---

* = non-FDA-approved use

PREGNANCY AND LACTATION: Pregnancy category B; similar drug, atenolol, frequently used in the third trimester for treatment of hypertension (many studies of efficacy and safety of atenolol in pregnancy-induced hypertension; long-term use has been associated with intrauterine growth retardation; enters breast milk in measurable amounts; observe for signs of β-blockade

SIDE EFFECTS/ADVERSE REACTIONS

CNS: Anxiety, *dizziness,* fatigue, hallucinations, *insomnia*

CV: AV block, bradycardia, chest pain, *CHF,* claudication, edema, hypotension, palpitation, tachycardia

EENT: Double vision, dry burning eyes, sore throat, *visual changes*

GI: Abdominal pain, diarrhea, *ischemic colitis, mesenteric arterial thrombosis,* nausea, vomiting

GU: Frequency, impotence

HEME: Agranulocytosis, purpura, thrombocytopenia

RESP: Bronchospasm, cough, *dyspnea,* rales

SKIN: Alopecia, pruritus, rash

MISC: Fever, joint pain, muscle pain

INTERACTIONS

Drugs

🔳 *Adenosine:* Bradycardia aggravated

• α-1 *adrenergic blockers:* Potential enhanced first dose response (marked initial drop in blood pressure) particularly on standing (especially prazocin)

• *Amiodarone:* Additive prolongation of atrioventricular (AV) conduction time; symptomatic bradycardia and sinus arrest

🔳 *Antacids:* Reduced pindolol absorption

🔳 *Calcium channel blockers:* See dihydropyridine calcium channel blockers and verapamil

🔳 *Cimetidine:* Renal clearance reduced; AUC increased with cimetidine coadministration

🔳 *Clonidine, guanabenz, guanfacine:* Exacerbation of rebound hypertension upon discontinuation of clonidine

🔳 *Cocaine:* Cocaine-induced vasoconstriction potentiated; reduced coronary blood flow

🔳 *Contrast media:* Increased risk of anaphylaxis

🔳 *Digitalis:* Enhances bradycardia

• *Digoxin:* Additive prolongation of atrioventricular (AV) conduction time

🔳 *Dihydropyridine calcium channel blockers:* Additive pharmacodynamic effects

• *Disopyramide:* Additive decreases in cardiac output

🔳 *Dipyridamole:* Bradycardia aggravated

• *Diltiazem:* Potentiates pharmacologic effects of β-adrenergic blocker, hypotension, left ventricular failure, and AV conduction disturbances reported; more likely in the elderly and in patients with left ventricular dysfunction, aortic stenosis, or large doses

🔳 *Epinephrine, isoproterenol, phenylephrine:* Potentiates pressor response; resultant hypertension and bradycardia

🔳 *Flecainide:* Additive negative inotropic effects

🔳 *Fluoxetine:* Increased β-blockade activity

🔳 *Fluoroquinolones:* Reduced clearance of pindolol

🔳 *Insulin:* Altered response to hypoglycemia; increased blood glucose concentrations; impair peripheral circulation

🔳 *Lidocaine:* Increased serum lidocaine concentrations possible

---

italic = common side effects   ***bold italic*** = life-threatening reactions

③ *Neostigmine:* Bradycardia aggravated

③ *Neuroleptics:*Both drugs inhibit each other's metabolism; additive hypotension

③ *NSAIDs:* Reduced antihypertensive effect of pindolol

③ *Physostigmine:* Bradycardia aggravated

③ *Prazosin:* First-dose response to prazosin may be enhanced by β-blockade

③ *Tacrine:* Bradycardia aggravated

② *Terbutaline:* Antagonized bronchodilating effects of terbutaline

② *Theophylline:* Antagonistic pharmacodynamic effects

③ *Verapamil:* Enhanced effects of both drugs; particularly AV nodal conduction slowing; reduced pindolol clearance

Labs

• *Alkaline phosphatase:* Increased serum levels

• *Aspartate aminotransferase:* Decreased serum levels

• *Bilirubin:* Decreased serum level

• *Creatine kinase:* Decreased serum level

SPECIAL CONSIDERATIONS

• Abrupt discontinuation may precipitate angina; taper over 1-2 wk

• Effective antihypertensive and probably antianginal agent (though not approved for this indication), especially for patients who develop symptomatic bradycardia with β-blockade

MONITORING PARAMETERS

• Angina: Reduction in nitroglycerin usage; frequency, severity, onset, and duration of angina pain; heart rate

• Hypertension: Blood pressure

• Toxicity: Blood glucose, bronchospasm, hypotension, bradycardia, depression, confusion, hallucination, sexual dysfunction

---

piperacillin; piperacillin/ tazobactam

(pi-per´a-sill-in; taz´o-bac-tam)

Rx: Pipracil (piperacillin); Zosyn, (piperacillin/tazobactam)

Chemical Class: Aminobenzyl penicillin, penicillin derivative/β-lactamase inhibitor (tazobactam)

Therapeutic Class: Antibiotic

CLINICAL PHARMACOLOGY

Mechanism of Action: Inhibits bacterial wall synthesis; bactericidal; tazobactam protects pipercillin from degradation by β-lactamase enzymes, extending the spectrum of activity

Pharmacokinetics

IM: Peak 30-50 min

IV: Peak 20-30 min

$t_{1/2}$ 0.7-1.33 hr; 33% protein bound; excreted in urine, bile; crosses placenta

INDICATIONS AND USES: Infections of the respiratory and genitourinary tract, bone; skin and intraabdominal infections; gonococcal infections; septicemia caused by susceptible organisms; combination with tazobactam effective against β-lactamase producing strains, moderate to severe nosocomial pneumonia

Antibacterial spectrum usually includes:

• Gram-positive organisms: *S. aureus, S. pyogenes, S. viridans, S. faecalis, S. bovis, S. pneumoniae, Clostridium perfringens, C. tetani*

• Gram-negative organisms: *N. gonorrhoeae, N. meningitidis, Bacteroides, Fusobacterium nucleatum, E. coli, Klebsiella, P. vulgaris, Proteus mirabilis, Morganella morganii, Enterobacter, Citrobacter, P seu-*

---

domonas aeruginosa, Serratia, Acinetobacter, Peptococcus, Peptostreptococcus, Eubacterium

• Anaerobes: *Bacteroides* sp., *Clostridium difficile*

DOSAGE

Adult

• *Systemic infections:* Piperacillin IM/IV 100-300 mg/kg/day in divided doses q4-6h; piperacillin/tazobactam IV INF 12-15 g/day given as 3.375 g q6hr over 30 min × 7-10 days

• *Prophylaxis of surgical infections:* IV 2 g ½-1 hr before procedure; may be repeated during surgery or after surgery

• *Uncomplicated gonorrhea:* IM 2 g as a single dose with 1 g probenecid 30 min before

• *Renal insufficiency:* Reduce dosage to degree of impairment; hemodialysis removes 40% of dose over 4 hr

Child >12 yr

• *Systemic infections:* IM/IV 100-300 mg/kg/day in divided doses q4-6h

• *Child* (doses are suggested but not established)

• IV 200-300 mg/kg/d (max daily dose 24 g) divided q4-6h

Neonate (term)

• IV 75 mg/kg q8h 1st week of life, q6h in 2nd week

Neonate (<36 wks)

• IV 75 mg/kg q12h 1st week of life, q8h in 2nd week

💲 AVAILABLE FORMS/COST OF THERAPY

Piperacillin:

• Inj, Lyphl-Sol—IM, IV: 2 g/vial: **$13.30;** 3 g/vial: **$19.44-$19.96;** 4 g/vial: **$26.62-$27.70**

Piperacillin/tazobactam:

• Inj, Sol—IV: 2 g/0.25 mg: **$10.80;** 3 g/0.375 mg: **$16.21;** 4 g/0.5 mg: **$21.61**

PRECAUTIONS: Hypersensitivity to cephalosporins; CHF; children <12 yr

PREGNANCY AND LACTATION: Pregnancy category B; excreted in breast milk in small concentrations

SIDE EFFECTS/ADVERSE REACTIONS

CNS: Anxiety, coma, depression, hallucinations, lethargy, seizures, twitching

GI: Abdominal pain, colitis, *diarrhea,* glossitis, increased AST, ALT; *nausea, vomiting*

GU: **Glomerulonephritis,** hematuria, *moniliasis,* oliguria, proteinuria, *vaginitis*

HEME: Anemia, **bone marrow depression,** increased bleeding time

METAB: Hypernatremia, hypokalemia

INTERACTIONS

Drugs

🔢 *Aminoglycosides:* Carbenicillin and other piperacillins can inactivate aminoglycosides in vitro and in certain patients with renal dysfunction

🔢 *Chloramphenicol:* Inhibited antibacterial activity of piperacillin; administer piperacillin 3 hr before chloramphenicol

🔢 *Macrolide antibiotics:* Inhibited antibacterial activity of piperacillin; administer piperacillin 3 hr before macrolides

🔢 *Methotrexate:* Piperacillin in large doses may increase serum methotrexate concentrations

🔢 *Oral contraceptives:* Occasional impairment of oral contraceptive efficacy; consider use of supplemental contraception during cycles in which piperacillin is used

🔢 *Tetracyclines:* Inhibited antibacterial activity of piperacillin; administer piperacillin 3 hr before tetracyclines

---

italic = common side effects   **bold italic** = life-threatening reactions

Labs
- *Cephalothin:* False positive serum
- *Penicillin G:* False positive serum
- *Protein:* False positive urine

SPECIAL CONSIDERATIONS
- Preferred over mezlocillin, more effective against *Pseudomonas;* reserve for carbenicillin- or ticarcillin-resistant *P. aeruginosa* infections in combination with an aminoglycoside

---

pirbuterol

(purr-byoo'ter-ole)
Rx: Maxair
Chemical Class: Sympathomimetic amine; β-adrenergic agonist
Therapeutic Class: Antiasthmatic, bronchodilator

CLINICAL PHARMACOLOGY
Mechanism of Action: Causes bronchodilation by β$_2$-stimulation, resulting in relaxation of bronchial smooth muscle; inhibits mast cell degranulation; stimulates cilia to remove secretions

Pharmacokinetics
INH: Onset 3 min, peak ½-1 hr, duration 5 hr, t$_{1/2}$ 2 hr

INDICATIONS AND USES: Prevention and reversal of bronchospasm including patients with asthma

DOSAGE
Adult and Child >12 yr
- MDI 1-2 puffs q4-6h, not to exceed 12 puffs/day

$ **AVAILABLE FORMS/COST OF THERAPY**
- MDI—INH: 0.2 mg/puff, 2.8 g: **$13.02;** 14 g: **$47.76;** 25.6 g: **$38.18**

PRECAUTIONS: Ischemic heart disease, cardiac dysrhythmias, hyperthyroidism, diabetes mellitus, prostatic hypertrophy, hypertension

PREGNANCY AND LACTATION:
Pregnancy category C

SIDE EFFECTS/ADVERSE REACTIONS
CNS: Anxiety, dizziness, drowsiness, hallucinations, headache, irritability, insomnia, restlessness, stimulation, tremors
CV: Angina, **dysrhythmias,** hypertension, hypotension, palpitations, tachycardia
EENT: Dry nose and mouth; irritation of nose, throat
GI: Anorexia, gastritis, nausea, vomiting
MS: Muscle cramps
RESP: **Bronchospasm,** coughing, dyspnea

INTERACTIONS
Drugs
❷ *Beta-blockers:* Decreased action of pirbuterol, cardioselective agents preferable if concurrent use necessary
❸ *Furosemide:* Potential for additive hypokalemia

SPECIAL CONSIDERATIONS
- No significant advantage over other selective β$_2$-agonists

PATIENT/FAMILY EDUCATION
- Initial and periodic reviews of metered dose inhaler technique

---

piroxicam

(peer-ox'i-kam)
Rx: Feldene
Chemical Class: Oxicam derivative
Therapeutic Class: NSAID with analgesic and antipyretic activity

---

CLINICAL PHARMACOLOGY
Mechanism of Action: Reversible cyclooxygenase (i.e., prostaglandin synthetase) inhibitor; nonselectively decreases the formation of both prostaglandins and thromboxane A2; var-

iable effects on lipoxygenase synthesis and subsequent leukotriene production; antiinflammatory, antipyretic, and analgesic activity; inhibits platelet aggregation

Pharmacokinetics

PO: Peak concentration 3-5 hr, analgesic onset 1 hr, duration 48-72 hr, antirheumatic onset 7-12 days, peak 2-3 wk, $t_{1/2}$ 30-86 hr; metabolized in liver, excreted in urine (metabolites); excreted in breast milk; 99% protein binding

INDICATIONS AND USES: Osteoarthritis, rheumatoid arthritis, ankylosing spondylitis,* prevention of cognitive decline,* prevention of colon cancer,* dysmenorrhea,* erythromelalgia,* acute gout,* pain* (dental, cancer, episiotomy, postoperative, sickle cell disease), soft tissue injury*

DOSAGE

Adult

• 20 mg qd or 10 mg bid

$ AVAILABLE FORMS/COST OF THERAPY

• Cap, Gel—Oral: 10 mg, 100's: **$118.77-$168.85;** 20 mg, 100's: **$203.92-$288.96**

CONTRAINDICATIONS: Bronchospasm, nasal polyps and angioedema precipitated by aspirin or other NSAIDs

PRECAUTIONS: History of GI ulceration, bleeding, or perforation; renal dysfunction, hypertension or cardiac conditions aggravated by fluid retention and edema, history of liver dysfunction, history of coagulation

PREGNANCY AND LACTATION: Pregnancy category B (avoid administration near term); excreted into breast milk; approximately 1% of mother's serum levels; should not present a risk to nursing infant

SIDE EFFECTS/ADVERSE REACTIONS

CNS: Anxiety, confusion, depression, dizziness, *drowsiness,* fatigue, *headache,* insomnia, tremors

CV: **Dysrhythmias,** palpitations, peripheral edema, tachycardia

EENT: Blurred vision, hearing loss, tinnitus

GI: Anorexia, **bleeding,** cholestatic hepatitis, constipation, cramps, *diarrhea,* dry mouth, flatulence, jaundice, *nausea,* **perforation, ulceration,** *vomiting*

GU: **Nephrotoxicity**

HEME: **Blood dyscrasias**

SKIN: Photosensitivity, pruritus, purpura, rash, sweating

INTERACTIONS

Drugs

⬛ *Aminoglycosides:* Reduced clearance with elevated aminoglycoside levels and potential for toxicity (especially indomethacin in premature infants; other NSAIDs probably)

⬛ *Anticoagulants:* Excessive hypoprothrombinemia, decreased platelet aggregation with increased risk of GI bleeding

⬛ *Antihypertensives (α-blockers, angiotensin-converting enzyme inhibitors, angiotensin II receptor blockers, β-blockers, diuretics):* Inhibition of antihypertensive and other favorable hemodynamic effects

⬛ *Corticosteroids:* Increased risk of GI ulceration

⬛ *Cyclosporine:* Increased nephrotoxicity risk

⬛ *Lithium:* Decreased clearance of lithium (mediated via prostaglandins) resulting in elevated serum lithium levels and risk of toxicity

⬛ *Methotrexate:* Decreased renal secretion of methotrexate resulting in elevated methotrexate levels and risk of toxicity

P

---

italic = common side effects   ***bold italic*** = life-threatening reactions

3 *Phenylpropanolamine:* Possible acute hypertensive reaction

3 *Potassium-sparing diuretics:* Additive hyperkalemia potential

3 *Triamterene:* Acute renal failure reported with addition of indomethacin; caution with other NSAIDs

SPECIAL CONSIDERATIONS
• Similar in efficacy to the other NSAIDs but has the advantage and disadvantage of an extended $t_{1/2}$

PATIENT/FAMILY EDUCATION

MONITORING PARAMETERS
• Initial hemogram and fecal occult blood test within 3 mo of starting regular chronic therapy; repeat every 6-12 mo (more frequently in high-risk patients (>65 years, peptic ulcer disease, concurrent steroids or anticoagulants); electrolytes, creatinine, and BUN within 3 mo of starting regular chronic therapy; repeat every 6-12 mo

---

plicamycin (mithramycin)

(plik-a-mi'sin)
Rx: Mithracin

Chemical Class: Crystalline aglycone
Therapeutic Class: Antineoplastic; antihypercalcemic

CLINICAL PHARMACOLOGY
Mechanism of Action: Inhibits DNA, RNA, protein synthesis; derived from *Streptomyces plicatus;* replication is decreased by binding to DNA; demonstrates calcium-lowering effect not related to its tumoricidal activity; also acts on osteoclasts and blocks action of parathyroid hormone

Pharmacokinetics
IV: Rapidly cleared from blood in 2 hr; 90% excretion in 24 hr; crosses blood-brain barrier

INDICATIONS AND USES: Testicular cancer; hypercalcemia and hypercalciuria of malignancy

DOSAGE
Adult
• *Testicular tumors:* IV 25-30 µg/kg/day × 8-10 days, not to exceed 30 µg/kg/day
• *Hypercalcemia/hypercalciuria:* IV 25 µg/kg/day × 3-4 days, repeat at intervals of 1 wk

$ **AVAILABLE FORMS/COST OF THERAPY**
• Inj, Lyphl-Sol—IV: 2.5 mg: **$85.56**

CONTRAINDICATIONS: Thrombocytopenia, bone marrow depression, bleeding disorders

PRECAUTIONS: Renal disease, hepatic disease, electrolyte imbalances

PREGNANCY AND LACTATION: Pregnancy category X

SIDE EFFECTS/ADVERSE REACTIONS
CNS: Depression, drowsiness, fever, flushing, headache, lethargy, weakness
GI: Anorexia, diarrhea, increased liver enzymes, *nausea, stomatitis, vomiting*
GU: Increased BUN, creatinine; proteinuria
HEME: **Hemorrhage, neutropenia, thrombocytopenia**
METAB: Decreased serum calcium, phosphate, potassium
SKIN: Cellulitis, extravasation, facial flushing, *rash*

INTERACTIONS
Drugs
3 *Bisphosphonates, calcitonin, foscarnet, glucagon:* Additive hypocalcemic effect

SPECIAL CONSIDERATIONS
• Effective but also toxic; use is therefore limited; additive with other calcium lowering therapies

MONITORING PARAMETERS
• CBC, differential, platelet count q wk; withhold drug if WBC is

---

<4000/mm^3 or platelet count is <50,000/mm^3

• Renal function studies: BUN, serum uric acid, urine CrCl, electrolytes, input and output ratio

• Liver function tests: bilirubin, AST, ALT, alk phosphatase before and during therapy

---

podofilox
(po-doe-fil′ox)
Rx: Condylox
Chemical Class: Podophyllum and Juniperus derivative
Therapeutic Class: Keratolytic

CLINICAL PHARMACOLOGY
Mechanism of Action: Exact mechanism unknown; results in necrosis of visible wart tissue
Pharmacokinetics
TOP: Application of 0.1-1.5 ml yields peak serum levels of 1-17 ng/ml in 1-2 hr; t$_{1/2}$ 1-4½ hr; no accumulation with multiple applications
INDICATIONS AND USES: Condyloma acuminatum (perianal, external genital)
DOSAGE
Adult
• TOP apply (cotton-tipped applicator) q12h for 3 consecutive days, then hold for 4 days; repeat 1 wk cycle until wart gone; if incomplete response after 4 cycles, consider alternate treatment; limit treatment to <10 cm^2 of wart tissue and no more than 0.5 ml of sol/day
$ **AVAILABLE FORMS/COST OF THERAPY**
• Sol—Top: 0.5%, 3.5 ml: **$83.80**
• Gel—Top: 0.5%, 3.5 g: **$83.80**
CONTRAINDICATIONS: Mucous membrane warts
PRECAUTIONS: External use only
PREGNANCY AND LACTATION: Pregnancy category C

SIDE EFFECTS/ADVERSE REACTIONS
CNS: Dizziness, insomnia, tingling
GI: Vomiting
GU: Hematuria
HEME: **Bleeding**
SKIN: Burning, chafing, crusting, edema, *erosion, inflammation, itching, pain,* scarring, tenderness, ulceration, vesicle formation
MISC: Malodor, pain with intercourse
SPECIAL CONSIDERATIONS
• Safety preferred over podophyllum resin

---

podophyllum
(poe-dah′fil-um)
Available in combination with benzoin
Rx: Podocon-25 (75% benzoin), Pododerm (10% benzoin)
Chemical Class: Podophyllum derivative
Therapeutic Class: Keratolytic

CLINICAL PHARMACOLOGY
Mechanism of Action: Arrests mitosis in metaphase by binding to tubulin, protein subunit of spindle microtubules
INDICATIONS AND USES: Condyloma acuminatum, multiple superficial epitheliomatoses and keratoses
DOSAGE
Adults
• *Warts:* TOP apply sparingly to wart using applicator, cover with wax paper, bandage for 1-4 hr, wash, may repeat qwk if needed
• *Keratosis, epitheliomatoses:* TOP apply qd with applicator, let dry, remove tissue, may reapply if needed
$ **AVAILABLE FORMS/COST OF THERAPY**
• Liq—Top: 25%, 5, 15, 30 ml: **$26.00-$38.00**/15 ml

---

italic = common side effects

bold italic = life-threatening reactions

CONTRAINDICATIONS: Bleeding warts or moles, birthmarks, moles with hair growing from them, poor blood circulation, diabetes

PRECAUTIONS: Avoid application on inflamed or irritated tissue

PREGNANCY AND LACTATION: Pregnancy category X; excretion into breast milk unknown, use caution in nursing mothers

SIDE EFFECTS/ADVERSE REACTIONS

CNS: Coma, confusion, dizziness, paresthesia, peripheral neuropathy, *seizures,* stupor

HEME: Leukopenia, thrombocytopenia

SKIN: Irritation of unaffected areas

MISC: Abdominal pain, diarrhea, nausea, vomiting

SPECIAL CONSIDERATIONS

• Not to be dispensed to the patient, professional application only

• Because of the potential for toxicity, cryotherapy should be attempted 1st or podofilox substituted

---

polymyxin B

(pol-ee-mix′in)

Rx: Aerosporin

Combinations

Rx: *Ophthal:* with bacitracin (Polysporin); with dexamethasone, neomycin (Dexacidin, Maxitrol); with hydrocortisone, neomycin (Cortisporin); with neomycin, bacitracin (Neosporin, Ocutricin); with neomycin, gramicidin (Neosporin); with oxytetracycline (Terak); with prednisolone, neomycin (Poly-Pred); with trimethoprim (Polytrim); *Topical:* with bacitracin, hydrocortisone, neomycin (Cortisporin); with dexamethasone, neomycin (Dioptrol, Maxitrol); with hydrocortisone, neomycin (Cortisporin)

OTC: *Topical:* with bacitracin (Bacimyxin, Polysporin); with bacitracin, neomycin (Neosporin, Triple Antibiotic); with bacitracin, neomycin, lidocaine (Lanabiotic, Spectrocin); with gramicidin (Polysporin); with gramicidin, lidocaine (Lidosporin, Polysporin Burn Formula); with gramicidin, neomycin (Neosporin)

Chemical Class: Polymyxin derivative

Therapeutic Class: Antibiotic; ophthalmic antibiotic

CLINICAL PHARMACOLOGY
Mechanism of Action: Interferes with membrane phospholipids and increases membrane permeability; bactericidal

---

Pharmacokinetics

PO: Not absorbed from the GI tract

IM/IV/IT (intrathecal): Repeated injections accumulate; tissue diffusion poor; does not cross blood-brain barrier; $t_{1/2}$ 4½-6 hr; excreted slowly in urine unchanged (60%)

INDICATIONS AND USES: Serious infections (bacteremia) caused by susceptible strains of *Pseudomonas aeruginosa, E. aerogenes, Klebsiella pneumoniae, E. coli, Haemophilus influenzae* when other antibiotics cannot be used; in meningeal infections, polymyxin B must be given intrathecally; ophth: superficial external ocular infections

DOSAGE

Adult

• IV INF 15,000-25,000 U/kg/day in divided doses q12h, or 25,000 U/kg/day in divided doses q4-8h; reduce dosage with renal dysfunction

• IM pain at inj site; reconstitute with procaine 1%; 25,000-30,000 U/kg/day divided q4-6h; reduce dosage with renal dysfunction

• IT 50,000 U qd for 3-4 days, then 50,000 qod for 2 wk after cultures negative and CSF glucose normalized

Child

• IV INF 15,000-25,000 U/kg/day in divided doses q12h, or 25,000 U/kg/day in divided doses q4-8h; infants <2 yr, up to 40,000 U/day

• IM not recommended, severe pain at inj site; reconstitute with procaine 1%; 25,000-30,000 U/kg/day q4-6h; reduce dosage with renal dysfunction; infants <2 yr up to 40,000 U/day

• IT 50,000 U qd for 3-4 days, then 50,000 qod for 2 wk after cultures negative and CSF glucose normalized; infants <2 yr up to 20,000U/

day × 3-4 days, then 25,000 U qod for 2 wk after cultures negative

🛇 AVAILABLE FORMS/COST OF THERAPY

• Inj, Dry-Sol—IM, IV, IT: 500,000 U/vial: **$5.32-$6.00**

CONTRAINDICATIONS: Severe renal disease

PRECAUTIONS: Renal dysfunction, neurologic or neuromuscular deficits

PREGNANCY AND LACTATION: Pregnancy category B

SIDE EFFECTS/ADVERSE REACTIONS

CNS: Coma, confusion, dizziness, drowsiness, headache, paresthesia, *seizures,* slurred speech, stiff neck, weakness

EENT: Overgrowth of nonsusceptible organisms, poor corneal wound healing, temporary visual haze

GU: Azotemia, hematuria, leukocyturia, proteinuria

*RESP: **Apnea** (concurrent use of other neurotoxic drugs or inadvertant overdosage)

SKIN: Urticaria

INTERACTIONS

Drugs

❷ *Anesthetics, neuromuscular blockers (e.g., gallamine, pancuronium, succinylcholine, tubocurarine):* Increased skeletal muscle relaxation

SPECIAL CONSIDERATIONS

• Generally replaced by the aminoglycosides or extended-spectrum penicillins for serious infections; still used for bladder irrigation and gut decontamination; used in combination with other antibiotics and/or corticosteroids topically to treat infections of the eye and skin

MONITORING PARAMETERS

• Intake and output, BUN, creatinine, urinalysis

P

---

italic = common side effects   ***bold italic*** = life-threatening reactions

polythiazide
(poly-thi'a-zide)
Rx: Renese
Combinations
  Rx: with prazosin (Mini-
    zide); with reserpine
    (Renese-R)
Chemical Class: Sulfonamide
derivative
Therapeutic Class: Thiazide
diuretic antihypertensive

CLINICAL PHARMACOLOGY
Mechanism of Action: Inhibits reabsorption of sodium and chloride
in cortical thick ascending limb of
the loop of Henle and the early distal tubules—increasing the urinary
excretion of sodium and chloride;
sulfonamide moiety provides some
carbonic anhydrase inhibition activity; other actions—increased potassium and bicarbonate excretion;
decreased calcium excretion; uric
acid retention; antihypertensive action dependent on sodium depletion, drop in peripheral vascular resistance, and reduction in extracellular volume
Pharmacokinetics
PO: Onset 2 hr, peak 6 hr, duration
24-48 hr, $t_{1/2}$ 25.7 hr
INDICATIONS AND USES: Edema
(CHF, hepatic cirrhosis, corticosteroid and estrogen therapy, nephrotic syndrome, acute glomerulonephritis), hypertension, calcium
nephrolithiasis,* prevention of osteoporosis,* diabetes insipidus*
DOSAGE
NOTE: Equivalent hydrochlorothiazide dose 2 mg = 50 mg
Adult
• 1-4 mg qd
**§ AVAILABLE FORMS/COST
  OF THERAPY**
• Tab, Uncoated—Oral: 1 mg, 100's:

$46.33; 2 mg, 100's: $60.63; 4 mg,
100's: $101.34
CONTRAINDICATIONS: Anuria,
renal decompensation
PRECAUTIONS: Fluid and electrolyte imbalance (including sodium,
potassium, magnesium calcium), renal disease, hepatic disease, gout,
COPD, lupus erythematosus, diabetes mellitus, hyperparathyroidism, vomiting, diarrhea, elevated
cholesterol/triglycerides, tartrazine
sensitivity
PREGNANCY AND LACTATION:
Pregnancy category D therapy for
preexisting hypertension can be continued throughout pregnancy with
minimal risk; initiating for simple
edema not recommended; few unequivocal indications for diuretic
therapy in pregnancy except for pulmonary edema or congestive heart
failure; excreted in breast milk in
low concentrations; compatible with
breast feeding
**SIDE EFFECTS/ADVERSE REAC-
  TIONS**
CNS: Dizziness, headache, paresthesias, vertigo, xanthopsia
CV: Arrhythmias, orthostatic hypotension
GI: Anorexia, constipation, cramping, diarrhea, gastric irritation, jaundice (intrahepatic cholestatic jaundice), nausea, *pancreatitis,* vomiting
HEME: ***Agranulocytosis, aplastic
anemia, leukopenia, thrombocytopenia***
METAB: Glycosuria, hyperglycemia,
hyperuricemia, lipid abnormalities
(increased total and LDL cholesterol, triglycerides)
MS: Muscle spasm, weakness
SKIN: Cutaneous vasculitis, necrotizing angitis, photosensitivity, purpura, rash, urticaria, vasculitis

* = non-FDA-approved use

INTERACTIONS
Drugs
❷ *Angiotensin-converting enzyme inhibitors:* Risk of postural hypotension when added to ongoing diuretic therapy; more common with loop diuretics; first dose hypotension possible in patients with sodium depletion or hypovolemia due to diuretics or sodium restriction; hypotensive response is usually transient; hold diuretic day of first dose

❸ *Calcium:* With large doses can result in milk-alkali syndrome

❸ *Carbenoxolone:* Additive potassium wasting; severe hypokalemia

❸ *Cholestyramine, colestipol:* Reduced absorption

❸ *Corticosteroids:* Concomitant therapy may result in excessive potassium loss

❸ *Diazoxide:* Hyperglycemia

❸ *Digitalis glycosides:* Diuretic-induced hypokalemia increases risk of digitalis toxicity

❸ *Hypoglycemic agents:* Increased dosage requirements due to increased glucose levels

❸ *Lithium:* Increased lithium levels, potential toxicity

❸ *Methotrexate:* Additive bone marrow suppression

❸ *Nonsteroidal antiinflammatory drugs:* Concurrent use may reduce diuretic and antihypertensive effects

Labs
• *False decrease:* Urine esriol

SPECIAL CONSIDERATIONS
• Doses above 1 mg provide no further blood pressure reduction, but are more likely to induce metabolic disturbance (i.e., hypokalemia, hyperuricemia, etc.)

• May protect against osteoporotic hip fractures

• Loop diuretics or metolazone more effective if CrCl <40-50 ml/min

PATIENT/FAMILY EDUCATION
• Will increase urination temporarily (approx. 3 wk); take early in the day to prevent sleep disturbance

• May cause sensitivity to sunlight; avoid prolonged exposure to the sun and other ultraviolet light

• May cause gout attacks; notify clinician if sudden joint pain occurs

MONITORING PARAMETERS
• Weight, urine output, serum electrolytes, BUN, creatinine, CBC, uric acid, glucose, lipids

---

poractant alfa
(poor-ak′tant)
Rx: Curosurf
Chemical Class: Phospholipid
Therapeutic Class: Porcine lung surfactant

CLINICAL PHARMACOLOGY
Mechanism of Action: Maintains lung inflation by lowering surface tension

Pharmacokinetics
Administered intratracheally; distributed to all lobes, distal airways, and alveolar spaces; biological $t_{1/2}$ 36 hr

INDICATIONS AND USES: Treatment (rescue) of respiratory distress syndrome (RDS) in premature infants

DOSAGE
Infant
• Intratracheal 100 mg/kg, followed by 2 additional 100 mg/kg doses at 12 and 24 hr in neonates still requiring mechanical ventilation with supplemental oxygen; a dose of 200 mg/kg within 10 min of delivery, followed prn by a 2nd mg/kg dose 6-24 hr later has been used for prophylaxis against neonatal RDS

💲 **AVAILABLE FORMS/COST OF THERAPY**
• Susp—Intratracheal: 120 mg/1.5

---

ml, vial: **$440.00;** 240 mg/3 ml, vial: **$762.00**

PRECAUTIONS: Infants born after >3 wk following ruptured membranes; intraventricular hemorrhage; major congenital malformations

SIDE EFFECTS/ADVERSE REACTIONS

CV: Patent ductus arteriosus, hypotension (transient)

RESP: Apnea

SKIN: Flushing

MISC: Antibody formation

SPECIAL CONSIDERATIONS

MONITORING PARAMETERS

• Continuous ECG and transcutaneous O_2 saturation; pCO_2; lung compliance; respiratory rate

---

potassium iodide

Rx: Pima, SSKI, Strong Iodine Solution (Lugol's Solution)

Chemical Class: Iodine product

Therapeutic Class: Expectorant; antithyroid agent

CLINICAL PHARMACOLOGY

Mechanism of Action: Reduces viscosity of mucus by increasing respiratory tract secretions; inhibits the release and synthesis of thyroid hormone

Pharmacokinetics

PO: Accumulates in thyroid gland; onset (antithyroid effects) 24-48 hr, peak effect (antithyroid effects) 10-15 days after continuous therapy; excreted mainly by the kidneys

INDICATIONS AND USES: Expectorant; preoperative reduction of thyroid gland vascularity prior to thyroidectomy, thyrotoxic crisis (in conjunction with other antithyroid agents), persistent or recurrent hyperthyroidism; radiation emergencies (to prevent uptake of radioactive isotopes of iodine); cutaneous sporotrichosis*

DOSAGE

Adult

• *Expectorant:* PO 300-650 mg tid-qid

• *Preoperative thyroidectomy:* PO 50-250 mg (1-5 gtt SSKI; 3-5 gtt Lugol's solution) tid for 10-14 days prior to surgery

• *Thyrotoxic crisis:* PO 300-500 mg (6-10 gtt SSKI; 1 ml Lugol's solution) tid

• *Cutaneous sporotrichosis:* PO 65-325 mg tid

• *Radiation emergency:* PO 130 mg qd for 10 days

Child

• *Expectorant:* PO 60-250 mg qid; max 500 mg/day

• *Preoperative thyroidectomy:* PO 50-250 mg (1-5 gtt SSKI; 3-5 gtt Lugol's solution) tid for 10-14 days prior to surgery

• *Thyrotoxic crisis:* PO <1 yr 65 mg qd for 10 days; older children 130 mg qd for 10 days

• *Radiation emergency:* PO <1 yr, 65 mg qd for 10 days; older children, 130 mg qd for 10 days

$ **AVAILABLE FORMS/COST OF THERAPY**

• Sol—Oral: 15 g/15 ml, 30 ml: **$6.60-$12.10**

• Syr—Oral: 325 mg/5 ml, 480 ml: **$19.90**

CONTRAINDICATIONS: Tuberculosis, acute bronchitis, hyperkalemia

PRECAUTIONS: Hypocomplementemic vasculitis, goiter, autoimmune thyroid disease, sulfite sensitivity (increased risk for iodine-induced adverse effects)

PREGNANCY AND LACTATION: Pregnancy category D; use of iodides as expectorants during pregnancy is contraindicated; concentrated in breast milk, may affect in-

---

* = non-FDA-approved use

fant's thyroid activity but considered compatible with breast feeding

SIDE EFFECTS/ADVERSE REACTIONS

CNS: Fever, headache

*CV: **Angioedema***

EENT: Rhinitis

GI: GI upset, metallic taste, soreness of teeth and gums

HEME: Cutaneous and mucosal hemorrhage, eosinophilia

METAB: Goiter, hypothyroidism

MS: Arthralgia

SKIN: Acne, urticaria

MISC: Lymph node enlargement

INTERACTIONS

Drugs

3 *Lithium:* Increased likelihood of hypothyroidism

SPECIAL CONSIDERATIONS

PATIENT/FAMILY EDUCATION

• Dilute sol with water or fruit juice to improve taste, drink sol through straw

• Administer with food or milk

MONITORING PARAMETERS

• Thyroid function tests if used for thyroid-related conditions

potassium salts

(po-taah'see-um)

Rx: *Potassium chloride:* Cena-K, Gen K, K+ Care, K+10, Kaochlor, Kaon-Cl, Kato, Kay Ciel, K-Dur, K-Lease, K-lor, Klor-Con, Klorvess, Klotrix, K·lyte/Cl, K-Norm, K-tab, Micro-K, Potasalan, Rum-K, Slow-K, Ten-K

Rx: *Potassium gluconate:* Kaon, Kaylixir, K-G Elixer

Rx: *Combinations of potassium salts:* Effer-K, K·Lyte, Klor-Con EF (as bicarbonate, citrate), K+ Care ET (as bicarbonate), Klorvess Effervescent Granules (as bicarbonate, chloride, citrate); K-Lyte/Cl (as bicarbonate, chloride), Kolyum (as chloride, gluconate); Tri-K, (as acetate, bicarbonate, citrate); Twin-K (as gluconate, citrate)

Chemical Class: Potassium salt

Therapeutic Class: Electrolyte supplement

P

CLINICAL PHARMACOLOGY

Mechanism of Action: Principal intracellular cation of most body tissues; necessary for maintenance of intracellular tonicity and proper relationships with sodium across cell membranes; needed for adequate nerve transmission, cardiac, skeletal, and smooth muscle contraction, renal function, and acid-base balance

Pharmacokinetics

PO/IV: Primarily renal excretion (90%); fecal (10%)

INDICATIONS AND USES: Prevention and treatment of hypokalemia;

---

italic = common side effects   ***bold italic*** = life-threatening reactions

with alkalosis (i.e., due to diuretics), use potassium chloride salt; when acidosis present, use potassium acetate, bicarbonate, citrate, or gluconate salts; hypertension*

DOSAGE

• Individualize dosage up to 400 mEq/day (usually not more than 3 mEq/kg/day): 10-30 mEq/day for prevention; 40-100 mEq/day for treatment

mEq/g of potassium salts

K⁺ Salt	mEq/g
gluconate	4.3
citrate	9.8
bicarbonate	10
acetate	10.2
chloride	13.4

Adult

• *Potassium acetate:* Serum potassium >2.5 mEq/L: IV INF up to 200 mEq/day in concentration <40 mEq/L at rate of 10 mEq/hr; serum potassium <2.0 mEq/L: IV INF up to 400 mEq/day in concentration <80 mEq/L and rate up to 40 mEq/hr

• *Potassium bicarbonate:* PO dissolve 25-50 mEq in water qd-bid up to 100 mEq/d

• *Potassium chloride:* PO 10-100 mEq/d divided qd-tid; IV serum potassium >2.5 mEq/L: IV up to 200 mEq/day in concentration <40 mEq/L at a rate not exceeding 10 mEq/hr; serum potassium <2.0 mEq/L: IV up to 400 mEq/day in concentration <80 mEq/L and rate of 40 mEq/hr

• *Potassium gluconate:* PO 20 mEq in divided doses bid-qid

Child

• *Potassium acetate:* IV up to 3 mEq/kg or 40 mEq/m² per day

• *Potassium chloride:* PO sol 15-40 mEq/m² or 1-3 mEq/kg/day in divided doses diluted in water or juice;

IV up to 3 mEq/kg or 40 mEq/m² per day

• *Potassium gluconate:* PO 20-40 mEq/m² or 2-3 mEq/kg per day in divided doses

💲 AVAILABLE FORMS/COST OF THERAPY

Potassium acetate

• Inj, Sol—IV: 2 mEq/ml, 20 ml: **$1.96-$5.23;** 4 mEq/ml, 50 ml: **$5.00-$6.46**

Potassium bicarbonate

• Tab, Effervescent—Oral: 25 mEq, 30's: **$6.06-$17.75**

Potassium chloride

• Cap, Gel, SUS Action—Oral: 8 mEq, 100's: **$10.75-$18.63;** 10 mEq, 100's: **$16.66-$20.48**

• Tab, Coated, SUS Action—Oral: 8 mEq, 100's: **$7.65-$20.40;** 10 mEq, 100's: **$37.55;** 20 mEq, 100's: **$42.25**

• Tab, Effervescent—Oral: 20 mEq, 30's: **$5.13-$28.00;** 25 mEq, 30's: **$7.09-$17.48;** 50 mEq, 30's: **$50.41**

• Liq—Oral: 20 mEq/15 ml, 480 ml: **$1.80-$46.62;** 30 mEq/15 ml, 480 ml: **$16.45;** 40 mEq/15 ml, 480 ml: **$2.80-$9.23**

• Powder, Reconst—Oral: 20 mEq/pkg, 30's: **$3.95-$50.71;** 25 mEq/pkg, 30's: **$7.41**

• Inj, Conc—Sol: 1.5 mEq/ml, 10 ml: **$4.36-$8.37;** 2 mEq/ml, 10 ml: **$2.74-$7.75**

Potassium gluconate

• Elixir—Oral: 20 mEq/15 ml, 480 ml: **$5.00-$27.34**

CONTRAINDICATIONS: Renal disease (severe), severe hemolytic disease, Addison's disease, hyperkalemia, acute dehydration, extensive tissue breakdown

PRECAUTIONS: Cardiac disease, potassium-sparing diuretic therapy, systemic acidosis

SIDE EFFECTS/ADVERSE REACTIONS

CNS: Confusion

---

* = non-FDA-approved use

*CV: **Arrest,*** bradycardia, cardiac depression, ***dysrhythmias,*** lowered R and depressed RST, peaking T waves, prolonged P-R interval, widened QRS complex

GI: Cramps, diarrhea, nausea, pain, ulceration of small bowel, *vomiting*

GU: Oliguria

SKIN: Cold extremities, rash

INTERACTIONS

3 *ACE inhibitors:* Hyperkalemia

3 *Disopyramide:* Increased potassium concentrations can enhance disopyramide effects

3 *Hypoglycemics:* Correction of hypokalemia may result in hypoglycemia

2 *Potassium-sparing diuretics:* Hyperkalemia

SPECIAL CONSIDERATIONS

• Avoid use of compressed tablets or enteric-coated tablets (i.e., non-sustained release or effervescent tablets for sol) due to significant ulcerogenic tendency and propensity to cause significant local tissue destruction

• Sol, powder, and oral susp: dilute or dissove in 120 ml cold water or juice

• Extended release caps and tabs: do not crush; take with food; swallow with full glass of liquid

• Injectable potassium products must be diluted prior to administration; direct inj of potassium concentrate may be fatal

• Central line preferable for IV infusions concentrated >40 mEq/L

MONITORING PARAMETERS

• ECG monitoring advisable for IV infusion rate >10 mEq/hr

• Normal serum potassium level 3.5-5.0 mEq/L (higher, to 7.7 mEq/L in neonates)

pralidoxime
(pra-li-dox′eem)
Rx: Protopam
Chemical Class: Quaternary ammonium derivative
Therapeutic Class: Anticholinesterase antidote

CLINICAL PHARMACOLOGY
Mechanism of Action: Reactivates cholinesterase inactivated by exposure to organophosphate pesticides or related compounds by displacing the enzyme from its receptor sites; most effective if administered within 24 hr of exposure

Pharmacokinetics
IM/IV: Peak 5-15 min, not bound to plasma proteins; metabolized in liver, excreted rapidly in urine (metabolite and unchanged drug); $t_{1/2}$ 1.7 hr (repeated doses may be needed)

INDICATIONS AND USES: Antidote in poisonings due to organophosphate pesticides and related compounds; control of overdosage by anticholinesterase drugs used to treat myasthenia gravis

DOSAGE
Use in conjunction with atropine
Adult

• *Organophosphate poisoning:* IM/IV 1-2 g, repeat in 1-2 hr if muscle weakness has not resolved, then at 10-12 hr intervals if cholinergic signs reappear

• *Anticholinesterase overdosage:* IV 1-2 g, followed by 250 mg q5 min until desired response

Child

• *Organophosphate poisoning:* IM/IV 20-50 mg/kg/dose, repeat in 1-2 hr if muscle weakness has not resolved, then at 10-12 hr intervals if cholinergic signs reappear

P

---

italic = common side effects   ***bold italic*** = life-threatening reactions

💲 AVAILABLE FORMS/COST OF THERAPY

• Inj, Lyphl-Sol—IM, IV, SC: 50 mg/ml, 20 ml: **$29.84**

PRECAUTIONS: Rapid IV inj, impaired renal function, myasthenia gravis, carbamate poisoning (less effective than with organophosphate poisoning)

PREGNANCY AND LACTATION: Pregnancy category C

SIDE EFFECTS/ADVERSE REACTIONS

CNS: Dizziness, drowsiness, headache

CV: Tachycardia

EENT: Blurred vision, diplopia, impaired accommodation

GI: Transaminase elevations (return to normal within 2 wk), nausea

MS: Muscular weakness

RESP: Hyperventilation

SKIN: Pain at inj site (IM)

SPECIAL CONSIDERATIONS MONITORING PARAMETERS

• CBC; plasma cholinesterase activity may help confirm diagnosis and follow course of illness

---

pramipexole

(pram-eh-pex′ol)

Rx: Mirapex

Chemical Class: Non-ergoline; a propylaminobenzothiazole
Therapeutic Class: Anti-Parkinson's agent, dopaminergic

CLINICAL PHARMACOLOGY

Mechanism of Action: Dopamine D_2-receptor agonist, with activity at both presynaptic and postsynaptic receptor sites; D_3-receptor subtype affinity greater than D_2-, D_4-receptor subtypes (different from other dopamine-receptor agonists); moderate affinity for alpha-2 adrenoceptors; low affinity for alpha-1, beta-adrenoceptors, serotonin, acetylcholine, and D_1 receptors; in Parkinson's disease, stimulates caudate neurons via D_3-receptor agonist mechanism

Pharmacokinetics

PO: Peak 1-3 hr; well absorbed (PO); minimally metabolized by liver, protein binding less than 20%, excreted renally, unchanged after 24 hr; $t_{1/2}$ 8-14 hr; crosses placenta

INDICATIONS AND USES: Treatment of signs and symptoms of idiopathic Parkinson's disease

DOSAGE

Adult

• *Parkinson's disease:* PO 0.125 mg tid initially increase gradually at 5-7 day intervals (max 1.5 mg tid); discontinue over a 1 wk period

• *Renal failure and geriatric patients:* Reduce dose according to CrCl; starting dose and (maximal dose) shown below

    CrCl >60 mL/min: 0.125 mg tid (1.5 mg tid)

    CrCl 35 to 59 mL/min: 0.125 mg bid (1.5 mg bid)

    CrCl 15 to 34 mL/min: 0.125 mg qd (1.5 mg qd)

    Ccr <15 mL/min and hemodialysis: avoid use of pramipexole

💲 AVAILABLE FORMS/COST OF THERAPY

• Tab—Oral: 0.125 mg, 63's: **$45.91;** 0.25 mg, 90's: **$87.05;** 0.5 mg, 90's: **$170.83;** 1 mg, 90's: **$170.83;** 1.5 mg, 90's **$170.83**

PRECAUTIONS: Hypersensitivity history or other untoward effects related to use of other dopamine agonists, psychotic disorders, dementia (potential for exacerbation), cardiovascular disease (postural hypotensive effects, increases in heart rate, and possibly hypertension), renal impairment (dose reductions are indicated), worsening of dyskinesia with advanced Parkinson's disease;

---

* = non-FDA-approved use

abrupt withdrawal of treatment (taper down over 1 wk)

PREGNANCY AND LACTATION:
Pregnancy category C; inhibits prolactin secretion; excretion into breast milk unknown

SIDE EFFECTS/ADVERSE REACTIONS

CNS: Akathesia, amnesia, asthenia, confusion, *dizziness, drowsiness,* dyskinesia, dystonia, hallucinations, hypesthesia, *insomnia,* restlessness, *somnolence (13%)*

CV: **Dysrhythmias,** chest pain, hypertension, *orthostatic hypotension* (domperidone may prevent), palpitations, syncope, tachycardia

EENT: Blurred vision

GI: Anorexia, *constipation (7%), dry mouth (10%),* dyspepsia, dysphagia, flatulence, *nausea (20%)*

GU: Impotence, urinary frequency

METAB: Decreases prolactin, thyrotropin levels; increases growth hormone, cortisol; peripheral edema, weight loss

MS: Increased CPK, leg cramps

SKIN: Diaphoresis, generalized rash, pruritus

INTERACTIONS

Drugs

3 *Cimetidine:* 50% increase in pramipexole AUC and 40% increase in $t_{1/2}$

3 *Dopamine antagonists (phenothiazines, butyrophenones, thioxanthenes, metoclopropamide):* May diminish effectiveness of pramipexole

3 *Levodopa:* 40% increase in levodopa concentrations

SPECIAL CONSIDERATIONS
• At least as effective as bromocriptine in the treatment of advanced parkinsonian patients with levodopa-related motor fluctuations; adverse effects similar in incidence and severity; appears to lack some of the toxicity seen with bromocriptine,

pergolide, and cabergoline (e.g., pleuropulmonary disease); may be a useful alternative in patients with intolerable adverse effects due to ergot derivatives

MONITORING PARAMETERS
• United Parkinson's Disease Rating Scale (UPDRS) useful for monitoring efficacy endpoints

---

pramoxine
(pra-mox'een)
OTC: Itch-X, PrameGel, Prax, ProctoFoam-NS, Tronolane, Tronothane
Chemical Class: Dyclonine derivative
Therapeutic Class: Topical anesthetic

CLINICAL PHARMACOLOGY
Mechanisms of Action: Decreases the neuronal membrane's permeability to sodium ions thus inhibiting depolarization; blocks initiation and conduction of nerve impulses

Pharmaconkinetics
TOP: Onset 2-5 min. duration may be several days

INDICATIONS AND USES: Temporary relief of pain and itching associated with dermatoses, minor burns, anogenital pruritus or irritation, anal fissures, hermorrhoids

DOSAGE
Adult
• TOP apply tid-qid: PR apply up to 5 times daily; apply 1 applicatorful of aerosol foam bid-tid after bowel movements

§ AVAILABLE FORMS/COST OF THERAPY
• Supp—Rect: 1%, 10's: **$3.41**
• Aer Foam Susp—Rect, Top: 1%, 15 g: **$22.15**
• Cre—Rect. Top: 1%, 30, 60g: **$3.05**/30 g
• Cre—Top: 1%, 30 g: **$10.80**

P

---

italic = common side effects   ***bold italic*** = life-threatening reactions

• Gel—Top:1%, 35.4,120 g: **$6.59/ 120 g**

• Lotion—Top: 1%, 15, 120, 240 ml: **$4.15**/15 ml

• Spray—Top: 1%, 59 ml: **$4.32**

PRECAUTIONS: Prolonged use, rectal bleeding, children, denuded skin

PREGNANCY AND LACTATION: Pregnancy category C; excretion into breast milk unknown

SIDE EFFECTS/ADVERSE REACTIONS

SKIN: Burning, irritation, rash, stinging

SPECIAL CONSIDERATIONS

• Cross-sensitization with other local anesthetics unlikely

PATIENT/FAMILY EDUCATION

• Do not use near eyes or nose

• Contact clinician if condition fails to improve after 3-4 days or worsens

• Do not apply to large areas

• Do not apply to unaffected areas

---

pravastatin
(prav-i-sta'tin)
Rx: Pravachol
Chemical Class: Substituted hexahydronaphthalene
Therapeutic Class: Antilipemic (HMG-CoA reductase inhibitor); "statin"

CLINICAL PHARMACOLOGY

Mechanism of Action: Competitively inhibits 3-hydroxy-3-methylglutaryl-coenzyme A (HMG-CoA) reductase, an early rate-limiting step in cholesterol biosynthesis; increases HDL cholesterol mildly [7%-12%], significant decreases in total and LDL cholesterol [16%-25%, 22%-34%, respectively], moderate lowering effect on triglycerides [11%-24%]

Pharmacokinetics

PO: Peak 1-1½ hr; absolute bioavailability 17%; 50% bound to plasma proteins; metabolized in liver, excreted in urine (20%) and feces (70%); t½ 77 hr

INDICATIONS AND USES: Primary hypercholesterolemia (heterozygous familial and nonfamilial hypercholesterolemia), mixed dyslipidemia (Fredrickson types IIa and IIb), primary prevention of coronary events, and secondary prevention of cardiovascular events

DOSAGE

Adult

• PO 10-20 mg qhs, may increase to 40 mg qhs if needed

$ AVAILABLE FORMS/COST OF THERAPY

• Tab, Uncoated—Oral: 10 mg, 100's: **$191.51;** 20 mg, 90's: **$204.59;** 40 mg, 90's: **$336.33**

CONTRAINDICATIONS: Active liver disease, unexplained persistent elevated liver function tests

PRECAUTIONS: History of liver disease, renal function impairment, elderly, children <18 yr, alcoholism; risk factors predisposing to the development of renal failure secondary to rhabdomyolysis (severe acute infection, trauma, hypotension, uncontrolled seizure disorder, severe metabolic disorders, electrolyte imbalance)

PREGNANCY AND LACTATION: Pregnancy category X; small amounts excreted in breast milk; should probably not be used by women who are nursing

SIDE EFFECTS/ADVERSE REACTIONS

CNS: Dizziness, headache
CV: Chest pain
GI: Abdominal pain, anorexia, cholestatic jaundice, cirrhosis, constipation, fatty change in liver, flatulence, heartburn, hepatitis, increased

---

* = non-FDA-approved use

serum transaminase levels, nausea, *pancreatitis,* vomiting
GU: Erectile dysfunction, loss of libido
MS: Arthralgia, localized pain, myalgia, myopathy, *rhabdomyolysis*
SKIN: Alopecia, photosensitivity, pruritus, rash
MISC: Fatigue, gynecomastia

INTERACTIONS
Drugs
❷ *Azole antifungals (fluconazole, itraconazole, ketoconazole, miconazole):* Increased plasma pravastatin levels via inhibition of metabolism with increased risk of rhabdomyolysis
❸ *Cholestyramine:* Reduced bioavailability of pravastatin
❸ *Clarithromycin:* Increased plasma pravastain levels via inhibition of metabolism with increased risk of rhabdomyolysis
❷ *Clofibrate:* Small increased risk of myopathy with combination
❸ *Colestipol:* Reduced bioavailability of pravastatin
❸ *Cyclosporine:* Concomitant administration increases risk of severe myopathy or rhabdomyolysis
❸ *Danazol:* Increased plasma pravastatin levels via inhibition of metabolism with increased risk of rhabdomyolysis
❸ *Erythromycin:* Increased pravastatin levels via inhibition of metabolism with increased risk of rhabdomyolysis
❸ *Fluoxetine:* Increased pravastatin levels via inhibition of metabolism with increased risk of rhabdomyolysis
❷ *Gemfibrozil:* Small increased risk of myopathy with combination, especially at high doses of statin
❸ *Isradipine:* Isradipine may decrease pravastatin plasma concentrations
❸ *Niacin:* Concomitant adminis-

tration increases risk of severe myopathy or rhabdomyolysis
❸ *Nefazodone:* May inhibit hepatic metabolism of pravastatin with risk of rhabdomyolysis
❸ *Troleandomycin:* Increased pravastatin levels via inhibition of metabolism with increased risk of rhabdomyolysis

SPECIAL CONSIDERATIONS
• Statin selection based on lipid-lowering prowess, cost, and availability

PATIENT/FAMILY EDUCATION
• Avoid prolonged exposure to sunlight and other UV light
• Promptly report any unexplained muscle pain, tenderness, or weakness, especially if accompanied by fever or malaise
• Strictly adhere to low cholesterol diet
• Take daily doses in the evening for increased effect

MONITORING PARAMETERS
• ALT and AST at baseline, and at 12 weeks of therapy. If no change at 12 weeks, no further monitoring necessary (discontinue if elevations persist at >3 times upper limit of normal)
• CPK in any patient complaining of diffuse myalgia, muscle tenderness, or weakness
• Fasting lipid profile

P

praziquantel
(pray-zi-kwon'tel)
Rx: Biltricide
Chemical Class: Pyrazinoisoquinoline derivative
Therapeutic Class: Anthelmintic

CLINICAL PHARMACOLOGY
Mechanism of Action: Increases cell membrane permeability in worm causing a loss of intracellular cal-

cium, massive contractions and paralysis of worm musculature leading to detachment of suckers from blood vessel walls and dislodgment; also results in vacuolization and disintegration of the schistosome in tegument, followed by attachment of phagocytes and death

Pharmacokinetics

PO: Rapidly absorbed, peak 1-3 hr; significant 1st-pass biotransformation; metabolites excreted primarily in urine; $t_{1/2}$ 0.8-1½ hr

INDICATIONS AND USES: Schistosomiasis caused by *Schistosoma* spp. pathogenic to humans, clonorchiasis and opisthorchiasis (liver flukes), cysticercosis,* tissue fluke infections,* intestinal fluke infections,* intestinal cestode (tapeworm) infections*

DOSAGE

Adult and Child

• *Schistosomiasis:* PO 20 mg/kg/dose 2-3 times/day for 1 day at 4-6 hr intervals

• *Clonorchiasis and opisthorchiasis:* PO 75 mg/kg/day divided q8h for 1-2 days

• *Cysticercosis:* PO 50 mg/kg/day divided q8h for 14 days (administer steroids prior to starting praziquantel for neurocysticercosis)

• *Cestodes:* PO 10-20 mg/kg as a single dose (25 mg/kg for *Hymenolepsis nana*)

$ **AVAILABLE FORMS/COST OF THERAPY**

• Tab, Plain Coated—Oral: 600 mg, 6's: **$66.74**

CONTRAINDICATIONS: Ocular cysticercosis

PRECAUTIONS: Children <4 yr, cerebral cysticercosis (hospitalize patient for duration of therapy)

PREGNANCY AND LACTATION: Pregnancy category B; do not nurse on day of treatment and during the subsequent 72 hr

SIDE EFFECTS/ADVERSE REACTIONS

CNS: Dizziness, drowsiness, fever, headache

GI: Abdominal discomfort, minimal increases in liver enzymes

SKIN: Urticaria

MISC: Malaise

INTERACTIONS

Drugs

3 *Chloroquine:* Reduces plasma level of praziquantel

3 *Cimetidine:* Increases plasma level of praziquantel

3 *Hydroxychloroquine:* Reduces plasma level of praziquantel

SPECIAL CONSIDERATIONS
PATIENT/FAMILY EDUCATION

• Swallow tablets unchewed with some liquid during meals

• May cause drowsiness

• Use caution driving or performing other tasks requiring alertness

---

prazosin

(pra'zoe-sin)

Rx: Minipress

Combinations

  Rx: with polythiazide (Minizide)

Chemical Class: Quinazoline derivative

Therapeutic Class: Alpha-1-adrenergic blocker: antihypertensive; symptomatic benign prostatic hypertrophy

CLINICAL PHARMACOLOGY

Mechanism of Action: Selectively blocks postsynaptic α_1-adrenergic receptors; dilates both arterioles and veins, reducing peripheral vascular resistance and blood pressure; no reflex tachycardia or changes in renin release; blockade of α_1-adrenoceptors in bladder neck and pros-

---

* = non-FDA-approved use

tate; relaxes smooth muscle, improving urine flow rates in benign prostatic hypertrophy

Pharmacokinetics

PO: Oral bioavailability 48%-68%, peak 1-3 hr, duration of antihypertensive effect 10 hr; 92%-97% bound to plasma proteins; extensively metabolized to active metabolites, excreted in bile (90%) and urine (10%); $t_{1/2}$ 2-3 hr

INDICATIONS AND USES: Hypertension, benign prostatic hypertrophy,* Raynaud's vasospasm,* refractory congestive heart failure*

DOSAGE

Adult

• PO 1 mg bid-tid, give 1st dose at bedtime; increase as needed to 6-15 mg/day in divided doses; doses >20 mg/day usually do not increase efficacy

Child

• PO 0.5-7 mg tid

[$] AVAILABLE FORMS/COST OF THERAPY

• Cap, Gel—Oral: 1 mg, 100's: **$8.03-$48.04;** 2 mg, 100's: **$35.10-$66.53;** 5 mg, 100's: **$60.00-$60.50**

PRECAUTIONS: Children, hepatic disease

PREGNANCY AND LACTATION: Pregnancy category C

SIDE EFFECTS/ADVERSE REACTIONS

CNS: Anxiety, asthenia, ataxia, depression, *dizziness,* fever, *headache,* hypertonia, insomnia, nervousness, paresthesia, somnolence

CV: Chest pain, dysrhythmia, edema, *"1st-dose" syncope,* flushing, palpitations, postural hypotension, tachycardia

EENT: Abnormal vision, tinnitus, vertigo

GI: Abdominal discomfort, constipation, diarrhea, dry mouth, flatulence, nausea, vomiting

GU: Incontinence, polyuria

MS: Arthralgia, myalgia

RESP: Dyspnea

SKIN: Pruritus, rash

INTERACTIONS

Drugs

[3] *ACE inhibitors:* Exaggerated first-dose response to prazosin

[3] β*-adrenergic blockers:* Exaggerated first-dose response to prazosin

[3] *NSAIDs:* Inhibits antihypertensive response to prazosin

[3] *Verapamil:* Reduces first pass metabolism of prazosin

Labs

• False positive urinary metabolites of norepinephrine and VMA

• No effect on prostate specific antigen (PSA)

SPECIAL CONSIDERATIONS

• Use as single antihypertensive agent, limited by tendency to cause sodium and water retention and increased plasma volume

PATIENT/FAMILY EDUCATION

• Alert patients to the possibility of syncopal and orthostatic symptoms, especially with the 1st dose ("1st-dose syncope")

• Initial dose should be administered at bedtime in the smallest possible dose

P

---

italic = common side effects   ***bold italic*** = life-threatening reactions

prednisolone

(pred-niss'oh-lone)

Rx: Prelone; (acetate) Key-Pred, Predacort, Key-Pred-SP (sodium phosphate), Pedia-pred; Ophthalmic: (acetate) Econopred, Econopred Plus, Pred Mild, Pred Forte; (sodium phosphate) AK-Pred, Inflamase Mild, Inflamase Forte, Prednisol

Chemical Class: Glucocorticoid
Therapeutic Class: Systemic corticosteroid; ophthalmic corticosteroid

CLINICAL PHARMACOLOGY
Mechanism of Action: Decreases inflammation by depressing migration of polymorphonuclear leukocytes and activity of endogenous mediators of inflammation; has many profound metabolic effects, possesses mineralocorticoid activity
Pharmacokinetics
PO: Peak 1-2 hr, duration 2 days
IM: Peak 3-45 hr
Metabolized in most tissues but primarily in liver, excreted in urine; $t_{1/2}$ 115-212 min (biologic 18-36 hr)
INDICATIONS AND USES: Anti-inflammatory or immunosuppressant agent in the treatment of a variety of diseases of hematologic, allergic, inflammatory, neoplastic, and autoimmune origin; (ophth) steroid-responsive inflammatory conditions of the palpebral and bulbar conjunctiva, lid, cornea, and anterior segment of the globe, corneal injury (chemical, radiation, or thermal burns or penetration of foreign bodies)
DOSAGE
Adult
• PO 5-60 mg/day; IM (acetate) 4-60 mg/day

• *Multiple sclerosis (acute exacerbations):* PO 200 mg qd for 1 wk, followed by 80 mg qod for 1 mo
• *OPHTH* apply 1gtt q1h during day, q2h during night until favorable response, then 1 gtt q4h
Child
• *Acute asthma:* PO 1-2 mg/kg/day divided 1-2 times/day for 3-5 days
• *Anti-inflammatory/immunosuppressive:* PO 0.1-2 mg/kg/day divided qd-qid
• *OPHTH* apply 1 gtt q1h during day, q2h during night until favorable response, then 1 gtt q4h
§ AVAILABLE FORMS/COST OF THERAPY
• Syr—Oral: 15 mg/5 ml, 30, 60, 120, 160, 240, 480 ml: **$11.81-$24.56**
• Liq—Oral (sodium phosphate): 5 mg/5 ml, 120 ml: **$18.46-$20.14**
• Tab, Uncoated—Oral: 5 mg, 100's: **$3.95-$13.75**
• Susp, Top—Ophth (acetate): 0.12%, 5, 10 ml: **$17.25-$20.05/5 ml**
• Susp—Ophth (acetate): 0.125%, 5, 10 ml: **$18.88/5 ml**, 1%, 5, 10 ml, 15 ml: **$1.80-$18.93/5 ml**
• Sol—Ophth (sodium phosphate): 0.125%, 5, 10 ml: **$1.72-$25.99/5 ml**; 1%, 5, 10, 15 ml: **$1.73-$25.99/5 ml**
• Inj, Susp—IM (acetate): 25 mg/ml, 10, 30 ml: **$6.50-$14.96/30 ml**; 50 mg/ml, 10, 30 ml: **$9.50-$11.50/30 ml**
CONTRAINDICATIONS: Systemic fungal infections; (ophth): acute superficial herpes simplex keratitis and other viral diseases of the cornea and conjunctiva; fungal diseases of ocular structures; ocular TB; following uncomplicated removal of a superficial corneal foreign body
PRECAUTIONS: Psychosis, cerebral malaria, elderly, AIDS, latent

tuberculosis or amebiasis (reactivation of disease), diabetes mellitus, glaucoma, osteoporosis, ulcerative colitis (intestinal perforation), CHF, myasthenia gravis, renal disease, esophagitis, peptic ulcer, hypertension; (ophth): infections of the eye, glaucoma

PREGNANCY AND LACTATION: Pregnancy category B; compatible with breast feeding

SIDE EFFECTS/ADVERSE REACTIONS

CNS: Depression, headache, *mood changes,* **seizures,** vertigo

CV: CHF, hypertension, tachycardia, **thromboembolism,** thrombophlebitis

EENT: Systemic: Cataracts, glaucoma, increased intraocular pressure, optic nerve damage, papilledema; Ophthalmic: Blurred vision, burning with administration, cataracts, corneal infection, decreased visual acuity and visual fields, glaucoma exacerbation, increased intraocular pressure, optic nerve damage, poor corneal wound healing, stinging with administration

GI: Abdominal distension, diarrhea, **GI hemorrhage,** increased appetite, *nausea,* **pancreatitis**

METAB: Cushingoid state, decreased glucose tolerance, growth suppression in children, *HPA axis suppression,* hypercalciuria, hypokalemia

MS: Aseptic necrosis of femoral and humeral heads, fractures, muscle mass loss, osteoporosis, weakness

SKIN: Acne, *ecchymosis,* petechiae, striae, *poor wound healing,* suppression of skin test reactions, *thin fragile skin*

INTERACTIONS
Drugs

3 *Aminoglutethamide:* Increased clearance of prednisolone; doubling of dose may be required

3 *Antidiabetics:* Increased blood glucose

3 *Barbiturates:* Increased clearance of prednisolone

3 *Cholestyramine, colestipol:* Reduced absorption of prednisolone

3 *Clarithromycin, erythromycin, troleandomycin, ketoconazole:* Possible enhanced steroid effect

3 *Estrogens, oral contraceptives:* Enhanced effects of corticosteroids

3 *Intrauterine devices:* Decreased contraceptive effect (possibly secondary inhibition of inflammatory reaction)

3 *Isoniazid:* Reduced plasma concentrations of isoniazid; (rapid isoniazid acetylators at increased risk)

3 *NSAIDs:* Increased risk GI ulceration

3 *Rifampin:* May reduce hepatic clearance of prednisolone

3 *Salicylates:* Increased salicylate clearance

Labs

• *False increase:* Cortisol, digoxin, theophylline

• *False decrease:* Urine glucose (Clinistix, Diastix only, Testape no effect)

• *False negative:* Skin allergy tests

SPECIAL CONSIDERATIONS
PATIENT/FAMILY EDUCATION

• May cause GI upset
• Take single daily doses in AM
• Increased dose of rapidly acting corticosteroids may be necessary in patients subjected to unusual stress
• Signs of adrenal insufficiency include fatigue, anorexia, nausea, vomiting, diarrhea, weight loss, weakness, dizziness, and low blood sugar
• Avoid abrupt withdrawal of therapy following high-dose or long-term therapy. Relative insufficiency may exist for up to 1 yr after discontinuation

P

---

italic = common side effects **bold italic** = life-threatening reactions

• Patients on chronic steroid therapy should wear Medical Alert bracelet

• Do not give live virus vaccines to patients on prolonged therapy

MONITORING PARAMETERS

• Potassium and blood sugar during long-term therapy

• Edema, blood pressure, cardiac symptoms, mental status, weight

• Observe growth and development of infants and children on prolonged therapy

• Check intraocular pressure and lens frequently during prolonged use of ophthalmic preparations

---

prednisone
(pred′ni-sone)
Rx: Deltasone, Liquid Pred, Meticorten, Pred-Pak 45, Pred-Pak 79, Prednisone Intensol Concentrate, Sterapred, Sterapred DS
Chemical Class: Glucocorticoid
Therapeutic Class: Systemic corticosteroid

CLINICAL PHARMACOLOGY
Mechanism of Action: Decreases inflammation by depressing migration of polymorphonuclear leukocytes and activity of endogenous mediators of inflammation; has many profound metabolic effects, possesses mineralocorticoid activity
Pharmacokinetics
PO: Absorption 78%; must be metabolized to prednisolone for activity, excreted in urine; $t_{1/2}$ 60 min (biologic 18-36 hr)
INDICATIONS AND USES: Anti-inflammatory or immunosuppressant agent in the treatment of a variety of diseases of hematologic, allergic, inflammatory, neoplastic, and autoimmune origin

DOSAGE
Adult
• PO 5-60 mg/day divided qd-qid
• *Physiologic replacement:* PO 4-5 mg/m²/day
• *Hepatic disease:* Conversion to active metabolite, prednisolone, may be impaired; use prednisolone at same dosage
Child
• *Anti-inflammatory/immunosuppressive:* PO 0.05-2 mg/kg/day divided qd-qid
• *Acute asthma:* PO 1-2 mg/kg/day divided qd-bid for 3-5 days
• *Asthma, long-term therapy:* PO <1 yr 10 mg qod, 1-4 yr 20 mg qod, 5-13 yr 30 mg qod, >13 yr 40 mg qod
• *Physiologic replacement:* PO 4-5 mg/m²/day

💲 AVAILABLE FORMS/COST OF THERAPY
• Sol—Oral: 5 mg/5 ml, 60, 120, 500 ml: **$7.02/60ml**
• Tab, Uncoated—Oral: 1 mg, 100's: **$3.53-$19.61;** 2.5 mg, 100's: **$3.70-$8.19;** 5 mg, 100's: **$3.50-$14.78;** 10 mg, 100's: **$5.23-$20.00;** 20 mg, 100's: **$10.00-$34.13**
• Syr—Oral: 5 mg/5 ml, 30 ml: **$15.42**

CONTRAINDICATIONS: Systemic fungal infections
PRECAUTIONS: Psychosis, cerebral malaria, elderly, AIDS, latent tuberculosis or amebiasis (reactivation of disease), diabetes mellitus, glaucoma, osteoporosis, ulcerative colitis (intestinal perforation), CHF, myasthenia gravis, renal disease, esophagitis, peptic ulcer, hypertension; (ophth): infections of the eye, glaucoma
PREGNANCY AND LACTATION: Pregnancy category B; compatible with breast feeding

---

* = non-FDA-approved use

SIDE EFFECTS/ADVERSE REACTIONS

CNS: Depression, headache, *mood changes,* psychosis, **seizures,** vertigo

CV: CHF, hypertension, tachycardia, **thromboembolism,** thrombophlebitis

EENT: Blurred vision, cataracts, increased intraocular pressure

GI: Abdominal distension, diarrhea, **GI hemorrhage** (esophagitis, peptic ulcer), increased appetite, *nausea,* **pancreatitis**

HEME: Leukocytosis

METAB: Cushingoid state, decreased glucose tolerance, decreased testosterone levels, growth suppression in children, **HPA axis suppression,** hypocalcemia, hypokalemia, metabolic alkalosis, Na and fluid retention

MS: Aseptic necrosis of femoral and humeral heads, fractures, muscle mass loss, osteoporosis, weakness

SKIN: Acne, bruising, ecchymosis, petechiae, poor wound healing, striae, suppression of skin test reactions, thin fragile skin

INTERACTIONS

Drugs

3 *Aminoglutethamide:* Increased clearance of prednisone; doubling of dose may be necessary

3 *Antidiabetics:* Increased blood glucose

3 *Barbiturates, carbamazepine:* Increased clearance of prednisone

3 *Cholestyramine, colestipol:* Possible reduced absorption of corticosteroids

3 *Cyclosporine:* Possible increased concentration of both drugs, seizures

3 *Erythromycin, troleandomycin, clarithromycin, ketoconazole:* Possible enhanced steroid effect

3 *Estrogens, oral contraceptives:* Enhanced effects of corticosteroids

3 *IUD's:* Inhibition of inflammation may decrease contraceptive effect

3 *Isoniazid:* Reduced plasma concentrations of isoniazid

3 *NSAIDs:* Increased risk GI ulceration

3 *Rifampin:* May reduce hepatic clearance of prednisone

3 *Salicylates:* Increased salicylate clearance

Labs

• *False increase:* Cortisol, digoxin, theophylline

• *False decrease:* Urine glucose (Clinistix, Diastix only, Testape no effect)

• *False negative:* Skin allergy tests

SPECIAL CONSIDERATIONS

PATIENT/FAMILY EDUCATION

• May cause GI upset, teach patient to take with meals or snacks

• May mask infections

• Take single daily doses in AM

• Increased dose of rapidly acting corticosteroids may be necessary in patients subjected to unusual stress

• Signs of adrenal insufficiency include fatigue, anorexia, nausea, vomiting, diarrhea, weight loss, weakness, dizziness, and low blood sugar

• Avoid abrupt withdrawal of therapy following high-dose or long-term therapy; relative insufficiency may exist for up to 1 yr after discontinuation

• Patients on chronic steroid therapy should wear medical alert bracelet

• Do not give live virus vaccines to patients on prolonged therapy

MONITORING PARAMETERS

• Serum K and glucose

• Edema, blood pressure, CHF symptoms, mental status, weight

• Growth in children on prolonged therapy

P

---

italic = common side effects   ***bold italic*** = life-threatening reactions

primaquine

(prim'a-kwin)

Rx: Primaquine

Chemical Class: 8-amino-quinoline derivative

Therapeutic Class: Antimalarial

CLINICAL PHARMACOLOGY

Mechanism of Action: Interferes with plasmodial DNA function

Pharmacokinetics

PO: Peak 1-3 hr; widely distributed in the body; rapidly metabolized in liver, excreted in urine (metabolites); $t_{1/2}$ 3.7-9.6 hr

INDICATIONS AND USES: Radical cure of vivax malaria, prevention of relapse in vivax malaria, following termination of chloroquine phosphate suppressive therapy in areas where vivax malaria is endemic, *Pneumocystis carinii* pneumonia (PCP) associated with AIDS (with clindamycin)*

DOSAGE

Adult

• *Vivax malaria:* PO 26.3 mg (15 mg base) qd for 14 days; patients suffering an attack of vivax malaria or having parasitized red blood cells should also receive a course of chloroquine phosphate; as follow-up therapy in areas where vivax malaria is endemic, begin therapy during the last 2 wk of, or following a course of, suppression with chloroquine or a comparable drug

• *PCP associated with AIDS:* PO 26.3-52.6 mg (15-30 mg base) qd (with clindamycin IV 1.8-3.6 g/day divided tid-qid or PO 1.2-3.6 g/day divided tid-qid) for 21 days

Child

• PO 0.5 mg/kg/day (0.3 mg base/kg/day; max 15 mg base/dose) for 14 days

💲 AVAILABLE FORMS/COST OF THERAPY

• Tab, Uncoated—Oral: 26.3 mg, 100's: **$72.23**

CONTRAINDICATIONS: Concomitant administration with quinacrine, acutely ill patients with a tendency to granulocytopenia (rheumatoid arthritis, systemic lupus erythematosus), concurrent administration of other potentially hemolytic drugs or bone marrow suppressants

PRECAUTIONS: G-6-PD deficiency, NADH methemoglobin reductase deficiency, large doses

PREGNANCY AND LACTATION: Pregnancy category C; if possible, withhold until after delivery; however, if prophylaxis or treatment is required, primaquine should not be withheld

SIDE EFFECTS/ADVERSE REACTIONS

CNS: Headache

EENT: Interference with visual accommodation

GI: Abdominal cramps, epigastric distress, *nausea, vomiting*

HEME: Hemolytic anemia in G-6-PD deficient patients, leukopenia, methemoglobinemia in NADH methemoglobin reductase-deficient patients

SKIN: Pruritus

SPECIAL CONSIDERATIONS
PATIENT/FAMILY EDUCATION

• Take with food if GI upset occurs, notify clinician if GI distress continues

• Urine may turn brown

MONITORING PARAMETERS

• CBC periodically during therapy, discontinue if marked darkening of urine or sudden decrease in hemoglobin concentrations or leukocyte count occurs

---

* = non-FDA-approved use

probenecid
(proe-ben'e-sid)
Rx: Benemid, Probalan
Combinations
   with colchicine (Colbenemid
   Proben-C); with ampicillin
   (Polycillin-PRB, Probam-
   pacin)
Chemical Class: Sulfonamide
derivative
Therapeutic Class: Antigout
agent; uricosuric

CLINICAL PHARMACOLOGY
Mechanism of Action: Uricosuric
inhibits tubular reabsorption of urate;
increasing urinary excretion of uric
acid; inhibits tubular secretion and
increases plasma concentrations of
most penicillins and cephalosporins
Pharmacokinetics
PO: Peak 2-4 hr; 85%-95% bound
to plasma proteins; hydroxylated in
liver to active metabolites, excreted
in urine (metabolites); $t_{1/2}$ 4-17 hr
INDICATIONS AND USES: Hyperuricemia associated with gout and
gouty arthritis, antibiotic adjuvant:
elevates and prolongs penicillin and
cephalosporin serum concentrations;
calcinosis,* diagnostic aid (differentiation between Parkinsonism and
depressive syndromes; drug-induced
nephrotoxicity chemo-protection)
DOSAGE
Adult
• *Hyperuricemia:* PO 250 mg bid
for 1 wk; increase to 500 mg bid;
increase q4 wk prn to max of 2-3
g/day; begin therapy 2-3 wk following acute gout attack
• *Penicillin or cephalosporin therapy:* PO 500 mg qid
Child 2-14 yr
• *Penicillin or cephalosporin therapy:* PO 25 mg/kg/dose initially; 40

mg/kg/day divided qid as mainte-
nance dose
**$ AVAILABLE FORMS/COST
   OF THERAPY**
• Tab, Plain Coated—Oral: 500 mg,
100's: **$9.00-$98.33**
• Combination Tab, Uncoated—
Oral: 0.5 mg colchicine/500 mg pro-
benecid 100's: **$84.34**
CONTRAINDICATIONS: Children
<2 yr, blood dyscrasias, uric acid
kidney stones, initiation of therapy
during acute gouty attack, moderate
to severe renal impairment (CrCl
<10 ml/min)
PRECAUTIONS: History of peptic
ulcer; renal insufficiency (CrCL
<30 ml/min)
PREGNANCY AND LACTATION:
Pregnancy category B; has been
used during pregnancy without caus-
ing adverse effects in fetus or infant
**SIDE EFFECTS/ADVERSE REAC-
   TIONS**
CNS: Dizziness, headache
GI: Anorexia, nausea, sore gums,
vomiting
GU: Costovertebral pain, hematuria, *nephrotic syndrome,* renal colic, uric acid stones, urinary frequency
HEME: Anemia, *aplastic anemia,
hemolytic anemia (possibly related
to G-6-PD deficiency)*
METAB: Exacerbation of gout
SKIN: Flushing, rash
MISC: Hypersensitivity reactions
INTERACTIONS
Drugs
3 *Dapsone:* Increased serum dapsone concentrations
3 *Dyphylline:* Increased serum dyphylline concentrations
2 *Methotrexate:* Marked increases
in serum methotrexate concentrations
3 *Salicylates:* Inhibition of uricosuric effect if used regularly

P

---

italic = common side effects   ***bold italic*** = life-threatening reactions

3 *Thiopental:* Prolonged anesthesia

3 *Zidovudine:* Increased plasma zidovudine concentrations

Labs

• *False positive:* Urine glucose (Ames Clinitest tablet, no effect on Ames Keto-Diastix, Diastix, Multistix, Clinistix)

• *False increase:* Free T_4 (Boehringer-Mannheim Enzymum procedure)

SPECIAL CONSIDERATIONS
PATIENT/FAMILY EDUCATION

• Avoid aspirin or other salicylates
• Take with food or antacids
• Drink 48-64 oz water daily to prevent development of kidney stones

MONITORING PARAMETERS

• Serum uric acid concentrations: continue the probenecid dose that maintains normal concentrations
• Renal function tests

---

procainamide
(proe-kane'a-mide)
Rx: Procan SR, Pronestyl, Pronestyl-SR
Chemical Class: P-aminobenzamide derivative
Therapeutic Class: Antidysrhythmic (Class IA)

CLINICAL PHARMACOLOGY
Mechanism of Action: Decreases myocardial excitability and conduction velocity; may depress myocardial contractility; increases threshold potential of ventricle, His-Purkinje system; prolongs effective refractory period and increases action potential duration in atrial and ventricular muscle; possesses anticholinergic properties, which may modify direct myocardial effects

Pharmacokinetics
IM: Onset 10-30 min, peak 15-60 min
PO: Peak 0.75-2.5 hr
15%-20% bound to plasma proteins; metabolized via acetylation in liver to N-acetyl procainamide (NAPA), which is a Class III antidysrhythmic; excreted in urine (25% as NAPA); $t_{1/2}$ 2.5-4.7 hr (NAPA 6-8 hr)

INDICATIONS AND USES: Life-threatening ventricular dysrhythmias, less severe but symptomatic ventricular dysrhythmias in select patients, maintenance of sinus rhythm following cardioversion in atrial fibrillation and/or flutter,* suppression of recurrent paroxysmal atrial fibrillation*

DOSAGE
Adult
• PO 250-500 mg q3-6h; PO SR 500-1000 mg q6h, usual dose 50 mg/kg/24 hr, max 4 g/24hr; IM 0.5-1 g q4-8h until PO therapy possible; IV 1 g INF over 25-30 min or 100-200 mg/day repeated q5 min as needed to total dose of 1 g as a loading dose, followed by continuous INF of 1-6 mg/min, titrate to patient response
Child
• PO 15-50 mg/kg/24 hr divided q3-6h, max 4 g/24 hr; IM 20-30 mg/kg/24 hr divided q4-6h, max 4 g/24 hr; IV 3-6 mg/kg INF over 5 min not to exceed 100 mg/day as a loading dose, then 20-80 µg/kg/min as a continuous INF, max 4 g/24 hr

$ **AVAILABLE FORMS/COST OF THERAPY**

• Cap, Gel—Oral: 250 mg, 100's: **$14.50-$69.67;** 375 mg, 30's: **$5.40;** 500 mg, 100's: **$11.00-$125.44**
• Tab, Sugar Coated—Oral: 250 mg, 100's: **$69.67;** 375 mg, 100's: **$96.61;** 500 mg, 100's: **$125.44**

* = non-FDA-approved use

• Tab, Coated, SUS Action—Oral: 250 mg, 100's: **$17.50-$35.69;** 500 mg, 100's: **$27.50-$83.30;** 750 mg, 100's: **$37.40-$47.25;** 1000 mg, 100's: **$47.50-$102.85**

• Inj, Sol—IM, IV: 100 mg/ml, 10 ml: **$4.00-$26.86;** 500 mg/ml, 2 ml: **$4.00-$26.86**

CONTRAINDICATIONS: Complete heart block, lupus erythematosus, torsade de pointes

PRECAUTIONS: Following MI, 1st-degree AV block (unless ventricular rate controlled by pacemaker), asymptomatic premature ventricular contractions, digitalis intoxication, CHF, myasthenia gravis, renal insufficiency, children

PREGNANCY AND LACTATION: Pregnancy category C; compatible with breast feeding, however long-term effects in nursing infant unknown

SIDE EFFECTS/ADVERSE REACTIONS

CNS: Depression, *dizziness,* giddiness, hallucinations, headache, psychosis, weakness

CV: Hypotension, **2nd-degree heart block, ventricular arrhythmias** (more common with IV administration)

GI: Abdominal pain, anorexia, bitter taste, diarrhea, hepatomegaly, nausea, vomiting

HEME: **Agranulocytosis, hemolytic anemia (rare), neutropenia, thrombocytopenia**

SKIN: **Angioneurotic edema,** flushing, pruritus, rash, urticaria

MISC: *Lupus erythematosus-like syndrome* (arthralgia, pleural or abdominal pain, arthritis, pleural effusion, pericarditis, fever, chills, rash) in up to 30% on long-term therapy

INTERACTIONS

Drugs

3 *Amiodarone, cimetidine, tri-methoprim:* Increased procainamide concentrations

3 *Cholinergic drugs:* Antagonism of cholinergic actions on skeletal muscle

3 *Procaine:* Interferes with procainamide concentration assay

Labs

• *False decrease:* Cholinesterase

• *False increase:* Potassium

SPECIAL CONSIDERATIONS
PATIENT/FAMILY EDUCATION

• Strict compliance to dosage schedule imperative

• Empty wax core from sustained release tablets may appear in stool; this is harmless

• Initiate therapy in facilities capable of providing continuous ECG monitoring and managing life-threatening dysrhythmias

MONITORING PARAMETERS

• CBC with differential and platelets qwk for 1st 3 mo, periodically thereafter

• ECG: R/O overdosage if QRS widens >25% or QT prolongation occurs; reduce dosage if QRS widens >50%

• ANA titer increases may precede clinical symptoms of lupoid syndrome

• Serum creatinine, urea nitrogen

• Plasma procainamide concentration (therapeutic range 3-10 µg/ml; 10-30 µg/ml NAPA)

---

procaine
(proe'kane)
Rx: Novocain, Mericaine
Chemical Class: Benzoic acid derivative
Therapeutic Class: Local anesthetic

CLINICAL PHARMACOLOGY
Mechanism of Action: Blocks generation and conduction of nerve im-

P

pulses; the order of loss of nerve function is: (1) pain, (2) temperature, (3) touch, (4) proprioception, and (5) skeletal muscle tone

Pharmacokinetics

INJ: Onset 2-5 min (15-25 min epidural), duration 0.25-1 hr (0.5-1.5 epidural); rapidly hydrolyzed by plasma pseudocholinesterase to *p*-aminobenzoic acid and diethylaminoethanol; excreted in urine; $t_{1/2}$ 7.7 min

INDICATIONS AND USES: Infiltration anesthesia, peripheral or sympathetic nerve block, spinal anesthesia, intractable pain (IV),* pruritus caused by jaundice (IV)*

DOSAGE

Dose varies with procedure, depth of anesthesia, vascularity of tissues, duration of anesthesia, and condition of patient

Adult

• *Infiltration anesthesia:* Inj 350-600 mg of 0.25%-0.5%

• *Peripheral nerve block:* Inj up to 200 ml of 0.5% or 100 ml of 1% or 50 ml of 2%

💲 AVAILABLE FORMS/COST OF THERAPY

• Inj, Sol—Infiltration: 1%, 30 ml: **$5.22-$20.43; 2%, 30 ml: $2.00-$20.43**

• Inj, Sol—IV: 10%, 2 ml: **$9.94**

CONTRAINDICATIONS: Myasthenia gravis (IV), severe shock, impaired cardiac conduction, inj into inflamed or infected tissue

PRECAUTIONS: Cardiac disease, hyperthyroidism, endocrine disease, liver disease, elderly, low plasma pseudocholinesterase concentrations, sulfite sensitivity, use in head and neck area, retrobulbar blocks

PREGNANCY AND LACTATION: Pregnancy category C; use caution in nursing mothers

SIDE EFFECTS/ADVERSE REACTIONS

CNS: Anxiety, disorientation, drowsiness, loss of consciousness, restlessness, *seizures,* shivering, tremors

CV: Bradycardia, *cardiac arrest, dysrhythmias,* fetal bradycardia, hypertension, hypotension, *myocardial depression*

EENT: Blurred vision, pupil constriction, tinnitus

GI: Nausea, vomiting

RESP: **Anaphylaxis, respiratory arrest**

SKIN: Allergic reactions, burning, edema, rash, skin discoloration at inj site, tissue necrosis, urticaria

DRUG INTERACTIONS

Drugs

❸ β-*blockers:* Acute discontinuation of β-blockers before local anesthesia increases the risk of hypertensive reactions

Labs

• *False increase:* CSF protein, urine porphobilinogen, urobilinogen

SPECIAL CONSIDERATIONS

• Esther-type local anesthetic

MONITORING PARAMETERS

• Blood pressure, pulse, respiration during treatment, ECG

• Fetal heart tones if used during labor

---

prochlorperazine

(proe-klor-per'a-zeen)

Rx: Compazine

Chemical Class: Piperazine phenothiazine derivative

Therapeutic Class: Antiemetic; antipsychotic

CLINICAL PHARMACOLOGY

Mechanism of Action: Dopamine antagonist directly affects medullary chemoreceptor trigger zone (CTZ); antipsychotic effects similar

---

* = non-FDA-approved use

to those of chlorpromazine; weak anticholinergic effects, moderate sedative effects, strong extrapyramidal effects

Pharmacokinetics

PO: Onset 30-40 min, duration 3-4 hr (extended release 10-12 hr)

IM: Onset 10-20 min, duration 12 hr

PR: Onset 60 min, duration 3-4 hr

Metabolized in liver, excreted in urine and through enterohepatic circulation

INDICATIONS AND USES: Severe nausea and vomiting, psychotic disorders

DOSAGE

Adult

• *Antiemetic:* PO 5-10 mg tid-qid, usual max 40 mg/day; PO extended release 10 mg bid or 15 mg qd; IM 5-10 mg q3-4h, usual max 40 mg/day; IV 2.5-10 mg q3-4h, max 10 mg/dose, 40 mg/day; PR 25 mg bid

• *Psychosis:* PO 5-10 mg tid-qid, increase dose prn, max 150 mg/day; IM 10-20 mg q4h prn, convert to PO as soon as possible

Child

• *Antiemetic:* PO/PR 9-14 kg: 2.5 mg q12-24h, max 7.5 mg/day; 14-18 kg: 2.5 mg q8-12h, max 10 mg/day; 18-39 kg: 2.5 mg q8h or 5 mg q12h, max 15 mg/day; IM 0.1-0.15 mg/kg/dose, convert to PO as soon as possible; IV not recommended

• *Psychosis:* PO/PR 2-12 yr: 2.5 mg bid-tid, increase dose prn, max 20 mg/day; 2-5 yr: 25 mg/day; IM 6-12 yr: 0.13 mg/kg/dose, convert to PO as soon as possible

💲 AVAILABLE FORMS/COST OF THERAPY

• Inj, Sol—IM, IV: 5 mg/ml, 2 ml: **$2.60-$8.46**

• Supp—Rect: 2.5 mg, 12's: **$29.50;** 5 mg, 12's: **$32.80;** 25 mg, 12's: **$34.00-$59.88**

• Syr—Oral: 5 mg/5 ml, 120 ml: **$22.45**

• Tab, Plain Coated—Oral: 5 mg, 100's: **$52.01-$65.55;** 10 mg, 100's: **$78.14-$97.25**

• Cap, Gel, SUS Action—Oral: 10 mg, 50's: **$59.95;** 15 mg, 50's: **$89.15**

CONTRAINDICATIONS: Severe toxic CNS depression, coma, subcortical brain damage, bone marrow depression, severe liver or cardiac disease, narrow-angle glaucoma, pediatric surgery

PRECAUTIONS: Children <5 yr, elderly, prolonged use, cardiovascular disease, epilepsy, hepatic or renal disease, glaucoma, prostatic hypertrophy, severe asthma, emphysema, hypocalcemia (increased susceptibility to dystonic reactions), thyrotoxicosis, tartrazine sensitivity

PREGNANCY AND LACTATION: Pregnancy category C; majority of evidence indicates safety for both mother and fetus if used occasionally in low doses; excretion into breast milk should be expected; sedation is a possible effect in nursing infant

SIDE EFFECTS/ADVERSE REACTIONS

CNS: Agitation, anxiety, catatonic-like behavioral states, confusion, depression, *drowsiness, EPS (pseudoparkinsonism, akathisia, dystonia,* tardive dyskinesia), euphoria, exacerbation of psychotic symptoms including hallucinations, *headache,* heat or cold intolerance, insomnia, lethargy, **neuroleptic malignant syndrome,** restlessness, **seizures,** vertigo

CV: ECG changes, hypertension, hypotension, tachycardia

EENT: Blurred vision, cataracts, dry eyes, *dry mouth,* glaucoma, pigmentation of retina or cornea, retinopathy

GI: Anorexia, *constipation,* diar-

P

---

italic = common side effects   ***bold italic*** = life-threatening reactions

rhea, dyspepsia, hypersalivation, *nausea,* vomiting
GU: Priapism, urinary retention
HEME: **Agranulocytosis,** anemia, **aplastic anemia, hemolytic anemia** leukocytosis, transient leukopenia
METAB: Breast engorgement, gynecomastia, hyperglycemia, hyperprolactinemia, hypoglycemia, hyponatremia, impotence, increased libido, lactation, mastalgia, menstrual irregularities
RESP: Bronchospasm, increased depth of respiration, laryngospasm
SKIN: Diaphoresis, loss of hair, maculopapular and acneiform skin reactions, photosensitivity
INTERACTIONS
Drugs
⊠ *Anticholinergics:* Inhibited therapeutic response to antipsychotic; enhanced anticholinergic side effects
⊠ *Antidepressants:* Increased serum concentrations of some cyclic antidepressants
⊠ *Attapulgite:* Inhibition of phenothiazine absorption
⊠ *Barbiturates:* Reduced effect of antipsychotic
⊠ *Beta-blockers:* Enhanced effects of both drugs (interaction less likely with atenolol, nadolol)
⊠ *Bromocriptine, lithium:* Reduced effects of both drugs
⊠ *Chloroquine, amodiaquine, pyrimethamine:* Possible increased phenothiazine concentrations
⊠ *Cigarettes:* Possible enhanced metabolism of neuroleptic
⊠ *Clonidine:* Possible enhanced hypotensive effect
⊠ *Epinephrine:* Reversed pressor response to epinephrine
⊠ *Ethanol:* Enhanced ethanol effects
⊠ *Guanethidine*: Inhibited antihypertensive response to guanethidine
⊠ *Indomethacin:* Possible in-

creased CNS effects, other NSAIDs less likely to have effect
❷ *Levodopa:* Inhibited effect of levodopa on Parkinson's disease
❸ *Narcotic analgesics:* Excessive CNS depression, hypotension, respiratory depression
❸ *Orphenadrine:* Reduced serum neuroleptic concentrations, excessive anticholinergic effects
❸ *Procarbazine:* Increased sedation, EPS effects
❸ *SSRIs:* Increased risk EPS effects
❸ *Trazadone:* Possible increased risk hypotension
Labs
• *False positive:* Phenylketones
SPECIAL CONSIDERATIONS
PATIENT/FAMILY EDUCATION
• Arise slowly from reclining position
• Do not discontinue abruptly
• Use a sunscreen during sun exposure to prevent burns; take special precautions to stay cool in hot weather
• May cause drowsiness
MONITORING PARAMETERS
• Observe closely for signs of tardive dyskinesia
• Treat acute dystonic reactions with parenteral diphenhydramine (2 mg/kg to max 50 mg) or benztropine (2 mg)
• Periodic CBC with platelets during prolonged therapy

---

procyclidine
(proe-sye′kli-deen)
Rx: Kemadrin
Chemical Class: Synthetic tertiary amine
Therapeutic Class: Anticholinergic, antiparkinson's agent

CLINICAL PHARMACOLOGY
Mechanism of Action: Blocks stri-

atal cholinergic receptors, which helps balance cholinergic and dopaminergic activity

Pharmacokinetics

PO: Peak 1.1-2 hr, $t_{1/2}$ 11.5-12.6 hr

INDICATIONS AND USES: Adjunctive treatment of all forms of Parkinson's disease; drug-induced extrapyramidal symptoms

DOSAGE

Adult

• *Parkinsonism:* PO 2.5 mg tid after meals initially, increase to 5 mg tid gradually; may occasionally administer additional dose hs if necessary

• *Drug-induced extrapyramidal symptoms:* PO 2.5 mg tid initially, increase by 2.5 mg/day increments until relief of symptoms obtained; usual dose 10-20 mg/day

💲 AVAILABLE FORMS/COST OF THERAPY

• Tab, Uncoated—Oral: 5 mg, 100's: **$56.50**

CONTRAINDICATIONS: Narrow-angle glaucoma, myasthenia gravis, GI/GU obstruction, peptic ulcer, megacolon, prostatic hypertrophy

PRECAUTIONS: Elderly, tachycardia, liver, kidney disease, drug abuse history, dysrhythmias, hypotension, hypertension, psychiatric patients, children, tardive dyskinesia

PREGNANCY AND LACTATION: Pregnancy category C; nursing infants may be particularly sensitive to anticholinergic effects

SIDE EFFECTS/ADVERSE REACTIONS

CNS: Anxiety, *confusion,* delusions, *depression,* dizziness, *hallucinations,* headache, incoherence, irritability, memory loss, restlessness, sedation

CV: Flushing, hypotension, mild bradycardia, palpitations, postural hypotension, tachycardia

EENT: Angle-closure glaucoma, blurred vision, difficulty swallowing, dilated pupils, dry eyes, *dry mouth,* increased intraocular tension, mydriasis, photophobia

GI: Abdominal distress, *constipation,* epigastric distress, nausea, *paralytic ileus,* vomiting

GU: Dysuria, erectile dysfunction, hesitancy, retention

MS: Cramping, muscular weakness

SKIN: Rash, urticaria, other dermatoses

MISC: Decreased sweating, heat stroke, hyperthermia, increased temperature, numbness of fingers

DRUG INTERACTIONS

Drugs

3 *Amantadine:* Potentiates CNS side effects of amantadine

3 *Anticholinergic:* Increased anticholinergic side effects

3 *Antipsychotic agents:* Possible worsening of psychosis, increased anticholinergic side effects

3 *Digoxin* (slow dissolution tab): Increased digoxin concentration

3 *Tacrine:* Reduced therapeutic effects of both drugs

SPECIAL CONSIDERATIONS

PATIENT/FAMILY EDUCATION

• Do not discontinue this drug abruptly

• Hard candy, frequent drinks, sugarless gum to relieve dry mouth

• Take with or after meals to prevent GI upset

• Use caution in hot weather, may increase susceptibility to heat stroke

P

---

italic = common side effects   ***bold italic*** = life-threatening reactions

progesterone

(proe-jess'ter-one)
Rx: Crinone (gel),
Progestasert, (IUD)
Chemical Class: Natural
progestin
Therapeutic Class: Progestin;
contraceptive

CLINICAL PHARMACOLOGY

Mechanism of Action: Exerts a progestational effect on the endometrium, alters cervical mucus, suppresses ovulation in some patients, renders the endometrium hostile to implantation

Pharmacokinetics

Hepatic metabolism, mostly renal excretion

IM: Rapidly absorbed, $t_{1/2}$ is a few minutes; Gel: Absorption $t_{1/2}$ 25-50 hr

INDICATIONS AND USES: Amenorrhea, dysfunctional uterine bleeding; as an intrauterine device (IUD) for contraception in women with at least 1 child in mutually monogamous relationships; Gel: Luteal phase deficiency in women undergoing assisted reproductive technology (ART) therapy for infertility

DOSAGE

Adult

• *Amenorrhea:* IM 5-10 mg qd for 6-8 days; if ovarian activity has produced a proliferative endometrium, expect withdrawal bleeding 48-72 hr after last inj

• *Dysfunctional uterine bleeding:* IM 5-10 mg qd for 6 doses; bleeding should cease within 6 days; when used with estrogen, begin progesterone after 2 wk of estrogen therapy; discontinue inj when menstrual flow begins

• *Contraception:* Insert 1 system into uterine cavity; replace after 1 yr

• *ART:* 1 applicator (90 g) in vagina QD (BID in ovarian failure) × 10-12 wk if pregnancy achieved

💲 **AVAILABLE FORMS/COST OF THERAPY**

• Inj, Sol—IM: 50 mg/ml, 10 ml: **$10.20-$26.80**

• Insert, SUS Action—Intrauterine: 38 mg: **$130.68**

• *Gel* (Crinone)—Vag: 8% 6 applicators **$60.00,** 4% 6 applicators, **$30.00**

CONTRAINDICATIONS: Active thrombophlebitis or thromboembolic disorders, cerebral hemorrhage, impaired liver function or disease, breast cancer, undiagnosed vaginal bleeding, missed abortion, use as a diagnostic test for pregnancy; *IUD:* patients at risk for pelvic infection, previous ectopic pregnancy, genital actinomycosis, increased susceptibility to infection (e.g., leukemia, diabetes, AIDS), IV drug use

PRECAUTIONS: Epilepsy, migraine, asthma, cardiac or renal dysfunction, depression, diabetes; (intrauterine system) history of menorrhagia or hypermenorrhea, valvular or congenital heart disease

PREGNANCY AND LACTATION: Pregnancy category D. Possible increase in limb reduction defects, hypospadias in male fetuses and mild virilization of female fetuses

SIDE EFFECTS/ADVERSE REACTIONS

CNS: Depression, fatigue, insomnia

CV: Fluid retention

GI: Increased weight, *nausea*

GU: Amenorrhea, breast changes, galactorrhea, breakthrough bleeding, spotting

IUD: Amenorrhea or delayed menses, anemia, cramping, difficult removal, dyspareunia, ***ectopic pregnancy,*** endometritis, intermenstrual spotting, pain, pelvic infection, ***per-***

foration of uterus and cervix, prolongation of menstrual flow, ***septic abortion, septicemia, spontaneous abortion,*** uterine embedment
METAB: Hyperglycemia
SKIN: Acne, irritation at inj site, melasma, rash, changes in hair growth

INTERACTIONS
Drugs
3 *Aminoglutethimide:* Possible decreased progestin effect
Labs
• *Increase:* Alk phosphatase, pregnanediol, liver function tests
• *Decrease:* Glucose tolerance test, HDL

SPECIAL CONSIDERATIONS
• Gel provides enhanced uterine delivery compared with IM administration

PATIENT/FAMILY EDUCATION
• Diabetic patients may note decreased glucose tolerance
• No evidence that use for habitual or threatened abortion is effective
• Notify clinician of abnormal or excessive bleeding, severe cramping, abnormal or odorous vaginal discharge, missed period (IUD)
• Cost and risk of infection (greatest in first months after insertion) less for non hormonal IUDs (e.g. ParaGard)

---

promethazine
(proe-meth'a-zeen)
Rx: Anergan, Autineus 50, Phenergan, Promet, Promacot, Promethegan, Prorex
Combinations
  Rx: with codeine (Phenergan with Codeine Syrup); with dextromethorphan (Phenergan with Dextromethorphan Syrup)
Chemical Class: Ethylamine phenothiazine derivative
Therapeutic Class: Antihistamine; antiemetic; sedative; antitussive; antivertigo agent

CLINICAL PHARMACOLOGY
Mechanism of Action: Acts as antihistamine by blocking H_1-receptors; antiemetic effects by inhibition of medullary chemoreceptor trigger zone (CTZ); anticholinergic activity produces sedation and antivertigo/motion sickness effects
Pharmacokinetics
PO/IM/PR: Onset 20 min, duration 6-12 hr (sedative effects 2-8 hr)
IV: Onset 3-5 min, duration 6-12 hr (sedative effects 2-8 hr)
Metabolized in liver, excreted in urine and feces (inactive metabolites)

INDICATIONS AND USES: Symptomatic treatment of various allergic conditions; active and prophylactic treatment of motion sickness; preoperative, postoperative, or obstetric sedation; nausea and vomiting associated with anesthesia and surgery; adjunct to analgesic for control of postoperative pain

DOSAGE
Adult
• *Antihistamine:* PO/PR 12.5 tid and 25 mg qhs; IM/IV 25 mg, repeated

---

in 2 hr if necessary, convert to PO as soon as possible

• *Antiemetic:* PO/IM/IV/PR 12.5-25 mg q4h prn

• *Motion sickness:* PO/PR 25 mg 30-60 min prior to departure, then q12h prn

• *Sedation:* PO/IM/IV/PR 25-50 mg/day

Child

• *Antihistamine:* PO/PR 0.1 mg/kg/dose q6h during the day and 0.5 mg/kg qhs prn

• *Antiemetic:* PO/IM/IV/PR 0.25-1 mg/kg q4-6h prn

• *Motion sickness:* PO/PR 0.5 mg/kg/dose 30-60 min prior to departure, then q12h prn

• *Sedation:* PO/IM/IV/PR 0.5-1 mg/kg/dose q6h prn

$ AVAILABLE FORMS/COST OF THERAPY

• Inj, Sol—IM, IV: 25 mg/ml, 1, 10 ml: **$0.40-$3.55**/ml; 50 mg/ml, 1, 10 ml: **$0.26-$4.27**/ml

• Supp—Rect: 12.5 mg, 12's: **$34.60;** 25 mg, 12's: **$39.68;** 50 mg, 12's: **$32.76-$50.81**

• Syr—Oral: 6.25 mg/5 ml, 120 ml, 480 ml, 3840 ml: **$1.80-$27.50**/480 ml; 25 mg/5 ml, 480 ml: **$57.26**

• Tab, Uncoated—Oral: 12.5 mg, 100's: **$6.50-$22.80;** 25 mg, 100's: **$3.96-$40.28;** 50 mg, 100's: **$5.98-$61.73**

CONTRAINDICATIONS: Narrow-angle glaucoma

PRECAUTIONS: Acute asthma, bladder neck obstruction, prostatic hypertrophy, predisposition to urinary retention, cardiovascular disease, glaucoma, hepatic function impairment, hypertension, history of peptic ulcer, seizure disorder, intestinal obstruction

PREGNANCY AND LACTATION: Pregnancy category C; passage of drug into breast milk should be expected

SIDE EFFECTS/ADVERSE REACTIONS

CNS: Anxiety, confusion, *dizziness, drowsiness,* EPS reactions, paradoxical hyperexcitability (children, relative overdose), euphoria, fatigue, poor coordination

CV: Hypotension, palpitations, tachycardia

EENT: Blurred vision, dilated pupils, dry nose, nasal stuffiness, tinnitus

GI: Anorexia, cholestatic jaundice, *constipation,* diarrhea, dry mouth, nausea, vomiting

GU: Amenorrhea, dysuria, galactorrhea, gynecomastia, impotence, *urinary retention*

HEME: **Agranulocytosis, hemolytic anemia, thrombocytopenia**

METAB: Hyperprolactinemia

RESP: Chest tightness, increased thick secretions, wheezing

SKIN: Photosensitivity, rash, urticaria

INTERACTIONS

Drugs

3 *CNS depressants:* Additive sedative action

Labs

• *False increase:* Tricyclic antidepressant

SPECIAL CONSIDERATIONS

PATIENT/FAMILY EDUCATION

• Avoid prolonged exposure to sunlight

---

propafenone

(proe-pa-fen'one)

Rx: Rythmol

Chemical Class: 3-Phenylpropiophenone derivative

Therapeutic Class: Antidysrhythmic (Class IC)

CLINICAL PHARMACOLOGY

Mechanism of Action: Local an-

---

esthetic effects and direct stabilizing action on myocardial membranes; reduces upstroke velocity (Phase O) of the monophasic action potential; reduces fast inward current carried by sodium ions in Purkinje fibers, and to a lesser extent myocardial fibers; increases diastolic excitability threshold, prolongs effective refractory period, reduces spontaneous automaticity, and depresses triggered activity; weak β-blocking activity

Pharmacokinetics

PO: Bioavailability 3.4%-10.6%; metabolized in liver to 5-hydroxy-propafenone and N-depropylpropafenone (active), excreted in urine; $t_{1/2}$ 2-10 hr in >90% of patients (10-32 hr in slow metabolizers)

INDICATIONS AND USES: Documented life-threatening ventricular dysrhythmias (e.g., sustained ventricular tachycardia), supraventricular tachycardias including atrial fibrillation and flutter,* dysrhythmias associated with Wolff-Parkinson-White syndrome*

DOSAGE

Adult

• PO 150 mg q8h initially; increase at 3-4 day intervals to 225 mg q8h and, if necessary, to 300 mg q8h; do not exceed 900 mg/day

$ AVAILABLE FORMS/COST OF THERAPY

• Tab, Coated—Oral: 150 mg, 100's: **$123.86;** 225 mg, 100's: **$176.57;** 300 mg, 100's: **$224.75**

CONTRAINDICATIONS: Uncontrolled CHF, cardiogenic shock, disorders of impulse generation or conduction in the absence of an artificial pacemaker, bradycardia, marked hypotension, bronchospastic disorders, manifest electrolyte imbalance

PRECAUTIONS: Non-life-threatening dysrhythmias, recent MI, hepatic and renal function impairment, elderly, children

PREGNANCY AND LACTATION: Pregnancy category C

SIDE EFFECTS/ADVERSE REACTIONS

CNS: Anxiety, ataxia, *dizziness,* drowsiness, fatigue, headache, insomnia, tremor

CV: Angina, atrial fibrillation, *AV block,* bradycardia, bundle branch block, chest pain, ***congestive heart failure*** (due to negative ionotrope effects), edema, hypotension, *intraventricular conduction delay,* palpitations, premature ventricular contractions, ***prodysrhythmia,*** syncope, ***ventricular tachycardia,*** widened QRS complex

EENT: Blurred vision, *unusual taste*

GI: Abdominal pain, anorexia, *constipation,* diarrhea, dry mouth, dyspepsia, flatulence, liver abnormalities, *nausea, vomiting*

HEME: ***Agranulocytosis, anemia, granulocytopenia,*** increased bleeding time, ***leukopenia,*** positive ANA, purpura, ***thrombocytopenia***

MS: Arthralgia, weakness

RESP: Dyspnea

SKIN: Diaphoresis, rash

INTERACTIONS

Drugs

❸ *Beta-blockers:* Increased metoprolol or propranolol concentrations

❸ *Cimetidine:* Increased propafenone concentrations

❸ *Digitalis glycosides:* Increased serum digoxin concentrations

❸ *Food:* Increased peak serum propafenone concentrations

❸ *Oral anticoagulants:* Increased serum warfarin concentrations, prolonged protime

❸ *Quinidine:* Increased propafenone concentrations but reduced concentrations of its active metabolite; net effect uncertain (toxicity vs reduced efficacy)

P

italic = common side effects   **bold italic** = life-threatening reactions

3 *Rifampin, phenobarbital, rifabutin:* Reduced serum propafenone concentrations

3 *Theophylline:* Increased plasma theophylline concentrations

SPECIAL CONSIDERATIONS
PATIENT/FAMILY EDUCATION
• Signs of overdosage include hypotension, excessive drowsiness, decreased heart rate, or abnormal heartbeat

MONITORING PARAMETERS
• ECG, consider dose reduction in patients with significant widening of the QRS complex or 2nd- or 3rd-degree AV block
• ANA, carefully evaluate abnormal ANA test, consider discontinuation if persistent or worsening ANA titers are detected

---

propantheline
(proe-pan'the-leen)
Rx: Propantheline
Chemical Class: Synthetic quaternary ammonium derivative
Therapeutic Class: GI antispasmodic; GI antiulcer agent (adjunctive)

CLINICAL PHARMACOLOGY
Mechanism of Action: Inhibits GI motility and diminishes gastric acid secretion

Pharmacokinetics
PO: Incompletely absorbed, extensive metabolism in upper small intestine prior to absorption; peak 2-6 hr; metabolized in GI tract/liver, excreted in urine; $t_{1/2}$ 1.6-9 hr

INDICATIONS AND USES: Peptic ulcer disease (in combination with other drugs); irritable bowel syndrome,* urinary incontinence due to uninhibited hypertonic neurogenic bladder*

* = non-FDA-approved use

DOSAGE
Adult
• PO 7.5-15 mg 30 min ac and 30 min hs
Child
• *Antisecretory:* PO 1.5 mg/kg/day divided tid-qid
• *Antispasmodic:* PO 2-3 mg/kg/day divided q4-6h and hs

$ **AVAILABLE FORMS/COST OF THERAPY**
• Tab, Sugar Coated—Oral: 15 mg, 100's: **$12.93-$23.68**

CONTRAINDICATIONS: Narrow-angle glaucoma, obstructive uropathy (e.g., bladder neck obstruction due to prostatic hypertrophy), obstructive disease of the GI tract (e.g., pyloroduodenal stenosis), paralytic ileus, intestinal atony, unstable cardiovascular status in acute hemorrhage, severe ulcerative colitis, toxic megacolon complicating ulcerative colitis, myasthenia gravis

PRECAUTIONS: Hyperthyroidism, CAD, dysrhythmias, CHF, ulcerative colitis, hypertension, hiatal hernia, hepatic disease, renal disease, urinary retention, prostatic hypertrophy, elderly

PREGNANCY AND LACTATION: Pregnancy category C; excretion into breast milk unknown, although would be expected to be minimal due to quaternary structure

SIDE EFFECTS/ADVERSE REACTIONS
CNS: Anxiety, confusion, dizziness, drowsiness, hallucination, headache, insomnia, stimulation (especially in elderly), weakness
CV: Palpitations, tachycardia
EENT: Blurred vision, cycloplegia, increased ocular tension, mydriasis, photophobia
GI: Absence of taste, *constipation, dry mouth,* dysphagia, heartburn, nausea, ***paralytic ileus,*** vomiting

GU: Hesitancy, impotence, retention

SKIN: Allergic reactions, anhidrosis, fever, pruritus, rash, urticaria

INTERACTIONS

Drugs

3 *Tricyclic antidepressants:* Additive anticholinergic effects

Labs

• *False increase:* Bicarbonate, chloride

SPECIAL CONSIDERATIONS

PATIENT/FAMILY EDUCATION

• Avoid driving or other hazardous activities until stabilized on medication

• Avoid alcohol or other CNS depressants

• Avoid hot environments, heat stroke may occur

• Use sunglasses when outside to prevent photophobia, may cause blurred vision

---

proparacaine

(proe-pare'a-kane)

Rx: Alcaine, Ocu-Caine, Ophthetic, Paracaine

Chemical Class: Benzoic acid derivative

Therapeutic Class: Ophthalmic local anesthetic

CLINICAL PHARMACOLOGY

Mechanism of Action: Blocks the generation and conduction of nerve impulses, presumably by increasing the threshold for electrical excitation in the nerve, slowing the propagation of the nerve impulse, and reducing the rate rise of the action potential

Pharmacokinetics

OPHTH: Onset 20 sec, duration 15 min or longer

INDICATIONS AND USES: Corneal anesthesia of short duration for tonometry, gonioscopy, removal of foreign bodies and sutures; short corneal and conjunctival procedures; cataract surgery; conjunctival and corneal scraping for diagnostic purposes; paracentesis of anterior chamber

DOSAGE

Adult

• *Deep anesthesia (e.g., cataract extraction):* 1 gtt q5-10 min for 5-7 doses

• *Removal of sutures or foreign bodies, tonometry:* 1-2 gtt 2-3 min before procedure

$ AVAILABLE FORMS/COST OF THERAPY

• Sol—Ophth: 0.5%, 2, 15 ml: **$7.49-$16.00**/15 ml

CONTRAINDICATIONS: Prolonged use, self-medication

PRECAUTIONS: Debilitated, elderly, acutely ill patients, reduced plasma esterase, cardiac disease, hyperthyroidism, children

PREGNANCY AND LACTATION: Pregnancy category C

SIDE EFFECTS/ADVERSE REACTIONS

EENT: Conjunctival congestion and hemorrhage, cycloplegia (rare), hyperallergic corneal reaction, local irritation, pupillary dilation (rare), softening and erosion of corneal epithelium, stinging

SPECIAL CONSIDERATIONS

• Because "blink" reflex is temporarily eliminated, covering eye with patch following instillation is recommended

SPECIAL CONSIDERATIONS

• Ester-type local anesthetic

PATIENT/FAMILY EDUCATION

• Avoid touching or rubbing eye until anesthesia has worn off, inadvertent damage to conjunctiva and cornea may occur

P

---

propoxyphene
(proe-pox'i-feen)
Rx: Darvon, Dolene;
Darvon-N
Combinations
  Rx: with acetaminophen
    (Darvocet, Propacet,
    Wygesic)
Chemical Class: Synthetic
opium alkaloid; diphenylhep-
tane derivative
Therapeutic Class: Narcotic
analgesic
DEA Class: Schedule IV

CLINICAL PHARMACOLOGY
Mechanism of Action: Narcotic agonist with activity at Mu receptors
(supraspinal analgesia, euphoria,
respiratory and physical depression,
miosis, and reduced GI motility),
Kappa receptors (pentazocine-like
spinal analgesia, sedation, and miosis), and Delta receptors (dysphoria, psychotomimetic effects [e.g.,
hallucinations] and respiratory and
vasomotor stimulation caused by
drugs with antagonist activity); compared to morphine, less analgesia,
respiratory depression, sedation,
emesis, and physical dependence
Pharmacokinetics
PO: Onset 15-60 min, peak 2-2½ hr
(3 hr napsylate), duration 4-6 hr;
metabolized in liver (25% to nor-
propoxyphene), excreted in urine;
$t_{1/2}$ 6-12 hr
INDICATIONS AND USES: Mild to
moderate pain
DOSAGE
Adult
• PO 65 mg (100 mg napsylate) q4h
prn; max 390 mg/day (600 mg/day
napsylate)
$ **AVAILABLE FORMS/COST**
  OF THERAPY
• Cap, Gel—Oral: 65 mg, 100's:
$6.61-$41.72 (hydrochloride)

• Tab, Uncoated—Oral: 100 mg,
100's: **$60.68** (napsylate)
PRECAUTIONS: History of drug
abuse, suicidal ideation, hepatic or
renal function impairment, children
PREGNANCY AND LACTATION:
Pregnancy category C (category D
if used for prolonged periods or in
high doses at term); withdrawal
could theoretically occur in infants
exposed *in utero* to prolonged maternal ingestion; compatible with
breast feeding
**SIDE EFFECTS/ADVERSE REAC-
  TIONS**
CNS: Dizziness, dysphoria, euphoria, headache, lightheadedness, *sedation*
EENT: Visual disturbances
GI: Abdominal pain, abnormal liver
function, constipation, *nausea*, reversible jaundice (rare), *vomiting*
RESP: Respiratory depression
SKIN: Rashes
MISC: Weakness
INTERACTIONS
Drugs
3 *Anticoagulants:* Potentiation of
warfarin's anticoagulant effect
3 *Antidepressants:* Increased cyclic antidepressant serum concentrations
3 *Antihistamines, chloral hydrate,
glutethimide, methocarbamol:* Enhanced depressant effects
3 *Barbiturates:* Additive respiratory and CNS depressant effects
3 *Beta-blockers:* Increased concentrations of highly metabolized
β-blockers (metoprolol, propranolol)
2 *Carbamazepine:* Marked increases in plasma carbamazepine
concentrations
3 *Ethanol:* Additive CNS effects
3 *Protease inhibitors:* Increased
respiratory and CNS depression

* = non-FDA-approved use

3 *Warfarin:* Increased hypoprothrombinemic response

Labs

• *False increase:* Amylase and lipase

SPECIAL CONSIDERATIONS
PATIENT/FAMILY EDUCATION

• May cause drowsiness, dizziness or blurred vision

• Use caution driving or engaging in other activities requiring alertness

• Avoid alcohol

---

propranolol

(proe-pran'oh-lole)
Rx: Betachron, Inderal, Inderal LA
Combinations
  Rx: with HCTZ (Inderide)
Chemical Class: Nonselective β-adrenergic blocker
Therapeutic Class: Antihypertensive; antianginal; antimigraine agent; antidysrhythmic (class II); postmyocardial infarction; antiglaucoma agent

CLINICAL PHARMACOLOGY
Mechanism of Action: PO competitive β-adrenergic antagonist; produces negative inotropic and chronotropic responses; slows AV nodal conduction; decreases heart rate; decreases myocardial oxygen consumption; antiarrhythmic effects (class II); reduction in platelet aggregation and blood viscosity; suppression of renin release; inhibition of central sympathetic outflow; decreases presynaptic receptor neurotransmitter release; no intrinsic sympathomimetic or membrane stabilizing activity; low to moderate lipid solubility; OPHTH: reduces intraocular pressure via reduction in production of aqueous humor

Pharmacokinetics
PO: Peak 60-90 min (L-A 6 hr), extensive 1st-pass effect
IV: Onset immediate
High lipid solubility; >90% bound to plasma proteins; metabolized in liver to active and inactive metabolites, excreted in urine; $t_{1/2}$ 4-6 hr (L-A 8-11 hr)

INDICATIONS AND USES: Glaucoma, migraine headache, hypertension, postmyocardial infarction, supraventricular arrhythmias (atrial fibrillation, atrial flutter, paroxysmal supraventricular tachycardia), ventricular arrhythmias, aggressive behavior,* angina pectoris, anxiety,* cataract extraction prophylaxis,* congestive heart failure,* hyperthyroidism,* neuroleptic-induced akathisia,* retinal detachment,* tremor, hypertrophic obstructive cardiomyopathy, hypertrophic subaortic stenosis, pheochromocytoma, portal hypertension, Wolff-Parkinson-White syndrome, Alzheimer's disease,* ascites,* carcinoid syndrome,* resistant giardiasis,* menopausal symptoms,* mitral valve prolapse,* priapism secondary to chronic antipsychotic medications,* restless leg syndrome,* schizophrenia,* tardive dyskinesia,* tetanus,* Tourette's syndrome,* withdrawal syndromes*

DOSAGE
Adult and Child >16 yr

• *Hypertension:* PO 40 mg bid (L-A 80 mg qd) initially, usual range 120-240 mg/day divided bid-tid (L-A 120-160 mg qd), max 640 mg/day

• *Dysrhythmias:* PO 10-30 mg tid-qid; IV (reserve for life-threatening situations or dysrhythmias occurring during anesthesia) 0.5-3 mg, at a rate not exceeding 1 mg/min, a 2nd dose may be administered after 2 min prn, additional doses at in-

---

italic = common side effects   ***bold italic*** = life-threatening reactions

tervals no less than 4 hr until desired response obtained

• *Angina pectoris:* PO 10-20 mg tid-qid (L-A 80 mg qd) initially, usual range 160-240 mg/day divided tid-qid, maximum 320 mg/day

• *Hypertrophic subaortic stenosis:* PO 20-40 mg tid-qid (L-A 80-160 mg qd)

• *Pheochromocytoma:* PO 30 mg/day in divided doses (in conjunction with α-adrenergic blocking agent)

• *Migraine prophylaxis:* PO 80 mg/day in divided doses (L-A 80 mg qd) initially, increase to optimal prophylaxis, usual range 160-240 mg/day

• *MI:* PO 180-240 mg/day divided bid-qid beginning 5-21 days after MI

• *Essential tremor:* PO 40 mg bid initially, usual range 120-320 mg/day divided tid

• *Gastrointestinal bleeding:* PO 40 to 360 mg qd titrated to reduce the resting heart rate by 25%

• *Thyroid storm:* IV 1 mg/min to max 10 mg; repeat in 4-6 hr; PO 40 to 80 mg q6h, following IV

Child

• *Dysrhythmias:* IV 0.1 mg/kg/dose up to a max of 1 mg/dose (slow infusion over 5 min); PO 2 to 6 mg/kg/day divided q6-8h (max 60 mg/day)

• *Hypertension:* PO 0.5-1 mg/kg/day divided q6-12h, increase dose at 3-7 day intervals, usual range 1-5 mg/kg/day

• *Migraine prophylaxis:* PO 0.6-1.5 mg/kg/day in divided doses

• *Tetralogy of Fallot* (acute treatment of spells): IV 0.15-0.25 mg/kg/dose (slowly—1 mg/min.); repeated once after 15 min; PO (maintenance) 1 to 2 mg/kg q6h; increase in increments; max 5 mg/kg

• *Thyrotoxicosis:* PO 2 mg/kg/day, given q6h

§ AVAILABLE FORMS/COST OF THERAPY

• Tab, Uncoated—Oral: 10 mg, 100's: **$2.25-$40.50;** 20 mg, 100's: **$2.50-$56.85;** 40 mg, 100's: **$3.00-$73.78;** 60 mg, 100's: **$4.25-$102.06;** 80 mg, 100's: **$3.75-$113.26**

• Cap, Gel, SUS Action—Oral: 60 mg, 100's: **$68.99-$104.08;** 80 mg, 100's: **$77.52-$121.71;** 120 mg, 100's: **$101.06-$150.85;** 160 mg, 100's: **$132.31-$197.51**

• Sol—Oral: 20 mg/5 ml, 500 ml: **$34.65;** 40 mg/5 ml, 500 ml: **$49.51;** 80 mg/ml, 30 ml: **$33.53**

• Inj, Sol—IV: 1 mg/ml, 1 ml: **$6.25-$15.49**

CONTRAINDICATIONS: Bronchial asthma, cardiogenic shock, overt cardiac failure, 2nd and 3rd degree AV block, severe sinus bradycardia

PRECAUTIONS: Anesthesia/surgery (myocardial depression), avoid abrupt withdrawal, bronchospastic airways, congestive heart failure, diabetes mellitus, hyperthyroidism/thyrotoxicosis (atenolol, unlike propranolol, does not decrease T_3 levels), concurrent clonidine (discontinue atenolol several days prior to withdrawal of clonidine), peripheral vascular disease, renal disease

PREGNANCY AND LACTATION: Pregnancy category C; similar drug, atenolol, frequently used in the third trimester for treatment of hypertension (many studies of efficacy and safety of atenolol in pregnancy-induced hypertension); long-term use has been associated with intrauterine growth retardation; milk levels approximately half of peak plasma levels; considered insignificant; compatible with breast feeding

---

* = non-FDA-approved use

SIDE EFFECTS/ADVERSE REACTIONS

CNS: Depression, *dizziness,* drowsiness, *fatigue,* hallucinations, insomnia, *lethargy,* memory loss, mental changes, strange dreams

CV: Bradycardia, **CHF,** cold extremities, postural hypotension, profound hypotension, **2nd or 3rd degree heart block**

EENT: Dry, burning eyes; sore throat; visual disturbances

GI: Diarrhea, dry mouth, elevated LFTs, **ischemic colitis, mesenteric arterial thrombosis,** *nausea,* vomiting

GU: Impotence, sexual dysfunction

HEME: **Agranulocytosis, thrombocytopenia**

METAB: Hyperglycemia, hyperlipidemia (increase TG, total cholesterol, LDL; decrease HDL), masked hypoglycemic response to insulin (sweating excepted)

RESP: **Bronchospasm,** dyspnea, wheezing

SKIN: Alopecia, pruritis, rash

INTERACTIONS

Drugs

🔳 *α-1 adrenergic blockers:* Potential enhanced first dose response (marked initial drop in blood pressure), particularly on standing (especially prazocin)

🔳 *Amiodarone:* Bradycardia, cardiac arrest, ventricular dysrhythmia shortly after initiation of β-blocker

🔳 *Antidiabetics:* Masked symptoms of hypoglycemia, prolonged recovery of normoglycemia

🔳 *Antipyrine:* Increased antipyrine concentrations

🔳 *Barbiturates, rifampin:* Reduced concentrations of propranolol

🔳 *β-agonists:* Antagonistic effects

🔳 *Calcium channel blockers:* Increased concentrations of propranolol; increased bioavailability of nifedipine

🔳 *Chlorpromazine:* Additive hypotensive effects and grand mal seizures; chlorpromazine decreases the clearance of oral propranolol by 25% to 32%, resulting in increased propranolol bioavailability

🔳 *Cimetidine, etintidine, fluoxetine, propoxyphene, propafenone, quinidine, quinolones:* Increased propranolol concentrations

🔳 *Clonidine, guanabenz, guanfacine:* Exacerbation of hypertension upon withdrawal of clonidine

🔳 *Cocaine:* Potentiation of cocaine-induced coronary vasospasm

🔳 *Contrast media:* Increased risk anaphylaxis

🔳 *Digitalis glycosides:* Increased digoxin concentrations

🔳 *Dihydroergotamine, ergotamine:* May result in excessive vasconstriction

🔳 *Fluvoxamine:* Increased propranolol serum concentrations; increased risk of bradycardia and hypotension

🔳 *Epinephrine:* Enhanced pressor response to epinephrine

🔳 *Flecainide:* Increased propranolol and flecainide concentrations; additive negative inotropic effects

🔳 *Hydralazine:* Increases oral bioavailability of propranolol (high clearance and lipophilic β-blockers) increasing risk of adverse effects

🔳 *Hydrochlorothiazide:* Exaggerated hyperglycemic response

🔳 *Lidocaine:* Increased lidocaine concentrations

🔳 *Local anesthetics:* Enhanced sympathomimetic side effects of epinephrine-containing local anesthetics

🔳 *Neostigmine, physostigmine, tacrine:* Additive bradycardia

🔳 *Neuroleptics:* Increased plasma concentrations of both drugs

P

---

italic = common side effects   ***bold italic*** = life-threatening reactions

3 *NSAIDs:* Reduced hypotensive effect of propranolol

3 *Phenylephrine:* Predisposition to acute hypertensive episodes

2 *Theophylline:* Increased theophylline concentrations; antagonistic pharmacodynamic effects

Labs

• *False increase:* Bilirubin

SPECIAL CONSIDERATIONS
PATIENT/FAMILY EDUCATION

• Do not discontinue abruptly, may require taper; rapid withdrawal may produce rebound hypertension or angina

MONITORING PARAMETERS

• Angina: Reduction in nitroglycerin usage; frequency, severity, onset, and duration of angina pain; heart rate

• Arrhythmias: Heart rate

• Congestive heart failure: Functional status, cough, dyspnea on exertion, paroxysmal nocturnal dyspnea, exercise tolerance, and ventricular function

• Hypertension: Blood pressure

• Migraine headache: Reduction in the frequency, severity, and duration of attacks

• Postmyocardial infarction: Left ventricular function, lower resting heart rate

• Toxicity: Blood glucose, bronchospasm, hypotension, bradycardia, depression, confusion, hallucination, sexual dysfunction

---

propylthiouracil (PTU)

(proe-pill-thye-oh-yoor'a-sill)
Chemical Class: Thioamide derivative
Therapeutic Class: Antithyroid agent

CLINICAL PHARMACOLOGY
Mechanism of Action: Inhibits synthesis of thyroid hormones by interfering with the incorporation of iodine into tyrosyl residues of thyroglobulin; does not inhibit action of already formed or exogenously administered thyroid hormones; partially inhibits peripheral conversion of T_4 to T_3

Pharmacokinetics

PO: Bioavailability 80%-95%; 75%-80% bound to plasma proteins; metabolized in liver, excreted in urine (35% unchanged); $t_{1/2}$ 1-2 hr

INDICATIONS AND USES: Hyperthyroidism, preparation for thyroidectomy or radioactive iodine therapy, thyrotoxic crisis, alcoholic liver disease*

DOSAGE

Adult

• PO 300-450 mg/day divided q8h initially (doses of 600-1200 mg/day may be required); maintenance dose 100-150 mg/day divided q8-12h

Child

• PO 5-7 mg/kg/day divided q8h initially; maintenance dose ⅓-⅔ of initial dose divided q8-12h

• Dose in renal impairment: PO CrCl 10-50 ml/min, decrease recommended dose by 25%; CrCl <10 ml/min, decrease recommended dose by 50%

$ **AVAILABLE FORMS/COST OF THERAPY**

• Tab, Uncoated—Oral: 50 mg, 100's: **$6.25-$13.13**

PRECAUTIONS: Infection, bone marrow depression, hepatic disease, children (hepatotoxicity has occurred), thyroid storm

PREGNANCY AND LACTATION: Pregnancy category D; considered drug of choice for medical treatment of hyperthyroidism during pregnancy; excreted into breast milk in low amounts; compatible with breast feeding

---

* = non-FDA-approved use

SIDE EFFECTS/ADVERSE REACTIONS

CNS: CNS stimulation, depression, drowsiness, headache, neuritis, neuropathies, paresthesias, vertigo
CV: Edema
GI: Epigastric distress, hepatitis, jaundice, loss of taste, nausea, sialadenopathy, vomiting
GU: Nephritis
*HEME: **Agranulocytosis, aplastic anemia, granulocytopenia, hypoprothrombinemia, leukopenia,*** lymphadenopathy, splenomegaly, ***thrombocytopenia***
METAB: Insulin autoimmune syndrome (may result in ***hypoglycemic coma***)
MS: Arthralgia, myalgia
RESP: Interstitial pneumonitis
SKIN: Abnormal hair loss, erythema nodosum, ***exfoliative dermatitis,*** lupus-like syndrome, pruritis, skin pigmentation, urticaria, rash

INTERACTIONS

Drugs
3 *Oral anticoagulants:* Reduced hypoprothrombinemic response to oral anticoagulants
3 *Theophylline:* Physiologic response to antithyroid drug will increase theophylline concentrations via decreased clearance
Labs
• *False increase:* Glucose

SPECIAL CONSIDERATIONS
PATIENT/FAMILY EDUCATION

• Notify clinician of fever, sore throat, unusual bleeding or bruising, rash, yellowing of skin, vomiting

MONITORING PARAMETERS

• CBC periodically during therapy (especially during initial 3 mo), TSH

---

protamine
(proe′ta-meen)
Rx: Protamine
Chemical Class: Basic protein
Therapeutic Class: Heparin antidote

CLINICAL PHARMACOLOGY

Mechanism of Action: Forms a stable salt with unfractionated heparin (strongly acidic) resulting in loss of anticoagulant activity of both drugs
Pharmacokinetics
IV: Rapid onset of action, unfractionated heparin neutralized within 5 min, duration 2 hr; metabolic fate of unfractionated heparin-protamine complex unknown

INDICATIONS AND USES: Unfractionated heparin overdose

DOSAGE

Adult and Child
• IV 1 mg neutralizes 90 USP units of lung tissue-derived unfractionated heparin and 115 USP units of intestinal mucosa-derived unfractionated heparin; administer slowly over 10 min (for SC unfractionated heparin overdose, a portion of the total protamine dose should be administered by continuous INF over 8-16 hr), do not exceed 50 mg in a 10 min period; dose requirement decreases rapidly with time elapsed since IV unfractionated heparin inj; guide dosage by blood coagulation studies

$ **AVAILABLE FORMS/COST OF THERAPY**
• Inj, Sol—IV: 10 mg/ml, 25 ml: **$4.06-$5.32/5 ml**

PRECAUTIONS: Rapid administration (hypotension, anaphylactoid reactions), previous protamine exposure, fish allergy

PREGNANCY AND LACTATION: Pregnancy category C

---

italic = common side effects   ***bold italic*** = life-threatening reactions

SIDE EFFECTS/ADVERSE REACTIONS

CNS: Lassitude
CV: Bradycardia, *circulatory collapse,* flushing, hypotension
GI: Nausea, vomiting
RESP: Dyspnea, *pulmonary edema, pulmonary hypertension*
MISC: Hypersensitivity reactions

SPECIAL CONSIDERATIONS
• Will not reliably inactivate low-molecular-weight heparin

MONITORING PARAMETERS
• Activated partial thromboplastin time (aPTT) or protamine activated clotting time (ACT) 15 min after dose, then in several hr

---

protriptyline
(proe-trip'ti-leen)
Rx: Vivactil
Chemical Class: Dibenzolcycloheptene derivative: secondary amine
Therapeutic Class: Tricyclic antidepressant

CLINICAL PHARMACOLOGY
Mechanism of Action: Inhibits the reuptake of norepinephrine (very high) and serotonin (moderate) at the presynaptic neuron; inhibition of histamine and acetylcholine activity; mild peripheral vasodilator effects and possible quinidine-like actions on cardiac conduction high anticholinergic activity; slight sedative and orthostatic hypotensive activity

Pharmacokinetics
PO: Peak 24-30 hr, therapeutic response 2-4 wk; metabolized by liver, excreted by kidneys; $t_{1/2}$ 67-89 hr

INDICATIONS AND USES: Depression, obstructive sleep apnea*

DOSAGE
Adult
• PO 15-40 mg/day divided tid-qid;

may increase to 60 mg/day; make increases in AM dosage (mild stimulant effect)

Geriatric/Adolescent
• PO 5 mg tid, increase gradually if needed; use caution if dose >20 mg/day

AVAILABLE FORMS/COST OF THERAPY
• Tab, Plain Coated—Oral: 5 mg, 100's: **$39.95-$53.33**; 10 mg, 100's: **$57.80-$77.28**

CONTRAINDICATIONS: Acute recovery phase of MI; concurrent use of MAOIs

PRECAUTIONS: Suicidal patients, seizure disorders, prostatic hypertrophy, increased intraocular pressure, narrow-angle glaucoma, urinary retention, cardiac disease, hepatic or renal disease, hyperthyroidism, electroshock therapy, elective surgery, elderly, abrupt discontinuation

PREGNANCY AND LACTATION: Pregnancy category C

SIDE EFFECTS/ADVERSE REACTIONS

CNS: Anxiety, confusion (especially in elderly), *dizziness,* extrapyramidal symptoms (elderly), fatigue, headache, increased psychiatric symptoms, insomnia, memory impairment, nervousness, nightmares, panic, sedation, stimulation, tremors, weakness
CV: **Dysrhythmias, ECG changes,** hypertension, *orthostatic hypotension,* palpitations, syncope, tachycardia
EENT: *Blurred vision, dry mouth,* mydriasis, nasal congestion, ophthalmoplegia, tinnitus
GI: *Constipation,* cramps, diarrhea, epigastric distress, hepatitis, increased appetite, jaundice, nausea, **paralytic ileus,** stomatitis, vomiting
GU: *Urinary retention*
HEME: **Agranulocytosis,** eosino-

---

* = non-FDA-approved use

philia, *leukopenia, thrombocytopenia*

SKIN: Photosensitivity, pruritus, rash, sweating, urticaria

INTERACTIONS

Drugs

3 *Altretamine:* Orthostatic hypotension

3 *Amphetamines:* Theoretical increase in effect of amphetamines, clinical evidence lacking

3 *Antidiabetics:* Monitor for enhanced hypoglycemia

3 *Barbiturates, rifampin, carbamazepine:* Reduced cyclic antidepressant concentrations

3 *Beta agonists (especially isoproterenol):* Cardiac arrhythmia risk increased

2 *Bethanidine, clonidine, guanethidine, guanabenz, guanfacine, guanadrel, debrisoquen:* Reduced antihypertensive effect

2 *Epinephrine, norepinephrine:* Markedly enhanced pressor response to IV administration

3 *Ethanol:* Additive impairment of motor skills; abstinent alcoholics may eliminate cyclic antidepressants more rapidly than non-alcoholics

3 *Fluoxetine, paroxetine:* Marked increases in cyclic antidepressant plasma concentrations

3 *H_2 blockers (especially cimetidine), calcium channel blockers:* Increased cyclic concentrations

3 *Lithium:* Increased risk neurotoxicity (especially in elderly)

3 *MAOIs:* Excessive sympathetic response, mania, or hyperpyrexia possible

3 *Neuroleptics:* Increased therapeutic and toxic effects of both drugs

3 *Phenylephrine:* Enhanced pressor response

3 *Propantheline:* Enhanced anticholinergic effects

3 *Propoxyphene:* Enhanced effect of cyclic antidepressants

3 *Quinidine:* Increased cyclic antidepressant serum concentrations

3 *Ritonavir, indinavir:* Possible increased cyclic concentrations, toxicity

Labs

• *Increase:* Serum bilirubin, blood glucose, alk phosphatase

• *Decrease:* VMA, 5-HIAA

• *False increase:* Urinary catecholamines

SPECIAL CONSIDERATIONS
PATIENT/FAMILY EDUCATION

• Therapeutic effects may take 2-3 wk

• Use caution in driving or other activities requiring alertness

• Avoid rising quickly from sitting to standing, especially elderly

• Avoid alcohol and other CNS depressants

• Do not discontinue abruptly after long-term use

• Wear sunscreen or large hat to prevent photosensitivity

MONITORING PARAMETERS

• CBC, weight, ECG, mental status (mood, sensorium, affect, suicidal tendencies)

P

---

italic = common side effects   ***bold italic*** = life-threatening reactions

pseudoephedrine

(soo-doe-e-fed'rin)
OTC: Cenafed, Decofed,
Efidac Genaphed, PediaCare
Infants' Decongestant,
Seudotabs, Sudafed, Sudafed
12 Hour Caplets
(Pseudoephedrine is available in many prescription
and over-the-counter
combinations; the following
list is not all-inclusive)

Rx: with azatadine (Trinalin
Repetabs); brompheniramine (Bromfed); carbinoxamine (Rondec); chlorpheniramine (Deconamine
SR, Novafed A); codeine
(Nucofed); guaifenesin and
codeine (Novagest
Expectorant); loratadine
(Claritin-D)

OTC: with acetaminophen
(Dristan Cold); chlorpheniramine (Chlor-Trimeton
12 Hour Relief); dexbrompheniramine (Drixoral
Cold and Allergy); dextromethorphan (Thera-Flu
Non-Drowsy Formula);
diphenhydramine (Actifed
Allergy); ibuprofen (Advil
Cold & Sinus, Dristan
Sinus); triprolidine
(Actifed)

Chemical Class: Sympathomimetic amine
Therapeutic Class: Decongestant

CLINICAL PHARMACOLOGY
Mechanism of Action: Directly-stimulates α-adrenergic receptors in respiratory tract mucosa causing vasoconstriction; direct stimulation of β-adrenergic receptors causes increased heart rate and contractility

Pharmacokinetics
PO: Onset 15-30 min, duration 4-6 hr (extended release 12 hr); partially metabolized in liver to inactive metabolite, excreted in urine (55%-75% unchanged)

INDICATIONS AND USES: Nasal decongestion associated with common cold, allergies, and sinusitis; promotes nasal or sinus drainage

DOSAGE
Adult
• PO 60 mg q4-6h; PO SUS REL 120 mg q12h or 240 mg qd (Efidac); max 240 mg/day
Child
• PO 6-11 yr 30 mg q4-6h, max 120 mg/day; 2-5 yr 15 mg q4-6h, max 60 mg/day; <2 yr 4 mg/kg/day divided q6h

$ AVAILABLE FORMS/COST OF THERAPY
• Syr—Oral: 30 mg/5 ml, 480 ml: **$1.80-$7.42**
• Drops—Oral: 7.5 mg/0.8 ml, 15 ml: **$3.65-$4.12**
• Tab, Uncoated—Oral: 30 mg, 100's: **$1.75-$11.16;** 60 mg, 100's: **$1.90-$20.38**
• Tab, Ext-Rel—Oral: 120 mg, 20's: **$6.44;** 240 mg, 12's: **$6.77**

CONTRAINDICATIONS: Hypersensitivity to sympathomimetics, severe hypertension, severe CAD

PRECAUTIONS: Heart disease, coronary insufficiency, dysrhythmias, angina, hyperthyroidism, diabetes mellitus, prostatic hypertrophy, increased intracranial pressure, hypovolemia, mild to moderate hypertension

PREGNANCY AND LACTATION: Pregnancy category C; compatible with breast feeding

SIDE EFFECTS/ADVERSE REACTIONS
CNS: Anxiety, confusion, dizziness, drowsiness, hallucinations, headache, insomnia, *tremors*

* = non-FDA-approved use

CV: Chest pain, *dysrhythmias,* palpitations, tachycardia
GI: Anorexia, nausea, *vomiting*
GU: Dysuria, urinary retention
METAB: Hyperglycemia
INTERACTIONS
Drugs
3 *Antacids:* Sodium bicarbonate doses sufficient to alkalinize urine can inhibit elimination of pseudoephedrine
A *MAOIs:* Hypertensive crisis
Labs
• *False increase:* Theophylline
SPECIAL CONSIDERATIONS
PATIENT/FAMILY EDUCATION
• May cause wakefulness or nervousness
• Take last dose 4-6 hr prior to hs, notify clinician of insomnia, dizziness, weakness, tremor, or irregular heart beat

---

psyllium
(sill'ee-yum)
OTC: Fiberall, Hydrocil, Konsyl, Metamucil, Modane Bulk, Perdiem Fiber, Reguloid, Serutan, Syllact, V-Lax
Combination
  OTC: with senna (Perdiem)
Chemical Class: Psyllium colloid
Therapeutic Class: Bulk laxative

CLINICAL PHARMACOLOGY
Mechanism of Action: Adsorbs water in intestine; promotes peristalsis and reduces GI transit time
Pharmacokinetics
PO: Generally not absorbed, onset 12-24 hr (may be as long as 2-3 days)
INDICATIONS AND USES: Constipation, irritable bowel syndrome, diverticular disease, spastic colon, hemorrhoids, hypercholesterolemia*

DOSAGE
Adult
• PO 1-2 rounded teaspoonfuls or 1-2 packets in 8 oz glass of liquid 1-4 times/day; 1-2 wafers with 8 oz glass of liquid 1-4 times/day
Child 6-11 yr
• PO ½ to 1 rounded teaspoonful in 4 oz glass of liquid 1-3 times/day
$ AVAILABLE FORMS/COST
  OF THERAPY
• Granules—Oral: 2.5-4.03 g/rounded teaspoon; 100, 180, 250, 480, 540 g: **$10.99/250 g**
• Powder—Oral: 50% psyllium and 50% dextrose/dose, 120, 396, 420, 480, 630 g: **$3.50-$8.86**
• Powder, Effervescent—Oral: 3.4 g/dose, 30's (packets) and 300 g (bulk): **$5.83-$7.60**
• Powder, Hydrophilic—Oral: 3.5 g/rounded teaspoon; 210, 300, 420, 630 g: **$5.83-$9.22**
• Wafer, Chewable—Oral: 1.7-3.4 g; 14's: **$3.66**
• Tab—Oral: 18's: **$4.68**
CONTRAINDICATIONS: Intestinal obstruction, fecal impaction
PRECAUTIONS: Phenylketonurics (sugar-free preparations may contain aspartame), abdominal pain, nausea or vomiting
PREGNANCY AND LACTATION: Pregnancy category C; not systemically absorbed; exposure of fetus or nursing infant unlikely
SIDE EFFECTS/ADVERSE REACTIONS
GI: Anorexia, bloating, constipation, cramping, diarrhea, *esophageal or bowel obstruction,* flatulence, nausea, vomiting
SPECIAL CONSIDERATIONS
PATIENT/FAMILY EDUCATION
• Maintain adequate fluid consumption
• Do not use in presence of abdominal pain, nausea, or vomiting
• Avoid inhaling dust from powder

---

italic = common side effects   ***bold italic*** = life-threatening reactions

preparations; can cause runny nose, watery eyes, wheezing

---

pyrantel
(pye-ran'tel)
OTC: Antiminth, Pin-Rid, Pin-X, Reese's Pinworm
Chemical Class: Pyrimidine derivative
Therapeutic Class: Anthelmintic

CLINICAL PHARMACOLOGY
Mechanism of Action: Spasmic paralysis of worm results from depolarizing neuromuscular blockade; worms expelled via normal peristalsis
Pharmacokinetics
PO: Poorly absorbed, achieves low systemic levels of unchanged drug; 50% excreted unchanged in feces, ≤7% found in urine (unchanged drug and metabolites)
INDICATIONS AND USES: Ascariasis (roundworm infection), enterobiasis (pinworm infection), hookworm infection,* trichostrongyliasis*
DOSAGE
Adult and Child
• *Roundworm, pinworm, trichostrongyliasis:* PO 11 mg/kg as a single dose; max 1 g/dose; repeat in 2 wk for pinworm infection
• *Hookworm:* PO 11 mg/kg qd for 3 days
💲 AVAILABLE FORMS/COST OF THERAPY
• Susp—Oral: 144 mg/ml, 30, 60, 240 ml: **$5.28-$7.30**/30 ml
• Tab—Oral: 180 mg, 24's: **$5.65**
CONTRAINDICATIONS: Hepatic disease
PRECAUTIONS: Child <2 yr
PREGNANCY AND LACTATION: Pregnancy category C

SIDE EFFECTS/ADVERSE REACTIONS
CNS: Dizziness, drowsiness, headache, insomnia
GI: Abdominal cramps, anorexia, diarrhea, elevated liver enzymes, *nausea, vomiting*
SKIN: Rash
INTERACTIONS
Drugs
❷ *Piperazine:* Mutual antagonism
SPECIAL CONSIDERATIONS
PATIENT/FAMILY EDUCATION
• Take with food or milk
• Using a laxative to facilitate expulsion of worms is not necessary
• All family members in close contact with patient should be treated
• Strict hygiene is essential to prevent reinfection
• Shake suspension well before pouring

---

pyrazinamide
(pye-ra-zin'a-mide)
Rx: Pyrazinamide
Chemical Class: Niacinamide derivative
Therapeutic Class: Antituberculosis agent

CLINICAL PHARMACOLOGY
Mechanism of Action: Converted to pyrazinoic acid (POA) by susceptible strains of *Mycobacterium tuberculosis;* POA has specific antimycobacterial activity against *M. tuberculosis* and may lower environmental pH below that necessary for growth of the organism
Pharmacokinetics
PO: Peak 2 hr (POA 4-8 hr); 17% bound to plasma proteins; widely distributed in body tissues and fluids; metabolized in liver to POA (active), excreted in urine (4%-14% unchanged); $t_{1/2}$ 9-10 hr
INDICATIONS AND USES: Active

---

tuberculosis (as part of a 6 mo regimen consisting of isoniazid, rifampin, and pyrazinamide given for 2 mo, followed by isoniazid and rifampin for 4 mo); after treatment failure with other primary drugs in any form of active tuberculosis

DOSAGE

Adult

• PO 15-30 mg/kg qd for 1st 2 mo of 6 mo regimen with isoniazid and rifampin or as part of an individualized regimen for drug-resistant disease, max 2 g/day; alternatively 50-70 mg/kg can be given twice weekly to improve compliance (base dosage calculations on lean body weight)

Child

• PO 15-40 mg/kg/day divided q12-24 hr, max 2 g/day; alternatively 50-70 mg/kg based on lean body weight twice weekly, max 3 g/dose

$ AVAILABLE FORMS/COST OF THERAPY

• Tab, Uncoated—Oral: 500 mg, 100's: **$101.43-$112.25**

CONTRAINDICATIONS: Severe liver disease, acute gout

PRECAUTIONS: History of gout, renal and hepatic function impairment, alcoholism, elderly, HIV infection (may require longer courses of therapy), diabetes mellitus

PREGNANCY AND LACTATION: Pregnancy category C; excreted into human milk

SIDE EFFECTS/ADVERSE REACTIONS

CNS: Fever

GI: Anorexia, hepatotoxicity, nausea, vomiting

GU: Dysuria, interstitial nephritis (rare)

HEME: Blood clotting abnormalities, increased serum iron concentration, porphyria, *sideroblastic anemia*, *thrombocytopenia*

METAB: Gout, hyperuricemia

MS: Arthralgia, *myalgia*

SKIN: Acne, photosensitivity, pruritus, rash, urticaria

INTERACTIONS

Drugs

3 *Cyclosporine:* Decreased concentrations cyclosporine

3 *Tacrolimus:* Decreased concentrations of tacrolimus

Labs

• *False positive:* Urine ketone tests

SPECIAL CONSIDERATIONS

PATIENT/FAMILY EDUCATION

• Compliance with full course is essential

• Notify clinician of fever, loss of appetite, malaise, nausea and vomiting, darkened urine, yellowish discoloration of skin and eyes, pain or swelling of joints

MONITORING PARAMETERS

• Liver function tests, serum uric acid at baseline and periodically throughout therapy

---

pyridostigmine

(peer-id-oh-stig'meen)

Rx: Mestinon, Mestinon Timespan, Regonol

Chemical Class: Synthetic quaternary ammonium compound

Therapeutic Class: Cholinergic

CLINICAL PHARMACOLOGY

Mechanism of Action: An acetylcholinesterase inhibitor; inhibits destruction of acetylcholine, facilitating transmission of impulses across myoneural junction

Pharmacokinetics

PO: Poorly absorbed, onset 30-45 min, duration 3-6 hr

IV: Onset 2-5 min, duration 2-3 hr

IM: Onset 15 min

Hydrolyzed by cholinesterases and

---

italic = common side effects   ***bold italic*** = life-threatening reactions

P

metabolized by microsomal enzymes in liver, excreted in urine

INDICATIONS AND USES: Myasthenia gravis, reversal of non-depolarizing neuromuscular blocking agents after surgery

DOSAGE

Adult

• *Myasthenia gravis:* PO 600 mg/day divided to provide max relief; usual range 60-1500 mg/day, individualize dosage; PO SUS REL 180-540 mg qd-bid, individualize dosage, use dosage intervals of at least 6 hr; IM/IV 1/30th PO dose, inj IV very slowly

• *Reversal of non-depolarizing neuromuscular blockade:* IV 10-20 mg; give atropine 0.6-1.2 mg IV immediately prior to pyridostigmine to minimize side effects

Child

• *Myasthenia gravis:* PO 7 mg/kg/day divided into 5-6 doses; IM/IV 0.05-0.15 mg/kg/dose; max 10 mg/dose, inj IV very slowly

• *Reversal of non-depolarizing neuromuscular blockade:* IV 0.1-0.25 mg/kg/dose preceded by atropine or glycopyrrolate

§ AVAILABLE FORMS/COST OF THERAPY

• Inj, Sol—IM; IV: 5 mg/ml, 2 ml: **$1.54-$5.04**

• Syr—Oral: 60 mg/5 ml, 480 ml: **$46.08**

• Tab, Uncoated—Oral: 60 mg, 100's: **$46.08**

• Tab, Coated, SUS Action—Oral: 180 mg, 30's: **$30.24**

CONTRAINDICATIONS: Mechanical obstruction of intestinal or urinary tracts, hypersensitivity to bromides (pyridostigmine bromide)

PRECAUTIONS: Seizure disorder, bronchial asthma, bradycardia, recent coronary occlusion, vagotonia, hyperthyroidism, cardiac dysrhythmias, peptic ulcer, large oral doses in megacolon and decreased GI motility (accumulation and toxicity may occur when motility is restored), anticholinesterase insensitivity (reduce or withhold dosages until patient again becomes sensitive)

PREGNANCY AND LACTATION: Pregnancy category C; would not be expected to cross the placenta because it is ionized at physiologic pH; although apparently safe for the fetus, may cause transient muscle weakness in the newborn; compatible with breast feeding

SIDE EFFECTS/ADVERSE REACTIONS

CNS: Dizziness, drowsiness, headache, incoordination, *loss of consciousness, paralysis, seizures*

CV: AV block, bradycardia, *cardiac arrest, dysrhythmias,* hypotension, nodal rhythm, non-specific ECG changes, syncope, tachycardia

EENT: Blurred vision, conjunctival hyperemia, diplopia, lacrimation, miosis, spasm of accommodation, visual changes

GI: Cramps, diarrhea, dysphagia, flatulence, *increased gastric secretions,* increased peristalsis, *increased salivation, nausea, vomiting*

GU: Frequency, incontinence, urgency

MS: Arthralgia, fasciculation, muscle cramps and spasms, weakness

RESP: Bronchospasm, dyspnea, increased secretions, *laryngospasm, respiratory arrest, respiratory depression*

SKIN: Rash, sweating, urticaria

INTERACTIONS

Drugs

§ *Beta blockers:* Additive bradycardia

§ *Tacrine:* Increased anticholinergic effects

Labs

• *False increase:* Serum bicarbonate, chloride

---

* = non-FDA-approved use

SPECIAL CONSIDERATIONS
PATIENT/FAMILY EDUCATION
• Do not crush or chew sustained release preparations

MONITORING PARAMETERS
• Therapeutic response: increased muscle strength, improved gait, absence of labored breathing (if severe)
• Appearance of side effects (narrow margin between 1st appearance of side effects and serious toxicity)
• Symptoms of increasing muscle weakness may be due to cholinergic crisis (overdosage) or myasthenic crisis (increased disease severity). If crisis is myasthenia, patient will improve after 1-2 mg edrophonium; if cholinergic withdraw pyridostigmine and administer atropine

---

pyridoxine (vitamin B$_6$)
(peer-i-dox'een)
Rx: Doxine, Rodex, Vitabee 6 (Injection); **OTC:** Nestrex
Chemical Class: B complex vitamin
Therapeutic Class: Vitamin; hydralazine/isoniazid antidote

CLINICAL PHARMACOLOGY
Mechanism of Action: Coenzyme in metabolism of protein, carbohydrates, and fat

Pharmacokinetics
PO: Readily absorbed; metabolized in liver to 4-pyridoxic acid, excreted in urine; biologic t$_{1/2}$ 15-20 days

INDICATIONS AND USES: Pyridoxine deficiency including inadequate diet and drug-induced (e.g., isoniazid, hydralazine, penicillamine, cycloserine, oral contraceptives); inborn errors of metabolism such as B$_6$-dependent seizures or B$_6$-responsive anemia; hydralazine or isoniazid poisoning,* premenstrual syndrome (PMS),* hyperoxaluria type I (and oxalate kidney stones); nausea and vomiting in pregnancy*; in conjunction with folic acid to reduce levels of homocysteine*

DOSAGE
Adult
• *Dietary deficiency:* PO 10-20 mg qd for 3 wk, then 2-5 mg/day
• *Drug-induced deficiency:* PO 100-200 mg/day
• *Prophylaxis of drug-induced deficiency:* PO 25-100 mg/day
• *Recommended daily allowance (RDA):* PO 1.6-2 mg
• *Isoniazid poisoning:* IV 4 g followed by 1 g IM q30 min to equal amount of isoniazid consumed; doses of 70-357 mg/kg have been administered without incident

Child
• *Dietary deficiency:* PO 5-25 mg/day for 3 wk, then 1.5-2.5 mg/day
• *Drug-induced deficiency:* PO 10-50 mg/day
• *Prophylaxis of drug-induced deficiency:* PO 1-2 mg/kg/day
• *Recommended daily allowance (RDA):* PO 1-3 yr 0.9 mg; 4-6 yr 1.3 mg; 7-10 yr 1.6 mg

💲 AVAILABLE FORMS/COST OF THERAPY
• Inj, Sol—IM, IV: 100 mg/ml, 10, 30 ml: **$4.20-$7.50**/10 ml
• Tab—Oral: 10, 25, 50, 100 mg, 200 mg, 250 mg, 500 mg, 100's: **$1.30-$12.50**

PREGNANCY AND LACTATION: Pregnancy category A (category C if used in doses above RDA); deficiency during pregnancy is common in unsupplemented women; excreted in human breast milk; RDA for lactating women is 2.3-2.5 mg

SIDE EFFECTS/ADVERSE REACTIONS
CNS: Awkwardness of hands, de-

---

italic = common side effects   ***bold italic*** = life-threatening reactions

creased sensation to touch/temperature/vibration, headache, numb feet, paresthesia, perioral numbness, *seizures* (following very large IV doses), sensory neuropathic syndromes, somnolence, unstable gait
GI: Increased AST, nausea
HEME: Low serum folic acid levels
RESP: Respiratory distress
SKIN: Burning or stinging at inj site
MISC: Allergic reactions

INTERACTIONS
Drugs
▪ *Levodopa:* Inhibited antiparkinsonian effect of levodopa; concurrent use of carbidopa negates the interaction
▪ *Phenytoin:* Reduced phenytoin concentrations

SPECIAL CONSIDERATIONS
PATIENT/FAMILY EDUCATION
• Avoid doses exceeding RDA unless directed by clinician
MONITORING PARAMETERS
• Respiratory rate, heart rate, blood pressure during large IV doses

---

pyrimethamine
(pye-ri-meth′a-meen)
Rx: Daraprim
Combination
  with sulfadoxine (Fansidar)
Chemical Class: Synthetic aminopyrimidine derivative
Therapeutic Class: Antimalarial

CLINICAL PHARMACOLOGY
Mechanism of Action: Inhibits dihydrofolate reductase, which catalyzes the reduction of dihydrofolate to tetrahydrofolate; highly selective against plasmodia and *Toxoplasma gondii*
Pharmacokinetics
PO: Peak 2-6 hr; 87% bound to plasma proteins; metabolized in liver, excreted in urine; $t_{1/2}$ 4 days (7 days for sulfadoxine) (suppressive concentrations are maintained for approximately 2 wk)

INDICATIONS AND USES: Chemoprophylaxis of malaria due to susceptible strains of plasmodia; toxoplasmosis (in combination with sulfonamide); combination therapy with quinine and sulfadiazine for uncomplicated attack of chloroquine-resistant *P. falciparum* malaria; initiation of transmission control and suppressive cure in conjunction with fast-acting schizonticide

DOSAGE
Adult
• *Malaria prophylaxis:* PO 25 mg qwk; begin 2 wk before entering areas where chloroquine-resistant *P. falciparum* exists, continue for at least 6-10 wk after leaving endemic area; in combination with sulfadoxine PO 1 tab qwk 1-2 days before departure, continue × 4-6 wk after return
• *Chloroquine-resistant P. falciparum malaria (with quinine and sulfadiazine):* PO 25 mg bid for 3 days or (use in combination with sulfadoxine) PO 2-3 tabs in single dose
• *Toxoplasmosis (with sulfadiazine):* PO 50-75 mg/day with 1-4 g of sulfonamide for 1-3 wk, reduce dose by 50% and continue for 4-5 wk; alternatively 25-50 mg/day for 3-4 wk
Child
• *Malaria prophylaxis:* PO 0.5 mg/kg qwk, do not exceed 25 mg/dose; begin 2 wk before entering areas where chloroquine-resistant *P. falciparum* exists, continue for at least 6-10 wk after leaving endemic area; in combination with sulfadoxine begin 1-2 days before departure, continue × 4-6 wk after return; PO ¾ tab qwk (9-14 yr), PO ½ tab qwk (4-8 yr), PO ¼ tab qwk (<4 yr)

- *Chloroqine-resistant P. falciparum malaria (with quinine and sulfadiazine):* PO <10 kg, 6.25 mg qd for 3 days; 10-20 kg 12.5 mg qd for 3 days; 20-40 kg 25 mg qd for 3 days or (in combination with sulfadoxine) PO 2 tabs in single dose (9-14 yr), PO 1 tab in single dose (4-8 yr), PO ½ tab in single dose (<4 yr)
- *Toxoplasmosis (with sulfadiazine):* PO 2 mg/kg/day divided q12h for 3 days followed by 1 mg/kg/day divided qd-bid for 4 wk

§ AVAILABLE FORMS/COST OF THERAPY

- Tab, Uncoated—Oral: 25 mg, 100's: **$43.42**
- Tab, Uncoated—Oral: 25 mg/500 mg sulfadoxine, 100's: **$337.08**

CONTRAINDICATIONS: Megaloblastic anemia secondary to folate deficiency; infants <2 mo

PRECAUTIONS: Malabsorption syndrome, alcoholism, pregnancy (increased risk folate deficiency); renal or hepatic function impairment; seizure disorder; G-6-PD deficiency

PREGNANCY AND LACTATION: Pregnancy category C; most studies have found pyrimethamine to be safe in pregnancy; folic acid supplementation should be given to prevent folate deficiency; compatible with breast feeding

SIDE EFFECTS/ADVERSE REACTIONS

CNS: Depression, fever, headache, insomnia, lightheadedness, *seizures*
CV: Cardiac rhythm disturbance (large doses)
EENT: Dry throat
GI: Anorexia, atrophic glossitis, diarrhea, dry mouth, *nausea, vomiting* (large doses)
GU: Hematuria (large doses)
HEME: Decreased folic acid, **hemolytic anemia, leukopenia, megaloblastic anemia, pancytopenia, thrombocytopenia**
RESP: Pulmonary eosinophilia
SKIN: Abnormal skin pigmentation, dermatitis, **Stevens-Johnson syndrome, toxic epidermal necrolysis**

INTERACTIONS
Drugs
❷ *Folic acid:* Decreased efficacy of pyrimethamine

SPECIAL CONSIDERATIONS

- Discontinue if folate deficiency develops; administer leucovorin 5-15 mg IM qd for ≥3 days when recovery slow

PATIENT/FAMILY EDUCATION

- Take with food
- Discontinue at 1st sign of rash

MONITORING PARAMETERS

- CBC with platelets semi-weekly during therapy for toxoplasmosis, less frequently for malaria-related indications

---

quazepam
(kway'ze-pam)
Rx: Doral
Chemical Class: Benzodiazepine
Therapeutic Class: Hypnotic
DEA Class: Schedule IV

CLINICAL PHARMACOLOGY
Mechanism of Action: CNS depressant via facilitation of inhibitory GABA at benzodiazepine receptor sites (BZ_1—associated with sleep; BZ_2—associated with memory, motor, sensory, and cognitive function); effects include muscle relaxation (spinal cord), anticonvulsant activity (brain stem), ataxia (cerebellum), emotional behavior (limbic and cortical areas), and anxiolytic effects (separate from general CNS depression); decreases sleep latency, the number of awakenings, and the time spent in stage 0 (awake)

---

italic = common side effects **bold italic** = life-threatening reactions

sleep; stage 2 (unequivocal sleep) is increased; in sum, sleep time increased

Pharmacokinetics
PO: Peak 2 hr; 95% bound to plasma proteins; metabolized in liver to 2-oxoquazepam and N-desalkyl-2-oxoquazepam (both active), excreted in urine (31%) and feces (23%); $t_{1/2}$ 25-41 hr (metabolites 40-114 hr)

INDICATIONS AND USES: Short-term management of insomnia

DOSAGE

Adult ≥18 yrs
• PO 7.5-15 mg hs; reduce dose after 1-2 nights if possible

💲 AVAILABLE FORMS/COST OF THERAPY
• Tab, Coated—Oral: 7.5 mg, 100's: **$221.32;** 15 mg, 100's: **$241.87**

CONTRAINDICATIONS: Narrow-angle glaucoma, psychosis, pregnancy

PRECAUTIONS: Elderly, debilitated, hepatic disease, renal disease, history of drug abuse, abrupt withdrawal, respiratory depression, prolonged use, sleep apnea

PREGNANCY AND LACTATION: Pregnancy category X; may cause fetal damage when administered during pregnancy; excreted into breast milk; may accumulate in breast-fed infants and is therefore not recommended

SIDE EFFECTS/ADVERSE REACTIONS
CNS: Abnormal thinking, agitation, amnesia, anxiety, apathy, *asthenia,* ataxia, decreased libido, decreased reflexes, emotional lability, falling (especially elderly), hangover, hostility, *hypokinesia,* **seizure,** sleep disorder, *somnolence,* stupor
CV: Palpitations, syncope
EENT: Ear pain; epistaxis, eye irritation, pain, pharyngitis, photophobia, rhinitis, sinusitis, swelling
GI: Abdominal pain, anorexia, constipation, diarrhea, heartburn, increased AST, jaundice, nausea, vomiting
HEME: Granulocytopenia, **leukopenia**
RESP: Dyspnea
SKIN: Dermatitis

INTERACTIONS

Drugs
🔳 *Cimetidine:* Increased plasma levels of quazepam
🔳 *Clozapine:* Isolated cases of cardiorespiratory collapse have been reported, causal relationship to benzodiazepines has not been established
🔳 *Disulfiram:* Increased serum quazepam concentrations
🔳 *Ethanol:* Enhanced adverse psychomotor side effects of benzodiazepines
🔳 *Levodopa:* Possible exacerbation of parkinsonism
🔳 *Neuroleptics:* Increased sedation, respiratory depression
🔳 *Omeprazole, macrolides, azole antifungals, isoniazid, digoxin, SSRI's, quinolones:* Possible increased benzodiazepine concentrations
🔳 *Rifampin:* Reduced serum quazepam concentrations

SPECIAL CONSIDERATIONS
PATIENT/FAMILY EDUCATION
• Avoid alcohol and other CNS depressants
• Do not discontinue abruptly after prolonged therapy
• May cause daytime sedation, use caution while driving or performing other tasks requiring alertness
• Inform clinician if planning to become pregnant, or are pregnant, or if you become pregnant while taking this medicine
• May be habit forming

quetiapine
(kwe-tye′a-peen)
Rx: Seroquel
Chemical Class: Dibenzothiazepine derivative
Therapeutic Class: Antipsychotic

CLINICAL PHARMACOLOGY
Mechanism of Action: Serotonin 5-HT$_2$ >dopamine (D$_2$)-receptor antagonist; activity at several neurotransmitter systems: selective antagonist at limbic dopamine receptors (D$_1$, D$_2$, D$_4$, D$_5$) and serotonin receptors (5-HT$_2$, 5-HT$_6$, 5-HT$_7$); antagonism at α_1-adrenergic receptors; and activity at muscarinic, histamine H$_1$, or nicotinic receptors; moderate sedation and orthostatic hypotension; minimal risk of extrapyrimadal symptoms or weight gain; no anticholinergic effects
Pharmacokinetics
PO: Peak 1.5 hr, onset of therapeutic effect 7-14 days, bioavailability 15%; metabolic pathways in humans have not been adequately studied; mainly eliminated unchanged in the urine; t$_{1/2}$ 3-3.5 hr

INDICATIONS AND USES: Schizophrenia
DOSAGE
Adult
• PO 25 mg tid for 1-2 days initially, titrate upward in increments of 25-50 mg/day to 225 mg bid or 150 mg tid; doses >750 mg/day have not been studied

§ AVAILABLE FORMS/COST OF THERAPY
• Tab, Uncoated—Oral: 25 mg, 100's: **$131.04;** 100 mg, 100's: **$238.49;** 200 mg, 100's: **$467.90**
CONTRAINDICATIONS: Severe CNS depression

PRECAUTIONS: Renal or hepatic impairment, cardiovascular disease, thyroid disorders, hyperprolactinemia
PREGNANCY AND LACTATION: Pregnancy category not available
SIDE EFFECTS/ADVERSE REACTIONS
CNS: Agitation, dizziness, dystonia and other extrapyramidal symptoms, *headache,* hostility, *insomnia, somnolence*
CV: Increased heart rate, orthostatic hypotension
GI: Abdominal pain, asymptomatic elevations of serum transaminases, constipation, *dry mouth,* dyspepsia
METAB: Weight gain
SPECIAL CONSIDERATIONS
• Limited clinical experience, but similar to clozapine and risperidone; may be effective for negative symptoms of schizophrenia; so far no agranulocytosis reported with quetiapine

quinapril
(kwin′na-pril)
Rx: Accupril
Chemical Class: Nonsulfhydryl angiotensin-converting enzyme (ACE) inhibitor
Therapeutic Class: Antihypertensive

CLINICAL PHARMACOLOGY
Mechanism of Action: Antihypertensive, hypoproliferative, and cardioprotective effects attributable to competitive inhibition of angiotensin-converting enzyme (ACE) yielding decreased plasma concentrations of angiotensin II, plasma aldosterone concentrations, systemic vascular resistance, blood pressure, preload, and afterload, not accompanied by changes in heart rate, pres-

Q

sor sensitivity to exogenous norepi-nephrine, or baroreceptor sensitiv-ity

Pharmacokinetics

PO: Onset 1 hr, duration 24 hr; has little pharmacologic activity until metabolized to active metabolite (quinaprilat), excreted in urine (60%) and feces (37%); $t_{1/2}$ (quinaprilat) 2 hr

INDICATIONS AND USES: Hypertension, CHF (left ventricular dysfunction), MI, erythrocytosis,* nephropathy,* retinopathy*

DOSAGE

Adult and Child >16 yr

• *Hypertension:* PO 10 mg qd (5 mg if on concomitant diuretics); titrate according to response at 2 wk intervals; usual dose, 20-80 mg in 1-2 divided doses

• *Congestive heart failure:* PO 5 mg initially, then, if tolerated (excessive hypotension or deterioration in renal function) 5 mg bid with further dose adjustments titrated at weekly intervals up to 20 mg bid

• *Renal insufficiency:* Usual dosing for CrCl >60 ml/min; 5 mg qd for CrCl 30-60 ml/min; 2.5 mg qd for CrCl 10-30 ml/min

§ AVAILABLE FORMS/COST OF THERAPY

• Tab, Uncoated—Oral: 5 mg, 90's: **$85.49;** 10 mg, 90's: **$85.49;** 20 mg, 90's: **$85.49;** 40 mg, 90's: **$85.49**

PRECAUTIONS: History of anaphylaxis, renal insufficiency (<30 ml/min), hypotension (CHF, elderly, volume depletion—diuretics, dialysis, cirrhosis), aortic stenosis, hyperkalemia (potassium supplements, potassium-sparing diuretics, renal disease, diabetes), neutropenia (autoimmune diseases, collagen vascular diseases, febrile illness, immunosuppressant drug therapy), pro-

teinuria, renal artery stenosis, surgery/anesthesia (excessive hypotension, correctable with fluids)

PREGNANCY AND LACTATION: Pregnancy category D; ACE inhibitors can cause fetal and neonatal morbidity and death when administered to pregnant women; when pregnancy is detected, discontinue ACE inhibitors as soon as possible

SIDE EFFECTS/ADVERSE REACTIONS

CNS: Dizziness, fatigue, *headache*

CV: Angina, palpitations, postural hypotension, syncope (especially with 1st dose)

GI: Abdominal pain, constipation, nausea, vomiting

GU: Decreased libido, impotence, increased BUN, creatinine

HEME: **Agranulocytosis, neutropenia, thrombocytopenia**

METAB: Hyperkalemia, hyponatremia, hypoglycemia

MS: Arthralgia, arthritis, myalgia

RESP: Asthma, bronchitis, cough

SKIN: Angioedema, pruritis, rash, sweating

INTERACTIONS

Drugs

❷ *Allopurinol:* Predisposition to hypersensitivity reactions

❸ *Alpha adrenergic blockers:* Exaggerated 1st dose hypotensive response

❸ *Aspirin:* Reduced hemodynamic effects; less likely with nonacetylated salicylates

❸ *Azathioprine:* Increased myelosuppression

❸ *Cyclosporine:* Renal insufficiency

❸ *Insulin:* Enhanced hypoglycemic response

❸ *Iron* (parenteral): Increased risk systemic reaction

❸ *Lithium:* Increased risk of serious lithium toxicity

* = non-FDA-approved use

3 *Loop diuretics:* Initiation of ACE inhibitor therapy may cause hypotension and renal insufficiency

3 *NSAIDs:* Inhibition of the antihypertensive response

3 *Potassium, potassium-sparing diuretics:* Increased risk for hyperkalemia

3 *Trimethoprim:* Additive risk of hyperkalemia, especially in patient predisposed to renal insufficiency
Labs
• ACE inhibition can account for approximately 0.5mEq/L rise in serum potassium

SPECIAL CONSIDERATIONS
PATIENT/FAMILY EDUCATION
• Caution with salt substitutes containing potassium chloride
• Rise slowly to sitting/standing position to minimize orthostatic hypotension
• Dizziness, fainting, lightheadedness may occur during 1st few days of therapy
• May cause altered taste perception or cough; persistent dry cough usually does not subside unless medication is stopped; notify clinician if these symptoms persist
MONITORING PARAMETERS
• BUN, creatinine, potassium within 2 wk after initiation of therapy (increased levels may indicate acute renal failure)

---

quinidine
(kwin'i-deen)
Rx: Quinaglute Dura-Tabs, Quinalan, (gluconate); Cardioquin (polygalacturonate); Quinidex Extentabs, Quinora (sulfate)
Chemical Class: Dextrorotatory isomer of quinine
Therapeutic Class: Antidysrhythmic (Class IA); antimalarial

CLINICAL PHARMACOLOGY
Mechanism of Action: Decreases the rate of rise of diastolic (Phase 4) depolarization, thereby depressing automaticity in ectopic foci; slows depolarization, repolarization, and amplitude of the action potential leading to an increase in the refractoriness of atrial and ventricular tissue; exerts indirect anticholinergic effects through blockade of vagal innervation, which may facilitate conduction in the atrioventricular junction
Pharmacokinetics
PO: Peak 3-4 hr (gluconate), 1-1½ hr (sulfate), 6 hr (polygalacturonate); duration 6-8 hr (EXT REL tab 12 hr)
IM: Peak ½-1½ hr
80%-90% bound to plasma proteins; metabolized in liver, excreted in urine (10%-50% unchanged); $t_{1/2}$ 6 hr
INDICATIONS AND USES: PO: Premature ventricular contractions, ventricular tachycardia (when not associated with complete heart block), junctional (nodal) dysrhythmias, AV junctional premature complexes, paroxysmal junctional tachycardia, premature atrial contractions, paroxysmal atrial tachycardia, atrial flutter, atrial fibrillation (chronic and paroxysmal); IM/IV when PO ther-

apy not feasible or when rapid therapeutic effect is required, life-threatening *Plasmodium falciparum* malaria

DOSAGE

Adult

• Give 200 mg test dose PO/IM several hr before full dosage to determine possibility of idiosyncratic reaction

• PO (sulfate) 100-600 mg q4-6h, initiate at 200 mg/dose and adjust dose to maintain desired therapeutic effect, max 3-4 g/d; SUS REL 300-600 mg q8-12h

• PO (gluconate) 324-972 mg q8-12h

• PO (polygalacturonate) 275 mg q8-12h

• IM 400 mg q4-6h

• IV 200-400 mg diluted and infused at a rate ≤10 mg/min

Child

• Give 2 mg/kg test dose PO/IM several hr before full dosage to determine possibility of idiosyncratic reaction

• PO (sulfate) 15-60 mg/kg/day divided into 4-5 doses or 6 mg/kg q4-6h; usual 30 mg/kg/day or 900 mg/m^2/day given in 5 doses/day

💲 AVAILABLE FORMS/COST OF THERAPY

• Tab, Uncoated—Oral (sulfate): 200 mg, 100's: **$9.25-$20.10:** 300 mg, 100's: **$18.62-$38.68**

• Tab, Coated, SUS Action—Oral (sulfate): 300 mg, 100's: **$74.53-$96.50**

• Tab, Uncoated—Oral (polygalacturonate): 275 mg, 100's: **$144.59**

• Tab, Uncoated, SUS Action—Oral (gluconate): 324 mg, 100's: **$25.99-$56.16**

• Inj, Sol—IM;IV (gluconate): 80 mg/ml, 10 ml: **$16.98**

CONTRAINDICATIONS: Digitalis intoxication manifested by AV condition disorders, complete AV block with an AV nodal or idioventricular pacemaker, left bundle branch block, or other severe intraventricular condition defects with marked QRS widening, ectopic impulses, and abnormal rhythms due to escape mechanisms, history of drug-induced torsade de pointes, history of long QT syndrome, myasthenia gravis

PRECAUTIONS: Treatment of atrial flutter without prior medication to control ventricular rate (e.g., digoxin, verapamil, diltiazem, beta-blocker), marginally compensated cardiovascular disease, incomplete AV block, digitalis intoxication, hyperkalemia, renal, or hepatic insufficiency

PREGNANCY AND LACTATION: Pregnancy category C; use during pregnancy has been classified in reviews of cardiovascular drugs as relatively safe for the fetus; high doses can produce oxytocic properties and potential for abortion; excreted in breast milk; compatible with breast feeding

SIDE EFFECTS/ADVERSE REACTIONS

CNS: Apprehension, ataxia, confusion, delirium, dementia, depression, *dizziness,* excitement, fever, *headache,* vertigo

CV: Angioedema, arterial embolism, *bradycardia,* **complete AV block,** *hypotension,* prolonged QT interval, syncope, *torsade de pointes,* ventricular extrasystoles, ventricular flutter, *ventricular tachycardia and fibrillation,* widening of the QRS complex

EENT: Disturbed hearing (tinnitus, decreased auditory acuity), disturbed vision (mydriasis, blurred vision, disturbed color perception, photophobia, diplopia, night blindness, scotomata), optic neuritis, reduced visual field

GI: Abdominal pain, anorexia, *diarrhea,* esophagitis, hepatotoxicity, nausea, vomiting

HEME: **Acute hemolytic anemia, agranulocytosis,** leukocytosis, **neutropenia, thrombocytopenia,** thrombocytopenic purpura

MS: Arthralgia, increase in serum skeletal muscle creatine phosphokinase, myalgia

SKIN: Abnormalities of pigmentation, cutaneous flushing with intense pruritus, eczema, exfoliative eruptions, photosensitivity, psoriasis, purpura, rash, urticaria, vasculitis

MISC: Cinchonism (tinnitus, headache, nausea, visual changes), lupus nephritis, positive ANA, systemic lupus erythematosus

INTERACTIONS

Drugs

3 *Acetazolamide, antacids, sodium bicarbonate:* Alkalinization of urine increases plasma quinidine concentrations

3 *Amiloride:* Increased risk of arrhythmias in patients with ventricular tachycardia

3 *Amiodarone, cimetidine, verapamil:* Increased plasma quinidine concentrations

3 *Azole antifungals:* Inhibition of quinidine metabolism (CYP3A4), increased concentrations

3 *Barbiturates, nifedipine, kaolinpectin, phenytoin, rifampin, rifabutin:* Decreased plasma quinidine concentrations

3 *Beta-blockers:* Increased concentrations of metoprolol, propranolol, and timolol

3 *Cholinergic agents:* Reduced therapeutic effects of cholinergic drugs

2 *Codeine:* Inhibition of codeine to its active metabolite, diminished analgesia

3 *Cyclic antidepressants:* Increased imipramine, nortriptyline and desipramine concentrations

3 *Dextromethorphan:* Increased dextromethorphan concentrations, toxicity may result

3 *Digitalis glycosides:* Increased digoxin and digitoxin concentrations, toxicity may result

3 *Encainide:* Increased encainide serum concentrations in rapid encainide metabolizers

3 *Haloperidol:* Increased haloperidol concentrations, toxicity

3 *Macrolides:* Increased quinidine concentrations with erythromycin, troleandomycin, clarithromycin due to CYP34A inhibition

3 *Mexiletine:* Increased mexiletine concentrations

3 *Neuromuscular blocking agents:* Enhanced effects of neuromuscular blocking agents

3 *Nifedipine:* Increased serum nifedipine concentrations

3 *Procainamide:* Marked increased procainamide concentrations

3 *Propafenone:* Increased propafenone concentrations and decreased concentrations of its active metabolite; net effect unknown

3 *Warfarin:* Enhanced anticoagulant response

Labs

• *False increase:* Urine 17-ketosteroids

SPECIAL CONSIDERATIONS

• 267 mg gluconate=275 mg polygalacturonate=200 mg sulfate

PATIENT/FAMILY EDUCATION

• Take with food to decrease GI upset

• Do not crush or chew sustained release tablets

MONITORING PARAMETERS

• Plasma quinidine concentration (therapeutic range 2-6 µg/ml)

- ECG
- Liver function tests during the 1st 4-8 weeks
- CBC periodically during prolonged therapy

---

quinine
(kwye'nine)

Rx: Quinine

Chemical Class: Cinchona alkaloid
Therapeutic Class: Antimalarial

CLINICAL PHARMACOLOGY
Mechanism of Action: Exact antimalarial mechanism of action unknown, appears to interfere with plasmodial DNA function; increases the refractory period of skeletal muscle by direct action on the muscle fiber, decreases the excitability of the motor endplate, and affects the distribution of calcium within the muscle fiber

Pharmacokinetics
PO: Peak 1-3 hr; 70% bound to plasma proteins; metabolized in liver, excreted in urine; $t_{1/2}$ 4-5 hr

INDICATIONS AND USES: Chloroquine-resistant *falciparum* malaria (alone or in combination with pyrimethamine and a sulfonamide or with a tetracycline),* alternative for chloroquine-sensitive strains of *P. falciparum, P. malariae, P. ovale* and *P. vivax,** nocturnal leg cramps*

DOSAGE
Adult
- *Chloroquine-resistant malaria:* PO 650 mg q8h for 5-7 days
- *Chloroquine-sensitive malaria:* PO 600 mg q8h for 5-7 days
- *Nocturnal leg cramps:* PO 260-300 mg hs

Child
- *Chloroquine-resistant malaria:* PO 25 mg/kg/day divided q8h for 5-7 days
- *Chloroquine-sensitive malaria:* PO 10 mg/kg q8h for 5-7 days

$ AVAILABLE FORMS/COST OF THERAPY
- Cap, Gel—Oral: 325 mg, 100's: **$7.01-$33.83**
- Cap, Gel—Oral: 200 mg, 100's: **$13.10**
- Cap, Gel—Oral: 300 mg, 100's: **$17.13**
- Tab, Uncoated—Oral: 260 mg, 100's: **$9.76-$63.00**

CONTRAINDICATIONS: G-6-PD deficiency, optic neuritis, tinnitus, history of blackwater fever, thrombocytopenic purpura (associated with previous quinine ingestion), pregnancy

PRECAUTIONS: Cardiac dysrhythmias, myasthenia gravis

PREGNANCY AND LACTATION: Pregnancy category X; excreted into breast milk; compatible with breast feeding; use caution in infants at risk for G-6-PD deficiency

SIDE EFFECTS/ADVERSE REACTIONS
CNS: Apprehension, confusion, fever, headache, restlessness, vertigo
CV: Anginal symptoms, syncope
EENT: Blurred vision, deafness, diminished visual field, *diplopia,* disturbed color vision, photophobia, tinnitus, visual disturbances
GI: Epigastric pain, **hepatitis,** nausea, vomiting
HEME: **Acute hemolysis, agranulocytosis, hypoprothrombinemia,** thrombocytopenic purpura
RESP: Asthmatic symptoms
SKIN: Cutaneous rashes, edema of the face, flushing, pruritus, sweating
MISC: Cinchonism (tinnitus, headache, nausea, disturbed vision)

---

* = non-FDA-approved use

INTERACTIONS
Drugs
3 *Digitalis glycosides:* Increased digoxin concentrations (especially at high quinine doses)

3 *Smoking:* Reduced serum quinine concentrations

Labs
• *False increase:* 17-ketosteroids

SPECIAL CONSIDERATIONS
PATIENT/FAMILY EDUCATION
• Take with food
• May cause blurred vision, use caution driving
• Discontinue drug if flushing, itching, rash, fever, stomach pain, difficult breathing, ringing in ears, visual disturbances occur

---

rabeprazole
(rab-eh-pra′zole)
Rx: Aciphex
Chemical Class: Substituted benzimidazole
Therapeutic Class: Gastrointestinal antiulcer agent

CLINICAL PHARMACOLOGY
Mechanism of Action: Suppresses gastric acid secretion by inhibiting the parietal cell H^+/K^+ ATP pump
Pharmacokinetics
PO: Peak 2-5 hr, bioavailability 52%; 96% bound to plasma proteins; extensively metabolized by CYP3A and 2C19; 90% eliminated as metabolites in the urine; $t_{1/2}$ 1-2 hr (increased with hepatic disease)

INDICATIONS AND USES: Short-term (4-8 wk) treatment of erosive or ulcerative gastroesophageal reflux disease (GERD); maintenance therapy in erosive or ulcerative GERD; short-term (up to 4 wk) treatment of duodenal ulcers; long-term treatment of pathological hypersecretory conditions, including Zollinger-Ellison syndrome

DOSAGE
Adult
• *GERD:* PO 20 mg qd for 4-8 wk; maintenance: 20 mg qd
• *Duodenal ulcer:* PO 20 mg qd after breakfast for 4 wk
• *Hypersecretory conditions:* PO 60 mg qd; dose may need to be adjusted prn; doses as high as 100 mg and 60 mg bid have been used

§ **AVAILABLE FORMS/COST OF THERAPY**
• Tab, delayed release—Oral: 20 mg, 30's: **$92.40**

PREGNANCY AND LACTATION: Pregnancy category B; excretion into breast milk unknown, use caution in nursing mothers

SIDE EFFECTS/ADVERSE REACTIONS
CNS: Headache, delirium, twitching, insomnia, anxiety, dizziness, depression, somnolence, hypertonia, neuralgia, vertigo, *seizure,* abnormal dreams, decreased libido, neuropathy, paresthesia, tremor, agitation, amnesia, confusion, extrapyramidal reaction, hyperkinesia
CV: Chest pain, hypertension, *myocardial infarction,* syncope, angina, bundle branch block, palpitation, bradycardia, tachycardia, SVT, *pulmonary embolus,* thrombophlebitis, vasodilation, QT prolongation, *ventricular tachycardia,* ecchymosis, lymphadenopathy, peripheral edema
EENT: Cataract, amblyopia, glaucoma, dry eyes, abnormal vision, tinnitus, otitis media, corneal opacity, blurred vision, eye pain, retinal degeneration, strabismus
GI: Diarrhea, nausea, abdominal pain, vomiting, dyspepsia, flatulence, constipation, dry mouth, eructation, gastroenteritis, rectal hemorrhage, melena, anorexia, cholelithiasis, stomatitis, dysphagia, gingivitis, cholecystitis, increased ap-

---

italic = common side effects   ***bold italic*** = life-threatening reactions

R

petite, colitis, esophagitis, glossitis, *pancreatitis,* proctitis, cholangitis, duodenitis, hepatitis, hepatic encephalopathy, fatty liver, salivary gland enlargement, increased transaminases

GU: Urinary frequency, cystitis, dysmenorrhea, dysuria, renal calculus, menorrhagia, polyuria, breast enlargement, impotence, hematuria, leukorrhea, orchitis, urinary incontinence

*HEME: **Agranulocytosis, hemolytic anemia, leukopenia, pancytopenia, thrombocytopenia,** anemia*

METAB: Hyperammonemia, elevated TSH, hyperthyroidism, hypothyroidism, gout

MS: Myalgia, arthritis, leg cramps, bone pain, bursitis

RESP: Dyspnea, asthma, epistaxis, laryngitis, hiccup, hyperventilation, apnea, hypoventilation

SKIN: Dermatologic eruptions, photosensitivity, rash, pruritus, sweating, urticaria, alopecia, dry skin, herpes zoster, psoriasis

MISC: Coma, jaundice, rhabdomyolysis, weakness, fever, chills, malaise, thirst, weight gain, dehydration, weight loss

INTERACTIONS
Drugs

3 *Cyclosporine:* Potential for increased cyclosporine concentrations

3 *Digoxin:* Increased serum concentrations of digoxin possible

3 *Ketoconazole:* Decreased bioavailability of ketoconazole

MONITORING PARAMETERS
• Symptom relief, mucosal healing

SPECIAL CONSIDERATIONS
• Symptomatic response does not rule out gastric malignancy

raloxifene
(ra-lox′-i-feen)
Rx: Evista
Chemical Class: Benzothiophene, selective estrogen receptor modulator (SERM)
Therapeutic Class: Antiosteoporotic

CLINICAL PHARMACOLOGY
Mechanism of Action: Binds to estrogen receptors, reducing resorption of bone, decreasing bone turnover. Estrogen-like effect on bone and lipids, lacks estrogen effects in uterine and breast tissues

Pharmacokinetics
PO: 60% of dose rapidly absorbed, undergoes extensive presystemic glucuronide conjugation. Absolute bioavailability 2%. Extensive protein binding but does not bind to sex steroid binding globulin. Not metabolized by cytochrome P450 pathways. Excreted in feces. $t_{1/2}$ 32 hr

INDICATIONS AND USES: Prevention and treatment of osteoporosis. Not indicated in premenopausal women.

DOSAGE
Adult
• PO 60 mg qd

AVAILABLE FORMS/COST OF THERAPY
• Tab, Coated—Oral: 60 mg, 100's: **$198.00**

CONTRAINDICATIONS: Pregnancy, women at risk for pregnancy, history of thromboembolism

PRECAUTIONS: Hepatic insufficiency

PREGNANCY AND LACTATION: Pregnancy category X. Abortion and fetal anomalies noted in animal studies. Unknown if excreted in milk.

SIDE EFFECTS/ADVERSE REACTIONS
CNS: Depression, insomnia

* = non-FDA-approved use

EENT: Sinusitis
GI: Nausea (8% incidence same as placebo), dyspepsia, vomiting
GU: Vaginitis, leukorrhea
*HEME: **Thromboembolism***
METAB: Weight gain, peripheral edema, decreased total cholesterol (6%), decreased LDL-C (11%), no effect on HDL-C or triglycerides
MS: Leg cramps (6%)
SKIN: Hot flashes (25%, vs 18% with placebo)

INTERACTIONS
Drugs
❷ *Cholestyramine:* Decreased absorption and enterohepatic cycling of raloxifene
❸ *Clofibrate, indomethacin, naproxen, ibuprofen, diazepam, diazoxide:* Possible displacement of these highly protein-bound drugs
❸ *Warfarin:* Decreased PT

SPECIAL CONSIDERATIONS
• Shown to preserve bone mass and increase bone mineral density relative to calcium alone at 24 mo, relationship to skeletal fracture rates not yet established
• Ensure adequate dietary or supplemental calcium, vitamin D
• Not associated with endometrial proliferation; however, investigate uterine bleeding
• Has not been adequately studied with concomitant use of estrogen or in women with prior history of breast cancer
• Risk of thromboembolic events greatest in first 4 mo, discontinue at least 72 hr prior to surgery involving immobilization. Resume when patient fully ambulatory

PATIENT/FAMILY EDUCATION
• May be taken without regard to meals
• Engage in weight-bearing exercises, do not smoke or use alcohol excessively
• Report leg pain or swelling, sudden chest pain, shortness of breath, vision changes
• Avoid restrictions of movement during travel. Discontinue if at bed rest.

MONITORING PARAMETERS
• Bone density tests (e.g., DEXA scan)

---

ramipril
(ram'i-pril)
Rx: Altace
Chemical Class: Nonsulfhydryl angiotensin-converting enzyme (ACE) inhibitor
Therapeutic Class: Antihypertensive

CLINICAL PHARMACOLOGY
Mechanism of Action: Antihypertensive, hypoproliferative, and cardioprotective effects attributable to competitive inhibition of angiotensin-converting enzyme (ACE) yielding decreased plasma concentrations of angiotensin II, plasma aldosterone concentrations, systemic vascular resistance, blood pressure, preload, and afterload, not accompanied by changes in heart rate, pressor sensitivity to exogenous norepinephrine, or baroreceptor sensitivity

Pharmacokinetics
PO: Onset 1-2 hr, duration 24 hr; 73% bound to plasma proteins; has little pharmacologic activity until metabolized to active metabolite (ramiprilat), excreted in urine (60%) and feces (40%); $t_{1/2}$ (ramiprilat) 13-17 hr

INDICATIONS AND USES: Hypertension, CHF (left ventricular dysfunction), MI (left ventricular function salvage), erythrocytosis,* nephropathy,* retinopathy*

DOSAGE
Adult and Child >16 yr
• *Hypertension:* PO 2.5 mg qd ini-

R

---

tially (1.25 mg if on concomitant diuretic); usual maintenance dose, 2.5-20 mg qd

• *Congestive heart failure (left ventricular dysfunction):* PO 1.25-2.5 mg bid; max daily dose, 10 mg, usually divided

• *Myocardial infarction:* PO 1.25 mg initially, followed by 2.5 mg 12 hr later and full titration to 10 mg qdd10 mg qd begun within 24 hr of MI

• *Dosage in renal failure:* PO 25%-50% dosage reduction for CrCl 10-50 ml/min; 50%-75% reduction for CrCl <10 ml/min

💲 AVAILABLE FORMS/COST OF THERAPY

• Cap, Gel—Oral: 1.25 mg, 100's: **$76.48;** 2.5 mg, 100's: **$89.79;** 5 mg, 100's: **$96.11;** 10 mg, 100's: **$111.36**

PRECAUTIONS: Renal insufficiency (<30 ml/min), hypotension (CHF, elderly, volume depletion—diuretics, dialysis, cirrhosis), aortic stenosis, hyperkalemia (potassium supplements, potassium-sparing diuretics, renal disease, diabetes), neutropenia (autoimmune diseases, collagen vascular, febrile illness, immunosuppressant drug therapy), proteinuria, renal artery stenosis, surgery/anesthesia (excessive hypotension, correctable with fluids)

PREGNANCY AND LACTATION: Pregnancy category D; ACE inhibitors can cause fetal and neonatal morbidity and death when administered to pregnant women; when pregnancy is detected, discontinue ACE inhibitors as soon as possible

SIDE EFFECTS/ADVERSE REACTIONS

CNS: Anxiety, dizziness, fatigue, *headache,* insomnia, paresthesia

CV: Angina, hypotension, palpitations, postural hypotension, syncope (especially with 1st dose)

GI: Abdominal pain, constipation, impaired taste sensation, nausea, pancreatitis, vomiting

GU: Decreased libido, impotence, renal insufficiency

HEME: **Agranulocytosis, neutropenia, thrombocytopenia**

METAB: Hyperkalemia, hyponatremia, hypoglycemia

MS: Arthralgia, arthritis, myalgia

RESP: Asthma, bronchitis, *cough,* dyspnea, sinusitis

SKIN: Angioedema, flushing, rash, sweating

INTERACTIONS

Drugs

❷ *Allopurinol:* Predisposition to hypersensitivity reactions

❸ *Alpha adrenergic blockers:* Exaggerated 1st dose hypotensive response

❸ *Aspirin:* Reduced hemodynamic effects; less likely with nonacetylated salicylates

❸ *Azathioprine:* Increased myelosuppression

❸ *Cyclosporine:* Renal insufficiency

❸ *Insulin:* Enhanced hypoglycemic response

❸ *Iron* (parenteral): Increased risk of systemic reaction

❸ *Lithium:* Increased risk of serious lithium toxicity

❸ *Loop diuretics:* Initiation of ACE inhibitor therapy may cause hypotension and renal insufficiency

❸ *NSAIDs:* Inhibition of the antihypertensive response to ACE inhibitors

❸ *Potassium, potassium-sparing diuretics:* Increased risk for hyperkalemia

❸ *Trimethoprim:* Additive risk of hyperkalemia, especially in patient predisposed to renal insufficiency

---

* = non-FDA-approved use

Labs
• ACE inhibition can account for approx 0.5mEq/L rise in serum potassium

SPECIAL CONSIDERATIONS
PATIENT/FAMILY EDUCATION
• Caution with salt substitutes containing potassium chloride
• Rise slowly to sitting/standing position to minimize orthostatic hypotension
• Dizziness, fainting, lightheadedness may occur during 1st few days of therapy
• May cause altered taste perception or cough; persistent dry cough usually does not subside unless medication is stopped; notify clinician if these symptoms persist

MONITORING PARAMETERS
• BUN, creatinine, potassium within 2 wk after initiation of therapy (increased levels may indicate acute renal failure)
• Potassium levels, although hyperkalemia rarely occurs

---

ranitidine
(ra-ni'ti-deen)
Rx: Zantac, Zantac EFFERdose, Zantac GELdose;
OTC: Zantac 75
Chemical Class: Aminoalkyl furan derivative
Therapeutic Class: Gastrointestinal antiulcer agent

CLINICAL PHARMACOLOGY
Mechanism of Action: Competitive, reversible inhibitor of histamine at gastric H_2-receptors; reduces gastric acid secretion

Pharmacokinetics
PO: Peak 1-3 hr
IM: Peak 0.25 hr
15% bound to plasma proteins; metabolized in liver, excreted in urine (30% of PO dose, 70% of IV dose unchanged) and bile; $t_{1/2}$ 2-2½ hr (prolonged in renal impairment)

INDICATIONS AND USES: Short-term treatment and maintenance of duodenal and benign gastric ulcers; pathological hypersecretory conditions (e.g., Zollinger-Ellison syndrome, systemic mastocytosis); gastroesophageal reflux disease (GERD); erosive esophagitis; heartburn, acid indigestion and sour stomach (OTC); stress ulcer prophylaxis,* chronic idiopathic urticaria (in combination with H_1-receptor antagonists),* acute upper GI bleeding*

DOSAGE
Adult
• *Duodenal and gastric ulcer:* PO 150 mg bid or 300 mg qhs for 4-8 wk, maintenance 150 mg qhs
• *GERD:* PO 150 mg bid
• *Erosive esophagitis:* PO 150 mg qid, maintenance 150 mg bid
• *Pathological hypersecretory conditions:* PO 150 mg bid initially, titrate to desired response up to 6 g/day; IV INF start at 1 mg/kg/hr, increase by 0.5 mg/kg/hr intervals q4h prn up to 2.5 mg/kg/hr
• IM/IV 50 mg q6-8h, do not exceed 400 mg/day; IV INF 6.25 mg/hr
• *Renal impairment (CrCl <50 ml/min):* PO 150 mg qd; IV/IM 50 mg q18-24 hr

Child
• PO 1.25-2.5 mg/kg q12h, max 300 mg/day; IM/IV 0.75-1.5 mg/kg q6-8h, max 6 mg/kg/day or 300 mg/day; IV INF 0.1-0.25 mg/kg/hr

ⓢ AVAILABLE FORMS/COST OF THERAPY
• Tab, Coated—Oral: 75 mg, 30's: **$9.23** (OTC); 150 mg, 100's: **$148.00-$178.07**; 300 mg, 100's: **$111.43-$321.02**
• Tab, Effervescent—Oral: 150 mg, 60's: **$101.52**

---

italic = common side effects   ***bold italic*** = life-threatening reactions

• Cap, Gel—Oral: 150 mg, 60's: **$101.52**; 300 mg, 30's: **$91.55**

• Granule, Effervescent—Oral: 150 mg, 60's: **$101.52**

• Syr—Oral: 15 mg/ml, 480 ml: **$198.18**

• Inj, Sol—IM, IV: 25 mg/ml, 2 ml: **$3.99**

PRECAUTIONS: Renal and hepatic function impairment, elderly, gastric malignancy, rapid IV administration, immunocompromised patients

PREGNANCY AND LACTATION: Pregnancy category B; compatible with breast feeding

SIDE EFFECTS/ADVERSE REACTIONS

CNS: Dizziness, insomnia, malaise, somnolence, vertigo

CV: Atrioventricular block, bradycardia, premature ventricular beats, tachycardia

GI: Abdominal discomfort or pain, constipation, diarrhea, hepatitis, increased liver function tests, nausea, pancreatitis (rare), vomiting

HEME: **Granulocytopenia, leukopenia, thrombocytopenia**

MS: Arthralgias, myalgias

SKIN: Alopecia, **erythema multiforme** (rare), rash

INTERACTIONS

Drugs

3 *Cefuroxine; cefpodoxime; enoxacin; ketoconazole:* Reduction in gastric acidity reduces absorption, decreased plasma levels, potential for therapeutic failure

3 *Glipizide; glyburide; tolbutamide:* Increased absorption of these drugs, potential for hypoglycemia

3 *Nifedipine, nitrendipine, nisoldipine:* Increased concentrations of these drugs

Labs

• *False positive:* Urine drugs of abuse screen

SPECIAL CONSIDERATIONS

• No advantage over other agents in this class, base selection on cost

PATIENT/FAMILY EDUCATION

• Stagger doses of ranitidine and antacids

• Dissolve effervescent tablets and granules in 6-8 oz water before drinking

MONITORING PARAMETERS

• Intragastric pH when used for stress ulcer prophylaxis, titrate dose to maintain pH >4

---

repaglinide
(re-pag'lih-nide)
Rx: Prandin
Chemical Class: Meglitinide
Therapeutic Class: Oral hypoglycemic agent

CLINICAL PHARMACOLOGY

Mechanism of Action: Stimulates insulin secretion via inhibition (closing) of ATP-sensitive potassium channels in β-cells (resultant increases in β-cell calcium influx)—lowers postprandial blood sugars

Pharmacokinetics

PO: Peak onset, 30-90 min (when administered 15 min ac); 4 hr duration, rapidly absorbed (PO bioavailability, 56%); >98% plasma protein bound; complete hepatic metabolism—CYP3A4 (no active metabolites); excreted predominantly in feces (unchanged after 24 hr); elimination $t_{1/2}$ <1 hr

INDICATIONS AND USES: Oral hypoglycemic adjunct to diet and exercise; as monotherapy and combination therapy with metformin in patients with type 2 diabetes mellitus; affects primarily postprandial blood glucose; minimal effects on fasting blood glucose were observed

---

* = non-FDA-approved use

DOSAGE
Adult and Child >16 yr
• 0.5 mg—4 mg tid (30 min ac); (0.5 mg initial dose when glycosylated hemoglobin <8%; 1-2 mg initial dose for patients who received other glucose-lowering agents (start morning after previous agent stopped) or had glycosylated hemoglobin >8%); max total daily dose should not exceed 16 mg; dosage adjustments should be made at intervals of at least 1 wk (slower in patients with moderate to severe hepatic failure)

💲 AVAILABLE FORMS/COST OF THERAPY
• Tab, Coated—Oral: 0.5 mg, 100's: **$57.34;** 1 mg, 100's: **$74.58;** 2 mg, 100's: **$83.00**

CONTRAINDICATIONS: Type 1 diabetes mellitus, ketoacidosis

PRECAUTIONS: Hypoglycemia; insulin replacement may be necessary during stress (infection, fever, trauma, surgery)

PREGNANCY AND LACTATION: Pregnancy category C

SIDE EFFECTS/ADVERSE REACTIONS
GI: Nausea, diarrhea, constipation, vomiting, dyspepsia
METAB: Hypoglycemia

INTERACTIONS
Drugs
3 *Aspirin, β-blockers, sulfa drugs, chloramphenicol, warfarin, MAO inhibitors:* hypoglycemia

3 *Ketoconazole, miconazole, erythromycin, troglitazone, rifampicin, carbamazepine, phenobarbital, butalbital, secobarbital, or primidone:* potential increased repaglinide metabolism secondary to cytochrome P450 enzyme induction

3 *Thiazide diuretics, calcium channel blockers, beta blockers, cough, cold, or hay fever medicines, estrogen, birth control pills, corticosteroids, thyroid medicine, phenytoin, isoniazid, or nicotinic acid:* hyperglycemia

SPECIAL CONSIDERATIONS
PATIENT/FAMILY EDUCATION
• Skip the dose of this medication if you skip a meal; take an extra dose with extra meal
• Recognize and treat hypoglycemia; maintain ready supply of glucose (glucose tablets or gel)

MONITORING PARAMETERS
• Blood glucose—biggest effect noted on postprandial values (50-75 mg/dL reductions expected); minimal effect on fasting blood glucose
• Glycosylated hemoglobin (1% to 2% reductions expected); hyperglycemia/hypoglycemia signs and symptoms

R

---

italic = common side effects   ***bold italic*** = life-threatening reactions

reserpine
(re-ser´peen)
Rx: Eskaserp, Lemiserp,
Reserpoid, Resine, Serpalan,
Serpasil, Unitensin-R
Combinations

  Rx: with thiazide diuretics:
  i.e., bendroflumethazide
  (flumethiazide), chlorothiazide, chlorthalidone (Re-
  greton), hydrochlorothiazide (Hydropres,
  Hydroserpalan, Hydroserpine, Mallopress), hydroflumethiazide (Salutensin),
  polythiazide (Reneese),
  quinethazone (Hydromox
  R), trichloromethiazide
  (Metatensin, Naquival),
  hydrochlorothiazide and
  hydralazine (Hyserp, Lo-
  Ten, Marpres, Ser-A-Gen,
  Seralazide, Ser-Ap-Es,
  Unipres, Uni-Serp)

Chemical Class: Rauwolfia
alkaloid
Therapeutic Class: Antihypertensive; postganglionic adrenergic neuron inhibitor antipsychotic

CLINICAL PHARMACOLOGY
Mechanism of Action: Depletes
stores of catecholamines and 5-
hydroxytryptamine in the CNS and
other organs; tissue catecholamines
restored slowly, thus accumulative
effect; blood pressure reduction results from a decrease in peripheral
resistance and reduced cardiac output; sedative and tranquilizing properties also related to depletion of
catecholamines and 5-hydroxytryp-
tamine from the brain in higher doses
Pharmacokinetics
PO: Peak serum concentration 3.5 hr;
slow onset of action (days), sustained duration of effect (1-6 wk;
persistent hypotensive effects post
discontinuation); 96% bound to
plasma proteins; extensive hepatic
metabolism; 90% excreted as metabolites—30% to 60% in feces, 1%
unchanged in urine; $t_{1/2}$ 50-100 hr
INDICATIONS AND USES: Hypertension, agitated psychotic states in
patients unable to tolerate phenothiazines, hyperthyroidism,* migraine,* progressive systemic sclerosis,* Raynaud's disease,* tardive
dyskinesia*
DOSAGE
Adult
• *Hypertension:* PO 0.05 mg qd for
1-2 wk, then 0.1-0.25 mg qd; higher
doses increase incidence of mental
depression and serious side effects
• *Psychotic states:* PO 0.5 mg qd,
range 0.1-1 mg/day
Child
• PO 20 µg/kg/day, max 0.25 mg/
day

**§ AVAILABLE FORMS/COST
OF THERAPY**
• Tab, Uncoated—Oral: 0.1 mg,
100's: **$2.95-$22.62;** 0.25 mg, 100's:
$3.50-$32.13
CONTRAINDICATIONS: Current
depression or history of depression,
active peptic ulcer, ulcerative colitis, patients receiving electroconvulsive therapy
PRECAUTIONS: History of peptic
ulcer (increases GI motility and secretion), history of gallstones, renal
function impairment, children
PREGNANCY AND LACTATION:
Pregnancy category C; excreted
into breast milk, no clinical reports
of adverse effects in nursing infants
have been located
**SIDE EFFECTS/ADVERSE REAC-
TIONS**
CNS: Depression, *dizziness, drowsiness,* dull sensorium, *fatigue,* head-

ache, *lethargy,* nervousness, nightmares, paradoxical anxiety, parkinsonian syndrome and other extrapyramidal tract symptoms (rare)
CV: Angina-like symptoms, *bradycardia, **dysrhythmias** (particularly when used concurrently with digitalis or quinidine), edema, syncope
EENT: Conjunctival injection, deafness, epistaxis, glaucoma, nasal congestion, optic atrophy, uveitis
GI: Anorexia, diarrhea, dryness of mouth, hypersecretion, nausea, vomiting
GU: Decreased libido, dysuria, impotence
METAB: Breast engorgement, elevated prolactin, gynecomastia, pseudolactation, weight gain
MS: Muscular aches
RESP: Dyspnea
SKIN: Pruritus, purpura, rash
INTERACTIONS
Drugs
3 *Non-selective MAOIs:* Hypertensive reactions
Labs
• *False increase:* Serum bilirubin, urine creatinine
• *False positive:* Guiacols spot test
SPECIAL CONSIDERATIONS
• Only remaining rauwolfia derivative available
PATIENT/FAMILY EDUCATION
• May cause drowsiness or dizziness, use caution driving or participating in other activities requiring alertness
• Therapeutic effect may take 2-3 wk
MONITORING PARAMETERS
• Blood pressure, edema, drowsiness, despondency or self-depreciation, early morning insomnia, CNS depression, hypothermia, extrapyradimal tract effects

reteplase
(reh'te-place)
Rx: Retavase
Chemical Class: Tissue plasminogen activator
Therapeutic Class: Antithrombotic

CLINICAL PHARMACOLOGY
Mechanism of Action: Promotes thrombolysis by converting endogenous plasminogen to plasmin
Pharmacokinetics
IV: Fibrinogen levels fall below 100 mg/dl 2 hr following double-bolus administration, mean fibrinogen level back to normal by 48 hr; coronary artery patency is usually achieved within 30-90 min; $t_{1/2}$ 13-16 min; cleared by liver and kidney
INDICATIONS AND USES: Acute myocardial infarction
DOSAGE
Adult
• IV: 10+10 U double-bolus injection, each bolus is administered over 2 min, 30 min apart
AVAILABLE FORMS/COST OF THERAPY
• Inj—Lyphl sol kit (2×10 U plus syringes, needles, etc.): **$2750.00**
CONTRAINDICATIONS: Active internal bleeding, history of cerebrovascular accident, recent intracranial or intraspinal surgery or trauma, intracranial neoplasm, arteriovenous malformation or aneurysm, known bleeding diathesis, severe uncontrolled hypertension
PRECAUTIONS: Recent major surgery, previous puncture of noncompressible vessels, cerebrovascular disease, recent gastrointestinal or genitourinary bleeding, recent trauma; hypertension: systolic BP ≥180 mm Hg and/or diastolic BP ≥110 mm Hg; high likelihood of left

R

heart thrombus; acute pericarditis, subacute bacterial endocarditis, hemostatic defects including those secondary to severe hepatic or renal disease, severe hepatic or renal dysfunction, pregnancy, diabetic hemorrhagic retinopathy or other hemorrhagic ophthalmic conditions, septic thrombophlebitis, advanced age, patients currently receiving oral anticoagulants, any other condition in which bleeding constitutes a significant hazard

PREGNANCY AND LACTATION: Pregnancy category C

SIDE EFFECTS/ADVERSE REACTIONS

*CV: **Cardiac tamponade, electromechanical dissociation, reinfarction***

*HEME: **Bleeding***

SKIN: Allergic reactions

MISC: Fever

INTERACTIONS

Drugs

❷ *Heparin, oral anticoagulants, drugs that alter platelet function (i.e., aspirin, dipyridamole, abciximab, eptifibitide, tirofiban):* May increase the risk of bleeding

SPECIAL CONSIDERATIONS

• No other IV medications should be administered in the same line

---

ribavirin

rye-ba-vye′rin

Rx: Virazole

Combinations

   Rx: with interferon alfa-26 (Rebetrom)

Chemical Class: Nucleoside analog

Therapeutic Class: Antiviral

CLINICAL PHARMACOLOGY

Mechanism of Action: Inhibits RNA and/or DNA synthesis by respiratory syncytial virus (RSV), in-

fluenza virus (types A and B), and many other RNA and DNA viruses

Pharmacokinetics

PO: Onset 30 min, peak 1-2 hr; well absorbed

INH: Aerosol has systemic absorption; respiratory tract secretion concentration much higher than plasma concentration; $t_{1/2}$ in respiratory tract secretion 1.4-2.5 hr

Metabolized in liver and erythrocytes; plasma $t_{1/2}$ 9.5 hr; accumulates in erythrocytes, concentration plateaus at 4 days; elimination $t_{1/2}$ from erythrocytes 40 days; excreted in urine and feces

INDICATIONS AND USES: Severe lower respiratory tract infection by RSV in children (if begun within 1st 3 days of infection), influenza A,* influenza B,* hepatitis C (combination with interferon alfa-26), Lassa fever,* hantavirus-associated hemorrhagic fever*

DOSAGE

Adult

• *Influenza A or B:* INH sol of 6 g in 300 ml additive free sterile water administered by small particle aerosol generator for 18 hr then 4 hr tid per day for 3 days

• *Lassa fever:* Treatment, IV 30 mg/kg load, then in 6 hr, 16 mg/kg q6h for 4 days, then 8 mg/kg q8h for 6 days; prevention in high-risk contacts, PO 500 mg q6h for 7-10 days

• *Hantavirus-associated hemorrhagic fever:* Treatment, IV 33 mg/kg (max 2000 mg) load, then in 6 hr, 16 mg/kg (max 1000 mg) q6h for 15 doses, then 8 mg/kg (max 500 mg) q8h for 9 doses

Child

• *RSV infection:* INH sol of 6 g in 300 ml additive free sterile water administered by small particle aerosol generator for 12-18 hr per day for 3-7 days

• *Lassa fever:* Prevention in high-risk contacts, age >9 yr, PO 500 mg q6h for 7-10 days; age 6-9 yr, PO 400 mg q6h for 7-10 days

💲 AVAILABLE FORMS/COST OF THERAPY

• Aer, Sol—INH: 6 g, 4's: **$5499.38**

CONTRAINDICATIONS: Pregnancy and females of childbearing age

PRECAUTIONS: Patients receiving mechanical ventilation

PREGNANCY AND LACTATION: Pregnancy category X, teratogenic in animals; contraindicated in lactating women

SIDE EFFECTS/ADVERSE REACTIONS

CNS: Headache, *seizures (systemic administration only)*

CV: **Cardiac arrest,** hypotension

EENT: Conjunctivitis

GI: Anorexia, increased transaminases (systemic administration only), nausea

HEME: Anemia, reticulocytosis

RESP: **Apnea,** bacterial pneumonia, **pneumothorax, worsening of respiratory status**

SKIN: Rash

SPECIAL CONSIDERATIONS
PATIENT/FAMILY EDUCATION

• Female health care workers who are pregnant or may become pregnant should avoid exposure to ribavirin

MONITORING PARAMETERS

• Hematocrit

---

rifabutin

(rif′a-byoo-ten)
Rx: Mycobutin
Chemical Class: Semisynthetic rifamycin S derivative
Therapeutic Class: Antibiotic

CLINICAL PHARMACOLOGY
Mechanism of Action: Inhibits DNA-dependent RNA polymerase in susceptible strains of *Escherichia coli* and *Bacillus subtilis* but not in mammalian cells; it is not known if DNA-dependent RNA polymerase is inhibited in *M. avium* complex (MAC) (*Mycobacterium avium* and *M. intracellulare*)

Pharmacokinetics

PO: Peak 2-4 hr; high lipophilicity; 85% bound to plasma proteins; metabolized to active and inactive metabolites, excreted in feces (30%) and urine (53%); $t_{1/2}$ 45 hr

INDICATIONS AND USES: Prevention of disseminated MAC disease in patients with advanced HIV infection; (not drug of choice; macrolides are first-line)

DOSAGE

Adult

• PO 300 mg qd; if GI upset occurs, can be administered 150 mg bid with food

Child

• PO 5 mg/kg/day has been administered to small numbers of HIV-positive children

💲 AVAILABLE FORMS/COST OF THERAPY

• Cap, Gel—Oral: 150 mg, 100's: **$425.11**

CONTRAINDICATIONS: Hypersensitivity to rifamycins

PRECAUTIONS: Active tuberculosis (may lead to resistant strains), children

PREGNANCY AND LACTATION: Pregnancy category B

SIDE EFFECTS/ADVERSE REACTIONS

GI: Abdominal pain, *anorexia,* dyspepsia, eructation, flatulence, hepatitis, *nausea,* taste perversion, *vomiting*

GU: Discolored urine (30%)

HEME: **Leukopenia, neutropenia, thrombocytopenia**

MS: Mylagia

SKIN: Rash

---

italic = common side effects   **bold italic** = life-threatening reactions

R

INTERACTIONS
Drugs
☒ *Acetaminophen:* Enhanced hepatotoxicity (overdoses and possibly large therapeutic doses)

☒ *Cyclosporine:* Reduced concentration of cyclosporine

☒ *Delavirdine:* Reduced concentration of delavirdine

☒ *Eprosartan:* Reduced concentration of eprosartan

☒ *Nifedipine:* Reduced nifedipine concentrations

☒ *Oral contraceptives:* Menstrual irregularities, contraceptive failure

☒ *Oral hypoglycemics:* Reduced hypoglycemic activity

☒ *Propafenone:* Lowered propafenone concentrations, loss of antiarrhythmic efficacy

❷ *Protease inhibitors:* Increased clearance (CYP3A4 induction) and decreased protease inhibitor efficacy

☒ *Quinidine:* Marked reduction quinidine levels

☒ *Tacrolimus:* Reduced concentration of tacrolimus

SPECIAL CONSIDERATIONS
• Has liver enzyme-inducing properties similar to rifampin although less potent
• Unlike rifampin, does not appear to alter the acetylation of isoniazid

PATIENT/FAMILY EDUCATION
• May discolor bodily secretions brown-orange, soft contact lenses may be permanently stained

MONITORING PARAMETERS
• Periodic CBC with differential and platelets
• Liver function tests

---

rifampin
(rye'fam-pin)
Rx: Rifadin, Rimactane
Chemical Class: Semisynthetic rifamycin B derivative
Therapeutic Class: Antituberculosis agent; antibiotic

CLINICAL PHARMACOLOGY
Mechanism of Action: Suppresses initiation of chain formation for RNA synthesis in susceptible bacteria by inhibiting DNA-dependent RNA polymerase
Pharmacokinetics
PO: Peak 2-4 hr; widely distributed into most body tissues and fluids; 84%-91% bound to plasma proteins; metabolized in liver to active metabolite, excreted mainly in bile; $t_{1/2}$ 3 hr

INDICATIONS AND USES: All forms of tuberculosis (in combination with at least 1 other antituberculosis drug), asymptomatic *Neisseria meningitidis* carriers, prophylaxis of meningitis due to *Hemophilus influenzae,** infections caused by *Staphylococcus aureus* and *S. epidermidis,** *Legionella* when not responsive to erythromycin,* leprosy (in combination with dapsone)* Antibacterial spectrum usually includes: *Mycobacterium tuberculosis, M. bovis, M. marinum, M. kansasii;* some strains of *M. fortuitum, M. avium,* and *M. intracellulare; Staphylococcus aureus, Hemophilus influenzae, Legionella pneumophilia*

DOSAGE
Adult
• *Tuberculosis:* PO/IV 600 mg in a single daily dose for 6-9 mo (in combination with at least 1 other antituberculosis agent)

---

* = non-FDA-approved use

• *Meningococcal carriers:* PO 600 mg bid for 2 days
• *H. influenzae prophylaxis:* PO 600 mg q24h for 4 days
Child
• *Tuberculosis:* PO/IV 10-20 mg/kg, not to exceed 600 mg/day
• *Meningococcal carriers:* PO (>1 mo) 10 mg/kg q12h for 2 days; (<1 mo) 5 mg/kg q12h for 2 days
• *H. influenzae prophylaxis:* PO (<1 mo) 10 mg/kg q24h for 4 days; (>1 month) 20 mg/kg q24h for 4 days; do not exceed 600 mg/dose

$ AVAILABLE FORMS/COST OF THERAPY
• Cap, Gel—Oral: 150 mg, 100's: **$147.51**; 300 mg, 100's: **$134.10-$211.20**
• Inj, Sol—IV: 600 mg/vial, 1's: **$79.38**

CONTRAINDICATIONS: Hypersensitivity to rifamycins
PRECAUTIONS: Hepatic dysfunction, porphyria, avoid extravasation
PREGNANCY AND LACTATION: Pregnancy category C; compatible with breast feeding

SIDE EFFECTS/ADVERSE REACTIONS
CNS: Ataxia, behavioral changes, confusion, dizziness, drowsiness, fatigue, fever, headache
EENT: Visual disturbances
GI: Abnormal liver function tests, anorexia, cramps, diarrhea, epigastric distress, flatulence, heartburn, hepatitis, jaundice, nausea, *pseudo-membranous colitis*, vomiting
GU: **Acute renal failure,** elevations in BUN, hematuria, hemoglobinuria, hemolysis, interstitial nephritis, menstrual disturbances, renal insufficiency
HEME: Eosinophilia, **hemolytic anemia, thrombocytopenia, transient leukopenia**
MS: Generalized numbness, muscular weakness, pains in extremities

SKIN: Pemphigoid reaction, pruritus, rash, urticaria
MISC: "Flu" syndrome (fever, chills, headache, dizziness, bone pain)
INTERACTIONS
Drugs
3 *Acetaminophen:* Enhanced hepatotoxicity (overdoses and possibly large therapeutic doses)
3 *Aminosalicylic acid:* Reduced serum concentrations of rifampin
3 *Antidiabetics:* Diminished hypoglycemic activity of sulfonylureas
3 *Azole antifungals, barbiturates, benzodiazepines, beta-blockers (except nadolol), calcium channel blockers, chloramphenicol, clofibrate, cyclic antidepressants, dapsone, digitalis glycosides, disopyramide, lorcainide, methadone, mexiletine, nortriptyline, phenytoin, pirmenol, propafenone, quinidine, tocainide, theophylline, zidovudine:* Reduced serum concentrations of these drugs
3 *Corticosteroids:* Reduced effect of corticosteroids
2 *Cyclosporine, tacrolimus:* Reduced concentrations of these drugs, possible therapeutic failure
3 *Isoniazid:* Increased hepatotoxic potential of isoniazid in slow acetylators or patients with pre-existing liver disease
2 *Oral anticoagulants:* Reduced hypoprothrombinemic effect of oral anticoagulants
3 *Oral contraceptives:* Menstrual irregularities, contraceptive failure
2 *Protease inhibitors:* Increased clearance (CYP3A4 induction) and decreased protease inhibitor efficacy
3 *Thyroid:* Increased elimination, increased thyroid requirements
Labs
• *Increase:* Liver function tests, uric acid

R

---

italic = common side effects   ***bold italic*** = life-threatening reactions

• *Interference*: Folate, vitamin B$_{12}$, BSP, gallbladder studies

• *False decrease:* Serum bilirubin, ALT, AST (by some methods), cholesterol, triglycerides

• *False increase:* Serum bilirubin (some methods, may also be true physiologic increase), glucose, iron, LDH, uric acid, metronidazole, phosphate, tetracycline, trimethoprim

• *False positive:* Clindamycin, erythromycin, polymyxin

SPECIAL CONSIDERATIONS
PATIENT/FAMILY EDUCATION

• Take on empty stomach, at least 1 hr before or 2 hr after meals

• May cause reddish-orange discoloration of bodily secretions, may permanently discolor soft contact lenses

MONITORING PARAMETERS

• Liver function tests at baseline and q2-4 wk during therapy

• CBC with differential and platelets at baseline and periodically throughout treatment

---

rifapentine

(rif-a-pen′-teen)
Rx: Priftin

Chemical Class: Semisynthetic rifamycin B derivative
Therapeutic Class: Antituberculous agent

CLINICAL PHARMACOLOGY

Mechanism of Action: Suppresses initiation of chain formation for RNA synthesis in susceptible bacteria by inhibiting DNA-dependent RNA polymerase; bactericidal for intracellular and extracellular *M. tuberculosis* organisms

Pharmacokinetics

PO: Peak 5 hr; 70% bioavailable, increased by food; 93%-98% protein bound; metabolized by liver to active metabolite, 25-desacetyl rifapentine; metabolites excreted in stool (70%) and urine (17%); t$_{1/2}$ 13 hr; crosses placenta

INDICATIONS AND USES: Pulmonary tuberculosis (combination therapy)

DOSAGE

Adult and Child >16 yr

• PO 600 mg twice weekly with at least 72 hr between doses. After 2 mo, selected patients (e.g., clinically stable, adherent, and not HIV coinfected) may go to weekly dosing

💲 AVAILABLE FORMS/COST OF THERAPY

• Tab, Coated—Oral: 150 mg, 32s: **$87.96**

CONTRAINDICATIONS: Hypersensitivity to any rifamycin (rifampin, rifabutin)

PRECAUTIONS: Alcoholism, liver disease, pregnancy (bleeding disorders in mother and newborn when taken in late pregnancy)

PREGNANCY AND LACTATION: Pregnancy category C (teratogenic in rats); excreted in breast milk, but compatible with breast feeding

SIDE EFFECTS/ADVERSE REACTIONS

CNS: Anorexia, headache, dizziness
CV: Hypertension
GI: Diarrhea, dyspepsia, *increased transaminases (20%),* nausea, vomiting
GU: Hematuria (13%), proteinuria (17%), pyuria, urinary casts
HEME: **Anemia, lymphopenia (16%), neutropenia (18%), thrombocytopenia**
MS: Arthralgia (9%)
SKIN: Rash (13%)

INTERACTIONS

Drugs

❸ *Acetaminophen:* Enhanced hepatotoxicity

❸ *Aminosalicylic acid:* Reduced

---

* = non-FDA-approved use

plasma concentrations of rifapentine

❸ *Azole antifungals, barbiturates, benzodiazepines, beta-blockers, calcium channel blockers, chloramphenicol, clofibrate, cyclic antidepressants, dapsone, digitalis glycosides, disopyramide, lorcainide, methadone, mexiletine, phenytoin, pirmenol, propafenone, quinidine, tocainide, theophylline, zidovudine:* Reduced plasma concentrations of these drugs

❸ *Corticosteroids:* Reduced effect of corticosteroids

❷ *Cyclosporine:* Reduced plasma concentration of cyclosporine

❸ *Isoniazid:* Increased hepatotoxic potential of isoniazid in slow acetylators or patients with preexisting liver disease

❸ *Oral contraceptives:* Reduced plasma levels of these drugs with menstrual irregularity and contraceptive failure

❷ *Protease inhibitors:* Increased clearance and decreased protease inhibitor efficacy

❸ *Sulfonylureas:* Diminished hypoglycemic activity of sulfonylureas

❷ *Tacrolimus:* Reduced plasma concentration of tacrolimus

❸ *Thyroid:* Increased clearance of thyroid hormone with increased dose requirement

❷ *Warfarin:* Reduced hypoprothrombinemic effect of warfarin

Labs

• *Interference:* Folate and vitamin B_{12} levels by microbiologic assay

SPECIAL CONSIDERATIONS
PATIENT/FAMILY EDUCATION

• Use an alternative method of contraception if taking oral contraceptives concurrently

• Avoid alcoholic beverages concurrently with this medication

• Rifapentine causes urine, stool, saliva, sputum, sweat, and tears to turn reddish-orange to reddish-brown and may also permanently discolor soft contact lenses; avoid wearing soft contact lenses

MONITORING PARAMETERS

• ALT, AST, alkaline phosphate, bilirubin, and CBC prior to treatment and monthly during treatment

---

riluzole
(rye'loo-zole)
Rx: Rilutek
Chemical Class: Benzothiazole derivative
Therapeutic Class: Amyotrophic lateral sclerosis (ALS) agent

CLINICAL PHARMACOLOGY
Mechanism of Action: Mode of action unknown, but may involve an inhibitory effect on glutamate release, inactivation of voltage-dependent sodium channels, and the ability to interfere with intracellular events that follow transmitter binding at excitatory amino acid receptors

Pharmacokinetics

PO: Bioavailability 60%, reduced by high-fat meal; 96% bound to plasma proteins; extensively metabolized (some metabolites active) by liver, excreted mainly in urine (90%) and feces (5%); $t_{1/2}$ 12 hr

INDICATIONS AND USES: Amyotrophic lateral sclerosis (ALS; Lou Gehrig's disease); extends survival and/or time to tracheostomy

DOSAGE
Adult

• PO 50 mg q12h on an empty stomach

💲 AVAILABLE FORMS/COST OF THERAPY

• Tab—Oral: 50 mg, 60's: **$807.63**

PRECAUTIONS: Abnormal liver function, renal insufficiency, elderly

PREGNANCY AND LACTATION:
Pregnancy category C; excretion into breast milk unknown, use caution in nursing mothers

SIDE EFFECTS/ADVERSE REACTIONS

CNS: Asthenia, circumoral paresthesia, *dizziness, headache,* malaise, somnolence

CV: Hypertension, peripheral edema, phlebitis, postural hypotension

EENT: Vertigo

GI: Abdominal pain, anorexia, diarrhea, dyspepsia, flatulence, *nausea,* oral moniliasis, stomatitis, tooth disorder, vomiting, AST/ALT elevation

HEME: Anemia, *neutropenia*

GU: Dysuria

MS: Arthralgia, back pain

RESP: Decreased lung function, increased cough, *rhinitis*

SKIN: Alopecia, eczema, *exfoliative dermatitis,* pruritus

INTERACTIONS

Drugs

3 *Caffeine, theophylline, amitriptyline, quinolones (CYP1A2 inhibitors):* Possible decreased riluzole elimination

3 *Cigarette smoking, rifampin, omeprazole (CYP1A2 inducers):* Possible increased riluzole elimination

SPECIAL CONSIDERATIONS
MONITORING PARAMETERS

• ALT, AST qmo for 3 mo, q3mo for 1 yr, then periodically thereafter; discontinue treatment if ALT or AST increases to >5 times upper limit of normal

---

rimantadine
(ri-man'ti-deen)
Rx: Flumadine
Chemical Class: Substituted amine
Therapeutic Class: Antiviral agent

CLINICAL PHARMACOLOGY

Mechanism of Action: Inhibits growth of influenza A virus, possibly by inhibiting the uncoating of the virus

Pharmacokinetics

PO: Onset 3 hr; peak 5-7 hr; 40% protein bound; metabolized by liver ($t_{1/2}$ doubled in severe hepatic dysfunction), 25% of dose excreted in urine as unchanged drug; $t_{1/2}$ 19-31 hr (20-48 hr if age >70 yr)

INDICATIONS AND USES: Prevention and treatment (within 48 hr of onset of illness) of influenza A

DOSAGE

Adult

• *Prevention:* PO 100 mg bid; if age >65 yr or with severe hepatic or renal dysfunction (CrCl ≤10 ml/min), reduce dose to 100 mg qd

• *Treatment:* PO 100 mg bid; if age >65 yr or with severe hepatic or renal dysfunction (CrCl ≤10 ml/min), reduce dose to 100 mg qd

Child

• *Prevention:* Age >10 yr, PO 100 mg bid; age <10 yr, 5 mg/kg qd as single dose (max dose 150 mg)

$ **AVAILABLE FORMS/COST OF THERAPY**

• Syr—Oral: 50 mg/5 ml, 240 ml: **$35.64**

• Tab, Plain Coated—Oral: 100 mg, 100's: **$161.74**

CONTRAINDICATIONS: Hypersensitivity to amantadine

PRECAUTIONS: Resistant strains

---

may develop during treatment (10%-30%), lactation

PREGNANCY AND LACTATION: Pregnancy category C; concentrated in breast milk

SIDE EFFECTS/ADVERSE REACTIONS

CNS: Asthenia, ataxia, depression, dizziness, insomnia, tremor

CV: Hypertension

GI: Abdominal pain, anorexia, constipation, diarrhea, nausea, vomiting

RESP: Bronchospasm, cough

SKIN: Rash

INTERACTIONS

Drugs

⑤ *Triamterene:* Increased concentrations, toxicity rimantadine

⑤ *Trihexyphenidyl:* Increased CNS effects

---

rimexolone
(rye-mex′o-lone)
Rx: Vexol
Chemical Class: Glucocorticoid
Therapeutic Class: Ophthalmic corticosteroid

CLINICAL PHARMACOLOGY

Mechanism of Action: Suppresses aspects of the inflammatory process such as hyperemia, cellular infiltration, vascularization, and fibroblastic proliferation

Pharmacokinetics

OPHTHAL: Absorbed systemically; extensively metabolized, excreted via feces (80%); $t_{1/2}$ 1-2 hr

INDICATIONS AND USES: Postoperative inflammation following ocular surgery; anterior uveitis

DOSAGE

Adult

• *Postoperative inflammation:* Instill 1-2 gtt in conjunctival sac of affected eye(s) qid beginning 24 hr after surgery; continue for 2 wk following surgery

• *Anterior uveitis:* Instill 1-2 gtt into conjunctival sac of affected eye(s) q1h during waking hours for 1 wk; reduce to 1 gtt q2h during waking hours of 2nd week then taper until symptoms resolve

💲 **AVAILABLE FORMS/COST OF THERAPY**

• Susp—Ophth: 1%, 5, 10 ml: **$32.00**/10 ml

CONTRAINDICATIONS: Epithelial herpes simplex keratitis, vaccinia, varicella, most viral diseases of the cornea and conjunctiva; mycobacterial infection of the eye; fungal diseases of the eye; acute purulent untreated infections of the eye

PRECAUTIONS: Prolonged use (may result in ocular hypertension/glaucoma, damage to optic nerve, defects in visual acuity and visual fields, and posterior subcapsular cataract formation)

PREGNANCY AND LACTATION: Pregnancy category C

SIDE EFFECTS/ADVERSE REACTIONS

EENT: Blurred vision, discharge, discomfort, elevated intraocular pressure, foreign body sensation, hyperemia, ocular pain, posterior subcapsular cataract formation, pruritis, secondary ocular infection

SPECIAL CONSIDERATIONS

PATIENT/FAMILY EDUCATION

• Do not discontinue use without consulting clinician

• Notify clinician if no improvement after 1 wk, if condition worsens, or if pain, itching, or swelling occurs

R

risedronate

(rih-she′dron-ate)
Rx: Actonel
Chemical Class: Synthetic analog of pyrophosphate
Therapeutic Class: Bisphosphonate; bone resorption inhibitor

CLINICAL PHARMACOLOGY
Mechanism of Action: Binds to hydroxyapatite at sites of bone resorption, inhibiting normal and abnormal bone resorption ("crystal poison"); minimal secondary reduction in bone formation (resorption coupled to formation)

Pharmacokinetics
PO: Peak 1 hr; (A significant decrease in, or normalization of, serum calcium has been reported after one week of oral risedronate administration in patients with primary hyperparathyroidism); poor PO absorption (1%); food reduces absorption further 50%; 60% bound to bone in 12-24 hr; not metabolized; remainder excreted in urine; $t_{1/2}$, 220 hr (representing dissociation of risedronate from bone surface)

INDICATIONS AND USES: Paget's disease, hyperparathyroidism,* hypercalcemia of malignancy,* osteoporosis,* osteoporosis—glucocorticoid induced*

DOSAGE
Adult and Child >16 yr
• Paget's Disease: PO 30 mg qd ×2 months
• Osteoporosis (prophylaxis): PO 2.5-5 mg qd
• Primary hyperparathyroidism: 20 mg qd

💲 **AVAILABLE FORMS/COST OF THERAPY**
• Tab, Coated—Oral: 30 mg, 30's: **$386.40**

CONTRAINDICATIONS: Hypocalcemia
PRECAUTIONS: Renal impairment, congestive heart failure, hyperphosphatemia (potential for increased tubular reabsorption of phosphate), liver disease, fever
PREGNANCY AND LACTATION: Pregnancy category C; breast milk excretion unknown
SIDE EFFECTS/ADVERSE REACTIONS
CV: Chest pain
EENT: Iritis, dry eyes
GI: Diarrhea (20%); epigastric pain (rarely)
MS: Arthralgias, myesthenia
INTERACTIONS
Drugs
3 *Antacids, calcium:* decreased absorption of risedronate
3 *Food:* decreases bioavailability of risedronate by 50%
SPECIAL CONSIDERATIONS
PATIENT/FAMILY EDUCATION
• Administer 30 minutes before the first food/beverage/medication of the day, with 6-8 oz plain water
MONITORING PARAMETERS
• Albumin-adjusted serum calcium; N-telopeptide, alkaline phosphatase, phosphorus, osteocalcin, DEXA scan, bone and joint pain, fractures on x-ray (osteoporosis, Paget's disease)

risperidone

(ris-per′i-done)
Rx: Risperdal
Chemical Class: Benzisoxazole derivative
Therapeutic Class: Antipsychotic

CLINICAL PHARMACOLOGY
Mechanism of Action: Serotonin 5-HT$_2$ >dopamine-(D$_2$-) receptor antagonist; activity against sev-

eral neurotransmitter systems: selective antagonist at limbic dopamine receptors (D_1, D_2, D_4, D_5) and serotonin receptors (5-HT_2, 5-HT_6, 5-HT_7); antagonism at α_1-adrenergic receptors; and activity at muscarinic, histamine H_1, or nicotinic receptors; minimal sedation, orthostatic hypotension, and weight gain; no anticholinergic effects; mild to moderate extrapyramidal symptoms (at higher doses, i.e., >10 mg) extrapyramidal reaction risk becomes similar to typical antipsychotics

Pharmacokinetics

PO: Peak level 1 hr; metabolized by liver to active metabolite, 9-hydroxyrisperidone (8% of Caucasians are poor metabolizers); mean elimination $t_{1/2}$ of total risperidone and 9-hydroxyrisperidone 20 hr; excreted in urine and feces; protein binding 85%

INDICATIONS AND USES: Psychotic disorders

DOSAGE

Adult

• PO: 1 mg bid, increase to 2 mg bid on 2nd day and 3 mg bid on 3rd day, then increase weekly as needed (usual effective dose 4-8 mg daily; max daily dose 16 mg; can be dosed either qd or bid); initial dose 0.5 mg bid increasing to 1.5 mg bid by 3rd day in elderly or those with severe renal or hepatic impairment

🔅 AVAILABLE FORMS/COST OF THERAPY

• Tab, Coated—Oral: 1 mg, 60's: **$146.16;** 2 mg, 60's: **$243.26;** 3 mg, 60's: **$287.28;** 4 mg, 60's: **$378.58**
• Sol—Oral: 1 mg/ml, 100 ml: **$286.54**

PRECAUTIONS: Neuroleptic malignant syndrome, tardive dyskinesia, prolonged QT interval, seizures

PREGNANCY AND LACTATION: Pregnancy category C; excreted in breast milk

SIDE EFFECTS/ADVERSE REACTIONS

CNS: Aggressive reaction, *anxiety, decreased libido,* dizziness, *EPS (frequency is dose related), increased dream activity,* insomnia, *somnolence*

CV: Orthostatic hypotension, tachycardia

EENT: Abnormal vision (accommodation), *dry mouth*

GI: Abdominal pain, *constipation, dyspepsia,* nausea, vomiting

GU: Menorrhagia, polyuria, sexual (erectile and orgasmic) dysfunction, urinary retention, vaginal dryness

HEME: Anemia

METAB: Amenorrhea, galactorrhea, gynecomastia, hyponatremia

MS: Arthralgia, back pain, chest pain

RESP: Cough, dyspnea, pharyngitis, *rhinitis,* sinusitis

SKIN: Dry skin, *increased pigmentation, photosensitivity,* rash, seborrhea

MISC: Fatigue, fever

INTERACTIONS

Drugs

3 *Levodopa, dopamine agonists:* Risperidone may antagonize effect

SPECIAL CONSIDERATIONS

PATIENT/FAMILY EDUCATION

• Risk of orthostatic hypotension, especially during the period of initial dose titration

• Do not operate machinery during dose titration period

R

---

italic = common side effects   ***bold italic*** = life-threatening reactions

ritonavir

(ri-tone'a-veer)
Rx: Norvir
Chemical Class: HIV Protease inhibitor
Therapeutic Class: HIV infection

CLINICAL PHARMACOLOGY
Mechanism of Action: Protease inhibitor of HIV; antiretroviral effects via interference with protease enzyme processing of Gag-Pol polyproteins, resulting in budding of immature noninfectious particles; inhibits both acutely and chronically infected cells

Pharmacokinetics
PO: Peak levels at 2-4 hr (>2 µg/ml at doses of 800 mg/day—*in vivo* effective vs. HIV-1); well absorbed; $t_{1/2}$ 3.5 hr

INDICATIONS AND USES: HIV-infected adults

DOSAGE
Adult
• *HIV infection:* PO 600 mg bid in combination with nucleoside analogues (to reduce nausea at initiation of therapy, prescribe 300 mg bid for 1 day, 400 mg bid for 2 days, 500 mg bid for 1 day, and finally 600 mg bid thereafter)
• Adjust dose when used with indinavir, nelfinavir, saquinavir

Child
• *HIV infection:* PO 400 mg/m^2 not to exceed 600 mg bid; start at 250 mg/m^2 and increase every 2-3 days by 50 mg/m^2 twice daily. If 400 mg/m^2 is not tolerated, the highest tolerated dose should be used for maintenance in combination with nucleoside analogues
• For latest treatment guidelines, see www.hivatis.org

* = non-FDA-approved use

$ **AVAILABLE FORMS/COST OF THERAPY**
• Cap—Oral: 100 mg, 120's: **$222.60**
• Sol—Oral: 80 mg/ml, 240 ml: **$311.65**
PRECAUTIONS: Liver disease
PREGNANCY AND LACTATION: Pregnancy category B; breast milk excretion unknown; breast feeding by HIV+ mothers not recommended
SIDE EFFECTS/ADVERSE REACTIONS
CNS: Abnormal dreams, *abnormal thinking,* agitation, amnesia, anxiety, aphasia, *asthenia (9%-14%),* ataxia, *circumoral paresthesia (15%),* confusion, convulsion, depression, diplopia, *dizziness,* euphoria, hallucinations, *headache,* hyperesthesia, incoordination, *insomnia, malaise,* nervousness, neuralgia, neuropathy, paralysis, personality disorder, peripheral neuropathy, *peripheral paresthesia (6%), somnolence,* tremor, vertigo
CV: Hemorrhage, hypotension, migraine, orthostatic hypotension, palpitations, peripheral vascular disorder, syncope, tachycardia, *vasodilation (2%)*
EENT: Abnormal electro-oculogram, abnormal electroretinogram, abnormal vision, blurred vision, blepharitis, eye pain, iritis, photophobia, uveitis, visual field defect
GI: Abdominal pain (7%), anorexia *(6%),* cheilitis, colitis, constipation, *diarrhea (12%-18%),* dry mouth, dyspepsia, dysphagia, elevations in liver transaminases (2%-15%), eructation, esophagitis, flatulence, gastritis, gastroenteritis, GI bleeding, gingivitis, hepatitis, hepatomegaly, ileitis, local throat irritation, *nausea (23%-26%),* oral candidiasis, pancreatitis, periodontal disease, *taste perversion (5%-10%), vomiting (12%-15%)*

GU: Decreased libido, dysuria, hematuria, impotence, kidney calculus, kidney failure, kidney pain, nocturia, polyuria, pyelonephritis, urethritis, urinary frequency, urinary retention

HEME: Anemia, ecchymosis, leukopenia, lymphadenophaty, lymphocytosis, thrombocytopenia

METAB: Avitaminosis, chills, dehydration, diabetes mellitus, edema, fever, gout, glycosuria, hypercholesterolemia, hyperlipidemia, hypothermia, increased phosphokinase, increased serum cholesterol, peripheral edema, sweating, thirst, triglycerides, weight loss

MS: Arthralgia, arthrosis, joint disorder, muscle cramps, muscle weakness, *myalgia,* myositis, twitching

RESP: Asthma, cough, dyspnea, epistaxis, hiccup, hypoventilation, interstitial pneumonia, *pharyngitis,* rhinitis

SKIN: Acne, contact dermatitis, dry skin, eczema, folliculitis, maculopapular rash, molluscum contagiosum, pruritus, psoriasis, *rash,* seborrhea, urticaria, vesiculobullous rash

INTERACTIONS

Drugs

⚠ *Amiodarone:* Increased plasma levels of amiodarone

⚠ *Astemizole:* Increased plasma levels of astemizole

3 *Barbiturates:* Increased clearance of ritonavir; reduced clearance of barbiturates

⚠ *Bepredil:* Increased plasma levels of bepredil

⚠ *Bupropion:* Increased plasma levels of bupropion

2 *Carbamazepine:* Increased clearance of ritonavir; reduced clearance of carbamazepine

⚠ *Cisapride:* Increased plasma levels of cisapride

2 *Clarithromycin:* Reduced clearance of ritonavir; ritonavir reduces clearance of clarithromycin; reduce clarithromycin dose for renal insufficiency

⚠ *Clorazepate:* Increased plasma levels of clorazepate

⚠ *Clozapine:* Increased plasma levels of clozapine

3 *Despiramine:* Ritonavir increases AUC of desipramine by 145%

⚠ *Diazepam:* Increased plasma levels of diazepam

⚠ *Encainide:* Increased plasma levels of encainide

⚠ *Ergot alkaloids:* Increased plasma levels of ergot alkaloids

3 *Erythromycin:* Reduced clearance of ritonavir; ritonavir reduces clearance of erythromycin

⚠ *Estazolam:* Increases plasma levels of estazolam

⚠ *Flecainide:* Increased plasma levels of flecainide

⚠ *Flurazepam:* Increased plasma levels of flurazepam

3 *Indinavir:* Increased plasma level of indinavir; reduce dose to 400 mg bid when ritonavir dose is 400 mg bid

3 *Ketoconazole:* Ritonavir reduces clearance of ketoconazole; reduce ketoconazole dose

⚠ *Lovastatin:* Ritonavir reduces clearance of lovastatin

⚠ *Meperidine:* Increased plasma levels of meperidine

3 *Methadone:* Ritonavir reduces methadone plasma concentration by 37%

⚠ *Midazolam:* Increased plasma levels of midazolam and prolonged effect

3 *Nelfinavir:* Increased plasma level of nelfinavir; reduce nelfinavir dose to 750 mg bid when ritonavir dose is 400 mg bid

3 *Oral contraceptives:* Ritonavir may reduce efficacy

R

---

italic = common side effects   ***bold italic*** = life-threatening reactions

■ *Phenytoin:* Increased clearance of ritonavir; reduced clearance of phenytoin

⚠ *Pimozide:* Increased plasma levels of pimozide

⚠ *Piroxicam:* Increased plasma levels of piroxicam

⚠ *Propafenone:* Increased plasma levels of propafenone

⚠ *Propoxyphene:* Increased plasma levels of propoxyphene

⚠ *Quinidine:* Increased plasma levels of quinidine

② *Rifabutin:* Increased clearance of ritonavir; reduced clearance of rifabutin; reduce rifabutin dose to 150 mg qod

■ *Rifampin:* Increased clearance of ritonavir

■ *Saquinavir:* Decreased clearance of saquinavir; reduce dose of Fortovase (saquinavir soft gel capsule) to 800 mg bid when ritonavir dose is 400 mg bid

⚠ *Simvastatin:* Ritonavir reduces clearance of simvastatin

⚠ *Terfenadine:* Increased plasma levels of terfenadine

■ *Theophylline:* Ritonavir reduces theophylline plasma concentration

⚠ *Triazolam:* Increased plasma levels of triazolam and prolonged effect

■ *Troleandomycin:* Reduced clearance of ritonavir; ritonavir reduces clearance of troleandomycin

⚠ *Zolpidem:* Increased plasma levels of zolpidem

SPECIAL CONSIDERATIONS
• As with other protease inhibitors, ritonavir will predominantly be used in combination regimens; the ability of ritonavir (alone or in combinations) to modify clinical endpoints (e.g., time to 1st AIDS-defining illness or death) will be important in determining the ultimate role of this agent in HIV; potential for drug interaction is troublesome; as with

other protease inhibitors, resistance has been problematic after several mo of treatment

PATIENT/FAMILY EDUCATION
• Store capsules in the refrigerator between 36° and 46° F (2°-8° C); protect from light; store oral sol in the refrigerator until it is dispensed; refrigeration of oral sol by the patient is not required if used within 30 days and stored below 77° F (25° C); avoid exposure to excessive heat; product should be stored in the original container and the cap tightly closed

MONITORING PARAMETERS
• Therapeutic: serum HIV-1 RNA, and CD4+ cell counts (every 2-4 wk)
• Take with food to improve tolerability
• Toxicity: complete blood counts, routine blood chemistry, liver function tests, and serum lipid and lipoprotein profiles

---

rizatriptan
(rize-a-trip'tan)
Rx: Maxalt; Maxalt MLT
Chemical Class: Serotonin derivative
Therapeutic Class: Antimigraine agent

CLINICAL PHARMACOLOGY
Mechanism of Action: Selectively activates vascular 5-HT$_1$-receptors in cranial arteries causing vasoconstriction and inhibition of proinflammatory neuropeptide release, actions correlating with the relief of migraine in humans
Pharmacokinetics
PO: 45% bioavailability, peak 1-1.5 hr
MLT (orally disintigrating tablet): Peak 1.6-2.5 hr
14% bound to plasma proteins; me-

tabolism mainly via oxidative deamination by MAO-A; 82% excreted in urine (14% unchanged), 12% in feces; $t_{1/2}$ 2-3 hr

INDICATIONS AND USES: Acute migraine headache with or without aura

DOSAGE

Adult

• PO 5-10 mg at first sign of headache; may repeat after 2 hr if partial response or headache returns (max 30 mg/24 hr)

§ AVAILABLE FORMS/COST OF THERAPY

• Tab, Compressed—PO 5 mg, 6's: **$81.00;** 10 mg, 6's: **$81.00**

• Tab, Orally Disintigrating—PO 5 mg, 6's: **$81.00;** 10 mg, 6's: **$81.00**

CONTRAINDICATIONS: Ischemic heart disease; hemiplegic or basilar migraine; Prinzmetal's angina; uncontrolled hypertension; within 24 hr of ergotamine-containing products or other 5-HT$_1$-receptor agonist; concurrent use of MAO inhibitor therapy (or within 2 wk of discontinuing an MAO inhibitor)

PRECAUTIONS: Atypical headache; dialysis patients or hepatic impairment; elderly; children; phenylketonuric patients (MLT formulation contains phenylalanine)

PREGNANCY AND LACTATION: Pregnancy category C; use caution in nursing mothers

SIDE EFFECTS/ADVERSE REACTIONS

CNS: Paresthesia, dizziness, fatigue, drowsiness, vertigo, tremors, cognitive function disorders, sleep disorders, equilibrium disorders

CV: Palpitations, increased blood pressure, tachyarrhythmias, abnormal ECG, syncope

EENT: Photophobia, blurred vision, tinnitus

GI: Nausea, hyposalivation, vomiting, dyspeptic symptoms, diarrhea, constipation

GU: Bladder inflammation, polyuria, diuresis

HEME: Increased white cells

METAB: Thirst, polydipsia, dehydration, fluid retention

MS: Muscle pain, arthralgia, articular rheumatism, muscle cramps/spasms, joint/muscle stiffness, tightness, rigidity

RESP: Bronchitis, cough, pneumonia

SKIN: Sweating, rash, pruritus, urticaria

MISC: Pain/pressure sensations in neck/throat/jaw; chills, fever

INTERACTIONS

Drugs

⚠ *Ergotamine-containing drugs:* Increased vasoconstriction

⚠ *MAO inhibitors:* Potential for decreased metabolism of rizatriptan

3 *Propranolol:* Propranolol has been shown to increase the plasma concentrations of rizatriptan by 70%; patients receiving propranolol should use 5 mg tablets (max 15 mg/24 hr)

2 *Sibutramine:* Increased risk of serotonin syndrome

SPECIAL CONSIDERATIONS

• Safety of treating, on average, more than 4 headaches in a 30-day period has not been established

• MLT does not provide faster absorption or onset of effect because almost the entire dose is swallowed with saliva and absorbed in the GI tract

PATIENT/FAMILY EDUCATION

• Use only to treat migraine headache, not for prevention

• MLT, administration with liquid is not necessary; orally disintegrating tablet is packaged in a blister within an outer aluminum pouch, do not remove the blister from the outer pouch until just prior to dosing; blister pack should then be

R

---

italic = common side effects   ***bold italic*** = life-threatening reactions

peeled open with dry hands and the orally disintegrating tablet placed on the tongue, where it will dissolve and be swallowed with the saliva

ropinirole
(ro-pin'i-role)
Rx: ReQuip
Chemical Class: Propylaminobenzothiazole (non-ergoline)
Therapeutic Class: Antiparkinson agent, dopaminergic

CLINICAL PHARMACOLOGY
Mechanism of Action: Selective dopamine-2 (D2) receptor agonist
Pharmacokinetics
PO: Peak 1-2 hr; $t_{1/2}$ 3-4 hr
INDICATIONS AND USES: Parkinson's disease
DOSAGE
Adult
• *Parkinson's disease:* Slow initiation titration necessary; titration kit available from company; dose titration schedule: Week 1, 0.25 mg tid; week 2, 0.5 mg tid; week 3, 0.75 mg tid; week 4, 1 mg tid; then increase by 1.5 mg/day weekly to a total of 24 mg/day if necessary
⑤ AVAILABLE FORMS/COST OF THERAPY
• Tab—Oral: 0.25 mg, 0.5 mg, 1 mg, 2 mg, 100's: **$93.10;** 5 mg, 100's: **$186.20**
PRECAUTIONS: Cardiovascular disease, breast feeding, pregnancy
PREGNANCY AND LACTATION: Pregnancy category D; inhibits lactation
SIDE EFFECTS/ADVERSE REACTIONS
CNS: Drowsiness, euphoria, somnolence
CV: Bradycardia, postural hypotension, supraventricular ectopy (rare)
GI: Nausea

INTERACTIONS
Drugs
⑧ *Ciprofloxacin, enoxacin, pefloxacin:* Addition increases ropinirole concentrations
⑧ *Dopamine antagonists:* Diminished anti-Parkinson's effect
⑧ *Estrogens:* Reduced ropinirole clearance, may need to decrease ropinirole if estrogen stopped
SPECIAL CONSIDERATIONS
• Domperidone 20 mg 1 hr prior to ropinirole prevents drug-induced postural effects
• Discontinue slowly over 1 wk

salicylic acid
(sal-i-sill'ik)
OTC: Compound W, DuoFilm, DuoPlant, Freezone, Gets-it, Gordofilm, Keralyt, Mediplast, Mosco, Occlusal-HP, Off-Ezy, Sal-Acid, Salactic Film, Sal-Plant, Trans-Ver-Sal, Wart Away, Wart Fix, Wart Remover
Combinations
  Rx: with sodium thiosulfate (Versiclear)
Chemical Class: Salicylate derivative
Therapeutic Class: Keratolytic

CLINICAL PHARMACOLOGY
Mechanism of Action: Produces desquamation of hyperkeratotic epithelium; dissolves intracellular cement substance
Pharmacokinetics
TOP: Peak 5 hr when occlusive dressing used; 50%-80% bound to plasma proteins; metabolized and excreted in urine
INDICATIONS AND USES: Removal of excessive keratin in hyperkeratotic skin disorders, including common and plantar warts, psoriasis, calluses, corns

* = non-FDA-approved use

DOSAGE
Adult and Child
• Gel: TOP apply thin layer to affected area(s) qd-bid
• Plaster: TOP cut to size that covers corn or callus, apply and leave in place for 48 hr; do not exceed 5 applications over 2 wk period
• Liq: TOP apply thin layer directly to wart qd as directed for 1 wk or until wart is removed

💲 AVAILABLE FORMS/COST OF THERAPY
• Liq—Top: 12%, 15 ml: **$2.39**; 17%, 10, 15 ml: **$4.58-$13.92**
• Gel—Top: 6%, 30 g: **$7.47**; 17%, 7.5, 15 g: **$4.58-$7.40**
• Film—Top: 15%, 10's **$9.83**; 17%, 18's: **$7.40**
• Plaster, Adhesive—Top: 40%, 25's: **$24.06**

CONTRAINDICATIONS: Prolonged use; diabetes; impaired circulation; use on moles, birthmarks, or warts with hair growing from them; genital or facial warts; warts on mucous membranes; irritated skin; infected skin

PRECAUTIONS: Children

PREGNANCY AND LACTATION: Pregnancy category C

SIDE EFFECTS/ADVERSE REACTIONS
SKIN: Burning, local irritation
MISC: Salicylism (tinnitus, hearing loss, dizziness, confusion, headache, hyperventilation)

SPECIAL CONSIDERATIONS
PATIENT/FAMILY EDUCATION
• For external use only; avoid contact with face, eyes, genitals, mucous membranes, and normal skin surrounding warts
• May cause reddening or scaling of skin
• Soaking area in warm water for 5 min prior to application may enhance effect (remove any loose tissue with brush, washcloth, or emery board and dry thoroughly prior to application)

---

salmeterol
(sal-me'te-rol)
Rx: Serevent, Serevent Diskus
Chemical Class: Sympathomimetic amine; β$_2$-adrenergic agonist
Therapeutic Class: Antiasthmatic, bronchodilator

CLINICAL PHARMACOLOGY
Mechanism of Action: Causes long-lasting bronchodilation by β$_2$-stimulation, resulting in relaxation of bronchial smooth muscle; inhibits mast cell degranulation; stimulates cilia to remove secretions; approximately 50 times more selective for β-$_2$-adrenergic receptors than albuterol

Pharmacokinetics
INH: Onset within 20 min, peak effect 2 hr, duration 12 hr; low systemic absorption; 94%-98% bound to plasma proteins; metabolized in liver, eliminated in feces; t$_{1/2}$ 3-4 hr

INDICATIONS AND USES: Maintenance of bronchodilation and prevention of symptoms of asthma, including nocturnal asthma; prevention of exercise-induced bronchospasm; maintenance treatment of bronchospasm associated with chronic bronchitis and emphysema (COPD)

DOSAGE
Adult and Child >12 yr
• *Asthma, COPD:* MDI 2 puffs q12h
• *Exercise-induced asthma:* MDI 2 puffs 30-60 min before exercise; do not repeat earlier than 12 hr following initial dose

💲 AVAILABLE FORMS/COST OF THERAPY
• MDI—INH: 21 µg/puffs, 6.5g:

S

$38.63 (60 puffs); 13 g: $61.88 (120 puffs)

• Powder, Disk—INH: 46 µg/INH, 28's: $42.00; 60's: $67.75

CONTRAINDICATIONS: Significantly worsening or acutely deteriorating asthma, acute symptoms

PRECAUTIONS: Cardiovascular disorders, coronary insufficiency, cardiac dysrhythmias, hypertension, convulsive disorders, thyrotoxicosis, children <12 yr, psychosis, diabetes, history of stroke

PREGNANCY AND LACTATION: Pregnancy category C

SIDE EFFECTS/ADVERSE REACTIONS

CNS: Anxiety, dizziness, headache, insomnia, nervousness, stimulation, tremors

CV: Cardiac arrest, dysrhythmias, hypertension, lengthened QT segment, palpitations, tachycardia

EENT: Throat irritation

GI: Bad taste, GI distress, nausea, vomiting

METAB: Hyperglycemia, hypokalemia

MS: Muscle cramps in extremities

RESP: Cough, dyspnea, *paradoxical bronchospasm*

INTERACTIONS

Drugs

❷ β-*blockers:* Decreased action of salmeterol, cardioselective β-blockers preferable if concurrent use necessary

❸ *Furosemide:* Potential for additive hypokalemia

SPECIAL CONSIDERATIONS

PATIENT/FAMILY EDUCATION

• Proper inhalation technique is vital

• Excessive use may lead to adverse effects

• Notify clinician if no response to usual doses, or if palpitations, rapid heartbeat, chest pain, muscle tremors, dizziness, headache occur

* = non-FDA-approved use

• **Do not use to treat acute symptoms or on an as-needed basis**

---

salsalate

(sal′sa-late)

Rx: Amigesic, Argesic-SA, Disalcid, Marthritic, Mono-Gesic, Salflex, Salsitab

Chemical Class: Salicylate derivative

Therapeutic Class: Nonnarcotic analgesic; NSAID

CLINICAL PHARMACOLOGY

Mechanism of Action: Inhibits prostaglandin synthesis; analgesic, anti-inflammatory, antipyretic actions

Pharmacokinetics

PO: Onset of anti-inflammatory action 3-4 days; 75%-90% bound to plasma proteins; hydrolyzed in liver to salicylic acid (active); excreted in urine; $t_{1/2}$ 7-8 hr

INDICATIONS AND USES: Mild to moderate pain, rheumatoid arthritis, osteoarthritis, related rheumatic disorders

DOSAGE

Adult

• PO 3 g/day divided bid-tid

$ AVAILABLE FORMS/COST OF THERAPY

• Cap, Gel—Oral: 500 mg, 100's: $59.64

• Tab, Coated—Oral: 500 mg, 100's: $11.90-$57.18; 750 mg, 100's: $9.30-$73.26

CONTRAINDICATIONS: Hypersensitivity to NSAIDs, hemophilia, bleeding ulcers, hemorrhagic states

PRECAUTIONS: Children or teenagers with chickenpox or influenza (association with Reye's syndrome), impaired hepatic or renal function, history of peptic ulcer disease, diabetes mellitus, gout, anemia, diabetes

PREGNANCY AND LACTATION:
Pregnancy category C; excreted into breast milk; use caution in nursing mothers due to potential adverse effects in nursing infant

SIDE EFFECTS/ADVERSE REACTIONS

CNS: Confusion, dizziness, drowsiness, headache

EENT: Dimness of vision, reversible hearing loss, tinnitus

GI: Acute reversible hepatotoxicity, anorexia, diarrhea, *dyspepsia,* epigastric discomfort, **GI bleeding,** heartburn, *nausea*

HEME: Decreased plasma iron concentration, **leukopenia,** shortened erythrocyte survival time, ***thrombocytopenia***

RESP: Hyperpnea, wheezing

SKIN: Angioedema, bruising, hives, rash, urticaria

MISC: Fever, thirst

INTERACTIONS

Labs

• *False increase:* Serum bicarbonate, CSF, protein, serum theophylline

• *False decrease:* Urine cocaine, urine estrogen, serum glucose, urine 17-hydroxycorticosteroids, urine opiates

• *False positive:* Urine ferric chloride test

SPECIAL CONSIDERATIONS

• Consider for patients with GI intolerance to aspirin or patients in whom interference with normal platelet function by aspirin or other NSAIDs is undesirable

MONITORING PARAMETERS

• AST, ALT, bilirubin, creatinine, CBC, hematocrit if patient is on long-term therapy

saquinavir
(sa-kwin'a-veer)
Rx: Fortovase, Invirase
Chemical Class: HIV protease inhibitor
Therapeutic Class: HIV infection

CLINICAL PHARMACOLOGY
Mechanism of Action: Inihibits HIV protease preventing cleavage of the viral polyproteins, resulting in the formation of immature noninfectious viral particles

Pharmacokinetics

PO: Absolute bioavailability 4%, increased by high-fat meal; 98% bound to plasma proteins; metabolized by hepatic cytochrome P450 enzymes, excreted in feces (88%) and urine (1%); mean residence time 7 hr

NOTE: Fortovase delivers more drug for prolonged periods compared to Invirase

INDICATIONS AND USES: Advanced HIV infection in combination with nucleoside analogues

DOSAGE

Adult

• Invirase PO 400 mg bid with ritonavir; Invirase otherwise not recommended

• Fortovase PO 1200 mg (6×200 mg caps) tid

• Adjust dose when used with delavirdine, efavirenz, nelfinavir, ritonavir

• For latest treatment guidelines, see www.hivatis.org

AVAILABLE FORMS/COST OF THERAPY

• Invirase Cap—Oral: 200 mg, 270's: **$603.95-$652.08**

• Fortovase Cap—Oral: 200 mg, 180's: **$207.71**

CONTRAINDICATIONS: Concurrent use of rifampin

PRECAUTIONS: Children <16 yr,

S

hepatic insufficiency; concurrent use of ritabutin

PREGNANCY AND LACTATION:
Pregnancy category B

SIDE EFFECTS/ADVERSE REACTIONS

CNS: Asthenia, dizziness, extremity numbness, headache, paresthesia, peripheral neuropathy

GI: Abdominal discomfort, abdominal pain, appetite disturbance, buccal mucosa ulceration, *diarrhea,* dyspepsia, mucosa damage, *nausea*

MS: Musculoskeletal pain, myalgia

SKIN: Pruritis, rash

INTERACTIONS

Drugs

⚠ *Astemizole:* Increased plasma levels of astemizole

🔟 *Barbiturates:* Increased clearance of saquinavir; reduced clearance of barbiturates

❷ *Carbamazepine:* Increased clearance of saquinavir, reduced clearance of carbamazepine

⚠ *Cisapride:* Increased plasma levels of cisapride

🔟 *Clarithromycin:* Reduced clearance of saquinavir; saquinavir reduces clearance of clarithromycin

🔟 *Delavirdine:* Decreased clearance of saquinavir; reduce dose of Fortovase (saquinavir soft gel capsule) to 800 mg tid

🔟 *Dexamethasone:* Reduced saquinavir level

⚠ *Efavirenz:* Reduced saquinavir level

⚠ *Ergot alkaloids:* Increased plasma levels of ergot alkaloids

🔟 *Erythromycin:* Reduced clearance of saquinavir; saquinavir reduces clearance of erythromycin

🔟 *Grapefruit juice:* Reduced saquinavir level

⚠ *Indinavir:* Decreased clearance of saquinavir

⚠ *Lovastatin:* Saquinavir reduces clearance of lovastatin

⚠ *Midazolam:* Increased plasma levels of midazolam and prolonged effect

🔟 *Nelfinavir:* Decreased clearance of saquinavir; reduce dose of Fortovase (saquinavir soft gel capsule) to 800 mg tid

🔟 *Oral contraceptives:* Saquinavir may reduce efficacy

🔟 *Phenytoin:* Increased clearance of saquinavir; reduced clearance of phenytoin

⚠ *Rifabutin:* Increased clearance of saquinavir

⚠ *Rifampin:* Increased clearance of saquinavir

🔟 *Ritonavir:* Decreased clearance of saquinavir; decreased saquinavir dose to 400 mg bid

⚠ *Simvastatin:* Saquinavir reduces clearance of simvastatin

⚠ *Terfenadine:* Increased plasma levels of terfenadine

⚠ *Triazolam:* Increased plasma levels of triazolam and prolonged effect

SPECIAL CONSIDERATIONS
• Invirase and fortovase not considered bioequivalent; no food effect on Invirase when taken with ritonavir; take Fortovase with large meal

---

scopolamine
(skoe-pol'a-meen)
Rx: *Transdermal:* Transderm-Scop
Ophth: Isopto Hyoscine
Oral: Scopace
Chemical Class: Belladonna alkaloid
Therapeutic Class: Mydriatic; cycloplegic; antiemetic; antivertigo agent; anticholinergic

---

CLINICAL PHARMACOLOGY
Mechanism of Action: Choliner-

gic receptor blocker decreases production of GI secretions and stomach acid; central muscarinic receptor blocker decreases involuntary movements; inhibition of vestibular input to the CNS, inhibits vomiting reflex; direct inhibitory effect on vomiting center in brain stem; ophth blocks cholinergic response of iris sphincter and accommodation of ciliary body to cholinergic stimulation resulting in dilation, paralysis of accommodation

Pharmacokinetics

SC/IM: Onset 30 min, duration 4 hr
IV: Peak 10-15 min, duration 4 hr
TRANSDERMAL: Onset 3 hr, duration, up to 72 hr
OPHTH: Peak 20-30 min, duration 3-7 days
Excreted in urine, bile, feces (unchanged), $t_{1/2}$ 8 hr

INDICATIONS AND USES: Systemic: Reduction of secretions before surgery; calm delirium; transdermal: motion sickness, vertigo; nausea and vomiting*; ophth: uveitis, iritis, cycloplegia, mydriasis

DOSAGE

• Geriatric and pediatric patients more sensitive to anticholinergic effects

Adult

• *Preoperatively:* SC/IM/IV 0.32-0.65 mg; dilute IV with sterile water; transderm 1.5 mg

• OPHTH instill 1-2 gtt before refraction or 1-2 gtt qd-tid for iritis or uveitis

• *Motion Sickness:* Place 1 patch behind ear 4-5 hr before travel; replace q72h prn

• *Nausea associated with analgesia and opiate anesthesia:* Transderm 1.5 mg q72h

Child

• OPHTH: instill 1 gtt bid × 2 days before refraction

• *Preoperatively:* SC 0.006 mg/kg or 0.2 mg/m^2

⑧ AVAILABLE FORMS/COST OF THERAPY

• Inj, Sol—IM, IV, SC: 0.4 mg/ml, 1 ml: **$1.76**; 1 mg/ml, 1 ml: **$1.76**
• Tab—Oral: 0.4 mg, 100's: **$29.95**
• Sol—Ophth: 0.25%, 5, 15 ml: **$14.00/5 ml**
• Film, CONTREL—Percutaneous: 0.5 mg, 4 discs: **$16.80**

CONTRAINDICATIONS: Narrow-angle glaucoma, increased intraocular pressure, adhesions between iris and lens, unstable cardiovascular status (tachycardia, myocardial ischemia), myasthenia gravis, GI or GU obstruction

PRECAUTIONS: Children, elderly, blondes, prostatic hypertrophy, Down's syndrome, debilitated COPD, asthma, CHF, hypertension, dysrhythmia, hiatal hernia

PREGNANCY AND LACTATION: Pregnancy category C; no reports of adverse effects reported; compatible with breast feeding

SIDE EFFECTS/ADVERSE REACTIONS

CNS: Anxiety, confusion, delirium, delusions, depression, dizziness, *drowsiness,* excitement, flushing, hallucinations, headache, incoherence, irritability, restlessness, sedation, weakness

CV: Palpitations, paradoxical bradycardia, postural hypotension, tachycardia

EENT: Blurred vision, difficulty swallowing, dilated pupils, nasal congestion, photophobia

GI: Abdominal distress, *constipation, dryness of mouth,* nausea, paralytic ileus, vomiting

GU: Hesitancy, retention

METAB: Decreased sweating, fever

SKIN: Urticaria

---

italic = common side effects   **bold italic** = life-threatening reactions

MISC: Nasal congestion, suppression of lactation

INTERACTIONS

Drugs

3️⃣ *Antihistamines, phenothiazines, tricyclics:* Additive anticholinergic effect

SPECIAL CONSIDERATIONS

PATIENT/FAMILY EDUCATION

• Avoid abrupt discontinuation (taper off over 1 wk)
• Wash hands thoroughly after handling transdermal patches before contacting eyes

---

secobarbital

(see-koe-bar´bi-tal)

Rx: Seconal
Combinations
  Rx: with amobarbital
    (Tuinal)
Chemical Class: Barbituric acid derivative
Therapeutic Class: Sedative/hypnotic; anesthesia adjunct; anticonvulsant
DEA Class: Controlled Substance Schedule II

CLINICAL PHARMACOLOGY

Mechanism of Action: CNS depressant: Depresses the sensory cortex, decreases motor activity, alters cerebellar function, produces drowsiness, sedation, and hypnosis; little analgesic action at subanesthetic doses (may increase reaction to painful stimuli); anticonvulsant activity in anesthetic doses; dose-dependent respiratory depression (hypnotic doses produce respiratory depression similar to physiologic sleep)

Pharmacokinetics

PO: Onset 10-15 min, duration 3-4 hr
IM: Onset 10-15 min, duration 3-4 hr

Metabolized by liver; excreted by kidneys (metabolites); $t_{1/2}$ 15-40 hr

INDICATIONS AND USES: Sedative, hypnotic; preanesthetic medication; status epilepticus,* acute tetanus convulsions*; acute psychotic agitation*

DOSAGE

Adult

• *Insomnia:* PO 100-200 mg hs
• *Sedation/preoperatively:* PO 200-300 mg 1-2 hr preoperatively

Child

• *Sedation/preoperatively:* PO 50-100 mg 1-2 hr preoperatively

💲 **AVAILABLE FORMS/COST OF THERAPY**

• Cap, Gel—Oral: 100 mg, 100's: **$22.64**

CONTRAINDICATIONS: Respiratory depression, severe liver impairment, porphyria

PRECAUTIONS: Anemia, hepatic disease, renal disease, hypertension, elderly, acute or chronic pain (paradoxical reaction to pain possible)

PREGNANCY AND LACTATION: Pregnancy category D; small amounts excreted in breast milk, drowsiness in infant reported; compatible with breast feeding

SIDE EFFECTS/ADVERSE REACTIONS

CNS: Ataxia, CNS depression, dependency, dizziness, *drowsiness, hangover, lethargy,* lightheadedness, mental depression, nightmares, paradoxical stimulation in the elderly and children, slurred speech

CV: Bradycardia, hypotension

GI: Constipation, diarrhea, nausea, vomiting

HEME: **Agranulocytosis, megaloblastic anemia** (long-term treatment), **thrombocytopenia**

---

* = non-FDA-approved use

RESP: **Apnea, bronchospasm,** hypoventilation, **laryngospasm**

SKIN: Abscesses at inj site, angioedema, pain, *rash,* **Stevens-Johnson syndrome,** thrombophlebitis, urticaria

MISC: Withdrawal symptoms, minor (anxiety, muscle twitching, tremor, weakness, dizziness, distortion in visual perception, nausea, vomiting, insomnia, orthostatic hypotension), major (**seizures,** delirium)

INTERACTIONS

Drugs

▣ *Acetaminophen:* Enhanced hepatotoxic potential of acetaminophen overdoses

▣ *Antidepressants:* Reduced serum concentration of cyclic antidepressants

▣ β-*adrenergic blockers:* Reduced serum concentrations of β-blockers which are extensively metabolized

▣ *Calcium channel blockers:* Reduced serum concentrations of verapamil and dihydropyridines

▣ *Chloramphenicol:* Increased barbiturate concentrations; reduced serum chloramphenicol concentrations

▣ *Corticosteroids:* Reduced serum concentrations of corticosteroids; may impair therapeutic effect

▣ *Cyclosporine:* Reduced serum concentration of cyclosporine

▣ *Digitoxin:* Reduced serum concentration of digitoxin

▣ *Disopyramide:* Reduced serum concentration of disopyramide

▣ *Doxycycline:* Reduced serum doxycycline concentrations

▣ *Estrogen:* Reduced serum concentration of estrogen

▣ *Ethanol:* Excessive CNS depression

▣ *Griseofulvin:* Reduced griseofulvin absorption

▣ *MAOIs:* Prolonged effect of barbiturates

▣ *Methoxyflurane:* Enhanced nephrotoxic effect

▣ *Narcotic analgesics:* Increased toxicity of meperidine; reduced effect of methadone; additive CNS depression

▣ *Neuroleptics:* Reduced effect of either drug

❷ *Oral anticoagulants:* Decreased hypoprothrombinemic response to oral anticoagulants

▣ *Oral contraceptives:* Reduced efficacy of oral contraceptives

▣ *Phenytoin:* Unpredictable effect on serum phenytoin levels

▣ *Propafenone:* Reduced serum concentration of propafenone

▣ *Quinidine:* Reduced quinidine plasma concentration

▣ *Tacrolimus:* Reduced serum concentration of tacrolimus

▣ *Theophylline:* Reduced serum theophylline concentrations

▣ *Valproic acid:* Increased serum concentrations of secobarbital

❷ *Warfarin:* See oral anticoagulants

Labs

• *Glucose:* Falsely low with Clinistix, Diastix

• *17-Ketosteroids:* Falsely increased in urine

• *Phenobarbital:* Falsely increased in serum

SPECIAL CONSIDERATIONS

• Compared to the benzodiazepine sedative hypnotics, secobarbital is more lethal in overdosage, has a higher tendency for abuse and addiction, and is more likely to cause drug interactions via induction of hepatic microsomal enzymes; few advantages if any in safety or efficacy over benzodiazepines

S

---

italic = common side effects   **bold italic** = life-threatening reactions

PATIENT/FAMILY EDUCATION

• Avoid driving and other dangerous activities

• Withdrawal insomnia may occur after short-term use; do not start using drug again, insomnia will improve in 1-3 nights

• May experience increased dreaming

---

selegiline

(seh-leg'ill-ene)
Rx: Atapryl, Carbex, Eldepryl, Selpak
Chemical Class: Phenethylamine derivative
Therapeutic Class: Anti-Parkinson's agent

CLINICAL PHARMACOLOGY
Mechanism of Action: Inhibition of monoamine oxidase, type B, which blocks the catabolism of dopamine, increasing the net amount of dopamine available; other less well understood mechanisms also lead to an increase in dopaminergic activity

Pharmacokinetics: Rapidly absorbed, peak ½-2 hr; rapidly metabolized (active metabolites: N-desmethyldeprenyl, $t_{1/2}$ 2 hr; amphetamine, $t_{1/2}$ 17.7 hr, methamphetamine, $t_{1/2}$ 20 ½ hr); metabolites excreted in urine (45% in 48 hr)

INDICATIONS AND USES: Adjunct management of Parkinson's disease in patients being treated with levodopa/carbidopa who have had a poor response to therapy; early Parkinson's disease to delay progression*; atypical depression,* Alzheimer's disease*

DOSAGE
Adult

• *Parkinson's disease:* PO 10 mg/day in divided doses 5 mg at breakfast and lunch; after 2-3 days, begin to reduce the dose of concurrent levodopa/carbidopa 10%-30%

$ **AVAILABLE FORMS/COST OF THERAPY**

• Cap—Oral: 5 mg, 60's: **$138.24-$153.60**

• Tab, Uncoated—Oral: 5 mg, 60's: **$49.80-$141.37**

CONTRAINDICATIONS: Concurrent use with meperidine

PRECAUTIONS: Doses above 10 mg/day (doses in the 30-40 mg/day range are associated with nonselective monoamine oxidase inhibition)

PREGNANCY AND LACTATION: Pregnancy category C; excretion in breast milk unknown

SIDE EFFECTS/ADVERSE REACTIONS

CNS: Anxiety, apathy, back and leg pain, blepharospasm, chorea, confusion, delusions, dizziness, dystonic symptoms, grimacing, hallucinations, headache, increased apraxia, increased bradykinesia, increased tremors, involuntary movements, lethargy, migraine, mood changes, muscle cramps, nightmares, numbness, overstimulation, personality change, restlessness, sleep disturbances, tardive dyskinesia, tiredness, vertigo

CV: Angina pectoris, *dysrhythmia,* edema, hypertension, hypotension, orthostatic hypotension, palpitations, sinus bradycardia, syncope, tachycardia

EENT: Blurred vision, diplopia, dry mouth, tinnitus

GI: Abdominal pain, anorexia, constipation, diarrhea, dysphagia, heartburn, nausea, poor appetite, rectal bleeding, vomiting, weight loss

GU: Frequency, hesitation, nocturia, prostatic hypertrophy, retention, sexual dysfunction, slow urination

RESP: Asthma, shortness of breath

---

* = non-FDA-approved use

SKIN: Alopecia, facial hair, hematoma, increased sweating, photosensitivity, rash

INTERACTIONS

Drugs

❷ *Antidepressants, serotonin reuptake inhibitors (fluoxetine, fluvoxamine, paroxetine, sertraline):* Serious, sometimes fatal, reactions including hyperthermia, autonomic instability and mental status changes

❷ *Dexfenfluramine, fenfluramine:* Increased risk of serotonin syndrome

❷ *Dextroamphetamine:* Severe hypertension

❷ *Dextromethorphan:* Increased risk of serotonin syndrome

❸ *Guanadrel, guanethidine:* May inhibit the antihypertensive effects of antihypertensive agents

❸ *Insulin:* Excessive hypoglycemia may occur when MAOIs are administered to patients with diabetes

❸ *Levodopa:* May precipitate hypertensive crisis

⚠ *Methylphenidate:* Increased risk of hypertensive reactions

❸ *Moclobemide:* Increased pressor effects of tyramine; increased risk of adverse drug or food interactions

❷ *Narcotic analgesics (meperidine):* Stupor, muscular rigidity, severe agitation, elevated temperature, hallucinations, and death

❸ *Narcotic analgesics (morphine):* Stupor, muscular rigidity, severe agitation, elevated temperature, hallucinations, and death

⚠ *Reserpine:* Loss of antihypertensive effects

⚠ *Sibutramine:* Increased risk of serotonin syndrome

❸ *Succinylcholine:* Prolonged muscle relaxation caused by succinylcholine

⚠ *Sympathomimetics (metaraminol, phenylpropanolamine, pseudoephedrine):* Additive pressor response to sympathomimetic

❸ *Sympathomimetics (norepinephrine, phenylephrine):* Additive pressor response to sympathomimetic

⚠ *Venlafaxine:* Increased risk of serotonin syndrome

Labs

• *False positive:* Urine ketones, urine glucose

• *False negative:* Urine glucose (glucose oxidase)

• *False increase:* Uric acid, urine protein

SPECIAL CONSIDERATIONS

• At low doses, irreversible type B MAOI; at higher doses is metabolized to amphetamine, inhibiting both A and B subtypes of MAO

• Several placebo-controlled studies have demonstrated a significant delay in the need to initiate levodopa therapy in patients who receive selegiline in the early phase of the disease

• May have significant benefit in slowing the onset of the debilitating consequences of Parkinson's disease

---

selenium sulfide
(see-leen´ee-um)

Rx: Exsel, Selsun

OTC: Selsun Blue

Chemical Class: Trace metal

Therapeutic Class: Antiseborrheic; antifungal

CLINICAL PHARMACOLOGY

Mechanism of Action: Antimitotic action reducing turnover of epidermal cells; additional local irritant, antibacterial, and antifungal activity

Pharmacokinetics

TOP: Absorption may be increased if applied to inflamed skin

---

italic = common side effects   ***bold italic*** = life-threatening reactions

INDICATIONS AND USES: Dandruff, seborrheic dermatitis, tinea versicolor
DOSAGE
Adult and child
• *Seborrheic dermatitis/dandruff:* TOP wash hair with 1-2 tsp, leave on 2-3 min, rinse, repeat; 2 applications/wk for control or as needed for maintenance
• *Tinea versicolor:* TOP apply to affected area (perhaps with small amount of water), allow to remain on skin for 10 min, rinse thoroughly, repeat daily × 7 days; repeat as needed for maintenance

$ AVAILABLE FORMS/COST OF THERAPY
• Lotion—Top: 1%, 240 ml: **$3.25-$3.31**
• Shampoo—Top: 1% 210 ml: **$4.57-$5.65** (OTC)
• Lotion/Shampoo—Top: 2.5% 120 ml: **$3.16-$15.46**

CONTRAINDICATIONS: Hypersensitivity to sulfur preparations
PRECAUTIONS: Infants, inflamed skin
PREGNANCY AND LACTATION: Pregnancy category C; excretion into breast milk unknown
SIDE EFFECTS/ADVERSE REACTIONS
SKIN: Alopecia, discoloration of hair (minimized with thorough rinsing), oiliness of hair and scalp, *skin irritation*

SPECIAL CONSIDERATIONS
PATIENT/FAMILY EDUCATION
• External use only; avoid contact with eyes
• May damage jewelry (remove before using)

senna
(sen′na)
OTC: Black Draught, Fletcher′s Castoria, Gentlax, Senexon, Senna-Gen, Senokot, Senokotxtra
Combinations
  OTC: with docusate (Senokot-S); with cascara sagrada (Herbal Laxative); with psyllium (Perdiem)
Chemical Class: Anthraquinone derivatives
Therapeutic Class: Stimulant laxative

CLINICAL PHARMACOLOGY
Mechanism of Action: Stimulates peristalsis by action on intramural nerve plexi; alters water and electrolyte secretion
Pharmacokinetics
PO: Onset 6-8 hr
PR: Onset 0.5-1 hr
Minimal absorption; metabolized by liver; fecal and/or renal elimination
INDICATIONS AND USES: Constipation; bowel evacuation or preparation for surgery or examination
DOSAGE
Adult
• PO up to 1600 mg/day; tabs (187-600 mg), 1-8 tabs/day; granules (163-1600 mg/½ tsp), ¼-½ tsp/day; syr (218 mg/5 ml), 5-20 ml/day; liq (33.3 mg/ml), 10-15 ml/day
• PR up to 1600 mg/day; supp (652 mg), 1-2/day
Child >6 yr; >27 kg
• Do not use Black Draught (granules) for children
• PO up to 800 mg/day; tabs (187-600 mg), 1-4 tabs/day; syr (218 mg/5 ml), 10-30 ml/day; liq (33.3 mg/ml), 10-15 ml/day
Child 2-5 yr
• PO up to 300-400 mg/day; liq 5-10 ml/day

Child 1 mo-1 yr
• PO up to 300-400 mg/day; syr 1.25-5 ml/day

$ AVAILABLE FORMS/COST OF THERAPY
• Tab—Oral: 187 mg, 100's: **$2.55-$16.61**; 217 mg, 100's: **$4.60**; 374 mg, 12's: 600 mg, 30's: **$1.31-$4.38**
• Granules—Oral: 326 mg/tsp, 168 g: **$15.82**
• Supp—Rect: 652 mg, 6's: **$14.35**
• Syr—Oral: 218 mg/5 ml, 240 ml: **$18.46**
• Liq—Oral: 33.3 mg/ml, 150 ml: **$5.27**

CONTRAINDICATIONS: GI bleeding, obstruction, fecal impaction, abdominal pain, nausea or vomiting, symptoms of appendicitis, acute surgical abdomen

PRECAUTIONS: Fluid and electrolyte imbalance can occur with abuse; abuse, dependency; children

PREGNANCY AND LACTATION: Pregnancy category C; not excreted into breast milk; compatible with breast feeding

SIDE EFFECTS/ADVERSE REACTIONS

GI: Anorexia, cramps, diarrhea, *nausea, vomiting*

METAB: Alkalosis, enteropathy, hypocalcemia, hypokalemia, tetany

SPECIAL CONSIDERATIONS
• Proposed laxative of choice for narcotic-induced constipation

---

sertraline
(sir'trall-een)
Rx: Zoloft
Chemical Class: Substituted nanphthalenamine derivative
Therapeutic Class: Selective serotonin reuptake inhibitor (SSRI) antidepressant

---

CLINICAL PHARMACOLOGY
Mechanism of Action: Inhibitor of CNS neuronal uptake of serotonin (5-HT); no significant activity for histaminergic α- or β-adrenergic, muscarinic, or dopaminergic receptors

Pharmacokinetics
PO: Peak 4.5-8.4 hr, extensive 1st pass metabolism; plasma protein binding 99%; elimination $t_{1/2}$ 26-65 hr; excreted in urine and feces

INDICATIONS AND USES: Major depression; obsessive-compulsive disorder, panic disorder

DOSAGE

Adult and Child >16 yrs
• PO 50 mg qd; may increase to a max of 200 mg/day; do not change dose at intervals of <1 wk; administer qd in AM or PM

Child (6-12 yrs)
• PO 25 mg qd; may increase to a max of 200 mg/day; do not change dose at intervals of <1 wk
• Reduce dose for hepatic or renal dysfunction

$ AVAILABLE FORMS/COST OF THERAPY
• Tab, Uncoated—Oral: 25 mg, 50's: **$109.98;** 50 mg, 100's: **$227.14;** 100 mg, 100's: **$233.70**

PRECAUTIONS: Weight loss, hepatic or renal disease, epilepsy

PREGNANCY AND LACTATION: Pregnancy category B

SIDE EFFECTS/ADVERSE REACTIONS

CNS: Agitation, ataxia, confusion, *dizziness, fatigue, headache, insomnia,* paresthesia, *somnolence, tremor,* twitching

CV: Chest pain, hypotension, palpitations

EENT: Vision abnormalities

GU: Male sexual dysfunction, micturition disorder

GI: Anorexia, constipation, *diarrhea, dry mouth,* dyspepsia, flatulence, *nausea,* vomiting

---

italic = common side effects   ***bold italic*** = life-threatening reactions

INTERACTIONS
Drugs

■ *Carbamazepine:* Inhibition of hepatic metabolism of carbamazepine, but the formation of carbamazepine epoxide is not inhibited, contributing to increased toxicity

■ *Cyproheptadine:* Serotonin antagonist may partially reverse antidepressant and other effects

❷ *Dexfenfluramine:* Duplicate effects on inhibition of serotonin reuptake; inhibition of dexfenfluramine metabolism (CYP2D6) exaggerates effect; both mechanisms increase risk of serotonin syndrome

❷ *Fenfluramine:* Duplicate effects on inhibition of serotonin reuptake; inhibition of dexfenfluramine metabolism (CYP2D6) exaggerates effect; both mechanisms increase risk of serotonin syndrome

■ *Lithium:* Neurotoxicity (tremor, confusion, ataxia, dizziness, dysarthria, and absence seizures) reported in patients receiving fluoxetine-lithium combination; mechanism unknown

▲ *MAOI's (isocarboxazid, phenelzine, tranylcypromine):* Increased CNS serotonergic effects has been associated with severe or fatal reactions with this combination

❷ *Selegiline:* Sporadic cases of mania and hypertension

■ *Tricyclic antidepressants (clomipramine, desipramine, doxepin, imipramine, nortriptyline, trazodone):* Marked increases in tricyclic antidepressant levels due to inhibition of metabolism (CYP2D6)

❷ *Tryptophan:* Additive serotonergic effects

■ *Warfarin:* Increased hypoprothrombinemic response to warfarin

SPECIAL CONSIDERATIONS
• SSRI of choice based on intermediate length $t_{1/2}$, linear pharmacokinetics, absence of appreciable age effect on clearance, substantially less effect on P450 enzymes, reducing potential for drug interactions
• Splitting 100 mg tablets to yield 50 mg dose cuts costs

---

sevelamer
(seh-vel'a-mer)
Rx: Renagel
Therapeutic Class: Phosphate adsorbent

CLINICAL PHARMACOLOGY
Mechanism of Action: Binds phosphate in GI tract, increases elimination
Pharmacokinetics
PO: Not systematically absorbed in healthy volunteers

INDICATIONS AND USES: Reduction of serum phosphorus in patients with end-stage renal disease (ESRD)

DOSAGE
Adult
• PO (serum phosphorus >6 and <7.5 mg/dL) 2 caps tid with meals; (serum phosphorus ≥7.5 and <9 mg/dL) 3 caps tid with meals; (serum phosphorus ≥9 mg/dL) 4 caps tid with meals; adjust dose to lower serum phosphorus to ≤6 mg/dL, increase or decrease dose by 1 cap/meal prn; max 30 caps/day

⚡ AVAILABLE FORMS/COST OF THERAPY
• Cap—Oral: 403 mg, 200's: **$110.40**

CONTRAINDICATIONS: Hypophosphatemia; bowel obstruction

PRECAUTIONS: Dysphagia, swallowing disorders, GI motility disorders, major GI tract surgery

PREGNANCY AND LACTATION: Pregnancy category C; use caution in nursing mothers due to potential for reductions in serum levels of various vitamins

SIDE EFFECTS/ADVERSE REACTIONS

CNS: Headache

CV: Hypertension, hypotension, ***thrombosis***

GI: Diarrhea, dyspepsia, vomiting, nausea, flatulence, constipation

INTERACTIONS

Drugs

3 *Antiarrhythmics, anticonvulsants:* Potential for decreased bioavailability of these drugs when concomitantly administered with sevelamer, administer >1 hr before or 3 hr after sevelamer

SPECIAL CONSIDERATIONS

• Has not been studied in ESRD patients not on hemodialysis

• Compared to calcium acetate, may reduce the risk of developing hypercalcemia

PATIENT/FAMILY EDUCATION

• A daily multivitamin supplement may prevent reduction in serum levels of vitamins D, E, K, and folic acid

• Do not chew or take caps apart prior to administration

MONITORING PARAMETERS

• Serum phosphorus, calcium, bicarbonate, and chloride levels

---

sibutramine

(sih-byoo'tra-meen)

Rx: Meridia

Chemical Class: Cyclobutane-methamine derivative

Therapeutic Class: Anorexiant

DEA Class: Schedule IV

CLINICAL PHARMACOLOGY

Mechanism of Action: Inhibits reuptake of norepinephrine, serotonin, and dopamine in the CNS

Pharmacokinetics

PO: Peak 1.2 hr, 77% absorption, extensive first pass metabolism in the liver; 97% bound to plasma proteins; metabolized in the liver by cytochrome P450(3A$_4$) to active desmethyl metabolites; excreted in urine (77%) and feces; t$_{1/2}$ 1.1 hr (14 and 16 hr for two active metabolites)

INDICATIONS AND USES: Management of obesity (initial body mass index ≥30 kg/m^2, or ≥27 kg/m^2 in the presence of other risk factors like hypertension, diabetes and dyslipidemia) in conjunction with a reduced calorie diet

DOSAGE

Adult

• PO 10 mg qd; may increase to 15 mg qd after 4 wk if inadequate results; safety and efficacy beyond 1 yr of therapy has not been determined

$ AVAILABLE FORMS/COST OF THERAPY

• Cap—Oral: 5, 10 mg, 100's: **$290.00;** 15 mg, 100's: **$375.00**

CONTRAINDICATIONS: Patients receiving MAO inhibitors or other centrally acting appetite suppressants; anorexia nervosa

PRECAUTIONS: Hypertension, CAD, CHF, arrhythmia, stroke, narrow angle glaucoma, seizure disorders, gallstones, renal or hepatic dysfunction

PREGNANCY AND LACTATION: Pregnancy category C; excretion into breast milk unknown, not recommended in nursing mothers

SIDE EFFECTS/ADVERSE REACTIONS

CNS: Anxiety, depression, dizziness, emotional lability, *headache, insomnia,* nervousness, paresthesia, somnolence, stimulation

CV: Generalized edema, hypertension, migraine, palpitation, tachycardia, vasodilation

EENT: Ear disorder, ear pain, taste perversion

---

italic = common side effects   ***bold italic*** = life-threatening reactions

S

GI: Anorexia, constipation, dry mouth, dyspepsia, gastritis, increased appetite, nausea, rectal disorder, vomiting
GU: Dysmenorrhea, metorrhagia
MS: Arthralgia, back pain, joint disorder, myalgia, tenosynovitis
RESP: Cough increase, laryngitis, pharyngitis, rhinitis, sinusitis
SKIN: Acne, rash, sweating
MISC: Abdominal pain, asthenia, chest pain, flu syndrome, neck pain, thirst

INTERACTIONS
Drugs
❷ *MAO inhibitors:* Potential for the development of serotonin syndrome; at least 14 days should elapse between administration of MAO inhibitors and sibutramine

SPECIAL CONSIDERATIONS
• Primary pulmonary hypertension and cardiac valve disorders have been associated with other centrally acting weight loss agents that cause release of serotonin from nerve terminals; although sibutramine has not been associated with these effects in pre-marketing clinical studies, patients should be informed of the potential for these side effects and monitored closely for their occurrence
• Substantially increases blood pressure in some patients
• Maintenance of weight loss beyond 1 yr has not been studied

MONITORING PARAMETERS
• Regular blood pressure monitoring

sildenafil
(sill-den′-a-fill)
Rx: Viagra
Chemical Class: cGMP-specific phosphodiesterase inhibitor
Therapeutic Class: Anti-impotence agent

CLINICAL PHARMACOLOGY
Mechanism of Action: Increases cGMP in the corpus cavernosum, causing smooth muscle relaxation and inflow of blood, resulting in penile erection
Pharmacokinetics
PO: Peak 30-120 min. Rapidly absorbed, metabolized by liver (cytochrome P450 3A4) to active metabolite, excreted in feces (80%) and urine (13%); $T_{1/2}$ 4 hr, rate of absorption decreased by fatty meal

INDICATIONS AND USES: Erectile dysfunction

DOSAGE
Adult
PO: 50 mg approx 1 hr before sexual activity. Dosage range 25-100 mg. Max recommended use once/day. Decrease dose in elderly (>65), hepatic dysfunction, renal insufficiency (CrCl <30 ml/min)

💲 **AVAILABLE FORMS/COST OF THERAPY**
• Tab, Coated—Oral: 25 mg, 100's: **$875.00;** 50 mg, 100's: **$875.00;** 75 mg, 100's: **$875.00**

CONTRAINDICATIONS: Concurrent nitrate use

PRECAUTIONS: Elderly, hepatic dysfunction, renal insufficiency, penile deformity, cardiac disease, conditions predisposing to priapism (sickle cell anemia, leukemia, multiple myeloma), bleeding disorders, active peptic ulcer disease, retinitis pigmentosa (some have disorders of

---

retinal phosphodiesterases), concurrent use of cytochrome P450 inhibitors

PREGNANCY AND LACTATION:
Pregnancy category B, use not recommended in women

SIDE EFFECTS/ADVERSE REACTIONS

CNS: Headache (16%), abnormal vision (11% at 100 mg dose, 3% at lower dose) including color tinge, photosensitivity, ataxia, hypertonia, neuropathy, paresthesia, tremor, vertigo, depression, insomnia, somnolence, abnormal dreams

CV: ***Cardiac arrest, death,*** angina, AV block, syncope, tachycardia, palpitations, hypotension, ***myocardial ischemia***

EENT: Dizziness, mydriasis, tinnitus, eye pain, ear pain

GI: Dyspepsia (17% at 100 mg dose, 7% at lower dose), diarrhea, vomiting, gastritis, esophagitis, stomatitis, abnormal LFTs

GU: Nocturia, frequency, breast enlargement, incontinence, abnormal ejaculation, anorgasmia, no cases of priapism reported

HEME: ***Anemia, leukopenia***

METAB: Hyperglycemia, hypoglycemia, hyperuricemia, hypernatremia

MS: Arthritis, synovitis, myalgia

RESP: Asthma, dyspnea, laryngitis, cough

SKIN: Flushing (10%), urticaria, pruritis, dermatitis

INTERACTIONS

Drugs

3 *Cimetidine, erythromycin, itraconazole, ketoconazole:* Increased sildenafil levels

⚠ *Nitrates:* Cardiac arrest, death

3 *Rifampin:* Decreased sildenafil levels

SPECIAL CONSIDERATIONS
• Tablets are priced the same re-

gardless of dose, 100-mg tablets can be broken in half

---

silver nitrate

Rx: Silver nitrate
Chemical Class: Heavy metal
Therapeutic Class: Antibiotic; cauterizing agent

CLINICAL PHARMACOLOGY

Mechanism of Action: Germicidal action via liberated silver ions, which precipitate bacterial proteins; also antiseptic, astringent, local epithelial stimulant, and caustic

INDICATIONS AND USES: Prevention, treatment of gonorrheal ophthalmia neonatorum; treatment of indolent wounds, ulcers, and fissures; cauterize vesicular, bullous, or aphthous lesions and provide styptic action; neurovascular helomas (10% oint, 10% sol); impetigo vulgaris (10% sol); pruritis, plantar warts (25% sol); granulation tissue, papillomatous growths, granuloma pyogenicum (50% sol); wet dressing in burns and acute dermatitis (0.1-0.5% sol)*

DOSAGE

Adult

• TOP (as wet dressing or irrigant) apply a cotton applicator dipped in sol to affected area 2-3 times/wk for approximately 2-3 wk prn; apply oint in an apertured pad on affected lesion or area for approximately 5 days prn; touch applicators to the bases of vesicular, bullous, or aphthous lesions

Neonate

• *Gonorrheal ophthalmia neonatorum:* Instill 2 gtt of 1% sol into each eye; do *not* follow with irrigation

---

italic = common side effects   ***bold italic*** = life-threatening reactions

$ AVAILABLE FORMS/COST OF THERAPY

• Applicators—Top: 100's: **$10.32-$120.00**

• Sol—Top: 0.5%, 960 ml: **$19.33**

• Sol—Top: 10%, 30 ml: **$22.30;** 25%, 30 ml: **$35.45;** 50%, 30 ml: **$51.25**

• Oint—Top: 10%, 30 g: **$34.40**

PRECAUTIONS: Antibiotic hypersensitivity; *not* effective for neonatal chlamydial conjunctivitis; caustic and irritating to skin

SIDE EFFECTS/ADVERSE REACTIONS

EENT: Discharge, edema, redness, swelling (chemical conjunctivitis)

METAB: Sodium and chloride depletion with chronic wet dressings

SKIN: Discoloration

SPECIAL CONSIDERATIONS
PATIENT/FAMILY EDUCATION

• Stains skin and utensils (removable with iodine tincture followed by sodium thiosulfate solution)

---

silver sulfadiazine
(sul-fa-dye'a-zeen)

Rx: Silvadene, SSD, SSD AF, Thermazene

Chemical Class: Sulfonamide derivative

Therapeutic Class: Topical antibiotic

CLINICAL PHARMACOLOGY

Mechanism of Action: Interferes with bacterial cell wall synthesis (bactericidal); broad antimicrobial activity including many gram-negative and gram-positive bacteria and yeast; *not* a carbonic anhydrase inhibitor, and may be useful in situations where such agents are contraindicated

Pharmacokinetics

TOP: Absorption varies depending on surface area covered and integrity of skin; appreciable serum concentrations obtainable with extensive use (8-12 µg/ml)

INDICATIONS AND USES: Adjunct for the prevention and treatment of wound sepsis in patients with 2nd and 3rd degree burns

DOSAGE

Adult and Child

• TOP apply to affected area qd-bid; burned area should be covered with cream at all times

$ AVAILABLE FORMS/COST OF THERAPY

• Cre—Top: 1%, 20, 25, 30, 50, 85, 400, 1000 g: **$25.40-$34.35**/400 g

CONTRAINDICATIONS: Child <2 mo

PRECAUTIONS: Impaired hepatic or renal function; G-6-PD deficiency

PREGNANCY AND LACTATION: Pregnancy category B; contraindicated in neonates (kernicterus)

SIDE EFFECTS/ADVERSE REACTIONS

GU: Crystalluria

*HEME: **Reversible leukopenia***

SKIN: Burning, brownish-gray skin discoloration, erythema, itching, pain, rash, skin necrosis, stinging, urticaria

INTERACTIONS

Drugs

3 *Proteolytic enzymes:* Silver may inactivate enzymes

SPECIAL CONSIDERATIONS

• Prior to application, burn wounds should be cleansed and debrided (following control of shock and pain)

• Use sterile glove and tongue blade to apply medication; thin layer (1.5 mm) to completely cover wound; dressing as required only

• Continue until no chance of infection

---

* = non-FDA-approved use

simethicone

(si-meth'i-kone)
OTC: Gas-X, Mylicon, Phazyme
Combinations
  OTC: with calcium carbonate (Titralac Plus); with aluminum hydroxide, magnesium hydroxide (Mylanta Gelisil, Maalox Extra Strength); with calcium carbonate, magnesium hydroxide (Tempo, Rolaids); with Magaldrate, (Riopan Plus); with charcoal (Charcoal Plus, Flatulex)

Therapeutic Class: Antiflatulent

CLINICAL PHARMACOLOGY
Mechanism of Action: Defoaming action, disperses and prevents formation of gas pockets in GI system
Pharmacokinetics
PO: Fecal elimination, unchanged
INDICATIONS AND USES: Relief of painful symptoms and pressure of excess gas in digestive tract; adjunct in conditions in which gas retention may be problematic (postoperatively, endoscopic examination, air swallowing, functional dyspepsia, peptic ulcer, spastic or irritable colon, diverticulosis); infant colic*
DOSAGE
Adult
• PO 40-125 mg qid pc, hs
Child 2-12 yr
• PO 40 mg qid
Child <2 yr
• PO 20 mg pc, hs (up to 240 mg/day)
  $ **AVAILABLE FORMS/COST OF THERAPY**
• Tab, Chewable—Oral: 40 mg,

100's: **$7.54;** 80 mg, 12's: **$1.61;**
100's: **$10.39;** 125 mg, 24's: **$3.62**
• Tab—Oral: 60 mg, 100's: **$15.34**
• Cap—Oral: 125 mg, 50's: **$10.07**
• Liq—Oral: 40 mg/0.6 ml, 30 ml: **$8.00-$10.36**
PREGNANCY AND LACTATION:
Pregnancy category C
SIDE EFFECTS/ADVERSE REACTIONS
GI: Belching, rectal flatus
SPECIAL CONSIDERATIONS
• Commonly prescribed, little evidence for any beneficial effect

simvastatin

(sim'va-sta-tin)
Rx: Zocor
Chemical Class: Substituted hexahydronaphthalene
Therapeutic Class: Antilipemic (HMG-CoA reductase inhibitor); "statin"

CLINICAL PHARMACOLOGY
Mechanism of Action: Competitively inhibits 3-hydroxy-3-methylglutaryl-coenzyme A (HMG-CoA) reductase, an early rate-limiting step in cholesterol biosynthesis; increases HDL cholesterol mildly [8%-12%], dramatically decreases total and LDL cholesterol [23%-36%, 14%-47%, respectively], moderate lowering effect on triglycerides [11%-24%]
Pharmacokinetics
PO: Peak 1-2½ hr, 85% absorbed; extensive 1st-pass metabolism (CYP3A4, active metabolites); 95% protein bound; excreted primarily in bile, feces (60%)
INDICATIONS AND USES: Reduction of elevated total and LDL cholesterol in patients with primary hypercholesterolemia, mixed dyslipidemia (types IIa and IIb and homozygous familial hyperlipidemia); re-

S

---

italic = common side effects   ***bold italic*** = life-threatening reactions

duction of morbidity and mortality in patients with coronary heart disease and hypercholesterolemia (secondary prevention)

DOSAGE

Adult

• PO 5-10 mg qd in PM initially, usual range 5-40 mg/day qd in PM; max daily dose 80 mg; dosage adjustments may be made in 4-wk intervals

🔰 AVAILABLE FORMS/COST OF THERAPY

• Tab, Plain Coated—Oral: 5 mg, 90's: **$160.26;** 10 mg, 90's: **$196.33;** 20 mg, 60's: **$228.33;** 40 mg, 60's: **$228.33;** 80 mg, 60's: **$228.33**

CONTRAINDICATIONS: Active liver disease

PRECAUTIONS: Past liver disease, alcoholism, severe acute infections, trauma, hypotension, uncontrolled seizure disorders, severe metabolic disorders, electrolyte imbalances

PREGNANCY AND LACTATION: Pregnancy category X; breast milk excretion unknown; other drugs in this class are excreted in small amounts; manufacturer recommends against breast feeding

SIDE EFFECTS/ADVERSE REACTIONS

CNS: Dizziness, headache, insomnia, memory loss, peripheral neuropathy, tremor, vertigo

GI: Abdominal pain, constipation, diarrhea, dyspepsia, flatus, heartburn, liver dysfunction, nausea, *pancreatitis,* vomiting

GU: Erectile dysfunction, gynecomastia, loss of libido

HEME: **Eosinophilia, hemolytic anemia, leukopenia, thrombocytopenia**

MS: Muscle cramps, myalgia, myositis, *rhabdomyolysis*

SKIN: Alopecia, pruritus, rash, *Stevens-Johnson syndrome*

INTERACTIONS

Drugs

❷ *Azole antifungals (fluconazole, itraconazole, ketoconazole, miconazole):* Increased simvastatin levels via inhibition of metabolism with increased risk of rhabdomyolysis

❸ *Cholestyramine, colestipol:* Reduced bioavailability of simvastatin

❸ *Cyclosporine:* Concomitant administration increases risk of severe myopathy or rhabdomyolysis

❸ *Danazol:* Inhibition of metabolism (CYP3A4) thought to yield increased simvastatin levels with increased risk of rhabdomyolysis

❷ *Fluoxetine:* Inhibits CYP3A4 hepatic metabolism with risk of rhabdomyolysis

❷ *Gemfibrozil:* Small increased risk of myopathy with combination, especially at high doses of statin

❸ *Isradipine:* Isradipine probably decreases simvastatin (like lovastatin) plasma concentrations minimally

❸ *Macrolide antibiotics (clarithromycin, erythromycin, troleandomycin):* Increased simvastatin levels via inhibition of metabolism with increased risk of rhabdomyolysis

❸ *Nefazadone:* Inhibit CYP3A4 hepatic metabolism (like lovastatin) with risk of rhabdomyolysis

❸ *Niacin:* Concomitant administration increases risk of severe myopathy or rhabdomyolysis

❸ *Warfarin:* Addition of simvastatin may increase hypoprothrombinemic response to warfarin via inhibition of metabolism (CYP2C9)

SPECIAL CONSIDERATIONS

• Superior to fibrates, cholestyramine, and probucol in lowering total and LDL cholesterol levels

• Statin selection based on lipid-lowering prowess, cost, and availability

PATIENT/FAMILY EDUCATION
• Report symptoms of myalgia, muscle tenderness, or weakness
• Take daily doses in the evening for increased effect

MONITORING PARAMETERS
• Cholesterol (max therapeutic response 4-6 wk)
• LFT's (AST, ALT) at baseline and at 12 wk of therapy; if no change, no further monitoring necessary (discontinue if elevations persist at >3× upper limit of normal)
• CPK in patients complaining of diffuse myalgia, muscle tenderness, or weakness

---

sirolimus
(sir-oh-leem′-us)
Rx: Rapamune
Chemical Class: Macrolide derivative
Therapeutic Class: Immunosuppressant

CLINICAL PHARMACOLOGY
Mechanism of Action: Inhibits a regulatory kinase involved in the cell cycle
Pharmacokinetics
PO: Peak 1-3 hr, low bioavailability (15%), extensively metabolized by cytochrome P450 in the liver, metabolites have <10% activity of parent compound, $T_{1/2}$ 60 hr

INDICATIONS AND USES: Prevention of organ rejection in renal transplantation (in combination with corticosteroids and cyclosporine)

DOSAGE
Adult and Child >16 yr
• PO 2-5 mg/m² qd or in 2 divided doses. Some suggest a loading dose 3× maintenance dose, not to exceed 60 mg. Follow trough levels to adjust dose. Reduce dose in hepatic insufficiency

💲 AVAILABLE FORMS/COST OF THERAPY
• Liq—Oral: 1, 2, 5, 60, 150 ml: **$205.50**/ml
• Tablet expected late 2000

PRECAUTIONS: Previous hypersensitivity to tacrolimus, infection, hyperlipidemia (especially hypertriglyceridemia), diabetes, coronary artery disease, myelosuppression, hepatic insufficiency, pregnancy

PREGNANCY AND LACTATION: No animal or human data; not recommended during pregnancy

SIDE EFFECTS/ADVERSE REACTIONS
CNS: Headache
CV: Peripheral edema
GI: Anorexia, weight loss, diarrhea, elevated transaminases
GU: Minimal nephrotoxicity in initial studies
HEME: ***Thrombocytopenia*** (dose related), ***leukopenia*** (nondose related, WBC <4800/mm³ in 20%)
METAB: *Hypertriglyceridemia, hyperlipidemia,* hyperglycemia
MS: Arthralgia

INTERACTIONS
Drugs
3 *Cyclosporine:* Increased sirolimus concentrations when given concurrently. Timing of cyclosporine dosing should remain consistent

SPECIAL CONSIDERATIONS
• Allows cyclosporine dose reduction
• Experience limited with use as rescue therapy
• Black patients had higher rejection rates (56% vs 13%) than nonblacks given same regimen
• Oral formulations with improved bioavailability and an IV formulation are under development

PATIENT/FAMILY EDUCATION
• Take medication the same each day with regard to timing of meals and other medications

S

---

italic = common side effects   **bold italic** = life-threatening reactions

MONITORING PARAMETERS

• Whole-blood sirolimus levels (drawn 1 hr prior to next dose), 5-7 days after initiation or dose change. Maintain levels at 10-15 ng/mL for first month, then consider increasing to 15-20 ng/mL, especially in patients receiving little cyclosporine

• CBC, platelets, lipids

---

sodium bicarbonate

Combinations
  OTC: with alginic acid, (AlOH, Mg Trisilicate Gastrocote); with sodium citrate (Citrocarbonate)
Chemical Class: Monosodium salt of carbonic acid
Therapeutic Class: Systemic/urinary alkalinizing agent; antacid; electrolyte supplement

---

CLINICAL PHARMACOLOGY

Mechanism of Action: Orally neutralizes gastric acid, which forms water, $NaCl$, CO_2; increases plasma bicarbonate, buffers H^+ ion concentration, raises pH, reverses acidosis

Pharmacokinetics

Excreted in urine and by lungs (CO_2)

INDICATIONS AND USES: Metabolic acidosis (e.g., renal disease, cardiac arrest, circulatory insufficiency); systemic and urinary alkalinization (renal calculi, treatment of drug intoxications); antacid; electrolyte replacement (diarrhea); sickle cell anemia treatment*

DOSAGE

Adult

• *Acidosis:* IV INF 100-350 mEq over 4-8 hr depending on CO_2 and pH

• *Cardiac arrest:* IV bolus 1 mEq/kg, then 0.5 mEq/kg q10min prn while arrest continues (based on ABGs)

• *Alkalinization of urine:* PO 325 mg-2 g qid

• *Antacid:* PO 300 mg-2 g chewed, taken with H_2O qd-qid

Child 6-12 yr

• *Acidosis:* IV INF 2-5 mEq/kg over 4-8 hr depending on CO_2 and pH

• *Cardiac arrest:* IV bolus 1 mEq/kg, then 0.5 mEq/kg q10 min prn while arrest continues (based on ABGs)

• *Alkalinization of urine:* PO 12-120 mg/kg/day

• *Antacid:* 520 mg; may repeat in 30 min

Infant

Acidosis: IV INF not to exceed 8 mEq/kg/day based on ABGs (4.2% sol)

💲 AVAILABLE FORMS/COST OF THERAPY

• Granules, Effervescent—Oral: 3 g: **$1.80**

• Inj, Sol—IV: 4.2%, 10 ml: **$7.44-$14.30;** 5%, 500 ml: **$39.23-$41.18;** 7.5%, 50 ml: **$7.46-$19.72;** 8.4%, 10 ml: **$7.44-$14.13**

• Tab, Coated—Oral: 325 mg, 100's: **$3.00;** 650 mg, 100's: **$1.44-$6.95**

CONTRAINDICATIONS: Continued losses from vomiting or GI suction; diuretic-induced hypochloremic alkalosis

PRECAUTIONS: CHF, cirrhosis, hypertension, hypocalcemia, toxemia, renal disease

PREGNANCY AND LACTATION: Pregnancy category C

SIDE EFFECTS/ADVERSE REACTIONS

CNS: Confusion, headache, *hyperreflexia,* irritability, *seizures* caused by alkalosis, stimulation, tetany, tremors, *twitching,* weakness

CV: Cardiac arrest, edema, irregular pulse, water retention, weight gain

---

* = non-FDA-approved use

GI: Acid rebound, *belching,* cramps, *distension,* flatulence, increased thirst, **paralytic ileus**

GU: Calculi

METAB: Alkalosis, hypercalcemia or milk-alkali syndrome, hypokalemia

RESP: **Apnea,** cyanosis, shallow, slow respirations

INTERACTIONS

Drugs

🔢 *Amphetamines:* Sodium bicarbonate inhibits the elimination and increases the effects of amphetamines

🔢 *Beta blockers:* Reduced absorption

🔢 *Cefpodoxime:* Reduced absorption

🔢 *Cefuroxime:* Reduced serum levels with reduced antibiotic efficacy

🔢 *Ephedrine:* Large doses of sodium bicarbonate increase the serum concentrations of ephedrine

🔢 *Flecainide:* Increased urine pH will increase flecainide serum concentration

🔢 *Glipizide:* Enhanced rate of glipizide absorption

🔢 *Glyburide:* Enhanced rate of glyburide absorption

🔢 *Iron:* Reduced absorption

🔢 *Ketoconazole:* Decreased absorption

🔢 *Lithium:* Sodium bicarbonate may lower lithium plasma concentrations

🔢 *Methenamine compound:* Sodium bicarbonate-induced urinary pH changes interfere with antibacterial activity of methenamine compounds

🔢 *Mexiletine:* Increased urine pH increases mexiletine concentrations

🔢 *Pseudoephedrine:* Sodium bicarbonate-induced urinary pH changes may markedly inhibit the elimination of pseudoephedrine

🔢 *Quinidine:* Sodium bicarbonate-induced urinary pH changes may increase quinidine concentrations

🔢 *Quinolones:* Reduced absorption

🔢 *Salicylates:* Sodium bicarbonate-induced urinary pH changes can decrease serum salicylate concentrations

🔢 *Tetracyclines:* Reduced absorption

Labs

• *Protein:* Falsely elevates urine protein

SPECIAL CONSIDERATIONS

PATIENT/FAMILY EDUCATION

• Milk-alkali syndrome (may result from excessive antacid use): confusion, headache, nausea, vomiting, anorexia, urinary stones, hypercalcemia

• To avoid drug interactions due to reduced absorption, separate intake by 2 hr

MONITORING PARAMETERS

• Electrolytes, blood pH, PO_2, HCO_3, during treatment

• ABGs frequently during emergencies

---

sodium chloride

OTC: *Nasal:* Afrin Saline Mist, Ayr, Breathe Free, Dristan Saline, HuMist, NāSal, Ocean, Pretz, SalineX, SeaMist

Ophth: Adsorbonac, AK-NaCl, Muro-128, Muroptic-5

Chemical Class: Sodium salt

Therapeutic Class: Electrolyte supplement; irrigant; moisturizing agent

---

CLINICAL PHARMACOLOGY

Mechanism of Action: Major electrolytes necessary for the maintenance of plasma tonicity; moisturizes dry mucous membranes; reduces corneal edema by osmosis of

---

italic = common side effects   ***bold italic*** = life-threatening reactions

water through the semipermeable corneal epithelium

INDICATIONS AND USES: Electrolyte replacement, flushing IV catheters, extracellular fluid replacement, abortifacient; prevention of muscle cramps and heat prostration; GU irrigation; nasal mucous moisturization; diluent for IV, IM, or SC injections; corneal edema (ophth)

DOSAGE

Adult

• *Electrolyte replacement:* IV sodium deficiency (mEq/kg) = [% dehydration (L/kg)/100 × 70 (mEq/L)] + [0.6(L/kg) × (140 − serum sodium)(mEq/L)]

• *Severe hyponatremia:* IV mEq sodium = [desired sodium (mEq/L] − [actual sodium (mEq/L) × 0.6 × wt (kg)]; for acute correction, use 125 mEq as the desired serum sodium; acutely correct serum sodium in 5 mEq/L dose increments; more gradual correction in increments of 10 mEq/L/day is indicated in the asymptomatic patient

• *Chloride maintenance electrolyte requirement in parenteral nutrition:* IV 2-4 mEq/kg/24 hr or 25-40 mEq/1000 kcal/24 hr; max 100-150 mEq/24 hr

• *Sodium maintenance electrolyte requirement in parenteral nutrition:* IV 3-4 mEq/kg/24 hr or 25-40 mEq/1000 kcal/24 hr; max 100-150 mEq/24 hr

• *Heat cramps:* PO 0.5-1 g with full glass of water (up to 4.8 g/day)

• *GU irrigant:* 1-3 L/day

• *Nasal:* prn

• *Corneal edema:* Instill 1-2 gtt q3-4h or ointment hs

• *Abortifacient:* 20% (250 ml) transabdominal intra-amniotic instillation

Child

• *Electrolyte replacement:* IV sodium deficiency (mEq/kg) = [% dehydration (L/kg)/100 × 70 (mEq/L)] + [0.6(L/kg) × (140 − serum sodium)(mEq/L)]

• *Nasal:* prn

• *Corneal edema:* Instill 1-2 gtt q3-4h or ointment hs

Newborn

• *Electrolyte requirement:* Premature, 2-8 mEq/kg/24 hr; term, 0-48 hr 0-2 mEq/kg/24 hr; >48 hr 1-4 mEq/kg/24 hr

$ AVAILABLE FORMS/COST OF THERAPY

• Sol, Bacteriostatic Diluent: 0.9%, 30 ml: **$0.49-$4.50**

• Sol, Electrolyte—IV: 0.45%, 1000 ml: **$10.88-$13.89;** 0.9%, 1000 ml: **$9.86-$14.16;** 3%, 500 ml: **$10.77-$13.78;** 5%, 500 ml: **$11.88-$15.18;** 14.6%, 20 ml (for dilution): **$2.26-$4.85;** 23.4%, 30 ml (for dilution): **$1.44-$2.39**

• Tab, Electrolyte—Oral: 250 mg, 200's: **$2.55;** 1 g, 100's: **$3.25-$5.86** Tab 250 mg 200's: **$2.55**

• Sol-Genitourinary Irrigant: 0.9% (isotonic), 2000 ml: **$11.00-$24.20;** 0.45%, 2000 ml (hypotonic): **$8.94-$14.05**

• Sol—Nasal 0.4%; 15 ml: **$3.38** 0.9%; 30 ml: **$3.54;** 45 ml-50 ml: **$1.65-$3.82**

• Sol, Isotonic—INH: 0.9%, 3 ml ×100: **$16.40-$24.20;** 0.45%, 3 ml ×100: **$24.20**

• Sol—Ophth: 2%, 15 ml: **$11.81-$14.63;** 5%, 15 ml: **$7.15-$17.06**

• Oint—Ophth: 5%, 3.5 g: **$7.78-$12.44**

CONTRAINDICATIONS: Hypernatremia, bacteriostatic solutions in newborns

PRECAUTIONS: Uncompensated cardiovascular, cirrhotic, or nephrotic disease; circulatory insufficiency; hypoproteinemia; hypervolemia; urinary tract obstruction; CHF; patients with concurrent edema and sodium retention, those receiving

---

* = non-FDA-approved use

corticosteroids, and those retaining salt

PREGNANCY AND LACTATION: Pregnancy category C

SIDE EFFECTS/ADVERSE REACTIONS

CNS: Coma, irritability, obtundation, restlessness, *seizures,* weakness

CV: **CHF,** hypervolemia

EENT: Stinging

GI: Abdominal cramps, diarrhea, nausea, vomiting

METAB: Sodium chloride excess or deficit

RESP: **Pulmonary edema**

MISC: Rapid infusion may cause local pain at inj site

INTERACTIONS

Drugs

3 *Lithium:* High sodium intake may reduce serum lithium concentrations, while restriction of sodium tends to increase serum lithium

SPECIAL CONSIDERATIONS
• One g of sodium chloride provides 17.1 mEq sodium and 17.1 mEq chloride

---

sodium citrate and citric acid
sodium citrate and potassium citrate

Rx: *Sodium citrate and citric acid:* Bicitra, Oracit
Sodium citrate and potassium citrate: Citrolith, Polycitra, Polycitra-K, Polycitra-LC

Therapeutic Class: Oral alkalinizing agents

CLINICAL PHARMACOLOGY
Mechanism of Action: Sodium citrate is absorbed and metabolized to sodium bicarbonate, thus acting as a systemic alkalinizer; the effects of these salts are essentially those of

chlorides before absorption and those of bicarbonates subsequently

Pharmacokinetics
PO: <5% of citrate is excreted unchanged

INDICATIONS AND USES: Alkalinizing agent; useful where long-term maintenance of an alkaline urine is desirable; alleviation of chronic metabolic acidosis (i.e., chronic renal insufficiency or the syndrome of renal tubular acidosis); buffers and neutralizes gastric acid

DOSAGE
Adult
• *Systemic alkalinization:* Sodium citrate and citric acid, PO 10-30 ml diluted pc, hs; sodium citrate and potassium citrate, PO 15-30 ml diluted pc, hs
• *Neutralizing buffer:* PO 15 ml diluted taken as a single dose

Child
• *Systemic alkalinization:* Sodium citrate and citric acid, PO 5-15 ml diluted pc, hs; sodium citrate and potassium citrate, PO 5-15 ml diluted pc, hs

$ **AVAILABLE FORMS/COST OF THERAPY**
Sodium Citrate/Citric Acid
• Sol—Oral: 480 ml: **$7.80-$15.02**
Sodium Citrate/Potassium Citrate
• Liq/Syr—Oral: 480 ml: **$18.46-$18.60**
• Tab—Oral: 50 mg-950 mg, 100's: **$9.70**

CONTRAINDICATIONS: Sodium-restricted diets; severe renal impairment

PRECAUTIONS: Low urinary output; patients with cardiac failure, hypertension, impaired renal function, peripheral and pulmonary edema, and toxemia of pregnancy

SPECIAL CONSIDERATIONS
PATIENT/FAMILY EDUCATION
• Sugar free
• Dilute adequately with water and,

---

italic = common side effects   ***bold italic*** = life-threatening reactions

preferably, take each dose after meals to avoid saline laxative effect

MONITORING PARAMETERS

• Serum electrolytes, particularly serum bicarb level

• NOTE: Sodium citrate and potassium citrate known as Sholl's Solution, sodium citrate and citric acid as modified Sholl's

---

sodium polystyrene sulfonate

(pol-ee-stye'reen)

Rx: Kayexalate, Kionex

Chemical Class: Cation exchange resin

Therapeutic Class: Antihyperkalemic

CLINICAL PHARMACOLOGY

Mechanism of Action: Removes potassium by exchanging sodium for potassium in body; occurs primarily in large intestine

Pharmacokinetics

PO/PR: Not absorbed from the GI tract

INDICATIONS AND USES: Hyperkalemia (in conjunction with other measures)

DOSAGE

Administer in approx 25% sorbitol susp or concurrently treat with 70% oral sorbitol syrup 10-20 ml q2h to produce 1 or 2 watery stools/day

Adult

• PO 15 g qd-qid

• PR 30-50 g/100 ml of sorbitol warmed to body temp q6h

Child

• PO/PR 1g/kg q6h

🟦 AVAILABLE FORMS/COST OF THERAPY

• Powder—Oral: 454 g: **$98.22-$166.69**

• Susp—Rect: 50 mg/200 mL 200 mL **$29.50**

• Susp—Oral: 15 g/60 ml, 60 mL: **$5.85-$8.65**

CONTRAINDICATIONS: Hypokalemia

PRECAUTIONS: Renal failure, CHF, severe edema, severe hypertension

PREGNANCY AND LACTATION: Pregnancy category C; excretion in breast milk not expected

SIDE EFFECTS/ADVERSE REACTIONS

CV: CHF

METAB: Alkalosis

GI: Anorexia, constipation, diarrhea (sorbitol), fecal impaction, gastric irritation, nausea, vomiting

METAB: Hypocalcemia, hypokalemia, hypomagnesemia, sodium retention

INTERACTIONS

Drugs

3 *Antacids:* Combined use of magnesium- or calcium-containing antacids with resin may result in systemic alkalosis

SPECIAL CONSIDERATIONS

• Exchange efficacy of resin is approx 33%; 1 g of resin (4.1 mEq of sodium) exchanges approximately 1 mEq of potassium

• Rectal route is less effective than oral administration

PATIENT/FAMILY EDUCATION

• Don't mix with orange juice

MONITORING PARAMETERS

• Serum K, Ca, Mg, Na, acid-base balance, bowel function, possibly ECG

---

* = non-FDA-approved use

somatropin/somatrem (growth hormone)

(soe-ma-troe'pin)

Rx: *Somatropin:* Genotropin, Norditropin, Nutropin, Nutropin AQ, Humatrope, Saizen, Serostim

Somatrem: Protropin

Chemical Class: Recombinant DNA product; somatropin is identical to human growth hormone, somatrem contains an additional amino acid

Therapeutic Class: Growth hormone; anticachexic

CLINICAL PHARMACOLOGY

Mechanism of Action: Stimulates skeletal growth in growth hormone deficiency, reduces fat stores, induces insulin resistance

Pharmacokinetics

SC: Peak 7.5 hr; localizes to highly perfused organs; metabolized by kidney, liver

INDICATIONS AND USES: Pituitary growth hormone deficiency; growth failure associated with chronic renal insufficiency (somatropin only); AIDS wasting or cachexia (Serostim); Turner's syndrome in girls (Neutropin only)

DOSAGE

Adult

• *AIDs wasting or cachexia:* SC >55 kg 6 mg qhs, 45-55 kg 5 mg qhs, 35-45 kg 4 mg qhs, <35 kg 0.1 mg/kg qhs

Child

Somatropin

• *Growth hormone inadequacy:* SC weekly dose of up to 0.3 mg/kg via daily injections (Nutropin); SC/IM up to 0.06 mg/kg 3 times /wk (Humatrope)

• *Chronic renal insufficiency:* SC weekly dose of up to 0.35 mg/kg via daily injections (Nutropin); therapy may be continued up to time of transplantation

• *Somatrem:* SC/IM up to 0.1 (0.26 IU) mg/kg 3 times/wk

💲 **AVAILABLE FORMS/COST OF THERAPY**

Somatropin

• Inj, Dry-Sol—IM, SC: 1.5 mg: **$63.00**; 4 mg: **$168.00**; 5 mg: **$210.01**; 5.8 mg: **$210.00**; 6 mg: **$252.00**; 8 mg: **$336.00**; 12 mg: **$504.00**; 24 mg: **$1008.00**

Somatrem

• Inj, Lyphl-Sol—IM, SC: 10 mg/vial: **$840.00**; 5 mg/vial: **$420.00**

CONTRAINDICATIONS: Hypersensitivity to benzyl alcohol, closed epiphyses, evidence of tumor activity and/or active neoplasia; sensitivity to m-cresol or glycerin (Humatrope)

PRECAUTIONS: Diabetes mellitus, hypothyroidism

PREGNANCY AND LACTATION: Pregnancy category C; excretion into breast milk unknown

SIDE EFFECTS/ADVERSE REACTIONS

CNS: Headache, *intracranial hypertension*

HEME: **Leukemia** (uncertain relationship)

METAB: Glycosuria, hypercalciuria, hypothyroidism, ketosis, mild hyperglycemia

SKIN: Inflammation at inj site, pain, rash, urticaria

MISC: Antibodies to growth hormone

SPECIAL CONSIDERATIONS MONITORING PARAMETERS

• Individualize doses for growth hormone inadequacy

• Check for hypothyroidism, malnutrition, antibodies or opportunistic infections (AIDs patients) if no response to initial dose

• TSH

S

- Evaluate if child limps
- Follow with fundoscopy (papilledema)

sorbitol

(sor'bi-tole)

Rx: Sorbitol

Chemical Class: Polyalcoholic sugar

Therapeutic Class: Osmotic laxative; osmotic diuretic

CLINICAL PHARMACOLOGY
Mechanism of Action: Hyperosmolar; acts as diuretic, laxative
Pharmacokinetics
PO/PR: Absorption poor, onset of action 15-60 min; when used as urologic irrigant, variable systemic absorption occurs; metabolized to CO_2 and dextrose by liver or excreted by kidneys

INDICATIONS AND USES: Irrigant sol during transurethral prostatic surgery; laxative*; facilitates passage of sodium polystyrene sulfonate through intestinal tract*

DOSAGE
Adult
- *Laxative:* PO 30-150 ml (70% sol)
- *Rectal enema:* 120 ml (25%-30% sol)
- *Adjunct to polystyrene sulfonate:* 15 ml (70% sol) until diarrhea, or 20-100 ml as oral vehicle for the resin
- *Irrigant:* Top 3.3% sol
Child 2-11 yr
- *Laxative:* PO 2 ml/kg (70% sol)
- *Rectal enema:* 30-60 ml (25%-30% sol)

$ AVAILABLE FORMS/COST OF THERAPY
- Sol—Irrigation: 3.3%, 4000 ml: **$28.35**
- Sol—Oral: 70%, 480 ml: **$5.25-$14.88**

CONTRAINDICATIONS: Anuria
PRECAUTIONS: Significant cardiopulmonary, renal dysfunction; diabetes mellitus, hyponatremia, hypovolemia
SIDE EFFECTS/ADVERSE REACTIONS
CNS: **Seizures,** vertigo
CV: Angina, **CHF,** hypotension
EENT: Blurred vision, rhinitis, thirst
GI: Colonic necrosis, diarrhea, nausea, vomiting
GU: Acidosis, diuresis, edema, fluid retention, urinary retention
METAB: Acidosis, hyperglycemia, hypernatremia, hyponatremia
MISC: Chills, urticaria

sotalol

(soe'ta-lole)

Rx: Betapace

Chemical Class: Nonselective β-adrenergic blocker

Therapeutic Class: Antidysrhythmic

CLINICAL PHARMACOLOGY
Mechanism of Action: PO Competitive β-adrenergic antagonist; produces negative inotropic and chronotropic responses; slows AV nodal conduction; decreases heart rate; decreases myocardial oxygen consumption; antiarrhythmic effects (class II); reduction in platelet aggregation and blood viscosity; suppression of renin release; inhibition of central sympathetic outflow; decreases presynaptic receptor neurotransmitter release; no intrinsic sympathomimetic or membrane stabilizing activity; low lipid solubility
Pharmacokinetics
PO: Onset 1-2 hr, peak effect 3-4 hr; $t_{1/2}$ 12 hr; excreted unchanged by kidney; low lipid solubility; not protein bound; absorption decreased 20%-30% by meals

INDICATIONS AND USES: Ventricular arrhythmias (tachycardia, fibrillation), angina pectoris,* hypertension,* postmyocardial infarction,* supraventricular arrhythmias,* congestive heart failure

DOSAGE

Adult and Child >16 yr

• *Arrhythmias (supraventricular and ventricular):* IV 0.2-1.5 mg/kg over 5 min; PO 80 mg bid (ac); increased q2-3 days in 40-80 mg increments to a total daily dose between 160-320 mg

NOTE: Gradually withdraw previous antiarrhythmic therapy prior to starting oral sotalol (2-3 half-lives); not a significant problem with lidocaine

• Renal failure adjustment: CrCl > 60 ml/min administer q12h; CrCl 30-60 ml/min administer q24h; CrCl 10-30 ml/min administer q36-48h; individualize dose for CrCl <10 ml/min; increase dose after 5-6 doses prn

§ AVAILABLE FORMS/COST OF THERAPY

• Tab, Coated—Oral: 80 mg, 100's: **$235.44;** 120 mg, 100's: **$314.13;** 160 mg, 100's: **$392.69;** 240 mg, 100's: **$510.50**

CONTRAINDICATIONS: Bronchial asthma, cardiogenic shock, overt cardiac failure, 2nd and 3rd degree AV block, severe sinus bradycardia

PRECAUTIONS: Anesthesia/surgery (myocardial depression), avoid abrupt withdrawal, bronchospastic airways, congestive heart failure, diabetes mellitus, hyperthyroidism/thyrotoxicosis, concurrent clonidine (discontinue atenolol several days prior to withdrawal of clonidine), peripheral vascular disease, renal disease

PREGNANCY AND LACTATION: Pregnancy category B; similar drug, atenolol, frequently used in the third trimester for treatment of hypertension (many studies of efficacy and safety of atenolol in pregnancy-induced hypertension); long-term use has been associated with intrauterine growth retardation; concentrated in breast milk (levels 3-5 times those of plasma); symptoms of β- blockade possible in infant, but considered compatible with breast feeding

SIDE EFFECTS/ADVERSE REACTIONS

CNS: Anxiety, confusion, depression, *dizziness,* drowsiness, *fatigue,* hallucinations, insomnia, nightmares, weakness

CV: Bradycardia, chest pain, ***CHF,*** hypotension, Raynaud's phenomena, ***ventricular dysrhythmias including torsade de points***

GI: Constipation, diarrhea, nausea, stomach discomfort, vomiting

GU: Sexual dysfunction

HEME: **Agranulocytosis**

RESP: **Bronchospasm,** cough, dyspnea

INTERACTIONS

Drugs

3 *Adenosine:* Bradycardia aggravated

3 *Alpha-1 adrenergic blockers:* Potential enhanced first dose response (marked initial drop in blood pressure), particularly on standing (especially prazocin)

3 *Amiodarone:* Combination yielded bradycardia and hypotension in case reports

3 *Antacids:* Reduced sotalol absorption

3 *Calcium channel blockers:* See dihydropyridine calcium channel blockers and verapamil

S

---

italic = common side effects   ***bold italic*** = life-threatening reactions

3 *Cimetidine:* Renal clearance reduced; AUC increased with cimetidine coadministration

3 *Cisapride:* Dual prolongation of QT interval; increased risk of ventricular tachyarrhythmias

3 *Clonidine, guanabenz, guanfacine:* Exacerbation of rebound hypertension upon discontinuation of clonidine

3 *Cocaine:* Cocaine-induced vasoconstriction potentiated; reduced coronary blood flow

3 *Contrast media:* Increased risk of anaphylaxis

3 *Digitalis:* Enhances bradycardia

3 *Dihydropyridine calcium channel blockers:* Additive pharmacodynamic effects

3 *Dipyridamole:* Bradycardia aggravated

3 *Epinephrine, isoproterenol, phenylephrine:* Potentiates pressor response; resultant hypertension and bradycardia

3 *Flecainide:* Additive negative inotropic effects; case report of bradycardia, AV block, and cardiac arrest following switch from flecainide to sotalol

3 *Fluoxetine:* Increased β-blockade activity

3 *Fluroquinolones:* Reduced clearance of sotalol

3 *Hypoglycemic agents:* Masked hypoglycemia, hyperglycemia

3 *Insulin:* Altered response to hypoglycemia; increased blood glucose concentrations; impaired peripheral circulation

3 *Lidocaine:* Increased serum lidocaine concentrations possible

3 *Neostigmine:* Bradycardia aggravated

3 *Neuroleptics:* Both drugs inhibit each other's metabolism; additive hypotension

3 *NSAIDs:* Reduced hemodynamic effects of sotalol

3 *Physostigmine:* Bradycardia aggravated

3 *Prazosin:* First-dose response to prazosin may be enhanced by β-blockade

3 *Tacrine:* Bradycardia aggravated

2 *Terbutaline:* Antagonized bronchodilating effects of terbutaline

2 *Theophylline:* Antagonistic pharmacodynamic effects

3 *Verapamil:* Enhanced effects of both drugs; particularly AV nodal conduction slowing; reduced sotalol clearance

Labs

• *Metanephrines total:* Falsely increases urine levels (may be double)

SPECIAL CONSIDERATIONS
PATIENT/FAMILY EDUCATION

• Do not discontinue abruptly; may require taper; rapid withdrawal may produce rebound hypertension or angina

MONITORING PARAMETERS

• Angina: Reduction in nitroglycerin usage; frequency, severity, onset, and duration of angina pain; heart rate

• Arrhythmias: Heart rate and rhythm; monitor QT intervals (discontinue or reduce dose if QT >550 msec)

• Congestive heart failure: Functional status, cough, dyspnea on exertion, paroxysmal nocturnal dyspnea, exercise tolerance, and ventricular function

• Hypertension: Blood pressure

• Toxicity: Blood glucose, bronchospasm, hypotension, bradycardia, depression, confusion, hallucination, sexual dysfunction

• Because of prodysrhythmic risk, begin and increase drug in setting with cardiac rhythm monitoring

* = non-FDA-approved use

sparfloxacin
(spar-floks'a-sin)
Rx: Zagam
Chemical Class: Fluoroquin-
olone derivative
Therapeutic Class: Antibiotic

CLINICAL PHARMACOLOGY
Mechanism of Action: Interferes
with the enzyme DNA gyrase needed
for the synthesis of bacterial DNA;
bactericidal
Pharmacokinetics
PO: Peak 3-6 hr; 45% bound to
plasma proteins, penetrates well into
body fluids and tissues; metabolized in liver (primarily by glucuronidation), excreted in feces (50%)
and urine (50%); $t_{1/2}$ 20 hr
INDICATIONS AND USES: Community-acquired pneumonia, acute
bacterial exacerbations of chronic
bronchitis caused by susceptible organisms
Antibacterial spectrum usually includes:
• Gram-positive organisms: *Staphylococcus aureus, Streptococcus
pneumoniae* (penicillin-susceptible
strains)
• Gram-negative organisms: *Enterobacter cloacae, Haemophilus influenzae, H. parainfluenzae, Klebsiella pneumoniae, Moraxella catarrhalis*
• Other organisms: *Chlamydia pneumoniae, Mycoplasma pneumoniae*
DOSAGE
Adult
• PO 400 mg × 1, then 200 mg qd
for 9 days; for CrCl <50 ml/min,
400 mg × 1, then 200 mg q48h for
9 days
**$ AVAILABLE FORMS/COST
OF THERAPY**
• Tab—Oral: 200 mg, 11's: **$76.65**
CONTRAINDICATIONS: History of

photosensitivity reactions, known
prolonged QT_c interval, children
<18 yr
PRECAUTIONS: Seizure disorder,
dehydration, renal impairment, hepatic impairment
PREGNANCY AND LACTATION:
Pregnancy category C; excretion
into breast milk unknown; due to
the potential for arthropathy and osteochondrosis, use extreme caution
in nursing mothers
**SIDE EFFECTS/ADVERSE REAC-
TIONS**
CNS: Anxiety, depression, dizziness,
fatigue, headache, insomnia, seizures, somnolence
CV: QT_c interval prolongation
EENT: Dizziness, visual disturbances
GI: Abdominal pain, anorexia, diarrhea, dry mouth, flatulence, heartburn, increased AST, ALT; *nausea,*
pseudomembranous colitis, vomiting
GU: Vaginal moniliasis
SKIN: Photosensitivity, pruritus, rash
INTERACTIONS
Drugs
3 *Aluminum:* Reduced absorption
of sparfloxacin; do not take within
4 hr of dose
3 *Antacids:* Reduced absorption of
sparfloxacin; do not take within 4 hr
of dose
3 *Antipyrine:* Inhibits metabolism
of antipyrine; increased plasma antipyrine level
3 *Calcium:* Reduced absorption of
sparfloxacin; do not take within 4 hr
of dose
3 *Diazepam:* Inhibits metabolism
of diazepam; increased plasma diazepam level
3 *Didanosine:* Markedly reduced
absorption of sparfloxacin; take sparfloxacin 2 hr before didanosine
3 *Foscarnet:* Coadministration increases seizure risk
3 *Iron:* Reduced absorption of

S

italic = common side effects   ***bold italic*** = life-threatening reactions

sparfloxacin; do not take within 4 hr of dose

■ *Magnesium:* Reduced absorption of sparfloxacin; do not take within 4 hr of dose

■ *Metoprolol:* Inhibits metabolism of metoprolol; increased plasma metoprolol level

■ *Phenytoin:* Inhibits metabolism of phenytoin; increased plasma phenytoin level

■ *Propranolol:* Inhibits metabolism of propranolol; increased plasma propranolol level

■ *Ropinirole:* Inhibits metabolism of ropinirole; increased plasma ropinirole level

■ *Sodium bicarbonate:* Reduced absorption of sparfloxacin; do not take within 4 hr of dose

■ *Sucralfate:* Reduced absorption of sparfloxacin; do not take within 4 hr of dose

■ *Warfarin:* Inhibits metabolism of warfarin; increases hypoprothrombinemic response to warfarin

■ *Zinc:* Reduced absorption of sparfloxacin; do not take within 4 hr of dose

SPECIAL CONSIDERATIONS
PATIENT/FAMILY EDUCATION
• Avoid direct or indirect sunlight during treatment and for 5 days after completion of therapy; drink fluids liberally

---

spectinomycin
(spek-ti-noe-mye′sin)
Rx: Trobicin
Chemical Class: Aminoglycoside derivative
Therapeutic Class: Antibiotic

CLINICAL PHARMACOLOGY
Mechanism of Action: Inhibits bacterial synthesis by binding to 30S subunit on ribosomes; bacteriostatic

Pharmacokinetics
IM: Peak 1-2 hr, duration 8 hr, $t_{1/2}$ 1-3 hr (10-30 hr if CrCl <20 ml/min); excreted in urine (unchanged); poor distribution into saliva

INDICATIONS AND USES: Gonorrhea (except pharyngeal infection) in patients who cannot take ceftriaxone

DOSAGE
Adult
• IM 2-4 g as single dose; 2 g q12h for disseminated infection

Child <45 kg
• IM 30-40 mg/kg as single dose

⚡ AVAILABLE FORMS/COST OF THERAPY
• Inj, Dry-Susp—IM: 400 mg/ml, 2 g: **$23.29**

CONTRAINDICATIONS: Infants (diluent contains benzyl alcohol)

PRECAUTIONS: Children

PREGNANCY AND LACTATION: Pregnancy category B; excretion into breast milk unknown

SIDE EFFECTS/ADVERSE REACTIONS
CNS: Anxiety, chills, dizziness, fever, headache, insomnia
GI: Nausea, vomiting
GU: Decreased urine output
HEME: Anemia
SKIN: Fever, *pain at inj site,* pruritus, rash, urticaria

SPECIAL CONSIDERATIONS
• Follow with doxycycline 100 mg bid for 7 days (erythromycin if pregnant or allergic)
• Ineffective against syphilis and may mask symptoms
• Give in gluteal muscle; dose >2 g must be divided in 2 gluteal injections

---

spironolactone

(speer-on-oh-lak'tone)

Rx: Aldactone
Combinations
   Rx: with hydrochlorothiazide
   (Aldactazide, Spirozide)
Chemical Class: Aldosterone
antagonist
Therapeutic Class: Potassium-
sparing diuretic, antihyperten-
sive

CLINICAL PHARMACOLOGY

Mechanism of Action: Competitive aldosterone inhibitor; interferes
with sodium reabsorption in the distal tubule, thus decreasing potassium secretion; weak diuretic and
antihypertensive effects when used
alone unless primary or secondary
hyperaldosteronism present (more
potent); other actions: interferes with
testosterone synthesis and conversion of testosterone to estradiol

Pharmacokinetics
PO: Peak serum concentration: 1-3
hr; peak effect, 48-72 hr; >90%
bound to plasma proteins; metabolized in liver, excreted in feces (50%)
urine (40%); crosses placenta; $t_{1/2}$
1.4 hr

INDICATIONS AND USES: Edema,
hypertension, CHF, diuretic-induced
hypokalemia, primary hyperaldosteronism, nephrotic syndrome, cirrhosis of the liver with ascites, polycystic ovary disease,* premenstrual
syndrome,* female hirsutism*

DOSAGE

Adult
• *Edema or hypertension:* PO 25-
200 mg/day in single or divided
doses
• *Hypokalemia:* PO 25-100 mg/day
in single or divided doses *CHF:* PO
25 mg/day
• *CHF:* PO 25 mg/day
• *Primary hyperaldosteronism di-*
agnosis: PO 400 mg/day for 4 days
(short test) or 4 wk (long test), then
100-400 mg/day maintenance
• *Polycystic ovary disease or hir-*
sutism: PO 100-200 mg/day

Child
• *Diuretic or antihypertensive or as-*
cites: PO 1-3 mg/kg/day in single
or divided doses

AVAILABLE FORMS/COST
OF THERAPY
• Tab, Plain Coated—Oral: 25 mg,
100's: **$6.25-$48.30;** 50 mg, 100's:
$72.74-$84.80; 100 mg, 100's:
$121.97-$142.18

CONTRAINDICATIONS: Anuria,
severe renal disease, hyperkalemia,
antikaliuretic therapy (including
angiotensin-converting enzyme inhibitors, angiotensin receptor blockers, and potassium supplements)

PRECAUTIONS: Dehydration, diabetes, hepatic disease, hyponatremia, renal insufficiency, potassium
supplements, menstrual abnormalities, gynecomastia, acidosis, elderly

PREGNANCY AND LACTATION:
Pregnancy category D; feminization occurs in male rat fetuses; active metabolite excreted in breast
milk; compatible with breast feeding but alternate options preferred;
therapy for existing hypertension
can be continued throughout pregnancy with minimal risk; initiating
for simple edema not recommended;
few unequivocal indications for diuretic therapy in pregnancy except
for pulmonary edema or congestive
heart failure

SIDE EFFECTS/ADVERSE REAC-
TIONS

CNS: Ataxia, confusion, drowsiness,
headache, lethargy
CV: Bradycardia, ***CHF,*** hypotension
GI: Anorexia, ***bleeding,*** constipation, cramps, *diarrhea,* gastritis, nausea, *vomiting*

---

italic = common side effects ***bold italic*** = life-threatening reactions

GU: Amenorrhea, deepening voice, gynecomastia, hirsutism, impotence, irregular menses, post-menopausal bleeding

METAB: Hyperchloremic metabolic acidosis, hyperkalemia, hyponatremia

SKIN: Pruritus, rash, urticaria

MISC: Breast cancer

INTERACTIONS
Drugs

3 *Ammonium chloride:* Combination may produce systemic acidosis

3 *Angiotensin-converting enzyme inhibitors:* Concurrent mechanisms to decrease potassium excretion; increased risk of hyperkalemia

3 *Angiotensin II receptor antagonists:* Concurrent mechanisms to decrease potassium excretion; increased risk of hyperkalemia

3 *Digitalis glycosides:* False or true increase in digoxin concentrations

3 *Disopyramide:* Increased potassium concentrations may enhance disopyramide effects on myocardial conduction

A *Mitotane:* Spironolactone antagonizes the activity of mitotane

2 *Potassium:* Increased risk of hyperkalemia

3 *Salicylates:* Decreased diuretic (not antihypertensive effect) due to decreased tubular secretion of active metabolite

Labs

• *Corticosteroids:* Marked false increase in plasma corticosteroids

• *Cortisol:* Falsely increased fluorometric methods of measurement

• *Digoxin:* False increases in digoxin concentrations

• *17-Hydroxycorticosteroids:* False increases in urine measurements

• *17-Ketogenic steroids:* Falsely increases urine concentrations

SPECIAL CONSIDERATIONS
MONITORING PARAMETERS

• When used for diagnosis of primary hyperaldosteronism, positive results are: (long test) correction of hyperkalemia and hypertension; (short test) serum potassium increases during administration, but falls upon discontinuation

• Blood pressure, edema, urine output, ECG (if hyperkalemia exists), urine electrolytes, BUN, creatinine, gynecomastia, impotence

---

stanozolol
(stan-oh'zoe-lole)
Rx: Winstrol
Chemical Class: Halogenated testosterone derivative
Therapeutic Class: Androgen; antiangioedema agent
DEA Class: Schedule III

CLINICAL PHARMACOLOGY
Mechanism of Action: Promotes body tissue-building processes and reverses catabolic processes when administered with adequate calories and protein; increases erythropoietin; increases C1 esterase inhibitor (deficient in hereditary angioedema) and resulting C2 and C4 concentrations; androgenic

INDICATIONS AND USES: Prophylaxis to decrease the frequency and severity of attacks of hereditary angioedema; possibly effective for aplastic anemia*

DOSAGE
Adult

• *Angioedema:* PO 2 mg tid, then decrease q1-3 mo to 2 mg qd or qod

• *Aplastic anemia:* PO 2 mg tid

Child

• *Angioedema:* PO up to 2 mg qd (6-12 yr); PO 1 mg qd (<6 yr)

• *Aplastic anemia:* PO up to 2 mg tid (6-12 yr); PO 1 mg bid (<6 yr)

* = non-FDA-approved use

AVAILABLE FORMS/COST OF THERAPY

• Tab, Uncoated—Oral: 2 mg, 100's: **$77.10**

CONTRAINDICATIONS: Severe renal disease, severe cardiac disease, severe hepatic disease, genital bleeding (abnormal), prostate cancer, male breast cancer, female breast cancer with hypercalcemia; nephrosis; enhancement of physical appearance or athletic performance

PRECAUTIONS: Diabetes mellitus, CV disease, or risk factors for atherosclerosis, hepatic disease, seizure disorder, headache, children

PREGNANCY AND LACTATION: Pregnancy category X (masculinization); excretion into breast milk unknown; use extreme caution in nursing mothers

SIDE EFFECTS/ADVERSE REACTIONS

CNS: Anxiety, carpal tunnel syndrome, dizziness, fatigue, flushing, headache, insomnia, lability, paresthesias, sweating, tremors

CV: Increased blood pressure, edema

EENT: Conjunctival edema, deepening of voice in women, nasal congestion

GI: Cholestatic jaundice, diarrhea, ***hepatocellular necrosis, hepatic tumors, peliosis hepatis,*** nausea, vomiting, weight gain

GU: Clitoral hypertrophy, decreased breast size, decreased libido, epididymitis, gynecomastia, hematuria, impotence, menstrual irregularities, oligospermia, phallic enlargement in prepubertal males, priapism, testicular atrophy, vaginitis

METAB: Abnormal glucose tolerance, decreased HDL, electrolyte imbalance

MS: Cramps, spasms, premature epiphyseal closure (children)

SKIN: Acneiform lesions; acne vulgaris, alopecia, flushing, hirsutism and male pattern baldness in women, oily hair, skin; rash, sweating

INTERACTIONS

Drugs

❷ *Oral anticoagulants:* Enhanced hypoprothrombinemic response

❸ *Antidiabetic agents:* Enhanced hypoglycemic response

❷ *Cyclosporine:* Increased cyclosporine concentrations

❸ *HMG-CoA reductase inhibitors (lovastatin, pravastatin):* Myositis risk increased

SPECIAL CONSIDERATIONS

• Anabolic steroids have potential for abuse, especially in the athlete

MONITORING PARAMETERS

• LFTs, lipids
• Growth rate in children (X-rays for bone age q6 mo)

---

stavudine (d4T)

stav'yoo-deen

Rx: Zerit

Chemical Class: Nucleoside analog

Therapeutic Class: Antiretroviral

CLINICAL PHARMACOLOGY

Mechanism of Action: Phosphorylated intracellularly to stavudine triphosphate, which inhibits HIV reverse transcriptase by competing with deoxythymidine triphosphate and inhibits viral DNA synthesis by causing DNA chain termination

Pharmacokinetics

PO: Peak 1 hr, bioavailability 85% (not affected by food); plasma $t_{1/2}$ 1½ hr, intracellular $t_{1/2}$ 3½ hr; not protein bound; only slightly metabolized; renal clearance by filtration and tubular secretion; urinary excretion of unchanged drug over 24 hr after oral dose 40%

INDICATIONS AND USES: Adults with advanced HIV infection who have received zidovudine therapy

---

italic = common side effects   ***bold italic*** = life-threatening reactions

DOSAGE

Adult

• *PO:* 40 mg q12h if weight ≥60 kg, 30 mg q12h if weight <60 kg; reduce dose by ½ if resuming therapy after resolution of side effect (neuropathy, transaminitis); adjust dose for renal insufficiency: CrCl 26-50 ml/min, 20 mg q12h if weight ≥60 kg, 15 mg q12h if weight <60 kg; CrCl 10-25 ml/min, 20 mg q24h if weight ≥60 kg, 15 mg q24h if weight <60 kg

• For latest treatment guidelines see www.hivatis.org

§ AVAILABLE FORMS/COST OF THERAPY

• Cap, Gel—Oral: 15 mg, 60's: **$235.64;** 20 mg, 60's: **$245.04;** 30 mg, 60's: **$255.65;** 40 mg, 60's: **$265.07**

• Sol—Oral: 1 mg/ml, 200 ml: **$57.85**

PRECAUTIONS: Peripheral neuropathy, pancreatitis, renal insufficiency, folate or vitamin B_{12} deficiency

PREGNANCY AND LACTATION: Pregnancy category C; excreted in breast milk

SIDE EFFECTS/ADVERSE REACTIONS

CNS: Dementia, headache, insomnia, *peripheral neuropathy* (15%-21%)

GI: Abdominal pain, diarrhea, *increased transaminases,* nausea, ***pancreatitis***

HEME: **Neutropenia**

MS: Myalgia

SKIN: Rash

MISC: Asthenia, fever

SPECIAL CONSIDERATIONS

PATIENT/FAMILY EDUCATION

• Report neuropathic symptoms (numbness, tingling, or pain in the feet or hands)

MONITORING PARAMETERS

• CBC, SGOT, SGPT

---

streptokinase
(strep-toe-kye'nase)
Rx: Kabikinase, Streptase
Chemical Class: Purified β-hemolytic streptococcus filtrate
Therapeutic Class: Thrombolytic

CLINICAL PHARMACOLOGY

Mechanism of Action: Promotes thrombolysis by promoting conversion of plasminogen to plasmin

Pharmacokinetics

IV/INTRACORONARY: Onset immediate; $t_{1/2}$ of streptokinase activator complex 23 min; mechanism of elimination unknown; no metabolites identified

INDICATIONS AND USES: Acute evolving transmural myocardial infarction; pulmonary embolism; deep venous thrombosis; arterial thrombosis or embolism; arteriovenous cannulae occlusion not responsive to heparin flush

DOSAGE

Adult

• *Acute evolving transmural MI:* IV INF 1,500,000 IU diluted to a volume of 45 ml; administer over 1 hr; intracoronary (IC) dilute 250,000 IU vial to total volume of 125 ml, give 20,000 IU (10 ml) by bolus followed by 2000 IU/min for 60 min for total dose 140,000 IU

• *Thrombosis or embolism:* IV INF 250,000 IU over ½ hr; then 100,000 IU/hr for 72 hr for deep vein thrombosis or 100,000 IU/hr for 24 hr for pulmonary embolism or 100,000 IU/hr for 24-72 hr for arterial thrombosis or embolism

• *Arteriovenous cannula occlusion:* IV INF 250,000 IU/2 ml sol into each occluded limb of cannula slowly; clamp for 2 hr; aspirate con-

---

* = non-FDA-approved use

tents; flush with saline sol and reconnect cannula

$ AVAILABLE FORMS/COST OF THERAPY

• Inj, Lyphl-Sol—Intracoronary; IV: 1,500,000 U/vial: **$511.75;** 750,000 U/vial:**$255.86;** 600,000 U/vial: **$160.00;** 250,000 U/vial: **$115.93**

CONTRAINDICATIONS: Active internal bleeding; recent (within 2 mo) CVA; intracranial or intraspinal surgery, intracranial neoplasm; severe uncontrolled hypertension

PRECAUTIONS: Recent (within 10 days) surgery, obstetrical delivery, organ biopsy, trauma including CPR; high likelihood of left heart thrombus (e.g., mitral stenosis with atrial fibrillation); subacute bacterial endocarditis; hemostatic defects; age ≥75 yr; diabetic hemorrhagic retinopathy; septic thrombophlebitis or infected occluded AV cannula at seriously infected site; recent streptococcal infection; repeat administration (between 5 days and 12 mo of prior streptokinase)

PREGNANCY AND LACTATION: Pregnancy category C; no data available for breast feeding

SIDE EFFECTS/ADVERSE REACTIONS

CNS: Fever, headache
CV: Hypotension, *reperfusion dysrhythmias*
EENT: Periorbital edema
GI: Nausea, vomiting
HEME: Anemia, *bleeding (GI, GU, intracranial, retroperitoneal, surface)*
RESP: Altered respirations, *bronchospasm, non-cardiogenic pulmonary edema,* shortness of breath
SKIN: Flushing, itching, phlebitis at IV INF site, rash, urticaria
MISC: Chills, sweating

INTERACTIONS

Drugs

3 *Heparin, oral anticoagulants,* *drugs that alter platelet function (i.e., aspirin, dipyridamole, abciximab, eptifibitide, tirofiben):* May increase the risk of bleeding

Labs

• *Fibrinogen:* False increase with certain methods
• *Lactate dehydrogenase isoenzymes:* False positive

---

streptomycin

(strep-toe-mye'sin)
Rx: Streptomycin
Chemical Class: Aminoglycoside
Therapeutic Class: Antibiotic; antituberculosis agent

CLINICAL PHARMACOLOGY

Mechanism of Action: Interferes with protein synthesis in bacterial cell by binding to ribosomal subunit, causing inaccurate peptide sequence to form in protein chain, causing bacterial death

Pharmacokinetics

IM: Onset rapid, peak 1-2 hr, plasma $t_{1/2}$ 2-2½ hr; not metabolized, excreted unchanged in urine; crosses placenta

INDICATIONS AND USES: In combination with other drugs (INH, rifampin, pyrazinamide) in the treatment of tuberculosis; also indicated when 1 or more of the above drugs contraindicated; part of multidrug treatment for *Mycobacterium avium* complex*; secondary choice for nontubercular infections caused by sensitive strains of gram-negative organisms: *Hemophilus influenzae* (with another agent); *H. ducreyi* (chancroid); *Klebsiella pneumoniae* pneumonia (with another agent); *Yersinia pestis* (plague); *Brucella* sp.; *Francisella tularensis* (tularemia); UTIs caused by *E. coli, Proteus* sp., *Klebsiella pneumonia;* gram-

S

---

italic = common side effects   ***bold italic*** = life-threatening reactions

positive organisms: *Streptococcus viridans* endocarditis (in combination with penicillin); *Enterococcus faecalis* (UTI and endocarditis); gram-negative bacillary bacteremia (with another agent); granuloma inguinale

DOSAGE

Adult

• *Tuberculosis:* IM 15 mg/kg/day (max 1 g qd); should ultimately be discontinued or reduced to 1 g 2-3 ×/wk; given in combination with other antitubercular drugs

• *Streptococcal endocarditis:* IM 1 g q12h for 1 wk with penicillin, then 500 mg bid for 1 wk; if >60 yr, give 500 mg bid for entire 2 wk

• *Enterococcal endocarditis:* IM 1 g q12h for 2 wk, then 500 mg q12h for 4 wk with penicillin

• *Tularemia:* IM 1-2 g qd in divided doses for 7-14 days or until afebrile for 5-7 days

• *Plague:* IM 2-4 g qd in divided doses until afebrile for 3 days

• *Moderate to severe infections:* IM 1-2 g qd in divided doses q6-12h, max 4 g qd

Child

• *Tuberculosis:* IM 20-40 mg/kg/day in divided doses q6-12h given with other antitubercular drugs, max 1 g/day

💲 AVAILABLE FORMS/COST OF THERAPY

• Inj, Sol—IM: 1 g: **$5.95**

CONTRAINDICATIONS: Severe renal disease

PRECAUTIONS: Neonates (renal immaturity) and especially those born to mothers on magnesium sulfate therapy (respiratory arrest), mild renal disease, hearing deficits, elderly

PREGNANCY AND LACTATION: Pregnancy category D; small amounts excreted into breast milk; compatible with breast feeding (oral absorption poor)

SIDE EFFECTS/ADVERSE REACTIONS

CNS: Confusion, depression, muscle twitching, neurotoxicity, numbness, *seizures,* tremors

CV: Hypotension, myocarditis, palpitations

EENT: Deafness, ototoxicity (especially vestibular toxicity), visual disturbances

GI: Anorexia, nausea, vomiting

GU: Azotemia, hematuria, ***nephrotoxicity,*** oliguria, ***renal damage, renal failure***

HEME: ***Agranulocytosis, eosinophilia, leukopenia, thrombocytopenia***

SKIN: Alopecia, burning, dermatitis, rash, urticaria

INTERACTIONS

Drugs

3 *Amphotericin B, cephalosporins, cyclosporine, NSAIDs:* Additive nephrotoxicity

3 *Carboplatin:* Additive ototoxicity

2 *Ethacrynic Acid:* Additive ototoxicity

3 *Extended-spectrum penicillins:* Inactivation of aminoglycoside

3 *Methoxyflurane:* Additive nephrotoxicity

2 *Neuromuscular blocking agents:* Respiratory depression

3 *Oral anticoagulants:* Enhanced hypoprothrombinemic response

Labs

• *Protein:* Falsely increases CSF-protein

• *Sugar:* Falsely increased urine levels via copper reduction methods

• *Urea Nitrogen:* Decreases serum levels

SPECIAL CONSIDERATIONS

• Not usually used for long term therapy secondary to nephrotoxicity and ototoxicity

---

* = non-FDA-approved use

MONITORING PARAMETERS

• Serum drug levels; therapeutic peak levels 20-30 µg/ml, toxic peak levels (1 hr after IM administration) >50 µg/ml

• Keep patient well hydrated

---

succimer

(sux′sim-mer)
Rx: Chemet
Chemical Class: Dimercaprol derivative
Therapeutic Class: Lead antidote

CLINICAL PHARMACOLOGY

Mechanism of Action: Forms water-soluble chelates with heavy metals that are excreted renally

Pharmacokinetics

PO: Rapidly but incompletely absorbed, peak 1-2 hr; metabolized to mixed succimer-cysteine disulfides; excreted in urine (mostly as metabolite) and feces; $t_{1/2}$ 2 days

INDICATIONS AND USES: Treatment of lead poisoning in children with blood levels >45 µg/dl; not for prophylaxis; may be of benefit in mercury* and arsenic* poisoning

DOSAGE

Adult and Child

• PO 10 mg/kg q8h for 5 days, then 10 mg/kg q12h for 14 days; may repeat if indicated by blood lead level; allow 2 wk between courses

💲 AVAILABLE FORMS/COST OF THERAPY

• Cap, Gel—Oral: 100 mg, 100's: **$405.33**

PRECAUTIONS: Reduced renal function, history of liver disease, children <1 yr

PREGNANCY AND LACTATION: Pregnancy category C; excretion in breast milk unknown; discourage mothers from breast feeding during therapy

SIDE EFFECTS/ADVERSE REACTIONS

CNS: Dizziness, drowsiness, headache, paresthesias
GI: Anorexia, diarrhea, metallic taste, nausea, vomiting
GU: Proteinuria, voiding difficulty
RESP: Cough
SKIN: Mucocutaneous eruptions, pruritus, rash
MISC: Chills, fever, flu-like symptoms

INTERACTIONS

Drugs

❷ *Other chelators (e.g., EDTA):* Coadministration not recommended

SPECIAL CONSIDERATIONS

PATIENT/FAMILY EDUCATION

• In children unable to swallow capsule, separate capsule and sprinkle beads on food or on spoon followed by fruit drink

MONITORING PARAMETERS

• Serum transaminases at start of therapy then qwk during therapy
• After therapy, monitor for rebound (because of redistribution of lead from bound stores to soft tissues, blood) qwk until stable

---

sucralfate

(soo-kral′fate)
Rx: Carafate
Chemical Class: Aluminum complex of sulfated sucrose
Therapeutic Class: Gastrointestinal antiulcer agent

CLINICAL PHARMACOLOGY

Mechanism of Action: Forms a complex that adheres to ulcer site, protects against acid, pepsin, bile salts

Pharmacokinetics

PO: Minimally absorbed, duration up to 5 hr; excreted in feces (90%)

---

italic = common side effects   ***bold italic*** = life-threatening reactions

INDICATIONS AND USES: Treatment and maintenance of duodenal ulcer; gastric ulcers*; reflux esophagitis*; NSAID-induced GI symptoms*; prevention of stress ulcers*; oral and esophageal radiation-induced ulcers (suspension)*

DOSAGE

Adult

• *Active ulcer:* PO 1 g qid 1 hr ac, hs for 4-8 wk

• *Maintenance:* PO 1 g bid

§ AVAILABLE FORMS/COST OF THERAPY

• Susp—Oral: 1 g/10 ml, 420 ml: **$35.58**

• Tab, Uncoated—Oral: 1 g, 100's: **$69.80-$85.26**

PRECAUTIONS: Renal failure, dialysis (small amounts aluminum absorbed with sucralfate)

PREGNANCY AND LACTATION: Pregnancy category B; little systemic absorption, so minimal, if any, excretion into milk expected

SIDE EFFECTS/ADVERSE REACTIONS

CNS: Dizziness, drowsiness, headache, vertigo

EENT: Laryngospasm

GI: Constipation, diarrhea, *dry mouth,* gastric pain, indigestion, nausea, vomiting

SKIN: Pruritus, rash, urticaria

INTERACTIONS

Drugs

3 *Ketoconazole:* Reduces plasma levels of antifungal

3 *Phenytoin:* Modest reduction in GI absorption of phenytoin

3 *Quinolones:* Reduced antibiotic levels

3 *Warfarin:* Isolated cases of reduced hypoprothrombinemic response to warfarin

SPECIAL CONSIDERATIONS
PATIENT/FAMILY EDUCATION

• Take antacids prn for pain relief,

but not within ½ hr before or after sucralfate

---

sulfacetamide

(sul-fa-see'ta-mide)

Rx: AK-Sulf, Bleph-10, Klaron, Ocu-Sul, Ocusulf-10, Sebizon, Sodium Sulamyd, Sulf-10, Sulfac
Combinations
  Rx: with prednisolone (Blephamide, Dioptimyd, Metamyd, Vasocidin, Isopto Cetapred); with sulfer (Sulfacet-R); with sulfabenzamide (Sulfathiazole, Sulfa-Gyn, Sulnac, Trysul); with phenylepherine (Vasosulf); with fluorometholone (FML-S)
Chemical Class: Sulfonamide derivative
Therapeutic Class: Antibiotic

CLINICAL PHARMACOLOGY
Mechanism of Action: Inhibits bacterial synthesis of dihydrofolic acid, which bacteria require for growth, through competitive inhibition of the enzyme dihydropteroate synthetase; bacteriostatic

Pharmacokinetics
OPHTH: Some systemic absorption; excreted mostly unchanged in urine; $t_{1/2}$ 7-13 hr

INDICATIONS AND USES: Conjunctivitis, corneal ulcer, superficial ocular infections, trachoma (adjunct to systemic sulfonamide therapy); seborrheic dermatitis, seborrhea sicca (dandruff); secondary bacterial infections of skin, acne vulgaris

DOSAGE

Adult and Child >2 mo (>12 yr for TOP lotion)

• *Conjunctivitis/corneal ulcer:* OPHTH instill 1 gtt in lower conjunctival sac(s) q1-3h according to

---

* = non-FDA-approved use

severity of infection; apply ¼ in ribbon of ointment to lower conjunctival sac(s) 1-4 times/day and hs
• *Trachoma:* Ophth instill 2 gtt of 30% sol q2h (in conjunction with systemic sulfonamide therapy)
• *Seborrheic dermatitis and dandruff:* TOP apply lotion hs and allow to remain overnight; may use bid for severe cases with crusting, heavy scaling, and inflammation
• *Acne:* Top apply 1-3 times/day

⑧ AVAILABLE FORMS/COST OF THERAPY
• Oint—Ophth: 10%, 3.5 g: **$5.09-$19.31**
• Sol—Ophth: 10%, 1, 2, 2.5, 5, 15 ml: **$1.45-$23.58**/15 ml; 15%, 5, 15 ml: **$2.10**/15 ml; 30%, 5, 15 ml: **$2.40-$25.01**/15 ml
• Lotion—Top: 10%, 60 ml: **$32.60;** 85 gm: **$23.72**

CONTRAINDICATIONS: Infants <2 mo; epithelial herpes simplex keratitis, vaccinia, varicella, and many other viral diseases of the cornea and conjunctiva; mycobacterial infection or fungal diseases of the ocular structures
PRECAUTIONS: Severe dry eye, children
PREGNANCY AND LACTATION: Pregnancy category B (category D if used near term); compatible with breast feeding in healthy, full-term infants
SIDE EFFECTS/ADVERSE REACTIONS
CNS: Fever, headache
EENT: Blurred vision (especially with ointment), browache, burning, conjunctival edema, itching, local irritation, reactive hyperemia, transient epithelial keratitis, transient stinging
METAB: **Bone marrow depression**
SKIN: **Exfoliative dermatitis,** photosensitivity, rash, **Stevens-Johnson**

syndrome, toxic epidermal necrolysis
INTERACTIONS
Drugs
❷ *Silver preparations:* Incompatible with sulfacetamide
SPECIAL CONSIDERATIONS
PATIENT/FAMILY EDUCATION
• May cause sensitivity to bright light
• Do not touch tip of container to any surface

---

sulfamethoxazole
(sul-fa-meth-ox′a-zole)
Rx: Gantanol
Combinations
  Rx: with trimethoprim, (Bactrim, Septra, Sulfaprim); see co-trimoxazol monograph
Chemical Class: Sulfonamide derivative
Therapeutic Class: Antibiotic

CLINICAL PHARMACOLOGY
Mechanism of Action: Inhibits bacterial synthesis of folic acid through competitive inhibition of the enzyme dihydropteroate synthetase; bacteriostatic
Pharmacokinetics
PO: Peak 3-4 hr; widely distributed into most body tissues; 50%-70% bound to plasma proteins; metabolized in liver by acetylation (inactive metabolite contributes to nephrotoxicity), excreted mainly in urine (20% unchanged, 70% acetylated metabolite); t₁/₂ 7-12 hr (prolonged in renal failure)
INDICATIONS AND USES: Chancroid, trachoma, inclusion conjunctivitis, nocardiosis, UTI, toxoplasmosis (adjunctive therapy with pyrimethamine), malaria (adjunctive therapy of chloroquine-resistant strains of *Plasmodium falciparum),*

S

meningococcal meningitis prophylaxis (when sulfonamide-sensitive group A strains prevail), acute otitis media due to *Hemophilus influenzae* (when used concomitantly with penicillin or erythromycin), pneumonia due to *pneumocystis carinii* Antibacterial spectrum usually includes:

• Gram-positive organisms: Some strains of staphylococci, streptococci, *Bacillus anthracis, Clostridium tetani, C. perfringens,* many strains of *Nocardia asteroides* and *N. brasiliensis*

• Gram-negative organisms: *Enterobacter, Escherichia coli, Klebsiella, Proteus mirabilis, P. vulgaris, Salmonella, Shigella*

• Miscellaneous organisms: *Pneumocystis carinii, Toxoplasma gondii, Plasmodium*

DOSAGE

Adult

• PO, mild to moderate infections, 2 g initially, then 1 g bid; or when combined with trimethoprim, 800 mg bid; severe infections, 2 g initially, then 1 g tid; dose modification for renal insufficiency: CrCl >30 ml/min: use normal dose; CrCl 15-30 ml/min: use one half of normal dose; CrCl <15 ml/min: use not recommended

Child >2 mo

• PO 50-60 mg/kg initially, then 25-30 mg/kg bid; do not exceed 75 mg/kg/day

$ AVAILABLE FORMS/COST OF THERAPY

• Tab, Uncoated—Oral: 500 mg, 100's: **$53.12**

• Tab, Uncoated—Oral: 400 mg combined with 80 mg trimethoprim, 100's: **$6.12-$78.18**

• Tab, Uncoated—Oral: 800 mg combined with 160 mg trimethoprim, 100's: **$8.93-$128.26**

CONTRAINDICATIONS: Infants <2 mo (except as adjunctive therapy with pyrimethamine for congenital toxoplasmosis), porphyria, megaloblastic anemia due to folate deficiency, pregnant women at term

PRECAUTIONS: Group A β-hemolytic streptococcal infections (do not use for treatment), renal or hepatic function impairment, allergy or asthma, G-6-PD deficiency

PREGNANCY AND LACTATION: Pregnancy category C (if used near term; may cause jaundice, hemolytic anemia, and kernicterus in newborns); excreted into breast milk in low concentrations; compatible with breast feeding in healthy, full-term infants

SIDE EFFECTS/ADVERSE REACTIONS

CNS: Apathy, ataxia, drowsiness, hallucinations, headache, insomnia, mental depression, peripheral neuropathy, *seizures,* transient lesions of posterior spinal column, transverse myelitis

CV: Allergic myocarditis

EENT: Conjunctival and scleral infection, hearing loss, tinnitus, vertigo

GI: Abdominal pains, anorexia, diarrhea, glossitis, hepatitis, *hepatocellular necrosis, nausea, pancreatitis, pseudomembranous colitis,* stomatitis, *vomiting*

GU: Crystalluria, elevated creatinine, hematuria, *nephrotic syndrome,* proteinuria, *toxic nephrosis with oliguria and anuria*

HEME: Agranulocytosis, aplastic anemia, hemolytic anemia, leukopenia, megaloblastic anemia, methemoglobinemia, purpura, *thrombocytopenia*

MS: Arthralgia

RESP: Pulmonary infiltrates, transient pulmonary changes

SKIN: Erythema multiforme, *exfo-*

liative dermatitis, photosensitivity, **Stevens-Johnson syndrome**

INTERACTIONS

Drugs

❷ *Para-aminobenzoic acid (PABA):* PABA may interfere with the antibacterial activity of sulfamethoxazole

❸ *Phenytoin:* Sulfamethoxazole increases phenytoin concentrations, requiring dosage adjustment

❸ *Warfarin:* Trimethoprim-sulfamethoxazole, sulfamethoxazole increase the hypoprothrombinemic response to warfarin via inhibition of metabolism

Labs

• α-*Amino-Nitrogen:* Increased in plasma
• *Clindamycin:* False positive
• *Colistin:* False positive
• *Creatinine-kinase:* Falsely decreases serum levels
• *Creatinine:* Falsely increases serum creatinine levels

SPECIAL CONSIDERATIONS
PATIENT/FAMILY EDUCATION

• Avoid prolonged exposure to sunlight
• Administer with full glass of water

MONITORING PARAMETERS

• CBC, renal function tests, urinalysis

---

sulfanilamide

(sul-fa-nil′a-mide)
Rx: AVC
Combinations
   Rx: with sulfabenzamide, sulfacetamide (Sultrin, Sulfa-Gyn, Sulnac, Trysol)
Chemical Class: Sulfonamide derivative
Therapeutic Class: Antifungal

CLINICAL PHARMACOLOGY
Mechanism of Action: Inhibits bacterial synthesis of folic acid through competitive antagonism of para-aminobenzoic acid (PABA); bacteriostatic

Pharmacokinetics

TOP: Absorbed through vaginal mucosa

INDICATIONS AND USES: *Candidia albicans* vulvovaginitis

DOSAGE

Adult

• VAG (supp) insert 1 suppository qd-bid, continue for 30 days; (cream) 1 applicatorful qd-bid, continued through 1 complete menstrual cycle

⑤ AVAILABLE FORMS/COST OF THERAPY

• Cre—Vag: 15%, 120 g: **$26.51-$37.48**
• Supp—Vag: 1.05 g, 16's: **$40.88**

CONTRAINDICATIONS: Kidney disease, pregnancy at term

PRECAUTIONS: Children

PREGNANCY AND LACTATION: Pregnancy category B (category D if used near term, may cause jaundice, hemolytic anemia, and kernicterus in newborns); excreted into breast milk in low concentrations, compatible with breast feeding in healthy, full-term infants

SIDE EFFECTS/ADVERSE REACTIONS

GU: Local irritation
HEME: **Agranulocytosis**
SKIN: **Stevens-Johnson syndrome** (rare)
MISC: Allergic reactions

SPECIAL CONSIDERATIONS
PATIENT/FAMILY EDUCATION

• Insert high into vagina
• Do not engage in vaginal intercourse during treatment
• Azoles are better choices

S

sulfasalazine
(sul-fa-sal'a-zeen)
Rx: Azaline, Azaline-EC,
Azulfidine, Azulfidine EN-Tabs
Chemical Class: Sulfonamide
derivative; salicylate derivative
Therapeutic Class: Gastrointestinal antiinflammatory;
disease-modifying arthritis
drug (DMARD)

CLINICAL PHARMACOLOGY
Mechanism of Action: Metabolized
in gut to sulfapyridine and 5-
aminosalicylic acid (mesalamine);
therapeutic action may be result of
antibacterial action of sulfapyridine
or antiinflammatory action of 5-
aminosalicylic acid on the colon;
5-aminosalicylic acid is the active
moiety in inflammatory bowel disease; in rheumatoid arthritis, intact
sulfasalazine and sulfapyridine both
have beneficial effects: sulfasalazine is thought to interact with the
mucosa-associated lymphoid tissue
in the gut whereas sulfapyridine primarily targets the synovium
Pharmacokinetics
PO: Unchanged drug 10%-15% absorbed, sulfapyridine rapidly absorbed, little 5-aminosalicylic acid
absorbed; peak 1.5-6 hr; sulfapyridine distributed to most body tissues and metabolized via acetylation in liver, excreted in urine (unchanged 15%, sulfapyridine and metabolites 60%, 5-aminosalicylic acid
and metabolites 20%-33%), unabsorbed 5-aminosalicylic acid excreted in feces; $t_{1/2}$ 8.4-10.4 hr
INDICATIONS AND USES: Ankylosing spondylitis,* atrophic balance,* collagenous colitis,* Crohn's
disease,* dermatitis herpetiformis,*
hypertrophic scars,* inflammatory
bowel disease,* juvenile arthritis,*
proctosigmoiditis—radiation induced,* psoriasis,* psoriatic arthritis,* pyoderma gangrenosum,* reactive arthritis,* Reiter's syndrome,*
rheumatoid arthritis, scleroderma,*
ulcerative colitis, urticaria*
DOSAGE
Adult
• PO 1 g tid-qid; do not exceed 6
g/day; maintenance 2 g/day divided
q6h
Child >2 yr
• PO 40-60 mg/kg/day in 3-6 divided doses; maintenance 30 mg/
kg/day in 4 divided doses; max dose
2 g/day
$ **AVAILABLE FORMS/COST
OF THERAPY**
• Tab, Uncoated—Oral: 500 mg,
100's: **$34.29**
• Tab, Enteric Coated—Oral: 500
mg, 100's: **$12.75-$28.61**
CONTRAINDICATIONS: Infants <2
yr, porphyria, intestinal or urinary
tract obstructions
PRECAUTIONS: Renal or hepatic
function impairment, allergy or
asthma, G-6-PD deficiency, blood
dyscrasias, slow acetylator pheno-
types
PREGNANCY AND LACTATION:
Pregnancy category B; excreted
into breast milk; should be given to
nursing mothers with caution because significant adverse effects
(bloody diarrhea) may occur in some
nursing infants
**SIDE EFFECTS/ADVERSE REAC-
TIONS**
CNS: Ataxia, cauda equina syndrome, drowsiness, fever, *Guillain-
Barré syndrome,* hallucinations,
headache, insomnia, mental depression, peripheral neuropathy, *seizures,*
transient lesions of the posterior spinal column, transverse myelitis, vertigo
CV: Allergic myocarditis, pericar-

---

* = non-FDA-approved use

ditis with or without tamponade, vasculitis

EENT: Conjunctival and scleral infection, hearing loss, periorbital edema, tinnitus

GI: Abdominal pains, *anorexia,* bloody diarrhea, diarrhea, *gastric distress, **hepatic necrosis,*** hepatitis, impaired folic acid absorption, *nausea,* neutropenic enterocolitis, ***pancreatitis,*** stomatitis, *vomiting*

GU: Crystalluria, hematuria, ***hemolytic-uremic syndrome,*** nephritis, nephrotic syndrome, proteinuria, *reversible oligospermia,* **toxic nephrosis with oliguria and anuria**

HEME: **Agranulocytosis, aplastic anemia, congenital neutropenia, Heinz body anemia, hemolytic anemia, hypoprothrombinemia, leukopenia,** megaloblastic anemia, **methemoglobinemia, myelodysplastic syndrome,** purpura, **thrombocytopenia**

MS: Arthralgias, ***rhabdomyolysis***

RESP: **Cyanosis,** fibrosing alveolitis, pleuritis, pneumonitis with or without eosinophilia

SKIN: Alopecia, ***epidermal necrolysis (Lyell's syndrome) with corneal damage,*** erythema multiforme, ***exfoliative dermatitis,*** parapsoriasis varioliformis acuta (Mucha-Habermann syndrome), photosensitization, pruritus, skin rash, ***Stevens-Johnson syndrome,*** urticaria

MISC: ***Anaphylaxis,*** polyarteritis nodosa, serum sickness syndrome

INTERACTIONS
Drugs

🔳 *Digoxin:* Sulfasalazine reduces digoxin serum concentrations

🔳 *Methenamine:* Combination of sulfadiazine and methenamine can result in crystalluria

🔳 *Phenytoin:* Some sulfonamides (sulfaphenazole, sulmethoxazole) increase phenytoin concentrations, requiring dosage adjustment

🔳 *Tolbutamide:* Several sulfonamides (sulfamethizole, sulfaphenazole, sulfisoxasole) can increase plasma sulfonylurea levels and enhance their hypoglycemic effects

🔳 *Warfarin:* Several sulfonamides (trimethoprim-sulfamethoxazole, sulfamethoxazole, sulfamethizole, sulfaphenazole) increase the hypoprothrombinemic response to warfarin via inhibition of metabolism

Labs
• *Bilirubin, conjugated:* Falsely increased in serum
• *Bilirubin, unconjugated:* Falsely decreased in serum
• *Creatinine:* Falsely increased in serum
• *Potassium:* Falsely decreased in serum
• *False positive:* Urinary glucose tests (Benedict's method)

SPECIAL CONSIDERATIONS
PATIENT/FAMILY EDUCATION
• Adequate hydration and urinary output are essential to prevent crystalluria and stone formation
• Avoid prolonged exposure to sunlight

MONITORING PARAMETERS
• Inflammatory bowel disease: Decrease in rectal bleeding or diarrhea in conjunction with mucosal healing
• Rheumatoid arthritis: Tender, swollen joints, visual analogue scale for pain; acute phase reactants (ESR, C-reactive protein), duration of early morning stiffness, preservation of function
• Baseline and periodic hematocrit, reticulocyte, platelet count and white blood cell count; urinalysis; renal and liver function tests

---

italic = common side effects   ***bold italic*** = life-threatening reactions

sulfathiazole/ sulfacetamide/ sulfabenzamide (triple sulfa)

(sul-fa-thye′a-zole/sul-fa-see′ta-mide/sul-fa-ben′za-mide)

Rx: Gyne-Sulf, Sultrin Triple Sulfa, Triple Sulfa, Trysul, V.V.S.

Chemical Class: Sulfonamide derivatives

Therapeutic Class: Antibiotic

CLINICAL PHARMACOLOGY

Mechanism of Action: Inhibits bacterial synthesis of folic acid through competitive antagonism of para-aminobenzoic acid (PABA); bacteriostatic

INDICATIONS AND USES: Bacterial vaginosis

DOSAGE

Adult

• VAG (cream) insert 1 applicatorful bid for 4-6 days, treatment can then be reduced 25%-50%, repeat prn

$ AVAILABLE FORMS/COST OF THERAPY

• Cre—Vag: 3.7% sulfabenzamide/ 2.86% sulfacetamide/3.42% sulfathiazole, 78, 82.5 g: **$5.37-$35.10**/78 g

CONTRAINDICATIONS: Kidney disease, pregnancy at term

PRECAUTIONS: Children

PREGNANCY AND LACTATION: Pregnancy category B (category D if used near term; may cause jaundice, hemolytic anemia, and kernicterus in newborns); excreted into breast milk in low concentrations; compatible with breast feeding in healthy, full-term infants

SIDE EFFECTS/ADVERSE REACTIONS

GU: Local irritation

HEME: Agranulocytosis

SKIN: Stevens-Johnson syndrome (rare)

MISC: Allergic reactions

SPECIAL CONSIDERATIONS

PATIENT/FAMILY EDUCATION

• Insert high into vagina

• Do not engage in vaginal intercourse during treatment

sulfinpyrazone

(sul-fin-pyr′a-zone)

Rx: Anturane

Chemical Class: Pyrazolidine derivative

Therapeutic Class: Antigout agent; uricosuric; antithrombotic agent

CLINICAL PHARMACOLOGY

Mechanism of Action: Uricosuric: Inhibits tubular reabsorption of uric acid; *Antithrombotic:* Prostaglandin synthetase inhibitor; lacks anti-inflammatory and analgesic properties

Pharmacokinetics

PO: Well absorbed; max plasma concentration, 1.6 hr; hepatic metabolism, 2 active metabolites, 98%-99% bound to plasma proteins; 50% excreted in urine unchanged; $t_{1/2}$ 2.2-3 hr

INDICATIONS AND USES: Chronic and intermittent gouty arthritis, prevention of recurrent MI (further study indicated),* prevention of systemic embolism in rheumatic mitral stenosis,* preservation of life of hemodialysis shunts

DOSAGE

Adult

• PO 200-400 mg/day in 2 divided doses initially, increase to 400-800 mg/day in 2 divided doses; use lowest dose that will control blood uric acid level

$ AVAILABLE FORMS/COST OF THERAPY

• Cap, Gel—Oral: 200 mg, 100's: **$48.51-$72.70**

* = non-FDA-approved use

• Tab, Uncoated—Oral: 100 mg, 100's: **$34.43-$45.15**

CONTRAINDICATIONS: Active peptic ulcer, symptoms of GI inflammation or ulceration, hypersensitivity to phenylbutazone or other pyrazoles, blood dyscrasias

PRECAUTIONS: Renal function impairment, healed peptic ulcer, dehydration, acute gout attack

PREGNANCY AND LACTATION: Pregnancy category C

SIDE EFFECTS/ADVERSE REACTIONS

GI: Aggravation or reactivation of peptic ulcer, *upper GI disturbances*
HEME: ***Agranulocytosis, aplastic anemia, anemia, leukopenia, thrombocytopenia***
GU: Interstitial nephritis, ***renal failure***
RESP: Bronchospasm (patients with aspirin-induced asthma)
SKIN: Rash

INTERACTIONS
Drugs
3 *Acetaminophen:* Increased metabolism of acetaminophen by about 20%; increased risk of acetaminophen toxicity
3 *Beta-blockers:* Reduced hypotensive effects of β-blockers
• *Heparinoids:* Risk of augmented bleeding and epidural or spinal hematomas is increased when used concurrently with another agent that affects hemostasis
2 *Methotrexate:* Increased methotrexate levels with subsequent increased effect and potential toxicity
2 *Oral anticoagulants:* Inhibit warfarin metabolism and possibly other oral anticoagulants, increasing prothrombin time response; concomitant antiplatelet effects further complicate combined therapy
3 *Salicylates:* Inhibited uricosuric effect of each other

Labs
• *Cyclosporine:* Falsely decreased serum levels

SPECIAL CONSIDERATIONS
PATIENT/FAMILY EDUCATION
• Take with food, milk, or antacids to decrease stomach upset
• Avoid aspirin and other salicylate-containing products
• Drink plenty of fluids
MONITORING PARAMETERS
• Serum uric acid concentrations, renal function, CBC

---

sulfisoxazole
(sul-fi-sox'a-zole)
Rx: Gantrisin
Combination
  Rx: with erythromycin
    (Pediazole, Sulfimycin)
Chemical Class: Sulfonamide derivative
Therapeutic Class: Antibiotic

CLINICAL PHARMACOLOGY
Mechanism of Action: Inhibits bacterial synthesis of folic acid (pteroylglutamic acid) from aminobenzoic acid through competitive inhibition of the enzyme dihydropteroate synthetase; bacteriostatic
Pharmacokinetics
PO: Peak 1-4 hr; 85% bound to plasma proteins; parent drug and acetylated metabolites excreted in urine; $t_{1/2}$ 4.6-7.8 hr
INDICATIONS AND USES: Chancroid, trachoma, inclusion conjunctivitis, nocardiosis, UTI, toxoplasmosis (adjunctive therapy with pyrimethamine), malaria (adjunctive therapy of chloroquine-resistant strains of *Plasmodium falciparum),* meningococcal meningitis prophylaxis (when sulfonamide-sensitive group A strains prevail), meningococcal meningitis, acute otitis me-

S

---

italic = common side effects   ***bold italic*** = life-threatening reactions

dia due to *Hemophilus influenzae* (when used concomitantly with penicillin or erythromycin), *H. influenzae* meningitis (adjunctive therapy with parenteral streptomycin), recurrent otitis media*

Antibacterial spectrum usually includes:

• Gram-positive organisms: some strains of staphylococci, streptococci, *Bacillus anthracis, Clostridium tetani, C. perfringens,* many strains of *Nocardia asteroides* and *N. brasiliensis*

• Gram-negative organisms: *Enterobacter, Escherichia coli, Klebsiella, Proteus mirabilis, P. vulgaris, Salmonella, Shigella*

• Miscellaneous organisms: *Toxoplasma gondii, Plasmodium*

DOSAGE
Adult
• PO 4-8 g/day in 4-6 divided doses
Child >2 mo
• PO 75 mg/kg initially, then 120-150 mg/kg/day in 4-6 divided doses; max 6 g/day

§ AVAILABLE FORMS/COST OF THERAPY
• Tab, Uncoated—Oral: 500 mg, 100's: **$7.88-$19.89**
• Sol—Ophth 4%: 15 ml: **$9.44**
• Susp—Oral: 500 mg/5 ml, 480 ml: **$42.21**

CONTRAINDICATIONS: Infants <2 mo, porphyria, megaloblastic anemia due to folate deficiency, pregnant women at term

PRECAUTIONS: Group A β-hemolytic streptococcal infections (do not use for treatment), renal or hepatic function impairment, allergy or asthma, G-6-PD deficiency

PREGNANCY AND LACTATION: Pregnancy category C (if used near term; may cause jaundice, hemolytic anemia, and kernicterus in newborns); excreted into breast milk in low concentrations; compatible with breast feeding in healthy, full-term infants

SIDE EFFECTS/ADVERSE REACTIONS
CNS: Apathy, ataxia, drowsiness, hallucinations, headache, insomnia, mental depression, peripheral neuropathy, *seizures,* transient lesions of posterior spinal column, transverse myelitis
CV: Allergic myocarditis
EENT: Conjunctival and scleral infection, hearing loss, tinnitus, vertigo
GI: Abdominal pains, anorexia, diarrhea, glossitis, hepatitis, *hepatocellular necrosis,* nausea, *pancreatitis, pseudomembranous colitis,* stomatitis, *vomiting*
GU: Crystalluria, elevated creatinine, hematuria, nephrotic syndrome, proteinuria, *toxic nephrosis with oliguria and anuria*
HEME: Agranulocytosis, aplastic anemia, hemolytic anemia, leukopenia, megaloblastic anemia, methemoglobinemia, purpura, *thrombocytopenia*
MS: Arthralgia
RESP: Pulmonary infiltrates, transient pulmonary changes
SKIN: Erythema multiforme, *exfoliative dermatitis,* photosensitivity, *Stevens-Johnson syndrome*

INTERACTIONS
Drugs
❷ *Para-aminobenzoicacid (PABA):* PABA may interfere with the antibacterial activity of sulfamethoxazole
❸ *Phenytoin:* Sulfamethoxazole increases phenytoin concentrations, requiring dosage adjustment
❸ *Tolbutamide:* Sulfisoxazole can increase plasma sulfonylurea levels and enhance their hypoglycemic effects

---

* = non-FDA-approved use

3 *Warfarin:* Trimethoprim-sulfamethoxazole, sulfamethoxazole increase the hypoprothrombinemic response to warfarin via inhibition of metabolism

Labs
• *Folate:* Falsely decreased serum levels
• *Protein:* Falsely increased in CSF
• *Urobilinogen:* Decreased falsely in feces

SPECIAL CONSIDERATIONS
PATIENT/FAMILY EDUCATION
• Avoid prolonged exposure to sunlight
• Administer with glass of water
MONITORING PARAMETERS
• CBC, renal function tests, urinalysis

---

sulindac
(sul-in′dak)
Rx: Clinoril
Chemical Class: Acetic acid derivative
Therapeutic Class: NSAID with analgesic and antipyretic activity

CLINICAL PHARMACOLOGY
Mechanism of Action: Reversible cyclooxygenase (i.e., prostaglandin synthetase) inhibitor; non-selectively decreases the formation of both prostaglandins and thromboxane A2; variable effects on lipoxygenase synthesis and subsequent leukotriene production; antiinflammatory, antipyretic, and analgesic activity; inhibits platelet aggregation
Pharmacokinetics
PO: Onset of antirheumatic action within 7 days, peak 1-2 wk, peak serum levels 2-4 hr; sulindac is inactive until metabolized to active sulfide metabolite, excreted in urine primarily in biologically inactive forms (may possibly affect renal

function to lesser extent than other NSAIDs), 25% excreted in feces; $t_{1/2}$ 7.8 hr (sulfide metabolite 16.4 hr)
INDICATIONS AND USES: Osteoarthritis, rheumatoid arthritis, ankylosing spondylitis, prevention of cognitive decline,* prevention of colon cancer,* colon polyposis,* acute gouty arthritis, pain—mild to moderate, tendonitis/bursitis, painful shoulder, amnioreduction,* cough—angiotensin-converting enzyme inhibitor,* diabetic neuropathy,* antihypertensive/diuretic requiring patient—less negating effects,* pain—cancer,* preterm labor,* soft tissue injuries,* SLE
DOSAGE
Adult
• PO 150-200 mg bid with food; max 400 mg/day
Child
• PO dose not established although 4 mg/kg/day divided bid has been used
$ **AVAILABLE FORMS/COST OF THERAPY**
• Tab, Uncoated—Oral: 150 mg, 100's: **$74.71-$112.34;** 200 mg, 100's: **$89.91-$138.05**
CONTRAINDICATIONS: Bronchospasm, nasal polyps, angioedema precipitated by aspirin or other NSAIDs
PRECAUTIONS: History of GI ulceration, bleeding, or perforation; renal dysfunction, hypertension or cardiac conditions aggravated by fluid retention and edema, history of liver dysfunction, history of coagulation
PREGNANCY AND LACTATION: Pregnancy category B (category D if used in 3rd trimester); could cause constriction of the ductus arteriosus *in utero*, persistent pulmonary hypertension of the newborn, or prolonged labor

---

italic = common side effects   ***bold italic*** = life-threatening reactions

S

SIDE EFFECTS/ADVERSE REACTIONS

CNS: Dizziness, headache, lightheadedness

CV: Chest pain, **CHF,** dysrhythmias, edema, hypertension, hypotension, palpitation, tachycardia

EENT: Dry eyes, hearing disturbances, photophobia, tinnitus, visual disturbances

GI: Abdominal cramps, constipation, diarrhea, *dyspepsia,* flatulence, **gastric or duodenal ulcer with bleeding or perforation,** hepatitis, **pancreatitis,** vomiting

GU: **Acute renal failure**

HEME: **Agranulocytosis,** eosinophilia, **leukopenia, neutropenia, pancytopenia, thrombocytopenia**

METAB: Hyperglycemia, hyperkalemia, hypoglycemia, hyponatremia

RESP: Bronchospasm, dyspnea, pulmonary infiltrates

SKIN: Photosensitivity, rash, urticaria

INTERACTIONS

Drugs

■ *Aminoglycosides:* Reduced clearance with elevated aminoglycoside levels and potential for toxicity (especially indomethacin in premature infants; other NSAIDs probably)

■ *Anticoagulants:* Excessive hypoprothrombinemia, decreased platelet aggregation with increased risk of GI bleeding

■ *Antihypertensives (α-blockers, angiotensin-converting enzyme inhibitors, angiotensin II receptor blockers, β-blockers, diuretics):* Inhibition of antihypertensive and other favorable hemodynamic effects

■ *Corticosteroids:* Increased risk of GI ulceration

■ *Cyclosporine:* Increased nephrotoxicity risk

■ *Lithium:* Decreased clearance of lithium (mediated via prostaglandins) resulting in elevated serum lithium levels and risk of toxicity

■ *Methotrexate:* Decreased renal secretion of methotrexate resulting in elevated methotrexate levels and risk of toxicity

■ *Phenylpropanolamine:* Possible acute hypertensive reaction

■ *Potassium-sparing diuretics:* Additive hyperkalemia potential

■ *Triamterene:* Acute renal failure reported with addition of indomethacin; caution with other NSAIDs

SPECIAL CONSIDERATIONS

• No significant advantage over other NSAIDs; cost should govern use

PATIENT/FAMILY EDUCATION

• Avoid aspirin and alcoholic beverages

• Take with food, milk, or antacids to decrease GI upset

• Antirheumatic action may not be apparent for several weeks

MONITORING PARAMETERS

• Initial hemogram and fecal occult blood test within 3 mo of starting regular chronic therapy; repeat every 6-12 mo (more frequently in high-risk patients >65 years, peptic ulcer disease, concurrent steroids or anticoagulants); electrolytes, creatinine, and BUN within 3 mo of starting regular chronic therapy; repeat every 6-12 mo

sumatriptan
(soo-ma-trip′tan)
Rx: Imitrex
Chemical Class: Serotonin derivative
Therapeutic Class: Antimigraine agent

CLINICAL PHARMACOLOGY
Mechanism of Action: Selectively

activates vascular 5-HT$_1$-receptors in cranial arteries causing vasoconstriction, and inhibiting proinflammatory neuropeptide release, actions correlating with the relief of migraine in humans

Pharmacokinetics

PO: Poor bioavailability (15%); onset 1-1½ hr, peak 2-2½ hr

SC: Onset within 1 hr, peak 12 min

Metabolized by microsomal monoamine oxidase (MAO), excreted in urine (60%) and feces (40%); t$_{½}$ 2½ hr

INDICATIONS AND USES: Acute migraine headache with or without aura; cluster headache

DOSAGE

Adult

• SC 6 mg at 1st sign of headache or after completion of aura; may repeat if partial relief after 1 hr; max 12 mg/24 hr

• PO 25-100 mg at 1st sign of headache; may repeat q2h prn up to 300 mg/24 hr max; no evidence that doses larger than 25 mg provide substantially greater relief

• PO following SC, single tablets (25-50 mg) may be repeated at 2 hr intervals up to 200 mg/24 hr max

• Nasal 5-20 mg at 1st sign of headache or after completion of aura; may repeat if partial relief after 2 hr, max 40 mg/24 hr

§ AVAILABLE FORMS/COST OF THERAPY

• Inj, Sol—SC: 6 mg/0.5 ml, 2's: **$91.43**

• Tab, Uncoated—Oral: 25 mg, 9's: **$133.46**; 50 mg, 9's: **$133.46**

• Spray, Sol—Nasal: 5 mg/spray, 6's: **$114.08**; 20 mg/spray, 6's: **$114.08**

CONTRAINDICATIONS: Hemiplegic or basilar migraine, IV inj (potential for coronary vasospasm), ischemic heart disease, Prinzmetal's angina, uncontrolled hypertension, within 24 hr of ergotamine-containing products

PRECAUTIONS: Atypical headache, renal or hepatic function impairment, elderly, children

PREGNANCY AND LACTATION: Pregnancy category C; excreted in breast milk in animals, no data in humans

SIDE EFFECTS/ADVERSE REACTIONS

CNS: Anxiety, *dizziness,* drowsiness, fatigue, headache

CV: Chest discomfort, **dysrhythmia,** hypertension, hypotension, **myocardial ischemia**

EENT: Sinus discomfort, throat discomfort, vertigo, vision alterations

GI: Diarrhea, discomfort of mouth and tongue, reflux

MS: Jaw discomfort, muscle cramps, myalgias, neck pain and stiffness, weakness

SKIN: Flushing, *inj site reaction,* sweating

MISC: Atypical sensations, (tingling, warm or hot sensation, burning sensation, feeling of heaviness, pressure sensation, feeling of tightness, numbness; feeling strange, tight feeling in head; cold sensation)

INTERACTIONS

Drugs

3 *Ergot-containing drugs:* Potential for prolonged vasospastic reactions and additive vasoconstriction, theoretical precaution

2 *Sibutramine:* Increased risk of serotonin syndrome

SPECIAL CONSIDERATIONS

• First inj should be administered under medical supervision

PATIENT/FAMILY EDUCATION

• Use only to treat migraine headache; not for prevention

---

italic = common side effects   **bold italic** = life-threatening reactions

suprofen
(soo-pro'fen)
Rx: Profenal
Chemical Class: Phenylal-
kanoic acid derivative
Therapeutic Class: Ophthal-
mic anti-inflammatory;
NSAID

CLINICAL PHARMACOLOGY
Mechanism of Action: Inhibits miosis induced during ocular surgery
by inhibiting the actions of prostaglandins that constrict the iris
sphincter independently of cholinergic mechanisms
INDICATIONS AND USES: Inhibi-
tion of intraoperative miosis
DOSAGE
Adult
• OPHTH 2 gtt in conjunctival sac
3, 2, and 1 hr prior to surgery; may
also instill 2 gtt q4h while awake the
day preceding surgery
**§ AVAILABLE FORMS/COST
OF THERAPY**
• Sol, Ophth—Top: 1%, 2.5 ml:
$10.00
CONTRAINDICATIONS: Epithelial herpes simplex keratitis
PRECAUTIONS: Known bleeding
tendencies, concurrent use of anti-
coagulants, children
PREGNANCY AND LACTATION:
Pregnancy category C
**SIDE EFFECTS/ADVERSE REAC-
TIONS**
EENT: Chemosis, discomfort, iritis,
irritation, itching, pain, photopho-
bia, punctate epithelial staining, red-
ness, transient burning and stinging

tacrine
(tack'rin)
Rx: Cognex
Chemical Class: Monoamine
acridine derivative
Therapeutic Class: Antidementia agent

CLINICAL PHARMACOLOGY
Mechanism of Action: Centrally
acting cholinesterase inhibitor; presumably elevates acetylcholine concentrations; a deficiency of acetylcholine may account for some clinical manifestations of mild to moderate dementia
Pharmacokinetics
PO: Rapidly absorbed; peak serum
concentrations 1-2 hr; 55% bound
to plasma proteins; metabolized by
cytochrome P450 system in liver;
elimination $t_{1/2}$ 2-4 hr
INDICATIONS AND USES: Treatment of mild to moderate dementia
of the Alzheimer's type
DOSAGE
Adult
• PO 10 mg qid for 4 wk, then 20
mg qid for 4 wk; increase at 4-wk
intervals, if patient tolerating drug
well, to dose of 120-160 mg/day in
divided doses qid
**§ AVAILABLE FORMS/COST
OF THERAPY**
• Cap, Gel—Oral: 10, 20, 30, 40
mg, 120's: **$147.01**
CONTRAINDICATIONS: Patients
treated with this drug who developed jaundice (total bilirubin >3
mg/dl)
PRECAUTIONS: Sick sinus syndrome, history of ulcers, GI bleeding, hepatic disease, bladder obstruction, asthma
PREGNANCY AND LACTATION:
Pregnancy category C; excretion
into breast milk unknown

SIDE EFFECTS/ADVERSE REACTIONS

CNS: Abnormal thinking, agitation, anxiety, ataxia, chills, confusion, depression, dizziness, fever, hallucinations, hostility, insomnia, somnolence, tremor

CV: Bradycardia, hypertension, hypotension

GI: Anorexia, diarrhea, dyspepsia, flatulence, **hepatotoxicity**, nausea, transaminase elevation, vomiting

GU: Frequency, incontinence, UTI

MS: Myalgia

SKIN: Flushing, rash

RESP: Asthma, cough, pharyngitis, rhinitis

INTERACTIONS

Drugs

3 *Anticholinergics:* Inhibits anticholinergic effect, centrally acting anticholinergics may inhibit effect of tacrine

3 *Beta-blockers:* Additive bradycardia

3 *Cholinergics:* Increased cholinergic effects

3 *Cimetidine:* Increased tacrine levels

3 *Levodopa:* Decreased levodopa effect

3 *Quinolones:* Inhibition of tacrine metabolism

3 *Serotonin reuptake inhibitors:* Increased tacrine concentrations

3 *Smoking:* Markedly reduces tacrine levels

3 *Theophylline:* Increased theophylline concentrations

SPECIAL CONSIDERATIONS

• Transaminase elevation is the most common reason for withdrawal of drug (8%); monitor ALT q wk for 1st 18 wk, then decrease to q 3 mo; when dose is increased, monitor q wk for 6 wk

• If elevations occur, modify dose as follows: ALT ≤3 times upper limit normal (ULN) continue current dose; ALT >3 to ≤5 times ULN reduce dose by 40 mg qd and resume dose titration when within normal limits; ALT >5 times ULN stop treatment; rechallenge may be tried if ALT is <10 times ULN

• Do not rechallenge if clinical jaundice develops

• Improvement in symptoms of dementia statistically, but perhaps not clinically significant; discontinue therapy if improvement not evident to family members and clinician

---

tacrolimus
(tak-roe-leem´us)
Rx: Prograf
Chemical Class: Macrolide derivative
Therapeutic Class: Immunosuppressant

CLINICAL PHARMACOLOGY

Mechanism of Action: Inhibits T-lymphocyte activation; suppresses humoral immunity and cell-mediated reactions such as allograft rejection

Pharmacokinetics

PO: Peak 1.5-3.5 hr, absolute bioavailability 14.4-17.4%, food reduces absorption and bioavailability; 75-99% bound to plasma proteins, crosses the placenta; extensively metabolized by liver; $t_{1/2}$ 11.7 hr

INDICATIONS AND USES: Prophylaxis of organ rejection in patients receiving allogenic liver transplants (in conjunction with adrenal corticosteroids); kidney, bone marrow, cardiac, pancreas, pancreatic island cell and small bowel transplantation*; autoimmune disease*; severe recalcitrant psoriasis*

DOSAGE

Adult

• IV 0.05-0.1 mg/kg/day as a continuous infusion; initiate no sooner

T

---

than 6 hr after transplantation; convert to oral therapy as soon as possible; PO 0.15-0.3 mg/kg/day divided q12h; initiate no sooner than 6 hr after transplantation or 8-12 hr after discontinuing IV infusion; titrate dose based on clinical assessments of rejection and tolerability

Child

• Initiate therapy at the high end of the recommended adult IV and PO dosing ranges (0.1 mg/kg/day IV and 0.3 mg/kg/day PO)

$ AVAILABLE FORMS/COST OF THERAPY

• Inj, Sol—IV: 5 mg/ml, **$115.62**
• Cap —Oral: 1 mg, 100's: **$280.48;** 5 mg, 100's: **$1,402.20**

CONTRAINDICATIONS: Hypersensitivity to HCO-60 polyoxyl 60 hydrogenated castor oil (used in vehicle for injection)

PRECAUTIONS: Impaired renal function

PREGNANCY AND LACTATION: Pregnancy category C; excreted in breast milk, avoid nursing

SIDE EFFECTS/ADVERSE REACTIONS

CNS: **Coma,** delirium, *neurotoxicity (tremor, headache, changes in motor function, mental status and sensory function),* paresthesia, **seizures**
CV: Hypertension, peripheral edema
GI: Abdominal pain, anorexia, constipation, diarrhea, elevated liver function tests, nausea, vomiting
GU: **Nephrotoxicity**
HEME: Anemia, leukocytosis, **thrombocytopenia**
METAB: Hyperglycemia, hyperkalemia (10-44%), hyperuricemia, hypokalemia, hypomagnesemia
MS: Back pain
RESP: Atelectasis, dyspnea, pleural effusion
SKIN: Pruritus, rash

MISC: **Anaphylaxis** (with injection), *asthenia, fever,* **lymphoma,** *pain*

INTERACTIONS

Drugs

3 *Antifungals, bromocriptine, calcium channel blockers, cimetidine, clarithromycin, danazol, erythromycin, methylprednisolone, metoclopramide:* Increased tacrolimus blood levels

3 *Carbamazepine, phenobarbital, phenytoin, rifamycins:* Decreased tacrolimus blood levels

2 *Nephrotoxic agents:* Potential for additive or synergistic nephrotoxicity (aminoglycosides, amphotericin B, cisplatin, cyclosporine)

2 *Potassium-sparing diuretics:* Increased risk of hyperkalemia

MONITORING PARAMETERS

• Regularly assess serum creatinine and potassium
• Whole blood tacrolimus concentrations as measured by ELISA may be helpful in assessing rejection and toxicity, median trough concentrations measured after the second week of therapy ranged from 9.8 to 19.4 mg/ml

---

tamoxifen

(ta-mox'i-fen)
Rx: Nolvadex
Chemical Class: Triphenylethylene derivative
Therapeutic Class: Antineoplastic

CLINICAL PHARMACOLOGY
Mechanism of Action: Competes with estrogen for receptor sites; nonsteroidal antiestrogen

Pharmacokinetics

PO: Extensively metabolized; peak 4-7 hr, $t_{1/2}$ 14 days (active metabolite); excreted primarily in feces

INDICATIONS AND USES: Adjuvant therapy of axillary node-negative breast cancer and of node positive cancer in post-menopausal women following mastectomy, axillary dissection, and breast irradiation; treatment of metastatic breast cancer in both women and men; most beneficial in estrogen receptor-positive tumors; reduction in incidence of breast cancer in high-risk women (defined as ≥35 yr with a 5-yr predicted risk of breast cancer ≥1.67% as calculated by the Gail Model); also used in mastalgia,* gynecomastia*

DOSAGE
Adult
• PO 10-20 mg bid
• *Gynecomastia/mastalgia:* PO 10 mg qd

💲 AVAILABLE FORMS/COST OF THERAPY
• Tab, Uncoated—Oral: 10 mg, 100's: **$149.30-$260.67**
• Tab—Oral: 20 mg, 100's: **$352.88**

PRECAUTIONS: Leukopenia, thrombocytopenia, cataracts, liver disease, hypercalcemia, undiagnosed abnormal vaginal bleeding

PREGNANCY AND LACTATION: Pregnancy category D; excretion into breast milk unknown

SIDE EFFECTS/ADVERSE REACTIONS
CNS: Depression, *headache, hot flashes, (33%) lightheadedness*
CV: Chest pain
EENT: Blurred vision (high doses), corneal opacity, ocular lesions, retinopathy
GI: Abnormal liver function tests, altered taste, anorexia, **hepatic necrosis,** *nausea, vomiting*
GU: **Endometrial cancer,** *menstrual changes (irregularity, oligomenorrhea, amenorrhea),* pruritus vulvae, vaginal bleeding
HEME: **Deep vein thrombosis, leukopenia, thrombocytopenia**
METAB: Hypercalcemia

RESP: **Pulmonary embolism**
SKIN: Alopecia, rash

INTERACTIONS
Drugs
❷ *Aminoglutethimide:* Reduces tamoxifen concentrations

SPECIAL CONSIDERATIONS
• Treatment duration >5 yr may provide no further benefit and increase risk of endometrial cancer for some women; reevaluate the need for continued therapy
• The Gail Model Risk Assessment Tool is available to health care professionals by calling (800) 456-3669 (ext. 3838)
• Premenopausal women should use nonhormonal contraception during treatment

MONITORING PARAMETERS
• Endometrial biopsy indicated for abnormal vaginal bleeding

---

tamsulosin
(tam-sool'o-sin)
Rx: Flomax
Chemical Class: Quinazoline
Therapeutic Class: α_1-adrenergic blocker: symptomatic benign prostatic hypertrophy

CLINICAL PHARMACOLOGY
Mechanism of Action: Selective and preferential postsynaptic alpha$_1$-adrenergic receptor blockade in lower urinary tract and prostate; results in smooth muscle relaxation in bladder neck and prostate without affecting bladder contractility; minimal effect on cardiovascular system (i.e., minimal hypotensive response)

Pharmacokinetics
PO: Peak 4-5 hr (6-7 hr with food) Absorption >90% fasting; food reduces peak concentrations by 40-70% and AUC by 30%; extensive hepatic metabolism; excreted in

urine as inactive metabolites; $t_{1/2}$ 9-13 hr

INDICATIONS AND USES: BPH, symptomatic relief of signs and symptoms

DOSAGE

Adult

• *BPH:* 0.4-0.8 mg qd (administered approx. 30 min following the same meal each day)

💲 AVAILABLE FORMS/COST OF THERAPY

• Cap—Oral: 0.4 mg 100's: **$149.98**

PRECAUTIONS: Like all alpha blockers, potential for "first-dose" phenomenon: marked hypotension with first couple of doses; elderly patients and those receiving calcium channel antagonists, diuretics, and β-blockers, have increased risks; anticipate the same effect if therapy is interrupted for several days

PREGNANCY AND LACTATION: Pregnancy category B; not indicated for use in women

SIDE EFFECTS/ADVERSE REACTIONS

CNS: Asthenia, dizziness, insomnia, somnolence, syncope, vertigo

CV: Orthostatic hypotension

GI: Bitter taste, elevations in ALT, AST; nausea, stomach discomfort

GU: Abnormal ejaculation, decreased libido

MS: Back pain

RESP: Cough, rhinorrhea

INTERACTIONS

Drugs

3 β-*blockers:* Enhanced "first-dose" phenomenon

SPECIAL CONSIDERATIONS
PATIENT/FAMILY EDUCATION

• Consider administration of first dose at bedtime; caution following first 12 hr after initiation or reinitiation of therapy for "first dose phenomenon"

---

tazarotene

(ta-zar'o-teen)

Rx: Tazorac

Chemical Class: Vitamin A derivative (retinoid prodrug)

Therapeutic Class: Antiacne, antipsoriatic agent

CLINICAL PHARMACOLOGY

Mechanism of Action: Prodrug, tazarotene rapidly converted to active metabolite, tazarotenic acid, following topical application; modulates differentiation and proliferation of epithelial tissue and exerts some antiinflammatory and immunological activity

Pharmacokinetics

TOP: Minimal (<1%) absorption of tazarotene and active metabolite (tazarotenic acid); retained in skin for prolonged periods (up to 3 months); eventually metabolized in liver with predominantly biliary excretion; active metabolite $t_{1/2}$ 18 hr

INDICATIONS AND USES: Acne (facial, mild to moderate); psoriasis (stable, plaque, ≤20% of body surface area)

DOSAGE

Adult and Child >16 yr

• *Acne:* TOP apply 0.05%-0.1% gel qd (evening)

• *Psoriasis:* TOP apply to plaques only qd (evening)

💲 AVAILABLE FORMS/COST OF THERAPY

• GEL—TOP: 0.05%, 30, 100 g: **$60.00**/30 g; 0.1%, 30, 100 g: **$63.75**/30 g

PRECAUTIONS: Eczema, concurrent use with other photosensitizers (thiazides, tetracyclines, fluoroquinolones, phenothiazines, sulfonamides)

PREGNANCY AND LACTATION: Pregnancy category X (some evidence to suggest potential increased safety margin vs. other retinoids based on minimal absorption and short half life); excreted into breast milk of rats; no human data

SIDE EFFECTS/ADVERSE REACTIONS

SKIN: Burning, desquamation, dry skin, erythema, fissuring, irritation, localized edema, *pruritus,* skin discoloration, skin pain, *stinging*

SPECIAL CONSIDERATIONS
• Attractive alternative to oral retinoid therapy in psoriasis (e.g., etretinate), primarily due to less toxicity. Structural changes to the basic retinoid structure (e.g., conformational rigidity) are claimed to enhance therapeutic efficacy and reduce the local toxicity associated with topical tretinoin (retinoic acid). However, place in therapy should await direct comparisons vs. standard regimens in terms of efficacy, toxicity, and cost

---

telmisartan
(tel-meh-sar'-tan)
Rx: Micardis
Chemical Class: Angiotensin II receptor antagonist
Therapeutic Class: Antihypertensive

CLINICAL PHARMACOLOGY
Mechanism of Action: Antihypertensive (inhibition of vasoconstrictor and aldosterone secretion), smooth muscle hypoproliferative, and cardioprotective effects are attributable to selective blockade of angiotensin II receptors found throughout the cardiovascular and renal systems; effects independent of angiotensin II synthesis
Pharmacokinetics
PO: Peak 0.5-1 hr; bioavailability, 42%, dose dependent, minimal food

effect; 99.5+% plasma protein bound (albumin and α_1-acid glycoprotein); <3% metabolized by liver, 97% excreted unchanged in urine; $t_{1/2}$ 24 hr
INDICATIONS AND USES: Hypertension, myocardial ischemia,* congestive heart failure (left ventricular dysfunction),* chronic renal failure,* diabetic nephropathy*

DOSAGE
Adult and Child >16 yr
• *Hypertension:* 20 to 80 mg PO qd

💲 AVAILABLE FORMS/COST OF THERAPY
• Tab—Oral: 40 mg, 28's: **$30.00**; 80 mg, 28's: **$30.00**

PRECAUTIONS: Angioedema (associated with aspirin and/or penicillin allergy), aortic or mitral valve stenosis, biliary cirrhosis or biliary obstruction, breast feeding period, coronary artery disease, elderly patients, hepatic dysfunction (adjust dose), hypertrophic cardiomyopathy, hypotension (sodium- or volume-depleted patients), pregnancy, renal artery stenosis, solitary kidney, or congestive heart failure

PREGNANCY AND LACTATION: Pregnancy category C, first trimester—category D, second and third trimesters; drugs acting directly on the renin-angiotensin-aldosterone system are documented to cause fetal harm (hypotension, oligohydramnios, neonatal anemia, hyperkalemia, neonatal skull hypoplasia, anuria, and renal failure); neonatal limb contractures, craniofacial deformities, and hypoplastic lung development

SIDE EFFECTS/ADVERSE REACTIONS
CNS: Headache, dizziness, insomnia, somnolence, migraine, vertigo, paresthesia, involuntary muscle contractions, and hypoesthesia (0.3%-1%)

---

italic = common side effects **bold italic** = life-threatening reactions

CV: Hypertension, chest pain, peripheral edema, palpitation, dependent edema, angina pectoris, tachycardia, leg edema, abnormal electrocardiogram, anxiety, depression, and nervousness (0.3%-1%)

EENT: Conjunctivitis

GI: Diarrhea (3%), dyspepsia, abdominal pain, nausea, flatulence, constipation, gastritis, vomiting, dry mouth, hemorrhoids, gastroenteritis, enteritis, gastroesophageal reflux, and toothache

GU: Impotence, urinary tract infection, increased frequency of urination, and cystitis (0.3%-1%)

MS: Back pain (3%), myalgia, arthritis, arthralgia, and leg cramps (0.3%-1%)

RESP: Angioedema (1 case in premarketing trials), upper respiratory tract infection (7%), sinusitis (7%), cough (1.6%), pharyngitis (1%), influenza-like symptoms, asthma, bronchitis, rhinitis, dyspnea, and epistaxis (0.3%-1%)

SKIN: Increased sweating, dermatitis, rash, eczema, and pruritus (0.3%-1%)

MISC: Angioedema

INTERACTIONS

Drugs

3 *Digoxin:* 49% increase in digoxin peak, 20% increase in trough digoxin concentrations

SPECIAL CONSIDERATIONS

• Potentially as or more effective than angiotensin-converting enzyme inhibitors, without cough; no evidence for reduction in morbidity and mortality as first-line agents in hypertension, yet; whether they provide the same cardiac and renal protection also still tentative; like ACE inhibitors, less effective in black patients

PATIENT/FAMILY EDUCATION

• Call your clinician immediately if note following side effects: wheezing; lip, throat, or face swelling; hives or rash

MONITORING PARAMETERS

• Baseline electrolytes, urinalysis, blood urea nitrogen and creatinine with recheck at 2-4 wk after initiation (sooner in volume-depleted patients); monitor sitting blood pressure; watch for symptomatic hypotension, particularly in volume-depleted patients

---

temazepam

(te-maz'e-pam)

Rx: Restoril

Chemical Class: Benzodiazepine

Therapeutic Class: Hypnotic

DEA Class: Schedule IV

CLINICAL PHARMACOLOGY

Mechanism of Action: CNS depressant via facilitation of inhibitory GABA at benzodiazepine receptor sites (BZ_1—associated with sleep; BZ_2—associated with memory, motor, sensory, and cognitive function); effects include muscle relaxation (spinal cord), anticonvulsant activity (brain stem), ataxia (cerebellum), emotional behavior (limbic and cortical areas), and anxiolytic effects (separate from general CNS depression); decreases sleep latency, the number of awakenings, and the time spent in stage 0 (awake) sleep; stage 2 (unequivocal sleep) is increased; in sum, sleep time increased

Pharmacokinetics: Onset 30-45 min, peak 2-4 hr, duration 6-8 hr; $t_{1/2}$ 9.5-10.4 hr; metabolized by liver to inactive metabolites; excreted by kidneys; crosses placenta, excreted in breast milk

INDICATIONS AND USES: Insomnia

---

* = non-FDA-approved use

DOSAGE
Adult

• PO 15-30 mg hs; 7.5 mg hs may be sufficient for elderly or debilitated patients

💲 AVAILABLE FORMS/COST OF THERAPY

• Cap, Gel—Oral: 7.5 mg, 100's: **$67.18-$80.63;** 15 mg, 100's: **$29.97-$87.64;** 30 mg, 100's: **$84.83-$98.01**

PRECAUTIONS: Anemia, hepatic disease, renal disease, suicidal individuals, drug abuse, elderly, depression, psychosis, children <18 yr, acute narrow-angle glaucoma, seizure disorders, lung disease

PREGNANCY AND LACTATION: Pregnancy category X; may cause sedation and poor feeding in nursing infant

SIDE EFFECTS/ADVERSE REACTIONS

CNS: Anxiety, confusion, *daytime sedation,* dizziness, *drowsiness,* headache, irritability, *lethargy,* lightheadedness, rebound insomnia

CV: Chest pain, hypotension, tachycardia

GI: Abdominal pain, anorexia, constipation, diarrhea, heartburn, nausea, vomiting

HEME: **Granulocytopenia** (rare), **leukopenia**

RESP: **Respiratory depression,** sleep apnea

INTERACTIONS
Drugs

3 *Cimetidine, disulfiram:* Increased benzodiazepine levels

3 *Clozapine:* Possible increased risk of cardiorespiratory collapse

3 *Ethanol:* Adverse psychomotor effects

3 *Rifampin:* Reduced benzodiazepine levels

SPECIAL CONSIDERATIONS

• Good benzodiazepine choice for elderly and patients with liver disease (phase II metabolism and lack of active metabolites)

PATIENT/FAMILY EDUCATION

• Withdrawal symptoms may occur if administered chronically and discontinued abruptly; symptoms include dysphoria, abdominal and muscle cramps, vomiting, sweating, tremor, and seizure

• May cause impairment the day following administration, exercise caution with hazardous tasks and driving

---

terazosin
(ter-a′zoe-sin)
Rx: Hytrin
Chemical Class: Quinazoline derivative
Therapeutic Class: α_1-adrenergic blocker; antihypertensive; symptomatic benign prostatic hypertrophy

CLINICAL PHARMACOLOGY

Mechanism of Action: Selectively blocks postsynaptic α_1-adrenergic receptors; dilates both arterioles and veins, reducing peripheral vascular resistance and blood pressure; no reflex tachycardia or changes in renin release; blockade of α_1-adrenoceptors in bladder neck and prostate relaxes smooth muscle, improving urine flow rates in benign prostatic hypertrophy

Pharmacokinetics

PO: Completely absorbed, peak 1 hr; 90%-94% bound to plasma proteins; $t_{1/2}$ 12 hr; excreted in urine (40%) and feces (60%), 70% as metabolites

INDICATIONS AND USES: Hypertension; benign prostatic hypertrophy (BPH), Raynaud's vasospasm,* refractory CHF*

---

italic = common side effects   ***bold italic*** = life-threatening reactions

DOSAGE
Adult
• *BPH:* PO 1 mg hs, increase to 2 mg, 5 mg, 10 mg/day (usual dose); not to exceed 20 mg/day; treatment at dose of 10 mg qd for 4-6 wk necessary to determine response
• *Hypertension:* PO 1 mg hs, increase to desired response; usual dose 1-5 mg qd, max 20 mg/day; measure BP at end of dosing interval to determine if bid dose needed

💲 **AVAILABLE FORMS/COST OF THERAPY**
• Cap, Gel—Oral: 1, 2, 5, 10 mg, 100's: **$160.38-$178.40**

PRECAUTIONS: Patients needing to perform hazardous tasks where syncope or dizziness could be dangerous

PREGNANCY AND LACTATION: Pregnancy category C; excretion into breast milk unknown

SIDE EFFECTS/ADVERSE REACTIONS
CNS: Depression, *dizziness, drowsiness,* fatigue, *headache,* paresthesia, syncope (especially 1st days of therapy), vertigo, weakness
CV: Edema, hypotension, palpitations, *postural hypotension*
EENT: Blurred vision, dry mouth, epistaxis, *nasal congestion,* red sclera, *sinusitis,* tinnitus
GI: Nausea
GU: Impotence, incontinence, urinary frequency
RESP: Dyspnea
MISC: Weight gain

INTERACTIONS
Drugs
🔢 *Angiotensin converting enzyme inhibitors (enalapril):* Potential for exaggerated first dose hypotensive episode when alpha blockers added
🔢 *Nonsteroidal antiinflammatory drugs (ibuprofen, indomethacin):* NSAIDs may inhibit antihypertensive effects
🔢 β-*adrenergic blockers:* Potential for exaggerated first dose hypotensive episode when alpha blockers added
Labs
• False positive urinary metabolites of norepinephrine and VMA
• No effect on prostate specific antigen (PSA)

SPECIAL CONSIDERATIONS
• Use as a single antihypertensive agent limited by tendency to cause sodium and water retention and increased plasma volume

PATIENT/FAMILY EDUCATION
• Alert patients to the possibility of syncopal and orthostatic symptoms, especially with the 1st dose ("1st dose syncope"); initial dose should be administered at bedtime in the smallest possible dose

---

terbinafine
(ter-been'a-feen)
Rx: Lamisil (tab)
OTC: Lamisil (cream)
Chemical Class: Synthetic allylamine derivative
Therapeutic Class: Antifungal

CLINICAL PHARMACOLOGY
Mechanism of Action: Inhibits fungal sterol biosynthesis, causing accumulation of squalene within the fungal cell and cell death
Pharmacokinetics
TOP: Variable systemic absorption
PO: Peak 2 hr
>99% bound to plasma proteins; distributed to sebum and skin; terminal $t_{1/2}$ 200-400 hr; extensively metabolized; eliminated via urine

INDICATIONS AND USES: Tinea cruris, tinea corporis, tinea pedis; onychomycosis due to dermatophytes; cutaneous candidiasis*; tinea versicolor; active against *Epidermophyton floccosum, Trichophyton*

mentagrophytes, Trichophyton rubrum

DOSAGE

Adult

• *Tinea pedis:* Top apply bid for 1-4 wk, until symptoms resolved

• *Tinea cruris, tinea corporis:* Top apply qd-bid for 1-4 wk

• *Onychomycosis:* PO 250 mg qd for 6 wk (fingernail) or 12 wk (toenail)

§ AVAILABLE FORMS/COST OF THERAPY

• Cre—Top: 1%, 15, 30 g: **$54.12/30 g**

• Tab—Oral: 250 mg, 30's: **$198.73**

CONTRAINDICATIONS: Pre-existing renal or hepatic disease (oral therapy)

PRECAUTIONS: Children <12 (safety and efficacy not established)

PREGNANCY AND LACTATION: Pregnancy category B; it is recommended that treatment of onychomycosis be delayed until after pregnancy; small amounts of terbinafine are excreted into breast milk when administered orally, not recommended in nursing mothers; avoid application to the breast when breast feeding

SIDE EFFECTS/ADVERSE REACTIONS

CNS: Headache

EENT: Visual disturbance

GI: Abdominal pain, diarrhea, dyspepsia, elevated transaminases, flatulence, nausea, taste disturbance

SKIN: Burning, dryness, irritation, itching

SPECIAL CONSIDERATIONS PATIENT/FAMILY EDUCATION

• Optimal clinical effect in onychomycosis may not be apparent for several mo following completion of therapy

---

terbutaline

(ter-byoo'te-leen)

Rx: Brethaire, Brethine, Bricanyl

Chemical Class: Sympathomimetic amine; β_2-adrenergic agonist

Therapeutic Class: Antiasthmatic, bronchodilator; tocolytic

CLINICAL PHARMACOLOGY

Mechanism of Action: Causes bronchodilation by β_2-stimulation, resulting in relaxation of bronchial smooth muscle; inhibits mast cell degranulation; stimulates cilia to remove secretions; relaxes uterine smooth muscle

Pharmacokinetics

PO: Onset ½ hr, peak 1-2 hr, duration 4-8 hr

SC: Onset 5-15 min, peak ½-1 hr, duration 1½-4 hr

INH: Onset 5-30 min, peak 1-2 hr, duration 3-6 hr

Metabolized in gut wall and liver; excreted in urine; $t_{1/2}$ 3-4 hr

INDICATIONS AND USES: Bronchial asthma; reversible bronchospasm associated with bronchitis and emphysema; premature labor*

DOSAGE

Adult

• *Bronchospasm:* MDI 2 puffs separated by 1 min q4-6h; PO 2.5-5 mg q8h to max 15 mg qd; SC 0.25 mg, may repeat once in 15-30 min

• *Premature labor:* SC 0.25 mg qh; IV INF 0.01 mg/min, titrate upward to max of 0.08 mg/min; maintain at minimum effective dose for 4 hr; PO 5 mg q4h for 48 hr, then 5 mg q6h as maintenance for above doses

Child

• MDI 1-2 puffs q 4-6h; PO 0.05 mg/kg/dose q8h, increased gradu-

T

---

italic = common side effects   **bold italic** = life-threatening reactions

ally to 0.15 mg/kg/dose to max daily dose 5 mg (<12 yr); SC 0.005-0.01 mg/kg/dose to max 0.4 mg/kg/dose q 15-20 min for 2 doses

$ AVAILABLE FORMS/COST OF THERAPY

• Inj, Sol—SC: 1 mg/ml, 1 ml: **$2.35-$3.17**
• MDI-INH: 0.2 mg/spray, 7.5 ml: **$19.34-$26.27**
• Tab, Uncoated—Oral: 2.5 mg, 100's: **$32.15;** 5 mg, 100's: **$46.25**

PRECAUTIONS: Ischemic heart disease, cardiac dysrhythmias, hyperthyroidism, diabetes mellitus, prostatic hypertrophy, hypertension

PREGNANCY AND LACTATION: Pregnancy category B; compatible with breast feeding

SIDE EFFECTS/ADVERSE REACTIONS

CNS: Anxiety, dizziness, headache, insomnia, *nervousness, shakiness, tremor*

CV: Angina, **cardiac arrest, dysrhythmias,** hypertension, *palpitations, tachycardia*

GI: Elevated liver enzymes, *nausea, vomiting*

INTERACTIONS

Drugs

❷ *Beta-blockers:* Decreased action of terbutaline, cardioselective beta-blockers preferable if concurrent use necessary; metoprolol inhibits terbutaline metabolism

❸ *Furosemide:* Potential for additive hypokalemia

---

terconazole

(ter-kon′a-zole)
Rx: Terazol 3, Terazol 7
Chemical Class: Triazole derivative
Therapeutic Class: Antifungal

CLINICAL PHARMACOLOGY
Mechanism of Action: Uncertain; may disrupt fungal cell membrane permeability

Pharmacokinetics: Systemic absorption 5%-16%

INDICATIONS AND USES: Local treatment of vulvovaginal candidiasis

DOSAGE

Adult

• VAG (cre) 5 g (1 applicator) qhs for 3 (0.8%) or 7 (0.4%) days
• VAG (supp) 1 qhs for 3 days

$ AVAILABLE FORMS/COST OF THERAPY

• Cre—Vag: 0.4%, 45 g: **$28.74;** 0.8%, 20 g: **$28.74**
• Supp—Vag: 80 mg, 3's: **$26.60**

PREGNANCY AND LACTATION: Pregnancy category C, systemic absorption occurs; excretion into breast milk unknown

SIDE EFFECTS/ADVERSE REACTIONS

CNS: Headache
GI: Abdominal pain
GU: Genital pain, *itching,* vulvovaginal burning
SKIN: Photosensitivity reactions with repeated application under artificial UV light

SPECIAL CONSIDERATIONS
• No significant advantage over less expensive OTC products

---

testosterone

(tess-toss'ter-one)

Rx: *Testosterone aqueous:*
Testamone-100, Testro AQ
Testosterone cypionate:
Depo-Testosterone, Depotest,
T-Cypionate, Virilon IM
Testosterone enanthate:
Delatestryl, Everone,
Testro-L.A.
Testosterone propionate:
Generics only
Transdermal System: Andro-
derm, Testoderm
Pellet: Testopel

Chemical Class: Testosterone
Therapeutic Class: Androgen;
antineoplastic

CLINICAL PHARMACOLOGY

Mechanism of Action: Promotes weight gain via retention of nitrogen, potassium, and phosphorous, increased protein anabolism and decreased catabolism; endogenous androgens essential for normal growth and development of male sex organs and maintenance of secondary sex characteristics

Pharmacokinetics

Testosterone: IM $t_{1/2}$ 10-100 min; transdermal peak 2-4 hr, returns to baseline 2 hr after removal (Testoderm)

Testosterone cypionate: IM $t_{1/2}$ 8 days; 98% protein bound; metabolized in liver; excreted in urine, breast milk; crosses placenta

INDICATIONS AND USES: Male primary and secondary hypogonadism (aqueous, transdermal, cypionate, enanthate, propionate); delayed puberty in males (enanthate, propionate); advanced metastatic breast cancer in women (enanthate, propionate), postpartum breast pain and engorgement (propionate); male contraceptive (enanthate)*

DOSAGE
Adult and Child

• *Hypogonadism:* IM 25-50 mg 2-3 times/wk (aqueous); 40-50 mg/m^2 monthly to initiate pubertal growth, increasing to 100 mg/m^2 monthly during terminal growth phase, maintenance dose 50-400 mg q2-4wk (propionate); 50-400 mg q2-4wk (enanthate, cypionate); transdermal 4-6 mg/day system applied to clean, dry, shaved scrotal skin, wear for 22-24 hr/day (Testoderm); 5 mg/day (2×2.5 mg/day systems) applied nightly to clean, dry area of upper back, arms, abdomen or thighs; adjust dose, based on patient response and serum testosterone levels, by increasing to 3 systems or decreasing to 1 system/day (Androderm)

• *Delayed puberty:* IM 40-50 mg/m^2 monthly for 6 months (propionate); 50-200 mg q2-4wk for a limited duration (enanthate, cypionate)

• Postpartum breast engorgement: IM 25-50 mg for 3-4 days starting at the time of delivery (propionate)

• *Breast cancer:* IM 50-100 mg 3 times/wk (propionate) or 200-400 mg q2-4wk (cypionate or enanthate)

💲 AVAILABLE FORMS/COST OF THERAPY

Testosterone

• Film, CONT REL—Percutaneous: 2.5 mg/24 hr, 60's: **$110.08-$120.13;** 4 mg/24 hr, 6 mg/24 hr, 30's: **$96.00;** 5 mg/24 hr, 30's: **$101.62-$110.08**

• Pellet—SC: 75 mg/pellet, 10's: **$150.00**

Testosterone aqueous

• Inj, Susp—IM: 50 mg/ml, 10 ml: **$8.50-$12.00;** 100 mg/ml, 10 ml: **$8.40-$16.10**

Testosterone cypionate

• Inj, Sol—IM: 100 mg/ml, 10 ml: **$11.59-$44.91;** 200 mg/ml, 10 ml: **$17.50-$80.58**

---

italic = common side effects   ***bold italic*** = life-threatening reactions

Testosterone enanthate
• Inj, Sol—IM: 200 mg/ml, 10 ml: **$12.00-$21.42**
Testosterone propionate
• Inj, Sol—IM: 100 mg/ml, 10 ml: **$8.40-$18.01**

CONTRAINDICATIONS: Severe renal disease, severe cardiac disease, severe hepatic disease, genital bleeding (abnormal), male breast cancer, prostate cancer

PRECAUTIONS: Diabetes mellitus, cardiovascular disease, risk factors for atherosclerosis, hepatic disease, seizure disorder, renal disease

PREGNANCY AND LACTATION: Pregnancy category X; excretion into breast milk unknown, use extreme caution in nursing mothers

SIDE EFFECTS/ADVERSE REACTIONS

CNS: Aggressive behavior, anxiety, depression, dizziness, emotional lability, fatigue, flushing, headache, insomnia, paresthesias, sweating, tremors

CV: **CHF,** edema, increased blood pressure

EENT: Conjunctival edema, deepening of voice, nasal congestion

GI: Cholestatic jaundice, constipation, **hepatocellular neoplasm,** nausea, vomiting, weight gain, **peliosis hepatis**

GU: Amenorrhea, clitoral hypertrophy, decreased breast size, gynecomastia, increased or decreased libido, priapism, testicular atrophy, vaginitis, virilization in females, oligospermia, menstrual irregularities

HEME: Polycythemia, suppression of clotting factors

METAB: Hypercalcemia (in breast cancer), hypercholesterolemia, hyperglycemia, increased potassium, premature epiphyseal closure (children)

SKIN: Acneiform lesions, acne vulgaris, alopecia, flushing, hirsutism, oily hair and skin, rash, sweating

MISC: Carpal tunnel syndrome

INTERACTIONS

Drugs

3 *Cyclosporine:* Increased cyclosporine concentrations

2 *Oral anticoagulants:* Increased hypoprothrombinemic response

SPECIAL CONSIDERATIONS

MONITORING PARAMETERS

• LFTs, lipids, Hct
• Growth rate in children (X-rays for bone age q6 mo)

---

tetracaine
(tet′ra-cane)
Rx: Opticaine, Pontocaine, Tetcaine HCL Ophthalmic
OTC: Pontocaine
Chemical Class: Benzoic acid derivative
Therapeutic Class: Local anesthetic

CLINICAL PHARMACOLOGY

Mechanism of Action: Decreases neuronal membrane permeability to sodium ions, blocking nerve impulses

Pharmacokinetics

INJ: Onset of action rapid, duration 2-3 hr

OPHTH: Onset of action 15 sec, duration 10-20 min

TOP: Peak 3-8 min, duration 30-60 min

Hydrolyzed by plasma esterases; excreted by kidney

INDICATIONS AND USES: TOP: pruritus, sunburn, toothache, sore throat, cold sores, oral pain, rectal pain and irritation; control of gagging prior to performing bronchoscopy, bronchography, and esophagoscopy; OPHTHAL: cataract extraction, tonometry, gonioscopy, removal of foreign objects, corneal suture removal, glaucoma surgery; INJ: spinal anesthesia

DOSAGE

Adult and Child

• TOP apply to affected area

• OPHTH instill 1-2 gtt before procedure

• INJ 0.2%-0.3% sol for spinal anesthesia; for prolonged anesthesia (2-3 hr) 1% sol

AVAILABLE FORMS/COST OF THERAPY

• Inj, Sol—IV: 1%, 2 ml: **$7.66**; 0.2%, 2 ml: **$7.46**; 0.3%, 5 ml: **$9.52**

• Sol—Ophth: 0.5%, 15 ml: **$3.54-$24.26**

• Sol—Top: 2%, 30 ml: **$27.00-$31.85**

• Cre—Top: 1%, 30 g: **$32.05** (OTC)

• Oint—Top: 1%, 30 g: **$32.05** (OTC)

CONTRAINDICATIONS: Hypersensitivity to ester anesthetics; infants less than 1 yr; application to large areas

PRECAUTIONS: Child <6 yr, sepsis, denuded skin

PREGNANCY AND LACTATION: Pregnancy category C; excretion into breast milk unknown

SIDE EFFECTS/ADVERSE REACTIONS

SKIN: Burning, irritation, rash, sensitization, stinging, tenderness

INTERACTIONS

Drugs

3 *Propranolol:* Enhanced sympathomimetic side effects resulting in hypertensive reactions; acute discontinuation of beta-blockers prior to local anesthesia may increase side effects of tetracaine

Labs

• *Interference:* CSF protein

SPECIAL CONSIDERATIONS

• Also used as a component of "Magic Numbing Solution" or TAC Sol (epinephrine 1 : 2,000, tetracaine 0.5%, cocaine 11.8%) and LET Sol (lidocaine 4%, epinephrine 0.1%, tetracaine 0.5%), which are used as topical anesthesia for repair of minor lacerations, especially in pediatric patients

---

tetracycline

(tet-ra-sye′kleen)

Rx: *Systemic:* Ala-Tet, Brodspec, Emtet-500, Panmycin, Sumycin, Tetra 500, Tetracap, Tetracon, Wesmycin
Topical: Topicycline
Peridontal fiber: Actisite

Chemical Class: Tetracycline
Therapeutic Class: Antibiotic

CLINICAL PHARMACOLOGY

Mechanism of Action: Inhibition of microbial protein synthesis; bacteriostatic

Pharmacokinetics

PO: Peak 2-3 hr, duration 6 hr; excreted in urine (60% unchanged); crosses placenta, excreted in breast milk; 20%-60% protein bound; $t_{1/2}$ 6-10 hr

INDICATIONS AND USES:

Systemic: Infections caused by Rickettsiae (Rocky Mountain spotted fever, typhus fever, Q fever, rickettsial pox and tick fever), *Mycoplasma pneumoniae,* agents of psittacosis and ornithosis, agents of lymphogranuloma venerium and granuloma inguinale, relapsing fever *(Borrelia recurrentis)*

Antimicrobial spectrum usually includes:

• Gram-positive organisms: streptococcus sp. (up to 44% of *S. pyogenes* and 74% of *S. faecalis* are resistant), *Diplococcus pneumoniae, Staph. aureus* (skin and soft tissue infections)

---

italic = common side effects   ***bold italic*** = life-threatening reactions

- Gram-negative organisms: *Hemophilus ducreyi* (chancroid), *Pasturella pestis, P. tularensis, Bartonella bacilliformis, Bacteroides* spp.; *Vibrio colera* and *V. fetus, Brucella* spp. (in combination with streptomycin); *Chlamydia trachomatis;* susceptibility should be demonstrated for *E. coli, Enterobacter aerogenes, Shigella* spp., *H. influenzae* (respiratory infections), *Klebsiella* spp. (respiratory and urinary infections)
- Anaerobic organisms: *Propionibacterium acnes* (acne)
- Alternative to penicillin for *Neisseria gonorrhoeae, Treponema pallidum,* and *T. pertenue* (syphilis and yaws); *Listeria monocytogenes, Clostridium* spp.; *Bacillus anthracis, Fugobacterium fusiforme* (Vincent's infection); *Actinomyces* spp.
Topical: Acne vulgaris
DOSAGE
Adult
- PO 250-500 mg q6h
- *Gonorrhea:* PO 1.5 g, then 500 mg qid for a total of 9 g
- *Chlamydia:* PO 500 mg qid for 7 days
- *Syphilis:* (Benzathine penicillin is the drug of choice for syphilis) PO 2-3 g in divided doses for 10-15 days; if syphilis duration >1 yr, must treat 30 days
- *Brucellosis:* PO 500 mg qid for 3 wk with 1 g streptomycin IM bid for 1 wk, and qd the 2nd wk
- *Acne:* PO 250 mg qid; maintenance 125-500 mg qd; TOP apply sol bid to affected area
Child >8 yr
- PO 25-50 mg/kg/d in divided doses q6h
$ **AVAILABLE FORMS/COST OF THERAPY**
- Cap, Gel—Oral: 250 mg, 100's: **$0.54-$14.88;** 500 mg, 100's: **$0.67-$11.35**

- Tab, Coated—Oral: 250 mg, 100's: **$6.31;** 500 mg, 100's: **$12.28**
- Susp—Oral: 125 mg/5 ml, 480 ml: **$6.00-$11.85**
- Sol—Top: 2.2 mg/ml, 70 ml: **$59.83**
- Fiber—Peridontal: 12.7 mg, 10's: **$240.00**
CONTRAINDICATIONS: Children <8 yr (systemic)
PRECAUTIONS: Renal disease, hepatic disease
PREGNANCY AND LACTATION: Pregnancy category D (systemic), category B (topical); systemic tetracycline excreted into breast milk in low concentrations; theoretically, dental staining could occur, but serum levels in infants undetectable, so considered compatible with breast feeding
SIDE EFFECTS/ADVERSE REACTIONS
CNS: Fever, headache, paresthesia, ***pseudotumor cerebri***
CV: Pericarditis
EENT: Dysphagia, esophagitis, oral candidiasis, oral ulcers
GI: Abdominal cramps, abdominal pain, anorexia, decreased calcification of deciduous teeth (children <8 yr), *diarrhea,* enterocolitis, epigastric burning, flatulence, glossitis, ***hepatotoxicity,*** *nausea,* stomatitis, *vomiting*
GU: Increased BUN, renal failure (associated with use of outdated products)
HEME: Eosinophilia, ***hemolytic anemia, neutropenia, thrombocytopenia***
SKIN: Angioedema, ***exfoliative dermatitis,*** *increased pigmentation, photosensitivity,* pruritus, *rash, stinging* (top), *urticaria*
INTERACTIONS
Drugs
3 *Antacids:* Reduced tetracycline concentrations

❷ *Bismuth subsalicylate:* Reduced tetracycline concentrations

❸ *Calcium:* Reduced tetracycline concentrations

❸ *Cholestyramine colestipol:* Reduced tetracycline concentrations

❸ *Digoxin:* Decreased digoxin concentrations due to reduced GI flora

❸ *Food:* Reduced tetracycline concentrations

❸ *Iron:* Reduced tetracycline concentrations

❸ *Magnesium:* Reduced tetracycline concentrations

❷ *Methoxyflurane:* Increased renal toxicity

❸ *Oral contraceptives:* Possible decreased contraceptive effect

❸ *Penicillin:* Impaired efficacy of penicillin

❸ *Sodium bicarbonate:* Reduced tetracycline concentrations

❸ *Zinc:* Reduced tetracycline concentrations

Labs

• *False negative:* Urine glucose with Clinistix or TesTape
• *False increase:* Serum glucose
• *False decrease:* Serum acetaminophen concentration, serum folate
• *Interference:* Plasma catecholamines, urinary porphyrins, CSF protein

SPECIAL CONSIDERATIONS
PATIENT/FAMILY EDUCATION
• Avoid milk products, antacids, or separate by 2 hr; take with a full glass of water
• Use in children ≤8 yr causes permanent discoloration of teeth, enamel hypoplasia, and retardation of skeletal development; risk greatest for children <4 yr and receiving high doses
• Side effects noted for systemic administration not observed with topical formulations

tetrahydrozoline
(tet-ra-hi-droz'o-leen)
Rx: *Nasal:* Tyzine, Tyzine Pediatric
OTC: *Ophthalmic:* Collyrium Fresh Eye Drops, Eyesine, Murine Plus Eye Drops, Optigene 3 Eye Drops, Visine Eye Drops
Chemical Class: Sympathomimetic amine
Therapeutic Class: Decongestant

CLINICAL PHARMACOLOGY
Mechanism of Action: Local α-adrenergic-mediated vasoconstriction dilated conjunctival and nasal mucosal blood vessels
Pharmacokinetics
TOP: Duration 2-3 hr
INDICATIONS AND USES: NASAL: Decongestion of nasal and nasopharyngeal mucosa; OPHTHAL: ocular congestion, irritation, itching, redness
DOSAGE
Adult
• NASAL, instill 2-4 gtt/sprays 0.1% sol in each nostril q4-8h
• OPHTH, instill 1-2 gtt in affected eye up to qid
Child (2-6 yr)
• NASAL, instill 2-3 gtt 0.05% sol in each nostril q4-6h
⟨$⟩ AVAILABLE FORMS/COST OF THERAPY
• Aer, Spray—Nasal: 0.1%, 15 ml: **$11.57**
• Sol—Nasal: 0.05%, 15 ml: **$11.39;** 0.1%, 30 ml: **$13.15**
• Sol—Ophth: 0.05%, 30 ml: **$2.50-$5.84**
CONTRAINDICATIONS: Narrow-angle glaucoma
PRECAUTIONS: Severe hypertension, diabetes, hyperthyroidism, el-

derly, severe arteriosclerosis, cardiac disease, infants, diabetes, asthma, CAD

PREGNANCY AND LACTATION: Pregnancy category C; excretion into breast milk unknown

SIDE EFFECTS/ADVERSE REACTIONS

CNS: Dizziness, headache, weakness

CV: **CV collapse, dysrhythmias,** hypertension, palpitation, reflex bradycardia, tachycardia

EENT: Blurred vision, conjunctival allergy, lacrimation, stinging

SPECIAL CONSIDERATIONS
• Manage rebound congestion by stopping tetrahydrozoline: one nostril at a time, substitute systemic decongestant, substitute inhaled steroid

PATIENT/FAMILY EDUCATION
• Do not use for >3-5 days or rebound congestion may occur

---

thalidomide
(thal-e-doe-mide)
Rx: Thalomid
Chemical Class: Glutamic acid derivative
Therapeutic Class: Leprostatic

CLINICAL PHARMACOLOGY
Mechanism of Action: Reduces inflammation by cytokine modulation. Reduces levels of tumor necrosis factor-alpha in patients with erythema nodosum leprosum

Pharmacokinetics
PO: Slowly absorbed from GI tract, peak 3-6 hr; highly protein bound; major metabolic pathway is nonenzymatic hydrolysis in plasma to multiple metabolites; minimal amount metabolized by liver; metabolites excreted in urine (1% unchanged after 24 hr); $t_{1/2}$ 5-7 hr

INDICATIONS AND USES: Erythema nodosum leprosum, discoid lupus erythematosus,* graft vs. host disease,* oral aphthous ulcers in immunocompromised patients*

DOSAGE
Adult
• *Aphthous ulceration:* PO 100-200 mg qd until response, then 50-100 mg qd
• *Discoid lupus erythematosus:* PO 400 mg qd until response, then 50-100 mg qd
• *Erythema nodosum leprosum:* PO 100-400 mg qd until response, then 25-100 mg qd
• *Graft vs. host disease:* PO 800-1600 mg qd until response, then taper by 25% every 2 wk

💲 AVAILABLE FORMS/COST OF THERAPY
• Cap—Oral: 50 mg, 14's: **$658.35**

CONTRAINDICATIONS: Women of child-bearing potential unless: 1. An effective form of contraception has been used for at least 1 mo before therapy, during therapy, and for 1 mo following discontinuation of therapy, and 2. Pregnancy has been definitely excluded through a negative pregnancy test within 2 wk prior to thalidomide therapy. Men must use barrier contraception if sexually active with women of child-bearing potential

PRECAUTIONS: Bradycardia, photosensitization

PREGNANCY AND LACTATION: Pregnancy category X; breast milk excretion unknown

SIDE EFFECTS/ADVERSE REACTIONS

CNS: Anxiety, *dizziness, headache (12%), neuropathy,* paresthesia, *somnolence (38%),* tremor, *vertigo*

CV: Edema

EENT: Dry mouth

GI: Anorexia, constipation, *elevated transaminase levels (10%),* nausea

GU: *Impotence*
HEME: *Anemia,* ***leukopenia (20%)***
METAB: *Hypothyroidism*
SKIN: *Pruritus, rash (25%)*
INTERACTIONS
Drugs
3 *Barbiturates:* Additive sedative effects
3 *Chlorpromazine:* Additive sedative effects
3 *Ethanol:* Additive sedative effects
3 *Reserpine:* Additive sedative effects
SPECIAL CONSIDERATIONS
PATIENT/FAMILY EDUCATION
• Teratogenic in human whether taken by male or female
• Sedation common; usually taken at bedtime
MONITORING PARAMETERS
• Pregnancy test (weekly during first mo of use, then monthly)
• ALT, AST
• CBC

---

theophylline
(thee-off'i-lin)
Rx: *Immediate release tabs:* Quibron-T, Slo-Phylline, Theolair
Liquids: Asmalix, Elixophyllin, Slo-Phyllin, Theolair, Truxophylline
Sustained release caps: Aerolate Slo-Bid Gyrocaps, Theo-24
Sustained release tabs: Quibron-T/SR, Respbid, Theochron, Theo-Dur, Theolair-SR, Theo-X, Uni-Dur, Theo-Time, T-Phyl, Uniphyl
Combinations
  Rx: with guaifenesin (Elixophyllin-GG, Quibron, Slo-Phyllin-GG); with potassium iodide (Elixophylline KI)
Chemical Class: Xanthine derivative
Therapeutic Class: Antiasthmatic, bronchodilator; COPD agent

CLINICAL PHARMACOLOGY
Mechanism of Action: Directly relaxes bronchial and pulmonary blood vessel smooth muscle; stimulates CNS; induces diuresis; increases gastric acid secretion, lowers lower esophageal sphincter pressure; is a central respiratory stimulant; exact mechanism unproven but may involve antagonism of pulmonary adenosine receptors
Pharmacokinetics
PO: Well absorbed from GI tract, absorption altered by food; peak 2 hr (immediate release), 4-6 hr (SUS REL); crosses placenta, excreted into breast milk; metabolized in liver; excreted (15% unchanged) in urine;

T

---

italic = common side effects   ***bold italic*** = life-threatening reactions

$t_{1/2}$ 3-15 hr in non-smokers, 4-5 hr in smokers, 1-9 hr in children, 20-30 hr in premature neonates (who may accumulate the caffeine metabolite)

INDICATIONS AND USES: Bronchial asthma; reversible bronchospasm of chronic bronchitis and emphysema; apnea and bradycardia of prematurity*

DOSAGE

(Based on ideal body weight) When converting to sustained release products, total daily dose remains the same but is divided q8h-q24h depending on product and dose (doses >1200 mg/day should be divided q8h, doses <1200 mg/day can be given q12h)

Adult

• *Acute symptoms:* PO 5 mg/kg load, maintenance 3 mg/kg q8h (non-smokers), 3 mg/kg q6h (smokers), 2 mg/kg q8h (older patients), 1-2 mg/kg q12h (CHF); IV 5 mg/kg load over 20 min, maintenance 0.2 mg/kg/hr (CHF, elderly), 0.43 mg/kg/hr (non-smokers), 0.7 mg/kg/hr (young adult smokers), measure serum level for patients currently receiving theophylline, approx 0.5 mg/kg theophylline increases serum level 1 µg/ml

• *Slow titration:* PO initial dose 16 mg/kg/24h or 400 mg/24 hr, whichever is less, doses divided q6-8h

• *PO dosage adjustment after serum theophylline measurement:*

• Serum level 5-10 µg/ml, increase dose by 25%, recheck level in 3 days

• Serum level 10-20 µg/ml, maintain dosage if tolerated, recheck level q6-12mo

• Serum level 20-25 µg/ml, decrease dose by 10%, recheck level in 3 days

• Serum level 25-30 µg/ml, skip next dose, decrease dose by 25%, recheck level in 3 days

• Serum level >30 µg/ml, skip next 2 doses, decrease dose by 50%, recheck level in 3 days

Child

• 9-16 yr: PO 5 mg/kg load, maintenance 3 mg/kg q6h; IV 5 mg/kg load over 20 min, maintenance 0.7 mg/kg/h

• 1-9 yr: PO 5 mg/kg load, maintenance 4 mg/kg q6h; IV 5 mg/kg load over 20 min, maintenance 0.8 mg/kg/hr

• Infants: PO [(0.2 × age in weeks) + 5] × kg = 24 hr dose in mg; divide into q8h dosing (6 wk-6 mo), q6h dosing (6-12 mo); IV 5 mg/kg load over 20 min, maintenance dose in mg/kg/hr [(.0008 × age in weeks) + 0.21]

• Premature infants: IV 1 mg/kg q12h (≤24 days postnatal), 1.5 mg/kg q12h (>24 days postnatal)

§ AVAILABLE FORMS/COST OF THERAPY

• Cap, Gel, SUS Action—Oral: 50 mg, 100's: **$24.65;** 65 mg, 100's: **$20.00;** 75 mg, 100's: **$27.20;** 100 mg, 100's, **$20.59-$33.02;** 125 mg, 100's: **$25.75-$37.22;** 130 mg, 100's: **$21.25;** 200 mg, 100's: **$30.60-$49.24;** 260 mg, 100's: **$23.00;** 300 mg, 100's: **$36.55-$57.35;** 400 mg, 100;s: **$85.03**

• Tab, Coated, SUS Action—Oral: 100 mg, 100's: **$4.80-$22.75;** 200 mg, 100's: **$6.20-$48.43;** 250 mg, 100's: **$34.24-$47.46;** 300 mg, 100's: **$8.15-$58.90;** 400 mg, 100's: **$85.51-$110.34;** 450 mg, 100's: **$53.45;** 500 mg, 100's: **$49.54-$70.86;** 600 mg, 100's: **$120.62-$123.52**

• Tab, Uncoated—Oral: 100 mg, 100's: **$21.73;** 125 mg, 100's:

---

* = non-FDA-approved use

$46.44; 200 mg, 100's: **$28.87;** 250 mg, 100's: **$72.06;** 300 mg, 100's: **$56.48**

• Elixir—Oral: 80 mg/15 ml, 480 ml: **$2.64-$87.74**
• Sol—Oral: 80 mg/15 ml, 480 ml: **$27.48**
• Syr—Oral: 80 mg/15 ml, 480 ml: **$24.98**
• Inj, Sol—IV: 0.4 mg/ml, 1000 ml: **$15.92;** 0.8 mg/ml, 1000 ml: **$17.14;** 1.6 mg/ml, 500 ml: **$15.24;** 2 mg/ml, 100 ml: **$13.18;** 3.2 mg/ml, 250 ml: **$19.74;** 4 mg/ml, 50 ml: **$15.26**

CONTRAINDICATIONS: Tachydysrhythmias; as sole treatment of status asthmaticus; active peptic ulcer disease; seizure disorders

PRECAUTIONS: Elderly, CHF, cor pulmonale, hepatic disease, diabetes mellitus, hyperthyroidism, hypertension, active alcoholism, children, neonates

PREGNANCY AND LACTATION: Pregnancy category C; no reports of malformations; compatible with breast feeding with precaution that rapidly absorbed preparations may cause irritability in the infant

SIDE EFFECTS/ADVERSE REACTIONS

CNS: Anxiety, *dizziness,* headache, insomnia, lightheadedness, muscle twitching, restlessness, **seizures**
CV: **Dysrhythmias,** fluid retention with tachycardia, hypotension, palpitations, pounding heartbeat, sinus tachycardia
GI: Anorexia, bitter taste, diarrhea, dyspepsia, gastroesophageal reflux, *nausea, vomiting*
GU: Urinary frequency
RESP: Increased rate
SKIN: Flushing, urticaria

INTERACTIONS
Drugs
❸ *Adenosine:* Inhibited hemodynamic effects of adenosine

❸ *Allopurinol, amiodarone, cimetidine, ciprofloxacin, disulfiram, erythromycin, interferon alfa, isoniazid, methimazole, metoprolol, norfloxacin, pefloxacin, pentoxyfylline, propafenone, propylthiouracil, radioactive iodine, tacrine, thiabendazole, ticlopidine, verapamil:* Increased theophylline concentrations

❸ *Aminoglutethamide, barbiturates, carbamazepine, moricizine, phenytoin, rifampin, ritonavir, thyroid hormone:* Reduced theophylline levels; decreased serum phenytoin concentrations

❸ *Beta-blockers:* Reduced bronchodilating response to theophylline

❷ *Enoxacin, fluvoxamine, mexiletine, propranolol, troleandomycin:* Markedly increased theophylline concentrations

❸ *Imipenem:* Some patients on theophylline have developed seizures following the addition of imipenem

❸ *Lithium:* Reduced lithium concentrations

❸ *Smoking:* Increased theophylline dosing requirements

Labs
• *False increase:* Serum barbiturate concentrations, urinary uric acid
• *False decrease:* Serum bilirubin
• *Interference:* Plasma somatostatin

SPECIAL CONSIDERATIONS
PATIENT/FAMILY EDUCATION
• Contents of beaded capsules may be sprinkled over food for children

MONITORING PARAMETERS
• Blood levels; therapeutic level is 10-20 μg/ml (6-14 μg/ml for apnea, bradycardia of prematurity); toxicity may occur with small increase above 20 μg/ml and occasionally at levels below this; obtain serum levels 1-2 hr after administration for immediate release products and 5-9

hr after the AM dose for sustained release formulations

• Recent evidence indicates that blood levels of 8-12 μg/ml may provide adequate therapeutic effect with a lower risk of adverse events

• Signs of toxicity include nausea, vomiting, anxiety, insomnia, seizures, ventricular dysrhythmias

---

thiabendazole

(thye-a-ben′da-zole)
Rx: Mintezol
Chemical Class: Benzimadazole derivative
Therapeutic Class: Anthelmintic

CLINICAL PHARMACOLOGY
Mechanism of Action: May inhibit the helminth-specific enzyme, fumarate reductase
Pharmacokinetics
PO: Peak 1-2 hr, metabolized completely to 5-hydroxy form, excreted in urine as glucuronide or sulfate conjugates, most within 24 hr
INDICATIONS AND USES: Vermicidal and/or vermifugal against *Enterobius vermicularis* (pinworm), *Ascaria lumbricoides* (roundworm), *Strongyloides stercoralis* (threadworm), *Trichuris trichiura* (whipworm), trichinosis, *Ancylostoma duodenale* (hookworm), *Necator americanus, Ancylostoma braziliense* (dog and cat hookworm)
DOSAGE
Adult and Child: PO 22 mg/kg/dose given bid for 2-7 days, not to exceed 3 g/day (strongyloidiasis 2 days; cutaneous larva migrans 2 days; visceral larva migrans 7 days; trichinosis 2-4 successive days per response; roundworms, including ascariasis, uncinariasis, and trichuriasis 2 days)

$ **AVAILABLE FORMS/COST OF THERAPY**
• Susp—Oral: 500 mg/5 ml, 120 ml: **$23.37**
• Tab, Chewable—Oral: 500 mg, 36's: **$40.25**
PRECAUTIONS: Severe malnutrition, hepatic disease, renal disease, anemia, severe dehydration, child <14 kg
PREGNANCY AND LACTATION: Pregnancy category C
SIDE EFFECTS/ADVERSE REACTIONS
CNS: Behavioral changes, dizziness, drowsiness, fever, flushing, headache, *seizures*
CV: Bradycardia, hypotension
EENT: Blurred vision, tinnitus, xanthopsia
GI: Anorexia, diarrhea, epigastric distress, increased AST, jaundice, liver damage, *nausea, vomiting*
GU: Abnormal smell of urine, enuresis, hematuria, *nephrotoxicity*
SKIN: Erythema, pruritus, rash, *Stevens-Johnson syndrome*
INTERACTIONS
Drugs
3 *Carbamazepine:* Decreased thiabendazole concentrations, therapeutic failure possible
3 *Theophylline:* May inhibit metabolism of xanthines, potentially elevating serum concentrations
SPECIAL CONSIDERATIONS
PATIENT/FAMILY EDUCATION
• Take after meals; chew before swallowing
• Proper hygiene after bowel movement, including handwashing technique; change bed linen

---

* = non-FDA-approved use

thiamine (vitamin B$_1$)

(thy′a-min)
Rx: Thiamine **OTC:** Thiamilate
Chemical Class: B complex vitamin
Therapeutic Class: Vitamin

CLINICAL PHARMACOLOGY

Mechanism of Action: Acts as co-enzyme, as an oxidation-reduction agent, or possibly as a mitochondrial agent in pyruvate metabolism

Pharmacokinetics

PO/IM: Rapid and complete absorption; widely distributed (highest concentrations in liver, brain, kidney, and heart); rapidly metabolized; excess excreted in urine; body depletion of vitamin B$_1$ can occur after approx 3 wk of total absence of thiamine in the diet

INDICATIONS AND USES: Vitamin B$_1$ deficiency syndromes including polyneuritis, beriberi, pellagra, Wernicke-Korsakoff syndrome; metabolic disorders (maple syrup urine disease, subacute necrotizing encephalitis); parenteral thiamine is recommended for alcoholic patients with altered sensorium admitted to the hospital and in all patients presenting with coma or hypothermia of unknown etiology; essential component of total parenteral nutrition therapy

DOSAGE

Adult

• *Beriberi:* IM/IV 10-500 mg tid × 2 wk, then 5-10 mg PO qd × 1 mo
• *Beriberi with cardiac failure:* IV 100-500 mg
• *Metabolic disorders:* PO 10-20 mg qd
• *Anemia or pellagra:* PO 100 mg qd
• *Wernicke's encephalopathy:* IV 100 mg, then 50-100 mg qd until patient is consuming a regular, well-balanced diet

Child

• *Beriberi:* IM 10-50 mg qd × 4-6 wk
• *Anemia or pellagra:* PO 10-50 mg qd
• *Beriberi with cardiac failure:* IV 100-500 mg

💲 AVAILABLE FORMS/COST OF THERAPY

• Inj, Sol—IM, IV: 100 mg/ml, 1 ml: **$0.75-$1.00**
• Tab—Oral: 50 mg, 100's: **$2.17-$7.00**; 100 mg, 100's: **$1.65-$4.68**; 250 mg, 100's: **$3.90**
• Tab, Enteric Coated—Oral: 20 mg, 100's: **$13.95**

PREGNANCY AND LACTATION: Pregnancy category A; excreted into breast milk; U.S. recommended daily allowance for thiamine during lactation is 1.5-1.6 mg; supplement women with inadequate intake; compatible with breast feeding

SIDE EFFECTS/ADVERSE REACTIONS

CNS: Restlessness, weakness
CV: **Collapse,** hypotension, **pulmonary edema**
EENT: Tightness of throat
GI: *Diarrhea,* hemorrhage, *nausea*
SKIN: Angioneurotic edema, cyanosis, pruritus, sweating, urticaria, warmth

SPECIAL CONSIDERATIONS

• Worsening of Wernicke's encephalopathy is possible following glucose administration, administer thiamine before or along with dextrose-containing fluids
• Single vitamin B$_1$ deficiency is rare—suspect multiple vitamin deficiencies

T

thiethylperazine
(thye-eth-il-per'azeen)
Rx: Torecan
Chemical Class: Piperazine phenothiazine derivative
Therapeutic Class: Antiemetic

CLINICAL PHARMACOLOGY
Mechanism of Action: Acts centrally by blocking chemoreceptor trigger zone and blocking vomiting center

Pharmacokinetics
PO: Onset 45-60 min, duration 4 hr; metabolized by liver; excreted by kidneys; crosses placenta

INDICATIONS AND USES: Nausea and vomiting

DOSAGE
Adult
• PO/IM 10 mg qd-tid

$ **AVAILABLE FORMS/COST OF THERAPY**
• Inj, Sol—IV: 5 mg/ml, 2 ml: **$4.48**
• Tab, Uncoated—Oral: 10 mg, 100's: **$54.30**

CONTRAINDICATIONS: Coma
PRECAUTIONS: Children <2 yr, elderly, sulfite sensitivity, bone marrow depression, seizure disorder

PREGNANCY AND LACTATION: Pregnancy category C; excretion into breast milk unknown, use caution in nursing mothers

SIDE EFFECTS/ADVERSE REACTIONS
CNS: Depression, drowsiness, *euphoria,* extrapyramidal symptoms, restlessness, *seizures*
CV: Circulatory failure, ECG changes, postural hypotension, tachycardia
GI: Anorexia, constipation, cramps, diarrhea, dry mouth, metallic taste, weight loss
GU: Dark urine, urinary retention
RESP: Respiratory depression

INTERACTIONS
Drugs
3 *Anticholinergics, antiparkinson drugs, antidepressants:* Increased anticholinergic action
3 *Barbiturates:* Induction, decreased effect of thiethylperazine
3 *Beta-blockers:* Augmented pharmacologic action of both drugs
3 *Bromocriptine:* Neuroleptic drugs inhibit bromocriptine's ability to lower prolactin concentration
3 *Epinephrine:* Reversed pressor response to epinephrine
3 *Levodopa:* Inhibited antiparkinsonian effect of levodopa
3 *Lithium:* Lowered serum concentration of both drugs in combination
3 *Narcotic analgesics:* Hypotension with meperidine, caution with other narcotic analgesics
3 *Orphenadrine:* Lower thiethylperazine concentration and excessive anticholinergic effects

SPECIAL CONSIDERATIONS
• Effective antiemetic agent for the treatment of postoperative nausea and vomiting, nausea and vomiting secondary to mildly emetic chemotherapeutic agents, and vomiting secondary to radiation therapy and toxins
• No comparisons with prochlorperazine
• More extrapyramidal reactions than chlorpromazine and promazine; thiethylperazine would be less desirable than these agents in patients where the occurrence of a dystonic reaction would be hazardous (i.e., head and neck surgery patients, patients with severe pulmonary disease, patients with a history of dyskinetic reactions)

* = non-FDA-approved use

PATIENT/FAMILY EDUCATION
• Avoid hazardous activities, activities requiring alertness

MONITORING PARAMETERS
• Respiratory status initially

---

thioridazine
(thye-or-rid'a-zeen)
Rx: Mellaril
Chemical Class: Piperidine phenothiazine derivative
Therapeutic Class: Antipsychotic

CLINICAL PHARMACOLOGY
Mechanism of Action: Dopamine receptor antagonist, with higher affinity for D_2 over D_1-receptors, and variable selectivity among the cortical dopamine tracts; also activity on nondopaminergic sites, i.e., cholinergic, α-adrenergic and histaminic receptors (explaining side effects); high rates of sedation, anticholinergic effects, and orthostatic hypotension; minimal risk of extrapyramidal reaction

Pharmacokinetics
PO: Onset erratic, peak 2-4 hr; metabolized by liver; excreted in urine; crosses placenta; $t_{1/2}$ 26-36 hr

INDICATIONS AND USES: Psychotic disorders; behavioral problems in children (combativeness, explosive hyperexcitable behavior); alcohol withdrawal as adjunct; short-term treatment of anxiety, major depressive disorders, organic brain syndrome

DOSAGE
Adult
NOTE: 100 mg equivalent to chlorpromazine 100 mg
• *Psychosis:* PO 25-100 mg tid, max dose 800 mg/day; dose is gradually increased to desired response, then reduced to maintenance
• *Depression, behavioral problems, organic brain syndrome:* PO 25 mg tid, range from 10 mg bid-qid to 50 mg tid-qid

Child 2-12 yr
• PO 0.5-3 mg/kg/day in divided doses

💲 AVAILABLE FORMS/COST OF THERAPY
• Conc—Oral: 30 mg/ml, 120 ml: **$39.57;** 100 mg/ml, 120 ml: **$103.26**
• Tab, Coated—Oral: 10 mg, 100's: **$36.62;** 15 mg, 100's: **$43.17;** 25 mg, 100's: **$51.53;** 50 mg, 100's: **$62.56;** 100 mg, 100's: **$73.45;** 150 mg, 100's: **$96.64;** 200 mg, 100's: **$112.88**
• Susp—Oral: 25 mg/5 ml, 480 ml: **$62.22;** 100 mg/5 ml, 480 ml: **$127.92**

CONTRAINDICATIONS: Coma, severe CNS depression, child <2 yr, brain damage, severe hypertension or hypotension

PRECAUTIONS: Seizure disorders, hypertension, hepatic disease, cardiac disease, COPD

PREGNANCY AND LACTATION: Pregnancy category C

SIDE EFFECTS/ADVERSE REACTIONS
CNS: Confusion, extrapyramidal symptoms (rare) including pseudoparkinsonism, akathisia, dystonia, tardive dyskinesia, *headache, seizures*
*CV: **Cardiac arrest,*** ECG changes, orthostatic hypotension, tachycardia
EENT: Blurred vision, dry eyes, glaucoma, pigmentary retinopathy
GI: Anorexia, *constipation,* diarrhea, *dry mouth;* increased ALT, AST, jaundice, *nausea, vomiting,* weight gain
GU: Amenorrhea, enuresis, galactorrhea, gynecomastia, impotence, urinary frequency, urinary retention

T

---

italic = common side effects   ***bold italic*** = life-threatening reactions

HEME: Agranulocytosis, anemia, *leukocytosis, leukopenia*
RESP: Dyspnea, *laryngospasm, respiratory depression*
SKIN: Dermatitis, photosensitivity, *rash*

INTERACTIONS
Drugs

3 *Anticholinergics, antiparkinson drugs, antidepressants:* Increased anticholinergic action

3 *Barbiturates:* Induction, decreased effect of thioridazine

3 *Beta-blockers:* Augmented pharmacologic action of both drugs

3 *Bromocriptine:* Neuroleptic drugs inhibit bromocriptine's ability to lower prolactin concentration; reverse not common

3 *Epinephrine:* Reversed pressor response

3 *Levodopa:* Inhibited antiparkinsonian effect

3 *Lithium:* Lowered serum concentration of both drugs in combination

3 *Narcotic analgesics:* Hypotension with meperidine, caution with other narcotic analgesics

3 *Orphenadrine:* Lower thioridazine concentration and excessive anticholinergic effects

3 *Phenylpropanolamine:* Patient on thioridazine died after single dose of phenylpropanolamine; a causal relationship was not established

Labs
• *False positive:* Pregnancy tests, serum tricyclic antidepressants screen

SPECIAL CONSIDERATIONS
• Phenothiazine with weak potency, low incidence of EPS, but high incidence of sedation, anticholinergic effects, and cardiovascular effects

PATIENT/FAMILY EDUCATION
• Arise slowly from reclining position
• Avoid abrupt withdrawal
• Use a sunscreen during sun exposure
• Caution with activities requiring complete mental alertness (e.g., driving), may cause sedation
• Provide full information on risks of tardive dyskinesia

---

thiothixene
(thye-oh-thix'een)
Rx: Navane
Chemical Class: Thioxanthene derivative
Therapeutic Class: Antipsychotic

CLINICAL PHARMACOLOGY
Mechanism of Action: Dopamine receptor antagonist, with higher affinity for D_2- over D_1-receptors, and variable selectivity among the cortical dopamine tracts; also activity on nondopaminergic sites, i.e., cholinergic, α-adrenergic and histaminic receptors (explaining side effects); minimal sedation and anticholinergic effects; moderate orthostatic hypotension; high risk of extrapyramidal reactions

Pharmacokinetics
PO: Onset slow, peak 2-8 hr, duration up to 12 hr
IM: Onset 15-30 min, peak 1-6 hr, duration up to 12 hr
Metabolized by liver, excreted in urine; crosses placenta; $t_{1/2}$ 34 hr

INDICATIONS AND USES: Psychotic disorders; acute agitation*

DOSAGE
NOTE: 4 mg equivalent to chlorpromazine 100 mg
Adult
• PO 2-5 mg bid-qid depending on severity of condition; dose gradu-

---

* = non-FDA-approved use

ally increased to 15-30 mg/day if needed; max 60 mg/day

• IM 4 mg bid-qid; max dose 30 mg/day; administer PO dose as soon as possible

💲 AVAILABLE FORMS/COST OF THERAPY

• Cap, Gel—Oral: 1 mg, 100's: **$13.43-$42.70;** 2 mg, 100's: **$16.58-$57.59;** 5 mg, 100's: **$20.12-$90.05;** 10 mg, 100's: **$33.26-$124.13;** 20 mg, 100's: **$174.16**

• Conc—Oral: 5 mg/ml, 120 ml: **$25.13-$91.88**

CONTRAINDICATIONS: Blood dyscrasias, child <12 yr, circulatory collapse, CNS depression, coma

PRECAUTIONS: Lactation, seizure disorders, hypertension, hepatic disease, cardiovascular disease, glaucoma, COPD

PREGNANCY AND LACTATION: Pregnancy category C

SIDE EFFECTS/ADVERSE REACTIONS

CNS: Akathisia, drowsiness, dystonia, *extrapyramidal symptoms* including pseudoparkinsonism, *headache, seizures,* tardive dyskinesia
*CV: **Cardiac arrest,*** ECG changes, hypertension, orthostatic hypotension, tachycardia
EENT: Blurred vision, glaucoma, mydriasis
GI: Anorexia, constipation, diarrhea, dry mouth; increased ALT, AST, jaundice, weight gain
GU: Amenorrhea, enuresis, galactorrhea, gynecomastia, impotence, urinary frequency, urinary retention
*HEME: **Agranulocytosis,*** anemia, ***leukocytosis, leukopenia***
RESP: Dyspnea, ***laryngospasm, respiratory depression***
SKIN: Dermatitis, photosensitivity, rash
*MISC: **Neuroleptic malignant syndrome***

INTERACTIONS
Drugs
3 *Anticholinergics, antiparkinson drugs, antidepressants:* Increased anticholinergic action
3 *Barbiturates:* Induction, decreased effect of thiothixene
3 *Beta-blockers:* Augmented pharmacologic action of both drugs
3 *Bromocriptine:* Thiothixene inhibits bromocriptine's ability to lower prolactin concentration, reverse not common
3 *Epinephrine:* Reversed pressor response
3 *Guanethidine:* Inhibited antihypertensive response to guanethidine
3 *Levodopa:* Inhibited antiparkinsonian effect
3 *Lithium:* Lowered serum concentration of both drugs in combination
3 *Narcotic analgesics:* Hypotension with meperidine, caution with other narcotic analgesics
3 *Orphenadrine:* Lower thiothixene concentration and excessive anticholinergic effects

SPECIAL CONSIDERATIONS
• High-potency antipsychotic with a relatively high incidence of EPS, but a low incidence of sedation, anticholinergic effects, and cardiovascular effects

PATIENT/FAMILY EDUCATION
• Informed consent regarding risks of tardive dyskinesia; orthostatic hypotension

T

---

italic = common side effects   ***bold italic*** = life-threatening reactions

---

thyroid
(thye´roid)
Rx: Armour Thyroid, Nature-
Throid, Westhroid
Chemical Class: Thyroid
hormone in natural state
Therapeutic Class: Thyroid
hormone

CLINICAL PHARMACOLOGY
Mechanism of Action: Increases
metabolic rate, increases cardiac output, O_2 consumption, body temperature, blood volume, growth, development at cellular level, metabolism of carbohydrates, lipids, and
proteins; exerts profound influence
on every organ system, especially
CNS
Pharmacokinetics
PO: Peak 12-48 hr, partially absorbed (48%-79%, $T_3 > T_4$); 99%
bound to plasma proteins; deiodi-
nated in liver, kidney; enterohepati-
cally circulated; neither T_3 or T_4
cross placenta; $t_{1/2}$ 6-7 days
INDICATIONS AND USES: Replacement or supplemental therapy
(hypothyroidism, cretinism, myxedema); pituitary TSH suppression
in the treatment or prevention of
various types of euthyroid goiters,
including thyroid nodules, subacute
or chronic lymphocytic thyroiditis
(Hashimoto's), multinodal goiter,
and in the management of thyroid
cancer; diagnostic agent in suppression tests to differentiate suspected
mild hyperthyroidism or thyroid
gland autonomy
DOSAGE
Adult
• *Hypothyroidism:* PO 30 mg qd,
increased by 15-30 mg q30d until
desired response; maintenance dose
65-120 mg qd
• *Myxedema:* After stabilization with

IV levothyroxine or liothyronine and
concurrent correction of electrolyte
disturbances and administration of
corticosteroids, switch to PO thyroid; initial PO 15 mg qd, double
dose q2wk, maintenance 65-120 mg/
day
• *Thyroid cancer, thyroid suppression therapy:* PO TSH should be
suppressed to low or undetectable
levels; therefore, larger doses of thyroid hormone than those used for
replacement therapy are required.
• *Geriatric:* PO 7.5-15 mg qd,
double dose q4-6wk until desired
response, maintenance dose
Child
• *Cretinism, juvenile hypothyroidism:* [age, mg/day (mg/kg/day)]: 0-6
mo, 15-30 mg (4.8-6 mg); 6-12 mo,
30-45 mg (3.6-4.8 mg); 1-5 yr, 45-60
mg (3-3.6 mg); 6-12 yr, 60-90 mg
(2.4-3 mg); >12 yr, >90 mg (1.2-
1.8 mg)
**💲 AVAILABLE FORMS/COST
OF THERAPY**
• Tab, Uncoated—Oral: 15 mg,
100's: **$7.00-$10.15;** 30 mg, 100's:
$9.50-$20.90; 60 mg, 100's: **$5.50-
$22.22;** 65 mg: **$1.92-$8.98;** 90 mg:
$5.00-$20.90; 120 mg, 100's: **$3.96-
$24.48;** 130 mg: **$3.10;** 180 mg,
100's: **$3.60-$38.84;** 240 mg, 100's:
$58.21-$72.17; 300 mg, 90's:
$172.51
CONTRAINDICATIONS: Adrenal
insufficiency (uncorrected), thyrotoxicosis, MI
PRECAUTIONS: Cardiovascular
disease, diabetes mellitus or insipidus, elderly
PREGNANCY AND LACTATION:
Pregnancy category A; little or no
transplacental passage at physiologic serum concentrations; excreted
into breast milk in low concentrations (inadequate to protect a hypothyroid infant; too low to inter-

---

* = non-FDA-approved use

fere with neonatal thyroid screening programs)

SIDE EFFECTS/ADVERSE REACTIONS

CNS: Headache, *insomnia, tremors*

CV: Angina, **cardiac arrest, dysrhythmias,** hypertension, *palpitations, tachycardia*

GI: Cramps, diarrhea, increased or decreased appetite, nausea

METAB: Bone demineralization (osteoporosis)

MISC: Fever, heat intolerance, menstrual irregularities, sweating, weight loss

INTERACTIONS

Drugs

⬛ *Carbamazepine, phenytoin, rifampin:* Increases elimination of thyroid hormones; may increase dosage requirements

⬛ *Bile acid sequestrants:* Reduced serum thyroid hormone concentrations

⬛ *Oral anticoagulants:* Thyroid hormones increase catabolism of vitamin K–dependent clotting factors; an increase or decrease in clinical thyroid status will increase or decrease the hypoprothrombinemic response to oral anticoagulants

⬛ *Theophylline:* Reduced serum theophylline concentrations with initiation of thyroid therapy

SPECIAL CONSIDERATIONS

• Although used traditionally, natural hormones less clinically desirable due to varying potencies, inconsistent clinical effects, and more adverse stimulatory effects; synthetic derivatives (i.e., levothyroxine) preferred

MONITORING PARAMETERS

• TSH yearly

---

tiagabine

(ti-ah-ga′bean)

Rx: Gabitril

Chemical Class: Nipecotic acid derivative

Therapeutic Class: Anticonvulsant

CLINICAL PHARMACOLOGY

Mechanism of Action: Gamma-aminobutyric acid (GABA) uptake inhibitor; inhibits uptake into neurons and glia with anticonvulsant, anxiolytic and analgesic effects

Pharmacokinetics

PO: Peak serum levels 0.5-1 hr with no accumulation with chronic dosing

Well absorbed (oral bioavailability, 95%; food reduces Cmax 40%, but not AUC); 95% plasma protein bound; metabolized by liver (CYP3A); undergoes enterohepatic recirculation; $t_{1/2}$ 7-9 hr

INDICATIONS AND USES: Adjunctive therapy in the treatment of refractive partial seizures (simple, complex, secondarily generalized)

DOSAGE

Adult

• PO 4 mg qd for first wk; then increase 4-8 mg/day, weekly up to maximum of 56 mg/day prn desired effect/tolerance

• (NOTE: no changes for patients with renal impairment or elderly patients; hepatic impairment may require reduced initial and maintenance doses)

Child >12 yr; <18 yr

• PO 4 mg qd for first wk; 4 mg bid second week; then increase 4-8 mg/day, weekly up to maximum of 32 mg/day prn desired effect/tolerance

💲 **AVAILABLE FORMS/COST OF THERAPY**

• Tab, Coated—Oral: 4 mg, 100's: **$110.26;** 12 mg, 100's: **$146.91;** 16

---

italic = common side effects   ***bold italic*** = life-threatening reactions

mg, 100's: **$195.89;** 20 mg, 100's: **$244.86**

PRECAUTIONS: Liver disease (dosage reductions may be necessary); concurrent neurologic disorders (Alzheimer's dementia, organic brain disease, stroke) given potential for exacerbation; withdrawal seizures with abrupt withdrawal

PREGNANCY AND LACTATION: Pregnancy category C

SIDE EFFECTS/ADVERSE REACTIONS

CNS: Confusion, dizziness, emotional lability, headache, *impaired concentration, speech or language,* memory impairment, *nervousness, sedation, somnolence*

EENT: Binds to eye and other melanin containing tissue

GI: Abdominal pain

SKIN: Rash

MISC: Generalized weakness

INTERACTIONS

Drugs

3 *Anticonvulsants (hepatic enzyme inducers—i.e., barbiturates, carbamazepine, phenytoin, primidone):* Decreased tiagabine levels and effect

3 *Rifampin:* Decreased tiagabine levels and effect via hepatic enzyme induction

3 *Valproate:* Increased tiagabine free blood levels

SPECIAL CONSIDERATIONS

• Patients should exercise caution with initiation and dosage titration when driving, operating hazardous machinery, or other activities requiring mental concentration; patients should be advised to take the medication with food, to delay peak effects to avoid many CNS adverse effects

---

ticarcillin ticarcillin/clavulanic acid

(tye-kar-sill'in)

Rx: *Ticarcillin:* Ticar
Ticarcillin/clavulanic acid: Timentin

Chemical Class: Penicillin derivative; β-lactamase inhibitor
Therapeutic Class: Antibiotic

CLINICAL PHARMACOLOGY

Mechanism of Action: Inhibits bacterial wall synthesis; bactericidal; clavulanate protects ticarcillin from degradation by β-lactamase enzymes

Pharmacokinetics

IM: Peak ½-1 hr, duration 4-6 hr
IV: Peak 30-45 min, duration 4 hr
$t_{1/2}$ 70 min; protein binding 45%; small amount metabolized in liver, excreted in urine (glomerular filtration and tubular secretion); addition of clavulanic acid doesn't affect pharmacokinetics of ticarcillin

INDICATIONS AND USES: Infections of the respiratory tract, skin and soft tissue, bones and joints, urinary tract, and bacterial septicemia; intra-abdominal and gynecological infections caused by susceptible organisms

Antibacterial spectrum usually includes:

• Gram-positive organisms: *Staphylococcus aureus, Streptococcus faecalis, Streptococcus pneumoniae*

• Gram-negative organisms: *Neisseria gonorrhoeae, Escherichia coli, Proteus mirabilis, Salmonella, Morganella morganii, Providencia rettgeri, Enterobacter, Pseudomonas aeruginosa, Serratia*

- Anaerobes: *Bacteroides* spp. including *Bacteroides fragilis; Fusobacterium* spp.; *Veillonella* spp.; *Clostridium; Eubacterium* spp.; *Peptococcus* spp.; *Peptostreptococcus* spp.

Ticarcillin/clavulanic acid: Addition of clavulanic acid expands spectrum to include bacteria caused by β-lactamase-producing strains of above organisms and also includes:
- Gram-positive organisms: *Staphylococcus epidermidis*
- Gram-negative organisms: *Klebsiella* spp., *Hemophilus influenzae, Citrobacter* spp., *Serratia marcescens*
- Anaerobes: *Bacteroides melaninogenicus*

DOSAGE

Adult
- Ticarcillin: IV/IM 12-24 g/day in divided doses q3-6h; infuse over ½-2 hr (usual dose 3 g q4h or 4 g q6h); dosage adjustments for decreased clearance: for CrCl (ml/min): >60, 3 g q4h; 30-60, 2 g q4h; 10-30, 2 g q8h; <10, 2 g q12h; <10 with hepatic dysfunction, 2 g q24h; peritoneal dialysis, 3 g q12h; hemodialysis, 2 g q12h supplemented with 3 g after each dialysis
- Ticarcillin/clavulanic acid: IV 3.1 g (contains 3 g ticarcillin, 100 mg clavulanic acid) q4-6h; for patients weighing ≤60 kg 200 mg-300 mg/kg/day (based on ticarcillin content) given in divided doses q4-6h

Child
- IV/IM 50-300 mg/kg/day in divided doses q4-8h

Neonates
- IV INF 75-100 mg/kg/8-12 hr

$ **AVAILABLE FORMS/COST OF THERAPY**
- Inj, Dry-Sol—IM, IV: 3 g/vial: **$13.43**
Ticarcillin/clavulanic acid:
- Inj, Dry-Sol—IV: 0.1 g/3 g: **$15.40**

PRECAUTIONS: Hypersensitivity to cephalosporins, renal and hepatic dysfunction

PREGNANCY AND LACTATION: Pregnancy category B; excreted into breast milk in low concentrations; compatible with breast feeding

SIDE EFFECTS/ADVERSE REACTIONS

CNS: Anxiety, coma, depression, hallucinations, lethargy, ***seizures,*** twitching

GI: Abdominal pain, *diarrhea,* glossitis, increased AST, ALT; *nausea,* ***pseudomembranous colitis,*** *vomiting*

GU: Glomerulonephritis, hematuria, *moniliasis,* oliguria, proteinuria, *vaginitis*

HEME: ***Bone marrow depression,*** increased bleeding

METAB: Hypokalemia

SKIN: Pruritus, rash, urticaria

MISC: Drug fever, local reactions (phlebitis)

INTERACTIONS

Drugs

3 *Aminoglycosides:* Inactivation of aminoglycosides *in vitro* and *in vivo,* reducing the aminoglycoside effect

Labs
- *False increase:* Urine glucose

SPECIAL CONSIDERATIONS
- Synergistic with aminoglycosides
- Sodium content, 5.2 mEq/g ticarcillin
- For reliable activity against *Pseudomonas,* must be dosed q4h

T

italic = common side effects   ***bold italic*** = life-threatening reactions

ticlopidine

(tye-klo'pa-deen)
Rx: Ticlid
Chemical Class: Thienpyridine derivative
Therapeutic Class: Antiplatelet agent

CLINICAL PHARMACOLOGY
Mechanism of Action: Selectively and irreversibly inhibits ADP-induced platelet aggregation by inhibiting the binding of ADP to its receptors on platelets, thereby affecting ADP-dependent activation of the glycoprotein IIb/IIIa complex, the major site of platelet-fibrinogen binding

Pharmacokinetics
PO: Peak 2 hr, rapidly absorbed (decreased 20% by meals); 98% bound to plasma proteins; extensively hepatically metabolized, excreted in urine (60%) and feces (23%); nonlinear pharmacokinetics (clearance decreases on repeated dosing); $t_{1/2}$ after a single 250 mg dose, 12.6 hr; with repeat dosing at 250 mg bid, $t_{1/2}$ rises to 4-5 days (steady state levels after approximately 14-21 days)

INDICATIONS AND USES: Reducing the risk of thrombotic stroke in aspirin intolerant patients or aspirin failures; prevention of thrombosis following intracoronary stent placement*; intermittent claudication*; chronic arterial occlusion*; sickle cell disease*

DOSAGE
Adult
• PO 250 mg bid with food

💲 AVAILABLE FORMS/COST OF THERAPY
• Tab, Uncoated—Oral: 250 mg, 60's: **$109.54**

CONTRAINDICATIONS: Current blood dyscrasia (neutropenia, thrombocytopenia); history of TTP; hemostatic disorder or active pathological bleeding (such as bleeding peptic ulcer or intracranial bleeding); patients with severe liver impairment

PRECAUTIONS: Past liver disease, renal disease, elderly, children, increased bleeding risk (trauma, surgery, or pathological conditions, dental procedures)

PREGNANCY AND LACTATION: Pregnancy category B; use caution in nursing mothers

SIDE EFFECTS/ADVERSE REACTIONS
GI (40% have GI effects): Cholestatic jaundice, *diarrhea, GI discomfort,* hepatitis; increased cholesterol, LDL, VLDL; *nausea, vomiting*
HEME: **Agranulocytosis,** bleeding (epistaxis, hematuria, conjunctival hemorrhage, GI bleeding), *neutropenia, thrombocytopenia*
SKIN: Pruritus, *rash*

INTERACTIONS
Drugs
🔳 *Cyclosporine:* Potential for reduction in blood cyclosporine concentrations
🔳 *Phenytoin:* Inhibition of hepatic metabolism (CYP2C9) of phenytoin; potential for development of phenytoin toxicity, reduction in phenytoin dose may be necessary
🔳 *Theophylline:* Increased theophylline level via inhibition of metabolism, increased risk of toxicity

SPECIAL CONSIDERATIONS
• Due to the risk of life-threatening neutropenia or agranulocytosis and cost, ticlopidine should be reserved for patients intolerant to aspirin or who fail aspirin

MONITORING PARAMETERS
• CBC q2wk for 1st 3 mo of therapy, then periodically thereafter

---

* = non-FDA-approved use

tiludronate

(ti-loo'dro-nate)
Rx: Skelid
Chemical Class: Synthetic analog of pyrophosphate
Therapeutic Class: Bisphosphonate

CLINICAL PHARMACOLOGY
Mechanism of Action: Binds to hydroxyapatite at sites of bone resorption, inhibiting normal and abnormal bone resorption ("crystal poison"); minimal secondary reduction in bone formation (resorption coupled to formation); suppresses the pagetic disease process

Pharmacokinetics
PO: Poorly absorbed, 3% bioavailability (reduced 90% by food), high affinity for bone, 90% protein bound, renal excretion, elimination $t_{1/2}$ 40-150 hr

INDICATIONS AND USES: Paget's disease, postmenopausal osteoporosis,* hyperparathyroidism,* bone pain in prostatic carcinoma and metastatic breast cancer,* hypercalcemia of malignancy*

DOSAGE
Adult
• *Paget's disease:* PO 400 mg qd for 3-6 months
• *Osteoporosis:* PO 100 mg qd for 6 months

💲 AVAILABLE FORMS/COST OF THERAPY
• Tab—Oral: 200 mg, 56's: **$420.89**

CONTRAINDICATIONS: Renal failure (CrCl <30 mL/min), due to lack of clinical experience
PRECAUTIONS: Esophageal, gastric disease, GERD
PREGNANCY AND LACTATION: Pregnancy category C; dose-related scoliosis; avoid exposure in children

SIDE EFFECTS/ADVERSE REACTIONS
CV: Chest pain, peripheral edema
GI: Diarrhea, dysphagia, esophageal ulcer, esophagitis, flatulence, gastric ulcer, nausea, vomiting
SKIN: Rash

INTERACTIONS
❷ *Food:* Reduces bioavailability 90%
Drugs
❷ *Antacids/calcium:* Reduces bioavailability 60-80%
❸ *Aspirin:* Decreases bioavailability of tiludronate by 50%
❸ *Indomethacin:* Bioavailability of NSAID increased 2-4 fold

SPECIAL CONSIDERATIONS
• Studies needed to assess place in therapy with other bisphosphonates
• Inhibition of bone loss in osteoporosis may persist up to 2 yr after 6 mo of treatment and discontinuation of drug

PATIENT/FAMILY EDUCATION
• Take with 6-8 oz plain water; do not take within 2 hr of food or other medications

timolol

(tim'oh-lole)
Rx: *Oral:* Blockadren, *Ophthalmic:* Betimol, Timoptic, Timoptic-XE
Combinations —Ophthalmic
  Rx: with dorzol amide (Cosopt)
Chemical Class: Nonselective, β-adrenergic blocker
Therapeutic Class: Antihypertensive; antianginal; antiglaucoma agent

CLINICAL PHARMACOLOGY
Mechanism of Action: PO: Competitive β-adrenergic antagonist; produces negative inotropic and chronotropic responses; slows AV

T

---

nodal conduction; decreases heart rate; decreases myocardial oxygen consumption; antiarrhythmic effects (class II); reduction in platelet aggregation and blood viscosity; suppression of renin release; inhibition of central sympathetic outflow; decreases presynaptic receptor neurotransmitter release; no intrinsic sympathomimetic or membrane stabilizing activity; low to moderate lipid solubility; OPHTH: reduces intraocular pressure via reduction in production of aqueous humor

Pharmacokinetics

OPHTH: Onset 0.5-20 min, peak 1-2 hr, duration 24 hr

PO: Peak 2 hr (0.5-3 hr); rapidly and completely absorbed; excreted 30%-45% unchanged, 60%-65% metabolized by liver; $t_{1/2}$ 4 hr

INDICATIONS AND USES: Aphakic glaucoma, glaucoma, migraine headache, hypertension, post-myocardial infarction, supraventricular arrhythmias (atrial fibrillation, atrial flutter, paroxysmal supraventricular tachycardia), aggressive behavior,* angina pectoris,* anxiety,* cataract extraction prophylaxis,* congestive heart failure,* hyperthyroidism,* neuroleptic-induced akathisia,* retinal detachment,* tremor*

DOSAGE

Adult

• OPHTH 1 gtt 0.25% sol in affected eye(s) bid, then 1 gtt qd for maintenance, may increase to 1 gtt 0.5% sol bid if needed

• *Hypertension:* PO 10 mg bid initially, usually maintenance 20-40 mg/day divided bid, not to exceed 60 mg/day

• *Post-MI prophylaxis:* PO 10 mg bid

• *Migraine:* 10 mg bid, up to 30 mg/day divided bid

• *Angina pectoris:* PO 10-60 mg daily (usually bid)

• *Arrythmias:* PO 20-30 mg daily (usually bid) for supraventricular arrythmias

⑤ AVAILABLE FORMS/COST OF THERAPY

• Sol—Ophth: 0.25%, 2.5, 5 ml: **$26.06-$33.39**/10 ml; 0.5%, 2.5, 5 ml: **$27.98-$39.66**/10 ml

• Gel—Ophth: 0.25%, 2.5, 5 ml: **$22.67-$25.19**/5 ml; 0.5%, 2.5, 5 ml: **$26.95-$29.94**/5 ml

• Tab, Uncoated—Oral: 5 mg, 100's: **$26.50-$49.01;** 10 mg, 100's: **$31.80-$60.61;** 20 mg, 100's: **$65.09-$111.83**

CONTRAINDICATIONS: Bronchial asthma, cardiogenic shock, overt cardiac failure, second and third degree AV block, severe sinus bradycardia

PRECAUTIONS: Anesthesia/surgery (myocardial depression), avoid abrupt withdrawal, bronchospastic airways, congestive heart failure, diabetes mellitus, hyperthyroidism/thyrotoxicosis, concurrent clonidine (discontinue timolol several days prior to withdrawal of clonidine), peripheral vascular disease, renal disease

PREGNANCY AND LACTATION: Pregnancy category C; similar drug, atenolol, frequently used in the third trimester for treatment of hypertension (many studies of efficacy and safety of atenolol in pregnancy induced hypertension; long term use has been associated with intrauterine growth retardation; mean milk:plasma ratio, 0.80 in one study; quantity of drug ingested by breast feeding infant unlikely to be therapeutically significant

---

* = non-FDA-approved use

SIDE EFFECTS/ADVERSE REACTIONS

CNS: Anxiety, confusion, depression, *dizziness,* fatigue, hallucinations, headache, insomnia, weakness

CV: Bradycardia, claudication, ***CHF, dysrhythmias,*** edema, ***heart block, hypotension, syncope***

EENT: Conjunctivitis, *double vision,* dry burning eyes, eye irritation, keratitis, sore throat, *visual changes*

GI: Abdominal pain, anorexia, diarrhea, dyspepsia, ***ischemic colitis, mesenteric arterial thrombosis,*** *nausea*

GU: Frequency, impotence

HEME: ***Agranulocytosis, purpura, thrombocytopenia***

METAB: Hyperglycemia, mask hypoglycemia

MS: Joint pain

RESP: ***Bronchospasm,*** cough, dyspnea, rales

SKIN: Alopecia, fever, pruritus, rash, urticaria

INTERACTIONS

Drugs

▪ *α-1 adrenergic blockers:* Potential enhanced first dose response (marked initial drop in blood pressure, particularly on standing (especially prazocin)

▪ *Amiodarone:* Combined therapy may lead to bradycardia, cardiac arrest, or ventricular dysrhythmia

▪ *Antidiabetics:* β-blockers increase blood glucose and impair peripheral circulation; altered response to hypoglycemia by prolonging the recovery of normoglycemia, causing hypertension, and blocking tachycardia

▪ *Clonidine:* Hypertension occurring upon withdrawal of clonidine may be exacerbated by timolol

▪ *Digoxin:* Additive prolongation of atrioventricular (AV) conduction time

▪ *Dihydropyridine calcium channel blockers:* Additive hypotension (kinetic and dynamic)

▪ *Diltiazem:* Potentiates β-adrenergic effects; hypotendion, left ventricular failure, and AV conduction disturbances problematic in elderly, patients with left ventricular dysfunction, aortic stenosis, or with large doses of either drug

▪ *Disopyramide:* Additive negative inotropic cardiac effects

▪ *Epinephrine:* Enhanced pressor response (hypertension and bradycardia)

▪ *Hypoglycemic agents:* Masked hypoglycemia, hyperglycemia

▪ *Isoproterenol:* Reduced isoproterenol efficacy in asthma

▪ *Methyldopa:* Potential for development of hypertension in the presence of increased catecholamines

▪ *Nonsteroidal anti-inflammatory drugs:* Reduced antihypertensive effects of timolol

▪ *Phenylephrine:* Potential for hypertensive episodes when administered together

▪ *Prazosin:* First-dose response to prazosin may be enhanced by β-blockade

▪ *Quinidine:* Increased timolol concentrations

▪ *Tacrine:* Additive bradycardia

▪ *Theophylline:* Antagonistic pharmacodynamic effects

▪ *Verapamil:* Potentiates β-adrenergic effects; hypotendion, left ventricular failure, and AV conduction disturbances problemmatic in elderly, patients with left ventricular dysfunction, aortic stenosis, or with large doses of either drug

T

---

italic = common side effects   ***bold italic*** = life-threatening reactions

SPECIAL CONSIDERATIONS
• Currently available β-blockers appear to be equally effective; cardioselective or combined α- and β-adrenergic blockade are less likely to cause undesirable effects and may be preferred

MONITORING PARAMETERS
• Angina: reduction in nitroglycerin usage; frequency, severity, onset, and duration of angina pain; heart rate
• Arrhythmias: heart rate
• Congestive heart failure: functional status, cough, dyspnea on exertion, paroxysmal nocturnal dyspnea, exercise tolerance, and ventricular function
• Hypertension: Blood pressure
• Migraine headache: reduction in the frequency, severity, and duration of attacks
• Post myocardial infaction: left ventricular function, lower resting heart rate
• Toxicity: blood glucose, bronchospasm, hypotension, bradycardia, depression, confusion, hallucination, sexual dysfunction

PATIENT/FAMILY EDUCATION
• Do not discontinue abruptly; may require taper; rapid withdrawal may produce rebound hypertension or angina

---

tioconazole
(tyo-con'a-zole)
OTC: Vagistat-1
Chemical Class: Imidazole derivative
Therapeutic Class: Antifungal

CLINICAL PHARMACOLOGY
Mechanism of Action: Alteration of the fungal cell membrane, which allows leakage of essential intracellular components; fungicidal against *Candida*

Pharmacokinetics
VAG: Negligible systemic absorption

INDICATIONS AND USES: Local treatment of vulvovaginal candidiasis

DOSAGE
Adult
• VAG 1 applicatorful hs × 1

💲 **AVAILABLE FORMS/COST OF THERAPY**
• Oint—Vag: 6.5%, 4.6 g single dose: **$14.39**

PRECAUTIONS: Discontinue if irritation or sensitization occurs; chronic or recurrent candidiasis may be a symptom of unrecognized diabetes or a compromised immune system

PREGNANCY AND LACTATION: Pregnancy category C; excretion into breast milk unknown

SIDE EFFECTS/ADVERSE REACTIONS
GU: Burning, desquamation, discharge, dryness of vaginal secretions, dysuria, irritation, itching, nocturia, vaginal pain, vulvar edema

SPECIAL CONSIDERATIONS
• Similar in efficacy to miconazole, econazole, and clotrimazole for the topical management of fungal skin infections; choice determined by cost and availability; additional efficacy vs. trichomoniasis with longer course of therapy

---

tiopronin
(tye-o-pro'nen)
Rx: Thiola
Chemical Class: Thiol derivative
Therapeutic Class: Anti-kidney stone agent

CLINICAL PHARMACOLOGY
Mechanism of Action: Undergoes thiol-disulfide exchange with cys-

---

* = non-FDA-approved use

teine to form a mixed, water-soluble disulfide of tiopronin-cysteine; the amount of sparingly soluble cysteine is reduced

Pharmacokinetics

PO: 48% appears in urine in 4 hr, 78% by 72 hr; reduction of urinary cysteine of 250-500 mg on 1-2 g/day may be expected; rapid onset and offset of action

INDICATIONS AND USES: Prevention of kidney stone formation in patients with severe homozygous cystinuria with urinary cysteine greater than 500 mg/day, who are resistant to conservative treatment

DOSAGE

Adult

• PO 800-1000 mg/day, given in divided doses tid at least 1 hr before or 2 hr after meals

Child

• PO 15 mg/kg/day, given in divided doses tid at least 1 hr before or 2 hr after meals

$ AVAILABLE FORMS/COST OF THERAPY

• Tab, Uncoated—Oral: 100 mg, 100's: **$71.25**

CONTRAINDICATIONS: History of agranulocytosis, thrombocytopenia, aplastic anemia on this medication

PRECAUTIONS: Goodpasture's syndrome, children <9 yr

PREGNANCY AND LACTATION: Pregnancy category C; excreted in breast milk and may cause adverse effects in nursing infant, mothers taking tiopronin should avoid nursing

SIDE EFFECTS/ADVERSE REACTIONS

METAB: Vitamin B_6 deficiency

SKIN: Erythema, lupus-like syndrome (fever, arthralgia, lymphadenopathy), maculopapular, pruritus, wrinkling skin

MISC: Blunting of taste, *drug fever*

SPECIAL CONSIDERATIONS

• May be associated with fever and less severe adverse reactions than d-penicillamine

---

tirofiban

(tye-roe-fye′ban)

Rx: Aggrastat

Chemical Class: Glycoprotein (GP) IIb/IIIa inhibitor

Therapeutic Class: Antiplatelet agent

CLINICAL PHARMACOLOGY

Mechanism of Action: Reversibly prevents fibrinogen, von Willebrand's factor, and other adhesion ligands from binding to platelet GP IIb/IIIa receptors, thereby inhibiting platelet aggregation

Pharmacokinetics

65% bound in human plasma; 65% cleared by renal excretion (significantly decreased in patients with creatinine clearance <30 ml/min, including patients requiring hemodialysis); $t_{1/2}$ 2 hr

INDICATIONS AND USES: Acute coronary syndromes in combination with heparin, including patients who are to be managed medically and those undergoing percutaneous transluminal coronary angioplasty (PCTA), or atherectomy

DOSAGE

Adult

• *Acute coronary syndrome:* IV administer in combination with heparin for 48-108 hr according to the schedule below; INF should be continued through angiography and for 12-24 hr after angioplasty or atherectomy

• Injection must first be diluted to same strength as injection premixed (50 mcg/ml)

Dosage adjustment of tirofiban by patient weight:

Most patients		
Patient weight (kg)	30 min loading rate (ml/hr)	Maintenance rate (ml/hr)
30-37	16	4
38-45	20	5
46-54	24	6
55-62	28	7
63-70	32	8
71-79	36	9
80-87	40	10
88-95	44	11
96-104	48	12
105-112	52	13
113-120	56	14
121-128	60	15
129-137	64	16
138-145	68	17
146-153	72	18

Severe renal impairment	
30 min loading rate (ml/hr)	Maintenance rate (ml/hr)
8	2
10	3
12	3
14	4
16	4
18	5
20	5
22	6
24	6
26	7
28	7
30	8
32	8
34	9
36	9

🔋 **AVAILABLE FORMS/COST OF THERAPY**

• Inj, Sol—IV: 250 mcg/ml, 50 ml (vial): **$420.00;** 50 mcg/ml, 500 ml (premixed): **$840.00**

CONTRAINDICATIONS: Active internal bleeding or history of bleeding diathesis within previous 30 days; history of stroke within 30 days; history of hemorrhagic stroke; major surgical procedure or severe physical trauma within previous month; systolic blood pressure >180 mm Hg or diastolic blood pressure >110 mm Hg; history of intracranial hemorrhage, intracranial neoplasm, arteriovenous malformation or aneurysm; history, symptoms or findings of aortic dissection, acute pericarditis

PRECAUTIONS: Platelet count <150,000/mm^3; hemorrhagic retinopathy; IM injections, urinary catheters, nasotracheal intubation, nasogastric tubes; elderly; severe renal insufficiency (creatinine clearance <30 ml/min)

PREGNANCY AND LACTATION: Pregnancy category B; use caution in nursing mothers

SIDE EFFECTS/ADVERSE REACTIONS

*HEME: **Bleeding** (major bleeding 1.4% to 2.2%, minor bleeding 10.5% to 12%)*

INTERACTIONS

Drugs

3 *Antithrombotics (aspirin, heparin, warfarin, ticlopidine, clopidogrel):* Increased risk of bleeding

SPECIAL CONSIDERATIONS

• When bleeding cannot be controlled with pressure discontinue INF

• Most major bleeding occurs at arterial access site for cardiac catheterization; prior to pulling femoral artery sheath, discontinue heparin for 3-4 hr and document activated clotting time (ACT) <180 sec or aPTT <45 sec; achieve sheath hemostasis ≥4 hr before discharge

• In clinical studies, patients received ASA unless it was contraindicated

• Tirofiban, eptifibitide, and abciximab can all decrease the incidence of cardiac events associated with acute coronary syndromes; direct comparisons are needed to establish which, if any, is superior; for angioplasty, until more data become available, abciximab appears to be the drug of choice

MONITORING PARAMETERS

• Platelet count, hemoglobin, hematocrit, PT/aPTT (baseline, within 6 hr following bolus dose, then daily thereafter)

---

tizanidine
(tye-zan′i-deen)
Rx: Zanaflex
Chemical Class: Imidazoline derivative
Therapeutic Class: Skeletal muscle relaxant

CLINICAL PHARMACOLOGY
Mechanism of Action: Centrally acting agonist at α_2-adrenergic receptor sites; presumably reduces spasticity by increasing presynaptic inhibition of motor neurons
Pharmacokinetics
PO: Peak 1.5 hr, bioavailability 40% due to extensive first-pass metabolism; 30% bound to plasma proteins; metabolized by liver to inactive metabolites, excreted in urine (60%) and feces (20%); half-life 2.5 hr

INDICATIONS AND USES: Acute and intermittent management of increased muscle tone associated with spasticity (e.g., with multiple sclerosis and spinal cord injuries)

DOSAGE
Adult
• PO 4-8 mg q4-6h prn; not to exceed 36 mg/day prn

$ AVAILABLE FORMS/COST OF THERAPY
• Tab—Oral: 4 mg, 150's: **$145.80**
PRECAUTIONS: Renal impairment, hypotension, impaired hepatic function, children
PREGNANCY AND LACTATION:
Pregnancy category C; lipid soluble, may pass into breast milk
SIDE EFFECTS/ADVERSE REACTIONS
CNS: Asthenia, dizziness, dyskinesia, nervousness, *somnolence,* speech disorder
CV: Hypotension, orthostatic hypotension
EENT: Blurred vision, pharyngitis, rhinitis
GI: Abnormal liver function tests, constipation, *dry mouth,* vomiting
GU: Urinary frequency
MS: Increased spasm or muscle tone
INTERACTIONS
Drugs
❷ *Clonidine, guanabenz, guanadrel, guanethidine, guanfacine:* Potential for hypotension, avoid concurrent use
❸ *Oral contraceptives:* Decreased clearance of tizanidine
PATIENT/FAMILY EDUCATION
• Arise slowly from a reclining position

T

---

tobramycin

(toe-bra-mye'sin)

Rx: *Systemic:* Nebcin
Ophthalmic: AKTob,
Tobralcon, Tobrex, Tomycine,
Tobrasol
Combinations
   Ophthalmic: **Rx:** with dexa-
   methasone (Tobradex)
Chemical Class: Aminoglyco-
side
Therapeutic Class: Antibiotic

CLINICAL PHARMACOLOGY

Mechanism of Action: Interferes
with protein synthesis in bacterial
cell by binding to ribosomal subunit, causing inaccurate peptide sequence to form in protein chain; bactericidal

Pharmacokinetics

IM: Onset rapid, peak 30-90 min
IV: Onset immediate, peak 1 hr
Not metabolized, excreted unchanged in urine (clearance propor-
tional to creatinine clearance);
crosses placental barrier; $t_{1/2}$ 2-3 hr

INDICATIONS AND USES: Severe
infections of CNS, respiratory, GI,
urinary tract, bone, skin, soft tissues, intra-abdominal infections,
septicemia caused by susceptible organisms

OPHTH: External infections of the
eye and its adnexa caused by susceptible bacteria

Antibacterial spectrum usually includes:

• Gram-positive aerobes: *S. aureus*
(Low order of activity against most
gram-positive organisms, including
Str. pyogenes, Str. pneumoniae, and
enterococci)

• Gram-negative aerobes: *Citrobacter* spp., *Enterobacter* spp., *Escherichia coli; Klebsiella* spp., *Morganella morgani, Pseudomonas
aeruginosa, Proteus mirabilis, P. vulgaris, Providencia* spp., *Serratia* spp.

DOSAGE

Base dosage calculations on lean
body weight

Adult

• IM/IV 3 mg/kg/day in divided
doses q8h; may give up to 5 mg/
kg/day in divided doses q6-8h; adjust dose according to serum peak
and trough concentrations; careful
monitoring of serum concentrations
and dose adjustment required in renal function impairment

Child

• IM/IV 6-7.5 mg/kg/day in 3-4
equal divided doses

Neonates <1 wk

• IM up to 4 mg/kg/day in divided
doses q12h; IV up to 4 mg/kg/day
in divided doses q12h

• OPHTH: Oint ¼ in ribbon to conjunctiva q8-12h; SOL: 1 gtt q4h

$ **AVAILABLE FORMS/COST
   OF THERAPY**

• Inj, Dry-Sol—IV: 80 mg/vial:
$7.76

• Sol—Ophth: 0.3%, 5 ml: **$4.04-
$24.06**

• Oint—Ophth, Top: 0.3%, 3.5 g:
$25.62

CONTRAINDICATIONS: Severe renal disease, hypersensitivity to
sulfites (contains sodium bisulfite)

PRECAUTIONS: Neonates, mild renal disease, myasthenia gravis, hearing deficits, Parkinson's disease, extensive burns (altered pharmacokinetics)

PREGNANCY AND LACTATION:
Pregnancy category D (ophth category B); excreted into breast milk;
given poor oral absorption, toxicity
minimal; limited to modification of
bowel flora and interference with
interpretation of culture results if
fever workup required

* = non-FDA-approved use

SIDE EFFECTS/ADVERSE REACTIONS

CNS: Confusion, depression, dizziness, muscle twitching, neurotoxicity, numbness, *seizures,* tremors, vertigo

CV: Hypertension, hypotension, palpitation

EENT: Deafness, ototoxicity, tinnitus

OPHTH: blurred vision, burning, stinging of eyes, visual disturbances

GI: Anorexia, hepatomegaly, hepatic necrosis, increased ALT, AST, bilirubin; nausea, splenomegaly, vomiting

GU: Azotemia, hematuria, *nephrotoxicity,* oliguria, renal damage, *renal failure*

HEME: **Agranulocytosis,** anemia, eosinophilia, **leukopenia, thrombocytopenia**

SKIN: Alopecia, burning, dermatitis, *rash,* urticaria

INTERACTIONS

Drugs

3 *Amphotericin B:* Synergistic nephrotoxicity

2 *Atracurium:* Tobramycin potentiates respiratory depression by atracurium

3 *Carbenicillin:* Potential for inactivation of tobramycin in patients with renal failure

3 *Carboplatin:* Additive nephrotoxicity or ototoxicity

3 *Cephalosporins:* Increased potential for nephrotoxicity in patients with preexisting renal disease

3 *Cisplatin:* Additive nephrotoxicity or ototoxicity

3 *Cyclosporine:* Additive nephrotoxicity

2 *Ethacrynic acid:* Additive ototoxicity

3 *Indomethacin:* Reduced renal clearance of tobramycin in premature infants

3 *Methoxyflurane:* Additve nephrotoxicity

2 *Neuromuscular blocking agents:* Tobramycin potentiates respiratory depression by neuromuscular blocking agents

3 *NSAIDs:* May reduce renal clearance of tobramycin

3 *Penicillins (extended spectrum):* Potential for inactivation of tobramycin in patients with renal failure

3 *Piperacillin:* Potential for inactivation of tobramycin in patients with renal failure

2 *Succinylcholine:* Tobramycin potentiates respiratory depression by succinylcholine

3 *Ticarcillin:* Potential for inactivation of tobramycin in patients with renal failure

3 *Vancomycin:* Additive nephrotoxicity or ototoxicity

2 *Vecuronium:* Tobramycin potentiates respiratory depression by vecuronium

SPECIAL CONSIDERATIONS

• Gentamicin is 1st-line aminoglycoside of choice; differences in toxicity between gentamicin and tobramycin not likely to be clinically important in most patients with normal renal function given short courses of treatment; consider tobramycin in patients who are more likely to develop toxicity (prolonged and/or recurrent aminoglycoside therapy, those with renal failure) and in patients infected with *Pseudomonas aeruginosa* because of increased antibacterial activity

• Has been administered via nebulizer to treat resistant pneumonia in patients with cystic fibrosis

MONITORING PARAMETERS

• Serum Ca, Mg, Na; serum concentrations, peak (30 min following IV INF or 1 hr after IM inj) and trough (just prior to next dose); prolonged concentrations above 12

---

italic = common side effects   ***bold italic*** = life-threatening reactions

µg/ml or trough levels above 2 µg/ml may indicate tissue accumulation; such accumulation, advanced age, and cumulative dosage may contribute to ototoxicity and nephrotoxicity; perform serum concentration assays after 2 or 3 doses, so that the dosage can be adjusted if necessary, and at 3- to 4-day intervals during therapy; in the event of changing renal function, more frequent serum concentrations should be obtained and the dosage or dosage interval adjusted according to more detailed guidelines

---

tocainide

(toe-kay′nide)
Rx: Tonocard
Chemical Class: Lidocaine derivative
Therapeutic Class: Antidysrhythmic (Class IB)

CLINICAL PHARMACOLOGY
Mechanism of Action: Decreases sodium and potassium conductance, resulting in decreased excitability of myocardial cells; no clinically significant changes in sinus nodal function, effective refractory periods or intracardiac conduction times; failure to respond to lidocaine predicts failiure to tocainide
Pharmacokinetics
PO: Peak ½-2 hr; oral bioavailability 100%; metabolized by liver (negligible 1st-pass metabolism), excreted in urine; $t_{1/2}$ 10-17 hr

INDICATIONS AND USES: Life-threatening ventricular dysrhythmias (i.e., sustained ventricular tachycardia)
DOSAGE
Adult
• PO initial 400 mg q8h; usual maintenance dose 1200 to 1800 mg/day divided tid

💲 AVAILABLE FORMS/COST OF THERAPY
• Tab, Plain Coated—Oral: 400 mg, 100's: **$88.31;** 600 mg, 100's: **$112.55**
CONTRAINDICATIONS: Hypersensitivity to amides, severe heart block (2nd or 3rd degree)
PRECAUTIONS: Children, renal disease, liver disease, CHF, respiratory depression, myasthenia gravis, blood dyscrasias
PREGNANCY AND LACTATION: Pregnancy category C
SIDE EFFECTS/ADVERSE REACTIONS
CNS: Confusion, dizziness, headache, involuntary movement, irritability, paresthesias, psychosis, restlessness, *seizures,* tremors
CV: Angina, bradycardia, *cardiovascular collapse,* chest pain, *CHF, heart block, prodysrhythmic effect,* PVCs, tachycardia
EENT: Blurred vision, hearing loss, tinnitus
GI: Anorexia, diarrhea, hepatitis, nausea, vomiting
HEME: Agranulocytosis, blood dyscrasias, hypoplastic anemia, leukopenia, thrombocytopenia
MS: Lupus-like illness, positive ANA
RESP: Dyspnea, *pulmonary fibrosis, respiratory depression*
SKIN: Edema, rash, swelling, urticaria
INTERACTIONS
Drugs
3 *Antacids:* Antacids which increase urinary pH may increase tocainide serum concentrations
3 *Rifampin:* Reduction of serum tocainide concentrations
SPECIAL CONSIDERATIONS
• Can be considered oral lidocaine; antidysrhythmic drugs have not been shown to improve survival in patients with ventricular dysrhythmias; class I antidysrhythmic drugs (e.g.,

tocainide) have increased the risk of death when used in patients with non-life-threatening dysrhythmias • Initiate therapy in facilities capable of providing continuous ECG monitoring and managing life-threatening dysrhythmias

MONITORING PARAMETERS

• Blood concentrations (therapeutic concentrations 4-10 μg/ml)

---

tolazamide
(tole-az'a-mide)
Rx: Tolinase
Chemical Class: Sulfonylurea (1st generation)
Therapeutic Class: Oral hypoglycemic

CLINICAL PHARMACOLOGY
Mechanism of Action: Decreases blood sugar via stimulation of insulin secretion and increased tissue responsiveness to insulin; initial hypoglycemic effects due to stimulation of pancreatic islets (dependent upon functioning β-cells); extrapancreatic effect predominantly due to inhibition of hepatic glucose production, but may also facilitate improved insulin-insulin receptor binding

Pharmacokinetics
PO: Onset 4-6 hr, peak 4-8 hr, duration 12-24 hr, completely absorbed by GI route; metabolized in liver, excreted in urine (active metabolites); highly protein bound; $t_{1/2}$ 7 hr

INDICATIONS AND USES: Type II (non-insulin-dependent) diabetes mellitus; adjunct to insulin in selected patients*

DOSAGE
Adult
• PO 100 mg/day for fasting blood sugar <200 mg/dl or 250 mg/day for fasting blood sugar >200 mg/dl; dose should be titrated to patient response; divide doses >500 mg/day bid; max dose 1 g/day

💲 AVAILABLE FORMS/COST OF THERAPY
• Tab, Uncoated—Oral: 100 mg, 100's: **$12.50-$40.21;** 250 mg, 100's: **$13.65-$84.88;** 500 mg, 100's: **$18.42-$162.83**

CONTRAINDICATIONS: Juvenile or brittle diabetes

PRECAUTIONS: Elderly, cardiac disease, thyroid disease, severe hypoglycemic reactions, renal disease, hepatic disease

PREGNANCY AND LACTATION: Pregnancy category C; inappropriate for use during pregnancy due to inadequacy for blood glucose control, potential for prolonged neonatal hypoglycemia, and risk for congenital abnormalities; insulin is the drug of choice for control of blood sugars during pregnancy; breast milk excretion data is not available—again, the potential for neonatal hypoglycemia dictates caution in nursing mothers

SIDE EFFECTS/ADVERSE REACTIONS
CNS: Dizziness, fatigue, headache, lethargy, weakness
EENT: Tinnitus, vertigo
GI: Constipation, diarrhea, gas, heartburn, ***hepatotoxicity,*** jaundice, *nausea, vomiting*
HEME: ***Agranulocytosis, aplastic anemia, hemolytic anemia, leukopenia, pancytopenia, thrombocytopenia***
METAB: Hypoglycemia
SKIN: Allergic reactions, eczema, erythema, photosensitivity, pruritus, rash, urticaria

INTERACTIONS
Drugs
3 *Anabolic steroids, chloramphenicol, clofibrate, cyclic antidepressants, MAOIs, sulfonamides:* Enhanced hypoglycemic effects

---

italic = common side effects   ***bold italic*** = life-threatening reactions

T

β-blockers: Alter response to hypoglycemia, increase blood glucose concentrations

Clonidine: Diminished symptoms of hypoglycemia

Ethanol: Altered glycemic control, usually hypoglycemia

Oral anticoagulants: Dicoumarol, not warfarin, enhances hypoglycemic response

Oral contraceptives: Impaired glucose tolerance

Rifampin: Reduced serum levels, reduced hypoglycemic activity

SPECIAL CONSIDERATIONS
• Similar clinical effect as 2nd generations (e.g., glyburide, glipizide); usually less expensive

PATIENT/FAMILY EDUCATION
• Home blood glucose monitoring
• Multiple drug interactions, including alcohol and salicylates
• Symptoms of hypoglycemia: tingling lips/tongue, nausea, confusion, fatigue, sweating, hunger, visual changes (spots)

MONITORING PARAMETERS
• Self-monitored blood glucoses; glycosolated hemoglobin q 3-6 mo

---

tolazoline
(toe-laz′a-leen)
Rx: Priscoline
Chemical Class: Imidoline derivative
Therapeutic Class: Direct peripheral vasodilator

CLINICAL PHARMACOLOGY
Mechanism of Action: Peripheral vasodilation occurs by direct relaxation of vascular smooth muscle; moderate α-adrenergic blocking properties; decreases peripheral resistance and increases venous capacity; other actions: sympathomimetic (cardiac stimulation), parasympathomimetic (GI tract stimu-

lation), histamine-like (gastric secretion and peripheral vasodilation)

Pharmacokinetics
IM/SC: Peak 30-60 min, duration 3-4 hr; excreted in urine; $t_{1/2}$ 3-10 hr

INDICATIONS AND USES: Persistent pulmonary hypertension of newborn; hypoxic pulmonary hypertension,* arterial trauma,* clonidine overdose,* cor pulmonale,* lumbar puncture headache,* peripheral vascular disease,* spasmodic torticollis*

DOSAGE
Newborn
• IV 1-2 mg/kg via scalp vein followed by IV INF 1-2 mg/kg/hr

AVAILABLE FORMS/COST OF THERAPY
• Inj, Repository—IV: 25 mg/ml, 4 ml: **$15.01**

PRECAUTIONS: Active peptic ulcer, mitral stenosis

PREGNANCY AND LACTATION: Pregnancy category C

SIDE EFFECTS/ADVERSE REACTIONS
CV: **Cardiovascular collapse, dysrhythmias,** edema, hypertension, *orthostatic hypotension,* tachycardia
GI: Diarrhea, **GI hemorrhage,** hepatitis, nausea, peptic ulcer, vomiting
GU: Hematuria, oliguria
HEME: **Leukopenia, thrombocytopenia**
RESP: **Pulmonary hemorrhage**
SKIN: Chills, *flushing,* increased pilomotor activity, rash, sweating, tingling

INTERACTIONS
Drugs
Epinephrine, norepinephrine, phenylephrine: Decrease blood pressure response; rebound hypertension

SPECIAL CONSIDERATIONS
MONITORING PARAMETERS
• Vital signs, oxygenation, acid-base status, fluid, and electrolytes

tolbutamide

(tole-byoo'ta-mide)
Rx: Orinase
Chemical Class: Sulfonylurea (1st generation)
Therapeutic Class: Oral hypoglycemic

CLINICAL PHARMACOLOGY

Mechanism of Action: Decreases blood sugar via stimulation of insulin secretion and increased tissue responsiveness to insulin; initial hypoglycemic effects due to stimulation of pancreatic islets (dependent upon functioning β-cells); extrapancreatic effect predominantly due to inhibition of hepatic glucose production, but may also facilitate improved insulin-insulin receptor binding

Pharmacokinetics
PO: Onset 30-60 min, peak 3-5 hr, duration 6-12 hr, completely absorbed by GI route, metabolized in liver, excreted in urine (active metabolites); 90%-95% plasma protein bound; $t_{1/2}$ 4-5 hr

INDICATIONS AND USES: PO diabetes mellitus type 2; IV diagnostic test (Fajan's test) for pancreatic islet cell adenoma

DOSAGE

Adult
• PO 1-2 g/day in divided doses, titrated to patient response, max 3 g/day
• *Diagnostic test:* IV 1 g at constant rate over 2-3 min

💲 **AVAILABLE FORMS/COST OF THERAPY**
• Tab, Uncoated—Oral: 500 mg, 100's: **$3.65-$37.56**
• Inj, Lyphl-Sol—IV: 1 g/vial, 20 ml: **$57.35**

CONTRAINDICATIONS: Diabetes mellitus, type 1; ketoacidosis

PRECAUTIONS: Elderly, cardiac disease, thyroid disease, severe hypoglycemic reactions, renal disease, hepatic disease

PREGNANCY AND LACTATION: Pregnancy category C; inappropriate for use during pregnancy due to inadequacy for blood glucose control, potential for prolonged neonatal hypoglycemia, and risk of congenital abnormalities; insulin is the drug of choice for control of blood sugars during pregnancy; milk-to-plasma ratio of 0.25 reported; the potential for neonatal hypoglycemia dictates caution in nursing mothers

SIDE EFFECTS/ADVERSE REACTIONS

CNS: Dizziness, *headache,* paresthesia, *weakness*
EENT: Tinnitus, vertigo
GI: Cholestatic jaundice, diarrhea, *fullness, heartburn,* **hepatotoxicity,** increased AST, ALT, alk phosphatase, *nausea,* taste alteration
HEME: **Agranulocytosis, aplastic anemia, leukopenia, thrombocytopenia**
METAB: **Hypoglycemia**
MS: Joint pains
SKIN: Allergic reactions, eczema, erythema, photosensitivity, pruritus, rash, urticaria

INTERACTIONS

Drugs
🔳 *Anabolic steroids, aspirin, chloramphenicol, MAOIs, sulfonamides:* Enhanced hypoglycemic effects
🔳 *β-blockers:* Alter response to hypoglycemia
⚠ *Ethanol:* Altered glycemic control, usually hypoglycemia; "Antabuse"-like reaction
🔳 *Fluconazole, halofenate, itraconazole, ketoconazole, miconazole:* Increased serum concentrations of tolbutamide and other sulfonylureas
🔳 *Oral anticoagulants:* Dicouma-

T

rol, not warfarin, enhances hypoglycemic response to tolbutamide

❷ *Phenylbutazone:* Increased hypoglycemic action

❸ *Rifabutin, rifampin:* Reduced serum levels, reduced hypoglycemic activity

Labs
• *False increase:* Serum AST, CSF protein
• *Interference:* Urinary albumin

SPECIAL CONSIDERATIONS
• Possible differences exist for tolbutamide (short duration of action, hepatic clearance), potential preferred choice in older patients with poor general physical status and renal impairment

PATIENT/FAMILY EDUCATION
• Multiple drug interactions, including alcohol and salicylates
• Symptoms of hypoglycemia: tingling lips/tongue, nausea, confusion, fatigue, sweating, hunger, visual changes (spots)

MONITORING PARAMETERS
• Self-monitored blood glucoses; glycosolated hemoglobin q 3-6 mo

---

tolcapone
(toll´ka-pone)
Rx: Tasmar
Chemical Class: Catechol-O-methyl-tranferase (COMT) inhibitor
Therapeutic Class: Anti-Parkinson's agent

CLINICAL PHARMACOLOGY
Mechanism of Action: Alters the plasma pharmacokinetics of levodopa; when given in combination with levodopa/carbidopa, plasma levels of levodopa are more sustained and result in more constant dopaminergic stimulation in the brain, leading to greater effects on the signs and symptoms of Parkinson's disease; may allow decrease in levodopa dose requirements

Pharmacokinetics
PO: Peak 2 hr; bioavailability 65% (decreased by food); >99.9% bound to plasma proteins (mainly albumin); almost completely metabolized prior to excretion; 60% excreted in urine, 40% in feces; $t_{1/2}$ 2-3 hr

INDICATIONS AND USES: As an adjunct to levodopa/carbidopa for the treatment of signs and symptoms of idiopathic Parkinson's disease

DOSAGE
Adult
• PO 100 mg tid, with or without food always as an adjunct to levodopa/carbidopa therapy (immediate or sustained release); in clinical trials the first dose of tolcapone was administered with the first levodopa/carbidopa dose of the day, and subsequent doses were given 6-12 hr later; doses of 200 mg should be used only if anticipated clinical benefit is justified (elevations in ALT may occur more frequently with 200 mg doses)
• Reduction of daily levodopa dose may be necessary, especially if levodopa dose >600 mg/day or in patients with severe dyskinesia before beginning treatment

💲 AVAILABLE FORMS/COST OF THERAPY
• Tab, Film Coated—Oral: 100 mg, 90's: **$166.86;** 200 mg, 90's: **$179.10**

CONTRAINDICATIONS: Clinical evidence of liver disease or ALT or AST values greater than twice upper limit of normal; retreatment in patients who develop evidence of hepatocellular injury during tolcapone therapy; history of nontraumatic rhabdomyolysis or hyperpy-

---

* = non-FDA-approved use

rexia and confusion possibly related to medication

PRECAUTIONS: Severe dystonia or dyskinesia; renal function impairment

PREGNANCY AND LACTATION: Pregnancy category C; use caution in nursing mothers

SIDE EFFECTS/ADVERSE REACTIONS

CNS: Dyskinesia, sleep disorder, dystonia, excessive dreaming, somnolence, confusion, dizziness, headache, hallucination

CV: Orthostatic complaints, chest pain, hypotension, chest discomfort

EENT: Sinus congestion

GI: **Hepatotoxicity,** *diarrhea, nausea,* anorexia, vomiting, constipation, dry mouth, abdominal pain, dyspepsia, flatulence

GU: Urine discoloration, micturition disorder

MS: Muscle cramps, stiffness, arthritis, neck pain

RESP: Dyspnea

SKIN: Increased sweating

MISC: Fatigue

INTERACTIONS

Drugs

❷ *Nonselective MAO inhibitors (phenelzine, tranycypromine):* Inhibition of the majority of the pathways responsible for normal catecholamine metabolism

❸ *Warfarin:* Possible increased hypoprothrombinemic effect of warfarin

SPECIAL CONSIDERATIONS

• Because of the risk of liver failure, use only in patients who are experiencing symptom fluctuations and are not responding to, or are not candidates for, other adjunctive therapies

• Withdraw drug from patients who fail to show substantial clinical benefit within 3 wk of initiation

• Consider having patients sign informed consent alerting them to potential risks and benefits of this drug

PATIENT/FAMILY EDUCATION

• Monitor for signs of liver disease (clay-colored stools, jaundice, dark urine, right upper quadrant tenderness, pruritus, fatigue, appetite loss, lethargy)

MONITORING PARAMETERS

• ALT/AST at baseline then q2 wk for first yr of therapy, q4 wk for next 6 mo, then q8 wk thereafter; repeat this cycle if dose increased to 200 mg tid; **discontinue tolcapone if ALT or AST exceeds upper limit of normal or if clinical signs and symptoms suggest onset of hepatic failure**

---

tolmetin

(tole′met-in)

Rx: Tolectin

Chemical Class: Acetic acid derivative

Therapeutic Class: NSAID with analgesic and antipyretic activity

---

CLINICAL PHARMACOLOGY

Mechanism of Action: Reversible cyclooxygenase (i.e., prostaglandin synthetase) inhibitor; nonselectively decreases the formation of both prostaglandins and thromboxane A2; variable effects on lipoxygenase synthesis and subsequent leukotriene production; antiinflammatory, antipyretic, and analgesic activity; inhibits platelet aggregation

Pharmacokinetics

PO: Peak 2 hr; metabolized in liver, excreted in urine (metabolites); 99% protein binding; $t_{1/2}$ 3-3½ hr

INDICATIONS AND USES: Osteoarthritis, rheumatoid arthritis, ankylosing spondylitis,* prevention of cognitive decline,* prevention of co-

---

italic = common side effects   ***bold italic*** = life-threatening reactions

lon cancer,* dysmenorrhea,* acute gout,* pain*

DOSAGE

Adult

• PO 400 mg tid-qid, not to exceed 2 g/day

Child >2 yr

• PO 15-30 mg/kg/day in 3 or 4 divided doses

💲 AVAILABLE FORMS/COST OF THERAPY

• Cap, Gel—Oral: 400 mg, 100's: **$78.45-$124.94**

• Tab—Oral: 200 mg, 100's: **$49.75-$60.74;** 600 mg, 100's: **$95.03-$151.62**

CONTRAINDICATIONS: Bronchospasm, nasal polyps, angioedema precipitated by aspirin or other NSAIDs

PRECAUTIONS: History of GI ulceration, bleeding, or perforation; renal dysfunction, hypertension or cardiac conditions aggravated by fluid retention and edema, history of liver dysfunction, history of coagulopathy

PREGNANCY AND LACTATION: Pregnancy category B (category D near term); small amounts excreted into breast milk, compatible with breast feeding

SIDE EFFECTS/ADVERSE REACTIONS

CNS: Anxiety, confusion, depression, dizziness, drowsiness, fatigue, insomnia, tremors

CV: **Dysrhythmias,** hypertension, palpitations, peripheral edema, tachycardia

EENT: Blurred vision, hearing loss, tinnitus

GI: Anorexia, **bleeding,** cholestatic hepatitis, constipation, cramps, diarrhea, dry mouth, flatulence, jaundice, nausea, peptic ulcer, perforation, ulceration, vomiting

GU: Azotemia, dysuria, hematuria, **nephrotoxicity,** oliguria, pseudoproteinuria

HEME: **Blood dyscrasias**

SKIN: Pruritus, purpura, rash, sweating

INTERACTIONS

Drugs

❸ *Aminoglycosides:* Reduced clearance with elevated aminoglycoside levels and potential for toxicity (especially indomethacin in premature infants; other NSAIDs probably)

❸ *Anticoagulants:* Excessive hypoprothrombinemia, decreased platelet aggregation with increased risk of GI bleeding

❸ *Antihypertensives (α-blockers, angiotensin-converting enzyme inhibitors, angiotensin II receptor blockers, β-blockers, diuretics):* Inhibition of antihypertensive and other favorable hemodynamic effects

❸ *Corticosteroids:* Increased risk of GI ulceration

❸ *Cyclosporine:* Increased nephrotoxicity risk

❸ *Lithium:* Decreased clearance of lithium (mediated via prostaglandins) resulting in elevated serum lithium levels and risk of toxicity

❸ *Methotrexate:* Decreased renal secretion of methotrexate resulting in elevated methotrexate levels and risk of toxicity

❸ *Phenylpropanolamine:* Possible acute hypertensive reaction

❸ *Potassium-sparing diuretics:* Additive hyperkalemia potential

❸ *Triamterene:* Acute renal failure reported with addition of indomethacin; caution with other NSAIDs

Labs

• *False positive:* Proteinuria (use dye-impregnated reagent strips), urinary drugs of abuse screen

SPECIAL CONSIDERATIONS
PATIENT/FAMILY EDUCATION
MONITORING PARAMETERS
• Initial hemogram and fecal occult blood test within 3 mo of starting regular chronic therapy; repeat every 6-12 mo (more frequently in high-risk patients [>65 years, peptic ulcer disease, concurrent steroids or anticoagulants]); electrolytes, creatinine, and BUN within 3 mo of starting regular chronic therapy; repeat every 6-12 mo

---

tolnaftate
(tole-naf'tate)
OTC: Aftate, NP-27, Tinactin, Ting
Chemical Class: Carbamothioic acid derivative
Therapeutic Class: Antifungal

CLINICAL PHARMACOLOGY
Mechanism of Action: Fungicidal
INDICATIONS AND USES: Topical fungal infections (tinea pedis, tinea manuum, tinea cruris, tinea corporis, tinea capitis, tinea versicolor) due to susceptible strains of the following dermatophytes: *Trichophyton rubrum, T. mentagrophytes, T. tonsurans, Microsporum canis, M. audouini Epidermophyton floccosum, Melassezia furfur*
DOSAGE
Adult and Child
• TOP apply to affected area bid for 2-6 wk

$ AVAILABLE FORMS/COST OF THERAPY
• Powder: 1%, 45, 90 g: **$1.92-$3.60**/45 g
• Powder, Aer—Top: 1%, 100, 150 g: **$4.88**/100 g
• Cre—Top: 1%, 15, 30 g: **$1.99-$5.28**/15 g
• Sol—Top: 10 ml: **$4.88**

• Spray—Top: 1%, 105, 120 ml: **$1.99-$4.88**/105 ml
PREGNANCY AND LACTATION:
Pregnancy category C
SIDE EFFECTS/ADVERSE REACTIONS
SKIN: Rash, stinging, urticaria
SPECIAL CONSIDERATIONS
• Non-prescription topical antifungal agent not effective in the treatment of deeper fungal infections of the skin, nor is it reliable in the treatment of fungal infections involving the scalp or nail beds; *Candida* is resistant; useful for patients desiring self-medication of mild tinea infections; patients must be advised of limitations
• Powders generally used as adjunctive therapy, but may be acceptable as primary therapy in very mild cases

---

tolteridine
(toll-ter'eh-deen)
Rx: Detrol
Chemical Class: Substituted amine
Therapeutic Class: Genitourinary muscle relaxant

CLINICAL PHARMACOLOGY
Mechanism of Action: Blocks urinary bladder muscle contraction by competitive muscarinic receptor antagonism
Pharmacokinetics
PO: Well absorbed, peak 1-2 hr; bioavailability increased by 53% with food; 96% protein bound; 98% metabolized by liver (CYP2D6 and CYP3A4 to active metabolite 5-hydroxymethyl tolteridine); 77% excreted in urine, 17% in stool; $t_{1/2}$ 2-4 hr
INDICATIONS AND USES: Overactive bladder with symptoms of urinary frequency, urgency, or urge incontinence

T

---

italic = common side effects   ***bold italic*** = life-threatening reactions

DOSAGE

Adult

• PO 2 mg bid; 1 mg bid for patients with liver disease or taking CYP3A4 inhibitors (see below)

💲 **AVAILABLE FORMS/COST OF THERAPY**

• Tab—Oral: 1 mg, 60's: **$72.00**
• Tab—Oral: 2 mg, 60's: **$73.88**

CONTRAINDICATIONS: Urinary retention, gastric retention, uncontrolled narrow-angle glaucoma

PRECAUTIONS: Bladder outflow obstruction, controlled narrow-angle glaucoma, liver disease, renal disease

PREGNANCY AND LACTATION: Pregnancy category C; probably excreted in breast milk. Not recommended during lactation

SIDE EFFECTS/ADVERSE REACTIONS

CNS: Anxiety, *headache (11%),* paresthesia, somnolence, *vertigo*

CV: Hypertension

EENT: Blurred vision, dry eyes, *dry mouth (40%)*

GI: Abdominal pain, constipation, dyspepsia

RESP: Bronchitis, cough

SKIN: Dry skin

INTERACTIONS

Drugs

3 *Clarithromycin:* Increased blood tolteridine concentration

3 *Erythromycin:* Increased blood tolteridine concentration

3 *Itraconazole:* Increased blood tolteridine concentration

3 *Ketoconazole:* Increased blood tolteridine concentration

SPECIAL CONSIDERATIONS
PATIENT/FAMILY EDUCATION

• Dry mouth occurs in 40% of treated patients at a dose of 2 mg bid; incidence is dose-dependent

---

topiramate

(toe-peer´a-mate)
Rx: Topamax
Chemical Class: Sulfamate-substituted monosaccharide derivative
Therapeutic Class: Anticonvulsant

CLINICAL PHARMACOLOGY

Mechanism of Action: Blocks voltage-dependent sodium and calcium channels and spread of seizure activity; does not affect reuptake or binding of neurotransmitters; weak carbonic anhydrase inhibitor

Pharmacokinetics

PO: Well absorbed; 75% bioavailable; peak 2-4 hr; excreted unchanged in urine; $t_{1/2}$ 20 hr

INDICATIONS AND USES: Adjunctive therapy for partial onset seizure treatment in adults

DOSAGE

Adult

• PO initiate at 50 mg/day and titrate upward, usual dose 200 mg bid, range 100-400 mg bid; maximum 1600 mg/day

💲 **AVAILABLE FORMS/COST OF THERAPY**

• Tab—Oral: 15 mg, 60's: **$68.74** 25 mg, 60's: **$72.67-$83.08;** 100 mg, 60's: **$170.38;** 200 mg, 60's: **$199.46**

PREGNANCY AND LACTATION: Pregnancy category C

SIDE EFFECTS/ADVERSE REACTIONS

CNS: Ataxia, cognitive dysfunction (83% in 1 study), *dizziness, nystagmus, paresthesia, sedation, visual disturbances*

GI: Constipation, decreased appetite, diarrhea, *dyspepsia, nausea, weight loss*

GU: Breast pain, dysmenorrhea, kidney stones

HEME: Leukopenia

INTERACTIONS

Drugs

3 *Phenytoin, carbamazepine, valproic acid:* Lowers topiramate concentrations

3 *Ethinyl estradiol:* Increased clearance of estrogen

SPECIAL CONSIDERATIONS
PATIENT/FAMILY EDUCATION

• Drink plenty of fluids to prevent kidney stone formation

---

torsemide

(tor′se-mide)

Rx: Demadex

Chemical Class: Pyridine-sulfonamide derivative

Therapeutic Class: Loop diuretic

CLINICAL PHARMACOLOGY

Mechanism of Action: Inhibits the $Na^+/K^+/Cl^-$ carrier system in the thick ascending portion of the loop of Henle where it increases urinary excretion of Na, Cl, and water, but does not significantly alter glomerular filtration rate, renal plasma flow, or acid-base balance

Pharmacokinetics

IV: Onset 10 min, peak 1 hr

PO: Onset 1 hr, peak 1-2 hr

Bioavailability 80%; minimal 1st-pass metabolism; volume of distribution 12-15 L (doubled in CHF, renal failure); cleared via hepatic metabolism (80%) and renal excretion (20%); $t_{1/2}$ 3½ hr

INDICATIONS AND USES: Edema (CHF, hepatic cirrhosis and chronic renal failure); hypertension

DOSAGE

Adult

NOTE: Because of high bioavailability, IV and PO doses are interchangeable

• *CHF, chronic renal failure:* PO/IV 10-20 mg qd, titrate upward to response (usually doubling) to max 200 mg/day

• *Cirrhosis:* PO/IV 5-10 mg qd (usually with aldosterone antagonist or potassium-sparing diuretic), titrate upward to response (usually by doubling) to max 40 mg/day

• *Hypertension:* 5-10 mg qd

$ AVAILABLE FORMS/COST OF THERAPY

• Inj, Sol—IV: 10 mg/ml, 2 ml: **$3.99**

• Tab, Uncoated—Oral: 5 mg, 100's: **$49.22;** 10 mg, 100's: **$54.55;** 20 mg, 100's: **$63.72;** 100 mg, 100's: **$236.18**

CONTRAINDICATIONS: Anuria, hepatic coma

PRECAUTIONS: Fluid and electrolyte imbalance (including sodium, chloride, potassium, magnesium, calcium), renal disease, hepatic disease (may precipitate hepatic encephalopathy), gout, COPD, lupus erythematosus, diabetes mellitus, hyperparathyroidism, vomiting, diarrhea, elevated cholesterol/triglycerides

PREGNANCY AND LACTATION: Pregnancy category B; cardiovascular disorders such as pulmonary edema, severe hypertension, or CHF are probably the only valid indications for loop diuretics during pregnancy

SIDE EFFECTS/ADVERSE REACTIONS

CNS: Asthenia, dizziness, *headache (7%),* insomnia, nervousness

CV: Atrial fibrillation, chest pain, ***ventricular tachycardia***

GI: Constipation, diarrhea, dyspepsia, edema

METAB: Hypocalcemia, hypokalemia, hypomagnesemia, increases in

---

italic = common side effects   ***bold italic*** = life-threatening reactions

T

BUN, creatinine, uric acid, glucose, total cholesterol
MS: Arthralgia, myalgia
RESP: Cough, rhinitis
SKIN: Rash
INTERACTIONS
Drugs
❷ *Aminoglycosides (gentamicin, kanamycin, neomycin, streptomycin):* Additive ototoxicity (ethacrynic acid > furosemide, torsemide, bumetanide)
❸ *Angiotensin converting enzyme inhibitors:* Initiation of ACEI with intensive diuretic therapy may result in precipitous fall in blood pressure; ACEIs may induce renal insufficiency in the presence of diuretic-induced sodium depletion
❸ *Barbiturates (phenobarbital):* Reduced diuretic response
❸ *Bile acid-binding resins (cholestyramine, colestipol):* Resins markedly reduce the bioavailability and diuretic response of furosemide
❸ *Carbenoxolone:* Severe hypokalemia from coadministration
❸ *Cephalosporins (cephaloridine, cephalothin):* Enhanced nephrotoxicity with coadministration
❷ *Cisplatin:* Additive ototoxicity (ethacrynic acid > furosemide, torsemide, bumetanide)
❸ *Clofibrate:* Enhanced effects of both drugs, especially in hypoalbuminemic patients
❸ *Corticosteroids:* Concomitant loop diuretic and corticosteroid therapy can result in excessive potassium loss
❸ *Digitalis glycosides (digoxin, digitoxin):* Diuretic-induced hypokalemia may increase risk of digitalis toxicity
❸ *Nonsteroidal antiinflammatory drugs (flurbiprofen, ibuprofen, indomethacin, naproxen, piroxicam, aspirin, sulindac):* Reduced diuretic and antihypertensive effects

❸ *Phenytoin:* Reduced diuretic response
❸ *Serotonin-reuptake inhibitors (fluoxetine, paroxetine, sertraline):* Case reports of sudden death; enhanced hyponatremia proposed; causal relationships not established
❸ *Terbutaline:* Additive hypokalemia
❸ *Tubocurarine:* Prolonged neuromuscular blockade
SPECIAL CONSIDERATIONS
• Offers potential advantages over other loop diuretics, including a longer duration of action and fewer adverse electrolyte and metabolic effects; available data not extensive or convincing enough at present to recommend replacement of standard loop diuretic (furosemide); considered alternative in refractory patients
MONITORING PARAMETERS
• Urine volume, creatinine clearance, BUN, electrolytes, reduction in edema, increased diuresis, decrease in body weight, reduction in blood pressure, glucose, uric acid, serum calcium (tetany), tinnitus, vertigo, hearing loss (especially in those at risk for ototoxicity—IV doses >120 mg; concomitant ototoxic drugs; renal disease)

---

tramadol
(traah′ma-doll)
Rx: Ultram
Chemical Class: Substituted-cyclohexanol derivative
Therapeutic Class: Centrally acting synthetic analgesic

CLINICAL PHARMACOLOGY
Mechanism of Action: Complementary binding to μ-opiate receptors and inhibition of reuptake of norepinephrine and serotonin

Pharmacokinetics

PO: Onset of analgesia/plasma concentrations 1 hr, peak plasma concentrations 2-3 hr, rapid/complete absorption; volume of distribution 2.6-2.9 L/kg; 20% protein binding; extensively metabolized, mostly inactive metabolites, 60% excreted in urine; $t_{1/2}$ 6-7 hr

INDICATIONS AND USES: Moderate to moderately severe pain management

DOSAGE

Adult

• PO 50-100 mg q4-6h, not to exceed 400 mg/day; not necessary to reduce dose for elderly (<300 mg/day suggested)

• *Renal impairment:* CrCl <30 ml/min, extend dosing interval q12h

• *Hepatic impairment:* (cirrhosis) 50 mg q12h

$ AVAILABLE FORMS/COST OF THERAPY

• Tab, Uncoated—Oral: 50 mg, 100's: **$74.50**

CONTRAINDICATIONS: Acute intoxication with alcohol, hypnotics, centrally acting analgesics, opioids or psychotropic drugs

PRECAUTIONS: Respiratory depression, increased intracranial pressure or head trauma, acute abdominal conditions, drug abuse and dependence, seizure disorder

PREGNANCY AND LACTATION: Pregnancy category C; small amounts excreted into breast milk

SIDE EFFECTS/ADVERSE REACTIONS

CNS: Anxiety, asthenia, CNS stimulation, confusion, coordination disturbance, dizziness, euphoria, headache, nervousness, *seizures,* sleep disorder, somnolence, vertigo

CV: Vasodilation

EENT: Visual disturbance

GI: Abdominal pain, anorexia, constipation, diarrhea, dry mouth, dyspepsia, flatulence, nausea, vomiting

GU: Menopausal symptoms, urinary retention and frequency

SKIN: Pruritus, rash

INTERACTIONS

Drugs

3 *Carbamazepine:* CNS depression; increased tramadol metabolism, may require significantly increased tramadol dosing for equianalgesic effects

3 *Ethanol, opioids, anesthetic agents, phenothiazines, tranquilizers, sedative-hypnotics:* CNS depression

3 *MAOIs:* Potential exaggerated norepinephrine and serotonin effects, as tramadol inhibits reuptake

3 *SSRIs:* Increased risk of seizures

SPECIAL CONSIDERATIONS

• Expensive, nonnarcotic, "narcotic"-tricyclic antidepressant combination analgesic; potential use in chronic pain; demonstrated efficacy in a variety of pain syndromes; minimal cardiovascular and respiratory side effects

• Does not completely bind to opioid receptors; caution in addicted patients

• Has more potential for abuse than previously thought

• Tolerance and withdrawal symptoms milder than with opiates

• Not chemically related to opiates

T

---

italic = common side effects   ***bold italic*** = life-threatening reactions

trandolapril

(tran-doe'la-pril)
Rx: Mavik
Combinations
   Rx: with verapamil (Tarka)
Chemical Class: Nonsulfhy-
dryl angiotensin-converting
enzyme (ACE) inhibitor
Therapeutic Class: Antihyper-
tensive

CLINICAL PHARMACOLOGY

Mechanism of Action: Antihypertensive, hypoproliferative, and cardioprotective effects attributable to
competitive inhibition of angiotensin-converting enzyme (ACE) yielding decreased plasma concentrations of angiotensin II, plasma aldosterone concentrations, systemic
vascular resistance, blood pressure,
preload, and afterload, not accompanied by changes in heart rate, pressor sensitivity to exogenous norepinephrine, or baroreceptor sensitivity

Pharmacokinetics

PO: Prodrug—peak 1 hr (4-10 hr
trandolaprilat), metabolized by liver
to active metabolite (trandolaprilat); 80% protein bound to plasma
proteins; eliminated in urine (30%)
and feces (66%); $t_{1/2}$ of trandolaprilat 10 hr

INDICATIONS AND USES: Hyper-
tension, CHF (left ventricular dysfunction),* MI (left ventricular salvage),* erythrocytosis,* nephropathy,* retinopathy*

DOSAGE

Adult and Child >16 yr

• *Hypertension:* PO initial dose: 0.5
mg qd (for renal or hepatic impairment or patients receiving diuretics), 1 mg qd (non-African American), 2 mg (African American pa-

tient); maintenance dose: titrate to 4
mg qd - 4 mg bid at 2 wk intervals
• *Dosage in renal failure:* CrCl
30-60 ml/min, initial dose 0.5 mg
qd; maximal dose 2 mg qd; patients
with CrCl <30 ml/min not recommended (resultant serum concentrations double)

💲 AVAILABLE FORMS/COST OF THERAPY

• Tab—Oral: 1 mg, 2 mg, 4 mg,
100's: **$54.30**

PRECAUTIONS: History of anaphylaxis, renal insufficiency (<30
ml/min), hypotension (CHF, elderly,
volume depletion—diuretics, dialysis, cirrhosis), aortic stenosis, hyperkalemia (potassium supplements,
potassium-sparing diuretics, renal
disease, diabetes), neutropenia (autoimmune diseases, collagen vascular, febrile illness, immunosuppressant drug therapy), proteinuria,
renal artery stenosis, surgery/anes-
thesia (excessive hypotension, correctable with fluids)

PREGNANCY AND LACTATION:
Pregnancy category C (1st trimester), category D (2nd and 3rd trimesters); ACE inhibitors can cause
fetal and neonatal morbidity and
death when administered to pregnant women; when pregnancy is detected, discontinue ACE inhibitors
as soon as possible

SIDE EFFECTS/ADVERSE REACTIONS

CNS: Anxiety, *dizziness, fatigue,
headache,* insomnia, paresthesia
CV: Angina, hypotension, palpitations, postural hypotension, syncope (especially with 1st dose)
GI: Abdominal pain, constipation,
melena, nausea, vomiting
GU: Decreased libido, impotence,
increased BUN, creatinine; urinary
tract infection
HEME: **Agranulocytosis, neutropenia**

---

* = non-FDA-approved use

METAB: Hyperkalemia, hyponatremia

MS: Arthralgia, arthritis, myalgia

RESP: Asthma, bronchitis, *cough,* dyspnea, sinusitis

SKIN: Angioedema, flushing, rash, sweating

INTERACTIONS

Drugs

3 *Azathioprine:* Increased myelosuppression

3 *Lithium:* Increased risk of serious lithium toxicity

3 *Loop diuretics:* Initiation of ACE inhibitor therapy in the presence of intensive diuretic therapy results in a precipitous fall in blood pressure in some patients; ACE inhibitors may induce renal insufficiency in the presence of diuretic-induced sodium depletion

3 *NSAIDs:* Inhibition of the antihypertensive response to ACE inhibitors

3 *Potassium-sparing diuretics:* Increased risk for hyperkalemia

3 *Trimethoprim:* Additive risk of hyperkalemia, especially in patient predisposed to renal insufficiency

Labs

• ACE inhibition can account for approximately 0.5mEq/L rise in serum potassium

SPECIAL CONSIDERATIONS
PATIENT/FAMILY EDUCATION

• Caution with salt substitutes containing potassium chloride

• Rise slowly to sitting/standing position to minimize orthostatic hypotension

• Dizziness, fainting, lightheadedness may occur during 1st few days of therapy

• May cause altered taste perception or cough; persistent dry cough usually does not subside unless medication is stopped; notify clinician if these symptoms persist

MONITORING PARAMETERS

• BUN, creatinine, potassium within 2 wk after initiation of therapy (increased levels may indicate acute renal failure)

---

tranylcypromine
(tran-ill-sip'roe-meen)
Rx: Parnate
Chemical Class: Substituted cyclopropylamine; nonhydrazine derivative
Therapeutic Class: Monoamine oxidase inhibitor (MAOI) antidepressant

CLINICAL PHARMACOLOGY

Mechanism of Action: MAOI resulting in increased endogenous concentrations of serotonin, norepinephrine, epinephrine, and dopamine in the CNS; chronic administration results in down regulation (desensitization) of α_2- or β-adrenergic and serotonin receptors, which may correlate with antidepressant activity

Pharmacokinetics

PO: Onset 10 days, well absorbed; metabolized by liver, excreted by kidneys (within 24 hr); monoamine oxidase activity is recovered in 3-5 days (possibly up to 10 days) after withdrawal

INDICATIONS AND USES: Atypical depression; bulimia*; panic disorder with agoraphobia*

DOSAGE

Adult

• PO 10 mg bid; may increase to 30 mg/day after 2 wk; max 60 mg/day

§ AVAILABLE FORMS/COST OF THERAPY

• Tab, Plain Coated—Oral: 10 mg, 100's: **$55.10**

CONTRAINDICATIONS: Hypertension, CHF, severe hepatic disease, pheochromocytoma, severe re-

---

italic = common side effects   ***bold italic*** = life-threatening reactions

nal disease, severe cardiac disease, cerebrovascular defects

PRECAUTIONS: Suicidal patients, convulsive disorders, severe depression, schizophrenia, hyperactivity, diabetes mellitus

PREGNANCY AND LACTATION: Pregnancy category C

SIDE EFFECTS/ADVERSE REACTIONS

CNS: Anxiety, confusion, *dizziness, drowsiness,* fatigue, headache, hyperreflexia, insomnia, mania, stimulation, tremors, weakness, weight gain

CV: **Dysrhythmias,** hypertension, **hypertensive crisis,** orthostatic hypotension

EENT: Blurred vision

GI: Anorexia, constipation, diarrhea, dry mouth, nausea, vomiting, weight gain

GU: Change in libido, urinary frequency

HEME: Anemia

METAB: Syndrome of inappropriate antidiuretic hormone release-like syndrome

SKIN: Flushing, increased perspiration, rash

INTERACTIONS

Drugs

⚠ *Amphetamines, ephedrine, metaraminol, phenylephrine, phenylpropanolamine, pseudoephedrine, tyramine-containing foods:* Severe hypertensive reactions

3 *Antidiabetics:* Prolonged hypoglycemia

3 *Barbiturates:* Prolonged effect of barbiturates

⚠ *Clomipramine, fluoxetine, fluvoxamine, paroxetine, sertraline:* Severe or fatal reactions, serotonin related

⚠ *Ethanol:* Hypertensive response with alcoholic beverages containing tyramine

3 *Guanethidine:* Inhibited antihypertensive response to guanethidine

3 *Levodopa:* Hypertensive response; carbidopa minimizes the reaction

2 *Lithium:* Hyperpyrexia with phenelzine

⚠ *Meperidine:* Serotonin accumulation—agitation, blood pressure elevations, hyperpyrexia, *seizures*

3 *Norepinephrine:* Increased pressor response to norepinephrine

3 *Reserpine:* Severe hypertensive reactions

⚠ *Sumatriptan:* Increased sumatriptan concentrations, possible toxicity

SPECIAL CONSIDERATIONS

• Irreversible nonselective MAOI effective for typical and atypical depression; equal efficacy to other MAOIs with quicker onset of action, and an amphetamine-like activity with a higher potential for abuse; no anticholinergic or cardiac effects

PATIENT/FAMILY EDUCATION

• Therapeutic effects may take 1-4 wk

• Avoid alcohol ingestion, CNS depressants, OTC medications (cold, weight loss, hay fever, cough syrup)

• Prodromal signs of hypertensive crisis are increased headache, palpitations; discontinue drug immediately

• Do not discontinue medication abruptly after long-term use

• Avoid high-tyramine foods (aged cheese, sour cream, beer, wine, pickled products, liver, raisins, bananas, figs, avocados, meat tenderizers, chocolate, yogurt)

---

* = non-FDA-approved use

trazodone

(tray´zoe-done)
Rx: Desyrel
Chemical Class: Triazolopyri-
dine derivative
Therapeutic Class: Antide-
pressant

CLINICAL PHARMACOLOGY
Mechanism of Action: Selective inhibition (high) of presynaptic serotonin uptake, prolonging neuronal
activity; slight anticholinergic, moderate orthostatic, and very high sedation side effects; cardiac conduction effects less pronounced than
those seen with tricyclic antidepressants

Pharmacokinetics
PO: Peak 1-2 hr, onset of therapeutic effect 2-4 wk; 85%-95% bound
to plasma proteins; extensively metabolized in liver, excreted mainly
in urine with some fecal elimination; $t_{1/2}$ 4-7½ hr

INDICATIONS AND USES: Depression, aggressive behavior,* panic
disorder,* agoraphobia with panic
attacks,* insomnia*

DOSAGE
Adult
• PO 150 mg/day divided tid initially, increase by 50 mg/day q3-4d;
adjust dose to lowest effective level;
max 400 mg/day (outpatients), 600
mg/day (inpatients)
Child 6-18 yr
• PO 1.5-2 mg/kg/day in divided
doses initially, increase gradually
q3-4d as needed; max 6 mg/kg/day
divided tid

$ AVAILABLE FORMS/COST
OF THERAPY
• Tab, Plain Coated—Oral: 50 mg,
100's: **$24.07-$189.36;** 100 mg,
100's: **$41.00-$330.90;** 150 mg,
100's: **$70.35-$285.07;** 300 mg,
100's: **$426.52-$507.38**

PRECAUTIONS: Pre-existing cardiac disease, initial recovery phase
of MI, children <18 yr, suicidal ideation, electroconvulsive therapy

PREGNANCY AND LACTATION:
Pregnancy category C; excreted
into human breast milk; effects on
nursing infant unknown, but of possible concern

SIDE EFFECTS/ADVERSE REAC-
TIONS
CNS: Agitation, akathisia, anger, confusion, decreased concentration, delusions, disorientation, *dizziness,*
drowsiness, excitement, extrapyramidal symptoms, fatigue, hallucinations, headache, hostility, hypomania, impaired memory, impaired
speech, incoordination, insomnia,
lightheadedness, mania, nervousness, nightmares or vivid dreams,
numbness, paresthesia, psychosis,
seizures, stupor, tardive dyskinesia,
tremors, weakness
CV: Atrial fibrillation, bradycardia,
cardiac arrest, chest pain, conduction block, ***dysrhythmias,*** edema,
hypertension, hypotension, ***MI,*** orthostatic hypotension, palpitations,
syncope, tachycardia, vasodilation,
ventricular ectopic activity
EENT: Blurred vision, diplopia, nasal and sinus congestion, red eyes,
tinnitus, vertigo
GI: Abdominal or gastric disorder,
bad taste in mouth, constipation, *diarrhea,* dry mouth, flatulence, hyperbilirubinemia, hypersalivation,
inappropriate antidiuretic hormone
syndrome, intrahepatic cholestasis,
jaundice, liver enzyme alterations,
nausea, vomiting
GU: Breast enlargement and engorgement, decreased or increased
libido, delayed urine flow, early menses, hematuria, increased urinary frequency, impotence, lactation, missed

T

italic = common side effects   **bold italic** = life-threatening reactions

periods, priapism, retrograde ejaculation, urinary incontinence or retention

MS: Aches and pains, ataxia, muscle twitches

RESP: Apnea, shortness of breath

SKIN: Alopecia, clamminess, pruritis, rash, sweating, urticaria

MISC: Decreased appetite, malaise, weight gain or loss

INTERACTIONS

Drugs

3 *Clonidine:* Inhibited antihypertensive response to clonidine

3 *Ethanol:* Additive impairment of motor skills; abstinent alcoholics may eliminate cyclic antidepressants more rapidly than non-alcoholics

3 *Fluoxetine:* Increased plasma trazodone concentrations

⚠ *MAOIs:* Potential for fatal serotonin syndrome

3 *Neuroleptics:* Additive hypotension

SPECIAL CONSIDERATIONS

• Very sedating antidepressant with minimal anticholinergic effects; good choice for elderly patients in whom sedating properties would be desirable

PATIENT/FAMILY EDUCATION

• Take with food

• Use caution driving or performing other tasks requiring alertness

---

tretinoin

(tret'i-noyn)

Rx: Topical: Avita, Retin-A, Renova

Oral: Vesanoid (Tretinoin/ Retinoic Acid)

Chemical Class: Vitamin A derivative

Therapeutic Class: Antiacne agent

CLINICAL PHARMACOLOGY

Mechanism of Action: Decreases cohesiveness of follicular epithelial cells with decreased microcomedone formation; stimulates mitotic activity and increases turnover of follicular epithelial cells causing extrusion of comedones

INDICATIONS AND USES: Topical treatment of acne vulgaris; lamellar ichthyosis,* mollusca contagiosa,* verrucae plantaris,* verrucae planae juveniles,* ichthyosis vulgaris,* bullous congenital icthyosiform and pityriasis rubra pilaris,* improvement of photoaged skin (especially wrinkling and liver spots)*; PO induction of remission in patients with acute promyelocytic leukemia (APL)

DOSAGE

Adult and Child >12 yr

• TOP apply qd before retiring; begin therapy with 0.025% cream or 0.01% gel and increase concentration as tolerated; if stinging or irritation develops, decrease frequency of application

• PO 45 mg/m^2/day divided bid until complete remission documented; discontinue 30 days after achievement of complete remission or after 90 days of treatment, whichever comes first; follow with standard consolidation and/or maintenance chemotherapy

💲 AVAILABLE FORMS/COST OF THERAPY

• Cre—Top: 0.025%, 20, 45 g: **$26.10-$30.78**/20 g; 0.05%, 20, 45 g: **$27.18-$34.56**/20 g; 0.10%, 20, 45 g: **$31.56**/20 g

• Gel—Top: 0.01%, 15, 45 g: **$26.88**/15 g; 0.025%, 15, 45 g: **$27.12**/15 g; 0.1%, 20, 45 g: **$33.96**/20 g

• Liq—Top: 0.05%, 28 ml: **$45.40**

• Cap—Oral: 10 mg, 100's: **$1,141.80**

PRECAUTIONS: Eczematous skin, sunburned skin (do not use until skin is fully recovered)

---

* = non-FDA-approved use

PREGNANCY AND LACTATION:
Pregnancy category B; teratogenic risk when used topically is thought to be close to zero; minimal absorption occurring after topical application probably precludes detection of clinically significant amounts in breast milk

SIDE EFFECTS/ADVERSE REACTIONS

CNS: Dizziness, fever, headache
CV: **CHF, dysrhythmia,** *hypertension*
EENT: Visual disturbance
GI: Constipation, diarrhea, dyspepsia, mucositis, nausea, vomiting
MS: Bone pain
SKIN: Alopecia, blistering, crusting, edema, *erythema, excessive dryness, increased sweating, initial acne flare-up, irritation,* photosensitivity, *pruritis, rash,* temporary hyperpigmentation or hypopigmentation

INTERACTIONS

Drugs

3 *Sulfur, resorcinol, benzoyl peroxide, salicylic acid:* Concomitant topical acne products may cause significant skin irritation

SPECIAL CONSIDERATIONS
• Oral therapy should be prescribed only by those knowledgeable in the treatment of APL

PATIENT/FAMILY EDUCATION
• Keep away from eyes, mouth, angles of nose, and mucous membranes
• Avoid exposure to ultraviolet light
• Acne may worsen transiently
• Normal use of cosmetics is permissible

triamcinolone
(trye-am-sin'oh-lone)
Rx: *Oral:* Aristocort, Aristopak
Injectable: Acetocot, Amcort, Aristocort, Aristocort Forte, Aristospan, Cinonide-40, Clinalog, TAC-3, Kenalog, Kenaject-40, Triam-A, Triam Forte, Triamcot, Tristoject *Inhalation:* Azmacort
Nasal: Nasacort, Nasacort AQ *Topical:* Aristocort, Cinalog, Cinolar, Kenalog, Kenalog in Orabase, Triacet, Triamcot

Chemical Class: Synthetic glucocorticoid
Therapeutic Class: Inhaled corticosteroid; systemic corticosteroid; topical corticosteroid, low potency (0.025%), intermediate potency (0.1%), high potency (0.5%)

CLINICAL PHARMACOLOGY

Mechanism of Action: Controls the rate of protein synthesis, depresses the migration of polymorphonuclear leukocytes and fibroblasts, reverses capillary permeability, and causes lysosomal stabilization at the cellular level to prevent or control inflammation

Pharmacokinetics

TOP: Absorbed through the skin (increased by inflammation and occlusive dressings)
IM: Peak within 8-10 hr
Metabolized in liver, excreted in urine and bile; biologic $t_{1/2}$ 18-36 hr

INDICATIONS AND USES: *Nasal:* Seasonal or perennial rhinitis, nasal polyps
Inhaled: Prophylaxis of asthma
Systemic: Anti-inflammatory or immunosuppressant agent in the treat-

T

ment of diseases of hematologic, allergic, inflammatory, neoplastic, and autoimmune origin

Topical: Psoriasis, eczema, contact dermatitis, pruritus, oral inflammatory and ulcerative traumatic lesions (dental paste)

Intraarticular: Synovitis, osteoarthritis

Intradermal: Keloids, alopecia areata, inflammatory skin lesions

DOSAGE

Adult

• PO 4-60 mg/day

• IM (diacetate) 40 mg per wk; (acetonide) 2.5-60 mg/day

• Intraarticular/intrasynovial/intralesional/sublesional (acetonide) 2.5-5 mg (small joints), 5-15 mg (large joints), 1 mg/inj site using only 3 mg/ml or 10 mg/ml strength (intradermal); (diacetate) 5-40 mg, do not use more than 12.5 mg/inj site, usual dose is 25 mg/lesion (intralesional or sublesional); (hexacetonide) 2-20 mg (intra-articular); 10-20 mg (large joints); 2-6 mg (small joints); up to 0.5 mg/in² of affected area (intralesional or sublesional)

• TOP apply to affected area bid-tid

• INH 2 inhalations tid-qid up to 16 INH/day

• NASAL 2 sprays in each nostril qd-bid

Child

• IM (acetonide or hexacetonide) 0.03-0.2 mg/kg at 1-7 day intervals

• INH 1-2 inhalation tid-qid up to 12 INH/day

• NASAL (6-11 yr) 2 sprays in each nostril qd (Nasacort AQ)

• Intra-articular/intrasynovial/intralesional/sublesional (acetonide) 2.5-15 mg, repeated prn

• TOP apply bid-tid

🔒 AVAILABLE FORMS/COST OF THERAPY

• Tab, Uncoated—Oral: 4 mg, 100's: **$131.23**

• Cre (acetonide)—Top: 0.025%, 15, 30, 60, 80, 454 g: **$3.31-$17.00**/80 g; 0.1%, 15, 30, 60, 80, 240, 454, 480 g: **$4.79-$15.39**/80 g; 0.5%, 15, 20 g: **$4.13-$29.48**/15 g

• Inj, Susp (acetonide)—Intraarticular, IM: 40 mg/ml, 5 ml: **$8.49-$30.68**

• Inj, Susp (diacetate)—Intraarticular, IM: 40 mg/ml, 5 ml: **$7.25-$15.95**

• Inj, Sol (acetonide)—IV: 40 mg/ml, 5 ml: **$8.49-$20.99**

• Inj, Sol (diacetate)—IV: 25 mg/ml, 5 ml: **$20.30**

• Inj, Sol (hexacetonide)—IV: 5 mg/ml, 5 ml: **$11.94;** 20 mg/ml, 5 ml: **$10.22-$18.40**

• Inj, Susp (acetonide)—Intraarticular, intradermal: 10 mg/ml, 5 ml: **$7.50**

• Inj, Susp (acetonide)—intradermal: 3 mg/ml, 5 ml: **$8.95**

• Inj, Sol (diacetate)—IM, IV, SC: 40 mg/ml, 5 ml: **$3.70-$18.85**

• Lotion (acetonide)—Top: 0.025%, 60 ml: **$34.51-$39.72;** 0.1%, 60 ml: **$8.76-$44.59**

• Oint (acetonide)—Top: 0.025%, 15, 30, 80, 454 g: **$2.80-$4.26**/80 g; 0.05%: **$25.00**/430 g; 0.1%, 15, 30, 60, 80, 240, 454 g: **$4.79-$27.48**/60 g; 0.5%, 15 g: **$4.13**/15 g

• Paste (acetonide)—Dental: 0.1%, 5 g: **$6.37-$23.33**

• Aer (acetonide)—INH: 100 μg/inh, 100 sprays: **$47.65-$58.44**

• Aer (acetonide)—Nasal: 55 μg/inh, 10 g: **$40.67-$46.60;** 16.5 g (AQ): **$38.71**

• Aer, Spray (acetonide)—Top: 0.147 mg/g, 63 g: **$32.98**

• Syr (diacetate)—Oral: 2 mg/5 ml, 120 ml: **$20.21;** 4 mg/5 ml, 120 ml: **$33.25**

---

* = non-FDA-approved use

CONTRAINDICATIONS: Systemic fungal infections, bacterial infection of nose (nasal); primary treatment of status asthmaticus (inhalation)

PRECAUTIONS: Psychosis, diabetes mellitus, glaucoma, osteoporosis, seizure disorders, ulcerative colitis (intestinal perforation), CHF, hypertension, myesthenia gravis (if used with anticholinesterase agents), renal disease, esophagitis, peptic ulcer, latent tuberculosis or amebiasis (reactivation of disease). Topical: use on face, groin, or axilla, ocular herpes simplex

PREGNANCY AND LACTATION: Pregnancy category C; excreted in breast milk and could interfere with infant's growth and endogenous corticosteroid production

SIDE EFFECTS/ADVERSE REACTIONS

CNS: Depression, headache, *mood changes,* **seizures,** vertigo (systemic)

CV: CHF, hypertension, tachycardia

EENT: Blurred vision, *Candida* infection of oral cavity, cataract; dysphonia, hoarseness, increased intraocular pressure, *sore throat* (inhalation); dryness, epistaxis, nasal irritation and stinging, rebound congestion, sneezing (nasal)

GI: Abdominal distension, diarrhea, **GI hemorrhage,** increased appetite, *nausea,* **pancreatitis**

METAB: Cushingoid state, decreased glucose tolerance, growth suppression in children, HPA suppression

MS: Aseptic necrosis of femoral and humeral heads, fractures, muscle mass loss, osteoporosis, weakness

SKIN: Acne, allergic contact dermatitis, atrophy, bruising, burning, dryness, ecchymosis, folliculitis, hypertrichosis, hypopigmentation, irritation, itching, miliaria, perioral dermatitis, petechiae, poor wound healing, secondary infection (topi-

cal), striae; suppression of skin test reactions; thin, fragile skin

MISC: Systemic absorption of topical corticosteroids has produced reversible HPA axis suppression (more likely with occlusive dressings, prolonged administration, application to large surface areas, liver failure, and in children)

INTERACTIONS

Drugs

▨ *Aminoglutethamide:* Increased clearance of steroid; doubling of dose may be necessary

▨ *Antidiabetics:* Increased blood glucose

▨ *Barbiturates, carbamazepine:* Reduced serum concentrations of corticosteroids

▨ *Cholestyramine, colestipol:* Possible reduced absorption of corticosteroids

▨ *Cyclosporine:* Possible increased concentration of both drugs, seizures

▨ *Erythromycin, troleandomycin, clarithromycin, ketoconazole:* Possible enhanced steroid effect

▨ *Estrogens, oral contraceptives:* Enhanced effects of corticosteroids

▨ *Isoniazid:* Reduced plasma concentrations of isoniazid

▨ *IUDs:* Inhibition of inflammation may decrease contraceptive effect

▨ *NSAIDs:* Increased risk of GI ulceration

▨ *Rifampin:* Reduced therapeutic effect of corticosteroids

▨ *Salicylates:* Increased elimination of salicylates

Labs

• *False increase:* Urinary amino acids

SPECIAL CONSIDERATIONS
PATIENT/FAMILY EDUCATION

• May cause GI upset, take with meals or snacks (systemic)

• Do not give live virus vaccines to

---

italic = common side effects   ***bold italic*** = life-threatening reactions

patients on prolonged systemic therapy

• Take PO as single daily dose in AM

• Signs of adrenal insufficiency include fatigue, anorexia, nausea, vomiting, diarrhea, weight loss, weakness, dizziness, and low blood sugar

• Avoid abrupt withdrawal of therapy following high-dose or long-term therapy

• Increased dose of rapidly acting corticosteroids may be necessary in patients subjected to unusual stress

• To be used on a regular basis, not for acute symptoms (nasal and inhalation)

• Use bronchodilators before oral inhaler (for patients using both)

• Rinse mouth to prevent oral candidiasis

• Nasal sol may cause drying and irritation of nasal mucosa, clear nasal passages prior to use

MONITORING PARAMETERS
• Serum K and glucose
• Growth of children on prolonged therapy

---

triamterene

(try-am'ter-een)
Rx: Dyrenium
Combinations
  Rx: with hydrochlorothiazide (Dyazide, Maxzide)
Chemical Class: Pteridine derivative
Therapeutic Class: Potassium-sparing diuretic, antihypertensive

CLINICAL PHARMACOLOGY
Mechanism of Action: Inhibits reabsorption of sodium ions in exchange for potassium and hydrogen ions directly in the distal renal tubule (not aldosterone inhibitor);

weak diuretic and antihypertensive effects when used alone
Pharmacokinetics
PO: Onset 2-4 hr, peak 3 hr, duration 7-9 hr; primarily metabolized to sulfate conjugate of hydroxytriamterene (active), 21% excreted in urine unchanged; $t_{1/2}$ 1½-2 hr
INDICATIONS AND USES: Edema (CHF, cirrhosis of the liver, nephrotic syndrome, steroid-induced, idiopathic, and secondary hyperaldosteronism); may be used alone or with other diuretics either for its added diuretic effect or its potassium-conserving potential
DOSAGE
Adult
• PO 100 mg bid pc; do not exceed 300 mg/day; when combined with other diuretics or antihypertensives, decrease total daily dosage initially and adjust to patient's needs
Child
• PO 2-4 mg/kg/day in 1-2 divided doses; max 6 mg/kg/day or 300 mg/day
⑤ AVAILABLE FORMS/COST OF THERAPY
• Cap, Gel—Oral: 50 mg, 100's: **$46.55;** 100 mg, 100's: **$58.45**
CONTRAINDICATIONS: Anuria, severe renal disease, hyperkalemia, antikaliuretic therapy (including angiotensin-converting enzyme inhibitors, angiotensin II receptor blockers, and potassium supplements)
PRECAUTIONS: Diabetes, renal function impairment, hepatic function impairment, children, electrolyte imbalance, renal stones, predisposition to gouty arthritis
PREGNANCY AND LACTATION: Pregnancy category B; therapy for preexisting hypertension can be continued throughout pregnancy with minimal risk; initiating for simple edema not recommended; few un-

---

* = non-FDA-approved use

equivocal indications for diuretic therapy in pregnancy except for pulmonary edema or congestive heart failure; may decrease placental perfusion; excreted in cow's milk, no human data

SIDE EFFECTS/ADVERSE REACTIONS

CNS: Dizziness, headache

GI: Diarrhea, dry mouth, jaundice, liver enzyme abnormalities, *nausea,* vomiting

GU: Elevated BUN and creatinine, has been found in renal stones, *interstitial nephritis*

HEME: Megaloblastic anemia, ***thrombocytopenia***

METAB: Electrolyte imbalance, hyperkalemia, hypokalemia

SKIN: Photosensitivity, rash

MISC: Fatigue, weakness

INTERACTIONS

Drugs

3 *ACE inhibitors:* Hyperkalemia in predisposed patients

3 *Amantadine:* Increased toxicity of amantadine

3 *Angiotensin II receptor antagonists:* Concurrent mechanisms to decrease potassium excretion; increased risk of hyperkalemia

3 *Cimetidine:* Increased triamterene bioavailability and decreased renal clearance

3 *NSAIDs:* Acute renal failure with indomethacin and possibly other NSAIDs

2 *Potassium preparation:* Concurrent use increases the risk of hyperkalemia

Labs

• *False increase:* Serum digoxin concentrations

• *Interference:* Urinary catecholamines

SPECIAL CONSIDERATIONS

PATIENT/FAMILY EDUCATION

• Take with meals

• Avoid prolonged exposure to sunlight

• Take single daily doses in AM

MONITORING PARAMETERS

• Blood pressure, edema, urine output, urine electrolytes, BUN, creatinine, ECG (if hyperkalemic), gynecomastia, impotence

---

triazolam

(trye-ay′zoe-lam)

Rx: Halcion

Chemical Class: Benzodiazepine

Therapeutic Class: Hypnotic

DEA Class: Schedule IV

CLINICAL PHARMACOLOGY

Mechanism of Action: CNS depressants via facilitation of inhibitory GABA at benzodiazepine receptor sites (BZ_1—associated with sleep; BZ_2—associated with memory, motor, sensory, and cognitive function); effects include muscle relaxation (spinal cord), anticonvulsant activity (brain stem), ataxia (cerebellum), emotional behavior (limbic and cortical areas), and anxiolytic effects (separate from general CNS depression); decreases sleep latency, the number of awakenings, and the time spent in stage 0 (awake) sleep; stage 2 (unequivocal sleep) is increased; in sum, sleep time increased

Pharmacokinetics

PO: Onset 15-30 min, peak 42 min, duration 6-7 hr; 89% bound to plasma proteins; extensively metabolized in liver, excreted in urine as unchanged drug and metabolites; $t_{1/2}$ 1.7-5 hr

INDICATIONS AND USES: Short-term treatment of insomnia (generally 7-10 days); use for more than

---

2-3 wk requires complete reevaluation of the patient

DOSAGE

Adult

• PO 0.125-0.5 mg hs

Elderly or debilitated patients

• PO 0.125-0.25 mg hs; initiate with 0.125 mg until individual response is determined

§ AVAILABLE FORMS/COST OF THERAPY

• Tab, Plain Coated—Oral: 0.125 mg, 100's: **$59.68-$94.45**; 0.25 mg, 100's: **$65.24-$103.39**

CONTRAINDICATIONS: Narrow-angle glaucoma, psychosis, children <18 yr

PRECAUTIONS: Elderly, debilitated, hepatic disease, renal disease, history of drug abuse, abrupt withdrawal, respiratory depression, prolonged use

PREGNANCY AND LACTATION: Pregnancy category X (according to manufacturer); no congenital anomalies have been attributed to use during human pregnancies; other benzodiazepines have been suspected of producing fetal malformations after 1st-trimester exposure

SIDE EFFECTS/ADVERSE REACTIONS

CNS: Abnormal thinking, agitation, anterograde amnesia, anxiety, apathy, *asthenia,* ataxia, decreased reflexes, early morning insomnia, emotional lability, hangover, hostility, *hypokinesia,* neuritis, **seizures,** sleep disorder, *somnolence,* stupor

CV: **Dysrhythmia,** syncope

EENT: Ear pain; epistaxis, eye irritation, pain, pharyngitis, photophobia, rhinitis, sinusitis, swelling

GI: Abdominal pain, decreased or increased appetite, dyspepsia, enterocolitis, flatulence, gastritis, increased AST, ALT, melena, mouth ulceration

GU: Decreased libido, frequent urination, hematuria, menstrual cramps, nocturia, oliguria, penile discharge, urinary hesitancy and urgency, urinary incontinence, vaginal discharge and itching

HEME: **Agranulocytosis**

MS: Back pain, lower extremity pain

RESP: Asthma, cough, dyspnea, hyperventilation

SKIN: Acne, dry skin, photosensitivity, urticaria

INTERACTIONS

Drugs

3 *Carbamazepine, phenytoin:* Reduced effect of triazolam

3 *Cimetidine, clarithromycin, disulfiram, erythromycin, fluvoxamine, grapefruit juice, isoniazid, troleandomycin:* Increased plasma triazolam concentrations

2 *Ethanol:* Enhanced adverse psychomotor effects of benzodiazepines

2 *Fluconazole, itraconazole, ketoconazole:* Increased plasma triazolam concentrations

SPECIAL CONSIDERATIONS

Prescriptions should be written for short-term use (7-10 days); drug should not be prescribed in quantities exceeding a 1 mo supply

PATIENT/FAMILY EDUCATION

• Avoid alcohol and other CNS depressants

• Do not discontinue abruptly after prolonged therapy

• May cause drowsiness or dizziness, use caution while driving or performing other tasks requiring alertness

• May be habit forming

trientine

(trye-en'teen)
Rx: Syprine
Chemical Class: Thiol derivative
Therapeutic Class: Copper antidote

CLINICAL PHARMACOLOGY
Mechanism of Action: Chelating agent that binds copper and facilitates its excretion from the body (cupriuresis)
INDICATIONS AND USES: Treatment of Wilson's disease in patients intolerant of penicillamine
DOSAGE
Adult
• PO 750-1250 mg/day divided bid-qid; may increase to max of 2 g/day
Child ≤12 yr
• PO 500-750 mg/day divided bid-qid; may increase to max of 1.5 g/day
$ **AVAILABLE FORMS/COST OF THERAPY**
• Cap, Gel—Oral: 250 mg, 100's: **$97.23**
CONTRAINDICATIONS: Cystinuria, rheumatoid arthritis, biliary cirrhosis
PRECAUTIONS: Iron deficiency anemia, children
PREGNANCY AND LACTATION: Pregnancy category C
SIDE EFFECTS/ADVERSE REACTIONS
GI: Epigastric pain, heartburn
HEME: Iron deficiency anemia
MS: Cramps, muscle pain
SKIN: Tenderness, thickening and fissuring of skin
MISC: Malaise, systemic lupus erythematosus
SPECIAL CONSIDERATIONS
PATIENT/FAMILY EDUCATION
• Take on empty stomach

MONITORING PARAMETERS
• Free serum copper (goal is <10 µg/dl); increase daily dose only when clinical response is not adequate or concentration of free serum copper is persistently above 20 µg/dl (determine optimal long-term maintenance dosage at 6-12 mo intervals)
• 24 hr urinary copper analysis at 6-12 mo intervals (adequately treated patients will have 0.5-1 mg copper/24 hr collection of urine)

trifluoperazine

(trye-floo-oh-per'a-zeen)
Rx: Stelazine
Chemical Class: Piperazine phenothiazine derivative
Therapeutic Class: Antipsychotic

CLINICAL PHARMACOLOGY
Mechanism of Action: Dopamine receptor antagonist, with higher affinity for D_2 over D_1 receptors, and variable selectivity among the cortical dopamine tracts; also activity on nondopaminergic sites, i.e., cholinergic, α_1-adrenergic and histaminic receptors (explaining side effects); high rates of extrapyramidal reactions; minimal sedation, anticholinergic effects and rates of orthostatic hypotension
Pharmacokinetics
PO: Peak 1½-4½ hr, duration ≥12 hr; ≥90% bound to plasma proteins; extensive liver metabolism, excreted in urine and bile; $t_{1/2}$ >24 hr with chronic use (7-18 hr after single dose)
INDICATIONS AND USES: Psychotic disorders, short-term treatment of non-psychotic anxiety (not drug of choice for most patients)

DOSAGE

NOTE: 5 mg equivalent to chlorpromazine 100 mg

Adult

• *Psychotic disorders:* PO 2-5 mg bid, most patients show optimum response with 15-20 mg/day, some may require ≥40 mg/day; IM (for prompt control of symptoms) 1-2 mg q4-6h prn, doses >6 mg/24 hr are rarely necessary

• *Non-psychotic anxiety:* PO 1-2 mg bid, do not administer >6 mg/day or for >12 wk

Child

• PO 1 mg qd-bid initially, usually not necessary to exceed 15 mg/day: IM 1 mg qd-bid (little experience in children)

💲 AVAILABLE FORMS/COST OF THERAPY

• Tab, Plain Coated—Oral: 1 mg, 100's: **$32.07-$69.90;** 2 mg, 100's: **$46.83-$103.10;** 5 mg, 100's: **$40.48-$129.75;** 10 mg, 100's: **$66.75-$195.55**

• Inj, Sol—IM: 2 mg/ml, 10 ml: **$56.85**

CONTRAINDICATIONS: Severe toxic CNS depression, coma, subcortical brain damage, bone marrow depression

PRECAUTIONS: Elderly, children <12 yr, prolonged use, severe cardiovascular disorders, epilepsy, hepatic or renal disease, glaucoma, prostatic hypertrophy, severe asthma, emphysema, hypocalcemia (increased susceptibility to dystonic reactions)

PREGNANCY AND LACTATION: Pregnancy category C; has been used as an antiemetic during normal labor without producing any observable effect on newborn; bulk of evidence indicates safety for mother and fetus

SIDE EFFECTS/ADVERSE REACTIONS

CNS: Agitation, anxiety, confusion, depression, *drowsiness,* euphoria, exacerbation of psychotic symptoms including hallucinations, catatonic-like behavioral states, *extrapyramidal symptoms (pseudoparkinsonism, akathisia, dystonia),* headache, insomnia, lethargy, **neuroleptic malignant syndrome,** restlessness, **seizures,** tardive dyskinesia

CV: ECG changes, hypertension, hypotension, tachycardia

EENT: Blurred vision, cataracts, dry eyes, glaucoma, pigmentation of retina or cornea, retinopathy, vertigo

GI: Anorexia, *constipation,* diarrhea, *dry mouth,* dyspepsia, hypersalivation, *nausea,* vomiting

GU: Gynecomastia, impotence, increased libido, menstrual irregularities, priapism, urinary retention

HEME: **Agranulocytosis,** anemia, **aplastic anemia, hemolytic anemia,** leukocytosis, minimal decreases in red blood cell counts, transient leukopenia

METAB: Breast engorgement, hyperglycemia, hypoglycemia, hyponatremia, lactation, mastalgia

RESP: **Bronchospasm,** increased depth of respiration, *laryngospasm*

SKIN: Diaphoresis, loss of hair, maculopapular and acneiform skin reactions, photosensitivity

MISC: Heat or cold intolerance

INTERACTIONS

Drugs

3 *Anticholinergics:* Inhibited therapeutic response to antipsychotic; enhanced anticholinergic side effects

3 *Antidepressants:* Increased serum concentrations of some cyclic antidepressants

3 *Barbiturates:* Reduced effect of antipsychotic

---

* = non-FDA-approved use

3 *Bromocriptine, lithium:* Reduced effects of both drugs

3 *Guanethidine:* Inhibited antihypertensive response to guanethidine

2 *Levodopa:* Inhibited effect of levodopa on Parkinson's disease

3 *Narcotic analgesics:* Excessive CNS depression, hypotension, respiratory depression

3 *Orphenadrine:* Reduced serum neuroleptic concentrations; excessive anticholinergic effects

Labs
• *False increase:* Urinary protein

SPECIAL CONSIDERATIONS
PATIENT/FAMILY EDUCATION
• Arise slowly from reclining position
• Do not discontinue abruptly
• Use a sunscreen during sun exposure; take special precautions to stay cool in hot weather

MONITORING PARAMETERS
• Observe closely for signs of tardive dyskinesia
• Periodic CBC with platelets during prolonged therapy

---

triflupromazine
(trye-floo-proe'ma-zeen)
Rx: Vesprin
Chemical Class: Aliphatic phenothiazine derivative
Therapeutic Class: Antipsychotic; antiemetic

CLINICAL PHARMACOLOGY
Mechanism of Action: Dopamine receptor antagonist, with higher affinity for D_2- over D_1-receptors, and variable selectivity among the cortical dopamine tracts; also activity on nondopaminergic sites, i.e., cholinergic, α_1-adrenergic and histaminic receptors (explaining side effects); high rates of sedation and anticholinergic effects; moderate risk of extrapyramidal reactions and orthostatic hypotension

Pharmacokinetics
IM: Onset 15-30 min, peak 1 hr, duration 4-6 hr; metabolized by liver, excreted in urine and feces

INDICATIONS AND USES: Psychotic disorders, control of severe nausea and vomiting

DOSAGE
NOTE: 25 mg equivalent to chlorpromazine 100 mg

Adult
• *Psychotic disorders:* IM 60 mg, up to max of 150 mg/day
• *Nausea and vomiting:* IV 1 mg up to a max total 3 mg/day; IM 5-15 mg as a single dose, may repeat q4h up to max of 60 mg/day

Elderly or debilitated patients
• *Nausea and vomiting:* IM 2.5 mg up to a max of 15 mg/day

Child >2 yr
• IM 0.2-0.25 mg/kg, up to max total dose of 10 mg/day

$ **AVAILABLE FORMS/COST OF THERAPY**
• Inj, Sol—IM, IV: 10 mg/ml, 10 ml: **$45.62;** 20 mg/ml, 1 ml: **$12.48**

CONTRAINDICATIONS: Severe toxic CNS depression, coma, subcortical brain damage, bone marrow depression, narrow-angle glaucoma

PRECAUTIONS: Elderly, prolonged use, severe cardiovascular disorders, epilepsy, hepatic or renal disease, glaucoma, prostatic hypertrophy, severe asthma, emphysema, hypocalcemia (increased susceptibility to dystonic reactions)

PREGNANCY AND LACTATION: Pregnancy category C; bulk of evidence indicates phenothiazines are safe for mother and fetus

SIDE EFFECTS/ADVERSE REACTIONS
CNS: Agitation, anxiety, confusion, depression, *drowsiness,* euphoria,

T

---

italic = common side effects   ***bold italic*** = life-threatening reactions

exacerbation of psychotic symptoms including hallucinations, catatonic-like behavioral states, *extrapyramidal symptoms (pseudoparkinsonism, akathisia, dystonia), headache,* insomnia, lethargy, **neuroleptic malignant syndrome,** restlessness, *seizures,* tardive dyskinesia

CV: ECG changes, hypertension, hypotension, tachycardia

EENT: Blurred vision, cataracts, dry eyes, glaucoma, pigmentation of retina or cornea, retinopathy, vertigo

GI: Anorexia, constipation, diarrhea, *dry mouth,* dyspepsia, hypersalivation, *nausea,* vomiting

GU: Gynecomastia, impotence, increased libido, menstrual irregularities, priapism, urinary retention

HEME: **Agranulocytosis,** anemia, **aplastic anemia, hemolytic anemia,** leukocytosis, minimal decreases in red blood cell counts, transient leukopenia

METAB: Breast engorgement, hyperglycemia, hypoglycemia, hyponatremia, lactation, mastalgia

RESP: **Bronchospasm,** increased depth of respiration, **laryngospasm**

SKIN: Diaphoresis, loss of hair, maculopapular and acneiform skin reactions, photosensitivity

MISC: Heat or cold intolerance

INTERACTIONS

Drugs

3 *Anticholinergics:* Inhibited therapeutic response to antipsychotic; enhanced anticholinergic side effects

3 *Barbiturates:* Reduced effect of antipsychotic

3 *Bromocriptine, lithium:* Reduced effects of both drugs

3 *Guanethidine:* Inhibited antihypertensive response to guanethidine

2 *Levodopa:* Inhibited effect of levodopa on Parkinson's disease

3 *Narcotic analgesics:* Excessive CNS depression, hypotension, respiratory depression

3 *Orphenadrine:* Reduced serum neuroleptic concentrations; excessive anticholinergic effects

SPECIAL CONSIDERATIONS
PATIENT/FAMILY EDUCATION

• Arise slowly from reclining position

---

trifluridine

(trye-flure'i-deen)

Rx: Viroptic

Chemical Class: Nucleoside analog

Therapeutic Class: Ophthalmic antiviral

CLINICAL PHARMACOLOGY

Mechanism of Action: Interferes with DNA synthesis in cultured mammalian cells; antiviral mechanism of action not completely known

Pharmacokinetics: Penetrates the intact cornea; systemic absorption following therapeutic dosing appears to be negligible

INDICATIONS AND USES: Primary keratoconjunctivitis and recurrent epithelial keratitis; epithelial keratitis; epithelial keratitis resistant to topical vidarabine; antiviral spectrum usually includes herpes simplex virus 1 and ·2 and vaccinia virus; some strains of adenovirus are also inhibited in vitro

DOSAGE

Adult

• OPHTH instill 1 gtt onto cornea of affected eye(s) q2h while awake until ulcer has completely reepithelialized, max 9 gtt/day; after reepithelialization, 1 gtt q4h while awake for an additional 7 days, minimum 5 gtt/day; do not exceed 21 days due to potential for ocular toxicity

---

💲 AVAILABLE FORMS/COST OF THERAPY

• Sol—Ophth: 1%, 7.5 ml: **$74.44**

PRECAUTIONS: Prolonged use (>21 days); not effective for bacterial, fungal, or chlamydial infections of the cornea or trophic lesions

PREGNANCY AND LACTATION: Pregnancy category C

SIDE EFFECTS/ADVERSE REACTIONS

EENT: Burning, epithelial keratopathy, hyperemia, hypersensitivity reaction, increased intraocular pressure, irritation, keratitis sicca, palpebral edema, stinging, stromal edema, superficial punctate keratopathy

SPECIAL CONSIDERATIONS PATIENT/FAMILY EDUCATION

• Notify clinician if no improvement after 7 days

---

trihexyphenidyl
(trye-hex-ee-fen'i-dill)

Rx: Artane
Chemical Class: Synthetic tertiary amine
Therapeutic Class: Anticholinergic, anti-Parkinson's agent

CLINICAL PHARMACOLOGY
Mechanism of Action: Blocks striatal cholinergic receptors, which helps balance cholinergic and dopaminergic activity

Pharmacokinetics
PO: Onset within 1 hr, peak effects last 2-3 hr, duration 6-12 hr; excreted in urine

INDICATIONS AND USES: Adjunctive treatment of all forms of Parkinson's syndrome; drug-induced extrapyramidal symptoms

DOSAGE
Adult
• *Parkinsonism:* PO 1-2 mg on 1st day, increase by 2 mg q3-5d to 6-10 mg/day divided tid-qid; postencephalitic patients may require 12-15 mg/day; when used with levodopa, 3-6 mg/day in divided doses is usually adequate

• *Drug-induced extrapyramidal symptoms:* PO 1 mg initially, progressively increase subsequent doses if reaction not controlled in a few hr; maintenance 5-15 mg/day in divided doses

💲 AVAILABLE FORMS/COST OF THERAPY

• Elixir—Oral: 2 mg/5 ml, 480 ml: **$20.00-$40.08**
• Tab, Uncoated—Oral: 2 mg, 100's: **$14.24-$19.39;** 5 mg, 100's: **$32.54-$39.64**

CONTRAINDICATIONS: Narrow-angle glaucoma, myasthenia gravis, GI or GU obstruction, peptic ulcer, megacolon, prostatic hypertrophy

PRECAUTIONS: Elderly, tachycardia, liver or kidney disease, drug abuse history, dysrhythmias, hypotension, hypertension, psychosis, children, tardive dyskinesia

PREGNANCY AND LACTATION: Pregnancy category C; nursing infants may be particularly sensitive to anticholinergic effects

SIDE EFFECTS/ADVERSE REACTIONS

CNS: Anxiety, confusion, delusions, depression, dizziness, hallucinations, headache, incoherence, irritability, memory loss, restlessness, *sedation*
CV: Flushing, hypotension, mild bradycardia, palpitations, postural hypotension, tachycardia
EENT: Angle-closure glaucoma, blurred vision, difficulty swallowing, dilated pupils, dry eyes, increased intraocular tension, mydriasis, photophobia
GI: Abdominal distress, *constipation, dry mouth,* epigastric distress, nausea, ***paralytic ileus,*** vomiting

---

italic = common side effects   ***bold italic*** = life-threatening reactions

T

GU: Dysuria, erectile dysfunction, hesitancy, retention
MS: Cramping, muscular weakness
SKIN: Dermatoses, rash, urticaria
MISC: Decreased sweating, heat stroke, hyperthermia, numbness of fingers

INTERACTIONS
Drugs

🔳 *Amantadine:* Potentiates the side effects of amantadine

🔳 *Anticholinergics:* Increased anticholinergic side effects

🔳 *Neuroleptics:* Inhibition of therapeutic response to neuroleptics; excessive anticholinergic effects

🔳 *Tacrine:* Reduced therapeutic effects of both drugs

Labs
• *False increase:* Serum T_3 and T_4

SPECIAL CONSIDERATIONS
PATIENT/FAMILY EDUCATION
• Do not discontinue abruptly
• Use caution in hot weather; drug may increase susceptibility to heat stroke

---

trimethadione
(trye-meth-a-dye'one)
Rx: Tridione
Chemical Class: Oxazolidinedione derivative
Therapeutic Class: Anticonvulsant

CLINICAL PHARMACOLOGY
Mechanism of Action: Decreases seizures in cortex, basal ganglia; decreases synaptic stimulation to low-frequency impulses
Pharmacokinetics
PO: Peak 30-120 min; demethylated in liver to active metabolite (dimethadione), excreted by kidneys; $t_{1/2}$ 16-24 hr (dimethadione 6-13 days)
INDICATIONS AND USES: Refractory absence (petit mal) seizures

DOSAGE
Adult
• PO 300-600 mg tid-qid; give 900 mg/day initially, increase by 300 mg at weekly intervals until therapeutic results are seen or toxicity appears
Child
• PO 300-900 mg/day divided tid-qid

💲 **AVAILABLE FORMS/COST OF THERAPY**
• Cap, Gel—Oral: 300 mg, 100's: **$44.19**
• Tab, Chewable—Oral: 150 mg, 100's: **$40.50**

PRECAUTIONS: Hepatic disease, renal disease, abrupt discontinuation, diseases of retina or optic nerve, intermittent porphyria, myasthenia gravis

PREGNANCY AND LACTATION: Pregnancy category D; has demonstrated both clinical and experimental fetal risk greater than other anticonvulsants; avoid use in pregnancy

SIDE EFFECTS/ADVERSE REACTIONS
CNS: Dizziness, *drowsiness,* fatigue, headache, insomnia, irritability, paresthesia
CV: Hypertension, hypotension
EENT: Diplopia, epistaxis, photophobia, retinal hemorrhage
GI: Abdominal pain, abnormal liver function tests, bleeding gums, *nausea, vomiting*
GU: Albuminuria, nephrosis, vaginal bleeding
HEME: **Agranulocytosis, aplastic anemia,** eosinophilia, **hemolytic anemia,** increased prothrombin time, **leukopenia, neutropenia, thrombocytopenia**
SKIN: Alopecia, erythema, **exfoliative dermatitis,** petechiae, rash
MISC: Lupus erythematosus

---

* = non-FDA-approved use

SPECIAL CONSIDERATIONS
PATIENT/FAMILY EDUCATION
• Take with food if GI upset occurs
• Avoid prolonged exposure to sunlight
MONITORING PARAMETERS
• CBC at baseline and qmo thereafter; satisfactory control usually occurs when serum dimethadione levels are ≥700 µg/ml

---

trimethobenzamide
(trye-meth-oh-ben′za-mide)
Rx: Benzacot, Stemetic, Tigan
Chemical Class: Ethanolamine derivative
Therapeutic Class: Antiemetic

CLINICAL PHARMACOLOGY
Mechanism of Action: Exact mechanism unknown; appears to directly affect the medullary chemoreceptor trigger zone (CTZ) by inhibiting stimuli at the CTZ
Pharmacokinetics
PO: Onset 10-40 min, duration 3-4 hr
IM: Onset 15-35 min, duration 2-3 hr
Exact metabolic fate unclear, 30%-50% excreted unchanged in urine
INDICATIONS AND USES: Nausea and vomiting
DOSAGE
Adult
• PO 250 mg tid-qid; PR/IM 200 mg tid-qid
Child
• PO (13.6-45 kg) 100-200 mg tid-qid; PR (<13.6 kg) 100 mg tid-qid; (13.6-45 kg) 100-200 mg tid-qid
💲 AVAILABLE FORMS/COST OF THERAPY
• Inj, Sol—IM: 100 mg/ml, 20 ml: **$12.95-$27.96**
• Cap, Gel—Oral: 100 mg, 100's: **$49.64;** 250 mg, 100's: **$27.00-$59.85**

• Supp—Rect: 100 mg, 10's: **$4.49-$15.05;** 200 mg, 10's: **$4.99-$22.64**
CONTRAINDICATIONS: Hypersensitivity to benzocaine or similar anesthetics; parenteral use in children; suppositories in premature infants or neonates
PRECAUTIONS: Acute febrile illness, encephalitis, Reye's syndrome, gastroenteritis, dehydration, electrolyte imbalance
PREGNANCY AND LACTATION: Pregnancy category C; has been used to treat nausea and vomiting during pregnancy
SIDE EFFECTS/ADVERSE REACTIONS
CNS: **Coma,** depression, disorientation, dizziness, *drowsiness,* dystonic reactions, headache, Parkinson-like symptoms, *seizures*
CV: Hypotenstion (IM)
EENT: Blurred vision
GI: Diarrhea, jaundice
HEME: ***Blood dyscrasias***
MS: Muscle cramps
SKIN: Allergic-type skin reactions, burning and stinging at inj site (IM)
INTERACTIONS
Labs
• *False positive:* Urinary amphetamine
SPECIAL CONSIDERATIONS
• Less effective than phenothiazines

---

italic = common side effects   ***bold italic*** = life-threatening reactions

trimethoprim

(trye-meth'oh-prim)
Rx: Proloprim, Trimpex
Combinations
  Rx: with sulfamethoxazole
    (see co-trimoxazole
    monograph); with poly-
    mixin B sulfate (Polytrim
    Ophthalmic)
Chemical Class: Synthetic
folate-antagonist
Therapeutic Class: Antibiotic

CLINICAL PHARMACOLOGY
Mechanism of Action: Selectively
interferes with bacterial biosynthesis of nucleic acids and proteins by
blocking production of tetrahydrofolic acid from dihydrofolic acid via
binding to and reversibly inhibiting
the required enzyme, dihydrofolate
reductase; binding much stronger for
bacterial enzyme than for corre-
sponding mammalian enzyme
Pharmacokinetics
PO: Peak 1-4 hr; widely distributed
into body tissues and fluids; 42%-
46% bound to plasma proteins; metabolized in liver to oxide and hydroxylated metabolites, excreted in
urine (80% unchanged); $t_{1/2}$ 8-11 hr
(prolonged in renal failure)
INDICATIONS AND USES: Acute
uncomplicated UTI, prophylaxis of
chronic and recurrent UTI,* *Pneumocystis carinii* pneumonia (in conjunction with dapsone or sulfamethoxazole),* travelers' diarrhea,*
otitis media, and chronic bronchitis
and shigella (with sulfamethoxazole)
Antibacterial spectrum usually includes:
• Gram-positive organisms: *Streptococcus pneumoniae,* group A β-
hemolytic streptococci, coagulase-
negative staphylococci
• Gram-negative organisms: *Acine-*

*tobacter, Citrobacter, Enterobacter,
Escherichia coli, Klebsiella pneumoniae, Proteus mirabilis, Salmonella, Shigella, Haemophilus influenzae*
DOSAGE
Adult
• PO 100 mg q12h or 200 mg q24h,
each for 10 days
• Dosing in renal failure (CrCl 15-30
ml/min): PO 50 mg q12h. Combination with sulfamethoxazole: see
co-trimoxazole

**$ AVAILABLE FORMS/COST
  OF THERAPY**
• Tab, Uncoated—Oral: 100 mg,
100's: **$14.93-$70.84;** 200 mg,
100's: **$22.10-$42.70**
CONTRAINDICATIONS: Megaloblastic anemia due to folate deficiency, infants <2 mo, CrCl <15 ml/
min
PRECAUTIONS: Renal or hepatic
impairment, children <12 yr, folate
deficiency (folates may be administered concurrently without interfering with antibacterial action)
PREGNANCY AND LACTATION:
Pregnancy category C; because trimethoprim is a folate antagonist,
caution should be used during the
1st trimester; excreted into breast
milk in low concentrations; compatible with breast feeding
**SIDE EFFECTS/ADVERSE REAC-
  TIONS**
CNS: Fever
GI: Elevation of serum transaminases and bilirubin, epigastric distress, glossitis, *hepatic necrosis,
nausea, vomiting*
GU: Increased BUN and serum creatinine
*HEME: Leukopenia, megaloblastic
anemia, methemoglobinemia, neutropenia, thrombocytopenia*
SKIN: Pruritus, rash, *Stevens-
Johnson syndrome, toxic epidermal necrolysis*

* = non-FDA-approved use

INTERACTIONS
Drugs
🔳 *Dapsone:* Increased serum concentrations of both drugs

🔳 *Phenytoin:* Increased serum phenytoin concentrations, potential for toxicity

🔳 *Procainamide:* Increased serum concentrations of procainamide and N-acetylprocainamide

SPECIAL CONSIDERATIONS
• Good alternative to co-trimoxazole in patients taking warfarin

---

trimipramine
(trye-mip'ra-meen)
Rx: Surmontil
Chemical Class: Dibenzazepine derivative: tertiary amine
Therapeutic Class: Tricyclic antidepressant

CLINICAL PHARMACOLOGY
Mechanism of Action: Inhibits the reuptake of norepinephrine and serotonin (slightly) at the presynaptic neuron prolonging neuronal activity; inhibition of histamine and acetylcholine activity; mild peripheral vasodilator effects and possible quinidine-like action on cardiac conduction; moderate anticholinergic and orthostatic hypotensive effects; high sedative activity

Pharmacokinetics
PO: Peak within 6 hr; 95% protein bound; metabolized in liver to desmethyltrimipramine, excreted in urine; $t_{1/2}$ 20-26 hr

INDICATIONS AND USES: Depression, chronic urticaria and angioedema,* nocturnal pruritus in atopic dermatitis*

DOSAGE
Adult
• PO 75-100 mg/day in divided doses initially, increase to 150-200 mg/day, max 300 mg/day
Adolescent and Elderly
• PO 50 mg/day initially, increase to 100 mg/day

💲 AVAILABLE FORMS/COST OF THERAPY
• Cap, Gel—Oral: 25 mg, 100's: **$81.96;** 50 mg, 100's: **$134.11;** 100 mg, 100's: **$194.96**

CONTRAINDICATIONS: Acute recovery phase of MI, concurrent use of MAOIs

PRECAUTIONS: Suicidal patients, seizure disorders, prostatic hypertrophy, psychiatric disease, severe depression, increased intraocular pressure, narrow-angle glaucoma, urinary retention, cardiac disease, hepatic disease, renal disease, hyperthyroidism, electroshock therapy, elective surgery, elderly, abrupt discontinuation

PREGNANCY AND LACTATION: Pregnancy category C; excreted into breast milk; effect on nursing infant unknown, but may be of concern

SIDE EFFECTS/ADVERSE REACTIONS
CNS: Anxiety, confusion (especially in elderly), *dizziness, drowsiness,* fatigue, headache, increased psychiatric symptoms, insomnia, memory impairment, nightmares, stimulation, tremors, weakness

CV: **Dysrhythmias,** ECG changes, hypertension, *orthostatic hypotension,* palpitations, tachycardia

EENT: *Blurred vision,* mydriasis, nasal congestion, ophthalmoplegia, tinnitus

GI: Constipation, cramps, diarrhea, *dry mouth,* epigastric distress, hepatitis, increased appetite, jaundice, nausea, *paralytic ileus,* stomatitis, vomiting

GU: Urinary retention

HEME: **Agranulocytosis,** eosino-

T

---

italic = common side effects   **bold italic** = life-threatening reactions

philia, *leukopenia, thrombocytopenia*

SKIN: Photosensitivity, pruritus, rash, sweating, urticaria

INTERACTIONS

Drugs

3 *Anticholinergics, propantheline:* Excessive anticholinergic effects

3 *Barbiturates, carbamazepine:* Reduced serum concentrations of cyclic antidepressants

3 *Cimetidine:* Increases trimipramine level

2 *Clonidine:* Reduced antihypertensive response to clonidine; enhanced hypertensive response with abrupt clonidine withdrawal

2 *Epinephrine, norepinephrine:* Markedly enhanced pressor response to IV epinephrine

3 *Ethanol:* Additive impairment of motor skills; abstinent alcoholics may eliminate cyclic antidepressants more rapidly than nonalcoholics

3 *Fluoxetine:* Marked increases in cyclic antidepressant plasma concentrations

2 *Guanadrel, guanethidine:* Inhibited antihypertensive response to guanethidine

A *MAOIs:* Excessive sympathetic response; mania or hyperpyrexia possible

2 *Moclobemide:* Potential association with fatal or non-fatal serotonin syndrome

3 *Phenylephrine:* Markedly enhanced pressor response to IV epinephrine

3 *Propoxyphene:* Enhanced effect of cyclic antidepressants

3 *Quinidine:* Increased cyclic antidepressant serum concentrations

SPECIAL CONSIDERATIONS

PATIENT/FAMILY EDUCATION

• Therapeutic effects may take 2-3 wk

• Avoid rising quickly from sitting to standing, especially elderly

• Do not discontinue abruptly after long-term use

MONITORING PARAMETERS

• CBC, ECG

---

trioxsalen

(trye-ox'a-len)

Rx: Trisoralen

Chemical Class: Psoralen derivative

Therapeutic Class: Pigmenting agent

CLINICAL PHARMACOLOGY

Mechanism of Action: Exact mechanism unknown; may involve increased tyrosinase activity in melanin-producing cells, which enhances melanin production; successful pigmentation requires the presence of functioning melanocytes

Pharmacokinetics

PO: Onset 1-2 hr, maximal effects 2-4 hr, duration 7-8 hr; 80% appears in urine within 8 hr as hydroxylated or glucuronide derivatives

INDICATIONS AND USES: Repigmentation in the treatment of vitiligo, in conjunction with UVA—treatment known as PUVA (psoralen plus ultraviolet light A); increasing tolerance to sunlight and enhancing pigmentation (in conjunction with controlled exposure to UVA light or sunlight)

DOSAGE

Adult and Child >12 yr

• *Idiopathic vitiligo:* PO 5-10 mg qd 2-4 hr before measured periods of sunlight or UVA exposure

• *Other uses:* PO 10 mg qd 2 hr before measured periods of sunlight or UVA exposure; do not exceed 14 days of therapy or 140 mg total dose

---

* = non-FDA-approved use

• Tab, Uncoated—Oral: 5 mg, 100's: **$228.78**
CONTRAINDICATIONS: Diseases associated with photosensitivity, melanoma, invasive squamous cell carcinoma, aphakia, children <12 yr
PRECAUTIONS: Cardiac disease, hepatic disease, contains tartrazine (FD&C #5), photosensitizing agents
PREGNANCY AND LACTATION: Pregnancy category C; excretion into breast milk unknown, use caution in nursing mothers

SIDE EFFECTS/ADVERSE REACTIONS
CNS: Depression, dizziness, headache, insomnia, malaise, nervousness
CV: Edema, hypotension
EENT: Cataract formation
GI: Nausea
MS: Leg cramps
SKIN: Basal cell epitheliomas, cutaneous tenderness, *erythema,* extension of psoriasis, folliculitis, hypopigmentation, *pruritus,* severe burns, urticaria, vesiculation and bullae formation

INTERACTIONS
Drugs
§ *Anthralin, coal tar, griseofulvin, phenothiazines, nalidixic acid, halogenated salicylanilides, sulfonamides, tetracyclines, thiazides:* Increased photosensitivity to these agents

SPECIAL CONSIDERATIONS
PATIENT/FAMILY EDUCATION
• Do not sunbathe during 24 hr prior to ingestion and UVA exposure
• Wear UVA-absorbing sunglasses for 24 hr following treatment to prevent cataract
• Avoid sun exposure for at least 8 hr after ingestion
• Avoid furocoumarin-containing foods (e.g., limes, figs, parsley, parsnips, mustard, carrots, celery)
• Repigmentation may begin after 2-3 wk but full effect may require 6-9 mo

---

tripelennamine
(tri-pel-enn'a-meen)
Rx: PBZ, PBZ-SR
Chemical Class: Ethylenediamine derivative
Therapeutic Class: Antihistamine

CLINICAL PHARMACOLOGY
Mechanism of Action: Decreases allergic response by blocking histamine at H_1-receptors
Pharmacokinetics
PO: Onset within 30 min, duration 4-6 hr (SUS REL 8 hr); metabolized in liver, excreted in urine

INDICATIONS AND USES: Perennial and seasonal allergic rhinitis; vasomotor rhinitis; allergic conjunctivitis due to inhalants, allergens and food; allergic skin manifestations of urticaria and angioedema; dermographism; adjunctive anaphylactic therapy

DOSAGE
Adult
• PO 25-50 mg q4-6h, max 600 mg/day; PO SUS REL 100 mg bid, may also be given q8h in difficult cases
Child
• PO 5 mg/kg/day or 150 mg/m²/day in 4-6 divided doses, max 300 mg/day

§ **AVAILABLE FORMS/COST OF THERAPY**
• Tab, Uncoated—Oral: 25 mg, 100's: **$17.91;** 50 mg, 100's: **$6.55-$27.20**
• Tab, Coated, SUS Action—Oral: 100 mg, 100's: **$44.71**

---

italic = common side effects   ***bold italic*** = life-threatening reactions

CONTRAINDICATIONS: Narrow-angle glaucoma, bladder neck obstruction

PRECAUTIONS: Liver disease, elderly, increased intraocular pressure, hyperthyroidism, cardiovascular disease, hypertension, urinary retention, renal disease, stenosed peptic ulcers

PREGNANCY AND LACTATION: Pregnancy category B; manufacturer considers the drug contraindicated in nursing mothers, possibly due to increased sensitivity of newborn or premature infants to antihistamines; anecdotal evidence indicates safety in pregnancy

SIDE EFFECTS/ADVERSE REACTIONS

CNS: Anxiety, confusion, *dizziness, drowsiness,* euphoria, fatigue, poor coordination

CV: Hypotension, palpitations, tachycardia

EENT: Blurred vision, dilated pupils, dry nose, throat, nasal stuffiness, tinnitus

GI: Anorexia, *constipation,* diarrhea, *dry mouth,* nausea, vomiting

GU: Dysuria, frequency, impotence, retention

HEME: **Agranulocytosis, hemolytic anemia, thrombocytopenia**

RESP: Increased thick secretions, wheezing

SKIN: Photosensitivity

---

triprolidine
(trye-proe′li-deen)
Combinations
  Rx: with pseudoephedrine, codeine (Triprolidine-C):
  OTC: with pseudoephedrine (Actifed)
Chemical Class: Alkylamine derivative
Therapeutic Class: Antihistamine

CLINICAL PHARMACOLOGY
Mechanism of Action: Decreases allergic response by blocking histamine at H_1-receptors
Pharmacokinetics
PO: Onset 20-60 min, duration 8-12 hr; metabolized in liver, excreted in urine

INDICATIONS AND USES: Perennial and seasonal allergic rhinitis and other allergic symptoms including urticaria

DOSAGE
Adult
• PO 2.5 mg q4-6h
Child 6-12 yr
• PO 1.25 mg q4-6h

$ **AVAILABLE FORMS/COST OF THERAPY**
• Syr—Oral: 1.25 mg/5 ml (with 30 mg pseudoephedrine and 10 mg codeine), 480 ml: **$12.25**
• Tab, Uncoated—Oral: 2.5 mg (with 60 mg pseudoephedrine), 100's: **$14.32**

CONTRAINDICATIONS: Narrow-angle glaucoma, bladder neck obstruction

PRECAUTIONS: Liver disease, elderly, increased intraocular pressure, hyperthyroidism, cardiovascular disease, hypertension, urinary retention, newborn or premature infants, renal disease, GI outlet obstruction

---

PREGNANCY AND LACTATION: Pregnancy category C (but no teratogenicity documented); excreted into breast milk; compatible with breast feeding

SIDE EFFECTS/ADVERSE REACTIONS

CNS: Anxiety, confusion, *dizziness, drowsiness,* euphoria, fatigue, poor coordination

CV: Hypotension, palpitations, tachycardia

EENT: Blurred vision, dilated pupils, dry nose, throat, nasal stuffiness; tinnitus

GI: Anorexia, *constipation,* diarrhea, *dry mouth,* nausea, vomiting

GU: Dysuria, frequency, impotence, retention

HEME: **Agranulocytosis, hemolytic anemia, thrombocytopenia**

RESP: Increased thick secretions, wheezing

SKIN: Photosensitivity

INTERACTIONS

Labs

• *False increase:* Urinary amino acids

---

tromethamine

(troe-meth′a-meen)

Rx: Tham

Chemical Class: Organic amine buffer

Therapeutic Class: Alkalinizing agent

CLINICAL PHARMACOLOGY

Mechanism of Action: Acts as a proton acceptor preventing or correcting acidosis by actively binding hydrogen ions (H^+); binds cations of fixed or metabolic acids, and hydrogen ions of carbonic acid, thus increasing bicarbonate anion (HCO_3^-); also acts as an osmotic diuretic, increasing urine flow, urinary pH, and excretion of fixed acids, carbon dioxide, and electrolytes

Pharmacokinetics

IV: Rapidly eliminated by kidney (75% or more appears in the urine after 8 hr), urinary excretion continues over a period of 3 days

INDICATIONS AND USES: Metabolic acidosis associated with cardiac bypass surgery and cardiac arrest; correction of acidity of acid citrate dextrose (ACD) blood in cardiac bypass surgery

DOSAGE

• Dosage may be estimated from the buffer base deficit of extracellular fluid (mEq/L) using the following formula as a general guide: ml of 0.3 M tromethamine solution = body weight (kg) × base deficit (mEq/L) × 1.1

Adult

• *Acidosis during cardiac bypass surgery:* IV INF total single dose of 500 ml (150 mEq or 18 g) is adequate for most adults; larger single doses (up to 1000 ml) may be required in severe cases; do not exceed individual doses of 500 mg/kg given over at least 1 hr

• *Acidity of ACD-priming blood:* Use from 0.5-2.5 g (15-77 ml) added to each 500 ml of ACD blood; 62 ml added to 500 ml of ACD blood is usually adequate

• *Acidosis associated with cardiac arrest:* IV 3.6-10.8 g (111-333 ml) into large peripheral vein; if chest is open, inject 2-6 g (62-185 ml) directly into ventricular cavity

$ **AVAILABLE FORMS/COST OF THERAPY**

• Inj, Sol—IV: 3.6 g/100 ml (0.3 M), 500 ml: **$154.80**

CONTRAINDICATIONS: Anuria, uremia

PRECAUTIONS: Respiratory depression, perivascular infiltration,

---

italic = common side effects   ***bold italic*** = life-threatening reactions

T

neonates, renal function impairment, children

PREGNANCY AND LACTATION: Pregnancy category C

SIDE EFFECTS/ADVERSE REACTIONS

*GI: **Hemorrhagic hepatic necrosis***

METAB: Hypovolemia, transient depression of blood glucose

*RESP: **Respiratory depression***

SKIN: Local reactions (febrile response, infection, venous thrombosis or phlebitis)

INTERACTIONS

Labs

• *False decrease:* Plasma ammonia, serum ionized calcium

SPECIAL CONSIDERATIONS

• Avoid overdosage and alkalosis

MONITORING PARAMETERS

• Pretreatment and subsequent blood gas values

• Urine output

• ECG

• Serum glucose and electrolytes before, during, and after administration

• Experience limited to short-term use; may administer for >1 day in life-threatening situation

---

tropicamide
(troe-pik′a-mide)
Rx: Mydral, Mydriacyl, Ocu-Tropic
Chemical Class: Tropic acid derivative
Therapeutic Class: Mydriatic; cycloplegic

CLINICAL PHARMACOLOGY
Mechanism of Action: Blocks responses of the sphincter muscle of the iris and the accommodative muscle of the ciliary body to stimulation by acetylcholine, dilation of the pu-

pil (mydriasis) and paralysis of accommodation (cycloplegia) result

Pharmacokinetics: Peak mydriasis 20-40 min, recovery 6 hr; peak cycloplegia 20-35 min, recovery <6 hr

INDICATIONS AND USES: Mydriasis and cycloplegia for diagnostic purposes

DOSAGE

Adult and Child

• *Refraction:* Instill 1-2 gtt of 1% sol into eye(s), repeat in 5 min; an additional gtt may be instilled after 20-30 min to prolong effect

• *Examination of fundus:* Instill 1-2 gtt of 0.5% sol 15-20 min prior to examination

§ AVAILABLE FORMS/COST OF THERAPY

• Sol—Ophth: 0.5%, 15 ml: **$8.93-$25.75;** 1%, 15 ml: **$9.38-$27.75**

CONTRAINDICATIONS: Hypersensitivity to belladonna alkaloids, adhesions between the iris and the lens, primary glaucoma, narrow anterior chamber angle

PRECAUTIONS: Elderly, small children, and infants

PREGNANCY AND LACTATION: Pregnancy category C

SIDE EFFECTS/ADVERSE REACTIONS

CNS: Confusion, fever, headache, somnolence, visual hallucinations

CV: Tachycardia, vasodilation

EENT: Blurred vision, edema, increased intraocular pressure, irritation, *photophobia*

GI: Abdominal distension in infants, decreased GI motility, dry mouth

GU: Urinary retention

SKIN: Dry skin, rash

SPECIAL CONSIDERATIONS

• Individuals with heavily pigmented irides may require larger doses

---

* = non-FDA-approved use

PATIENT/FAMILY EDUCATION
• Do not drive or engage in any hazardous activities while pupils are dilated
• May cause sensitivity to light; protect eyes from bright light
• To minimize systemic effects, compress the lacrimal sac for several min following instillation

---

trovafloxacin/ alatrovafloxacin

(troh-vah-floks'-uh-sin)
Rx: Trovan
Combinations:
  Rx: with azithromycin (Trovan/Zithromax compliance pak)
Chemical Class: Fluoroquinolone derivative
Therapeutic Class: Antibiotic

CLINICAL PHARMACOLOGY
Mechanism of Action: Inhibtis DNA gyrase and topoisomerase 4, which are needed for the synthesis of bacterial DNA. Alatrovafloxacin is the L-alanyl prodrug of trovafloxacin
Pharmacokinetics
IV (alatrovafloxacin): Rapidly converted to trovafloxacin, peak plasma level 1 hr, $t_{1/2}$ 9-11 hr
PO (trovafloxacin): Bioavailability 88%, not affected by food; peak plasma level 1-2 hr; widely distributed (concentrated in lung, bile, and urine), 76% protein bound; 51% metabolized by conjugation in the liver (CYP450 independent), excreted unchanged in stool (43%), urine (6%), and as metabolites in urine; $t_{1/2}$ 9-12 hr
INDICATIONS AND USES: Serious life- or limb-threatening infections of the following types: Acute bacterial exacerbations of chronic bronchitis; acute sinusitis; cellulitis; diabetic foot infections; gonorrhea (urethral in males; endocervical and rectal in females); gynecologic and pelvic infections; intraabdominal infections; nongonococcal urethritis (female) and cervicitis; pelvic inflammatory disease; pneumonia, community or hospital acquired; bacterial prostatis; urinary tract infection (cystitis) caused by susceptible organisms. **Based on FDA advisory June 9, 1999 (see precautions), patients should receive their initial therapy in an inpatient health care facility.**
Antibacterial spectrum usually includes:
• Gram-positive organisms: *Enterococcus faecalis* (many strains are only moderately susceptible), *Staphylococcus aureus* (methicillin-susceptible strains), *S. epidermidis* (methicillin-susceptible strains), *Streptococcus pneumoniae, S. pyogenes, Viridans*-group *streptococci*
• Gram-negative organisms: *Citrobacter freundii, Enterobacter aerogenes, Escherichia coli, Gardnerella vaginalis, H. influenzae, H. parainfluenza, Klebsiella pneumoniae, Moraxella catarrhalis, Morganella morganii, N. gonorrhoeae, Proteus mirabilis, P. vulgaris, Pseudomonas aeruginosa*
• Other: *Chlamydia pneumoniae, Chlamydia trachomatis, Legionella pneumophila, Mycoplasma hominis, Mycoplasma pneumoniae;* Anaerobes: *Bacteroides fragilis, Bacteroides distasonis, Clostridium perfringens, Peptostreptococcus species*
DOSAGE
Adult
• *Acute bacterial exacerbations of chronic bronchitis:* PO 100 mg qd × 7-10 days

---

italic = common side effects   ***bold italic*** = life-threatening reactions

- *Acute sinusitis:* PO 200 mg qd × 10 days
- *Cellulitis (uncomplicated):* PO 100 mg qd × 7-10 days
- *Cellulitis (complicated) including diabetic foot infections:* PO 200 mg qd × 10-14 days
- *Gonorrhea (urethral in males):* PO 100 mg (single dose)
- *Gonorrhea (endocervical and rectal in females):* PO 200 mg qd × 5 days
- *Gynecologic and pelvic infections:* IV 300 mg, then PO 200 mg qd × 7-14 days
- *Intraabdominal infections:* IV 300 mg, then PO 200 mg qd × 7-14 days
- *Nongonococcal urethritis (female) and cervicitis:* PO 200 mg qd × 5 days
- *Pelvic inflammatory disease:* PO 200 mg qd × 14 days
- *Pneumonia, community acquired:* PO 200 mg qd × 7-14 days
- *Pneumonia, hospital acquired:* IV 300 mg, then PO 200 mg qd × 10-14 days
- *Chronic bacterial prostatitis:* PO 200 mg qd × 28 days
- *Cystitis:* PO 100 mg qd × 3 days
- *Prophylaxis of infection associated with elective colorectal surgery or hysterectomy:* IV 200 mg or PO 200 mg
- Dose change for renal disease: none
- Dose change for hepatic disease (mild-moderate cirrhosis): for 300 mg IV, substitute 200 mg IV; for 200 mg IV or PO, substitute 100 mg IV or PO; for 100 mg PO, no change

💲 AVAILABLE FORMS/COST OF THERAPY
- Inj, Sol—IV (alatrovafloxacin): 200 mg/40 ml, 1's: **$36.79**
- Tab—Oral (trovafloxacin): 100 mg, 30's: **$177.69;** 200 mg, 30's: **$215.09**

PRECAUTIONS: Pregnancy, lactation, age <18 yr, chronic liver disease (e.g., cirrhosis), **reported to cause unpredictable life-threatening hepatotoxicity, which is more common with therapy longer than 14 days (see http://www.fda.gov/cder/news/trovan/trovan-advisory.htm for more information)**

PREGNANCY AND LACTATION: Pregnancy category C; excreted in breast milk

SIDE EFFECTS/ADVERSE REACTIONS

CNS: Anxiety, dizziness (11%), headache, light-headedness

GI: Abdominal pain, diarrhea, *elevated transaminases (9% with 28-day course),* **hepatic failure (1 per 25,000 patients receiving trovafloxacin),** nausea (8%), vomiting

GU: Vaginitis

HEME: Prolonged INR (even if not taking warfarin)

MS: Arthralgia, tendinitis

SKIN: Photosensitivity, rash

INTERACTIONS

Drugs

3 *Aluminum:* Reduced absorption of trovafloxacin; do not take within 4 hr of dose

3 *Antacids:* Reduced absorption of trovafloxacin; do not take within 4 hr of dose

3 *Antipyrine:* Inhibits metabolism of antipyrine; increased plasma antipyrine level

3 *Calcium:* Reduced absorption of trovafloxacin; do not take within 4 hr of dose

3 *Diazepam:* Inhibits metabolism of diazepam; increased plasma diazepam level

3 *Didanosine:* Markedly reduced absorption of trovafloxacin; take trovafloxacin 2 hr before didanosine

3 *Foscarnet:* Coadministration increases seizure risk

3 *Iron:* Reduced absorption of trovafloxacin; do not take within 4 hr of dose

3 *Magnesium:* Reduced absorption of trovafloxacin; do not take within 4 hr of dose

3 *Metoprolol:* Inhibits metabolism of metoprolol; increased plasma metoprolol level

3 *Morphine:* Reduced absorption of trovafloxacin; do not take within 2 hr of dose

3 *Pentoxifylline:* Inhibits metabolism of pentoxifylline; increased plasma pentoxifylline level

3 *Phenytoin:* Inhibits metabolism of phenytoin; increased plasma phenytoin level

3 *Propranolol:* Inhibits metabolism of propranolol; increased plasma propranolol level

3 *Ropinirole:* Inhibits metabolism of ropinirole; increased plasma ropinirole level

3 *Sodium bicarbonate:* Reduced absorption of trovafloxacin; do not take within 4 hr of dose

3 *Sucralfate:* Reduced absorption of trovafloxacin; do not take within 4 hr of dose

3 *Warfarin:* Inhibits metabolism of warfarin; increases hypoprothrombinemic response to warfarin

3 *Zinc:* Reduced absorption of trovafloxacin; do not take within 4 hr of dose

SPECIAL CONSIDERATIONS
PATIENT/FAMILY EDUCATION
• Do not take antacids (aluminum, calcium, or magnesium-containing) or iron within 2 hr of taking trovafloxacin. Take at bedtime or with food to minimize dizziness associated with trovafloxacin. Avoid excessive sunlight during treatment

MONITORING PARAMETERS
• Transaminases if given for more than 7 days

undecylenic acid
(un-de-sye-len'ik)
OTC: Caldesene, Cruex, Desenex, Fungoid Topical Solution, Protectol
Chemical Class: Hendecenoic acid derivative
Therapeutic Class: Antifungal

CLINICAL PHARMACOLOGY
Mechanism of Action: Interferes with fungal cell membrane permeability; fungistatic
Pharmacokinetics: Improvement may be seen within 1 wk
INDICATIONS AND USES: Tinea cruris, tinea pedis, tinea corporis, diaper rash
DOSAGE
Adult and Child
• TOP apply to affected areas bid for 2-4 wk

$ **AVAILABLE FORMS/COST OF THERAPY**
• Tincture—Top: 2%, 30 ml: **$10.50**
• Cre—Top: 1%, 15 g: **$5.28**
• Oint—Top: 15, 30 g: **$1.80-$7.40**/30 g
• Powder—Top: 45, 60, 120 g: **$2.10-$5.15**/60 g
• Spray—Top: 2%, 85 g: **$4.64-$4.93**
PRECAUTIONS: Impaired circulation; diabetes mellitus; broken, pustular skin; puncture wounds; children <2 yr
PREGNANCY AND LACTATION: Problems not documented in breast feeding
SIDE EFFECTS/ADVERSE REACTIONS
SKIN: Skin irritation
SPECIAL CONSIDERATIONS
• Newer topical antifungals more effective
• Powders are generally used as adjunctive therapy, but may be useful for primary therapy in very mild cases

U

---

italic = common side effects   ***bold italic*** = life-threatening reactions

urea

(yoor-ee'a)

Rx: *Parenteral:* Ureaphil
Topical: Gordon's Urea 40%;
OTC: *Topical:* Aqua Care,
Carmol, Gormel, Lanaphilic
Ultramide, Nutraplus,
Ureacin

Chemical Class: Carbonic
acid diamide salt
Therapeutic Class: Osmotic
agent; antiglaucoma agent

CLINICAL PHARMACOLOGY
Mechanism of Action: Systemic;
elevates plasma osmolality, increasing flow of water from tissues into
blood, including the brain and the
eye; Topical: promotes hydration;
removes excess keratin

Pharmacokinetics
IV: Onset of action 10 min, peak
effect 1-2 hr, duration of action 3-10
hr (diuresis and decreased CSF pressure), 5-6 hr (reduced intraocular
pressure); excreted in urine; crosses
placenta; excreted in breast milk
INDICATIONS AND USES: Parenteral: cerebral edema, glaucoma; has
been used for induction of abortion
by intra-amniotic injection; topical:
emollient, hydration, and removal
of hyperkeratotic skin
DOSAGE
Adult and Child >2 yr
• IV 0.5-1.5 g/kg as 30% sol in 5%
or 10% dextrose over ½-2 hr at rate
not exceeding 4 ml/min, max 2 g/kg/
day
• TOP apply bid-qid
Child <2 yr
• IV 0.1-1.5 g/kg as sol as described
and administered for adults
**💲 AVAILABLE FORMS/COST
OF THERAPY**
• Inj, Dry-Sol—IV: 40 g: **$88.66**

• Lotion—Top: 10%, 180/240/480
ml: **$5.89-$7.95**/240 ml; 15%, 120
g: **$5.90**; 25%, 105/240 ml: **$15.50**/
240 ml
• Cre—Top:10%, 75/90/454 g:
$5.78/75 g; 20%, 75/90/120/454/
22% g: **$6.35**/90 g, 22%, 30 g:
$13.75; 30%, 60 g: **$6.50**; 40%,
30/90 g: **$19.48-$24.95**/30 g
• Paste—Top: 50%, 60 g: **$14.28**
• Oint—Top: 10%, 180/454/480 g:
$3.85/180 g; 20%, 454/480 g: **$7.50**/
480 g
CONTRAINDICATIONS: Severe renal disease, active intracranial bleeding (except during craniotomy), severe dehydration, liver failure
PRECAUTIONS: Hepatic disease,
renal disease, electrolyte imbalances,
cardiac disease, CHF, hypovolemia
PREGNANCY AND LACTATION:
Pregnancy category C; no data on
breast feeding available
SIDE EFFECTS/ADVERSE REACTIONS
For systemic use:
CNS: Disorientation, dizziness, fever, *headache,* syncope
CV: Postural hypotension, tachycardia, venous thrombosis
GI: Nausea, vomiting
HEME: **Hemolysis, intraocular
bleeding**
METAB: Dehydration, hypokalemia,
hyponatremia
SKIN: Extravasation, phlebitis

SPECIAL CONSIDERATIONS
• Do not infuse into lower extremity veins
• Monitor for extravasation, tissue
necrosis may occur

urokinase

(yoor-oh-kine'ase)
Rx: Abbokinase, Abbokinase Open-Cath (not for systemic administration)
Chemical Class: Renal enzyme
Therapeutic Class: Thrombolytic

CLINICAL PHARMACOLOGY
Mechanism of Action: Promotes thrombolysis by directly converting plasminogen to plasmin
Pharmacokinetics: Onset of fibrinolysis is rapid, duration ≥4 hr; cleared by liver, small amount excreted in urine and bile; unknown if crosses placenta or if excreted in breast milk; $t_{1/2}$ 10-20 min

INDICATIONS AND USES: Massive pulmonary embolism (PE); arteriovenous cannula occlusion; acute myocardial infarction; thrombotic stroke*; arterial thrombosis,* arterial embolism*

DOSAGE
Adult and Child
• *Pulmonary embolism and arterial or venous thrombosis:* IV 4400 IU/kg over 10 min followed by 4400 IU/kg/hr for 12 hr; after thrombin time has decreased to less than twice normal control value (approx 3-4 hr), begin heparin (no loading dose)
• *Venous catheter occlusion:* Instill into catheter a volume of urokinase (5000 IU/ml) equal to the internal volume of catheter over 1-2 min; aspirate from catheter 1-4 hr later, flush catheter with saline, may repeat with 10,000 U/ml sol if not cleared
• *Acute myocardial infarction (adult):* Intracoronary (following IV heparin bolus of 2500 to 10,000 units) 6000 IU/min for up to 2 hr

(average dose 500,000 IU); repeat angiography q15min until artery maximally opened; continuing heparin therapy recommended

$ AVAILABLE FORMS/COST OF THERAPY
• Inj, Lyphl-Sol—IV: 5000 U/ml, 1 ml: **$59.59** (not for systemic administration); 9000 U/vial: **$103.91** (not for systemic administration); 250,000 U/vial: **$467.78**

CONTRAINDICATIONS: (Systemic therapy only, no contraindications to use for declotting catheter); active bleeding, intraspinal surgery, CNS neoplasms; ulcerative colitis, enteritis; coagulation defects; rheumatic valvular disease; cerebral embolism, thrombosis, hemorrhage within 2 mo; intra-arterial diagnostic procedure, surgery, or trauma within 10 days; severe hypertension

PRECAUTIONS: Moderate hypertension, recent lumbar puncture, patients receiving IM medications, renal disease, hepatic disease, childbirth within 10 days, diabetic retinopathy, age >75 yr

PREGNANCY AND LACTATION: Pregnancy category B; no data available on breast feeding

SIDE EFFECTS/ADVERSE REACTIONS
CV: MI, tachycardia, transient hypertension or hypotension
GI: Nausea, vomiting
HEME: Internal bleeding (GI, GU, vaginal, IM, retroperitoneal or intracranial sites), surface bleeding
METAB: Acidosis
RESP: Bronchospasm, dyspnea, hypoxemia
SKIN: Rash
MISC: Chills, fever

INTERACTIONS
Drugs
▪ *Heparin, oral anticoagulants, drugs that alter platelet function (i.e.,*

---

italic = common side effects   ***bold italic*** = life-threatening reactions

aspirin, dipyridamole, abciximab, eptifibitide, tirofiban): May increase the risk of bleeding

---

ursodiol
(your-soo'dee-ol)
Rx: Actigall, Urso
Chemical Class: Ursodeoxycholic acid
Therapeutic Class: Cholelitholytic

CLINICAL PHARMACOLOGY
Mechanism of Action: Decreases cholesterol content of bile and gallstones by reducing hepatic cholesterol secretion and reabsorption of cholesterol by the intestine
Pharmacokinetics
PO: 90% absorption from small bowel; 1st-pass hepatic clearance; conjugates secreted into bile; peak concentration 1-3 hr, $t_{1/2}$ 100 hr
INDICATIONS AND USES: Dissolution of radiolucent, non-calcified gallbladder stones (<20 mm in diameter) for which surgery is not indicated; chronic cholestatic liver disease*
DOSAGE
Adult
• PO 8-10 mg/kg/day in 2-3 divided doses; perform gallbladder ultrasound q6mo to determine if stones have dissolved; if so, continue therapy, repeat ultrasound within 1-3 mo; maintenance therapy 250 mg qhs for 6-12 mo; safety beyond 24 mo not established
Child
• *Cholestatic liver disease:* PO 10-18 mg/kg/day
🚺 **AVAILABLE FORMS/COST OF THERAPY**
• Cap, Gel—Oral: 300 mg, 100's: **$262.52**
• Tab—Oral: 250 mg, 100's: **$194.64**

CONTRAINDICATIONS: Calcified cholesterol stones, radiopaque stones, stones >20 mm in diameter, bile pigment stones, patients with compelling reasons for cholecystectomy (cholangitis, biliary obstruction)
PRECAUTIONS: Children, chronic liver disease, non-visualizing gallbladder
PREGNANCY AND LACTATION: Pregnancy category B; excretion into breast milk unknown
SIDE EFFECTS/ADVERSE REACTIONS
CNS: Anxiety, depression, fatigue, headache, insomnia
EENT: Metallic taste, rhinitis
GI: Abdominal pain, constipation, diarrhea, dyspepsia, flatulence, nausea, stomatitis, vomiting
MS: Arthralgia, back pain, myalgia
RESP: Cough
SKIN: Alopecia, dry skin, pruritus, rash, sweating, urticaria
SPECIAL CONSIDERATIONS
• Complete dissolution may not occur; likelihood of success is low if partial stone dissolution not seen by 12 mo
• Stones recur within 5 yr in 50% of patients
PATIENT/FAMILY EDUCATION
• Administer with food to facilitate dissolution in the intestine

---

valacyclovir
(val-a-sye'kloe-ver)
Rx: Valtrex
Chemical Class: Acyclovir derivative
Therapeutic Class: Antiviral

CLINICAL PHARMACOLOGY
Mechanism of Action: Converted to acyclovir triphosphate, causing decreased viral DNA synthesis

---

* = non-FDA-approved use

Pharmacokinetics

PO: Rapidly absorbed from GI tract and converted to acylovir by 1st-pass intestinal or hepatic metabolism; bioavailability 55% not altered by food; plasma protein binding 14%-18%; excreted in urine (89%) and feces; $t_{1/2}$ of acyclovir 2.5-3.3 hr (14 hr in end-stage renal disease)

INDICATIONS AND USES: Herpes zoster in immunocompetent adults; initial episode and episodic treatment of recurrent genital herpes in immunocompetent adults; suppression of recurrent episodes of genital herpes in immunocompetent adults

DOSAGE

• *Herpes zoster:* PO 1 g tid for 7 days within 72 hr of onset of rash; for CrCl 30-49 ml/min 1 g q12h, CrCl 10-29 ml/min 1 g q24h, CrCl <10 ml/min 500 mg q24h

• *Initial episode genital herpes:* PO 1 g bid for 10 days; for CrCl 10-29 ml/min 1 g qd, CrCl <10 ml/min 500 mg qd

• *Recurrent genital herpes:* PO 500 mg bid for 5 days; for CrCl <30 ml/min, 500 mg qd

• *Chronic suppression of genital herpes:* PO 500-1000 mg qd (if <9 attacks per year, start with 500 mg); for CrCl <30 ml/min, 500 mg q48h

⑧ AVAILABLE FORMS/COST OF THERAPY

• Cap—Oral: 500 mg, 42's: **$127.07-$194.46**

PRECAUTIONS: Renal insufficiency, hepatic insufficiency, elderly, children

PREGNANCY AND LACTATION: Pregnancy category B; acyclovir excreted into breast milk, safety not established but should be compatible with breast feeding

SIDE EFFECTS/ADVERSE REACTIONS

CNS: Dizziness, headache

GI: Abdominal pain, anorexia, constipation, diarrhea, nausea, vomiting

GU: Renal dysfunction

*HEME: **Anemia, thrombocytopenia***

SPECIAL CONSIDERATIONS

• Acyclovir 400 mg PO bid less expensive for chronic suppression of genital herpes

---

valproate/divalproex

(val-proe′ate)

Rx: *Valproate Sodium:* Depacon
Valproic acid: Depakene
Divalproex: Depakote, Depakote Sprinkle

Chemical Class: Carboxylic acid derivative
Therapeutic Class: Anticonvulsant

CLINICAL PHARMACOLOGY

Mechanism of Action: Increases levels of gamma-aminobutyric acid (GABA), inhibitory neurotransmitter in brain; divalproex dissociates to the valproate ion in the GI tract

Pharmacokinetics

PO: Onset 15-30 min, peak 1-5 hr (slower absorption with sprinkles and food), $t_{1/2}$ 6-16 hr (shorter with younger age and serum levels lower in polytherapy; 40-60 hr in newborns)

RECT: Onset slow, duration 4-6 hr, $t_{1/2}$ 6-16 hr

Metabolized by liver, excreted by kidneys and in feces; crosses placenta; excreted into breast milk

INDICATIONS AND USES: Simple, complex (petit mal) absence, mixed, tonic-clonic (grand mal) seizures, mania in bipolar disorders in adults (divalproex sodium), prophylaxis of adult migraine (divalproex sodium)

V

---

italic = common side effects   ***bold italic*** = life-threatening reactions

DOSAGE
Adult
Epilepsy:

• PO for monotherapy 5-15 mg/kg/day divided in 1-3 doses, may increase by 5-10 mg/kg/day qwk; for polytherapy, initial dose 10-30 mg/kg/day, if dose exceeds 250 mg qd, divide into 2 or more doses, max 60 mg/kg/day; IV same as PO; administer as 60 min infusion at a rate not exceeding 20 mg/min

Mania: (Divalproex sodium)

• PO 750 mg/day in divided doses; increase until desired effect or plasma concentration at trough of 50-125 µg/ml; max 60 mg/kg/day

Migraine:

• PO 250 mg bid; dose may be increased up to 1000 mg/d if necessary

Child

• PO same as adult; children receiving polytherapy may require doses up to 100 mg/kg/day in 3-4 divided doses

• RECT dilute syr 1:1 with water; give loading dose 17-20 mg/kg once as retention enema; maintenance 10-15 mg/kg/day q8h

💲 AVAILABLE FORMS/COST OF THERAPY

Valproic acid:

• Cap, Elastic—Oral: 250 mg, 100's: **$36.10-$154.14**

• Syr—Oral: 250 mg/5 ml, 480 ml: **$29.00-$162.26**

Divalproex sodium:

• Cap, Enteric Coated (Sprinkle)—Oral: 125 mg, 100's: **$42.45**

• Tab, Enteric Coated—Oral: 125 mg, 100's: **$42.24;** 250 mg, 100's: **$82.93;** 500 mg, 100's: **$152.94**

Valproate sodium:

• Inj—IV: 100 mg/ml, 5 ml: **$9.85**

CONTRAINDICATIONS: Hepatic disease

PRECAUTIONS: Renal disease, Addison's disease, blood dyscrasias; children <2 yr, patients with organic brain disease, and patients on multiple anticonvulsants (polytherapy) at increased risk of hepatotoxicity

PREGNANCY AND LACTATION: Pregnancy category D; teratogenic; increased risk of neural tube defects (1%-2% when used between day 17-30 after fertilization); compatible with breast feeding

SIDE EFFECTS/ADVERSE REACTIONS

CNS: Ataxia, behavioral changes, *coma,* depression, diplopia, dizziness, *drowsiness, encephalopathy,* hallucinations, headache, incoordination, nystagmus, paresthesia, *sedation,* tremors

GI: Anorexia, *constipation,* cramps, *diarrhea, heartburn, hepatic failure,* nausea, *pancreatitis,* stomatitis, *vomiting*

GU: Amenorrhea, breast enlargement, enuresis, galactorrhea, irregular menses

HEME: Anemia, hypofibrinogenemia, leukopenia, lymphocytosis, *thrombocytopenia*

METAB: Abnormal thyroid function tests, carnitine deficiency, hyperammonemia, hyperglycemia, hyponatremia, syndrome of inappropriate antidiuretic hormone release

SKIN: Alopecia, *erythema multiforme,* pruritis, *rash, Stevens-Johnson syndrome*

INTERACTIONS
Drugs

3 *Carbamazepine, phenytoin:* Increase, decrease, or no effect on carbamazepine and phenytoin concentrations

3 *Cholestyramine, colestipol:* Reduced absorption of valproic acid

3 *Clarithromycin, erythromycin, troleandomycin:* Increased valproic acid concentrations

---

* = non-FDA-approved use

3 *Clonazepam:* Absence seizure reported with concurrent use

3 *Clozapine:* Reduced serum clozapine concentrations

3 *Felbamate:* Increased valproic acid concentrations

3 *Isoniazid:* Increased valproic acid concentrations

3 *Lamotrigine:* Increased plasma lamotrigine concentrations; decreased valproic acid concentrations

3 *Nimodipine:* Increased nimodipine area under the plasma concentration-time curve

3 *Phenobarbital, primidone:* Increased phenobarbital levels

3 *Salicylates:* Increased valproate levels

3 *Zidovudine:* Increased zidovudine levels

Labs

• *False increase:* Serum free fatty acids

• *False positive:* Urinary ketones

SPECIAL CONSIDERATIONS
PATIENT/FAMILY EDUCATION

• Administer with food to decrease GI side effects

• Do not administer with carbonated beverages or milk

MONITORING PARAMETERS

• Therapeutic levels (draw just before next dose) 50-100 µg/ml

• ALT, AST, coagulation studies, and platelet count prior to and during therapy, especially 1st 6 mo

• Minor elevations in ALT, AST are frequent and dose related

valsartan
(val-sar′tan)
Rx: Diovan
Combinations
  Rx: with hydrochlorothiazide (Diovan HCT)
Chemical Class: Angiotensin II receptor antagonist
Therapeutic Class: Antihypertensive

CLINICAL PHARMACOLOGY
Mechanism of Action: Antihypertensive (inhibition of vasoconstriction and aldosterone secretion), smooth muscle hypoproliferative, and cardioprotective effects are attributable to selective blockade of angiotensin II (AT1) receptors found throughout the cardiovascular and renal systems; effects independent of angiotensin II synthesis

Pharmacokinetics
PO: Peak 2-4 hr, duration 24 hr; steady state maximal reduction in blood pressure 2-4 wk; bioavailability approx 25%; food decreases exposure significantly; elimination as unchanged drug in feces (83%) and urine (13%); $t_{1/2}$ 6 hr

INDICATIONS AND USES: Hypertension; CHF,* myocardial infarction,* diabetic nephropathy

DOSAGE
Adult
• *Hypertension:* PO 80-320 mg qd

💲 **AVAILABLE FORMS/COST OF THERAPY**

• Caps—Oral: 80 mg, 100's: **$121.00;** 160 mg, 100's: **$121.00**

• Caps—Oral (with hydrochlorothiazide): 12.5 mg-80 mg, 100's: **$121.00;** 12.5 mg-160 mg, 100's: **$121.00**

PRECAUTIONS: Angioedema (associated with aspirin and/or penicillin allergy), aortic or mitral valve

V

---

italic = common side effects   **bold italic** = life-threatening reactions

stenosis, biliary cirrhosis or biliary obstruction, breast feeding period, coronary artery disease, elderly patients, hepatic dysfunction (adjust dose), hypertrophic cardiomyopathy, hypotension (sodium- or volume-depleted patients), pregnancy, renal artery stenosis, solitary kidney, or congestive heart failure

PREGNANCY AND LACTATION: Pregnancy category C, first trimester—category D, second and third trimesters; drugs acting directly on the renin-angiotensin-aldosterone system are documented to cause fetal harm (hypotension, oligohydramnios, neonatal anemia, hyperkalemia, neonatal skull hypoplasia, anuria, and renal failure); neonatal limb contractures, craniofacial deformities, and hypoplastic lung development

SIDE EFFECTS/ADVERSE REACTIONS

CNS: Dizziness, headaches
CV: Palpitations
GI: Abdominal pain, constipation, diarrhea, dyspepsia, flatulence, liver function test abnormalities
GU: Impotence
METAB: Hyperkalemia
MS: Back pain, muscle cramps, myalgia
RESP: Cough, dyspnea, pharyngitis, rhinitis, sinusitis
SKIN: Pruritus and rash
MISC: Anemia, fatigue, angioedema

SPECIAL CONSIDERATIONS

• Potentially as or more effective than angiotensin-converting enzyme inhibitors, without cough; no evidence for reduction in morbidity and mortality as first-line agents in hypertension, yet; whether they provide the same cardiac and renal protection also still tentative; like ACE inhibitors, less effective in black patients

PATIENT/FAMILY EDUCATION

• Call your clinician immediately if note following side effects: wheezing; lip, throat, or face swelling; hives or rash

MONITORING PARAMETERS

• Baseline electrolytes, urinalysis, BUN and creatinine with recheck at 2-4 wk after initiation (sooner in volume-depleted patients); monitor sitting blood pressure; watch for symptomatic hypotension, particularly in volume-depleted patients

---

vancomycin

(van-koe-mye′sin)
Rx: Lyphocin, Vancocin, Vancoled
Chemical Class: Tricyclic glycopeptide derivative
Therapeutic Class: Antibiotic

CLINICAL PHARMACOLOGY

Mechanism of Action: Inhibits bacterial cell wall synthesis, cell membrane permeability, and RNA synthesis; bactericidal against Gram-positive organisms, except bacteriostatic against enterococci

Pharmacokinetics

PO: Absorption poor
IV: 15 mg/kg over 60 min yields mean plasma concentration of 63, 23, and 8 µg/ml immediately, 2 hr, and 8 hr after INF; penetrates inflamed meninges, and into inflamed pleural, pericardial, ascitic, and synovial fluids, urine, peritoneal dialysis fluid, atrial appendage tissue, and bile; 55% protein bound; $t_{1/2}$ 4-8 hr; excreted in urine (active form); linearly associated with creatinine clearance; therapeutic serum concentrations, peak 25-40 µg/ml, trough <5-10 µg/ml

INDICATIONS AND USES: Serious or severe Gram-positive infections not treatable with other antimicro-

---

bials, including penicillins and cephalosporins, caused by susceptible organisms (e.g., endocarditis, osteomyelitis, pneumonia, and pseudomembranous colitis)

Antibacterial spectrum usually includes:

• Gram-positive organisms: Staphylococci, streptococci, *enterococcus*

• Anaerobes: *C. difficile*

DOSAGE

Note: Administer IV doses over 60 min; prevents "red-neck syndrome"

Adult

• *Serious staphylococcal infections:* IV 500 mg q6h or 1 g q12h

• *Pseudomembranous, staphylococcal enterocolitis:* PO 500 mg to 2 g/day in 3-4 divided doses for 7-10 days

• *Dosage adjustment for renal impairment:* After initial loading dose of 750 mg to 1 g, CrCl 50-80 ml/min 1 g q1-3d, CrCl 10-50 ml/min 1 g q3-7d, CrCl <10 1 g q7-14d; guided by serum vancomycin concentrations

Child

• *Serious staphylococcal infections:* IV 40 mg/kg/day divided q6h

Neonates

• *Serious staphylococcal infections:* IV 15 mg/kg initially followed by 10 mg/kg q8-12h

• *Pseudomembranous, staphylococcal enterocolitis:* PO 40 mg/kg/day divided q6h, not to exceed 2 g/day

$ **AVAILABLE FORMS/COST OF THERAPY**

• Inj, Conc-Sol—IV: 500 mg/vial: **$7.80-$8.92;** 1 g/vial: **$16.08-$17.73**

• Cap, Gel—Oral: 125 mg, 20's: **$107.56;** 250 mg, 20's: **$215.13**

CONTRAINDICATIONS: Decreased hearing

PRECAUTIONS: Renal disease, elderly, neonates

PREGNANCY AND LACTATION: Pregnancy category C (oral), B (IV); excreted into breast milk, milk level 4 hr after steady state dose, 12.7 µg/ml (similar to mother's trough level); poorly absorbed orally, systemic absorption not expected; problems limited to modification of bowel flora, allergic sensitization, and interference with interpretation of culture results during fever workup

SIDE EFFECTS/ADVERSE REACTIONS

*CV: **Cardiac arrest, vascular collapse***

EENT: Ototoxicity, permanent deafness, tinnitus

HEME: Eosinophilia, ***leukopenia, neutropenia***

GI: Nausea

*GU: **Nephrotoxicity***

RESP: Dyspnea, wheezing

SKIN: Chills, fever, necrosis with extravasation (red man's syndrome or "red-neck syndrome"), pruritus, rash, thrombophlebitis at inj site, urticaria

INTERACTIONS

Drugs

⚅ *Aminoglycosides:* Enhanced nephrotoxicity

⚅ *Indomethacin:* Increased vancomycin in neonates, possible vancomycin toxicity

⚅ *Methotrexate:* Reduced methotrexate concentrations with oral vancomycin

Labs

• *False increase:* CSF protein

SPECIAL CONSIDERATIONS
MONITORING PARAMETERS

• Audiograms, BUN, creatinine, serum vancomycin concentrations

V

---

italic = common side effects   ***bold italic*** = life-threatening reactions

vasopressin

(vay-soe-press'in)
Rx: Pitressin
Chemical Class: Arginine
vasopressin
Therapeutic Class: Antidiuretic; hemostatic

CLINICAL PHARMACOLOGY
Mechanism of Action: A posterior pituitary hormone product; has ADH activity (promotes renal tubular reabsorption of water) and vasopressor activity (vascular smooth muscle contraction)

Pharmacokinetics

IM/SC: Antidiuretic activity duration 2-8 hr

Metabolized or destroyed in liver, kidneys; excreted in urine; t₁/₂ 15 min

INDICATIONS AND USES: Neurogenic diabetes insipidus, treatment of abdominal distension postoperatively, prior to abdominal x-rays to dispel interfering gas shadows, bleeding esophageal varices*

DOSAGE
Adult

• *Diabetes insipidus:* IM/SC 5-10 U bid-tid as needed

• *Abdominal distension:* IM 5 U, increasing to 10 U after 3-4 hr if needed

• *Abdominal x-rays:* IM/SC 10 U given 2 hr and then ½ hr prior to x-rays

• *Esophageal varices:* IV or selective intra-arterial: 0.2 U/min initially, increased to 0.4 U/min if bleeding continues (max 0.9 U/min)

Child

• *Diabetes insipidus:* IM/SC 2.5-10 U bid-qid as needed

💲 AVAILABLE FORMS/COST OF THERAPY

• Inj, Sol—IM, SC: 20 U/ml, 2 ml: **$8.50**

CONTRAINDICATIONS: Chronic nephritis

PRECAUTIONS: Vascular disease (especially CAD), epilepsy, migraine, asthma, CHF

PREGNANCY AND LACTATION: Pregnancy category C; breast feeding reported without complications

SIDE EFFECTS/ADVERSE REACTIONS

CNS: Drowsiness, flushing, headache, lethargy, tremor, vertigo

CV: Angina, *cardiac arrest,* circumoral pallor, decreased cardiac output, *dysrhythmias,* gangrene, hypertension, *MI,* peripheral vasoconstriction

GI: Cramps, flatus, heartburn, nausea, vomiting

GU: Uterine cramping, vulvar pain

METAB: Hyponatremia

RESP: Bronchial constriction

SKIN: Sweating, urticaria, vasoconstriction or necrosis with extravasation

SPECIAL CONSIDERATIONS

• For diabetes insipidus, vasopressin sol for injection may be administered intranasally on cotton pledgets, by nasal spray or by dropper; dose must be individualized

PATIENT/FAMILY EDUCATION

• Common adverse effects (skin blanching, abdominal cramps, and nausea) may be reduced by taking 1-2 glasses of water with the dose of vasopressin; self-limited in minutes

MONITORING PARAMETERS

• ECG, fluid and electrolyte status

• Extravasation may cause tissue necrosis

---

* = non-FDA-approved use

venlafaxine

(ven-la-fax´een)
Rx: Effexor, Effexor XR
Chemical Class: Phenethylamine derivative
Therapeutic Class: Antidepressant

CLINICAL PHARMACOLOGY

Mechanism of Action: Potentiation of neurotransmitter activity in the CNS by strong inhibition of neuronal serotonin and norepinephrine reuptake and weak inhibition of dopamine reuptake; no anticholinergic, sedation, or orthostatic hypotensive activity

Pharmacokinetics

PO: Peak level 1-2 hr, steady state level of drug and active metabolites achieved in 3 days; absorption 92% (no change with food); protein binding 27%; metabolized by cytochrome p450 system in liver, unchanged drug and metabolites excreted in urine; elimination $t_{1/2}$ 3-7 hr for drug, 9-13 hr for active metabolites; clearance of drug and active metabolites reduced by 50% in cirrhotics, reduced by 25% if CrCl 10-70 ml/min, and reduced by 60% in dialysis patients

INDICATIONS AND USES: Depression, obsessive-compulsive disorder,* generalized anxiety disorder

DOSAGE

Adult

• PO starting dose 75 mg/day, given bid or tid (qd for SUS REL); increase daily dose by 75 mg up to 225 mg/day, given bid or tid (qd for SUS REL) (375 mg/day for severe depression) at intervals of no less than 4 days

• Reduce total daily dose 25% in patients with mild to moderate renal impairment, by 50% in patients with severe renal impairment; dialysis patients should receive dose after dialysis; reduce total daily dose by 50% in patients with moderate hepatic impairment

• When discontinuing drug, taper over 2 wk

💲 **AVAILABLE FORMS/COST OF THERAPY**

• Tab, Uncoated—Oral: 25 mg, 100's: **$112.83;** 37.5 mg, 100's: **$116.20;** 50 mg, 100's: **$119.66;** 75 mg, 100's: **$126.88;** 100 mg, 100's: **$134.48**

• Cap, SUS REL—Oral: 37.5 mg, 100's: **$200.46;** 75 mg, 100's: **$224.53;** 150 mg, 100's: **$244.56**

CONTRAINDICATIONS: Concurrent use of MAOIs (at least 14 days should elapse between discontinuation of an MAOI and initiation of venlafaxine; at least 7 days should be allowed after stopping venlafaxine before starting an MAOI), age <18 yr

PRECAUTIONS: Hypertension, anxiety, seizures, aggravation of bipolar disorder (0.5%)

PREGNANCY AND LACTATION: Pregnancy category C; excretion into breast milk unknown

SIDE EFFECTS/ADVERSE REACTIONS

*CNS: Anxiety, dizziness, insomnia, nervousness, **seizures (0.3%),** somnolence, tremor

CV: Hypertension (dose dependent; frequency 3%-13%), *vasodilation*

EENT: Blurred vision, dry mouth, dysgeusia, mydriasis, tinnitus

GI: Anorexia, dyspepsia, *nausea,* vomiting

GU: Abnormal ejaculation or orgasm; impotence, urinary retention

RESP: Yawning

SKIN: Sweating

MISC: Asthenia

SPECIAL CONSIDERATIONS

• Do not stop abruptly

---

italic = common side effects   ***bold italic*** = life-threatening reactions

verapamil
(ver-ap'a-mill)
Rx: Calan, Calan SR, Covera HS, Isoptin, Isoptin SR, Verelan
Combinations
  Rx: with trandolapril (Tarka)
Chemical Class: Phenylalkylamine
Therapeutic Class: Calcium channel blocker, antihypertensive; antianginal; antidysrhythmic (Class IV)

CLINICAL PHARMACOLOGY
Mechanism of Action: Inhibits calcium ion influx across cell membrane during cardiac depolarization; produces relaxation of coronary vascular smooth muscle; dilates coronary arteries; slows SA/AV node conduction; dilates peripheral arteries; hemodynamics: decreases myocardial contractility and peripheral vascular resistance; can decrease or increase cardiac output
Pharmacokinetics
IV: Onset 3 min, peak 3-5 min, duration 10-20 min
PO: Onset variable (30 min for non-sustained-release preparations), peak serum concentration 1-2.2 hr, duration 17-24 hr, 90% absorption; extensive 1st-pass metabolism; bioavailability 20%-35%; 83%-90% protein bound; metabolized by liver to norverapamil (20% activity of verapamil), excreted in urine (96% as metabolites); $t_{1/2}$ (biphasic) 4 min, 3-7 hr (terminal)
INDICATIONS AND USES: Chronic stable angina pectoris, vasospastic angina, unstable angina, dysrhythmias (atrial flutter, atrial fibrillation, paroxysmal supraventricular tachycardia [PSVT]), hypertension, prophylaxis of migraine headaches,* cardiomyopathy (diastolic dysfunction)
DOSAGE
Adult
• *Angina:* PO initial 80-120 mg tid; titrate to 480 mg/day based on response (adjust dose weekly)
• *Dysrhythmias (atrial fibrillation/digitalized):* PO 240-320 mg/day in tid or qid dosage
• *Dysrhythmias (supraventricular tachycardia):* IV bolus initial 5-10 mg over 2 min; repeat dose 10 mg, 30 min after 1st if ineffective
• *Hypertension:* PO 80 mg bid initially, increase as need to 480 mg/d divided bid; SUS REL 180-240 mg qd initially, increase as need up to 360 mg/day
Child 0-1 yr
• *Dysrhythmias (PSVT):* IV bolus 0.1-0.2 mg/kg over >2 min with ECG monitoring; repeat if necessary in 30 min
Child 1-15 yr
• *Dysrhythmias (PSVT):* IV bolus 0.1-0.3 mg/kg over >2 min; repeat in 30 min; not to exceed 10 mg in a single dose
⑤ AVAILABLE FORMS/COST OF THERAPY
• Inj, Sol—IV: 2.5 mg/ml, 2 ml: **$2.44-$12.99**
• Tab ER—Oral: 120 mg, 100's: **$86.21-$112.14**
• Tab, Coated, SUS REL—Oral: 180 mg, 100's: **$99.80-$142.11;** 240 mg, 100's: **$114.14-$170.44;**
• Tab, Plain Coated—Oral: 40 mg, 100's: **$27.25-$41.45;** 80 mg, 100's: **$9.19-$59.62;** 120 mg, 100's: **$12.30-$80.63**
• Cap, SUS REL—120 mg, 100's: **$129.05-$145.00;** 100 mg, 100's: **$135.00;** 180 mg, 100's: **$135.16-$151.86;** 200 mg, 100's: **$162.50;**

* = non-FDA-approved use

240 mg, 100's: **$152.54-$171.39; 300 mg, 100's: $225.00; 360 mg, 100's: $209.94-$235.89**

CONTRAINDICATIONS: Sick sinus syndrome, 2nd or 3rd degree heart block, hypotension less than 90 mm Hg systolic, cardiogenic shock, severe CHF

PRECAUTIONS: CHF, hypotension, hepatic injury, children, renal disease, concomitant IV β-blocker therapy, cirrhosis, Duchenne's muscular dystrophy

PREGNANCY AND LACTATION: Pregnancy category C; excreted in breast milk (approx 25% of maternal serum); compatible with breast feeding

SIDE EFFECTS/ADVERSE REACTIONS

CNS: Asthenia, dizziness, headache, lightheadedness

CV: **AV block,** bradycardia, **CHF,** edema, hypotension, palpitations

GI: Constipation, nausea

GU: Nocturia, polyuria

SKIN: Rash

INTERACTIONS

Drugs

🔳 *Amiodarone:* Cardiotoxicity with bradycardia and decreased cardiac output

🔳 *Barbiturates:* Reduced plasma concentrations of verapamil

🔳 *Benzodiazepines:* Marked increase in midazolam concentrations, increased sedation likely to result

🔳 *Beta-blockers:* β-blocker serum concentrations increased *(atenolol, metoprolol, propranolol);* increased risk of bradycardia, hypotension, AV conduction, and myocardial contractility

❷ *Carbamazepine:* Increased carbamazepine toxicity when verapamil added to chronic anticonvulsant regimens; reduced metabolism

🔳 *Cimetidine:* Increased verapamil concentrations and effect by cimetidine

🔳 *Cyclosporine, tacrolimus:* Increased concentrations of these drugs, nephrotoxicity possible

🔳 *Dantrolene:* Hyperkalemia and myocardial depression may occur; consider a dihydropyridine calcium blocker

🔳 *Diclofenac:* Reduced verapamil concentrations

🔳 *Digitalis glycosides:* Increased digoxin concentrations by approximately 70%

🔳 *Doxazosin, prazosin, terazosin:* Enhanced hypotensive effects

🔳 *Doxorubicin:* Increased doxorubicin concentrations

🔳 *Encainide:* Increased encainide concentrations

🔳 *Ethanol:* Increased ethanol concentrations, prolonged and increased levels of intoxication

🔳 *Fentanyl:* Severe hypotension or increased fluid volume requirements

🔳 *Histamine H_2-antagonists:* Increased blood levels of verapamil with cimetidine

🔳 *Hydantoins:* Serum verapamil levels may fall if used concurrently

🔳 *Imipramine:* Increased imipramine concentrations

🔳 *Lithium:* Potential for neurotoxicity

🔳 *Neuromuscular blocking agents:* Prolonged neuromuscular blockade

🔳 *Quinidine:* Quinidine toxicity via inhibition of metabolism

🔳 *Rifampin, rifabutin:* Induced metabolism; reduced verapamil concentrations

🔳 *Sulfinpyrazone:* Increased clearance of verapamil

🔳 *Theophylline:* Verapamil inhibits metabolism, increases theophylline levels

V

italic = common side effects   ***bold italic*** = life-threatening reactions

3 *Vitamin D:* Therapeutic efficacy of verapamil may be reduced

SPECIAL CONSIDERATIONS

• Dihydropyridine calcium channel blockers preferred over verapamil and diltiazem in patients with sinus bradycardia, conduction disturbances, and for combination with a β-blocker

• Differentiate PSVT from narrow complex ventricular tachycardia prior to IV administration; failure to do so has resulted in fatalities

---

vidarabine

(vye-dare'a-been)

Rx: Vira-A

Chemical Class: Nucleoside analog

Therapeutic Class: Antiviral

CLINICAL PHARMACOLOGY

Mechanism of Action: Inhibits bacterial and viral replication by preventing DNA synthesis

Pharmacokinetics

OPHTH: Minimal systemic absorption

INDICATIONS AND USES: Acute keratoconjunctivitis and recurrent epithelial keratitis; superficial keratitis caused by susceptible organisms

Antiviral spectrum usually includes herpes simplex virus 1 and 2, varicella zoster, and vaccinia viruses, except for rhabdovirus and oncornavirus; minimal activity against other RNA or DNA viruses

DOSAGE

Adult and Child

• OPHTH: ½ inch ribbon to lower lid 5 times daily (q3h); after re-epithelialization, treat for 7 more days at bid

💲 AVAILABLE FORMS/COST OF THERAPY

• Oint—Ophth: 3%, 3.5g: **$24.81**

PREGNANCY AND LACTATION:
Pregnancy category C

SIDE EFFECTS/ADVERSE REACTIONS

EENT: Burning, pain, photophobia, stinging, temporary visual haze

INTERACTIONS

Drugs

3 *Allopurinol:* Increased vidarabine toxicity

SPECIAL CONSIDERATIONS

• Trifluridine is more effective; vidarabine is not the drug of choice in any viral infection; however, it may be a useful alternative in patients who cannot tolerate or have failed other antiviral therapy

---

vitamin A

Rx: Aquasol A

Chemical Class: Fat soluble vitamin

Therapeutic Class: Vitamin

CLINICAL PHARMACOLOGY

Mechanism of Action: Involved in bone and tooth development, visual dark adaptation, skin disease, mucosa tissue repair, assists in production of adrenal steroids, cholesterol, RNA

Pharmacokinetics

PO/IM: Stored in liver, kidneys, fat; transported in plasma as retinol, bound to retinol-binding protein, excreted (metabolites) in bile bound to glucuronide and small amount in urine

INDICATIONS AND USES: Vitamin A deficiency

DOSAGE

Adult and Child >8 yr

• PO 100,000-500,000 IU qd × 3 days, then 50,000 qd × 2 wk; dose based on severity of deficiency; maintenance 10,000-20,000 IU qd for 2 mo

---

Child 1-8 yr
• IM 5,000-15,000 IU qd × 10 days; then maintenance as follows:
Child 4-8 yr
• IM 15,000 IU qd × 2 mo
Child <4 yr
• IM 10,000 IU qd × 2 mo
Infants <1 yr
• IM 5,000-15,000 IU × 10 days

💲 **AVAILABLE FORMS/COST OF THERAPY**
• Cap, Elastic—Oral: 25,000 U, 100's: **$4.50-$50.07**; 50,000 U, 100's: **$5.50-$87.10**
• Inj, Sol—IM: 50,000 U/ml, 2 ml: **$22.17**

CONTRAINDICATIONS: Malabsorption syndrome (PO)
PRECAUTIONS: Impaired renal function
PREGNANCY AND LACTATION: Pregnancy category A; safety of exceeding 5000/6000 IU PO/IV recommended daily allowance (RDA) not established; naturally present in breast milk, deficiency rare, RDA during lactation is 6000 IU; danger of higher doses unknown
SIDE EFFECTS/ADVERSE REACTIONS
CNS: Headache, increased intracranial pressure, intracranial hypertension, lethargy, malaise
EENT: Exophthalmos, gingivitis, inflammation of tongue and lips, papilledema
GI: Abdominal pain, anorexia, jaundice, nausea, vomiting
METAB: Hypercalcemia, hypomenorrhea
MS: Arthralgia, hard areas on bone, retarded growth
SKIN: Alopecia, drying of skin, increased pigmentation, night sweats, pruritus
INTERACTIONS
Drugs
③ *Acitretin, etretinate:* Large doses

of vitamin A should be avoided with these retinoids
SPECIAL CONSIDERATIONS
PATIENT/FAMILY EDUCATION
• Administer with food for better PO absorption
• Foods high in vitamin A: yellow and dark green vegetables, yellow and orange fruits, A-fortified foods, liver, egg yolks

---

vitamin D (cholecalciferol, vitamin D₃; ergocalciferol, vitamin D₂)

(cole'ee-cal-sif'er-ol; er'go-cal-sif'erol)
Rx: Calciferol, Drisdol
OTC: Calciferol, Drisdol
Chemical Class: Fat soluble vitamin
Therapeutic Class: Vitamin

CLINICAL PHARMACOLOGY
Mechanism of Action: Participates in regulation of calcium, phosphate, bone development, parathyroid activity, neuromuscular functioning; synthesis in two steps: hydroxylation in the liver (to 25-hydroxy vitamin D) and in the kidneys (to 1,25-dihydroxy vitamin D); parathyroid hormone is responsible for regulation of metabolism in the kidneys
Pharmacokinetics
PO/INJ: Lag of 10 to 24 hr between the administration of vitamin D and the initiation of its action in the body due to the necessity of synthesis of active metabolites; max hypercalcemic effects at 4 wk, duration 2 mo, readily absorbed from small intestine (bile is essential for adequate absorption), t₁/₂ 7-12 hr; stored in liver; excreted in bile (metabolites) and urine

V

---

italic = common side effects   ***bold italic*** = life-threatening reactions

INDICATIONS AND USES: Dietary supplement, vitamin D deficiency, refractory rickets, renal osteodystrophy, hypoparathyroidism, hypophosphatemia, hypocalcemic tetany, osteoporosis

DOSAGE

NOTE: The range between therapeutic and toxic doses is narrow; calcium intake must be adequate; cholecalciferol 1 mg provides 40,000 U vitamin D activity; ergocalciferol 1.25 mg provides 50,000 IU of vitamin D activity

Adult

• Dietary supplementation (including prevention of osteoporosis): PO 400-800 IU qd

• *Vitamin D deficiency:* PO/IM 12,000 IU qd, then increase to 500,000 IU qd

• *Vitamin D-resistant rickets:* PO/IM 12,000 to 500,000 IU qd

• *Hypoparathyroidism:* PO/IM 25,000 to 200,000 IU qd concomitantly with calcium lactate 4 g, administered 6 times/day

• Refractory rickets: PO/IM 12,000-500,000 IU qd (with phosphate supplements)

• Familial hypophosphatemia: PO/IM 10,000-80,000 IU qd (with 1-2 g/day elemental phosphorous)

Child

• Dietary supplementation: PO 400 IU qd

• *Vitamin D deficiency:* PO/IM 1500-5000 IU qd × 2-4 wk, may repeat after 2 wk or 600,000 IU as single dose

• *Hypoparathyroidism:* PO/IM 50,000-200,000 IU qd (with calcium supplements)

• Refractory rickets: PO/IM 400,000-800,000 IU qd (with phosphate supplements)

§ AVAILABLE FORMS/COST OF THERAPY

• Cap, Elastic—Oral: 50,000 U D_2, 100's: **$5.78-$108.68**

• Liq—Oral: 8000 U/ml D_2, 60 ml (OTC): **$47.50-$73.14**

• Tab—Oral: 400 IU D_3, 100's: **$2.08**

• Inj—IM: 500,000 IU/ml, D_2, 1 ml amp: **$25.96**

CONTRAINDICATIONS: Hypercalcemia, renal dysfunction, hyperphosphatemia, abnormal sensitivity to the toxic effects of vitamin D and hypervitaminosis D

PRECAUTIONS: Cardiovascular disease, renal calculi, elderly

PREGNANCY AND LACTATION: Pregnancy category A (400 IU/d); category D (doses above recommended daily allowance) associated with supravalvular aortic stenosis, elfin facies, and mental retardation; caution should be exercised when ergocalciferol is administered to nursing women; vitamin D and metabolites appear in breast milk; compatible with breast feeding, but infant should be monitored for hypercalcemia if doses exceed recommended daily allowance

SIDE EFFECTS/ADVERSE REACTIONS

CNS: Drowsiness, fatigue, headache, psychosis, *seizures,* weakness, anorexia

CV: Dysrhythmias, hypertension, vascular calcification

GI: Constipation, cramps, diarrhea, dry mouth, metallic taste, nausea, vomiting, *pancreatitis,* elevated ALT/AST

GU: Albuminuria, decreased libido, hematuria, nocturia, polyuria, reversible azotemia

METAB: Hypercholesterolemia, mild acidosis

MS: Bone pain, muscle pain, weakness

---

* = non-FDA-approved use

SKIN: Photophobia, pruritus

MISC: Weight loss

INTERACTIONS

Labs

• *Interference:* Serum cholesterol

SPECIAL CONSIDERATIONS

• IM therapy should be reserved for patients with GI, liver, or biliary disease associated with vitamin D malabsorption

• Ensure adequate calcium intake; maintain serum calcium levels between 9-10 mg/dL

MONITORING PARAMETERS

• Serum calcium and phosphorus levels (vitamin D levels also helpful, although less frequently)

• Height and weight in children

• X-ray bones monthly until condition is corrected and stabilized

• Periodically determine magnesium and alk phosphatase

• Serum calcium times phosphorous should not exceed 70 mg/dL to avoid ectopic calcification

---

vitamin E

OTC: Aquasol E, E-400, Gordon's Vite E

Chemical Class: Fat soluble vitamin

Therapeutic Class: Vitamin

CLINICAL PHARMACOLOGY

Mechanism of Action: Involved in digestion and metabolism of polyunsaturated fats, decreases platelet aggregation, decreases blood clot formation, promotes normal growth and development of muscle tissue, prostaglandin synthesis

Pharmacokinetics

PO: Metabolized in liver, excreted in bile

INDICATIONS AND USES: Vitamin E deficiency, impaired fat absorption,* hemolytic anemia in premature neonates,* prevention of retrolental fibroplasia,* sickle cell anemia,* supplement in malabsorption syndrome*; reduction of the risk of second MI in patients with CAD*

DOSAGE

Adult

• *Vitamin E deficiency:* PO/IM 60-75 IU qd, not to exceed 300 IU/day

• *Secondary prevention of MI:* PO 400-800 IU/d

Child

• *Vitamin E deficiency:* PO/IM 1 IU/kg/day

AVAILABLE FORMS/COST OF THERAPY

• Cap, Gel—Oral: 100 IU, 100's: **$1.75-$82.04;** 200 IU, 100's: **$2.20-$3.78;** 400 IU, 100's: **$2.90-$12.00;** 600 IU, 100's: **$9.45;** 1000 IU, 100's: **$12.98**

• Sol, Drops—Oral: 50 IU/ml, 12 ml: **$22.51**

PREGNANCY AND LACTATION: Pregnancy category A (C if used above recommended daily allowance doses); recommended daily allowance in pregnancy is 15 IU; excreted into breast milk, 5 times richer in vitamin E than cow's milk; U.S. recommended daily allowance of vitamin E during lactation is 16 IU

SIDE EFFECTS/ADVERSE REACTIONS

CNS: Fatigue, headache

EENT: Blurred vision

GI: Cramps, diarrhea, nausea

GU: Gonadal dysfunction

METAB: Altered metabolism of thyroid, pituitary, and adrenal hormones

MS: Weakness

SKIN: Contact dermatitis, sterile abscess

INTERACTIONS

Drugs

⬛ *Iron:* Impaired hematological response to iron in children with iron-deficiency anemia

⬛ *Oral anticoagulants:* Vitamin E increases hypoprothombinemic re-

V

sponse to oral anticoagulants, especially in doses >400 IU/day
SPECIAL CONSIDERATIONS
• Recommended daily allowance adult male 15 IU, adult female 12 IU

---

warfarin

(war'far-in)
Rx: Coumadin, Warfilone
Chemical Class: Coumarin derivative
Therapeutic Class: Oral anticoagulant

CLINICAL PHARMACOLOGY

Mechanism of Action: Interferes with hepatic synthesis of vitamin K-dependent clotting factors, causing depression in the activity of factors II, VII, IX, X and proteins C and S in a dose-dependent manner; has no direct effect on established thrombus, but prevents further extension of formed clot

Pharmacokinetics

PO: Rapidly and completely absorbed, peak activity 1½-3 days, duration 2-5 days; 97%-99% bound to plasma proteins; metabolized by hepatic microsomal enzymes; excreted in urine and feces (inactive metabolites); $t_{1/2}$ 36 hr

INDICATIONS AND USES: Prophylaxis and treatment of: venous thrombosis; pulmonary embolism; atrial fibrillation with embolism; thromboembolic complications associated with cardiac valve replacement; and death, recurrent MI, and systemic embolism after MI; recurrent transient ischemic attack,* hypercoagulable states*

DOSAGE

Adult

• PO initiate with 5 mg qd for 2-4 days; adjust dosage according to INR determinations; make dose adjustments in 5-20% increments based on weekly dose of warfarin; usual maintenance dose 2-10 mg qd based on INR determinations

Child

• PO 0.1 mg/kg/day with a range of 0.05-0.34 mg/kg/day; adjust dosage according to INR determinations; consistent anticoagulation may be difficult to maintain in children <5 yr

AVAILABLE FORMS/COST OF THERAPY

• Sol, Inj—IV; 5 mg, **$18.73**
• Tab, Uncoated—Oral: 1 mg, 100's: **$50.87-$56.52;** 2 mg, 100's: **$53.08-$58.98;** 2.5 mg, 100's: **$54.76-$60.84;** 3 mg, 100's: **$57.67-$61.08;** 4 mg, 100's: **$55.13-$61.26;** 5 mg, 100's: **$55.51-$61.68;** 6 mg, 100's: **$82.57-$87.48;** 7.5 mg, 100's: **$81.43-$90.48;** 10 mg, 100's: **$84.46-$93.84**

CONTRAINDICATIONS: Active bleeding, hemorrhagic blood dyscrasias; hemorrhagic tendencies, history of bleeding diathesis, recent cerebral hemorrhage; active ulceration of the GI tract; ulcerative colitis; open traumatic or surgical wounds; recent or contemplated brain, eye, spinal cord surgery, or prostatectomy; regional or lumbar block anesthesia; bacterial endocarditis; pericarditis; visceral carcinoma; severe or malignant hypertension; eclampsia or pre-eclampsia; threatened abortion; emaciation; pregnancy; history of warfarin-induced skin necrosis; uncooperative patient

PRECAUTIONS: Trauma, infection, renal insufficiency, hypertension, vasculitis, indwelling catheters, severe diabetes, active tuberculosis, postpartum, protein C deficiency, hepatic insufficiency, elderly, children, hyperthyroidism, hypothyroidism,

---

* = non-FDA-approved use

CHF, polyarteritis, diverticulitis, antibiotic therapy, malnutrition

PREGNANCY AND LACTATION: Pregnancy category X; use in 1st trimester carries significant risk to the fetus; exposure in the 6th-9th wk of gestation may produce a pattern of defects termed the fetal warfarin syndrome with an incidence up to 25% in some series; compatible with breast feeding for normal, full-term infants

SIDE EFFECTS/ADVERSE REACTIONS

GI: Anorexia, cholestatic jaundice, *hepatotoxicity,* mouth ulcers, nausea, paralytic ileus, sore mouth, vomiting

GU: Albuminuria, anuria, red-orange urine, *renal tubular necrosis*

HEME: *Hemorrhage, leukopenia*

SKIN: Alopecia, dermatitis, *exfoliative dermatitis, necrosis or gangrene of skin and other tissues,* urticaria

MISC: Systemic cholesterol microembolization ("purple toe" syndrome)

INTERACTIONS

Drugs

3 *Acetaminophen:* Repeated doses of acetaminophen may increase the hypoprothrombinemic response to warfarin

3 *Allopurinol, amiodarone, ciprofloxacin, clarithromycin, erythromycin, fluconazole, fluorouracil, fluvastatin, fluvoxamine, glucagon, isoniazid, itraconazole, ketoconazole, lovastatin, miconazole, nalidixic acid, neomycin (oral), norfloxacin, ofloxacin, propafenone, propoxyphene, quinidine, sertraline, sulfonamides, sulfonylureas, thyroid hormones, triclofos, troleandomycin, vitamin E, zafirlukast:* Enhanced hypoprothrombinemic response to warfarin

3 *Aminoglutethimide, carbamazepine, cyclophosphamide, ethchlorvynol, griseofulvin, mercaptopurine, methimazole, mitotane, nafcillin, propylthiouracil, vitamin K:* Reduced hypoprothrombinemic response to warfarin

2 *Aspirin:* Increased risk of bleeding complications

2 *Azathioprine, chloramphenicol, cimetidine, clofibrate, co-trimoxazole, danazole, dextrothyroxine, disulfiram, gemfibrozil, metronidazole, sulfinpyrazone, testosterone derivatives:* Enhanced hypoprothrombinemic response to warfarin

2 *Barbiturates, glutethimide, rifampin:* Reduced hypoprothrombinemic response to warfarin

3 *Bile acid-binding resins:* Variable effect on hypoprothrombinemic effect of warfarin

2 *Cephalosporins:* Enhanced hypoprothrombinemic response to warfarin with moxalactam, cefoperazone, cefamandole, cefotetan, and cefmetazole

3 *Chloral hydrate:* Transient increase in hypoprothrombinemic response to warfarin

3 *Ethanol:* Enhanced hypoprothrombinemic response to warfarin with acute ethanol intoxication

3 *Heparin:* Prolonged activated partial thromboplastin time in patients receiving heparin; prolonged prothrombin times in patients receiving warfarin

3 *Mesalamine:* Warfarin effect inhibited in one case report

2 *NSAIDs:* Increased risk of bleeding in anticoagulated patients

2 *Oral contraceptives:* Increase or decrease in anticoagulant response; increased risk of thromboembolic disorders

3 *Phenytoin:* Transient increase in hypoprothrombinemic response to

w

warfarin with initiation of phenytoin therapy, followed within 1-2 wk by inhibition of hypoprothrombinemic response to warfarin

3 *Salicylates:* Increased risk of bleeding in anticoagulated patients; enhanced hypoprothrombinemic response to warfarin with large salicylate doses

Labs

• *Interference:* May cause orange-red discoloration of urine, which may interfere with some lab tests

SPECIAL CONSIDERATIONS

• Avoid use of initial doses >5 mg
• INR during 1st 5 days of therapy does not correlate with degree of anticoagulation
• Anticoagulant effect of warfarin may be reversed by administration of vitamin K or fresh frozen plasma; should only use in situations where INR is severely elevated >10, or when patient is actively bleeding

PATIENT/FAMILY EDUCATION

• Strict adherence to prescribed dosage schedule is necessary
• Avoid alcohol, salicylates, and drastic changes in dietary habits
• Do not change from one brand to another without consulting clinician

MONITORING PARAMETERS

• Dosage of anticoagulants must be individualized and adjusted according to INR determinations; it is recommended that INR determinations be performed prior to initiation of therapy, at 24-hr intervals while maintenance dosage is being established, then once or twice weekly for the following 3-4 wk, then at 1-4 wk intervals for the duration of treatment
• Maintain INR at 2-3 (2.5-3.5 for mechanical valves, recurrent systemic thromboembolism)

---

xylometazoline
(zye-loe-met-az'oh-leen)
OTC: Otrivin
Chemical Class: Imidazoline derivative
Therapeutic Class: Decongestant

CLINICAL PHARMACOLOGY
Mechanism of Action: Local α-adrenergic-mediated vasoconstriction on dilated nasal mucosal blood vessels

Pharmacokinetics
NASAL: Onset 5-10 min, duration 5-6 hr, occasionally enough drug is absorbed to produce systemic effects

INDICATIONS AND USES: Relief of nasal congestion associated with acute or chronic rhinitis, common cold, sinusitis, and hay fever or other allergies

DOSAGE
Adult
• INSTILL 2-3 gtt or sprays of 0.1% sol into each nostril q8-10h; do not exceed 3 administrations in 24 hr; should not be used for longer than 3-5 days

Child 2-12 yr
• INSTILL 2-3 gtt of 0.05% sol into each nostril q8-10h; do not exceed 3 administrations in 24 hr; should not be used for longer than 3-5 days

$ AVAILABLE FORMS/COST OF THERAPY
• Sol, Drops—Nasal: 0.05%, 25 ml: **$5.89;** 0.1%, 25 ml: **$6.84**
• Sol, Spray—Nasal: 0.1%, 20 ml: **$5.36**

CONTRAINDICATIONS: Angle-closure glaucoma

PRECAUTIONS: Children <2 yr, hyperthyroidism, heart disease, hypertension, diabetes mellitus

---

PREGNANCY AND LACTATION: Pregnancy category C

SIDE EFFECTS/ADVERSE REACTIONS

CNS: Dizziness, headache, nervousness, weakness

CV: Cardiac irregularities, hypertension

EENT: Anosmia; dryness, rebound congestion and hyperemia, sneezing, stinging, transient burning, ulceration of nasal mucosa

GI: Nausea

SKIN: Sweating

SPECIAL CONSIDERATIONS
• Manage rebound congestion by stopping xylometazoline: one nostril at a time, substitute systemic decongestant, substitute inhaled steroid

PATIENT/FAMILY EDUCATION
• Do not use for >3-5 days or rebound congestion may occur

---

yohimbine
(yoe-him'been)
Rx: Actibine, Aphrodyne, Dayto-Himbin, Testomar, Yocon, Yohimar, Yohimex, Yoman

Chemical Class: Indolalkylamine derivative
Therapeutic Class: Anti-impotence agent

CLINICAL PHARMACOLOGY
Mechanism of Action: Blocks presynaptic α_2-adrenergic receptors; increases parasympathetic (cholinergic) and decreases sympathetic (adrenergic) activity in peripheral autonomic nervous system; may increase penile blood inflow, decrease penile blood outflow, or both

Pharmacokinetics
No data available

INDICATIONS AND USES: No FDA-sanctioned indications; impotence of vascular or diabetic origins (data are sparse),* sexual dysfunction caused by selective serotonin reuptake inhibitors,* orthostatic hypotension*

DOSAGE
Adult
• *Impotence:* PO 5.4 mg tid
• *Orthostatic hypotension:* PO 12.5 mg/day in divided doses

💲 **AVAILABLE FORMS/COST OF THERAPY**
• Tab, Uncoated—Oral: 5.4 mg, 100's: **$7.00-$23.95**

CONTRAINDICATIONS: Renal disease, children

PRECAUTIONS: History of gastric or duodenal ulcer; generally not for use in females

PREGNANCY AND LACTATION: Do not use during pregnancy

SIDE EFFECTS/ADVERSE REACTIONS

CNS: Central excitation, dizziness, headache, increased motor activity, irritability, nervousness, tremor

CV: Increased or decreased blood pressure, increased heart rate

GI: Nausea, vomiting

GU: Antidiuresis

SKIN: Skin flushing, sweating

---

zafirlukast
(za-feer'loo-kast)
Rx: Accolate

Chemical Class: Tolylsulfonyl benzamide derivative
Therapeutic Class: Antiasthmatic; leukotriene receptor antagonist

---

CLINICAL PHARMACOLOGY
Mechanism of Action: Competitive and reversible antagonist of the leukotriene D_4 receptor; leukotriene D_4 increases airway reactivity and vascular permeability and causes bronchoconstriction

Pharmacokinetics

PO: Onset 1 hr, peak 2-4 hr, duration 12-14 hr; metabolized in liver by cytochrome 3A4 and 2C9, elimination $t_{1/2}$ 2 hr

INDICATIONS AND USES: Asthma (maintenance treatment), exercise-induced asthma*

DOSAGE

Adult and Child ≥12 yr

• *Asthma:* PO 20 mg bid on an empty stomach

• *Exercise-induced asthma:* PO 20 mg, taken 2 hr before exercise

$ **AVAILABLE FORMS/COST OF THERAPY**

• Tab—Oral: 20 mg, 60's: **$59.77**

PRECAUTIONS: Liver disease, severe asthma

PREGNANCY AND LACTATION: Pregnancy category C; breast milk excretion unknown

SIDE EFFECTS/ADVERSE REACTIONS

CNS: Headache (18%), somnolence, weakness

EENT: Pharyngitis (20%), rhinitis *(9%)*

GI: Dry mouth, elevated transaminase levels, gastritis

RESP: Cough, exacerbation of asthma

INTERACTIONS

Drugs

3 *Astemizole, terfenadine:* Zafirlukast inhibits drug metabolism with potential for cardiac dysrhythmias

3 *Warfarin:* Zafirlukast increases hypoprothrombinemic effect

SPECIAL CONSIDERATIONS

PATIENT/FAMILY EDUCATION

• Take regularly, even during symptom-free periods

MONITORING PARAMETERS

• ALT, AST, CBC

---

zalcitabine (ddC)

(zal-site'a-been)

Rx: Hivid

Chemical Class: Nucleoside analog

Therapeutic Class: Antiretroviral

CLINICAL PHARMACOLOGY

Mechanism of Action: Converted to active metabolite, dideoxycytidine 5'-triphosphate (ddCTP), by cellular enzymes; ddCTP serves as an alternative substrate to deoxycytidine triphosphate (dCTP) for HIV reverse transcriptase and inhibits the *in vitro* replication of HIV-1 by inhibition of viral DNA synthesis; incorporation into growing DNA chain leads to premature chain termination; ddCTP serves as a competitive inhibitor of the natural substrate, dCTP, for the active site of DNA polymerase, further inhibiting viral and cellular DNA synthesis

Pharmacokinetics

PO: Peak serum level 0.8 hr; bioavailability 80% (reduced by food); <4% bound to plasma proteins; phosphorylated intracellularly to ddCTP; excreted in urine; $t_{1/2}$ 1-3 hr

INDICATIONS AND USES: Combination therapy with zidovudine in advanced HIV infection (CD4 cell count ≤300/mm^3 with significant clinical or immunologic deterioration); monotherapy for advanced HIV in patients who are either intolerant to zidovudine or have disease progression while receiving zidovudine

DOSAGE

Adult and Children >12 yr, >30 kg

• PO 0.75 mg with 200 mg zidovudine q8h; for monotherapy 0.75 mg q8h; interrupt therapy with zalcitabine if signs or symptoms of pe-

---

ripheral neuropathy appear, reinstitute at 0.375 mg q8h if all findings related to peripheral neuropathy improve to mild symptoms

• *Renal function impairment:* PO (CrCl 10-40 ml/min) 0.75 mg q12h; (CrCl <10 ml/min) 0.75 mg q24h

• For latest treatment guidelines, see www.hivatis.org

$ **AVAILABLE FORMS/COST OF THERAPY**

• Tab, Uncoated—Oral: 0.375 mg, 100's: **$188.02;** 0.75 mg, 100's: **$235.67**

PRECAUTIONS: Low CD4 cell counts (<50/mm^3), existing peripheral neuropathy, history of pancreatitis, ethanol abuse, cardiomyopathy, CHF, renal or hepatic function impairment, children <13 yr

PREGNANCY AND LACTATION: Pregnancy category C

SIDE EFFECTS/ADVERSE REACTIONS

CNS: Dizziness, fever, headache, *peripheral neuropathy (28%)*

EENT: Pharyngitis

GI: Abdominal pain, anorexia, constipation, diarrhea, dry mouth, dyspepsia, dysphagia, esophageal ulcers, exacerbation of hepatic dysfunction, glossitis, nausea, *oral ulcers,* **pancreatitis,** vomiting

MS: Arthralgia, myalgia

SKIN: Night sweats, pruritus, rash

MISC: Fatigue, weight decrease

SPECIAL CONSIDERATIONS

• Consult the most recent guidelines for HIV antiviral therapy prior to prescribing

MONITORING PARAMETERS

• Periodic CBC, serum chemistry tests, transaminase levels

• Serum amylase and triglyceride concentrations in patients with history of elevated amylase, pancreatitis, ethanol abuse, or receiving parenteral nutrition

---

zidovudine

(zyde-o'vue-deen)
Rx: Retrovir
Combinations
  Rx: with lamivudine (Combivir)
Chemical Class: Nucleoside analog
Therapeutic Class: Antiretroviral

CLINICAL PHARMACOLOGY

Mechanism of Action: Converted by cellular thymidine kinase to zidovudine monophosphate, which is further converted to diphosphate by cellular thymidylate kinase and to triphosphate derivative by other cellular enzymes; triphosphate interferes with the HIV reverse transcriptase thus inhibiting viral replication

Pharmacokinetics

PO: Peak 30-90 min; 25%-38% bound to plasma proteins; metabolized in liver to inactive metabolites, 63%-95% excreted in urine as metabolites and unchanged drug; terminal $t_{1/2}$ 60 min

INDICATIONS AND USES: Treatment of HIV infection when antiretroviral therapy is indicated (should not be used as monotherapy); prevention of maternal-fetal HIV transmission

DOSAGE

Adult

• PO 600 mg/d in divided doses in combination with other antiretroviral agents; IV 1 mg/kg/dose infused over 1 hr q4h while awake (5 mg/kg/day)

• *Maternal-fetal HIV transmission:* Maternal dose (>14 wk of pregnancy) PO 100 mg 5 times/day until start of labor; during labor and delivery, IV zidovudine should be ad-

z

---

ministered at 2 mg/kg (total body weight) over 1 hr followed by continuous IV INF of 1 mg/kg/hr (total body weight) until clamping of the umbilical cord; infant dose PO 2 mg/kg q6h starting within 12 hr after birth and continuing through 6 wk of age; IV 1.5 mg/kg, infused over 30 min q6h

• For latest treatment guidelines see www.hivatis.org

Child 3 mo-12 yr

• PO 180 mg/m^2 taken q6h, max 200 mg q6h; IV INF 0.5-1.8 mg/kg/hr; IV 100 mg/m^2/dose q6h

• For latest treatment guidelines see www.hivatis.org

$ AVAILABLE FORMS/COST OF THERAPY

• Cap, Gel—Oral: 100 mg, 100's: **$168.68-$183.18**
• Tab—Oral: 300 mg, 60's: **$303.64**
• Inj, Conc, w/Buffer—IV: 10 mg/ml, 20 ml: **$18.24**
• Syr—Oral: 50 mg/5 ml, 240 ml: **$40.49-$45.52**

PRECAUTIONS: Bone marrow compromise (granulocyte count <1000 cells/mm^3 or Hgb <9.5 g/dl); hepatomegaly, hepatitis, or other known risk factor for liver disease; severely impaired renal or hepatic function; children

PREGNANCY AND LACTATION: Pregnancy category C; indicated for pregnant women >14 wk gestation for prevention of maternal-fetus HIV transmission

SIDE EFFECTS/ADVERSE REACTIONS

CNS: Anxiety, chills, confusion, depression, dizziness, emotional lability, fever, *headache, insomnia,* loss of mental acuity, paresthesia, *somnolence,* tremor, twitching

EENT: Hearing loss, photophobia, vertigo

GI: Anorexia, cholestatic hepatitis, constipation, cramps, *diarrhea, dys-*pepsia, dysphagia, flatulence, mouth ulcer, *nausea,* taste change, vomiting

GU: Dysuria, polyuria, urinary frequency or hesitancy

HEME: **Anemia, granulocytopenia, leukopenia, thrombocytopenia**

MS: Arthralgia, muscle spasm, *myalgia*

RESP: Dyspnea

SKIN: Acne, diaphoresis, pigmentation of nails (blue), pruritus, *rash,* urticaria

MISC: Malaise

INTERACTIONS

Drugs

3 *Food:* Taking zidovudine with meals lowers plasma concentrations

A *Ganciclovir:* Increased hematologic toxicity

3 *Interferon:* Increased plasma concentrations of zidovudine

3 *Probenecid:* Increased plasma concentration of zidovudine

3 *Rifampin:* Reduced plasma concentrations of zidovudine

SPECIAL CONSIDERATIONS

• Consult the most recent guidelines for HIV antiviral therapy prior to prescribing

PATIENT/FAMILY EDUCATION

• Close monitoring of blood counts is extremely important; does not reduce risk of transmitting HIV to others through sexual contact or blood contamination

MONITORING PARAMETERS

• CBC with differential and platelets q2wk initially for 2 mo, then q4-8 wk

zileuton

(zi-loo'ton)
Rx: Zyflo
Chemical Class: Not available
Therapeutic Class: Antiasthmatic; lipoxygenase inhibitor

CLINICAL PHARMACOLOGY
Mechanism of Action: Specific inhibitor of 5-lipoxygenase, the 1st enzymatic step in conversion of arachidonic acid to leukotrienes
Pharmacokinetics
PO: Onset 30 min, peak 1-3 hr, duration of effect 5-8 hr, oral absorption rapid; extensive 1st-pass metabolism primarily by glucuronidation with renal excretion of inactive metabolites; elimination $t_{1/2}$ 2-3 hr
INDICATIONS AND USES: Asthma (maintenance treatment); aspirin-induced wheezing,* allergic rhinitis,* ulcerative colitis*
DOSAGE
Adult and child ≥12 yr
• *Asthma:* PO 600 mg qid
$ AVAILABLE FORMS/COST OF THERAPY
• Tab—Oral: 600 mg, 120's: **$82.53**
CONTRAINDICATIONS: Active liver disease, unexplained transaminase elevation
PRECAUTIONS: Renal insufficiency, hepatic insufficiency
PREGNANCY AND LACTATION: Pregnancy category C; breast milk excretion unknown
SIDE EFFECTS/ADVERSE REACTIONS
CNS: Dizziness, fatigue, *headache,* insomnia, paresthesia
GI: Abdominal pain, *dyspepsia (8%),* elevated transaminase levels, nausea
SKIN: Rash, urticaria

SPECIAL CONSIDERATIONS
PATIENT/FAMILY EDUCATION
• Must be taken regularly, even during symptom free periods
• Not a bronchodilator, do not use to treat acute episodes of asthma
MONITORING PARAMETERS
• CBC, renal function, and transaminase levels periodically during 1st year of prolonged therapy

zinc sulfate/zinc acetate

Rx: Injection: Zinca-Pak
Oral: Galzin, Zincate
OTC: Oral: Orazinc 110, Orazinc 220, Verazinc, Zinc Sulfate 15, Zinc 15, Zinc 220
Ophthalmic: Eye-Sed
Chemical Class: Zinc salt
Therapeutic Class: Ophthalmic astringent; trace element; chelating agent

CLINICAL PHARMACOLOGY
Mechanism of Action: Vasoconstriction occurs by action on conjunctiva; needed for adequate healing, bone and joint development; in patients with Wilson's disease induces the production of metallothronein in the enterocyte, a protein that binds copper thereby preventing its transfer into the blood, the bound copper is then lost in the stool following desquamation of the intestinal cells
Pharmacokinetics
PO: Poorly absorbed, excreted mainly through the intestine
INDICATIONS AND USES: Dietary supplement, treatment or prevention of zinc deficiency; temporary relief of minor eye irritation (ophthalmic); chelation therapy maintenance in Wilson's disease (zinc acetate)

z

italic = common side effects   ***bold italic*** = life-threatening reactions

DOSAGE

Zinc sulfate:

Adult

• PO 110-220 mg (15-50 mg zinc) qd, recommended daily allowance 66 mg (15 mg zinc) qd; IV 2.5-4 mg/day in metabolically stable adults (add 2 mg/day for acute catabolic states)

• *Minor eye irritation:* Instill 1 gtt bid-tid

Child

• PO 0.3 mg/kg/day

• *Minor eye irritation:* Instill 1 gtt bid-tid

Zinc acetate:

Adult

• PO 50 mg tid; 25 mg tid may be appropriate in children >10 or pregnant women

$ AVAILABLE FORMS/COST OF THERAPY

Zinc sulfate:

• Sol—Ophth: 0.25%, 15 ml: **$2.72**

• Tab—Oral: 66 mg (15 mg zinc), 100's: **$1.45**; 110 mg (25 mg zinc), 100's: **$3.89**; 200 mg (45 mg zinc), 1000's: **$10.73**

• Cap, Gel—Oral: 220 mg, (50 mg zinc), 100's: **$6.92-$26.51**

• Inj, Sol—IV: 1 mg/ml, 10 ml: **$1.19-$2.50**; 5 mg/ml, 5 ml: **$2.46-$5.00**

Zinc acetate:

• Cap—Oral: 25 mg, 250's: **$154.80**; 50 mg, 250's: **$258.00**

PRECAUTIONS: Narrow-angle glaucoma (ophthalmic), excessive doses

PREGNANCY AND LACTATION: Pregnancy category A (in doses not exceeding recommended daily allowance); for zinc acetate, zinc has appeared in breast milk and zinc-induced copper deficiency may occur, nursing not recommended

SIDE EFFECTS/ADVERSE REACTIONS

EENT: Burning (ophthalmic), eye irritation

GI: Nausea, vomiting

INTERACTIONS

Drugs

3 *Ciprofloxacin, enoxacin, norfloxacin:* Reduced serum concentrations of these drugs

3 *Tetracycline:* Reduced serum tetracycline concentrations

SPECIAL CONSIDERATIONS

• Acetate not recommended for initial therapy of symptomatic Wilson's disease (should be treated initially with chelating agents)

PATIENT/FAMILY EDUCATION

• Take acetate on an empty stomach

MONITORING PARAMETERS

• 24 hr urine copper, LFTs (acetate)

---

zolmitriptan

(zohl-mih-trip'tan)

Rx: Zomig, Papimeh

Chemical Class: Serotonin derivative

Therapeutic Class: Antimigraine agent

CLINICAL PHARMACOLOGY

Mechanism of Action: Selectively activates vascular 5-HT$_1$ receptors in cranial arteries causing vasoconstriction and inhibition of proinflammatory neuropeptide release, actions correlating with the relief of migraine in humans

Pharmacokinetics

PO: Well absorbed, peak 2 hr (2-3 hr for active metabolite), absolute bioavailability 40%; 25% bound to plasma proteins; converted to an active N-desmethyl metabolite with 2 to 6 times the potency of the parent compound; excreted in urine (65%) and feces (30%); t$_{1/2}$ 3 hr (mean of parent drug and active metabolite)

INDICATIONS AND USES: Treatment of acute migraine with or without aura

DOSAGE

Adult

• PO 1.25-2.5 mg at first sign of headache; may repeat initial dose after 2 hr; max 10 mg/24 hr period; the safety of treating an average of more than 3 headaches in a 30 day period has not been established

$ AVAILABLE FORMS/COST OF THERAPY

• Tab, Film-coated—Oral: 2.5 mg, 6's: **$81.74**; 5 mg, 3's: **$46.48**

CONTRAINDICATIONS: Ischemic heart disease, coronary artery vasospasm, significant underlying cardiovascular disease; uncontrolled hypertension; use within 24 hr of another 5-HT$_1$ agonist, or an ergotamine-containing or ergot-type medication (e.g. dihydroergotamine or methysergide); hemiplegic or basilar migraine; within 2 weeks MAO inhibitor therapy; symptomatic Wolff-Parkinson-White syndrome

PRECAUTIONS: Hypertension, hypercholesterolemia, smokers, obesity, diabetes, strong family history of early CAD, peripheral vascular disease, impaired hepatic function (initiate therapy with low dose)

PREGNANCY AND LACTATION: Pregnancy category C; excretion into breast milk unknown, use caution in nursing mothers

SIDE EFFECTS/ADVERSE REACTIONS

CNS: Agitation, anxiety, depression, dizziness, emotional lability, insomnia, somnolence, vertigo

CV: Bradycardia, chest pain, ***dysrhythmia;*** edema, extrasystoles, hypertension, palpitations; postural hypotension, pressure or heaviness; syncope, tightness

EENT: Dry eyes, ear pain, eye pain, tinnitus

GI: Dry mouth, dyspepsia, dysphagia, nausea

GU: Hematuria, polyuria, urinary frequency, urinary urgency

MS: Myalgia, myasthenia

RESP: ***Bronchospasm,*** hiccup, laryngitis, yawning

SKIN: Pruritus, rash, sweating, urticaria

MISC: Asthenia; hyperesthesia, neck, throat, jaw pain, paresthesia, pressure or tightness, warm or cold sensations

INTERACTIONS

Drugs

3 *Cimetidine:* Increased zolmitriptan concentration

3 *Ergot-containing drugs:* Potential for prolonged vasospastic reactions and additive vasoconstrictions, theoretical precaution

2 *MAO inhibitors:* Increased zolmitriptan concentrations, increased potential for serotonin-related toxicity

2 *Sibutramine:* Increased risk for serotonin syndrome

SPECIAL CONSIDERATIONS

• Alternative to sumatriptan for the treatment of migraine headache; has not been compared head-to-head with sumatriptan; choice should be based on cost and availability

• First dose should be administered in medical office in case cardiac symptoms occur; take great care to exclude the possibility of silent cardiovascular disease prior to prescribing

• Doses >2.5 mg were not associated with more headache relief, but were associated with increased side effects; if no relief is obtained after first dose, a second dose is unlikely to provide any benefit

z

---

italic = common side effects   ***bold italic*** = life-threatening reactions

zolpidem
(zole-pi'dem)
Rx: Ambien
Chemical Class: Imidazopyridine derivative
Therapeutic Class: Hypnotic
DEA Class: Schedule IV

CLINICAL PHARMACOLOGY
Mechanism of Action: Subunit modulation of the GABA receptor is responsible for pharmacologic effects: sedative, anticonvulsant, anxiolytic, and myorelaxant properties; selective binding to the BZ, or omega, receptor may explain the preservation of deep sleep (stages 3 and 4) and the relative absence of myorelaxant and anticonvulsant effects
Pharmacokinetics
PO: Peak 1.6 hr (delayed by food); 92% bound to plasma proteins; converted in liver to inactive metabolites, eliminated primarily by renal excretion; $t_{1/2}$ 2½ hr
INDICATIONS AND USES: Short-term treatment of insomnia
DOSAGE
Adult
• PO 5-10 mg immediately before hs; do not exceed 10 mg/day
$ **AVAILABLE FORMS/COST OF THERAPY**
• Tab, Uncoated—Oral: 5 mg, 100's: **$173.84;** 10 mg, 100's: **$213.83**
PRECAUTIONS: Psychiatric disorders, elderly and/or debilitated patients, depression, abrupt discontinuation, concomitant systemic illness, compromised respiratory function, hepatic impairment, history of drug abuse, children <18 yr
PREGNANCY AND LACTATION: Pregnancy category B; excreted into breast milk in small amounts

SIDE EFFECTS/ADVERSE REACTIONS
CNS: Amnesia, anxiety, confusion, daytime drowsiness, dizziness, *headache,* irritability, lethargy, lightheadedness, poor coordination
CV: Chest pain, palpitation
GI: Abdominal pain, constipation, diarrhea, heartburn, nausea, vomiting
HEME: Granulocytopenia (rare), leukopenia
SPECIAL CONSIDERATIONS
PATIENT/FAMILY EDUCATION
• Take immediately prior to retiring
• Avoid alcohol
• Use caution driving or performing other tasks requiring alertness

---

* = non-FDA-approved use

Appendix A

Comparative Tables

The following comparative drug tables were developed by the authors to assist providers in choosing medications of a given therapeutic class. These tables allow clinicians to compare drugs on the basis of important pharmacologic or clinical characteristics. Whenever possible, the information is based on definitive drug data and should help the reader obtain maximal therapeutic effect with minimal adverse effects. When applicable, accepted clinical practice guidelines have been incorporated into the tables.

Tables:

Acid Secretion Inhibitors

Drug Name	Trade Name	Usual Adult Starting Oral Dose	Nonprescription Strength	Cost	Drug Interactions/ Comments	Dose Adjustment in Renal Dysfunction
H2 Blockers						
Cimetidine	Tagamet, Tagamet HB	300 mg qid or 800 mg hs	100 mg	$1.50 (300 mg)	Amiodarone, benzodiazepines, calcium channel blockers, carbamazepine, carmustine, cisapride, clozapine, flecainide, glipizide, glyburide, itraconazole, ketoconazole, lidocaine, lomustine, melphalan, meperidine, narcotic analgesics, phenytoin, praziquantel, procainamide, propafenone, quinidine, tacrine, theophylline, tolbutamide, tricyclic antidepressants, warfarin	Yes (CrCl <30 ml/min)
Famotidine	Pepcid, Pepcid AC	20 mg bid or 40 mg hs	10 mg	$1.77 (20 mg)	Cefpodoxime, cefuroxime, dihydropyridine calcium channel blockers, glipizide, glyburide, itraconazole, ketoconazole, quinolone antibiotics, tolbutamide	Yes (CrCl <50 ml/min)
Nizatidine	Axid, Axid AR	150 mg bid or 300 mg hs	NA	$1.78 (150 mg)	Cefpodoxime, cefuroxime, dihydropyridine calcium channel blockers, glipizide, glyburide, itraconazole, ketoconazole, quinolone antibiotics, tolbutamide	Yes (CrCl <50 ml/min)
Ranitidine	Zantac, Zantac 75	150 mg bid or 300 mg hs	NA	$1.48 (150 mg)	Cefpodoxime, cefuroxime, dihydropyridine calcium channel blockers, glipizide, glyburide, itraconazole, ketoconazole, quinolone antibiotics, tolbutamide	Yes (CrCl <50 ml/min)
Proton Pump Inhibitors						
Lansoprazole	Prevacid	15-30 mg qd	NA	$3.66 (15 mg); $3.73 (30 mg)	Cefpodoxime, cefuroxime, dihydropyridine calcium channel blockers, diazepam, digoxin, food, glipizide, glyburide, iron, itraconazole, ketoconazole, methotrexate, phenytoin, quinolone antibiotics, tolbutamide, warfarin	No
Omeprazole	Prilosec	20 mg qd	NA	$3.98 (20 mg)	Same as lansoprazole	No
Pantoprazole	Pantozol	40 to 80 mg qd	NA	NA	Same as lansoprazole but magnitude may be less; available in IV form	No
Rebeprazole	Aciphex	20 mg qd	NA	$3.70	Same as lansoprazole but magnitude may be less	No

Nonnarcotic Analgesics

Drug Name	Trade Name	Usual Adult Dose (mg)	Maximum Adult Daily Dose (mg)	Oral Dose Forms (mg)	Nonprescription Strength (mg)	Chemical Class	Comment
Acetaminophen	Tylenol	325–650 q4-6h	4000	80, 160, 325, 500, 650	All forms	Aminophenol	Hepatotoxicity if overdosed and in persons with cirrhosis (limit dose to 2000 mg/day in cirrhotics)
Salicylates							
Acetylsalicylic acid	Aspirin	325–975 q4h	6000	81, 165, 325, 500, 650, 975	All forms	Salicylate	Antagonizes effect of probenecid; increases effect of sulfonylureas; reduces renal clearance of methotrexate
Choline magnesium trisalicylate	Trilisate	500–1000 q12h	3000	500, 750, 1000	NA	Salicylate	Antagonizes effect of probenecid; increases effect of sulfonylureas; reduces renal clearance of methotrexate
Salsalate	Disalcid	500–1000 q8h 750–1500 q12h	3000	500, 750, 1000	NA	Salicylate	Antagonizes effect of probenecid; increases effect of sulfonylureas; reduces renal clearance of methotrexate
Short-acting NSAIDs							
Diclofenac	Cataflam	50 tid	200	25, 50	NA	Acetic acid	Formulation is immediate release
Diclofenac	Voltaren, Voltaren SR	25–75 bid-tid	200	25, 50, 75	NA	Acetic acid	Formulation is delayed release; also available in qd dose form
Fenoprofen	Nalfon	300–600 q6h	3200	200, 300, 600	NA	Propionic acid	Highly protein bound (to albumin); greater renal toxicity
Ibuprofen	Motrin, Rufen	400–600 q6h	3200	200, 300, 400, 600, 800	200	Propionic acid	Also approved for primary dysmenorrhea; available in combination with hydrocodone (Vicoprofen)

Continued

Nonnarcotic Analgesics—cont'd

Drug Name	Trade Name	Usual Adult Dose (mg)	Maximum Adult Daily Dose (mg)	Oral Dose Forms (mg)	Nonprescription Strength (mg)	Chemical Class	Comment
Indomethacin	Indocin, Indocin SR	25-50 q8h or 75 q12h (sustained release)	200	25, 50, 75 (sustained release)	NA	Acetic acid	Available in suppository, suspension, and sustained-release forms
Ketoprofen	Orudis, Oruvail	50-75 q6-8h	300	12.5, 25, 50, 75; 100, 150, 200 (sustained release)	12.5	Propionic acid	High rate of dyspepsia (11%), available in sustained-release form
Ketorolac	Toradol	10 q4-6h	40	10	NA	Acetic acid	100% bioavailable; indicated only as continuation of parenteral ketorolac, short term
Meclofenamate	Meclomen	50-100 q6h	400	50, 100	NA	Anthranilic acid	High rate of diarrhea (10%-33%)
Mefenamic acid	Ponstel	500, then 250 q6h	1000	250	NA	Anthranilic acid	Also approved for primary dysmenorrhea
Tolmetin	Tolectin	400 q6-8h	2000	200, 400, 600	NA	Acetic acid	High rate of nausea (11%)
Intermediate-acting NSAIDs							
Celecoxib	Celebrex	100-200 bid	400	100, 200	NA	NA	Cyclo-oxygenase 2 (COX-2) selective; rate of GI side effects equal to placebo
Diflunisal	Dolobid	500 q12h	1500	250, 500	NA	Salicylate derivative	Not metabolized to salicylate; increases acetaminophen level by 50% when coadministered
Etodolac	Lodine, Lodine XL	200-400 bid-qid	1200	200, 300	NA	Acetic acid	Antacids reduce peak concentration by 20%; long-acting form available

						Phenylalkanoic acid	May cause CNS stimulation
Flurbiprofen	Ansaid	50-100 bid-tid	300	50, 100	NA		
Naproxen	Naprosyn, Naprelan	250-500 q8-12h	1250	220, 250, 375, 500	220	Propionic acid	Approved for acute gout; may increase effect of protein-bound drugs such as phenytoin, sulfonylureas, and warfarin; available in qd dose form
Naproxen	Anaprox, Anaprox DS	275-550 q8-12h	1375	275, 550	220	Propionic acid	Approved for acute gout; may increase effect of protein-bound drugs such as phenytoin, sulfonylureas, and warfarin
Sulindac	Clinoril	150-200 q12h	400	150, 200	NA	Acetic acid	Approved for acute gout; less renal toxicity
Long-acting NSAIDs							
Nabumetone	Relafen	500-750 bid; 1000-1500 qd	1500	500, 750	NA	Nonacidic	High rate of diarrhea (14%); metabolized to active agent
Piroxicam	Feldene	10-20 qd	20	10, 20	NA	Oxicam	High rate of dyspepsia (20%); may increase effect of protein-bound drugs such as phenytoin, sulfonylureas, and warfarin
Oxaprozin	Daypro	1200 qd	1800	600	NA	Proprionic acid	
Rofecoxib	Vioxx	12.5-50 qd	12.5, 25, 50	50	NA	NA	Cyclo-oxygenase 2 (COX-2) selective; rate of GI side effects equal to placebo
Parenteral NSAID							
Ketorolac	Toradol	30 or 60 initially, then 15-30 q6h (all IM)	150 1st day, then 120 qd	15, 30, 60	NA	Acetic acid	Total duration of treatment should not exceed 5 days; 30 mg equal to 6-12 mg morphine sulfate but 10 times as expensive

Narcotic and Narcotic-Like Analgesics

Drug Name	Trade Name	Usual Adult Dose (mg) and Routes	Parenteral Dose (mg) Equal to 10 mg Morphine Sulfate IM	Oral Dose (mg) Equal to Listed Parenteral Dose	Comment
Narcotic-like agents					
Buprenorphine	Buprenex	0.3 q6h IM	0.3	NA	Mixed agonist-antagonist; schedule V controlled substance
Butorphanol	Stadol	1-4 q3-4h IM, Nasal	2-3	NA	Mixed agonist-antagonist; not a controlled substance
Nalbuphine	Nubain	10 q6h IM, IV, or SC	10	NA	Mixed agonist-antagonist; not a controlled substance
Tramadol	Ultram	50-100 q4-6h PO	NA	NA	100 mg equianalgesic to 60 mg codeine; long term use may cause dependence and withdrawal syndromes; toxicity includes seizures
Narcotics					
Fentanyl	Sublimaze, Duragesic (transdermal)	0.05-0.1 q1-2h IM or IV; 25-100 µg/h transdermal (base dose on total morphine dose); 0.2-0.4 as lozenge	0.125	NA	Primary use is IV or epidural for perioperative or patient-controlled analgesia; transdermal form available but costly
Oxymorphone	Numorphan	1-1.5 q4-6h IM; 5 q4-6h PR	1	NA	Major use is perioperative
Hydromorphone	Dilaudid	2 q4-6h PO; 1-2 q4-6h IM; 3 q6-8h PR	1.5	7.5	High abuse potential

Levorphanol	Levo-Dromoran	2 q6-8h PO	NA	4	Long acting
Methadone	Dolophine	5-10 q4-6h PO	NA	20	Different $t_{1/2}$ for analgesia and prevention of opiate withdrawal
Morphine sulfate	Roxanol	5-20 q4h IM; 5-20 q6h PR; 10 q4h SL; 10-30 mg q4h PO	10	60 (single dose)	Oral bioavailability poor; sublingual form useful for breakthrough pain
Morphine, sustained release	MS Contin	15-60 q6-12h PO	NA	30 (repeated doses)	Not appropriate for prn use
Oxycodone	Percocet, Percodan, Tylox, Oxycontin, Roxicodone	5-10 q4-6h PO	NA	25	Often combined with aspirin (Percodan) or acetaminophen (Percocet, Tylox); available in long-acting form (Oxycontin)
Hydrocodone	Vicodin, Vicoprofen	5-10 q4-6h PO	NA	30	Only available combined with acetaminophen, aspirin, ibuprofen, or decongestants
Pentazocine	Talwin	30-60 q3-4h IM; 50-100 q4h PO	45	135	Mixed narcotic agonist-antagonist
Meperidine	Demerol	50-125 q3-4h IM; 50-100 q4h PO	75	250	May be used IV; metabolite normeperidine may accumulate with prolonged use causing excitation or seizures
Codeine	Codeine	15-60 q4h PO	130	200	Schedule II unless combined with acetaminophen or aspirin; used as cough suppressant
Propoxyphene	Darvon	32-100 q4h PO	180	360	Less abuse potential than codeine at usual doses

Cephalosporin Antibiotics

Drug Name (Generation in Parentheses)	Trade Name	Usual Adult Dose (g)	Adjust Dose for Renal Insufficiency	Comment
Oral				
Cefadroxil (1)	Duricef	0.5-1.0 q12-24h	Y	
Cephalexin (1)	Keflex	0.25-0.5 q6h	Y	Cheapest in its therapeutic class
Cephradine (1)	Velosef	0.5 q6h	Y	
Cefaclor (2)	Ceclor	0.25-0.5 q8h	N	
Cefpodoxime proxetil (2)	Vantin	0.1-0.4 q12h	Y	
Cefprozil (2)	Cefzil	0.25-0.5 q12h	Y	
Cefuroxime axetil (2)	Ceftin	0.25-0.5 q12h	Y	
Loracarbef (2)	Lorabid	0.2-0.4 q12h	Y	Carbacephem derivative rather than true cephalosporin
Ceftibuten (3)	Cedax	0.4 q24h	Y	
Cefixime (3)	Suprax	0.4 q24h	Y	Single dose therapy for gonococcal genital and pharyngeal infections
Parenteral (IV/IM)				
Cefazolin (1)	Ancef, Kefzol	1-2 q6-8h	Y	
Cephalothin (1)	Keflin	1-2 q4-6h	Y	

Cephapirin (1)	Cefadyl	1 q4-6h	Y	
Cefamandole (2)	Mandol	0.5-1.0 q4-8h	Y	
Cefmetazole (2)	Zefazone	2 q6-12h	Y	
Cefonicid (2)	Monocid	1-2 q24h	Y	May be useful in outpatient therapy of endocarditis
Ceforanide (2)	Precef	0.5-1.0 q12h	Y	
Cefotetan (2)	Cefotan	1-2 q12h	Y	Covers GI anaerobes
Cefoxitin (2)	Mefoxin	1-2 q4-6h	Y	Covers GI anaerobes
Cefuroxime (2)	Zinacef	0.75-1.5 q8h	Y	Crosses blood-brain barrier
Cefepime (3)	Maxipime	0.5-2.0 q12h	Y	
Cefoperazone (3)	Cefobid	1-2 q8-12h	N	
Cefotaxime (3)	Claforan	1-2 q4-6h	Y	Crosses blood-brain barrier
Ceftazidine (3)	Fortaz	1-2 q6-8h	Y	
Ceftizoxime (3)	Cefizox	1-2 q6-8h	Y	Crosses blood-brain barrier
Ceftriaxone (3)	Rocephin	1-2 q12-24h	N	May be useful in outpatient therapy of endocarditis; single-dose (250 mg IM) therapy for gonococcal genital and pharyngeal infections; crosses blood-brain barrier

Macrolide Antibiotics

Drug Name	Trade Name	Usual Adult Dose (mg)	Comment
Azithromycin	Zithromax	500, followed by 250 q24h	Single dose therapy for chlamydial urethritis or cervicitis (1000 mg); antibacterial spectrum includes *Hemophilus influenzae*; indicated to prevent *Mycobacterium avium-intracellulare* infection (1200 mg qwk); available in parenteral form
Clarithromycin	Biaxin	250-500 q12h	Antibacterial spectrum includes *H. influenzae*; used to treat *Helicobacter pylori* and to prevent *Mycobacterium avium-intracellulare* infection; multiple drug interactions
Dirithromycin	Dynabac	500 q24h	Antibacterial spectrum includes *H. influenzae*
Erythromycin	Erythromycin	250-500 q6-12h	Available as combination product with sulfisoxazole (extends spectrum to include *H. influenzae*); coating does not decrease GI side effects; available in parenteral form; multiple drug interactions

Penicillin Antibiotics

Drug Name	Trade Name	Usual Adult Dose (g)	Comment
ORAL			
Penicillin V	Penicillin VK	0.25-0.5 q6h	
Broad Spectrum Penicillins			
Amoxicillin	Amoxicillin	0.25-0.5 q8h	May take with meals
Amoxicillin-Potassium Clavulanate	Augmentin	One tablet (0.25 or 0.5 amoxicillin/0.125 clavulanate) q8h, or one tablet (0.875 mg amoxicillin/0.125 clavulanate) q12h	Spectrum extended to include beta-lactamase producers such as *Hemophilus influenza, Moraxella catarrhalis, Staphylococcus aureus* (except **MRSA**), and *Escherichia coli*
Ampicillin	Ampicillin	0.5-1.0 q6h	Do not take with food
Bacampicillin	Spectrobid	0.4-0.8 q12h	Gives higher and more sustained serum levels of ampicillin
Penicillinase Resistant Penicillins			
Cloxacillin	Tegopen	0.25-0.5 q6h	Oral penicillin of choice for *S. aureus* (except **MRSA**)
Dicloxacillin	Dycill	0.25-0.5 q6h	Oral penicillin of choice for *S. aureus* (except **MRSA**)
PARENTERAL (IV)			
Penicillin G	Penicillin	1-3 million U q4-6h	Procaine and benzathine forms available for IM use
Broad Spectrum Penicillins			
Ampicillin	Ampicillin	1-2 q4-6h	
Ampicillin-Sulbactam	Unasyn	1-2/0.5-1.0 q6h	Spectrum extended to include beta-lactamase producers such as *H. influenza. M. catarrhalis. S. aureus* (except **MRSA**). and *E. coli*

Continued

Penicillin Antibiotics—cont'd

Drug Name	Trade Name	Usual Adult Dose (g)	Comment
Carbenicillin	Geopen, Geocillin	4-5 q4-6h	Carbenicillin indanyl sodium available for oral use
Ticarcillin	Ticar	2-3 q4-6h	
Ticarcillin-Potassium Clavulanate	Timentin	3.1 (3.0 ticarcillin, 0.1 potassium clavulanate) q4-6h	Spectrum extended to include beta-lactamase producers such as *S. aureus* (except MRSA), *E. coli, Klebsiella* spp., and *Bacteroides fragilis*
Azlocillin	Azlin	2-3 q4-6h	Spectrum includes enterococci, *Klebsiella, Enterobacter,* and *Serratia* spp.
Mezlocillin	Mezlin	2-4 q4-8h	Spectrum includes enterococci, *Klebsiella, Enterobacter,* and *Serratia* spp.
Piperacillin	Pipracil	3-4 q4-6h	Spectrum includes enterococci, *Klebsiella, Enterobacter, Acinetobacter,* and *Serratia* spp.
Piperacillin-Tazobactam	Zosyn	3.375 (3.0 piperacillin, 0.375 tazobactam) q4-6h	Spectrum includes enterococci, *Klebsiella, Enterobacter, Acinetobacter,* and *Serratia* spp; extended to include beta-lactamase producers such as *S. aureus* (except MRSA) and *B. fragilis*
Penicillinase Resistant Penicillins			
Methicillin	Methicillin	1-2 q4-6h	Parenteral penicillin of choice for *S. aureus* (except MRSA)
Nafcillin	Nafcillin	0.5-2.0 q4-6h	Parenteral penicillin of choice for *S. aureus* (except MRSA)
Oxacillin	Oxacillin	0.5-2.0 q4-6h	Parenteral penicillin of choice for *S. aureus* (except MRSA)

NOTE: MRSA = Methicillin resistant *S. aureus.*

Quinolone Antibiotics

Drug Name	Trade Name	Usual Adult Dose (mg)	Cost (10 Days of Oral Therapy)	Comment
Cinoxacin	Cinobac	PO: 250 q6h or 500 q12h	$49	Approved only to treat UTIs; *Enterococcus*, *Staphylococcus*, and *Pseudomonas* spp. are resistant
Ciprofloxacin	Cipro	PO: 250–750 q12h IV: 200–400 q12h	$72	Available for ophthalmic use; useful in oral therapy of osteomyelitis; approved for *Campylobacter*, *Salmonella*, and *Shigella* infections; antibacterial spectrum includes *Mycobacterium avium-intracellulare*
Enoxacin	Penetrex	PO: 400 q12h	$64	Approved only to treat UTIs
Grepafloxacin	Raxar	PO: 400–600 q24h	$61	Enhanced activity against gram-positive cocci; removed from market, October, 1999
Levofloxacin	Levaquin	PO: 250–500 q24h	$73	Levo-form of ofloxacin
Lomefloxacin	Maxaquin	PO: 400 q24h	$64	Not effective for *Pseudomonas aeruginosa* infections outside of the urinary tract
Norfloxacin	Noroxin	PO: 400 q12h	$63	Available for ophthalmic use; approved only to treat UTIs and conjunctivitis
Ofloxacin	Floxin	PO: 200–400 q12h IV: 200–400 q12h	$86	Available for ophthalmic use
Sparfloxacin	Zagam	PO: 200–400 load, then 100–300 q24h	$74	Enhanced activity against gram-positive cocci and anaerobes
Trovafloxacin	Trovan	PO: 100–200 q24h	$60	Enhanced activity against gram-positive cocci and anaerobes; rare reports of fatal hepatitis

Systemic Antifungal Antibiotics

Drug Name	Trade Name	Usual Adult Dose	Common Indications	Comment
Amphotericin B	Abelcet, Amphotec, Fungizone	IV: 0.4-0.6 mg/kg/d for 8-10 wk	Histoplasmosis, blastomycosis, candidiasis, cryptococcosis, coccidioidomycosis, aspergillosis, mucormycosis	Used topically in bladder; causes multiple electrolyte abnormalities (hypokalemia, renal tubular acidosis, hypomagnesemia, azotemia); give 1 mg test dose prior to giving full dose; also available in lipid-complexed forms
Fluconazole	Diflucan	PO or IV: 100-400 qd	Blastomycosis, histoplasmosis, candidiasis, coccidioidomycosis	Increases serum rifabutin levels and toxicity; increases effect of cyclosporine, terfenadine, astemizole, warfarin, sulfonylureas, and others; single dose oral treatment for vaginal infection
Flucytosine	Ancobon	PO: 12.5-37.5 mg/kg q6h	Cryptococcosis, candidiasis, chromoblastomycosis	Usually used in combination with amphotericin B (allows lower dose); converted to 5-fluorouracil in fungal cell
Griseofulvin	Fulvicin, Gris-PEG	PO: 500 mg qd-bid (microcrystalline) PO: 330 mg qd-bid (ultra microcrystalline)	Dermatophytes	Cytochrome P450 inducer; absorption enhanced when taken with fatty foods
Itraconazole	Sporanox	PO: 100-200 mg qd-bid	Onychomycosis, blastomycosis, histoplasmosis, candidiasis, coccidioidomycosis, sporotrichosis, cryptococcosis, aspergillosis	Cytochrome P450 3A inhibitor—affects cyclosporine, terfenadine, astemizole, warfarin, sulfonylureas, and others
Ketoconazole	Nizoral	PO: 200-400 mg qd-bid	Blastomycosis, histoplasmosis, candidiasis, coccidioidomycosis, dermatophytes	Cytochrome P450 3A inhibitor—affects cyclosporine, terfenadine, astemizole, warfarin, sulfonylureas, and others; requires acid pH for absorption; reduces testosterone synthesis; available in topical form
Miconazole	Monistat	IV: 200-1200 mg q8h	Coccidioidomycosis, candidiasis, cryptococcosis	Increases warfarin and sulfonylurea effect; used topically for cutaneous and vaginal infections
Terbinafine	Lamisil	PO: 250 mg qd	Onychomycosis	Hepatic clearance increased by rifampin, decreased by cimetidine

Selective Serotonin Reuptake Inhibitor (SSRI) Antidepressants

Drug Name	Brand Name	Usual Adult Dose (mg/d)	Drug and Active Metabolite ($t_{1/2}$ (hr))	Serotonin Reuptake Inhibition	Anticholinergic Effect	Drowsiness	Degree of Cytochrome P450 System Inhibition	Comment
Citalopram	Celexa	20-40	35	4+	0	0	0	Dose up to 80 mg/d occasionally needed
Fluoxetine	Prozac	20-40 (starting dose 10 in elderly)	24-72 (acute); 96-144 (chronic); (norfluoxetine: 96-384)	4+	0-1+	0	3+	Up to 60 mg/d for obsessive-compulsive disorder
Fluvoxamine	Luvox	50-300	15-26 (no active metabolite)	4+	0-1+	1+	2+	Indicated only for obsessive-compulsive disorder
Paroxetine	Paxil	20-50 (starting dose 10 in elderly)	21 (no active metabolite)	4+	0	1+	2+	May cause weight gain
Sertraline	Zoloft	50-200 (starting dose 12.5-25 in elderly)	26 (desmethylsertraline: 62-104)	4+	0	0	1+	Metabolite weakly active

Tricyclic and Tetracyclic Antidepressants

Drug Name	Brand Name	Usual Adult Dose (mg) for Acute Therapy (Maintenance Dose is $\frac{1}{2}$–$\frac{2}{3}$ of this; lower doses recommended for elderly persons)	Relative Sedation	Relative Anticholinergic Effect	Relative Delay of Cardiac Conduction	Relative Postural Hypotension	Comment
Tricyclic							
Amitriptyline	Elavil	75–300	3+	2+	3+	3+	Used for chronic pain
Clomipramine	Anafranil	25–250	2+	2+	2+	2+	Primary use is for obsessive-compulsive disorder; may lower seizure threshold; may increase plasma concentration of protein bound drugs (e.g., digoxin, warfarin)
Desipramine	Norpramin	75–300	1+	1+	3+	1+	Used for chronic pain; metabolite of imipramine
Doxepin	Sinequan	75–300	3+	3+	1+	3+	Potent antihistamine
Imipramine	Tofranil	50–300	2+	2+	3+	2+	Used for chronic pain, panic disorder, and headache
Nortriptyline	Pamelor	50–150	1+	1+	2+	2+	Used for chronic pain, panic disorder, and headache; metabolite of amitriptyline

Protriptyline	Vivactil	15-60	0+	2+	2+	1+	
Trimipramine	Surmontil	50-300	2+	2+	3+	2+	
Tetracyclic							
Amoxapine	Asendin	200-600	2+	1+	1+	1+	Metabolite has neuroleptic side effect
Maprotiline	Ludiomil	75-300	2+	1+	1+	1+	May lower seizure threshold
Heterocyclic							
Nefazodone	Serzone	200-600	2+	1+	0+	1+	Divided doses on bid schedule; do not administer with astemizole, cisapride, lovastatin, or simvastatin; may increase plasma concentration of protein bound drugs (e.g., digoxin, warfarin); cytochrome 3A4 inhibitor
Trazodone	Desyrel	150-600	3+	1+	0+	2+	Risk of priapism in males and similar phenomenon in females; may increase plasma concentration of protein bound drugs (e.g., digoxin, warfarin); should be given in divided doses

Miscellaneous Antidepressants, Including Foods that Interact with MAOIs

Drug Name	Brand Name	Usual Adult Dose (mg/d)	Anticholinergic Effect	Drowsiness	Orthostatic Hypotension	Cardiac Dysrhythmias	Comment
Bupropion	Wellbutrin, Zyban	300-450	1+	1+	1+	1+	Single dose should not exceed 150 mg; inhibits dopamine reuptake; given bid or tid; FDA-approved as an aid to smoking cessation
Mirtazapine	Remeron	15-45	2+	3+	0	0-1+	Do not use with MAOIs
Venlafaxine	Effexor, Effexor XR	75-375	0	1+	0	1+	Inhibits serotonin and norepinephrine reuptake; given bid or tid or as long-acting form
Monoamine oxidase inhibitors (MAOIs)							Avoid foods rich in amines (see below) and selected medications while taking MAOI and for 14 days after last dose
Isocarboxazid	Marplan	10-30	1+	1+	2+	1+	May be given as single daily dose
Phenelzine	Nardil	15-90	1+	1+	2+	1+	Given in divided doses
Tranylcypromine	Parnate	30-60	1+	1+	1+	1+	Given in divided doses

Avoid the following foods if taking MAOIs (contain tyramine and other amines, often as a result of aging or fermenting): broad beans; red wines; yeast extracts; beer with yeast; chicken or beef liver; caviar, anchovies, and pickled herring; fermented sausages (bologna, pepperoni, salami, and summer sausage); and aged cheeses (Boursault, Brie, Camembert, cheddar, Emmenthaler, Gruyere, mozzarella, parmesan, romano, Roquefort, and Stilton).

Systemic Antihistamines

Drug Name	Trade Name	Usual Adult Dose (mg)	Cost per Dose	Comment
First-Generation Agents				
Acrivastine	Semprex-D	8 qid	$0.75	Only available in combination with pseudoephedrine
Azatadine	Optimine, Rynatan, Trinalin	1 bid	$1.11	
Bromodiphenhydramine	Ambenyl and others	12.5–25.0 qid	$0.83	Only available as a syrup and in combination with codeine phosphate
Brompheniramine	Dimetane	4 q4h	$0.03	Also available as syrup, extended release capsule, and in combination with decongestants
Carbinoxamine	Rondec and others	4 qid	$0.16	Only available in combination with pseudoephedrine; available as syrup and extended release tablet
Chlorpheniramine	Chlor-Trimeton and others	4 qid	$0.02	Also available as syrup, extended release capsule, and in combination with decongestants
Clemastine	Tavist and others	1.34 bid	$0.33	Also available as syrup and in combination with decongestants
Cyproheptadine	Periactin and others	4 qid	$0.06	Also available as syrup
Diphenhydramine	Benadryl and others	25–50 qid	$0.02	Also available as syrup
Hydroxyzine	Atarax, Vistaril	10–75 qid	$0.07	Also available as syrup
Pheniramine	Triaminic and others	4 qid	$0.40	Only available in combination with phenylpropanolamine and pyrilamine; available as syrup and extended release tablet
Pyrilamine	Triaminic and others	4 qid	$0.25	Only available in combination with phenylpropanolamine and pheniramine; available as syrup and extended release tablet
Tripelennamine	PBZ and others	25–50 qid	$0.07	Also available as sustained action tablet
Triprolidine	Actifed and others	2.5 qid	$0.05	Also available in combination with pseudoephedrine; also available as syrup

Continued

Systemic Antihistamines—cont'd

Drug Name	Trade Name	Usual Adult Dose (mg)	Cost per Dose	Comment
Second-Generation Agents				
Astemizole	Hismanal	10 qd	$2.07	Removed from market in U.S., 1999, because of potential for QT interval prolongation; non-sedating agent; potential drug interaction with macrolides and azole antifungals
Cetirizine	Zyrtec	10 qd	$1.85	Less-sedating agent; prescription required in U.S.; no drug interaction with macrolides and azole antifungals; QT interval prolongation not reported; available as syrup; antipruritic
Fexofenadine	Allegra	60 bid	$0.99	Non-sedating agent; prescription required in U.S.; potential drug interaction with macrolides and azole antifungals; QT interval prolongation not reported; available in combination with pseudoephendrine
Loratadine	Claritin	10 qd	$2.24	Non-sedating agent; prescription required in U.S.; potential drug interaction with macrolides and azole antifungals; QT interval prolongation not reported; available in combination with pseudoephedrine and as syrup
Terfenadine	Seldane	60 bid	$0.94	Removed from market in U.S., 1999, because of potential for QT interval prolongation; non-sedating agent; potential drug interaction with macrolides and azole antifungals
Miscellaneous Agents				
Doxepin	Sinequan	10-50 qd-tid	$0.04	Sedating tricyclic antidepressant
Promethazine	Phenergan	12.5 tid-qid	$0.06	Phenothiazine derivative; well tolerated by children; available as syrup

Systemic Corticosteroids

Drug Name	Trade Name	Oral or Parenteral Dose for Equivalent Glucocorticoid Effect (mg)*	Relative Mineralocorticoid Effect	Biologic Half-life (hrs)†
Betamethasone	Celestone	0.75	0	36-54
Cortisone	Cortone	25	1	8-12
Dexamethasone††	Decadron, Dexone, Hexadrol	0.75	0	36-54
Hydrocortisone	Cortef, Solu-Cortef	20	1	8-12
Methylprednisolone	Medrol	4	0	18-36
Prednisolone	Delta-Cortef	5	0.5	18-36
Prednisone	Deltasone, Orasone	5	0.5	18-36
Triamcinolone	Aristocort, Atolone, Kenacort	4	0	18-36

*Not all preparations are suitable for IV injection.

†Because chemical half-life of all agents is 0.5-4.0 hrs, endogenous cortisol level can be measured 24 hrs after last corticosteroid dose (*JAMA* 1999; 282:671-676).

††Dexamethasone is only corticosteroid that does not cross-react with cortisol assay.

Inhaled Antiinflammatory Drugs

Drug Name	Trade Name	Dose per inhalation	Usual adult dose	Maximum adult daily dose (#inhalations)
Respiratory Corticosteroids				
Beclomethasone	Beclovent, Vanceril	42 µg	84 µg tid-qid or 168 µg bid	840 µg (20)
Beclomethasone	Vanceril Double Strength	84 µg	168 µg bid	840 µg (10)
Budesonide	Pulmicort	200 µg	200-800 µg bid	1600 µg (8)
Fluticasone	Flovent	44, 110, 220 µg	88-220 µg bid	880 µg (4-20)
Flunisolide	AeroBid	250 µg	500 µg bid	2000 µg (8)
Triamcinolone	Azmacort	100 µg	200 µg tid-qid or 400 µg bid	1600 µg (16)
Intranasal Corticosteroids				
Beclomethasone	Beconase, Vancenase (metered dose inhaler)	42 µg	42 µg each nostril bid-qid	336 µg (8)
Beclomethasone	Beconase AQ, Vancenase AQ (solution with metering pump)	42 µg	42 µg each nostril bid-qid	336 µg (8)

Budesonide	Rhinocort	32 µg	64 µg each nostril bid	256 µg (8)
Dexamethasone	Decadron Phosphate Turbinaire	84 µg	168 µg each nostril bid-tid	1008 µg (12)
Flunisolide	Nasalide (metered dose inhaler); Nasarel (solution with metering pump)	25 µg	50 µg each nostril bid	400 µg (16)
Fluticasone	Flonase	50 µg	100 µg each nostril qd	200 µg (4)
Mometasone	Nasonex	50 µg	100 µg each nostril qd	200 µg (4)
Triamcinolone	Nasacort (metered dose inhaler); Nasacort AQ (solution with metering pump)	55 µg	110 µg each nostril qd	440 µg (8)
Noncorticosteroids				
Cromolyn (inhaled)	Intal	800 µg	1600 µg qid	6400 µg (8)
Cromolyn (intranasal)	Nasalcrom	5.2 mg	5.2 mg each nostril q 3-6h	62.4 mg (12)
Nedocromil (inhaled)	Tilade	1.75 mg	3.5 mg bid-qid	14 mg (8)

*NA = Not available

Inhaled Bronchodilators

Drug Name	Trade Name	Dose per Inhalation with Metered Dose Inhaler	Usual Adult Dose
Albuterol	Proventil, Proventil-HFA, Ventolin, Combivent (with ipratropium)	90 µg	1-2 inhalations q 4-6h
Bitolterol	Tomalate	370 µg	2-3 inhalations q 4-6 h (max 12 per day)
Epinephrine	Medihaler-Epi, Primatene	160 µg	1-2 inhalations q 3-4 h (max 12 per day)
Ipratropium	Atrovent, Combivent (with albuterol)	18 µg	2 inhalations q 4-6 h (max 12 per day)
Isoetharine	Bronkometer	340 µg	1-2 inhalations q 4h
Isoproterenol	Medihaler-Iso	80 µg	1-2 inhalations q 4-6h
Metaproterenol	Alupent, Metaprel	650 µg	2-3 inhalations q 3-4 h (max 12 per day)
Pirbuterol	Maxair	200 µg	1-2 inhalations q 4-6 h (max 12 per day)
Salmeterol	Serevent	25 µg	2 inhalations q 12h
Terbutaline	Brethaire	200 µg	2 inhalations q 4-6h

Noncontraceptive Estrogens

Drug Name	Trade Name	Available Strengths	Usual Adult Dose	Comment
Systemic				
Conjugated estrogens, oral	Premarin	0.3 mg, 0.625 mg, 0.9 mg, 1.25 mg, 2.5 mg	0.625-1.25 mg qd	Available in IV form; available in combination with medroxyprogesterone acetate (2.5 mg-Prempro; 5 mg Premphase); dose for bone loss prevention 0.625 mg qd
Esterified estrogens	Estratab, Menest	0.3 mg, 0.625 mg, 1.25 mg, 2.5 mg	0.625-1.25 mg qd	Contains 80% sodium estrone sulfate
Estradiol oral	Estrace	0.5 mg, 1 mg, 2 mg	0.5-2 mg qd	Dose for bone loss prevention 0.5 mg qd
Estradiol transdermal systems	Vivelle, Climara, Estraderm	0.0375 mg/24 hr 0.05 mg/24 hr 0.075 mg/24 hr 0.1 mg/24 hr	0.05-0.1 mg/24 hr	Estraderm and Vivelle applied twice weekly; Climara applied weekly; dose for bone loss prevention 0.05 mg qd
Estradiol valerate in oil	Delestrogen, Dioval, Estra-L, Gynogen LA	10 mg/ml; 20 mg/ml; 40 mg/ml	10-20 mg q 4 weeks	Oil suspension gives long action
Estrone	Aquest, Kestrone	2 mg/ml; 5 mg/ml	0.1-2 mg per week in single or divided doses	Aqueous solution of estrone

Continued

Noncontraceptive Estrogens—cont'd

Drug Name	Trade Name	Available Strengths	Usual Adult Dose	Comment
Estropipate	Ortho-Est, Ogen	0.75 mg, 1.5 mg, 3 mg	0.75-1.5 mg qd	0.75 mg estropipate equivalent to 0.625 mg conjugated estrogens; dose for bone loss prevention 0.75 mg qd
Ethinyl estradiol	Estinyl	0.02 mg, 0.05 mg, 0.5 mg	0.02-0.05 mg qd	
Topical				
Conjugated estrogens	Premarin	0.625 mg conjugated estrogens per g	0.5-2 g cream qd	
Dienestrol	Ortho Dienestrol	0.01% cream	1 applicatorful qd-bid	
Estradiol	Estrace	0.1 mg estradiol per g	2-4 g cream qd	
Estradiol	Estring	2 mg estradiol	Insert vaginal ring and leave in place for 90 days	
Estropipate	Ogen	1.5 mg estropipate per g	2-4 g cream qd	

Oral Hypoglycemic Agents

Drug Name	Trade Name	Equipotent Dose *or* Usual Dose Range (mg)	Usual Adult Dose Schedule	Adjust Dose in Renal Insufficiency	Cost per Dose	Comment
First-Generation Sulfonylurea						
Acetohexamide	Dymelor	500	qd-bid	Yes	$0.37	Do not use if CrCl <50 ml/min
Chlorpropamide	Diabinese	250	qd	Yes	$0.05	Do not use if CrCl <50 ml/min
Tolazamide	Tolinase	250	qd-bid	Yes	$0.12	Do not use if CrCl <50 ml/min
Tolbutamide	Orinase	1000	bid-tid	No	$0.08	Do not use if CrCl <50 ml/min
Second-Generation Sulfonylurea						
Glimepiride	Amaryl	2	qd	Yes	$0.40	Duration of action 24 hrs
Glipizide	Glucotrol	10	bid	Yes	$0.50	Do not use if CrCl <10 ml/min; available as qd formulation (Glucotrol XL); absorption delayed by food
Glyburide, micronized	Glynase	3	qd-bid	Yes	$0.50	More rapid onset than nonmicronized form
Glyburide, nonmicronized	DiaBeta, Micronase	5	qd-bid	Yes	$0.52	Do not use if CrCl <10 ml/min
Thiazolidinedione						
Pioglitazone	Actos	15-45	qd	No	$4.56 (30 mg)	Monitor for drug-induced hepatitis; baseline ALT (SGPT), q 2 months during first year, and q 3 months afterwards

Continued

Oral Hypoglycemic Agents—cont'd

Drug Name	Trade Name	Equipotent Dose or Usual Dose Range (mg)	Usual Adult Dose Schedule	Adjust Dose in Renal Insufficiency	Cost per Dose	Comment
Rosiglitazone	Avandia	4-8	qd-bid	No	$2.50 (4 mg)	Monitor for drug-induced hepatitis: baseline ALT (SGPT), q 2 months during first year, and q 3 months afterwards
Troglitazone	Rezulin	200-600	qd	No	$2.98 (200 mg)	Monitor for drug-induced hepatitis: baseline ALT (SGPT), q month during first year, and q 3 months afterwards
Intestinal Alpha-Glucosidase Inhibitor						
Acarbose	Precose	25-100	tid	No	$0.46 (50 mg)	Minimally absorbed; take dose at the start of each meal; delays glucose absorption and lowers postprandial hyperglycemia
Miglitol	Glyset	25-100	tid	No	$0.58 (50 mg)	Nearly completely absorbed; excreted renally; take dose at the start of each meal; delays glucose absorption and lowers post-prandial hyperglycemia
Miscellaneous						
Metformin	Glucophage	500-850	bid-tid	Yes	$0.46 (500 mg)	Do not use if serum creat >1.4 mg/dl (male) or >1.3 mg/dl (female); max daily dose 2550 mg
Repaglinide	Prandin	0.5-4.0	tid	No	$0.75 (1 mg)	Take with meals

Insulins

Drug Name	Time to Onset of Effect (hr) for SC	Time to Peak Effect (hr) for SC	Duration of Effect (hr) for SC	Routes of Administration
Insulin lispro	¼	1	4	SC
Regular insulin (SC)	½-1	3-8	6-12	SC
Regular insulin (IV)	⅙-½	¼-½	½-1	IV, IM
NPH insulin	2-4	4-12	24	SC
Lente insulin	1-3	5-14	24	SC
Protamine zinc insulin (PZI)	4-8	14-24	36	SC
Ultralente insulin	4-8	10-30	36	SC
50/50 insulin	½-1	4-8	24	SC
70/30 insulin	½-1	4-8	24	SC

NOTES: 1. Most insulin types are available as beef, pork, or human types. Onset of action is faster and duration is shorter with human insulin preparations.
2. Insulin is available in U-100 (100 units per ml) and U-500 (500 units per ml) forms.
   Duration of action of U-500 forms is longer than U-100 forms.

Lipid Lowering Agents

Drug Name	Trade Name	Usual Adult Dose	Maximum Effect on Serum Lipid Levels	Cost ($) per Dose
Bile Acid Binding Resins			LDL–cholesterol reduced 20%–35% HDL–cholesterol not changed Triglycerides increased 5%–20%	
Cholestyramine	Questran	8 g bid-tid		1.33 (4 g); available in bulk form
Colestipol	Colestid	10 g bid-tid		1.63 (5 g); available in bulk form
Niacin	Niacin	1-2 g bid-tid	LDL–cholesterol reduced 20% HDL–cholesterol increased 20% Triglycerides reduced 40%	0.04 (500 mg)
Fibric Acid Derivatives			LDL–cholesterol reduced 10% HDL–cholesterol increased 10%–25% Triglycerides reduced 40%–60%	
Clofibrate	Atromid-S	500 qid		0.85 (500 mg)
Fenofibrate	Tricor	67 qd-tid with meals		0.70 (67 mg)
Gemfibrozil	Lopid	600 bid		1.03 (600 mg)

HMG Co A Reductase Inhibitors			LDL-cholesterol reduced 20%–40% HDL-cholesterol increased 5%–15% Triglycerides reduced 5%–25%*	
Atorvastatin*	Lipitor	10–20 qd (hs administration unnecessary)		1.87 (10 mg)
Cerivastatin	Baycol	0.2–0.3 qhs		1.42 (200 mg)
Fluvastatin	Lescol	20–40 qhs		1.25 (40 mg)
Lovastatin	Mevacor	20–40 qhs		2.54 (20 mg)
Pravastatin	Pravachol	20–40 qhs		1.82 (20 mg)
Simvastatin	Zocor	10–20 qhs		2.18 (10 mg)

*Atorvastatin at maximum dose reduces LDL-cholesterol by 60% and triglycerides by 50%

Topical Steroids

Potency Category	Drug Name	Trade Name	Type of Preparation	Comment
1 (most potent)	Betamethasone dipropionate (0.05%)	Diprolene AF (cream) Diprolene (ointment)	Cream, ointment	
	Clobetasol propionate (0.05%)	Temovate	Cream, ointment	Least expensive in potency group
	Diflorasone diacetate (0.05%)	Psorcon	Ointment	
	Halobetasol propionate (0.05%)	Ultravate	Cream, ointment	
2	Fluocinonide (0.05%)	Lidex Lidex-E (cream)	Cream, gel, ointment, solution	
	Halcinonide (0.1%)	Halog Halog-E (cream)	Cream, gel, ointment, solution	
	Betamethasone dipropionate (0.05%)	Alphatrex (ointment) Diprosone (ointment) Maxivate (cream, ointment)	Cream, ointment	Least expensive in potency group
3	Betamethasone valerate (0.1%)	Betatrex (ointment) Valisone (ointment)	Ointment	Least expensive in potency group
	Triamcinolone acetonide (0.5%)	Aristocort (cream, ointment) Kenalog (cream, ointment) Trymex (cream)	Cream, ointment	
	Betamethasone dipropionate (0.05%)	Alphatrex (cream, lotion) Diprosone (cream) Maxivate (lotion)	Cream, lotion	

4	Fluocinolone acetonide (0.025%)	Fluonide (ointment) Synalar (ointment)	Cream, ointment	
	Fluocinolone acetonide (0.2%)	Synalar-HP (cream)	Cream	
	Halcinonide (0.025%)	Halog (cream, ointment)	Cream, ointment	
	Triamcinolone acetonide (0.1%)	Aristocort (ointment) Kenalog (ointment) Trymex (ointment)	Ointment	Least expensive in potency group
5	Hydrocortisone butyrate (0.1%)	Locoid (cream, ointment)	Cream, ointment	
	Betamethasone valerate (0.1%)	Beta-Val (cream) Betatrex (cream, lotion) Valisone (cream, lotion)	Cream, lotion	Least expensive in potency group
	Triamcinolone acetonide (0.1%)	Aristocort (cream) Kenalog (cream, lotion) Trymex (cream)	Cream, lotion	
	Fluocinolone acetonide (0.025%)	Fluonid (cream) Synalar (cream) Synemol (cream)	Cream	
6	Desonide (0.05%)	Des Owen (cream) Tridesilon (cream)	Cream	
	Dexamethasone (0.01%, 0.04%)	Aeroseb-Dex Decaspray	Aerosol	
	Fluocinolone acetonide (0.01%)	Fluonid (cream, solution) Synalar (cream, solution)	Cream, solution	
	Triamcinolone acetonide (0.025%)	Aristocort (cream) Kenalog (cream, lotion) Trymex (cream)	Cream, lotion	Least expensive in potency group
7	Betamethasone valerate (0.01%)	Valisone (cream)	Cream	
	Hydrocortisone (2.5%, 1%)	Hytone (cream, ointment)	Cream, ointment	Available without prescription; least expensive in potency group

Topical Antifungal Agents

Drug Name	Trade Name	Usual Adult Dose	Spectrum/Comment
Vaginal Preparations for Candidiasis			
Butoconazole	Femstat	2% vaginal cream, 5 g qhs × 3d (6d if pregnant)	Pregnancy category C
Clotrimazole	FemCare, Gyne-Lotrimin, Mycelex	1% vaginal cream, 1 applicatorful qhs × 7d; 100 mg vaginal tablet qhs × 7d; 500 mg vaginal tablet × 1	Pregnancy category B
Miconazole	Monistat	1% vaginal cream, 1 applicatorful qhs × 7d; 100 mg vaginal tablet qhs × 7d; 200 mg vaginal tablet × 3	Pregnancy category C
Nystatin	Mycostatin	100,000 units vaginal tablet qd × 14d	Pregnancy category A
Terconazole	Terazol	0.8% vaginal cream 1 applicatorful (5g) or 80 mg vaginal suppositories qhs × 3d	Pregnancy category C
Tioconazole	Vagistat	6.5% vaginal ointment, 1 applicatorful qhs × 1	Pregnancy category C
Dermatologic Preparations			
Amphotericin	Fungizone	3% cream, lotion, ointment	Candida
Butenafine	Mentax	1% cream	Tinea
Ciclopirox	Loprox	1% cream, ointment	Tinea, Candida, Tinea versicolor

Generic	Trade	Formulation	Uses
Clioquinol	Vioform	3% cream, ointment	Tinea
Clotrimazole	Lotrimin, Mycelex	1% cream, lotion, solution	OTC-Tinea; Rx-Tinea, Candida, Tinea versicolor
Econazole	Spectazole	1% cream	Tinea, Candida, Tinea versicolor
Haloprogin	Halotex	1% cream, solution	Tinea, Tinea versicolor
Iodoquinol			
Ketoconazole	Nizoral	2% cream, shampoo	Tinea, Candida, Tinea versicolor; scalp seborrheic dermatitis
Miconazole	Micatin, Monistat-Derm	2% cream, powder, spray	Tinea, Candida, Tinea versicolor
Naftifine	Naftin	1% cream, gel	Tinea, Candida
Nystatin	Mycostatin, Nilstat, Nystex	100,000 units per gram, cream, ointment, powder	Candida
Oxiconazole	Oxistat	1% cream, lotion	Tinea, Candida, Tinea versicolor
Selenium sulfide	Selsun Blue, Exsel	1%, 2.5% lotion, shampoo	Tinea versicolor; scalp seborrheic dermatitis
Sulconazole	Exelderm	1% cream, solution	Tinea, Candida, Tinea versicolor
Terbinafine	Lamisil	1% cream	Tinea, Candida, Tinea versicolor
Tolnaftate	Aftate, Tinactin, Desenex	1% cream, gel, powder, solution, spray liquid, spray powder	Tinea, Tinea versicolor
Undecylenic acid	Cruex, Desenex, Pedi-Pro, Caldesene, Protectol	8-20% cream, foam, ointment, powder, soap	Tinea

Nucleoside Reverse Transcriptase Inhibitor Antiretroviral Drugs

Drug Name	Trade Name	Usual Adult Dose (mg)	Dose Change in Renal Insufficiency	Drug Interactions	Comment
Abacavir	Ziagen	300 q12h	No	Ampenavir	Hypersensitivity in 2-5% of recipients; rechallenge may be fatal; penetrates into CSF
Didanosine (ddI)	Videx	125-200 q12h on empty stomach (pills)	Reduce dose if CrCl <60 ml/min	Dapsone, ganciclovir, itraconazole, quinolones	Take 2 pills at a time to ensure adequate buffering; available as a powder (not bioequivalent to pills); penetrates into CSF
Lamivudine (3TC)	Epivir, Combivir	150 q12h	Reduce dose if CrCl <50 ml/min	Trimethoprim-sulfamethoxazole	Available as oral solution; penetrates into CSF; available in combination with zidovudine
Stavudine (D4T)	Zerit	30-40 q12h	Reduce dose if CrCl <50 ml/min	Additive neuropathic effect with dapsone, isoniazid, metronidazole, phenytoin, vincristine	Antagonism with zidovudine penetrates into CSF; associated with lipodystrophy
Zalcitabine (ddC)	Hivid	0.75 q8h	Reduce dose if CrCl <40 ml/min	Antacids, amphotericin, foscarnet, aminoglycosides, probenecid, cimetidine, pentamidine	Penetrates into CSF
Zidovudine (AZT)	Retrovir, Combivir	100-200 q8h or 300 q12h	Reduce dose if CrCl <10 ml/min	Ganciclovir, interferon, probenecid, rifampin, valproic acid	Available as syrup, injection; penetrates into CSF; available in combination with lamivudine

Non-Nucleoside Reverse Transcriptase Inhibitors

Drug Name	Trade Name	Usual Adult Dose (mg)	Dose Change in Renal Insufficiency	Drug Interactions	Comment
Delavirdine	Rescriptor	400 tid	No	Antacids, astemizole, barbiturates, carbamazepine, cisapride, clarithromycin, dapsone, didanosine, ergotamines, H2 blockers, indinavir, midazolam, nelfinavir, nifedipine, phenytoin, proton pump inhibitors, quinidine, rifabutin, rifampin, saquinavir, terfenadine, triazolam, warfarin, zidovudine	Do not use as monotherapy due to resistance induction; separate dosing with didanosine or antacids by 1 hour; cytochrome P4503A4 inhibitor; coadministration with astemizole, cisapride, ergotamines, H2 blockers, lovastatin, midazolam, proton pump inhibitors, rifabutin, rifampin, simvastatin, terfenadine, triazolam not recommended
Efavirenz	Sustiva	600 qd	No	Amprenavir, astemizole, barbiturates, carbamazepine, cisapride, clarithromycin, ergotamines, ethinyl estradiol, indinavir, lovastatin, midazolam, nelfinavir, nifedipine, phenytoin, rifabutin, rifampin, ritonavir, saquinavir, simvastatin, terfenadine, triazolam, warfarin	Do not use as monotherapy due to resistance induction; CNS side effects very frequent; cytochrome P450 mixed inducer and inhibitor; coadministration with astemizole, cisapride, clarithromycin, ergotamines, midazolam, saquinavir, terfenadine, triazolam not recommended
Nevirapine	Viramune	200 qd for 14d, then 200 bid	No	Clarithromycin, erythromycin, indinavir, ketoconazole, methadone, nelfinavir, rifabutin, rifampin, ritonavir, saquinavir	Do not use as monotherapy due to resistance induction; cytochrome P4503A4 inducer; coadministration with ketoconazole, rifampin not recommended; may affect methadone dose needed

Protease Inhibitor Antiretroviral Drugs

Drug Name	Trade Name	Usual Adult Dose (mg)	Dose Change in Renal Insufficiency	Selected Drug Interactions (see individual monographs for complete list)	Comment
Amprenavir	Agenerase	1200 q12h	No	Astemizole, cisapride, ergot alkaloids, lovastatin, midazolam, rifampin, simvastatin, terfenadine, triazolam	Capsules of amprenavir contain 109 IU of vitamin E; liquid contains 46 IU per mL
Indinavir	Crixivan	800 q8h (400 mg tablets)	No	Astemizole, cisapride, ergot alkaloids, lovastatin, midazolam, rifampin, saquinavir, simvastatin, terfenadine, triazolam	Do not take with large meal; associated with nephrolithiasis
Nelfinavir	Viracept	750 tid	No	Astemizole, cisapride, ergot alkaloids, lovastatin, midazolam, rifampin, simvastatin, terfenadine, triazolam	Diarrhea most common side effect
Ritonavir	Norvir	600 q12h (100 mg tablets)	No	Amiodarone, astemizole, bepredil, bupropion, cisapride, clorazepate, clozapine, diazepam, encainide, ergot alkaloids, estazolam, flecainide, flurazepam, lovastatin, meperidine, midazolam, pimozide, piroxicam, propafenone, propoxyphene, simvastatin, terfenadine, triazolam, zolpidem	Take with food; start with 300 mg q12h, increase in 100 mg increments to 600 mg q12h
Saquinavir	Invirase (hard capsule), Fortovase (soft capsule)	Hard capsule: 400 q12h with ritonavir; soft capsule: 1200 q8h	No	Astemizole, cisapride, efavirenz, ergot alkaloids, indinavir, lovastatin, midazolam, rifabutin, rifampin, simvastatin, terfenadine, triazolam	Take with high fat meal to enhance bioavailability; available in more bioavailable gel capsule form (Fortovase)

Appendix B

Bibliography

1. Mosby's GenRx, 9th ed., St. Louis, Mosby, 1999.
2. Briggs GG, Freeman RK, Yaffe SJ. Drugs in pregnancy and lactation, 5th ed. Baltimore, Williams and Wilkins, 1998.
3. Shepard TH. Catalog of teratogenic agents, 8th ed. Baltimore, Johns Hopkins University Press, 1995.
4. Hansten PD, Horn JR. Drug interactions analysis and management. Vancouver, Washington, Applied Therapeutics Incorporated, 1999.
5. Drug facts and comparisons. St. Louis, Facts and Comparisons, Incorporated, 1999.
6. McEvoy, GK, American Hospital Formulary Service: Drug information, Bethesda, American Society of Hospital Pharmacists, 1999.
7. Doherty MC. Drug topics red book 1999. Montvale, NJ, Medical economics data production company, 1999.
8. Young DS. Effects of Drugs on Clinical Lab Tests, 4th ed. Washington D.C., 1995, American Association for Clinical Press.

Therapeutic Index

Abortion
carboprost, 154-155
dinoprostone, 316-317
methotrexate, 626-628
misoprostol, 667
oxytocin, 752-753
sodium chloride, 905-907
Acetaminophen poisoning
acetylcysteine, 12
Acidosis, metabolic
sodium bicarbonate, 904-905
sodium citrate and citric acid,
907-908
tromethamine, 1009-1010
Acne
adapalene, 15
azelaic acid, 86-87
benzoyl peroxide, 100-101
clindamycin, 226-227
co-trimoxazole, 250-252
demeclocycline, 273-275
doxycycline, 336-337
erythromycin, 365-368
isotretinoin, 526-528
metronidazole, 652-654
minocycline, 663-665
tazarotene, 938-939
tetracycline, 947-949
tretinoin, 990-991
Acromegaly
bromocriptine, 119-120
octreotide, 725-726
pergolide, 774
Actinomycosis
amoxicillin, 51-52
ampicillin, 57-59
clindamycin, 226-227
doxycycline, 336-337
erythromycin, 365-368
minocycline, 663-665
penicillin, 764-767
tetracycline, 947-949
Addison's disease
betamethasone, 105-107
corticotropin (ACTH), 247-248

cortisone, 248-249
cosyntropin, 249-250
dexamethasone, 282-284
fludrocortisone, 408-409
hydrocortisone, 482-484
methylprednisolone, 641-643
prednisolone, 820-822
prednisone, 822-823
Adrenocortical function
corticotropin (ACTH),
247-248
cosyntropin, 249-250
Aggression
acebutolol, 4-5
bisoprolol, 113-115
esmolol, 370-371
metoprolol, 650-652
nadolol, 680-682
propranolol, 839-842
Alcohol withdrawal
acebutolol, 4-5
atenolol, 76-78
bisoprolol, 113-115
carbamazepine, 148-151
chloral hydrate, 192-193
chlordiazepoxide, 195-197
clonidine, 236-237
clorazepate, 239-240
disulfiram, 323-324
hydroxyzine, 491-492
labetalol, 541-543
lithium, 568-570
lorazepam, 574-575
mesoridazine, 609-610
metoprolol, 650-652
nadolol, 680-682
naloxone, 688
naltrexone, 688-689
oxazepam, 742-743
propranolol, 839-842
pindolol, 798-800
thiamine, 954-956
thioridazine, 957-958
Alkalosis
ammonium chloride, 46-47

The therapeutic index is arranged by condition/disorder. *Italics* indicate category of drug.

Index

A

AA HC Otic, 9
abacavir, 1
Abbokinase, 1015-1016
Abbokinase Open-Cath, 1015-1016
abciximab, 1-3
Abelcet (ABLC), 55-57
acarbose, 3
Accolate, 1033-1034
Accupril, 855-857
Accuretic, 477-479
Accutane, 526-528
acebutolol, 4-5
Acediur, 477-479
Acephen, 6-7
Aceta, 243-244
acetaminophen (APAP), 6-7
Acetasol, 9
Acetasol HC, 9
acetazolamide, 7-8
acetic acid, 9
Acetocot, 991-994
acetohexamide, 9-10
acetohydroxamic acid (AHA), 10-11
Acetoxyl, 100-101
acetylcholine, 11
acetylcysteine, 12
Aci-Jel, 9
Aciphex, 861-862
acitretin, 12-13
Aclovate, 19-20
Acne-10, 100-101
Acnomel, 100-101
Acthar Gel, H.P., 247-248
Actibine, 1033
Acticin, 774-775
Actidose-Aqua, 191
Actidose with sorbitol, 191
Actifed, 846-847, 1008-1009
Actifed Allergy, 846-847
Actifed Plus, 6-7
Actigall, 1016

Actimmune, 512
Actiq, 398-400
Actisite, 947-949
Activase, 25-26
Actonel, 878
Actron, 537-539
Acular, 539-541
Acular PF, 539-541
Acutrim, 789-790
acyclovir, 13-15
Adalat, 708-709
Adalat CC, 708-709
adapalene, 15
Adapin, 334-335
Adderall, 54-55
Adenocard, 15-16
adenosine, 15-16
Adipex-P, 784-785
Adipost, 778-779
Adrenalin, 356-358
Adrenaline, 356-358
Adsorbonac, 905-907
Advanced Formula Oxy Sensitive, 100-101
Advil, 493-495
Advil Cold & Sinus, 846-847
AeroBid, 410-411
Aerolate Slo-Bid Gyrocaps, 951-954
Aerosporin, 806-807
Afrin 12-Hour, 748
Aftate, 981
Agenerase, 60-61
Aggrastat, 969-971
Aggrenox, 72-75
Agrylin, 64
AH-Chew D, 786-787
Airet, 18-19
Akarpine, 796-797
AK-Con, 691
Ak-Dex Ophthalmic, 282-284
AK-Dilate, 788-789
AK-Fluor, 413

Entries can be identified as follows: generic name, Trade Name.

Entries can be identified as follows: generic name, Trade Name.

Entries can be identified as follows: generic name, Trade Name.

Entries can be identified as follows: generic name, Trade Name.

Entries can be identified as follows: generic name, Trade Name.

Entries can be identified as follows: generic name, Trade Name.

Entries can be identified as follows: generic name, Trade Name.

Entries can be identified as follows: generic name, Trade Name.

Entries can be identified as follows: generic name, Trade Name.

Entries can be identified as follows: generic name, Trade Name.

Entries can be identified as follows: generic name, Trade Name.

Entries can be identified as follows: generic name, Trade Name.

Entries can be identified as follows: generic name, Trade Name.

Entries can be identified as follows: generic name, Trade Name.

Entries can be identified as follows: generic name, Trade Name.

Entries can be identified as follows: generic name, Trade Name.

Entries can be identified as follows: generic name, Trade Name.

Entries can be identified as follows: generic name, Trade Name.

Entries can be identified as follows: generic name, Trade Name.

Entries can be identified as follows: generic name, Trade Name.

Entries can be identified as follows: generic name, Trade Name.

Entries can be identified as follows: generic name, Trade Name.

Entries can be identified as follows: generic name, Trade Name.

Entries can be identified as follows: generic name, Trade Name.

Entries can be identified as follows: generic name, Trade Name.

Entries can be identified as follows: generic name, Trade Name.

Entries can be identified as follows: generic name, Trade Name.

Entries can be identified as follows: generic name, Trade Name.

Entries can be identified as follows: generic name, Trade Name.

Entries can be identified as follows: generic name, Trade Name.

Entries can be identified as follows: generic name, Trade Name.

Entries can be identified as follows: generic name, Trade Name.

IDEAL BODY WEIGHT (IBW)

ADULTS (>18 YRS):
Male IBW (kg) = 50 + 2.3 for each inch over 60 inches
Female IBW (kg) = 45.5 + 2.3 for each inch over 60 inches

CHILDREN:
Age 1 to 18 yrs, height <60 inches: IBW (kg) = $[1.65 \times height^2 (cm)]/1000$

BODY MASS INDEX (BMI)

$$BMI = \frac{weight\ (kg)}{height^2\ (m)}$$

Normal range:
    Male: 21.9-22.4
    Female: 21.3-22.1

CREATININE CLEARANCE CALCULATION

ADULTS (AGE >18; SERUM CREAT <5 MG/DL AND NOT CHANGING RAPIDLY):

$$CrCl\ (ml/min) = \frac{(140 - age)\ (weight\ in\ kg)}{(serum\ creat\ [mg/dl])\ (72)}$$

NOTES: 1. Multiply by 0.85 for females
        2. Use the following value for weight:
          a. If actual weight <IBW, use actual weight
          b. If actual weight is 100%-130% of IBW, use IBW
          c. If actual weight >130% of IBW, easiest approximation is by using IBW + (actual weight − IBW)/3
        3. Accuracy reduced in muscle wasting diseases (e.g., neuromuscular disease) and amputees

CHILDREN:
CrCl $(ml/min/1.73m^2) = [0.48 \times height\ (cm)]/serum\ creat\ (mg/dl)$

Conversion Information

WEIGHTS AND MEASURES

PREFIXES FOR FRACTIONS
deci = 10^{-1}
centi = 10^{-2}
milli = 10^{-3}
micro = 10^{-6}
nano = 10^{-9}
pico = 10^{-12}

TEMPERATURE MEASURES
°C = 5/9 × (°F −32)
°F = 9/5 × (°C) + 32

PERCENTAGE EQUIVALENTS
0.1% solution contains: 1 mg per ml
1% solution contains: 10 mg per ml
10% solution contains: 100 mg per ml

MILLIEQUIVALENT CONVERSIONS
1 mEq Na = 23 mg Na = 58.5 mg NaCl
1 g Na = 2.54 g NaCl = 43 mEq Na
1 g NaCl = 0.39 g Na = 17 mEq Na

1 mEq K = 39 mg K = 74.5 mg KCl
1 g K = 1.91 g KCl = 26 mEq K
1 g KCl = 0.52 g K = 13 mEq K

1 mEq Ca = 20 mg Ca
1 g Ca = 50 mEq Ca

1 mEq Mg = 0.12 g $MgSO_4 \cdot 7H_2O$
1 g Mg = 10.2 g $MgSO_4 \cdot 7H_2O$ = 82 mEq Mg

10 mmol P_i = 0.31 g P_i = 0.95 g PO_4
1 g P_i = 3.06 g PO_4 = 32 mmol P_i